Clinical Practice

Principles and Practice of Ophthalmology

SECTION EDITORS

R. Rand Allingham, M.D.

A. Robert Bellows, M.D.

Frederick A. Jakobiec, M.D., D.Sc.(Med.)

Claudia U. Richter, M.D.

Daniel J. Townsend, M.D.

John J. Woog, M.D.

Clinical Practice

Principles and Practice of Ophthalmology

Volume 3

DANIEL M. ALBERT, M.D.
Frederick A. Davis Professor and Chairman,
Department of Ophthalmology,
University of Wisconsin Medical School,
Madison, Wisconsin

FREDERICK A. JAKOBIEC, M.D., D.Sc.(Med.)
Henry Willard Williams Professor of Ophthalmology,
Professor of Pathology, and Chairman,
Department of Ophthalmology,
Harvard Medical School;
Chief, Department of Ophthalmology, and
Surgeon in Ophthalmology,
Massachusetts Eye and Ear Infirmary,
Boston, Massachusetts

NANCY L. ROBINSON, A.B.
Managing Editor

W.B. SAUNDERS COMPANY
A Division of Harcourt Brace & Company
Philadelphia   London   Toronto   Montreal   Sydney   Tokyo

W.B. SAUNDERS COMPANY
A Division of Harcourt Brace & Company

The Curtis Center
Independence Square West
Philadelphia, Pennsylvania 19106

Library of Congress Cataloging-in-Publication Data

Principles and practice of ophthalmology : clinical practice / [edited by]
Daniel M. Albert, Frederick A. Jakobiec.

    p.   cm.

ISBN 0–7216–3418–4 (5 v. set)

1. Ophthalmology.   I. Albert, Daniel M.   II. Jakobiec,
Frederick A.

[DNLM: 1. Eye Diseases.   2. Ophthalmology.   WW 140
P957 1994] RE46.P743 1994

617.7—dc20

DNLM/DLC   93–7247

PRINCIPLES AND PRACTICE OF OPHTHALMOLOGY: ISBN Volume 3 0–7216–6595–0
CLINICAL PRACTICE   5-Volume Set 0–7216–3418–4

Printed in the United States of America.

Last digit is the print number: 9   8   7   6   5   4   3   2   1

Contributors

Daniel M. Albert, MD
Frederick A. Davis Professor and Chairman,
Department of Ophthalmology, University of Wisconsin
Medical School, Madison, Wisconsin

Robert C. Allen, MD
Associate Professor of Ophthalmology, University of
Virginia, and University of Virginia Health Sciences
Center, Charlottesville, Virginia

R. Rand Allingham, MD
Assistant Professor of Ophthalmology, University of
Texas Southwestern Medical Center; Active Attending
Ophthalmologist and Assistant Surgeon, Zale Lipshy
University Hospital and Parkland Memorial Hospital,
Dallas, Texas

Claudia A. Arrigg, MD
Clinical Instructor in Ophthalmology, Harvard Medical
School; Assistant Surgeon, Massachusetts Eye and Ear
Infirmary, Boston; Chief of Ophthalmology, Lawrence
General Hospital and Holy Family Medical Center,
Lawrence, Massachusetts

Isaac Ashkenazi, MD, MSc
Lecturer in Ophthalmology, Sackler School of Medicine,
Tel-Aviv University; Goldschleger Eye Institute, Tel
Hashomer, Israel

Ann Sullivan Baker, MD
Associate Professor of Medicine (Ophthalmology),
Harvard Medical School; Director, Infectious Disease
Unit, Massachusetts Eye and Ear Infirmary; Physician,
Infectious Disease Unit, Massachusetts General
Hospital, Boston, Massachusetts

C. Davis Belcher, III, MD
Assistant Clinical Professor of Ophthalmology, Harvard
Medical School; Assistant Surgeon, Massachusetts Eye
and Ear Infirmary; Attending Ophthalmologist,
Hahnemann Hospital, Boston, Massachusetts

A. Robert Bellows, MD
Assistant Clinical Professor of Ophthalmology, Harvard
Medical School; Assistant Surgeon, Massachusetts Eye
and Ear Infirmary, Boston, Massachusetts

Stanley J. Berke, MD, FACS
Ophthalmology and Visual Sciences, Albert Einstein
College of Medicine, New York; Attending, Long Island
Jewish Medical Center, Mercy Medical Center, Nassau
County Medical Center, Franklin Hospital Medical
Center, South Nassau Communities Hospital,
Hempstead General Hospital, and Queens Hospital
Medical Center, New York

Frank G. Berson, MD
Assistant Professor of Ophthalmology, Harvard Medical
School; Chief of Ophthalmology and Surgeon, Beth
Israel Hospital; Associate Surgeon in Ophthalmology,
Massachusetts Eye and Ear Infirmary, Boston,
Massachusetts

Charles K. Beyer-Machule, MD
Associate Clinical Professor, Department of
Ophthalmology, Harvard Medical School; Surgeon,
Massachusetts Eye and Ear Infirmary, Boston,
Massachusetts; Honorary Professor, Ludwig-Maximilians
University, and Consulting Surgeon, University Eye
Clinic, Munich, Germany

Gary E. Borodic, MD
Assistant Clinical Professor in Ophthalmology, Harvard
Medical School; Director of Oculoplastics Service,
Boston University Hospital; Assistant Surgeon,
Massachusetts Eye and Ear Infirmary, Boston,
Massachusetts

Joseph F. Burke, Jr., MD
Clinical Assistant, Harvard Medical School; Clinical
Instructor, Tufts Medical School; Attending,
Massachusetts Eye and Ear Infirmary and Tufts New
England Medical Center, Boston; Charlton Memorial
Hospital, Fall River; and St. Lukes Hospital, New
Bedford, Massachusetts

David G. Campbell, MD
Professor of Surgery (Ophthalmology), Dartmouth
Medical School, Hanover, New Hampshire

David M. Chacko, MD, PhD
Assistant Professor, University of Nebraska Medical
School; Attending, University of Nebraska Medical
Center, Clarkson Hospital, and Omaha Veterans
Hospital, Omaha, Nebraska

Jean-Bernard Charles, MD
Assistant in Ophthalmology, Massachusetts Eye and Ear Infirmary, Boston, Massachusetts

M. Ronan Conlon, MB, BCh
Fellow, Oculoplastics, Orbital Reconstructive Surgery, and Oncology, University of Iowa Hospitals and Clinics, Department of Ophthalmology, Iowa City, Iowa

Marshall N. Cyrlin, MD
Clinical Associate Professor, Oakland University Eye Research Institute, Rochester; Director, Glaucoma Service, Sinai Hospital of Detroit, Detroit; Chief, Glaucoma Division, Beaumont Eye Institute, Royal Oak, Michigan

Richard L. Dallow, MD
Assistant Clinical Professor of Ophthalmology, Harvard Medical School; Surgeon in Ophthalmology, Massachusetts Eye and Ear Infirmary, Boston, Massachusetts

Richard K. Dortzbach, MD, FACS
Clinical Professor of Ophthalmology, University of Wisconsin Medical School; Active Staff, University Hospital and Meriter Hospital; Consultant, Veterans Administration Hospital, Madison, Wisconsin

Michael V. Drake, MD
Associate Professor of Ophthalmology, University of California, San Francisco; Attending Physician, University of California, San Francisco; Hospital and Clinics, San Francisco General Hospital, and San Francisco Veterans Administration Hospital, San Francisco, California

David K. Dueker, MD
Associate Professor of Ophthalmology, University of Missouri, Columbia, Missouri

David A. Echelman, MD
Physician, MetroWest Medical Center, Framingham, Massachusetts

David L. Epstein, MD
Professor and Chairman of Ophthalmology, Duke University Medical Center; Chief of Ophthalmology, Duke University Eye Center, Durham, North Carolina

Philip M. Fiore, MD
Clinical Assistant Professor of Ophthalmology, University of Medicine and Dentistry of New Jersey : New Jersey Medical School, Newark, New Jersey

Ramon L. Font, MD
Director, Ophthalmic Pathology Laboratory, Cullen Eye Institute; Professor of Pathology and Ophthalmology, Baylor College of Medicine; Consultant in Pathology, The Methodist Hospital, Baylor College of Medicine, and M. D. Anderson Hospital and Tumor Institute, Texas Medical Center, Houston, Texas

Craig E. Geist, MD
Assistant Clinical Professor of Ophthalmology, George Washington University, Washington, DC

A. Tyrone Glover, MD
Assistant Clinical Professor of Ophthalmology, University of California, Davis; Surgeon, Eye Plastic and Orbital Surgery, Kaiser Foundation Hospital and University of California, Davis, Medical Center, Sacramento, California

Linda J. Greff, MD
Clinical Fellow, Massachusetts Eye and Ear Infirmary, Harvard Medical School, and New England Glaucoma Research Foundation, Boston, Massachusetts; Staff Ophthalmologist, Cincinnati Eye Institute, Cincinnati, Ohio

Arthur S. Grove, Jr., MD
Assistant Clinical Professor of Ophthalmology, Harvard Medical School; Surgeon in Ophthalmology, Massachusetts Eye and Ear Infirmary, Boston, Massachusetts

Ahmed A. Hidayat, MD
Staff Pathologist, Department of Ophthalmic Pathology, Armed Forces Institute of Pathology, Walter Reed Army Medical Center, Washington, DC

Eve Juliet Higginbotham, MD, SM
Associate Professor of Ophthalmology, University of Michigan, Kellogg Eye Center, Ann Arbor, Michigan

B. Thomas Hutchinson, MD
Associate Clinical Professor of Ophthalmology, Harvard Medical School; Surgeon in Ophthalmology, Massachusetts Eye and Ear Infirmary; Consultant, Massachusetts General Hospital, Boston, Massachusetts

Frederick A. Jakobiec, MD, DSc(Med)
Henry Willard Williams Professor of Ophthalmology, Professor of Pathology, and Chairman, Department of Ophthalmology, Harvard Medical School; Chief, Department of Ophthalmology, and Surgeon in Ophthalmology, Massachusetts Eye and Ear Infirmary, Boston, Massachusetts

Douglas H. Johnson, MD
Associate Professor of Ophthalmology, Mayo Medical School and Clinic; Consultant in Ophthalmology, Rochester Methodist Hospital and St. Mary's Hospital, Rochester, Minnesota

Murray A. Johnstone, MD
Clinical Instructor, University of Washington, Department of Ophthalmology; Glaucoma Consultant, Swedish Hospital Medical Center, Seattle, Washington

Jemshed A. Khan, MD
Associate Professor of Ophthalmology, Kansas University School of Medicine; Director of Oculoplastic Surgery, Kansas University Medical Center, Kansas City, Kansas

Jan W. Kronish, MD
Assistant Clinical Professor of Ophthalmology, University of Miami, Bascom Palmer Eye Institute, Miami, Florida

Joseph H. Krug, Jr., MD
Former Instructor in Ophthalmology, Harvard Medical School, Boston, Massachusetts; Attending, Presbyterian Hospital, Charlotte, North Carolina

Kathleen A. Lamping, MD
Associate Clinical Professor of Ophthalmology, Case Western Reserve University Medical School; Director, Glaucoma Service, Mt. Sinai Medical Center, Cleveland; Director, Glaucoma Service, Meridia Hillcrest Hospital, Mayfield Heights, Ohio

Mark A. Latina, MD
Instructor in Ophthalmology, Harvard Medical School, and Assistant Clinical Professor of Ophthalmology, Tufts University Medical School; Assistant Surgeon, Massachusetts Eye and Ear Infirmary, Boston, Massachusetts

David Anson Lee, MD, MS
Associate Professor of Ophthalmology, UCLA School of Medicine and Medical Center; Chief, Glaucoma Division, Jules Stein Eye Institute, Los Angeles, California

Paul P. Lee, MD, JD
Assistant Professor of Ophthalmology, University of Southern California School of Medicine; Active Staff, Doheny Eye Institute, University Hospital, and Los Angeles County Hospital, Los Angeles, California

Leonard A. Levin, MD, PhD
Clinical Fellow in Ophthalmology, Harvard Medical School; Fellow in Neuro-Ophthalmology, Massachusetts Eye and Ear Infirmary, Boston, Massachusetts

David B. Lyon, MD
Clinical Assistant Professor of Ophthalmology, University of Wisconsin, Madison, Wisconsin

Robert A. Lytle, MD
Instructor in Ophthalmology, Harvard Medical School; Assistant Surgeon, Massachusetts Eye and Ear Infirmary, Boston, Massachusetts

Curtis E. Margo, MD
Professor of Ophthalmology and Pathology, University of South Florida College of Medicine; Chief, Section of Ophthalmology, Veterans Medical Center, Tampa, Florida

Marlon Maus, MD
Instructor, Thomas Jefferson University, Thomas Jefferson University Hospital, and Wills Eye Hospital, Philadelphia, Pennsylvania

John A. McDermott, MD
Assistant Clinical Professor of Ophthalmology, New York Medical College; Associate Attending Surgeon, The New York Eye and Ear Infirmary, New York, New York

Peter J. McDonnell, MD
Associate Professor of Ophthalmology, University of Southern California; Staff Physician, Doheny Eye Institute and USC University Hospital, Los Angeles, California

Shlomo Melamed, MD
Associate Professor of Ophthalmology, Sackler School of Medicine, Tel Aviv University; Goldschleger Eye Institute, Tel Hashomer, Israel

Peter A. Netland, MD, PhD
Instructor in Ophthalmology, Harvard Medical School; Assistant in Ophthalmology, Massachusetts Eye and Ear Infirmary, Boston, Massachusetts

Randall Ozment, MD
Active Staff, St. Josephs Hospital and Crawford Long Hospital of Emory University, Atlanta, Georgia

Steven G. Pratt, MD
Director, Ocular Plastics Service, Department of Ophthalmology, University of California, San Diego, School of Medicine, San Diego, California

Thomas M. Richardson, MD
Assistant Clinical Professor of Ophthalmology, Harvard Medical School; Assistant Surgeon, Massachusetts Eye and Ear Infirmary, Boston, Massachusetts

Claudia U. Richter, MD
Clinical Assistant in Ophthalmology, Harvard Medical School; Assistant Surgeon in Ophthalmology, Massachusetts Eye and Ear Infirmary, Boston, Massachusetts

Klaus G. Riedel, MD
Professor, Augen Klinik Herzog Carl Theodor, Munich, Germany

I. Rand Rodgers, MD
Director, Ophthalmic Plastic and Reconstructive Surgery, North Shore University Hospital, Cornell University Medical College, Manhasset, New York; Attending Physician, Department of Ophthalmology, Mount Sinai Medical Center, New York, New York

Robert C. Rosenquist, MD
Assistant Professor of Ophthalmology, Loma Linda University, Loma Linda, California

Peter A. D. Rubin, MD
Instructor in Ophthalmology, Harvard Medical School; Associate Director, Eye Plastics and Orbit Service, Massachusetts Eye and Ear Infirmary, Boston, Massachusetts

Joseph W. Sassani, MD
Associate Professor of Ophthalmology, Pennsylvania State University School of Medicine; Staff, Milton S. Hershey Medical Center, Pennsylvania State University, Hershey, Pennsylvania

Joel S. Schuman, MD, FACS
Assistant Professor of Ophthalmology, Tufts University School of Medicine; Ophthalmologist, New England Eye Center, New England Medical Center; Assistant in Ophthalmology, Massachusetts Eye and Ear Infirmary, Boston, Massachusetts

Kevin R. Scott, MD
McLean, Virginia

M. Bruce Shields, MD
Professor of Ophthalmology, Duke University Medical Center; Attending, Duke University Eye Center, Durham Veterans Administration Hospital, and Asheville Veterans Administration Hospital, Durham, North Carolina

Bradford J. Shingleton, MD
Clinical Instructor in Ophthalmology, Harvard Medical School; Clinical Associate Professor of Ophthalmology, Tufts University School of Medicine; Associate Surgeon in Ophthalmology, Massachusetts Eye and Ear Infirmary; Surgeon in Ophthalmology, Boston Eye Surgery and Laser Center; Associate Staff in Ophthalmology, New England Medical Center, Boston, Massachusetts

John W. Shore, MD, FACS
Assistant Professor of Ophthalmology, Harvard Medical School; Associate Chief of Ophthalmology, Massachusetts Eye and Ear Infirmary, Boston; Consultant in Ophthalmology, Emerson Hospital, Concord, Massachusetts

Richard J. Simmons, MD
Associate Clinical Professor of Ophthalmology, Harvard Medical School; Surgeon, Massachusetts Eye and Ear Infirmary; Chief of Ophthalmology, Hahnemann Hospital, Boston, Massachusetts

Omah S. Singh, MD
Assistant Clinical Professor of Ophthalmology, Tufts New England Medical School; Surgeon in Ophthalmology, Hahnemann Hospital, Beverly Hospital, and The Hunt Center, Boston, Massachusetts

Neal G. Snebold, MD
Clinical Assistant in Ophthalmology, Harvard Medical School; Assistant in Ophthalmology, Massachusetts Eye and Ear Infirmary, Boston, Massachusetts

Sandra J. Sofinski, MD
Clinical Glaucoma Fellow, Massachusetts Eye and Ear Infirmary, New England Glaucoma Research Foundation, Harvard Medical School, Boston, Massachusetts; Attending Staff Ophthalmologist, Torrance Memorial Medical Center, Torrance, California

Francis C. Sutula, MD
Clinical Instructor in Ophthalmology, Harvard Medical School; Associate Director, Oculoplastics Service, and Assistant Surgeon in Ophthalmology, Massachusetts Eye and Ear Infirmary; Associate Clinical Professor, Tufts Medical School, Boston, Massachusetts

John V. Thomas, MD
Clinical Instructor in Ophthalmology, Harvard Medical School; Clinical Assistant in Ophthalmology, Massachusetts Eye and Ear Infirmary, Boston, Massachusetts

David P. Tingey, MD
Assistant Professor of Ophthalmology, University of Western Ontario, Ivey Institute of Ophthalmology, London, Ontario

Daniel J. Townsend, MD
Instructor in Ophthalmology, Harvard Medical School; Active Staff, Massachusetts Eye and Ear Infirmary and New England Deaconess Hospital; Consultant, Spaulding Rehabilitation Hospital, Boston; Consultant, Nantucket Cottage Hospital, Nantucket, Massachusetts

Nicholas J. Volpe, MD
Clinical Instructor in Ophthalmology, Harvard Medical School; Director, Eye Emergency and Trauma Service, and Associate Chief of Ophthalmology, Massachusetts Eye and Ear Infirmary, Boston, Massachusetts

Martin Wand, MD
Associate Clinical Professor of Ophthalmology, University of Connecticut School of Medicine, Farmington; Senior Staff, Hartford Hospital, Hartford, Connecticut

David P. Wellington, MD
Active Staff, Swedish Hospital Medical Center, Seattle, Washington

Christopher T. Westfall, MD, FACS
Chairman, Department of Ophthalmology, and Chief of Oculoplastic Surgery Service, Wilford Hall U.S. Air Force Medical Center, San Antonio, Texas; Chief Consultant in Ophthalmology to the Air Force Surgeon General

William L. White, MD
Clinical Assistant Professor of Ophthalmology, The University of Texas Health Science Center at San Antonio; Associate Director, Ophthalmic Plastic and Reconstructive Surgery, Ophthalmology Service, Brooke Army Medical Center, Ft. Sam Houston, Texas

Janey L. Wiggs, MD, PhD
Instructor in Ophthalmology, Massachusetts Eye and Ear Infirmary, Harvard Medical School, Boston, Massachusetts

A. Sydney Williams, MD
Department of Ophthalmology, Stanford University, Stanford, California

M. Roy Wilson, MD, MS
Associate Professor of Ophthalmology, Jules Stein Eye Institute, University of California, Los Angeles; Associate Professor of Ophthalmology and Chief of Ophthalmology, Charles R. Drew University of Medicine and Science; Staff, UCLA Center for Health Sciences and King/Drew Medical Center, Los Angeles, California

John J. Woog, MD
Assistant Clinical Professor, Tufts University School of Medicine; Clinical Instructor, Harvard Medical School; Assistant Surgeon, Massachusetts Eye and Ear Infirmary, Boston, Massachusetts

To Ellie

D.M.A.

Preface

"INCIPIT." The medievel scribe would write this Latin word, meaning *so it begins,* to signal the start of the book he was transcribing. It was a dramatic word that conveyed promise of instruction and delight. In more modern times INCIPIT has been replaced by the PREFACE. It may be the first thing the reader sees, but it is, in fact, the last thing the author writes before the book goes to press. I appreciate the opportunity to make some personal comments regarding **Principles and Practice of Ophthalmology.**

One of the most exciting things about writing and editing a book in a learned field is that it puts the authors and editors in touch with those who have gone before. Each author shares with those who have labored in past years and in past centuries the tasks of assessing the knowledge that exists in his or her field, of determining what is important, and of trying to convey it to his or her peers. In the course of the work the author experiences the same anticipation, angst, and ennui of those who have gone before. He or she can well envision the various moments of triumph and despair that all authors and editors must feel as they organize, review, and revise the accumulating manuscripts and reassure, cajole, and make demands of their fellow editors, authors, and publisher.

This feeling of solidarity with early writers becomes even more profound when one is a collector and reviewer of books, and conversant with the history of one's field. In Ecclesiastes it is stated, "of the making of books, there is no end" (12:12). Indeed, there are more books than any other human artifact on earth. There is, however, a beginning to the "making of books" in any given field. The first ophthalmology book to be published was Benvenuto Grassi's *De Oculis* in Florence in 1474. Firmin Didot in his famous *Bibliographical Encyclopedia* wrote that Grassus, an Italian physician of the School of Solerno, lived in the 12th century and was the author of two books, *Ferrara Quarto* (1474) and the *Venetian Folio* (1497). Eye care in the 15th century was in the hands of itinerant barber-surgeons and quacks, and a treatise by a learned physician was a remarkable occurrence. The next book on the eye to appear was an anonymous pamphlet written for the layperson in 1538 and entitled *Ein Newes Hochnutzliches Büchlin von Erkantnus der Kranckheyten der Augen.* Like **Principles and Practice of Ophthalmology,** the *Büchlin* stated its intention to provide highly useful knowledge of eye diseases, the anatomy of the eye, and various remedies. It was illustrated with a full-page woodcut of the anatomy of the eye (Fig. 1). At the conclusion of the book, the publisher, Vogtherr, promised to bring more and better information to light shortly, and indeed, the next year he published a small book by Leonhart Fuchs (1501–1566) entitled *Alle Kranckheyt der Augen.*

Fuchs, a fervent Hippocratist, was Professor first of Philosophy and then of Medicine at Ingolstadt, Physician of the Margrave Georg of Brandenburg, and finally Professor at Tübingen for 31 years. Like the earlier *Büchlin,* his work begins with an anatomic woodcut (Fig. 2), then lists in tabular form various eye conditions, including strabismus, paralysis, amblyopia, and nictalops. The work uses a distinctly Greco-Roman terminology, presenting information on the parts of the eye and their affections, including conjunctivitis, ophthalmia, carcinoma, and "glaucoma." The book concludes with a remedy collection similar to that found in the *Büchlin.* Most significant in the association of Leonhart Fuchs with this book is the fact that a properly trained and

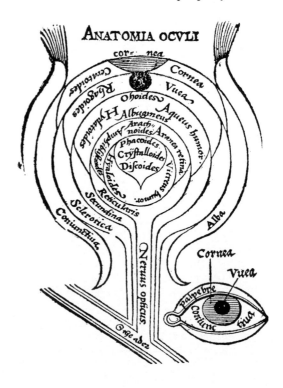

xi

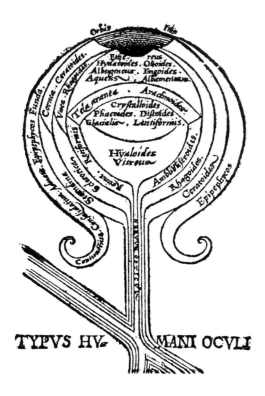

well-recognized physician addressed the subject of oph-thalmology.

Julius Hirschberg, the ophthalmic historian, noted that Fuch's *Alle Kranckheyt,* along with the anonymous *Büchlin,* apparently influenced Georg Bartisch in his writing of *Das ist Augendienst.* This latter work, published in 1583, marked the founding of modern ophthalmology. Bartisch (1535–1606) was an itinerant barber-surgeon but nonetheless a thoughtful and skillful surgeon, whose many innovations included the first procedure for extirpation of the globe for ocular cancer. Bartisch proposed standards for the individual who practices eye surgery, noting that rigorous training and concentration of effort were needed to practice this specialty successfully.

By the late 16th century, eye surgery and the treatment of eye disease began to move into the realm of the more formally trained and respected surgeon. This is evidenced by Jacques Guillemeau's *Traité des Maladies de l'Oeil,* published in 1585. Guillemeau (1550–1612) was a pupil of the surgical giant Ambroise Paré, and his book was an epitome of the existing knowledge on the subject.

The transition from couching of cataracts to the modern method of treating cataracts by extraction of the lens, as introduced by Jacques Daviel in 1753, further defined the skill and training necessary for the care of the eyes. The initiation of ophthalmology as a separate specialty within the realm of medicine and surgery was signaled by the publication of George Joseph Beer's two-volume *Lehre von den Augenkrankheiten* in 1813–1817. Beer (1763–1821) founded the first eye hospital in 1786 in Vienna, and his students became famous ophthalmic surgeons and professors throughout Europe.

In England, it was not only the demands of cataract surgery but also the great pandemic of trachoma following the Napoleonic wars that led to the establishment of ophthalmology as a recognized specialty. Benjamin Travers (1783–1858) published the earliest treatise in English on diseases of the eye, *A Synopsis of the Diseases of the Eye,* in 1820. In the United States, acceptance of ophthalmology as a specialty had to await the description of the ophthalmoscope by Helmholtz in 1851, and the additional need of special skills that using the early primitive "Augenspiegel" required.

As the complexity of ophthalmology increased and as subspecialization began to develop in the 19th century, multiauthored books began to appear. This culminated in the appearance in 1874 of the first volume of the Graefe-Saemisch *Handbuch.* The final volume of this great collective work, of which Alfred Carl Graefe (1830–1899) and Edwin Theodor Saemisch (1833–1909) were editors, appeared in 1880. The definitive second edition, which for more than a quarter of a century remained the most comprehensive and authoritative work in the field, appeared in 15 volumes between 1899 and 1918. The great French counterpart to the Graefe-Saemisch *Handbuch* was the *Encyclopédie Française d'Ophtalmologie,* which appeared in 9 volumes (1903–1910), edited by Octave Doin, and filled a similar role for the French-speaking ophthalmologist.

In 1896, the first of 4 volumes of Norris and Oliver's *System of Diseases of the Eye* was published in the United States. The senior editor, Dr. William Fisher Norris (1839–1901), was the first Clinical Professor of Diseases of the Eye at the University of Pennsylvania. Charles A. Oliver (1853–1911) was his student. Norris considered the *System* to be his monumental work. For each section he chose an outstanding authority in the field, having in the end more than 60 American, British, Dutch, French, and German ophthalmologists as contributors. Almost 6 years of combined labor on the part of the editors was needed for completion of the work. In 1913, Casey A. Wood (1856–1942) introduced the first of his 18 volumes of the *American Encyclopedia and Dictionary of Ophthalmology.* The final volume appeared in 1921. Drawn largely from the Graef-Saemisch *Handbuch* and the *Encyclopédie Française d'Ophtalmologie,* Wood's *Encyclopedia* provided information on the whole of ophthalmology through a strictly alphabetic sequence of subject headings.

The book from which the present work draws inspiration is Duke-Elder's *Textbook of Ophthalmology* (7 volumes; 1932) and particularly the second edition of this work entitled *System of Ophthalmology* (15 volumes, published between 1958 and 1976). The *System of Ophthalmology* was written by Sir Stewart Duke-Elder (1898–1978) in conjunction with his colleagues at the Institute of Ophthalmology in London. In 1976, when the last of his 15 volumes appeared, Duke-Elder wrote in the Preface:

> The writing of these two series, the *Textbook* and the *System,* has occupied all my available time for half a century. I cannot deny that its completion brings me relief on the recovery of my freedom, but at the same time it has left some sadness for I have enjoyed writing it. As

Edward Gibbon said on having written the last line of *The Decline and Fall of the Roman Empire:* "A sober melancholy has spread over my mind by the idea that I have taken everlasting leave of an old and agreeable companion."

Duke-Elder adds a final line that I hope will be more apropos to the present editors and contributors. "At the same time the prayer of Sir Francis Drake on the eve of the attack of the Spanish Armada is apposite: 'Give us to know that it is not the beginning but the continuing of the same until it is entirely finished which yieldeth the true glory.'" The void that developed as the Duke-Elder series became outdated has been partially filled by many fine books, notably Thomas Duane's excellent 5-volume *Clinical Ophthalmology.*

Inspiration to undertake a major work such as this is derived not only from the past books but from teachers and role models as well. For me, this includes Francis Heed Adler, Harold G. Scheie, William C. Frayer, David G. Cogan, Ludwig von Sallmann, Alan S. Rabson, Lorenz E. Zimmerman, Frederick C. Blodi, Claes H. Dohlman, and Matthew D. Davis.

Whereas the inspiration for the present text was derived from Duke-Elder's *Textbook* and *System* and from teachers and role models, learning how to write and organize a book came for me from Adler's *Textbook of Ophthalmology,* published by W. B. Saunders. This popular textbook for medical students and general practitioners was first produced by Dr. Sanford Gifford (1892–1945) in 1938. Francis Heed Adler (1895–1987), after writing the 6th edition, published in 1962, invited Harold G. Scheie (1909–1989); his successor as Chairman of Ophthalmology at the University of Pennsylvania, and myself to take over authorship. We completely rewrote this book and noted in the Preface to the 8th edition, published in 1969: "This book aims to provide the medical student and the practicing physician with a concise and profusely illustrated current text, organized in a convenient and useable manner, on the eye and its disorders. It is hoped that the beginning, or even practicing, ophthalmologist may find it of value."

In 1969 it was apparent that even for the intended audience, contributions by individuals expert in the subspecialties of ophthalmology were required. The book was published in Spanish and Chinese editions and was popular enough to warrant an updated 9th edition, which appeared in 1977. One of the high points of this work was interacting with John Dusseau, the Editor-in-Chief for the W. B. Saunders Company. As a 10th edition was contemplated, I became increasingly convinced that what was needed in current ophthalmology was a new, comprehensive, well-illustrated set of texts intended for the practicing ophthalmologist and written by outstanding authorities in the field. I envisioned a work that in one series of volumes would provide all of the basic clinical and scientific information required by practicing ophthalmologists in their everyday work. For more detailed or specialized information, this work should direct the practitioner to the pertinent journal articles or more specialized publications. As time pro-

gressed, a plan for this work took shape and received support from the W. B. Saunders Company.

Memories of the formative stages of the **Principles and Practice of Ophthalmology** remain vivid: Proposing the project to Fred Jakobiec in the cafeteria of the Massachusetts Eye and Ear Infirmary in early 1989. Having dinner with Lew Reines, President and Chief Executive Officer, and Richard Zorab, Senior Medical Editor, at the Four Seasons Hotel in May 1989, where we agreed upon the scope of the work. My excitement as I walked across the Public Garden and down Charles Street back to the Infirmary, contemplating the work we were to undertake. Finalizing the outline for the book in Henry Allen's well-stocked "faculty lounge" in a dormitory at Colby College during the Lancaster Course. Meeting with members of the Harvard Faculty in the somber setting of the rare-book room to recruit the Section Editors. Persuading Nancy Robinson, my able assistant since 1969, to take on the job of Managing Editor. The receipt of our first manuscript from Dr. David Cogan.

We considered making this work a departmental undertaking, utilizing the faculty and alumni of various Harvard programs. However, the broad scope of the series required recruitment of outstanding authors from many institutions. Once the Section Editors were in place, there was never any doubt in my mind that this work would succeed. The Section Editors proved a hard-working and dedicated group, and their choice of authors reflects their good judgment and persuasive abilities. I believe that you will appreciate the scope of knowledge and the erudition.

The editorship of this book provided me not only with an insight into the knowledge and thinking of some of the finest minds in ophthalmology but also with an insight into their lives. What an overwhelmingly busy group of people! Work was completed not through intimidation with deadlines but by virtue of their love of ophthalmology and their desire to share their knowledge and experience. The talent, commitment, persistence, and good humor of the authors are truly what made this book a reality.

It was our intent to present a work that was at once scholarly and pragmatic, that dealt effectively with the complexities and subtleties of modern ophthalmology, but that did not overwhelm the reader. We have worked toward a series of volumes that contained the relevant basic science information to sustain and complement the clinical facts. We wanted a well-illustrated set that went beyond the illustrations in any textbook or system previously published, in terms of quantity and quality and usefulness of the pictures.

In specific terms, in editing the book we tried to identify and eliminate errors in accuracy. We worked to provide as uniform a literary style as is possible in light of the numerous contributors. We attempted to make as consistent as possible the level of detail presented in the many sections and chapters. Related to this, we sought to maintain the length according to our agreed-upon plan. We tried, as far as possible, to eliminate repetition and at the same time to prevent gaps in information. We worked to direct the location of information into a logical and convenient arrangement. We attempted to separate the basic science chapters to the major extent into the separate **Basic Sciences** volume, but at the same time to integrate basic science information with clinical detail in other sections as needed. These tasks were made challenging by the size of the work, the number of authors, and the limited options for change as material was received close to publishing deadlines. We believe that these efforts have succeeded in providing ophthalmologists and visual scientists with a useful resource in their practices. We shall know in succeeding years the level of this success and hope to have the opportunity to improve all these aspects as the book is updated and published in future editions. Bacon wrote: "Reading maketh a full man, conference a ready man, and writing an exact man." He should have added: *Editing maketh a humble man.*

I am personally grateful to a number of individuals for making this book a reality. Nancy Robinson leads the list. Her intelligent, gracious, and unceasing effort as Managing Editor was essential to its successful completion. Mr. Lewis Reines, President of the W. B. Saunders Company, has a profound knowledge of publishing and books that makes him a worthy successor to John Dusseau. Richard Zorab, the Senior Medical Editor, and Hazel N. Hacker, the Developmental Editor, are thoroughly professional and supportive individuals with whom it was a pleasure to work. Many of the black-and-white illustrations were drawn by Laurel Cook Lhowe and Marcia Williams; Kit Johnson provided many of the anterior segment photographs. Archival materials were retrieved with the aid of Richard Wolfe, Curator of Rare Books at the Francis A. Countway Library of Medicine, and Chris Nims and Kathleen Kennedy of the Howe Library at the Massachusetts Eye and Ear Infirmary.

The most exciting aspect of writing and editing a work of this type is that it puts one in touch with the present-day ophthalmologists and visual scientists as well as physicians training to be ophthalmologists in the future. We hope that this book will establish its own tradition of excellence and usefulness and that it will win it a place in the lives of ophthalmologists today and in the future.

"EXPLICIT," scribes wrote at the end of every book. EXPLICIT means *it has been unfolded.* Olmert notes in *The Smithsonian Book of Books,* "the unrolling or unfolding of knowledge is a powerful act because it shifts responsibility from writer to reader. . . . Great books endure because they help us interpret our lives. It's a personal quest, this grappling with the world and ourselves, and we need all the help we can get." We hope that this work will provide such help to the professional lives of ophthalmologists and visual scientists.

DANIEL M. ALBERT, M.D.
MADISON, WISCONSIN

To my beloved family, both living and elsewhere;
To my cherished teachers and trainees, both past and present;
To my incomparable patients, both cured and uncured;
And to my supportive colleagues and friends, all insufficiently
  celebrated in my preface.

F.A.J.

Preface

Because of the pellucid beauty of the organ and tissues it studies, ophthalmology affords many pleasures and allurements. Although it might be more of a confessional than a verifiable statement, I have always believed that many individuals are also attracted to ophthalmology with the inchoate fantasy (later found to be erroneous) that it is an encapsulated and somewhat secessionist medical specialty one can totally master; this may indeed be an expression of the ophthalmic temperament's constitutive tropism toward control. Ophthalmology, furthermore, has long been a discipline that has generated exquisite teaching aids; most of the diseases and tissues we contend with are amenable to photographic documentation and elegant analysis by modern imaging and angiographic techniques. The quest for mastery in ophthalmology is marked by the periodic appearance of comprehensive textbooks, an example of which is the present enterprise.

If one person certainly could not do it today, is it possible for multiple authors to create a *Summa Ophthalmologica?* In my professional lifetime the most bruited effort was Duke-Elder's *System of Ophthalmology,* which encompassed 15 volumes, appearing ad seriatim from 1958 to 1976. As a resident-in-training, I remember anticipating the arrival of each new volume, and of devouring it from cover to cover because of the spectacular tour d'horizon that was provided. Early in my career, I was privileged to become involved with the orbit section of Duane's 5-volume *Clinical Ophthalmology* and subsequently with the anatomy, embryology, and teratology section of his 3-volume *Biomedical Foundations of Ophthalmology,* both of which were intended to supersede Duke-Elder. Now, having acquired more experience and maturity, I am aware that it is impossible for an ophthalmic diorama to rival the timelessness of Thomas Aquinas' *Summa Theologica,* Immanuel Kant's *Kritiken,* or Bertrand Russell's *Principia Mathematica,* all of which self-reflexively proceed from deductions based on a priori axioms. Ophthalmology is a contingent, empirical, and nonoracular discipline, and its intellectual artifacts necessarily reflect the imperfections and messiness of human inductive knowledge. At their best, the present and predecessor efforts to produce comprehensive ophthalmic textbooks are temporary codifications, inventories, and snapshots of an everunfolding field, much as sequential photograph albums reveal the fructifying growth and evolution of families over generations.

Why, then, was the present project undertaken, and what are its distinctive features? Dan Albert and I began jointly planning this work in early 1989, shortly after I arrived in Boston from New York City to become Chief of Ophthalmology at the Massachusetts Eye and Ear Infirmary and Chairman of the Department of Ophthalmology at the Harvard Medical School. We felt the time was right for a new gesamtwerk for ophthalmology, fraught as it might be with the limitations alluded to previously. We believed that the Harvard environment would be especially conducive to producing an outstanding work of scholarship. Initially the **Principles and Practice of Ophthalmology** textbook carried the subtitle "The Harvard System"; this was reflected in the contract signed with the publisher as well as in the stationery that was used throughout the project in correspondence with the contributors. Whereas it is true that all of the section editors and the vast majority of the 440 contributors are by design either present or past faculty or trainees of the Harvard Medical School, the Massachusetts Eye and Ear Infirmary, or the Schepens Eye Research Institute (now formally affiliated with the Harvard Department of Ophthalmology), it quickly became apparent that there was no single "Harvard" or systematic way of thinking about the various topics covered in these volumes. Even within the Harvard Department there are manifold approaches to basic science and clinical problems. Therefore, we were led to abandon the subtitle. Nonetheless, I personally am unabashedly proud that the high quality and erudition of the chapters derive from the intellectual formation that many contributors received from their association with the greater Harvard ophthalmic environment; well represented within this cadre are recent residents and fellows.

Of the 6 volumes, the longest **(Basic Sciences)** deals with the basic sciences of ophthalmology in ten sections. It is in this realm that one will expect the most rapid changes in subject matter in the immediate years ahead; on the other hand, this may be the most fecund and valuable of all the volumes, because there has not been a recent effort to synthesize the burgeoning of knowledge that has attended the revolutions in morphologic investigations, pharmacology, cell biology, immunology, and, lately, molecular genetics. Not every topic in the visual basic sciences could be covered: For example, an extensive and conventional repetition of the facts of embryology and anatomy has not been essayed, since there already exist serviceable references for these comparatively static subjects. The focus instead was on investigations that had been particularly rewarding and luminous over the past 10 years. My advice to readers is to approach each chapter in this volume as if it were an article in the *Scientific American* and to derive both knowledge and pleasure from these lapidary syntheses.

The 5 clinical volumes have been organized along the lines of standard anatomic and tissue-topographic demarcations. Additionally, there are systematic approaches to some established and newly emerging nodal points of knowledge: neuroophthalmology; the eye and systemic disease; pediatric ophthalmology; ocular oncology; ophthalmic pathology; trauma; diagnostic imaging; optical principles and applications; and psychological, social, and legal aspects of ophthalmology. Efforts were made to reduce unnecessary duplication from section to section in the coverage of various subjects; however, when it was felt that it would be profitable to have the same disease or topic covered from several perspectives, this was permitted. We are aware that, despite the length of our present undertaking, the end result is one of comprehensiveness but not exhaustiveness. It should be remembered that there already exist many published and revised multivolume treatises on subjects covered herein. What we have aimed for is to provide the generalist with a digestible up-to-date overview of ophthalmology and also to provide the superspecialist with readily accessible introductions to topics outside of his or her intensive areas of expertise.

Another distinctive feature of the present volumes is the prodigious number of illustrations, totaling well over 6000 if one includes tables, diagrams, and graphs. About half of these are in color, which enhances the aesthetic and teaching value of the entire project. The bibliographies are often daunting and will serve as pathfinders into the larger universe of their subjects. I would particularly like to thank Ms. Kit Johnson of the Infirmary for providing many of the color illustrations for diseases of the eyelids, conjunctiva, and anterior segment of the eye. For voluptuaries of ophthalmology, these and the fundus illustrations should provide a sumptuous feast.

It staggers the mind to contemplate the quotidian and oppressive amount of effort expended on this project— the incalculable atomistic acts of assemblage, the gently hectoring telephone calls, the background acquisition and scope of the basic science and clinical knowledge, the multiple textual revisions, the amassing of bibliographies and illustrations, and so on—and indeed the formidable cost of producing each of the individual chapters, much of which was borne by the authors themselves. Even as we are hopeful that these volumes will make a major positive impression on American and international ophthalmology, modesty in the face of our challenging task rather than arrogance has inspired the lofty goals that sustained the creation of the **Principles and Practice of Ophthalmology.** Still, I have no doubt that many of the chapters contained in these volumes are the most incandescent, scholarly, and useful summary presentations of their subjects that have been crafted up to now. In a many-authored textbook there

will be some unevenness, the result of the idiosyncrasies of the contributors as well as the state of development of their subject matter. My own criterion for the success of this enterprise is a simple one: that 50 percent or more of the chapters will have achieved the status of being the best overviews and introductions for their subjects. Regarding topics that should have been covered but were somehow missed or that were surveyed inadequately, the chief editors, the section editors, the authors, and the publisher will look forward to hearing from readers and reviewers about any constructive criticisms on how to improve the textbook in its next edition. We are also exploring various mechanisms for issuing supplemental chapters to rectify some of these perceived and real deficiencies before the next edition.

Based on my familiarity with ophthalmic texts, I think the present work is the largest ophthalmic publication ever to appear *all at once as a complete set.* The W. B. Saunders Company is consequently to be congratulated for having maintained the highest standards of production in terms of copy editing, printing, paper quality, indexing, and reproduction of color and black-and-white illustrations. Mr. Richard Zorab, Senior Medical Editor, was a tireless and relatively humane flogger of myself and the other contributors to meet realistic deadlines; Mrs. Hazel N. Hacker was our highly expert Developmental Editor, and Mrs. Linda R. Garber kept the movement of manuscripts and galleys on schedule with minimal breakage. Ms. Nancy Robinson was a compassionate, patient, and effective intradepartmental Managing Editor. I particularly applaud the ability of the publisher to keep the price of the 6 volumes, with all their color illustrations, at a respectable level so that they are within the reach of trainees, basic scientists, and clinicians in an era of highly competitive National Institutes of Health funding and when ophthalmic reimbursements are being ratcheted down.

It is my compressed personal philosophy that we live to feel, think, and act and that the highest emanations of these faculties are enthusiasm, creativity, and love. This textbook is a manifestation of all six of these capacities, served up in superabundance. May the response of the ophthalmic community be commensurate with the spiritual and intellectual largesse lavished by the contributors on these volumes. Finally, although I somewhat iconoclastically do not fully subscribe to the notion of role models (because I believe that each person should construct his or her unique identity and excellence by cultivating one's intrinsic gifts while at the same time selectively interiorizing the finest qualities of many exemplars), I would like to thank my many professional friends and colleagues who have played salutary roles in the parturition of my own career, and who have taught me and/or supported me to this point in my professional life so that I could participate in this magnificent and bracing academic adventure: Dean S. James Adelstein, Dr. Henry Allen, Dr. Myles Behrens, Mr. Alexander Bernhard, Dr. Frederick Blodi, Dr. Sheldon Buckler, Dr. Alston Callahan, Dr. Charles J. Campbell, Dr. H. Dwight Cavanaugh, Mr. Melville Chapin, Dr.

David Cogan, Dr. D. Jackson Coleman, Dr. Brian Curtin, Dr. Donald D'Amico, Dr. Arthur Gerard DeVoe, Dr. Jack Dodick, Dr. Claes Dohlman, Dr. Anthony Donn, Dr. Thomas Duane, Dr. Howard Eggers, Dr. Robert Ellsworth, Dr. Andrew Ferry, Dr. Ben Fine, Dr. Ramon L. Font, Dr. Max Forbes, Dr. Ephraim Friedman, Mr. J. Frank Gerrity, Dr. Gabriel Godman, Dr. Evangelos Gragoudas, Dr. W. Richard Green, Dr. Winston Harrison, the late Dr. Paul Henkind, Dr. George M. Howard, Dr. Takeo Iwamoto, Dr. Ira Snow Jones, Mrs. Diane Kaneb, Dr. Donald West King, Dr. Daniel M. Knowles, Dr. Raphael Lattes, Dr. Simmons Lessell, Dr. Harvey Lincoff, Mr. Martin Lipton, Dr. Richard Lisman, Mr. Richard MacKinnon, Dr. Ian McLean, Dr. Julian Manski, Dr. Norman Medow, Mr. August Meyer, Dr. George (Bud) Merriam, Jr., Dr. Karl Perzin, Dr. Kathryn Stein Pokorny, Dr. Elio Raviola, the late Dr. Algernon B. Reese, Mr. William Renchard, Dr. Rene Rodriguez-Sains, Dr. Evan Sacks, Dr. Charles Schepens, Dr. James Schutz, the late Dr. Sigmund Schutz, Dr. Jesse Sigelman, Mr. F. Curtis Smith, Dr. William Spencer, Ms. Cathleen Douglas Stone, Dr. R. David Sudarsky, Dr. Myron Tannenbaum, Dr. Elise Torczynski, Dean Daniel Tosteson, Dr. Arnold Turtz, Dr. Robert Uretz, the late Dr. Sigmund Wilens, Dr. Marianne Wolff, Dr. Myron Yanoff, and Dr. Lorenz E. Zimmerman.

I hope that this textbook will touch the lives of those who read it as much as these individuals have influenced my own.

Ad Astra Per Aspera!

FREDERICK A. JAKOBIEC, M.D., D.SC.(MED.)
BOSTON, MASSACHUSETTS

Contents

VOLUME 1

VOLUME 2

VOLUME 3

VOLUME 4

SECTION X

Ophthalmic Pathology, 2099
Edited by DANIEL M. ALBERT, THADDEUS P. DRYJA, and
FREDERICK A. JAKOBIEC

SECTION XI

Neuroophthalmology, 2387
Edited by JOSEPH F. RIZZO III and SIMMONS LESSELL

SECTION XII

Pediatric Ophthalmology, 2715
Edited by RICHARD M. ROBB and DAVID S. WALTON

VOLUME 5

SECTION VII

Glaucoma

Edited by
R. RAND ALLINGHAM, A. ROBERT BELLOWS,
and CLAUDIA U. RICHTER

Chapter 110

—■—

Overview

R. RAND ALLINGHAM

The glaucomas constitute a diverse group of disorders associated with elevated intraocular pressure that culminate in a characteristic pattern of optic atrophy and loss of visual field. In the past decade there have been vast improvements in diagnosis, management, and basic understanding of the pathophysiology of this group of diseases. This section has been written to serve as a useful resource for the diagnosis and management of patients with glaucoma.

Glaucoma is typically associated with painless and progressive loss of vision that may escape detection by the patient or by the attending physician for long periods. A carefully directed history (see Chap. 111) and physical examination (see Chap. 112) are essential for the correct diagnosis and proper management of a disease that may have many causes. Various diagnostic modalities (see Chaps. 113 to 116) are used routinely in the evaluation of a patient with glaucoma. Visual field assessment, which is certainly the most commonly performed ancillary test in the management of patients with glaucoma, is discussed in Chapter 113. Other diagnostic tests that may be more commonly used in the future are discussed in the chapter on optic nerve imaging (see Chap. 114). The measurement of intraocular pressure, tonometry, tonography, and the clinical assessment of aqueous outflow facility are discussed in Chapter 115. Provocative tests used for the evaluation and assessment of patients with both open and narrow-angle glaucoma are discussed in Chapter 116.

Glaucomas are often divided into primary and secondary types as well as closed-angle types. Chapters 117 to 119 deal with primary open-angle glaucoma, juvenile open-angle glaucoma, and low-tension glaucoma. A discussion of congenital glaucoma is found in Chapter 221 on pediatric ophthalmology. Primary angle-closure glaucoma may occur acutely or insidiously. Primary angle-closure glaucoma and plateau iris syndrome are discussed in Chapter 120. Perhaps the most commonly misdiagnosed form of glaucoma, combined-mechanism glaucoma, is discussed in Chapter 121.

The secondary glaucomas occur in association with a wide variety of ocular and systemic disorders. The first group of chapters is related to disorders associated with an anatomically open angle. Both common syndromes such as pseudoexfoliation syndrome (see Chap. 122), pigment dispersion syndrome (see Chap. 123), and traumatic glaucomas (see Chap. 125), as well as uncommon causes of secondary open-angle glaucoma such as iridocorneal endothelial syndrome (see Chap. 127), the

phakomatoses (see Chap. 128), and elevated episcleral venous pressure (see Chap. 130) are discussed. The next group of chapters is related to the secondary angle-closure glaucomas. These glaucomas have an equally diverse group of causes. Neovascular glaucoma, perhaps the most common secondary form of angle-closure glaucoma, is discussed in Chapter 132. Other less common forms are discussed in subsequent chapters including the type associated with cataract surgery (see Chap. 133), unusual forms of angle-closure glaucoma such as malignant glaucoma (see Chap. 134), and nanophthalmos (see Chap. 135) are discussed. Glaucoma following penetrating keratoplasty or association with retinal and choroidal surgery or diseases are discussed in Chapters 136 and 137, respectively.

The therapeutic approach to glaucoma of course depends on its specific cause. The management of almost all glaucomas is initiated with medical therapy (see Chap. 138). Laser therapy has become increasingly important in the management of both open-angle glaucoma (see Chap. 139), angle-closure glaucoma (see Chap. 140), and may, in the future, replace many forms of traditional glaucoma surgery (see Chap. 141). Despite the advances of medical and laser therapy, surgical therapy is still an important approach to patients who otherwise have uncontrollable glaucoma. In patients for whom laser therapy is ineffective in establishing an iridectomy or in whom the anterior chamber remains shallow and requires deepening, a surgical approach may be required (see Chap. 142). Filtration surgery is still an important approach to patients with glaucoma that does not respond to more conservative treatment (see Chap. 143). Both cataracts and glaucoma are associated with aging. Issues regarding the management of these diseases when they occur concomitantly is discussed in Chapter 144. Although filtration surgery has a high degree of success in most cases, a variety of complications may occur in association with these procedures (see Chap. 145). In cases in which filtration surgery has failed in the past or the likelihood of success is very low, the placement of setons has become increasingly common and is frequently successful (see Chap. 146). In children, and in some selected cases of juvenile open-angle glaucoma, goniotomy or trabeculotomy has been successful (see Chap. 221). When filtration surgery or placement of a seton does not appear to be practical, the use of cycloablative procedures is often considered (see Chap. 147). In the future, new surgical techniques (see Chap. 148) will improve our management of patients with glaucoma.

CLINICAL EXAMINATION

■

Chapter 111

■

History

FRANK G. BERSON

A thorough and accurate history, which is always an essential component of good medical practice, is especially important for diagnosing and managing glaucoma. When a patient presents with signs of glaucoma, the past general medical history and the past ocular history often help to establish the cause of the condition and facilitate treatment.

Regarding primary open-angle glaucoma, it is particularly important to determine risk factors in the history—that is, family history of open-angle glaucoma, cardiovascular disease, or diabetes mellitus. Additional risk factors, including age, race, cup:disc ratio, high myopia, central retinal vein occlusion, and elevated intraocular pressure (IOP),[1-3] may be determined at the time of clinical examination.

FAMILY HISTORY OF GLAUCOMA

The prevalence of primary open-angle glaucoma increases among relatives of patients with glaucoma, but the genetic basis is still unclear. Inheritance is usually described as multifactorial, and a positive family history has been found in up to 50 percent of patients with primary open-angle glaucoma.[4] Furthermore, evidence suggests that a positive maternal family history is a stronger risk factor than a positive paternal family history.

Family history is less useful in establishing the risk of angle-closure glaucoma in a patient with a narrow angle.[3] The ocular history is more conclusive in terms of symptoms suggestive of previous angle-closure attacks or the clinical judgment of the ophthalmologist determining the occludability of an angle in the individual patient.

SYSTEMIC DISEASES

Cardiovascular diseases, including hypertension, arteriosclerotic cardiovascular disease, cardiac failure from various causes, hypercoagulability, and hypercholesterolemia, potentially diminish optic nerve head perfusion and are more common in patients with open-angle glaucoma, particularly in those with low-tension glaucoma.

A severe hypotensive episode, perhaps related to a major blood loss, can temporarily compromise optic nerve head perfusion and result in optic atrophy and subsequent glaucomatous cupping at relatively modest pressure elevations or even at normal pressures.

Diabetes mellitus is an endocrine disorder that is strongly associated with the development of open-angle glaucoma.[5] In addition, patients with diabetes who have developed proliferative diabetic retinopathy are at risk for neovascularization of the anterior segment and secondary glaucoma.

Various forms of arthritis are associated with the development of uveitis, which in turn can cause a secondary glaucoma. Ocular inflammation is particularly common in ankylosing spondylitis and monarthric juvenile rheumatoid arthritis and is less common in Reiter's syndrome and adult rheumatoid arthritis.[6]

Sarcoidosis is a systemic inflammatory disease that causes granulomatous uveitis, in which synechia formation is common. Extensive posterior synechiae can lead to seclusion of the pupil, iris bombé, and secondary angle-closure requiring iridectomy.

MEDICATIONS

Various topical or systemic drugs previously used by the patient may have caused elevated IOP or other adverse reactions. Use of these agents may be documented as part of a complete ocular and general medical history.

A number of systemic medications have sympathomimetic or cholinergic activity and are contraindicated for use in patients with a history of glaucoma. However, this warning is relevant only to the patient with anatomically narrow angles in whom partial pupil dilatation could effect a pressure rise or a full-blown attack of angle-closure glaucoma. The patient with a history of angle-closure glaucoma almost invariably has undergone an iridectomy, in which case these drugs are not contraindicated. Similarly, these agents can be prescribed for the patient with a history of open-angle glaucoma, because dilatation should not induce a pressure rise.

Corticosteroids, commonly administered for a variety of ocular, dermatologic, or systemic conditions, can induce substantial IOP elevations in susceptible individuals with open angles.[7] The patients who are most at risk are those with a history of open-angle glaucoma, diabetes mellitus, and high myopia. Approximately 4 percent of "normal" individuals experience a substantial pressure rise to greater than 30 mmHg after 4 to 6 wk of topical corticosteroid administration; 30 percent of the population has a less dramatic, albeit significant, elevation.[8] The pressure elevation induced by corticosteroids in certain individuals usually abates within weeks of discontinuation but may persist. Thus, previous, long-term usage may manifest as normal or elevated IOP with or without glaucomatous optic atrophy.

Corticosteroids can be administered for a variety of conditions by a number of possible routes. These routes include topical ocular preparations for chronic conjunctivitis, periocular skin applications for dermatitis that may reach the conjunctiva, periocular "depot" injections for chronic uveitis, and systemic administration for a variety of inflammatory diseases.

It is important to obtain a history of allergic reactions to medications. In particular, carbonic anhydrase inhibitors are contraindicated for use in patients who have had previous adverse reactions to sulfonamides. A previous reaction to fluorescein is a relative contraindication to use of intravenous fluorescein in connection with a work-up for optic atrophy or ocular vascular occlusion.

PAST OCULAR HISTORY

Trauma is a common cause of both acute and chronic glaucoma. Whereas a blunt injury commonly results in an acute pressure rise due to blood, iritis, or trabecular dysfunction, late-onset glaucoma may be seen after perforating and nonperforating injuries. Many patients relate a history of an eye "injury." Although such injuries are often trivial, a history of profound, transient loss of vision, intraocular bleeding with or without hospitalization, or treatment with surgery indicates increased risk of subsequent glaucoma.

The degree of angle recession can predict the risk of future glaucoma and can help to explain the cause of glaucoma with antecedent blunt trauma, usually in association with a hyphema. Recession less than 180 degrees does not appear to be a significant risk factor, but if two thirds or more of the angle is recessed, up to 10 percent of patients may have persistent or late-onset glaucoma.[9, 10]

A traumatic vitreous hemorrhage can lead to ghost-cell glaucoma, which can be difficult to manage. Severe pressure rises may persist for days to weeks and require repeat anterior chamber washouts or vitrectomy for definitive treatment. The sequela of this condition may be optic atrophy.

If a patient has had a perforating injury, usually requiring surgical repair, late glaucoma is a common sequela from peripheral anterior synechia. These synechia may result from a flat anterior chamber or from a severe intraocular inflammation.

Surgery can induce significant pressure elevations that are usually brief and self-limited but that can be severe and prolonged. This can occur with various types of anterior and posterior segment surgery in eyes with or without a history of preexistent glaucoma. Self-limited pressure elevations are common following cataract extraction and intraocular lens implantation. Causes of acute postoperative glaucoma include trabecular deformation in the area of the incision as well as inflammatory products, viscoelastics, and blood that temporarily compromise trabecular outflow. "Enzyme glaucoma," resulting from the use of α-chymotrypsin during intracapsular surgery, was a common event; however, α-chymotrypsin is no longer used in extracapsular surgery. Glaucoma occurring days to weeks after surgery can result from pupillary block, posterior aqueous diversion, and prolonged use of corticosteroids in susceptible individuals. Subsequent clinical examination may not reveal any of these causes, with optic nerve head atrophy as the only sequela.

Glaucoma is a common complication of penetrating keratoplasty.[3, 6, 10] The cause may be a pupillary block in the absence of a functional iridectomy. Other causes are believed to be iris swelling, angle compression, and choroidal detachment, which can lead to extensive peripheral anterior synechiae. These cases present subsequently as chronic angle-closure glaucoma.

Scleral buckling procedures for retinal detachment can also cause chronic glaucoma as a result of peripheral anterior synechia. Acutely, the buckle may occlude vortex veins, causing congestion and anterior ciliary body rotation. Peripheral choroidal detachments are often seen with shallowing of the anterior chamber.[6, 10] Intravitreal silicone oil, used in conjunction with vitrectomy and scleral buckling, can cause acute pupillary block or persistent open-angle glaucoma.

Inflammation, which occurs as a result of both trauma and surgery, can occur spontaneously. Inflammatory glaucoma can compromise the optic nerve head without other sequelae. Other pathologic changes, including peripheral anterior synechiae and posterior synechiae,[3, 10] may result from chronic inflammation. The use of corticosteroids to treat ocular inflammation may induce or aggravate IOP elevations.

Optic neuropathy from various causes mimics glaucomatous optic atrophy or presents an additional risk factor for further damage at a given IOP. In ischemic optic neuropathy due to giant cell arteritis, initial pale swelling of the disc can be followed months later by glaucomatous cupping. There is less prominent cupping in the nonarteritic cases that are presumably caused by arteriosclerosis.[3, 10–12] Other conditions include compressive tumors and demyelinating disease. Toxins and drugs, such as methyl alcohol or ethambutol, can result in optic atrophy.

Previous glaucoma treatments and diagnostic tests constitute extremely valuable and sometimes crucial historical information for the ophthalmologist caring for a patient with a history of glaucoma. Since the patient is often unaware of or cannot recall much of this information, efforts should be made to obtain medical records or reports of previous care.

The IOP level at which treatment was initiated as well as the pressure at which further disc damage or field loss may have occurred should be known. Optic disc photographs, drawings, and descriptions as well as previous fields are important for future management. Topical and systemic medications that may have been nonefficacious or poorly tolerated because of side effects or allergic reactions should be documented along with exact dosages. For example, a patient who is thought to be intolerant of carbonic anhydrase inhibitors may never have been placed on a lower dosage that may have significantly lowered the IOP. Similarly, a patient with a history of pilocarpine intolerance may have been given a 4 percent solution in both eyes, whereas a weaker solution in one eye may have been more effective.

If a patient previously underwent either laser or incisional glaucoma surgery, details of the methodology and postoperative course should be obtained. In the case of laser trabeculoplasty, one should know the exact clock hours of the trabecular meshwork treated, because laser application to a previously untreated area is much safer than re-treatment. It is often impossible to ascertain gonioscopically the location of a previous treatment. Conversely, if a cyclodestructive procedure is planned, care should be taken not to treat the entire remainder of the untreated clock hours of the ciliary body. In this case, to avoid hypotony re-treatment is safer than 360-degree treatment. Finally, when previous incisional surgery has been performed, one should be aware of the techniques used and the complications, if any, to maximize the success of future surgery.

OCULAR SYMPTOMS

Patients with primary open-angle glaucoma are usually asymptomatic, even when the IOP is very high. The lack of symptoms is a major contributing factor to late diagnosis; in fact, the diagnosis is most commonly established during a routine evaluation and screening or when the patient presents with an unrelated complaint. Certainly, an advanced field defect or a compromise of central visual acuity may be noted by a particular patient. In addition, if IOP is high enough to cause corneal edema or bullous keratopathy, the patient may have pain or diminished visual acuity.

With angle-closure glaucoma, intermittent pain, photophobia, and colored haloes around lights often indicate rapid pressure elevations, which may resolve spontaneously. Visual blurring, varying in severity in subacute angle-closure, can mimic amaurosis fugax seen with vascular insufficiency. Severe pain around the eye accompanied by nausea and vomiting are highly suggestive of acute angle-closure.

Symptoms in glaucomatocyclitic crisis can be similar to those seen in acute angle-closure glaucoma. Clinical examination, with particular emphasis on gonioscopy, is essential for establishing an accurate diagnosis.

Secondary open-angle glaucomas such as corticosteroid glaucoma, pseudoexfoliative glaucoma, and pigmentary glaucoma also are generally asymptomatic as in primary open-angle glaucoma. A notable exception is seen in a few patients with pigment dispersion syndrome. In those cases, exercise can provoke an acute pressure rise, resulting in blurred vision and colored haloes around lights.[10]

Patients with secondary glaucoma associated with uveitis usually present with pain, photophobia, and blurred vision. The extent of the pressure rise varies considerably. The blurring may be related to either an acute pressure rise causing corneal edema or corneal decompensation secondary to heavy keratic precipitation on the central endothelium (e.g., granulomatous uveitis).

Patients with neovascular glaucoma present with ocular symptoms similar to those seen in uveitic glaucoma. However, the angle is more likely to be closed, and the IOP is higher. Therefore, pain and blurred vision predominate over photophobia. The patient may be less aware of an acute change in vision because there is often pre-existent fundus pathology (e.g., proliferative diabetic retinopathy, central retinal vein occlusion).

RISK FACTORS

When risk factors have been determined by both the history and the clinical examination, patients with normal IOPs should be reevaluated at least annually and perhaps more frequently. If the patient develops elevated IOP, treatment is usually initiated. Conversely, in the patient who presents with a mild-to-moderate elevation of IOP (i.e., the glaucoma suspect or ocular hypertensive), the establishment of one or more additional risk factors usually determines whether or not the IOP is treated and to what extent. As with low-tension glaucoma, treatment may be initiated when IOP is not elevated if other risk factors are sufficiently compelling.

REFERENCES

1. Kass MA, Hart WM, Gordon M, Miller JP: Risk factors favoring the development of glaucomatous visual field loss in ocular hypertension. Surv Ophthalmol 25:155, 1980.
2. Hoskins HD, Kass MA (eds): Becker-Shaffer's Diagnosis and Therapy of the Glaucomas, 7th ed. St Louis, CV Mosby, 1988, pp 293–296.
3. Shields MB: Textbook of Glaucoma, 2nd ed. Baltimore, Williams & Wilkins, 1987, pp 81–349.
4. Shin DH, Becker B, Kolker AE: Family history in primary open-angle glaucoma. Arch Ophthalmol 95:598, 1977.
5. Becker B: Diabetes mellitus and primary open angle glaucoma. Am J Ophthalmol 71:1, 1971.
6. Ritch R, Shields MB, Krupin T (eds): The Glaucomas. St. Louis, CV Mosby, 1989, pp 1052–1347.
7. Becker B, Hahn KA: Topical corticosteroids and heredity in primary open-angle glaucoma. Am J Ophthalmol 57:543, 1964.
8. Becker B: Intraocular pressure responses to topical corticosteroids. Invest Ophthalmol 4:198, 1965.
9. Kaufman JH, Tolpin DW: Glaucoma after traumatic angle recession: A ten year prospective study. Am J Ophthalmol 78:648, 1974.
10. Epstein DL: Chandler and Grant's Glaucoma. Philadelphia, Lea & Febiger, 1986, pp 99–410.
11. Hayreh SS: Pathogenesis of cupping of the optic disc. Br J Ophthalmol 58:863, 1974.
12. Quigley H, Anderson DR: Cupping of the optic disc in ischemic optic neuropathy. Trans Am Acad Ophthalmol Otolaryngol 83:755, 1977.

Chapter 112

■

Ocular Examination of Patients With Glaucoma

DAVID K. DUEKER

GENERAL CONSIDERATIONS

A simple linear progression from complaint to history to examination rarely suffices when evaluating a patient with glaucoma. Frequently, particularly with primary open-angle glaucoma (POAG), a patient's presenting complaint has little or no connection with the yet undiscovered glaucoma. Instead, a patient presents requesting stronger bifocals, is concerned about a floater, or simply has scheduled a routine check-up. Abnormalities suggestive of glaucoma are uncovered during the examination, leading to a more detailed history taking that, in turn, may suggest additional areas for examination.

In this common scenario, on discovery of asymptomatic glaucoma, the focus of the clinical visit rapidly shifts from the "minor" presenting complaint to the more serious problem. It is important to remember that this discovery is often shocking to patients. Even though the physician rightly believes that by detecting glaucoma he or she renders a crucial service, the patient, who perhaps came prepared only for new glasses, suddenly must adjust to the possibility of having a chronic, potentially blinding disease. Clear communication is important during this difficult time for a patient. Listening well and responding to a patient's problems help to develop the trust and commitment necessary for successful long-term treatment of glaucoma.

Because the time scheduled for a routine office visit is often inadequate to evaluate newly discovered glaucoma, one may explain the initial findings to patients and schedule a follow-up visit for further testing to confirm the diagnosis and initiate any necessary treatment. This approach is preferable to making a diagnosis based on incomplete information and starting treatment without offering thorough instructions and support. Of course, this option must be tempered by consideration of the urgency to begin treatment and the type of glaucoma involved.

MEDICAL HISTORY AND GENERAL HEALTH

The general health of a patient is relevant to a broad range of ocular diseases, and the glaucomas have multiple interactions with systemic disease. Many elements of the medical history obtained during a routine ocular examination relate directly or indirectly to glaucoma and its management. For example, diabetes mellitus is a risk factor for several different forms of glaucoma

through separate and distinct mechanisms—for example, POAG, neovascular glaucoma, ghost cell glaucoma, and pseudophakic pupillary block glaucoma.

Sickle cell anemia/trait is another systemic disorder with multiple links to glaucoma. Retinal ischemia caused by the disease may lead to anterior segment neovascularization and neovascular glaucoma. Glaucoma secondary to traumatic hyphema is also more likely to occur in a patient who has a tendency to develop sickle cell anemia. Furthermore, when glaucoma does occur, the eye is much less able to tolerate even moderate pressure elevations because of the tendency to develop vascular occlusions. Finally, the treatment options are limited; two of the standard medications for acute glaucoma, acetazolamide and mannitol, are contraindicated because they can cause acidosis and hemoconcentration.

Clearly, multiple pathways may link systemic illness with various glaucomas (Table 112–1). For this reason, a comprehensive medical history is an essential part of the glaucoma evaluation. It is also wise to communicate directly with a patient's primary physician and to update the medical status (e.g., surgery, drug changes) routinely.

OCULAR HISTORY

The ocular history in POAG may be largely noncontributory. Myopia is more common among these patients than in the general population (whereas hyperopia is decidedly more common in POAG). In addition, because glaucoma tends to develop in older patients, presbyopia is frequently present. To eliminate other mechanisms for glaucoma, one should inquire specifically about prior trauma (including surgery), inflammation (including use of steroids), or infection. Recollection of these historical events is often triggered or reemphasized during the examination. For example, a patient may not recall serious trauma, yet the examination reveals a recessed chamber angle. Further careful questioning may uncover a childhood injury forgotten during the initial inquiry.

Many forms of secondary glaucoma have distinctive ocular histories, information about which will be forthcoming in the course of routine questioning about ocular health. A sudden, profound, and lasting visual decrease after central retinal vein occlusion, a predisposing event for neovascular glaucoma, is usually reported by patients. Hazing of vision on vigorous exercise may be symptomatic of pigmentary glaucoma (from sudden release of pigment into the aqueous). Because vision clears

Table 112–1. PATHWAYS LINKING SYSTEMIC ILLNESS WITH GLAUCOMA

	Causal link	
	←————————→	
	Treatment	
Systemic Disorder	←————————→	Glaucoma
	Genetic link	
	←————————→	

The importance of the medical history in a patient with glaucoma is seen in the ways glaucoma may be linked with systemic illness.

Causal link: A pathologic derangement caused by a systemic disease leads directly or indirectly to glaucoma (e.g., homocystinuria with lens subluxation and angle-closure).

Treatment: The treatment of a systemic disease causes or aggravates glaucoma, or conversely, the glaucoma treatment causes a systemic side effect (e.g., corticosteroid therapy may cause or worsen glaucoma; carbonic anhydrase inhibition may cause kidney stones).

Genetic link: The tendency for glaucoma to be inherited along with other systemic abnormalities (e.g., Axenfeld-Rieger syndrome).

within hours, patients may not mention this spontaneously but respond if asked specifically. The pain and blurred vision characteristic of angle-closure glaucoma are often distinctive points in an ocular history. However, some patients with angle-closure are so impressed by their headache during an attack that this becomes their predominant memory. Further careful, pointed questions, in this case triggered by finding a narrow angle on clinical examination, may lead to a more accurate description of the symptoms. The evaluation process should be continued in this recursive fashion, from history to examination, back to history and so on, until the best possible agreement between history and examination findings is established.

FAMILY HISTORY

The family history is important for several reasons. First, a positive family history is an important risk factor for POAG. In addition, several of the childhood glaucomas have well-described hereditary patterns that can be helpful in diagnosis and genetic counseling. Finally, a positive family history often has important psychosocial overtones.

Patients who have a family member with glaucoma, particularly with a complicated case, are usually more anxious when confronted with their own disease process. A personal experience such as this can have a positive effect by encouraging careful adherence to treatment; however, if treatment was unsuccessful for the patient's relative, the patient may feel discouraged and unmotivated. Clearly, it is important to develop an understanding of an individual patient's perception of glaucoma, dispel unreasonable fears, and work toward a firm commitment to therapy.

EXTERNAL EXAMINATION

In POAG, the external appearance of the eyes and adnexa is generally unremarkable. In other circumstances, however, the periocular structures may provide obvious or subtle clues that suggest coexisting glaucoma. For example, a hemangioma of the upper lid frequently is associated with open-angle glaucoma of the ipsilateral eye in patients with Sturge-Weber syndrome. Dilatation of the episcleral veins, a less obvious vascular abnormality, may signal glaucoma caused by an arteriovenous malformation that increases the episcleral venous pressure. In addition to noting specific glaucoma-related findings such as these, the external examination should include a search for signs of previous trauma, proptosis, restriction of movement, photophobia and tearing, and hyperemia.

The pupillary responses are generally normal in POAG, but an afferent defect may be present if severe nerve damage has occurred. Other glaucomas may show more distinct pupillary signs, such as a fixed midposition pupil in acute angle-closure; a miotic pupil in acute iritis; an irregular pupil bound down by posterior synechiae in a case of previous inflammation; displaced or multiple pupils in the iridocorneoendothelial (ICE) syndrome; and color change in Fuchs's heterochromic iridocyclitis. Therefore, in addition to direct and consensual responsiveness, the pupils should be evaluated for size, number, shape and equality (preferably in both light and dark), and color.

SLIT-LAMP BIOMICROSCOPY

A slit-lamp biomicroscope is invaluable in the ocular clinical examination; findings associated with the glaucomas demonstrate its versatility. Observation of subtle elements in the anterior segment requires both the magnified stereo view provided by the slit lamp and the great variability in lighting afforded by this instrument. In addition, through use of auxiliary optic devices, a slit-lamp biomicroscope offers one of the best ways to examine the anterior chamber angle and the optic nerve head.

The conjunctiva is usually normal in appearance in POAG as well as in other types of glaucoma. Dilated episcleral veins, specifically associated with glaucoma, already have been mentioned. A single dilated anterior vein (sentinel vessel) is an important sign of an anteriorly located tumor, which presents with glaucoma. More generalized hyperemia is a nonspecific sign of inflammation or irritation and may be associated with several types of secondary glaucoma.

Although initially normal, the conjunctiva may be altered later in the course of glaucoma by an allergic reaction to drug treatment or through accumulation of drug deposits (adrenochrome) after long-term epinephrine instillation. Histologic signs of long-term toxicity from topical glaucoma drug therapy have been described, but these changes do not appear to have specific biomicroscopic correlates. Of course, the conjunctiva is an important tissue in the context of filtering surgery. Slit-lamp biomicroscopy is used preoperatively to select an optimal "filtering bed" (mobile and free from scarring); postoperatively, conjunctival hypovascularity, translucency, and surface microcysts are useful signs of bleb function.

CORNEAL SLIT-LAMP EXAMINATION

Biomicroscopic corneal examination should include an assessment of clarity, size, and vascularity, as well as attention to each tissue layer. Specific corneal findings, some of which are subtle and must be specifically sought, are helpful in diagnosing several secondary glaucomas.

Not surprisingly, the cornea is generally normal for age in POAG, unless the intraocular pressure (IOP) is sufficiently high to cause corneal edema, which is rare at the usually moderate pressure levels of POAG. Rapid development of extremely high pressures (>50 mmHg) is more likely to cause marked corneal edema, such as in acute angle-closure or neovascular glaucoma. Lower pressures may cause corneal edema in cases in which the corneal endothelium is compromised, such as with inflammatory precipitates or in the ICE syndrome.

Corneal stromal scars are useful markers of prior trauma, infection, or inflammation. Careful inspection of the stroma for signs of old interstitial keratitis (midstromal scarring and ghost vessel) is valuable, because these otherwise quiet eyes may develop glaucoma as a late complication. When the cornea is of normal thickness, it is a useful gauge of anterior chamber depth: Normal chamber depth is approximately four to five times the central corneal thickness. When chamber depth varies (e.g., progressive shallowing after filtration surgery) and one wishes to chart its progress, a sequential record of depth by corneal thickness can be extremely helpful. Corneal thickness is used in the periphery of the anterior chamber to gauge the distance between the anterior surface of the peripheral iris and the posterior surface of the peripheral cornea. A space less than one fourth of the corneal thickness is highly suggestive of a dangerously narrow angle.

Abnormalities of Descemet's membrane are not frequent in glaucomas. In infantile glaucoma, sudden stretching of the globe caused by elevated pressure may result in rupture of the membrane. Overlying edema that clears as the endothelium heals over the rupture is thus created, leaving curved, usually horizontal, ridges (Haab's striae) on the posterior surface. Descemet's membrane is also the site of the major pathologic changes in posterior polymorphous dystrophy, which is attended by glaucoma in 15 percent of cases.

Several forms of glaucoma are associated with characteristic alterations in or on the endothelial surface of the cornea. Material suspended in the aqueous humor tends to deposit on the endothelium. For example, in pigment dispersion and pigmentary glaucoma, a narrow spindle of deposited pigment builds up on the central cornea posteriorly (Krukenberg's spindle). In glaucoma associated with intraocular inflammation, cells deposit on the endothelium sometimes in typical formations. These keratic precipitates (KPs) may be small round mounds; large juicy clumps (mutton-fat KP of granulomatous disease); or delicate stellate (typical of heterochromic iridocyclitis) deposits. With time, these deposits tend to become pigmented. It must be emphasized that inflammation sufficient to cause glaucoma may not produce marked signs of anterior chamber inflammation and numerous KPs. In fact, KPs associated with glaucoma may be restricted to the chamber angle, as discussed later under Gonioscopy.

In ICE syndrome, the primary pathology is abnormal corneal endothelial cells, with secondary glaucoma and iris distortion and atrophy resulting from posterior migration of these abnormal cells. Because the iris and chamber angle changes may be minimal in one subcategory of this disorder (Chandler's syndrome), careful slit-lamp examination of the corneal endothelium may be crucial to the diagnosis. The cells are large and irregular, and the endothelial surface has a beaten silver appearance in specular illumination. A specular microscope is a useful adjunct in suspected cases.

The normal anterior chamber is four to five corneal thicknesses deep, with its posterior extent defined by the lens and a relatively flat iris plane; its anterior extent is determined by the corneal endothelial surface. The normal aqueous humor is optically clear. The depth of the peripheral chamber must be assessed separately, because a deep central chamber does not ensure depth in the periphery. The surface contour of the iris is normally flat or slightly bowed forward. Moderate forward bowing may be associated with increased relative pupillary block or lens enlargement. Marked forward bowing of the iris is seen with iris bombé. Backward bowing (peripheral concavity of the iris) is a frequent finding in pigmentary glaucoma.

The iris itself is examined for abnormal surface deposits (e.g., pigment in pigmentary dispersion; pigment or exfoliation material in exfoliation syndrome), pigmented nodules (ICE syndrome), lens or peripheral corneal adhesions (secondary to inflammation), and abnormal surface vessels (rubeosis). The iris may be atrophied in sectors (status postacute angle-closure), patches (ICE syndrome), or diffusely (heterochromic iridocylitis). Iris transillumination may reveal characteristic defects in the pigment epithelial layer: transillumination along the pupillary margin in exfoliation syndrome, transillumination in a spoke-wheel pattern in pigmentary glaucoma.

Through abnormalities in its fixation, size, location, and integrity, the lens is the primary cause of several glaucomas. If the lens zonules are weak because of either metabolic abnormality or trauma, the lens may move forward into the pupil, causing pupillary block, a shallow anterior chamber, and angle-closure glaucoma. A lens with loose zonules shows a slight tremulousness, particularly after a refixation movement or blink when observed on biomicroscopy with a slit of light focused across the anterior lens surface. With greater degrees of dislocation, the lens decenters and an edge may become visible along one section of the pupillary margin.

The lens surface often provides useful clues to pathologic processes. Synechiae may form to the lens during inflammation, and the iris later breaks free spontaneously or because of cycloplegic therapy, leaving an incomplete circle of pigment on the anterior lens surface near the pupil as a marker of prior inflammation. In exfoliation syndrome, the lens surface is coated with variable amounts of fine, ashen-gray, irregular flakes that are pathognomonic. The typical distribution of this material suggests that the moving pupil scrapes off material wherever it makes contact with the lens, resulting in an undisturbed central round zone that is lightly coated with material, outside of which is a fairly even circle of lens surface free of exfoliation material and an irregular wreath of material in the far periphery. These features are best appreciated with a dilated pupil.

As the lens enlarges during cataract formation, relative pupillary block is increased and the danger of angle-closure rises. If a lens becomes sufficiently large, it may force the angle closed by direct pressure. In addition, with full or nearly full cataract maturation, the capsule may lose its integrity and begin to leak lens material in the aqueous, causing a phacolytic glaucoma. Slit-lamp examination reveals an aqueous flare, often with fragments of suspended lens material, and various degrees of cellular response.

GONIOSCOPY

Gonioscopy, visual inspection of the anterior chamber angle, is a valuable and essential tool for evaluating virtually all glaucomas. Initial evaluation of any newly diagnosed case is complete only if it includes a gonioscopic examination. In addition, proper long-term glaucoma management requires gonioscopy at appropriate intervals because the condition of the angle is not static through life—that is, it is influenced by pupil size, ciliary tone, lens size, and other changeable factors. In absolutely stable, easily controlled cases, gonioscopy should be repeated every 2 to 3 yr. However, any time that a patient has an erratic course (e.g., marked fluctuations in pressure, lack of response to previously effective medications), reexamination of the chamber angle is indicated.

Unfortunately, angle examination is not simply a matter of redirecting the slit-lamp biomicroscope. Light leaving the chamber angle strikes the cornea-air interface at such an oblique angle that it is reflected internally: No image can form outside the eye. To overcome this, various lenses have been designed to allow imaging of the angle by first neutralizing the cornea-air interface and then providing a less oblique angle of incidence at the surface where light from the angle enters the air. Numerous optical devices have been designed for gonioscopy, all of which can be categorized as either direct or indirect, and there are several useful instruments in each group.

It is not advisable to select one form of gonioscopy and use it to the exclusion of all others; each has advantages in specific circumstances. Chandler and Grant advocate careful laboratory dissection of the anterior chamber angle of an enucleated eye to enhance one's understanding of gonioscopic findings. This is an instructive exercise for beginning gonioscopists. Repetition of this exercise after gaining some clinical experience usually allows understanding that is not possible initially. Direct gonioscopy with a Koeppe's lens provides the most natural clinical correlate to this laboratory experience and an excellent introduction to the technique.

The image of the angle may be viewed directly or indirectly; both types of gonioscopy have their advantages. In the direct form of gonioscopy, a contact lens with a large spherical front surface is used, allowing the image to leave the eye by eliminating the cornea-air interface and then to leave the lens by allowing the light to strike the lens-air interface almost perpendicularly. A typical direct gonioscopic set-up includes the contact lens designed by Koeppe used with a hand-held binocular microscope and a Barkan's light (a high-intensity hand-held illuminating source). Direct ophthalmoscopy is advantageous because all the angle features are seen in their normal spatial relationship. A broad panoramic view of the angle contours is obtained with great flexibility in viewing angle and lighting. For direct surgical intervention in the angle, the direct view is the only practical approach. Several specialized surgical lenses have been designed to allow simultaneous instrumentation and viewing of the angle.

Goldmann designed a gonioscopy lens that allows the image to leave the eye by providing a cornea-lens interface and then redirecting the image with a small mirror to the slit lamp for viewing (indirect gonioscopy). Because of the mirror, the observer sees a reversed image of the angle. With experience, use of this lens is usually not a problem, but beginners at gonioscopy find this more challenging than the direct view afforded by a Koeppe's lens. Because the mirrored lens can be used at the slit lamp, all of the advantages of the slit lamp are incorporated into this technique—that is, both the patient and the physician are already familiar with the examination position and no special rearrangement of the examining room is necessary. The slit lamp affords stable and well-focused illumination coupled with high-magnification optics. Slit-lamp–based gonioscopy is also directly compatible with slit-lamp–based lasers.

An extremely useful variation of indirect gonioscopy is the Zeiss four-mirror lens, which is mounted in a metal fork (Posner's and Sussman's lenses are effective alternatives). This is an indirect lens with four mirrors that allows observation of four quadrants without turning the lens. However, the most useful aspect of the lens is its small, central, and relatively flat area of contact with the cornea. Because the lens curve closely matches the corneal curve, no specific gonioscopic fluids are used, and the normal tear film provides optical coupling of the lens to the cornea. Because the area of the contact is small and central, slight pressure on the lens indents the central cornea, forcing aqueous fluid into the periphery of the chamber. This particular maneuver is useful to assess the degree of synechial closure of a very narrow angle. Frequently, an angle is so narrow in appearance that it is not clear by usual gonioscopy whether the angle is actually closed by synechiae or merely extremely narrow or even touching but without synechia formation. By gentle indentation of the central cornea with the four-mirror lens, the chamber can be transiently deepened in the periphery, and this differentiation can be made. If the need for iridotomy is questionable in a narrow-angle situation, clear demonstration of early synechia formation by indention gonioscopy resolves the question in favor of iridotomy.

All patients with elevated pressures should undergo gonioscopy to make this important distinction. Different systems for grading the narrowness of the angle have been developed to help clinicians define the appearance of the angle and predict the threat of angle-closure. In a widely used grading system proposed by Shaffer, a wide-open angle (an angle of approximately 30 to 40 degrees between iris and peripheral cornea) is graded 3 to 4. An angle that is somewhat narrow but still allows a view of the scleral spur (approximately 20 degrees) is graded 2. A grade 1 angle is considered to be at significant risk for closure, with the angle between the iris and the peripheral cornea approximately 10 degrees. In grade 1, because of the forward bowing of the peripheral iris, the scleral spur cannot be seen and only Schwalbe's line and some of the trabecular meshwork is visible. A grade 0 angle is considered to be closed and allows no view of any angle structures.

Spaeth suggested a somewhat more complex grading system that includes the capability for recording not only the angle between the iris and the cornea but also an estimate of the height of iris insertion and the general shape of the iris contour. Such variations emphasize the difficulty of reducing the variability of angle appearance to a single numerical value. Even though it may be useful to sort out gonioscopic appearance initially on the basis of four of five angle grades, the duty of a gonioscopist does not stop there. Features such as the peripheral iris contour, the distribution of pigmentation, and the consistency of appearance from one region to the next all demand careful attention.

It is not impossible to produce a simple and short list of gonioscopic findings that separate normality from pathology. Some discrete and obvious findings are clearly evident, including foreign bodies in the angle, large peripheral synechiae, and proliferation of new vessels. Many other findings are more subtle and are readily apparent only to an observer who has an extensive background in the appearance and variations of the normal angle. For this reason, gonioscopy should be performed frequently, not only in patients for whom it is absolutely essential but also in a number of normal persons, to gain a sense of the clinical appearance of the chamber angle. For example, the chamber angle of normal infants differs from an adult's angle. If an examiner has not observed a number of infants' angles (which can be done, for example, during strabismus surgery), it is difficult to appreciate the unique abnormality of a congenital glaucoma angle. Practitioners can

achieve full benefits from gonioscopy only by being comfortable and proficient with the technique.

OPTIC NERVE HEAD

Glaucoma reduces visual function by damaging the optic nerve as it enters the eye. Examination of the nerve is helpful in making the initial diagnosis, setting a goal for treatment, and monitoring its success. Clinical visible nerve head damage may take the form of relatively discrete focal damage or a more generalized, diffuse loss of axons. The two modes of damage may occur together.

A normal nerve head consists of approximately 1.2 million nerve axons and their supporting tissues, including glia, blood vessels, and connective tissue. The axons enter the eye in multiple bundles traveling through openings in the lamina cribrosa and then, within the eye, spread out to all regions of the retina. This divergence of axons from the optic nerve head to the retina usually leaves a small depression or "cup" in the center of the optic nerve head. Between this cup and the edge of the optic disc is the neural rim, a band of orange-pink neural tissue.

The major retinal vessels travel within the optic nerve into the eye; within the eye they travel on or near the surface of the nerve head and nerve fiber layer. In this way, the vessels mark the surface topography of the nerve head. Because the nerves are packed together at the nerve head before spreading out over the retina, the neural rim usually is elevated somewhat above the level of the retina; gentle curves in the vessel paths as the nerves cross the neural rim reflect this.

A normal optic disc has a slightly oval shape, the vertical dimension being greatest. The normal optic cup is nearly circular, though it may be a slightly oval. The size of the cup directly reflects the ratio between the size of the disc and the number of nerve fibers; in normal persons, the number of nerve fibers is not highly variable; disc area may vary four to five times. Therefore, most of the variability in the size of the normal cup reflects the size of the optic disc; larger discs have larger cups, and smaller discs, smaller cups. Clearly, the size of the cup alone or the ratio of cup size to disc size has little meaning without considering the absolute size of the disc.

The question of cup size is important in glaucoma, because the cup increases in size as nerve fibers are lost to the disease. Generalized, diffuse axon loss produces uniform cup enlargement; focal loss of axons produces localized cup enlargement. The whole process also may be stated in terms of the neural rim, which is perhaps more meaningful because the neural rim contains the functional tissue. From that perspective, generalized loss produces uniform narrowing of the neural rim, whereas focal loss produces focal narrowing of the rim.

A large circular cup may be a sign of glaucoma (a population of glaucoma patients generally has larger optic nerve cups and smaller neural rim areas than normal controls), but it also may be a normal variant. If the disc is small and the cup is large, the index of suspicion is higher. Of course, extremely large cups are also more suspect. On a single observation, however, cup size by itself is not highly specific for glaucoma.

A single look at circular cups can be more specific if inequality between the two eyes of a patient is noted. If the eyes are otherwise similar, the cups should be similar (within 0.1 cup:disc ratio). A difference greater than 0.2 cup:disc ratio is highly unusual in normal eyes and probably represents acquired damage.

Identifying pathologic damage in a circular cup is far simpler if a change occurs over time. Although a slow, age-related loss of axons probably occurs, this progression is not detectable by the usual clinical means. Therefore, detection of such change is clear evidence of an uncontrolled pathologic process.

As noted, glaucoma may selectively damage certain areas of the nerve head. The two most likely foci for early selective damage are the superior and inferior poles of the nerve, with the latter at somewhat greater risk than the former. Early loss of neural tissue at the poles leads to a change in the shape of the optic cup from circular to oval because of vertical elongation of the cup. A slightly oval cup may be found in normals, but a marked difference in vertical versus horizontal dimension suggests glaucoma, even on a single examination. Of course, vertical cup elongation is a sign of active pathology.

Selective loss at one or both poles may lead to focal narrowing of the neural rim, sometimes referred to as a *notch*. The cup in this region extends locally toward the scleral rim and may ultimately reach it.

As cupping progresses, the vertical cup elongation produced by moderate damage may revert to a circular shape as the horizontal dimension of the cup expands because of increasing loss of temporal, then nasal, axons. A small group of nasal axons usually survives in the late stages of damage, subserving a small island of vision in the temporal field. As the cup widens and deepens, the openings in the lamina cribrosa may be exposed to view.

Throughout this process, the surface vessels, with a few notable exceptions discussed later, shift with the diminishing nerve substance and provide a helpful guide to the altered contours of a damaged nerve. Tracing the path of individual vessels provides useful clues to overall nerve head contours; comparison of the vascular paths on sequential photographs can be a sensitive indicator of change. The vessels are particularly useful as markers in cases in which the clinical view of the nerve is gradually obscured, as with an advancing contact.

Occasionally, a vessel does not shift as the nerve beneath it atrophies, with the separation between the nerve and the previously adjacent vessel often marking pathologic change. A vessel that follows the rim of the optic cup is termed a *circumlinear vessel*. If the cup expands and the vessel remains in place, a space develops between the vessel and the cup (baring of a circumlinear vessel). Unfortunately, this sign is sometimes seen in normal eyes, so it is not specific for glaucoma. However, documented acquired baring, like other observable increases in cupping, is a specific sign of active pathology.

The small vessels of the upper and lower poles of the nerve occasionally bleed, giving rise to splinter hemorrhages on the disc. This finding is very rare in normal populations; it is most commonly associated with glaucoma but also may be seen with posterior vitreous detachment, ischemic optic neuropathy, or a bleeding diathesis. These small superficial hemorrhages occur in POAG and more frequently in normal-tension glaucoma. They are often associated with focal thinning of the nerve and sometimes may presage later field defects. These hemorrhages are important because they signal an active pathologic process, with glaucoma high on the list of causes.

Loss of axons, which present at the nerve head as changes in the cup and neural rim, also can be detected over the retina. The retinal nerve fiber layer may be seen as a uniform pattern of closely packed fine bundles radiating from the disc. Glaucomatous damage produces defects in these parallel bundles that appear as radiating dark flat stripes. The red free light on the slit lamp or ophthalmoscope increases the visibility of these defects, and specialized photographic techniques provide even more detail. This finding may be helpful in glaucoma screening and management. Unfortunately, the nerve fiber layer is more difficult to visualize in older patients and in the presence of cataracts.

METHODS

The nerve head examination is clearly a procedure that must be performed repeatedly and with great care. Many of the signs of active damage are subtle (e.g., small hemorrhages, focal thinning of the nerve rim, vessel shifts). A direct ophthalmoscope provides excellent magnification and good illumination (with the newer light sources), but the view is monocular, making assessment of subtle contour changes more difficult.

For examiners who wish a stereo view, several methods are available. The disc can be imaged in stereo at high magnification and in normal orientation using either a fundus contact lens or a Hruby's lens and the slit-lamp biomicroscope. The contact lens has the advantage of providing some lid and globe stability. It has the disadvantage of requiring a viscous coupling fluid. An alternative is to use a high-diopter indirect lens (78 to 90 D) with the slit lamp. This combination also provides a well-magnified stereo view, but the image is inverted. Once an examiner adjusts to the image inversion, this examination method is highly satisfactory. The standard binocular indirect ophthalmoscope does not provide sufficient magnification for routine careful nerve head examination.

RECORDS

The nerve head changes caused by glaucoma generally occur gradually over several years. Therefore, it is useful to have accurate records of nerve head status on several occasions. An ideal method is high-magnification stereo disc photos. Subtle but definite changes can frequently be seen in photographs even when no suspicion is raised on clinical examination, reflecting the ease with which fine details can be studied and compared. It also is helpful to make frequent drawings of the nerve head.

These cannot replace the precision of photographs, but drawings do force examiners to focus their observations and usually capture the major features of the nerve head. Of course, in the absence of photographic capability, careful drawings are mandatory.

Chapter 113

■

Glaucomatous Visual Field Loss

MICHAEL V. DRAKE

Visual field evaluation has been an integral part of the diagnosis and management of glaucoma for over a century. Although many methods have been introduced to assess visual function in glaucoma and in patients suspected of having glaucoma, perimetric evaluation of the glaucomatous visual field is the most important.

In the 1980s, many academic institutions and large practices in the industrialized Western world converted to automated perimetry for visual field testing in glaucoma. Several dozen automated perimeters were commercially available at that time,[1, 2] the precise workings of which are explained in hundreds of articles and several books.

DETECTING EARLY VISUAL FIELD LOSS

For decades, glaucoma has been diagnosed through the classic triad of elevated intraocular pressure (IOP), "glaucomatous" optic atrophy or cupping, and visual field loss.[3] An elevated IOP or a suspicious cup:disc ratio usually is noted first, and the visual field examination follows. However, the visual field examination is the factor that actually determines the diagnosis of glaucoma. A patient with a high IOP and a normal or suspicious cup:disc ratio generally is classified as an ocular hypertensive or glaucoma suspect if the visual field examination is normal. If the field examination is abnormal the patient is diagnosed as having glaucoma. Although most patients with glaucoma have an abnormal IOP, cup:disc ratio, and visual field examination, if the visual field shows typical damage the diagnosis is made, even if only one of the other two examinations is abnormal. Examples of this are patients with low-tension glaucoma[4-7] in whom the cup:disc ratio and visual field are abnormal but in whom the IOP falls within the statistically normal range, and glaucomatous optic atrophy in patients with congenitally small discs who have high IOP and glaucomatous field loss, but no increased cup:disc ratio.[8]

There are two main reasons to conduct a visual field examination in patients with glaucoma or in patients suspected of having glaucoma:(1) to detect or establish the diagnosis[9] and (2) for follow-up and to determine visual field stability.

Most glaucoma is treatable but not curable, thus, the diagnosis usually remains with the patient for a lifetime and should not be made lightly. In addition to the nuisance, expense, and possible morbidity of extended treatment, the knowledge that they have a lifelong and potentially blinding disease may be psychologically devastating for some patients. Because of the importance of visual field examinations in establishing the diagnosis of glaucoma, they must possess a high degree of specificity—that is, a low false-positive rate. If the test specificity is good, a high degree of correlation exists between visual field loss characteristic of glaucoma and the presence of the disease.[10] If specificity is poor, an unacceptably large number of normal patients produce visual field results characteristic of glaucoma.

Ample evidence indicates that visual loss is best avoided when glaucoma is treated early.[11-13] A significant degree of optic nerve atrophy occurs before field loss is detected by Goldmann perimetry.[14, 15] Thus, "early" visual field loss is not characteristic of the initial stages of glaucoma but rather takes a substantial period of time to develop. If chances of preserving vision are best when we treat glaucoma early, then visual field examinations must be sensitive enough to reliably detect glaucoma. Failure to detect glaucomatous visual field loss represents a false-negative finding: a normal test generated by a patient who has the disease. The relationship between specificity and sensitivity—the ability to keep both false-positive and false-negative results acceptably low—is extremely important in determining the value of a given method of visual field examination.

OTHER PSYCHOPHYSICAL TESTS

For many years, investigators have studied the effects of glaucoma on contrast sensitivity and color vision.[16-20] Evidence that Goldmann perimetry was not abnormal until 30 to 50 percent of the optic nerve was lost to atrophy prompted several investigators to reexamine the feasibility of contrast-sensitivity testing and color-vision testing as alternatives to visual examination for glaucoma detection.

Many investigators have found decreased contrast sensitivity in patients with glaucoma compared with normal control subjects.[21–23] Mean contrast sensitivity also is decreased in ocular hypertensive or glaucoma-suspect patients compared with normal subjects. In these studies, the glaucoma-suspect patients had risk factors characteristic of glaucoma (usually elevated IOP) but did not have glaucomatous visual field loss. However, they did have visual loss (in this case, contrast-sensitivity loss) that correlated highly with glaucoma. The presence of contrast-sensitivity loss without visual field loss in glaucoma-suspect patients led the authors to conclude that contrast-sensitivity loss might be a more sensitive method of detecting glaucomatous visual loss. Unfortunately, at this time contrast-sensitivity tests lack sufficient specificity for routine use as a diagnostic modality in patients suspected of having glaucoma. A great degree of overlap exists between the contrast-sensitivity scores of patients with confirmed glaucoma, confirmed normal patients, and patients suspected of having glaucoma. No reliable cut-off point exists that allows one to categorize a patient based on the results of a contrast-sensitivity examination alone.

As with contrast-sensitivity testing, color vision defects, particularly in the blue/yellow axis, appear more frequently in patients with glaucoma and glaucoma suspects than in normal subjects.[19, 24] Abnormal color-vision tests in glaucoma suspects suggest that blue/yellow color testing is more sensitive than visual field testing for detecting early glaucomatous visual loss. However, practical use of color-vision testing in early glaucoma has yet to be established. For many years, some of the difficulty in establishing reliable color perimetry and color-vision testing for patients with glaucoma was due to problems in instrument standardization. However, even with more standardized instrumentation, results vary substantially among investigators. Hart, using conventional manual kinetic Goldmann perimetry and manual kinetic color-contrast perimetry to compare 19 eyes of 15 patients with open-angle glaucoma, found that color-contrast defects in all patients could be detected simultaneously by the conventional method.[25] He also found that defects mapped with conventional perimetry had more distinct topographic features than did those mapped with color-contrast perimetry. Johnson and associates[26] compared patients with early glaucomatous field loss with those with ocular hypertension and normal control subjects. They performed perimetry using both a blue test stimulus on a yellow background and a standard white-on-white test, with the former detecting up to 10 percent more abnormalities in the ocular hypertensive patients than the latter test. In patients with early glaucomatous field loss, the blue-on-yellow test detected up to 15 percent more abnormalities. They concluded that a blue test object projected on a yellow background was more sensitive for detecting early damage caused by glaucoma than was a white target on a white background.

The visual defects that are evident after psychophysical testing, as well as nerve fiber layer photography[27, 28] and quantitative computer imaging of the optic disc,[29] correlate well with the presence of established glaucoma. The presence of a substantial number of abnormalities in patients with elevated IOP and normal visual fields indicates that these abnormalities are predictive of later visual field change. However, none of these methods currently possesses sufficient specificity to induce most ophthalmologists to begin treatment in the absence of classical visual field defects.

EARLIEST VISUAL FIELD LOSS IN GLAUCOMA

Over the past century, many investigators have studied the location and characteristics of the earliest visual field loss in glaucoma.[30–33] The location of this field loss and the nature of defects that qualify for early glaucoma loss depend highly on the methodology used for examining the visual field.

Before the early 1980s, most of the careful quantitative visual field studies were performed manually, using either the tangent screen or the Goldmann perimeter.[34] Alhorn and Harms and others used the Tubingen perimeter for detailed static perimetric evaluation of the central visual field, but the difficulty of performing these tests meant that they were relegated mainly to research institutions. The facility with which automated perimeters perform static perimetry led to the abandonment of manual Tubingen perimetry under all except the most unusual circumstances.

Previously, early glaucoma defects were characterized as being either shallow pericentral scotomas, nasal steps, or a general collapsing of the isopters,[35] currently referred to as localized or diffuse loss (Figs. 113–1 and 113–2). Manual perimetric examinations for early localized visual field loss found that the early paracentral scotoma was the most characteristic type of shallow or perhaps fleeting visual field loss in early glaucoma.[36, 37] In a study of 53 patients who developed visual field loss while under study, Werner and Drance found that localized defects often were preceded by inconsistent responses in the region that subsequently would develop the scotoma.[38] Hart and Becker[31] found that 53 percent of the initial defects in 800 patients with glaucoma were found in the superior or inferior arcuate region extending from the blind spot to the horizontal raphe in an arc that was between 5 and 15 degrees from fixation.

A potential source of bias is inherent in manual perimetric glaucoma detection, because the examiners often know that the patients are glaucoma suspects, and, therefore, concentrate on testing areas that are expected to show glaucoma defects. The chance of discovering a defect is increased by careful examination of the area in question. Furthermore, because the parameters for detecting diffuse loss with manual perimetry are less well defined, a fair number of patients with early diffuse loss possibly had visual field examinations that were interpreted as normal, and the prevalence of diffuse field loss in early glaucoma was underestimated.

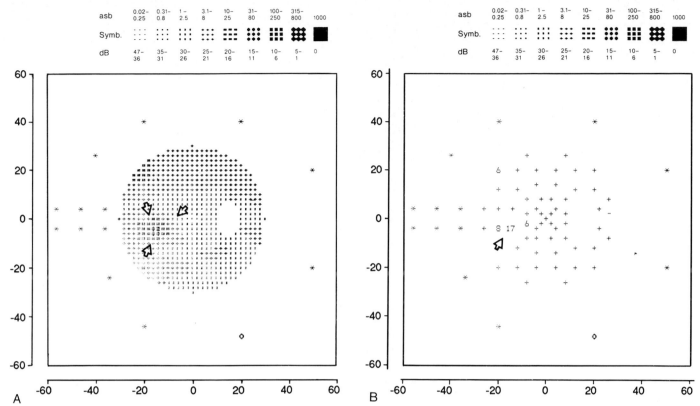

Figure 113–1. *A* and *B,* Octopus fields from the right eye of a 59-year-old man with open-angle glaucoma. Note the localized depression (*arrows*) just nasal to fixation, representative of an early paracentral scotoma.

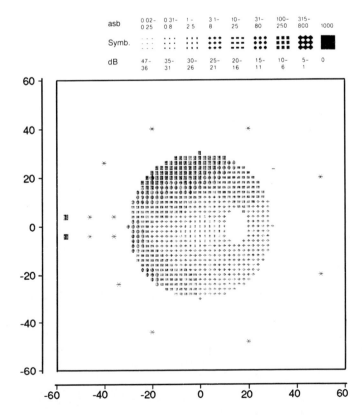

Figure 113–2. A 76-year-old man with mild to moderate diffuse depression superiorly and mild midperipheral depression nasally. He has elevated intraocular pressure and an increased cup:disc ratio, but it is difficult to state that his field loss is entirely glaucomatous.

Automated perimetric examinations, which have been performed with increased frequency since 1980, usually test pertinent areas of the visual field equally, and they are not subject to observer bias.[39–41] Early studies of the frequency of glaucomatous loss in various areas of the visual field using automated perimetry confirmed that the greatest loss was in the arcuate region, but distribution of the defects was somewhat different from that which has been determined by manual perimetry.[33] Early-generation automated perimeters generally used symmetric test grids that purposely did not emphasize any particular area of the visual field (Fig. 113–3).[42] One reason for using symmetric grids was the developer's knowledge that observer bias could play a role in determining the sites that were the most frequently affected by initial glaucoma defects. A computer-generated testing program that examined all areas of the test field equally should generate a more accurate display of the frequency distribution of the earliest glaucoma defects. Data from these early symmetric programs, combined with data from manual perimetric examinations, have been used to develop more glaucoma-specific grids, such as the "G1" program for the Octopus perimeters (Fig. 113–4),[43, 44] that concentrate test points in areas more likely to be affected early in the glaucomatous process.

DIFFUSE VERSUS LOCALIZED DEFECTS

In the mid-1980s, Flammer introduced visual field indices,[45] the basic concept of which is that visual field loss can be divided into two types of defects: localized and diffuse. A visual field with more localized loss is

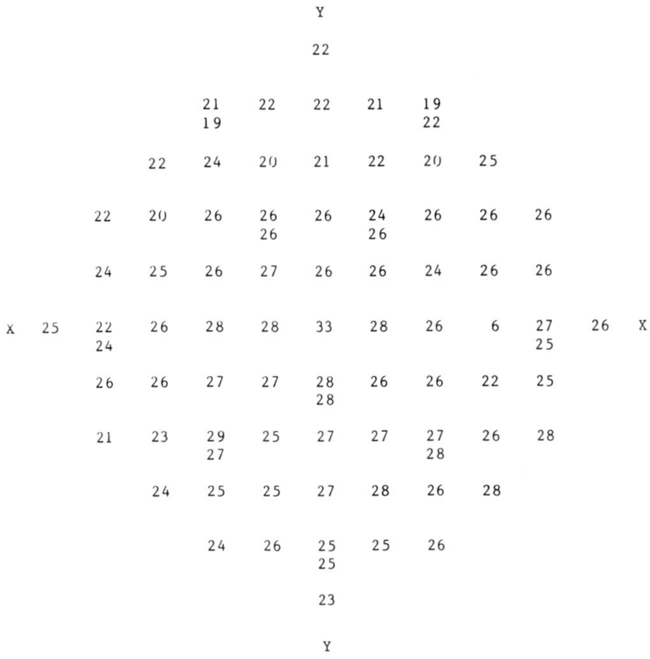

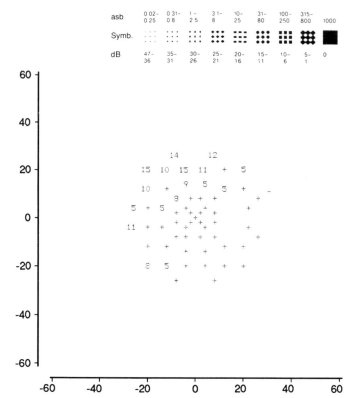

Figure 113–4. The test pattern used by the Octopus GI program. Note that the test points are packed tightly in the center of the field, with wider spacing toward the periphery. The crosses indicate that the patient's response was within normal expected limits. The numbers indicate depth of depression (in decibels).

characterized by the presence of isolated, discrete, abnormal areas within normal or near-normal regions. The spatial scatter (or the degree of local nonuniformity) of measured threshold values is relatively high. The values of individual given test points might vary considerably from their neighbors (Fig. 113–5). Conversely, a field with diffuse or uniform loss has many or most test points depressed. Areas of normal function tend to be clustered, as are areas of depressed function. Such fields have relatively little spatial scatter and exhibit a great degree of uniformity. The values of individual test points tend to be similar to the values of their neighbors (Fig. 113–6).

Visual field indices were developed in part to assist clinicians in segregating the effects of increased media opacity from glaucomatous progression. For example, in a patient with cataract and glaucoma, if the glaucoma were stable as the cataract deteriorated, one would expect the degree of localized loss to remain relatively constant, while the degree of generalized loss increased. Conversely, in a patient with uncontrolled glaucoma but stable cataract, one might expect the localized component of the field loss to increase at a faster rate than the diffuse field loss. To simplify interpreting this information, several manufacturers (Octopus, Humphrey) have empowered the computer associated with their field machines to calculate a numerical "index" that corresponds to the amount of diffuse or localized loss present.[46, 47] These visual field indices produce a value

Figure 113–3. Octopus 31 test from 1985 illustrating the on-axis 6-degree spacing that was the preferred method for visual field assessment in our clinic at the time.

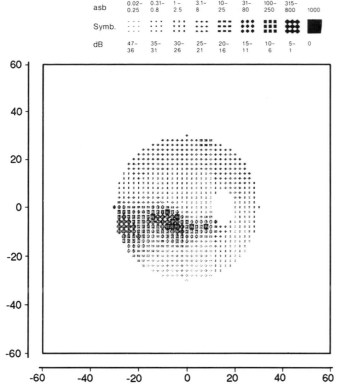

Figure 113–5. The printout shows a dense localized defect largely surrounded by a normal area.

and range of normal for the diffuse component of the loss and for the localized component of the loss. The mean deviation or mean defect (MD) is the index sensitive to the diffuse component of the loss; the loss variance (LV) (Octopus) or pattern standard deviation (PSD) (Humphrey) is the index sensitive to localized loss (Fig. 113–7). In practice, a value for short-term

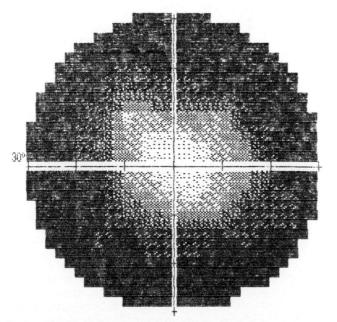

Figure 113–6. A Humphrey visual field showing severe generalized depression.

GLOBAL INDICES

MD	-22.14 DB	P < 0.5%
PSD	10.03 DB	P < 0.5%
SF	1.98 DB	
CPSD	9.77 DB	P < 0.5%

Figure 113–7. Visual field indices from the Humphrey visual field shown in Figure 113–6. The *P* values indicate that the values for the mean difference or mean defect (MD), PSD, and corrected pattern standard deviation (CPSD) are quite depressed. The short-term fluctuation (SF) value is within the normal range.

fluctuation (SF) or measurement error also is calculated. A sophisticated mathematical adjustment places the SF in both the numerator and denominator of the equation used to calculate the localized index, thus canceling out the effect of measurement error. The resultant indices are referred to as the corrected loss variance (CLV on the Octopus) or corrected pattern standard deviation (CPSD on the Humphrey) (Fig. 113–8).

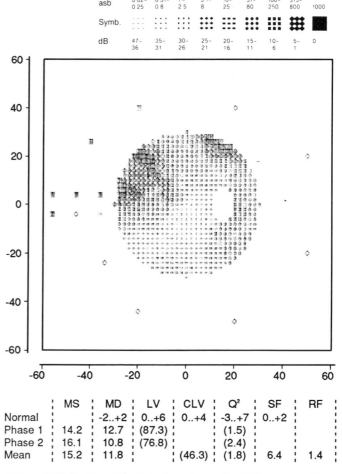

	MS	MD	LV	CLV	Q²	SF	RF
Normal		-2..+2	0..+6	0..+4	-3..+7	0..+2	
Phase 1	14.2	12.7	(87.3)		(1.5)		
Phase 2	16.1	10.8	(76.8)		(2.4)		
Mean	15.2	11.8		(46.3)	(1.8)	6.4	1.4

Figure 113–8. Visual field indices from the Octopus machine. The loss variance (LV) was very high in phases 1 (first test) and 2 (second test, performed during the same examination session). In this case, the short-term fluctuation (SF), similar to measurement error, was also high. When the LV is mathematically corrected for the highly abnormal SF, the resultant corrected loss variance (CLV) is much lower than the LV. In other words, the LV in this case was elevated substantially by measurement error; the corrected value gives a more accurate indication of the level of pathology.

Visual field indices make it easier for investigators studying glaucomatous visual field loss to routinely look at diffuse and localized loss.[48] An interesting result of having these data available is that patients with early glaucoma and without media opacity were found to segregate into groups with predominantly diffuse or predominantly localized visual field loss.[49–51] Diffuse loss had been recognized for years as a classic early glaucoma defect. Using kinetic fields, the pattern was a generalized collapsing of the isopters, a type of field defect relatively nonspecific and difficult to quantitate. It was not studied as intensively as arcuate scotomas, paracentral depressions, or other localized defects. However, with an automated threshold test, a computerized index can be generated indicating whether or not the visual field shows statistically significant diffuse depression. Caproli and associates examined 15 patients—eight with diffuse depression of the differential light sensitivity without localized scotomas and seven with localized scotomas without diffuse depression.[52] They found that patients with diffuse depression had higher mean IOPs than did those with localized defects. This finding was consistent with observations that patients with normal or low-tension glaucoma have deeper, steeper, and more localized defects than do patients with glaucoma and elevated IOP.[53, 54] Drance and coworkers conducted a study of 61 patients with normal-tension glaucoma (24 patients) or elevated IOP and glaucoma (37 patients) and with localized defects limited to one hemifield.[55] They found that the patients with chronic open-angle glaucoma had twice as much diffuse loss in the opposite hemifield as did patients with low-tension glaucoma, which supported the concept that higher pressures lead to more diffuse damage than do lower pressures. More recently, Chauhan and Drance studied IOP and visual field damage in normal-tension and high-tension glaucoma.[56] In their study, 40 pairs of patients with normal-tension and high-tension glaucoma were matched for the extent of visual field damage, pupil size, and visual acuity. Their final analysis was based on defining patients with normal-tension and high-tension glaucoma as individuals whose IOP either never had pressures that exceeded 18 mmHg, or had pressures of at least 41 mmHg on one or more occasion, respectively. Using these widely disparate definitions, they found a highly significant correlation between the type of loss present and the level of IOP. More diffuse field loss was evident in patients in the high-tension glaucoma group than in the low-tension glaucoma group. However, even defining high- and low-tension glaucoma in the extreme terms used in their study, they still found that approximately 25 percent of the patients with normal-tension glaucoma had more diffuse loss than did patients with high-tension glaucoma. They concluded that multiple factors affecting visual field loss in patients with glaucoma are likely to be present and that pressure is only one of them.

Caprioli and associates[52] suggested that very high IOP alone is enough to prompt careful visual field evaluation and thus facilitate the finding of diffuse visual field loss. Patients with low or normal IOP generally are not subjected to visual field examination unless their optic nerve shows suspicious defects. Localized visual field loss correlates with localized disc notching or with vertical elongation of the optic nerve head, both of which are easier to detect by routine ophthalmoscopy than the more saucerized depression associated with diffuse visual field loss.[28] A patient with a pressure of 18 mmHg with a localized optic disc notch likely will undergo visual field examination, and a localized defect may be found. However, if a patient with a pressure of 18 mmHg has a more saucerized optic nerve, it is likely to be regarded as normal on many ophthalmic examinations; visual field study is not performed, and associated diffuse visual field loss is missed. There is a selection bias in favor of patients with low-tension glaucoma who have localized visual field defects and a selection bias in favor of patients with high-tension glaucoma who have diffuse visual field loss. Careful study is needed to resolve this issue.

PERIPHERAL VERSUS CENTRAL DEFECTS

Practical considerations such as time and patient fatigue limit the visual field area that can be examined at any given time. However, limiting the examination to too small an area results in significant glaucoma defects being missed simply because the region of the field in which they occurred is not examined. The tangent screen sees its greatest utility within the central 30 degrees, and when tangent screen study was the primary mode of visual field assessment in glaucoma, examiners rarely found peripheral defects in the absence of central defects. The popularization of the Goldmann perimeter allowed more careful peripheral examination, and peripheral nasal step and temporal defects in the absence of central defects were discovered as the first visual field loss in some patients with glaucoma.[31] The pendulum has swung back toward concentrating on the central 30 degrees when computerized automated perimeters are used and sensitive threshold measurements are made. Several authors have found that peripheral defects in the absence of central defects are relatively rare, on the order of 5 to 10 percent.[57–59]

Most glaucomatologists believe that it is reasonable to concentrate on the central 30 degrees and to deemphasize but not ignore the periphery.[60] Some instrument manufacturers have designed programs that allow the examiner to test the central 30 degrees with a full threshold strategy and the peripheral with either a screening protocol or kinetic isopter test.[61]

IDENTIFYING EARLY GLAUCOMATOUS VISUAL FIELD LOSS

In addition to being appropriately sensitive and specific, a quality visual field examination must also be reliable. For serial visual field examinations, patient and examiner reliability is important. Patient reliability is usually assessed by the examiner during the test, and is influenced by factors such as understanding the test, response consistency, and general attentiveness. Examiner reliability is harder to measure but includes the level of training, choice of technique, and performance during the test. Examiner fatigue or inattentiveness can be at least as important as poor patient reliability in producing an unreliable manual test.

Reliability considerations for automated perimeters are somewhat different. The first and most obvious difference is that examiner reliability is largely eliminated from consideration because the computer is administering the test. However, there are a host of examiner-dependent factors, such as patient instruction, pupillary dilatation, and use of proper refractive correction that can affect examination reliability. These test parameters must also be addressed appropriately to produce a reliable manual parametric examination. A benefit of computerized perimetry is that the test itself is the same from one year to another; examiner variability is at a minimum.[62]

Computerized perimeters also allow more consistent methods for evaluating patient reliability. The most commonly used reliability factors are the number of false-positive and false-negative patient responses, and the number of fixation losses.[63, 64] False-positive patient responses occur when an auditory or other stimulus is given in the absence of a visual stimulus and the patient responds as though a visual stimulus had been detected. A false-negative response is generated when a patient fails to respond to an extremely bright stimulus in an area in which he or she responded to a much less intense stimulus earlier during the same examination. The "fluctuation" value generated by many machines is an attempt to measure the intratest physiologic variability or measurement error. The percentage of fixation losses during a given examination is another commonly used reliability factor (for machines such as the Humphrey Field Analyzer, which uses an image projected on the blind spot to check for fixation losses). For most purposes, a fixation loss percentage of more than 20 percent is considered unacceptably high. Machines such as the Octopus perimeter measure iridocorneal reflectivity to assess fixation and are programmed to disregard responses generated when the patient has lost fixation. Thus, the patient's test results are assumed to exclude data generated during fixation losses.

SCREENING VERSUS THRESHOLD FIELDS

A fair degree of controversy has existed over the years regarding the use of screening versus threshold field strategies for detection of glaucoma.[65, 66] In simple terms, a screening examination is one that produces qualitative information of test normality or abnormality. A threshold examination produces quantitative information, the level of sensitivity at the test point. As such, screening tests seem well suited for the initial visual field examination for detecting glaucoma, and practitioners have used them successfully for this purpose. However, two problems arise with using these examinations. The first occurs when an unselected population is examined, such as when all patients seen in a given care facility undergo a visual field examination to screen for glaucoma. Patients with abnormal field results are referred to the glaucoma-suspect group; other patients are considered normal. The problem is that the incidence of glaucomatous visual field damage in an unselected population is low, approximately 2 percent.[67, 68] Furthermore, most of these patients already know that they have glaucoma, thus the incidence of unsuspected glaucomatous visual field loss is even lower. If the false-positive rate for a screening test is 1 percent (specificity) and the false-negative rate is 0 (sensitivity), given a 2 percent glaucoma prevalence, a patient with an abnormal field result still has only a 50 percent chance of actually having glaucoma. The sensitivity and specificity figures in the example are unrealistically optimistic. In practice, when an unselected population is screened, the number of false-positive results exceeds the number of true-positive results by several fold. For this reason, it is more practical to perform visual field examinations in patients whose history or physical examination indicates risk for glaucoma.

The second problem with using screening fields for glaucoma detection occurs when testing patients known to be at risk for glaucoma. A screening field examination can determine with reasonable certainty whether glaucomatous field damage exists, but a full threshold examination is superior for establishing a reliable baseline for future comparison. Threshold examinations usually take approximately 7 to 8 min longer per eye than do screening examinations; however, in our experience this has been time well spent.

REPEATING THE VISUAL FIELD EXAMINATION

The proper interval between the initial visual field examination and the follow-up examination depends on the results of the initial examination and on the patient's clinical condition. For example, when managing a patient with a completely normal field, a small cup:disc ratio, and a pressure of 22 mmHg, we repeat the visual field testing at 6- to 12-mo intervals initially. If the patient remained stable through several of these examinations, we would reexamine the patient as infrequently as annually or biannually. If the field is normal, the pressures are elevated into the upper 20s or 30s, and the optic nerve head shows more substantial cupping, we repeat our initial field within a few weeks to months and then again at every few months until the patient is stable with or without therapy. Conversely, if we find visual field results that are worse than expected, considering the patient's pressure and optic nerve appearance, we repeat the field quickly to confirm the initial test findings. The final circumstance in which we repeat visual fields in the near term is when we are considering surgical intervention based on the visual field results.

The inherent variability of visual field testing makes it prudent to avoid basing irreversible therapeutic interventions on a single examination.[69–71]

FOLLOW-UP VISUAL FIELDS: GLAUCOMATOUS PROGRESSION

Visual field study is extremely useful in following glaucoma progression. Paracentral scotomas coalesce to form arcuate scotomas that then break through into the periphery and encroach on fixation (Fig. 113–9). Regardless of the initial site at which visual field loss is detected, the defects tend to enlarge and deepen and follow the nerve fiber bundle pattern as they progress. Although generalized depression can be a sign of early visual loss due to glaucoma, localized nerve fiber defects superimposed on this generalized depression are a more commonly recognized sign of progression. By late stage, the contribution of localized and generalized depression cannot be separated meaningfully. Severe visual loss exists throughout the field. (Table 113–1).

Sensitivity and specificity are essential considerations in the detection phase of glaucomatous field evaluation; reliability and reproducibility are key in performing follow-up fields. The reproducibility of the field examination refers primarily to the examiner's ability to subject the patient to the same test over time. If, when tested with the proper refraction, a controlled pupil size, or the same test program, the patient shows visual field

Table 113–1. TYPICAL GLAUCOMATOUS VISUAL FIELD DEFECTS

Generalized peripheral and central depression
Shallow localized paracentral scotomas
Isolated shallow peripheral or midperipheral nasal step defects
Arcuate or nerve fiber bundle defects that progress from incomplete to complete and from single (see Fig. 113–5) to double (see Fig. 113–9)
Persistent retention of the central field until the late stage of the disease
Loss of the central island with retention of a small temporal island of vision
Loss of light perception

progression, it is appropriate to consider that the progression is real. If the testing parameters, examination strategy, or machine manufacturer change, it is difficult to determine whether a slight variation in patient response is due to pathologic progression or to artifact.

In late-stage glaucoma, the advantage of using computerized perimetry in the detection and early follow-up phases of glaucoma disappears. When a patient has only a small central island of vision, a program that concentrates on areas of the visual field in which all sensitivity is lost wastes time and can be extremely discouraging. A manual test, particularly one with a tangent screen, quickly and precisely delineates the margins of a central visual island, and under many circumstances this test may be the preferred follow-up method. In addition, a tangent screen examination allows the examiner to move the patient 2 meters or more away from the screen, which substantially enlarges the size of the preserved island of vision. Although the visual angle remains constant, an island of central vision is much larger in centimeters when the patient is tested further from the screen. Using an appropriately intense stimulus, this large central island can be mapped carefully. On follow-up examinations, relatively subtle decreases in the size of the island should be more readily apparent.

Visual field study assumes further importance in very late-stage glaucoma because psychophysical tests (e.g., color vision and contrast sensitivity) and physical examinations (e.g., evaluation for the cup:disc ratio or the retinal nerve fiber layer) are relatively insensitive. The latter can be useful to detect visual loss before the visual field is abnormal, but in an advanced stage of disease, the patient's performance on color-vision and contrast-sensitivity tests and the appearance of the disc and nerve fiber layer are so poor that a small change is difficult to ascertain. If the patient only has minimal vision, a small change in the nerve appearance can represent a substantial degree of visual loss.

SUMMARY

Visual field testing remains a mainstay of diagnosis and follow-up of glaucoma. Fields used for the initial diagnosis of glaucoma must be sufficiently sensitive to detect abnormality and must be sufficiently specific to

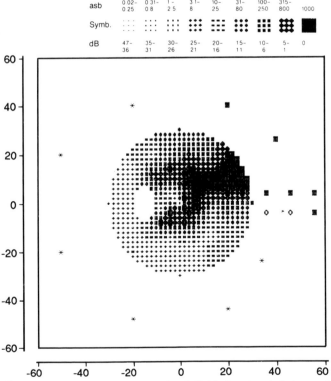

Figure 113–9. Glaucomatous visual field showing inferior and superior arcuate scotomas, superior nasal step, and superior nasal peripheral breakthrough. Central fixation and the temporal and inferior periphery are spared.

ensure that an abnormal test is likely to predict the presence of the disease. Both manual and automated perimetric methods are capable of detecting glaucoma reliably. The former tend to be tedious and require a well-trained technician or physician to administer them. Even under optimal circumstances, examiner variability can have a negative impact on test reliability and reproducibility. For these reasons and others, computerized automated perimetry has become increasingly popular since 1980. In addition to its ability to decrease examiner variability by eliminating the examiner during the actual testing procedure, computerized perimeters can process data statistically and help the examiner to interpret the results more reliably and consistently. The disadvantages are that computerized perimeters are expensive to purchase and maintain, and they are not as flexible as manual perimeters in performing quick, patient-specific examinations. However, in most clinical circumstances, the advantages of computerized perimeters outweigh the disadvantages.

Although some psychophysical tests and physical examinations may claim superiority in detecting glaucoma, visual field examinations continue to be the best way to assess the impact of the glaucomatous process on the patient's visual system and to help the physician to determine the appropriate therapy.

REFERENCES

1. Keltner JL, Johnson CA: Comparative material on automated and semiautomated perimeters—1983. Ophthalmology 90 (Suppl): 34, 1983.
2. Keltner JL, Johnson CA: Comparative material on automated and semiautomated perimeters—1985. Ophthalmology 92 (Suppl):34, 1985.
3. Hoskins HD, Kass MA: Becker Shaffer's Diagnosis of Glaucoma. St Louis, CV Mosby, 1989, p 2.
4. Caprioli J, Spaeth GL: Comparison of optic nerve head in high and low tension glaucoma. Arch Ophthalmol 103:1145, 1985.
5. Lewis RA, Hayreh SS, Phelps CD: Optic disc and visual field correlations in primary open angle and low tension glaucoma. Am J Ophthalmol 96:148, 1983.
6. Levene RA: Low tension glaucoma: A critical review and new material. Surv Ophthalmol 104:577, 1987.
7. Drance SM, Douglas GR, Airaksinen PJ, et al: Diffuse visual field loss in chronic open-angle and low-tension glaucoma. Am J Ophthalmol 104:577, 1987.
8. Jonas JB, Fernandez MC, Naumann COH: Glaucomatous optic nerve atrophy in small discs with low cup-to-disc ratios. Ophthalmology 97:1211, 1990.
9. Sommer A, Euger C, Witt K: Screen for glaucomatous visual field loss with automated threshold perimetry. Am J Ophthalmol 103:681, 1987.
10. Sommer A, Duggan C, Auer C, Abbey H: Analytic approaches to the interpretation of automated threshold perimetric data for the diagnosis of early glaucoma. Trans Am Ophthalmol Soc 83:250, 1985.
11. Grant WM, Burke JF: Why do some people go blind from glaucoma? Arch Ophthalmol 89:991, 1982.
12. Spaeth GL: The effect of change in intraocular pressure on the natural history of glaucoma. III: Lowering intraocular pressure in glaucoma can result in improvement of visual fields. Trans Ophthalmol Soc UK 104:256, 1985.
13. Spaeth GL: Reversibility of optic disc cupping. Arch Ophthalmol 107:1583, 1989.
14. Quigley HA, Green WR: The histology of human glaucoma cupping and nerve damage: Clinicopathologic correlation in 21 eyes. Ophthalmology 10:803, 1979.
15. Quigley HA, Holman RM, Addiche EM, et al: Morphologic changes in the laminal cribrosa correlated with neural loss in open angle glaucoma Am J Ophthalmol 95:673, 1983.
16. Stamper RL, Hsu-Winges C, Sopher M: Arden contrast sensitivity testing in glaucoma. Arch Ophthalmol 100:947, 1982.
17. Hitchings RA, Powell DJ, Arden GB, Carter RM: Contrast sensitivity gradings in glaucoma family screening. Br J Ophthalmol 65:518, 1981.
18. Arden GB, Jacobson JJ: A simple grading test for contrast sensitivity: Preliminary results indicate value for screening in glaucoma. Invest Ophthalmol Vis Sci 17:23, 1978.
19. Sample PA, Weinreb RN, Bornton RM: Acquired dyschromatopsia in glaucoma. Surv Ophthalmol 31:54, 1986.
20. Drance SM, Lakowski R, Schulzer M, Douglas GR: Acquired color vision changes in glaucoma. Arch Ophthalmol 99:829, 1981.
21. Bodes-Wollner I: Electrophysiological and psychophysical testing of vision in glaucoma. Surv Ophthalmol 33 (Suppl):301, 1989.
22. Regan D, Neiman D: Low contrast letter charts in early diabetic retinopathy, ocular hypertension glaucoma, and Parkinson's disease. Br J Ophthalmol 68:885, 1989.
23. Tytla ME, Trobe JE, Bunic VR: Flicker sensitivity in treated ocular hypertension. Ophthalmology 97:36, 1990.
24. Adams AJ, Nodic R, Husted R, Stamper R: Spectrosensitivity in color discrimination changes in glaucoma and glaucoma suspect patients. Invest Ophthalmol Vis Sci 23:516, 1982.
25. Hart WM: Blue/yellow color contrast perimetry in patients with established glaucomatous visual field defects. In Heijl A (ed): Perimetry Update 1988/89. Amsterdam, Kugler & Ghedini, 1989, pp 23–30.
26. Johnson CA, Adams AJ, Lewis RA: Automated perimetry of short wavelength-sensitive mechanisms in glaucoma and other hypertension: Preliminary findings. In Heijl A(ed): Perimetry Update 1988/89. Amsterdam, Kugler & Ghedini, 1989, pp 31–38.
27. Airaksinen PJ, Lakowski R, Drance SM, Price M: Color vision and retinal nerve fiber layer in early glaucoma. Am J Ophthalmol 98:566, 1984.
28. Airaksinen PJ, Drance SM, Douglas GR, et al: Diffuse and localized nerve fiber loss in glaucoma. Am J Ophthalmol 98:566, 1984.
29. Takamoto T, Schwartz B: Reproducibility of photogrammetric optic disc cup measurements. Invest Ophthalmol Vis Sci 26:814, 1985.
30. Aulhorn E, Harms H: Early visual field defects in glaucoma. In Leydhecker W (ed): Glaucoma: Tutzing Symposium, 1966. Basel, Karger, 1967, pp 151–186.
31. Hart WM, Becker B: The onset and evolution of glaucomatous visual field defects. Ophthalmology 89:268, 1982.
32. Harrington DO: The Bjerrum scotoma. Trans Am Ophthalmol Soc 62:324, 1964.
33. Heijl A, Lunqvist L: The frequency distribution of earliest glaucomatous visual field defects documented by automated perimetry. Acta Ophthalmol 62:658, 1984.
34. Armaly MF: Selective perimetry for glaucomatous defects in ocular hypertension. Arch Ophthalmol 87:518, 1972.
35. Harrington DO, Drake MV: The Visual Field. St Louis, CV Mosby, 1990, pp 179–218.
36. Harrington DO: The pathogenesis of the glaucomatous visual field. Am J Ophthalmol 47:177, 1958.
37. Drance SM: The early field defect in glaucoma. Invest Ophthalmol 8:84, 1969.
38. Werner EB, Drance SM: Early visual field disturbances in glaucoma. Arch Ophthalmol 95:1173, 1977.
39. Drake MV: Design parameters of automated perimeters. Trans Pac Coast Oto-ophthalmol Soc 66:297, 1985.
40. Whalen W, Spaeth G (eds): Computerized Visual Fields: What They are and How to Use Them. Thorofare, NJ, Slack, 1985.
41. Greve EL: Performance of computer assisted perimeters. Doc Ophthalmol 53:343, 1982.
42. Frankhauser F: Problems related to the design of automatic perimeters. Doc Ophthalmol 47:89, 1979.
43. Flammer J, Drance SM, Jenni A, et al: JO and STATJO programs for investigating the visual field with the Octopus perimeter. Am J Ophthalmol 18:115, 1983.
44. Flammer J, Drance SM, Augustiny L, et al: Quantification of glaucomatous visual field defects with automated perimetry. Invest Ophthalmol Vis Sci 26:176, 1985.

45. Flammer J: The concept of visual field indices. Graefes Arch Clin Exp Ophthalmol 224:389, 1986.
46. Flammer J, Drance SM, Augustiny L, Frankhauser A: Quantification of glaucomatous visual field defects with automated perimetry. Invest Ophthalmol Vis Sci 26:176, 1985.
47. Heijl A, Lindgren G, Olsson J: A package for the statistical analysis of visual fields. Doc Ophthalmol Proc Ser 49:153, 1987.
48. Dannheim F: First experiences with the new Octopus GI program in chronic simple glaucoma. Doc Ophthalmol Proc Ser 49:321, 1987.
49. Glowazki A, Flammer J: Is there a difference between glaucoma patients with rather localized visual field damage and patients with more diffuse visual field damage? Doc Ophthalmol Proc Ser 49:317, 1987.
50. Drance SM, Douglas GR, Airaksinen PJ, et al: Diffuse visual field loss in chronic open angle glaucoma and low tension glaucoma. Am J Ophthalmol 104:577, 1987.
51. Chauhan BC, Drance SM, Douglas GR, Johnson CA: Visual field damage in normal and high tension glaucoma. Am J Ophthalmol 108:636, 1989.
52. Caprioli J, Sears M, Miller JM: Patterns of early visual field loss in open angle glaucoma and low tension glaucoma. Am J Ophthalmol 103:512, 1987.
53. Caprioli J, Spaeth GL: Comparison of visual field defects in the low tension glaucomas with high tension glaucomas. Am J Ophthalmol 103:512, 1987.
54. Anderson S, Hitchings RA: A comparative study of visual fields of patients with low tension glaucoma and those with chronic simple glaucoma. In Greve EL, Heijl T (eds): 5th International Field Symposium. The Hague, Junk, 1983, pp 97–99.
55. Drance SM, Douglas CR, Aukamen PJ, et al: Diffuse visual field loss in chronic open angle and low tension glaucoma. Am J Ophthalmol 104:577, 1987.
56. Chauhan BC, Drance SM: The influence of intraocular pressure on visual field damage in patients with normal tension and high tension glaucoma. Invest Ophthalmol Vis Sci 31:2367, 1990.
57. Seamone C, LeBlanc RP, Rubillowicz MC, Orr A: The value of indices in the central and peripheral visual fields for the detection of glaucoma. Am J Ophthalmol 106:180, 1988.
58. Drake MV: Peripheral static testing in early glaucoma. Ophthalmology 94 (Suppl):253, 1987.
59. Stuart WC, Shields MB, Ollie AR: Peripheral visual field testing by automated kinetic testing in glaucoma. Arch Ophthalmol 106:202, 1988.
60. Caprioli J: Automated perimetry in glaucoma. Am J Ophthalmol 109:235, 1991.
61. Miller KN, Shields MB, Ollie AR: Automated kinetic perimetry with two peripheral isopters in glaucoma. Arch Ophthalmol 107:1316, 1989.
62. Harrington DO, Drake MV: The Visual Fields. St Louis, CV Mosby, 1990, pp 35–55.
63. Katz J, Sommer A: Screening for glaucomatous visual field loss: The effect of patient reliability. Ophthalmology 97:1032, 1990.
64. Heijl A, Lindgren G, Olsson J: Reliability parameters in computerized perimetry. Doc Ophthalmol Proc Ser 49:593, 1987.
65. Mills R: A comparison of Goldmann, Fieldmaster 200, and Dicon AP2000 perimeters used in a screening mode. Ophthalmology 91:347, 1984.
66. Drake MV: Discussion of Mills RP: A comparison of Goldmann, Fieldmaster 200, and Dicon AP2000 perimeters used in a screening mode. Ophthalmology 91:354, 1984.
67. Leske MC: The epidemiology of open angle glaucoma: A review. Am J Epidemiol 118:166, 1983.
68. Wilson MR: Epidemiological features of glaucoma. Int Ophthalmol Clin 30:153, 1990.
69. Hoskins HD, Magee SD, Drake MV, Kidd MN: A system for the analysis of automated visual fields using the Humphrey visual field analyser. Doc Ophthalmol Proc Ser 49:145, 1987.
70. Wilensky JT: Automated perimetry. Arch Ophthalmol 107:185, 1989.
71. Frankhauser F, Bebie H: Threshold fluctuations, interpolations, and spatial resulution in perimetry. Doc Ophthalmol Proc Ser 19:295, 1979.

Chapter 114

■

Optic Nerve Head Imaging

DAVID A. ECHELMAN and M. BRUCE SHIELDS

The clinical appearance of the optic disc and peripapillary retina provides the only objective evidence of the presence and progression of glaucomatous damage. Despite this, less technology routinely has been applied to the development of clinical methods for direct measurement of optic nerve head (ONH) status than to measurements of intraocular pressure (IOP) or visual field. Consequently, the practitioner currently must evaluate subtle, but extremely important physical findings using only the office fundus examination and fundus photographs.

More sensitive methods to detect glaucomatous optic atrophy should improve our ability to make an early diagnosis and help to monitor subsequent progressive change during the course of therapy. For example, we know that significant nerve fiber loss can occur before a glaucomatous visual field defect can be detected and that significant additional loss occurs during the course

of therapy before a progressive change is recognized.[1] We often do not know whether the IOP in a particular patient is low enough to prevent gradual progressive damage and must base our clinical decisions on limited IOP readings, visual field testing, and the clinical appearance of the optic disc and peripapillary retina, underscoring the need for more sensitive methods of documenting progressive optic atrophy in glaucoma management.[2]

Efforts to develop more sophisticated manual techniques for documenting ONH status have failed to achieve widespread clinical acceptance, either because they lacked sufficient reliability and sensitivity for detecting subtle pathologic change or because they were too time-consuming to be clinically practical. However, with the application of computer technology to ONH imaging, the potential exists for clinically useful, sensitive documentation of glaucomatous optic atrophy. Although first-generation image analyzers failed to satisfy the requirements for practical office ONH analyzer,[3, 4] continued research promises to make this a reality. Many image-analysis tasks, such as pallor and topography determination, performed manually in the past, readily can be performed today by computers with good reliability. Laser tomographic scanning, an emerging computer-based technology that is still in its infancy, also offers promise for the future. This chapter reviews what we have learned from past and present techniques of ONH imaging. After assessing the capabilities and limitations of various approaches, we will speculate on the future of this exciting field.

PRINCIPLES OF ONH IMAGING

Photographic Considerations

The introductions of the direct ophthalmoscope and the indirect ophthalmoscope[5] led to classical descriptions of glaucomatous ONH damage principally in terms of observed cupping, pallor, and nerve fiber layer (NFL) defects.[6, 7] Subsequent improvements in slit-lamp design[8] and the introduction of the 90-diopter lens have facilitated high-resolution stereoscopic clinical evaluation of the magnified ONH.

Meanwhile, the development of the fundus camera[9] has aided documentation on ONH status. Because fundus cameras use the principle of indirect ophthalmoscopy, their magnification, field of view, resolution, and depth of field are dependent on the real image created by their front ophthalmoscopic lens.[9] Stereoscopic documentation of ONH topography can be performed in a nonsimultaneous fashion by shifting the camera laterally between photos or by using an Allen separator to provide a more reproducible stereo base.[10] Cameras also have been developed that produce simultaneous stereophotos by using prisms to provide twin perspectives of the real image created by the front ophthalmoscopic lens.[11] The constant stereo base of these simultaneous stereocameras provides superior reproducibility for stereoscopic documentation of ONH topography.[12–14] Because stereoscopic reproducibility is improved further when the relative direction of subject fixation is constant, this approach seems to be most reliable when using a stereocamera modified to target the corneal reflex at the time of photography.[15, 16]

The lateral and axial magnification produced by a given ophthalmoscopic system depends on the optics of the imaging system as well as several patient-related factors.[17, 18] Given this calibration problem, ONH measurements generally require correction factors to convert from relative to absolute scaling. Although several magnification correction formulas have been proposed, one population study[19] found that correction for refractive error[20] generally agreed closely with correction for both refractive error and anterior corneal curvature.[21] However, these methods differed slightly from formulas correcting for a combination of refractive error, anterior corneal curvature, and axial length.[21] Other factors, such as posterior corneal curvature, corneal thickness, anterior chamber depth, anterior and posterior lens curvature, and lens thickness do not significantly influence the magnification error.[21]

Because axial magnification is a squared function of lateral magnification in many imaging systems, errors in lateral magnification are squared in vertical depth measurements.[5] Errors in lateral magnification also are squared in two-dimensional area measurements. Because these errors in depth and area measurements are multiplied in three-dimensional volume measurements, errors in lateral magnification are raised to the fourth power in volume measurements.[22] In contrast, proportional measurements of cup:disc ratio or cup area:disc area ratio are relatively independent of lateral magnification.

These considerations become important when the lateral magnification of an imaging system is uncalibrated and can only be approximated. One proposed measurement system calibrates linear magnification by photographing an interference fringe pattern projected on the fundus.[22] Although it has not been applied to photographic imaging, another calibration method corrects for the effect of refractive error on linear magnification in indirect ophthalmoscopy by measuring real image dimensions in the principal plane of the ophthalmoscopic lens.[23]

Digital Imaging Systems

Ophthalmic imaging systems traditionally have used photographic film to capture images for storage, retrieval, and analysis. Recent technologic developments have made video camera-based ophthalmic imaging systems practical, in which images are digitally captured, stored, retrieved, analyzed, and displayed.[24, 25] The availability of low-cost video cameras for high-speed, high-resolution, black-and-white imaging has made direct digital image acquisition particularly practical for fluorescein angiographic systems.[26] These all-digital systems avoid film processing, provide lower cost per image, and allow excess images to be edited out after examination without the cost of wasting film.

However, the original video images have lower resolution than color film, which can capture a continuous range of hue, saturation, and brightness at a spatial resolution of about 7 μ.[27] When higher resolution digital imaging is needed, economical desktop slide scanners permit color slides to be digitized at the spatial resolution of the film. These scanners convert each slide image into a large two-dimensional array of picture elements, or "pixels." Because they use red, green, and blue filters to numerically measure the color at each pixel in terms of 256 or more shades of each red, green, and blue primary color, over 16 million possible colors can be numerically distinguished. Although digitizing a 35-mm color slide at such high-resolution corresponds to creating a table of millions of primary color intensities that represent the image with a spatial resolution exceeding distinctions that can be visually perceived, practical image analysis can be performed using smaller monochromatic image arrays after cropping the image and reducing it to an acceptable resolution.

Digital images can even be acquired without going through a conventional photographic or videographic medium. In laser tomographic scanning, for example, a three-dimensional object is imaged one point at a time, using microprocessor control to vary the x, y, and z coordinates of the point imaged by the optical system. Regardless of whether the original image was digitized directly or later digitized from film, computerized image analysis occurs by performing numerical operations on the pixel array. Because each high-resolution image might be represented in terms of a million or more pixels, sophisticated image-analysis techniques that would have overwhelmed the capabilities of older computers have been made practical by recent advances in the speed, capacity, and affordability of computers and their associated input/output devices. For purposes of low-cost image archiving with rapid random-access image storage and retrieval, magnetooptical drives can inscribe thousands of images (depending on the resolution) on each reusable, removable CD-like disc. Digitized color images can be recreated with high-resolution, red-green-blue display monitors, slide makers, or printers. High-resolution color images can also be viewed in three dimensions in a flicker-free stereoscopic fashion when wearing lightweight glasses with a liquid crystal shutter over each eye operating at 60 Hz. When using this stereoscopic display mode, a modified display monitor alternates between the left and right perspective images at a rate of 120 Hz while appropriately synchronizing these liquid crystal shutters with an infrared controller.[28]

Image Analysis Techniques

Digital image-analysis techniques can improve on ophthalmoscopic imaging and facilitate recognition of various image features. Relatively straightforward array operations and digital filtering readjust image magnification and boundaries, as well as regional image brightness, contrast, and sharpness.[26, 29] Other techniques have been used to provide edge enhancement and aid boundary determination for ONH features,[29, 30] enhance visibility of NFL striations,[31] or partially compensate for image degradation by cataracts.[32] More sophisticated image-analysis techniques now being used in artificial visual systems in other fields could also improve the feature recognition capabilities of ophthalmic imaging systems.[33] When data on pallor distribution and ONH topography are available, the ONH may be represented in three dimensions as a shaded surface[34, 35] that can be rotated and undergo changes in perspective.

Image analysis has also facilitated detailed comparison of similar ophthalmoscopic images that might differ chronologically or stereoscopically. Here, each compared image pair first must be brought into gross registration before comparing smaller regions. Although image registration can be performed using operator-defined "special points," this shortcut can result in operator-dependent registration errors.[29, 36, 37] Alternatively, the disparity between corresponding regions in the two images can be calculated grossly to provide image registration,[38] before proceeding to finer disparity calculations for smaller regions that may have shifted chronologically or stereoscopically.

Once brought into gross registration, corresponding points in successive images can be matched, for example, in a fluorescein angiogram, allowing the relative observed fluorescence at specific intravascular or extravascular points of interest to be followed over time.[38] Other techniques can be used to detect and measure small localized shifts in image position over time, although the reproducibility of these methods is sensitive to parallax-related shifts due to variation in image perspective from visit to visit. One method flickers between the image pair to detect changes subjectively.[39] In another technique, shifts in vessel position over time can be detected using digital subtraction to compare local intensity levels.[40] Changes in ONH topography over time also can be assessed using stereochronometry, in which changes in two time-separated images creates stereopsis. Although this method can produce large quantitative measurement errors when the two compared images were obtained using different perspectives,[41] the reproducibility of this approach can be improved using a stereocamera modification that targets the corneal reflex at the time of photography.[15, 16]

When evaluating paired stereoscopic images, depth calculations can be inferred from measurements of the disparity between corresponding points (Fig. 114–1). In general terms, because all stereoscopic methods use some localized features of the paired images to match corresponding regions or points, measurements of the disparity between corresponding points become less reliable when matching regions with little image detail. To provide additional image detail for more reliable measurements of horizontal disparity in stereoscopic matching, stereocameras have been modified to project vertical stripes of light on the ONH during photography. This approach has proved to be useful both for manual photogrammetric[42] and automated[36] disparity measurements.

A commonly used stereoscopic matching technique identifies each pair of corresponding points by the similarity of a window of intensity values around the two points; that is, for a given window of intensity values around a point of interest in one image, this intensity window is translated across possible corresponding locations in other image until the best appropriate intensity correlation is found. After performing this cross-correlation operation to match corresponding points in a gridlike fashion (Fig. 114–2), a smooth surface is interpolated between points that were matched with a good correlation of their intensity windows.[29, 37] When detailed matching of corresponding points is based on these regional comparisons, disparity measurements can be calculated with a fraction of the pixel size, allowing relative disparity resolution to exceed the spatial resolution of each image.[43]

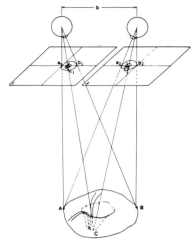

Figure 114–1. Corresponding points in a stereo image pair represent a particular site of the original surface, as viewed from two perspectives. The disparity between corresponding points is related to the depth of that site and the geometry of the optical system creating the stereo images, including the stereo base (b). (From Schwartz B: New techniques for the examination of the optic disc and their clinical application. Trans Am Acad Ophthalmol Otolaryngol 81:227, 1976.)

These automated methods use a different approach from that believed to result in depth perception, apparently involving cooperative phenomena of large arrays of parallel processors in the visual cortex.[44] Although artificial visual systems are only beginning to approximate this "biologic approach,"[33] limited efforts have been made at improving matching reliability by enhancing image features before cross-correlation[36, 39] and by identifying corresponding points on the basis of a more sophisticated multiresolution description of local image structure (Fig. 114–3).[33, 45]

ONH IMAGING APPROACHES

Pallor Distribution

Assessments of pallor distribution evaluate the ONH cup and neural rim in terms of color differences. Pallor

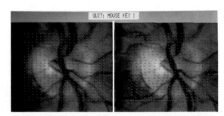

Figure 114–2. In this example from the Humphrey Retinal Analyzer, a grid of points selected in the left stereo image was matched to corresponding points in the right stereo image, using a cross-correlation operation that identifies pairs of corresponding points by the similarity of a window of intensity values around each point. After matching 400 to 650 pairs of corresponding points that have a good correlation of their intensity windows (shown with *red crosses*), a smooth surface is interpolated. (From Dandona L, Quigley HA, Jampal DH: Variability of depth measurements of the optic nerve head and peripapillary retina with computerized image analysis. Arch Ophthalmol 107:1786, 1989. Copyright 1989, American Medical Association.)

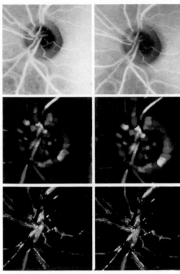

Figure 114–3. The top two images are gray scale representations of intensity values in an original pair of digitized stereo images. The middle and bottom pairs of stereo images represent digitally filtered versions of these original stereo images, with each column corresponding to the same perspective. For each location in the original stereo image pair, a series of directional filters at a given level of spatial resolution was used to evaluate the magnitude and direction of local intensity gradients at the level of spatial resolution. In these images, false colors represent these local intensity gradient direction values, and intensities represent these local gradient magnitude values. The middle pair of images was obtained at low spatial resolution, and the bottom pair of images was obtained at high spatial resolution. Note that some features of the original image are enhanced in the low-resolution images (e.g., the rim of the optic disc and larger vessels), whereas other features of the original image are enhanced in the high-resolution images (e.g., the smaller vessels). This type of multiresolution description of local image structure has been used to construct an artificial visual system. (From Coggins JM: A multi-scale description of image structure for segmentation of biomedical images. Proceedings of the Conference on Visualization in Biomedical Computing. Atlanta, May 22, 1990, pp 123–130.)

distribution should be distinguished from topographic descriptions that evaluate the ONH cup and rim in structural terms, even though there is often a close correspondence between ONH pallor distribution and topography.[6] Early quantitative approaches to evaluating pallor distribution generally began by manually identifying or tracing cup and rim boundaries in projected monoscopic color slides. Analog devices like a planimeter then used these boundaries to measure the two-dimensional areas and dimensions of the cup and rim.[46–48] Whether using manual or automated techniques, an unrecognized pigmented crescent within the neural rim[49] or a peripapillary zone of pigment disturbance could perturb boundary determination in pallor evaluation.

Automated approaches have also been used to evaluate pallor distribution in digitized monoscopic images. When using red, green, and blue filters to describe the color at each pixel in terms of red, green, and blue primary colors, the red intensities from the red-filtered image are most useful for automated boundary determination of the disc margin, and green intensities from the green-filtered image are most useful for automatic boundary determination of the cup margin. In fact, by using histogram methods to pick a red-intensity threshold for the disc margin and a green-intensity threshold for the cup margin, ellipses fitted to these boundaries can measure pallor cup:disc ratios with good reproducibility.[50] Alternatively, by combining these red and green intensities in pallor index, particular pallor index histogram thresholds could approximate the disc and cup margins.[18, 51–53]

Rather than determine cup and disc margins with histograms generated using the entire image, or impose a geometric shape on the cup and disc, these boundaries can be determined locally by using image analysis. One approach uses a boundary-tracking algorithm to follow the edge of the cup and disc, while ignoring edges due to crossing vessels which are excluded by a set of local curvature constraints (Fig. 114–4).[30] When this boundary-tracking approach used the red-filtered image for disc margin determination and the green-filtered image for cup margin determination, measurements of the pallor cup area:disc area ratio had a standard deviation that was only 2 percent of its mean value.[47] This reliability index was not affected by changes in exposure but was sensitive to photographic image defocusing or decentration. In fact, using this reliability index, this boundary-tracking method under these poor conditions was slightly more reliable than using conventional manual planimetry by an experienced planimetrist under optimal photographic conditions. The reliability of manual planimetry was even worse when performed by an inexperienced planimetrist or when exposure was varied.[47]

Although little is known about changes in pallor distribution over time, limited longitudinal studies have been performed using this boundary-tracking pallor determination method. A longitudinal study of untreated patients with ocular hypertension (OHTN) noted a significant increase in the pallor cup area:disc area ratio,[54] and a longitudinal study of patients with OHTN with asymmetric cupping observed less change in cup volume or pallor in eyes with initially large cup volume or pallor.[55] A longitudinal study of 59 patients with glaucoma and 96 patients with OHTN followed for an average of 9 yr showed a strong correlation between initial measurements of neuroretinal rim area in terms of pallor and topography, as well as a strong correlation of changes of these two types of rim area. In 55 percent of glaucomatous eyes, the neural rim area changed more in topography than pallor, whereas the neural rim area changed more in pallor than in topography in only 9 percent of glaucomatous eyes. In contrast, these percentages were 42 percent and 29 percent, respectively, in the 35 patients with OHTN who eventually developed early glaucoma. Based on these relative findings, the authors believed that larger changes in the topographic area of the neuroretinal rim were more characteristic of advanced glaucoma, whereas larger changes in the pallor area of the neuroretinal rim were less characteristic of advanced glaucoma than early glaucoma.[56]

In a different approach, an optical system with twin projectors sharing a beam splitter was used to manually superimpose two monoscopic color slide images of a well-centered optic disc and then to flicker between them. In a longitudinal study of 131 eyes with OHTN followed at 3-mo intervals with fundus photos and automated perimetry for an average of 40 mo, these flicker comparisons detected definite or highly suspected optic disc changes in 10 of 12 eyes that developed visual field defects and in four of 119 eyes that did not develop visual field defects.[57] Because automated registration of digitized images for flicker comparison is relatively straightforward,[39] this study suggests that following ONH pallor using subjective flicker comparison of digitized color images should be surprisingly sensitive to ONH damage over time.

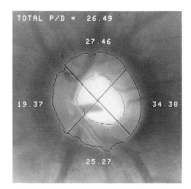

Figure 114–4. A boundary-tracking algorithm followed the edge of the cup and disc, while ignoring edges due to crossing vessel, which are excluded by a set of local curvature constraints. The optic disc margin was determined with the red-filtered image, and the pallor margin was determined with the green-filtered image. Pallor area-to-disc area ratios were computed for each of the four illustrated quadrants and for the entire disc. (From Nagin P, Schwartz B, Nanba K: The reproducibility of computerized boundary analysis for measuring optic disc pallor in the normal optic disc. Ophthalmology 92:243, 1985.)

Surface Topography

Stereoscopic Approaches. Although various subjective scoring systems have been devised for topographically evaluating glaucomatous damage, clinical estimation of ONH cupping has been unsatisfactory in sensitivity and reliability.[58, 59] An early approach to quantitative evaluation of ONH topography manually measured perceived depth while viewing a pair of stereophotos with a photogrammetric plotter. Each time that the operator uses this analog device to position a floating mark in space on the perceived surface, a set of surface coordinates is entered into the computer database.[12, 18, 60–63] Reliable depth readings can be obtained by an experienced photogrammetrist using this approach with appropriate standardization and magnification correction.[13, 64–67] When performed under these optimum conditions with about 300 depth readings per eye, a study using relative scaling obtained median coefficients of variation for cup area/disc area and cup volume/disc

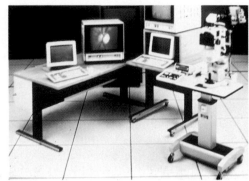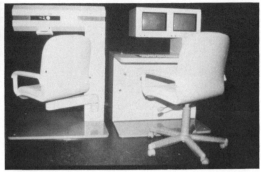

A   B

Figure 114–5. *A,* The PAR IS-2000, later known as the Topcon Imagenet, was the first commercial system allowing automated stereoscopic evaluation of optic disc topography. (Courtesy of George Spaeth, M.D.) *B,* The Heidelberg Laser Tomographic Scanner was the first confocal scanning optical microscope designed to evaluate optic disc topography using an automatically obtained series of evenly spaced focal plane images. (Courtesy of Robert Weinreb, M.D.)

area of about 5 percent in patients with glaucoma.[68] To improve the reliability of photogrammetric depth measurements by providing additional ONH image detail, manual photogrammetry also has been performed with simultaneous stereophotos created while projecting equidistant parallel stripes on the disc with a laser interferometer.[42]

A depth reading can also be obtained with stereoscopic imaging by photographing the disc while obliquely projecting a parallel stripe pattern.[69] When these stripes are vertical in orientation, the angle between the stripe projector and the camera in the horizontal plane is responsible for the deviation of the stripes with variation in surface depth. When this approach was compared to photogrammetry with nonsimultaneous stereophotos, manually obtained surface profiles had qualitatively comparable reliability.[60]

The first commercial system allowing automated stereoscopic evaluation of optic disc topography was the PAR IS-2000, which is now available as the Topcon Imagenet (Topcon Instruments, Paramus, NJ),[70, 71] an unusually versatile ONH imaging system that can be combined with evaluation of fluorescein angiography (Fig. 114–5A).[76] This Topcon system can digitize simultaneous stereoimages either directly with video cameras or from 35-mm color slides. After using algorithms for image registration and cross-correlation to calculate depth values at well-matched corresponding points, a three-dimensional ONH surface is interpolated. This topographic data can be represented in terms of numerical depth maps, color-coded depth maps, contour maps, radial cross-sectional profiles, or three-dimensional "wire basket" plots (Fig. 114–6).[2, 29]

The Topcon system defines the disc margin with an elliptical approximation based on four user-determined points on the disc margin and defines the cup margin by points on the sloping wall that are 120 μ down from the optic disc margin. These definitions are used to calculate a battery of "basic ONH statistics," including vertical cup:disc ratio, horizontal cup:disc ratio, cup area:disc ratio, neuroretinal rim area:disc area ratio, and cup volume. Other features include a histogram-based method for defining the pallor margin and computing pallor area:disc area, edge enhancement, and a "vessel shift" program that superimposes color-coded vessel margins.[2, 29, 40]

The Humphrey Retinal Analyzer (Allergan Humphrey, San Leandro, CA) uses a similar approach to the Topcon system, although digital input must be obtained directly with a red-free stereoscopic video camera (Fig. 114–7).[37] The Humphrey system defines the disc margin in a slightly different fashion, working from at least eight user-determined points on the disc margin. After fitting these points with a low-order Fourier series to determine a general oval or egg-shaped approximation for the disc margin, an edge-enhancement operation is performed before refining the preliminary disc margin by searching radially for a nearby intensity gradient or edge.[37]

The Rodenstock Optic Nerve Head Analyzer (Rodenstock Instruments, Danbury, CT) uses a similar approach to the Topcon system, although a 150-μ vertical "cup-drop" is standard. Unlike the Topcon system, topographic analysis requires directly obtaining digital

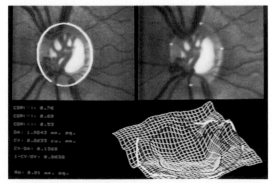

Figure 114–6. In this example from the Topcon Imagenet, a pair of stereo images are shown at the top with four operator-provided control points on the right image, and the calculated cup margin and elliptical disc margin are superimposed on the left image. The three-dimensional wire basket plot was interpolated from calculated depth values and is shown with the superimposed blue cup margin determined by the cup-drop method. Using the cup-and-rim model, the optic nerve head is described in terms of several calculated statistics. (From Varma R, Spaeth GL: The PAR IS 2000: A new system for retinal digital image analysis. Ophthalmic Surg 19:183, 1988.)

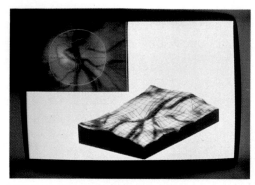

Figure 114–7. In this example from the Humphrey Retinal Analyzer, the three-dimensional wire basket plot was interpolated from calculated depth values and is shown with image intensity superimposed on a shaded surface. The green optic disc margin has an oval shape, and the red cup margin is determined by the cup-drop method. (From Dandona L, Quigley HA, Jampal DH: Variability of depth measurements of the optic nerve head and peripapillary retina with computerized image analysis. Acta Ophthalmol 107:1786, 1989.)

input with a stereoscopic video camera while projecting two sets of seven evenly spaced vertical stripes on the ONH.[36] Because these stripes provide useful image detail for reliable measurements of horizontal disparity in stereoscopic matching, depth values are calculated at 140 points along each of the 14 vertical stripes, and a surface is interpolated between the stripes (Fig. 114–8).[72] The value of projecting multiple vertical stripes during stereoscopic video imaging recently has been evaluated in the Topcon system.[73]

Based on their definitions of disc margin and topographic cup margin, the PAR, Rodenstock, and Humphrey systems generate the same battery of basic ONH statistics described above. The cup-drop method of defining the cup margin in these systems tends to underestimate large cups and overestimate small cups, perhaps

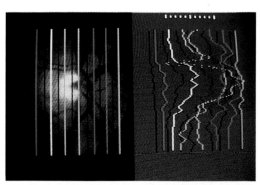

Figure 114–8. In this example from the Rodenstock Optic Nerve Head Analyzer, the vertical stripes superimposed on the left image correspond to the vertical depth profiles shown on the right. After projecting two sets of seven vertical stripes on the optic nerve head during imaging, depth values are calculated at 140 points along each of the 14 stripes, and a surface is interpolated between the stripes. The seven color-coded stripes represent one set of these vertical stripes. (From Shields MB, Martone JF, Shelton AR, et al: Reproducibility of optic disk topographic measurements with the Rodenstock Optic Nerve Head Analyzer. Am J Ophthalmol 106:696, 1988. Published with permission from The American Journal of Ophthalmology. Copyright by The Ophthalmic Publishing Company.)

because the elevation of the disc margin is lower in eyes with large cups due to NFL loss, and higher in eyes with small cups.[74] Using a cup-drop of 150 μ proved superior to 100 μ or 300 μ in sorting early glaucoma from ocular hypertension and normals, perhaps because values of 100 μ and 300 μ define the cup margin in a region too close to or too far from the disc margin to aid distinction of early glaucoma from ocular hypertension and normals.[75] The optimal cup-drop value for correlation with clinical estimation of cup:disc ratio seems to be about 140 μ.[76]

Given their multiple common features, it is not surprising that the Topcon,[77] Rodenstock,[78–80] and Humphrey systems[81] have grossly comparable reproducibility of their basic ONH statistics. It is reassuring that automated measurements of these statistics are strongly correlated with their manual measurement from stereophotos.[82] Accuracy studies with a model eye have shown good qualitative correspondence of calculated and actual depth profiles,[83] and in vivo measurements of disc area in glaucomatous monkeys, when corrected for corneal curvature and axial length, have shown good quantitative correspondence with postmortem anatomic measurements of disc area.[84] However, magnification determination remains an approximate science. This partially may explain why optic disc area correlated with axial length in one ONH imaging study,[85] even though this was not observed in eyes from eye bank.[86] Because errors in linear magnification could affect several measurements, this may contribute to the correlation observed between magnification-corrected measurements of disc area with cup area, rim area, and cup volume.[87]

Several specific sources of possible variability have been examined in these stereoscopic systems, using their basic ONH statistics for comparison. Reliability is improved when using simultaneous stereophotos rather than nonsimultaneous stereophotos,[14] although calculated ONH statistics were dependent on the stereobase used in the simultaneous stereocamera.[88] Reliability was unaffected when using a slide scanner to enter photographic images rather than direct video input,[77] although calculated ONH statistics from the same slides with the same commercial system depended on the center at which the image analysis was performed.[88] Contrast-enhancement techniques did not affect observer variability,[77, 89] although image exposure did affect the variability of calculated ONH statistics.[77] The variability of calculated ONH statistics was the same for patients with glaucoma and normal people, with the greatest source of variability relating to instrument variability in imaging the same eye multiple times, rather than observer variability in evaluating the same image multiple times.[78] The variability of calculated ONH statistics depended on the disc appearance and could be substantial for one observer,[77, 81] whereas the variability in evaluating the same image multiple times with the same observer was less than the variability with different observers.[77, 78] Despite these problems, the variability of various calculated ONH statistics was much less than for clinical estimation.[58, 77]

The reproducibility of regional depth values has also been evaluated in these stereoscopic systems. Studies using the optic disc margin for reference plane determination have shown relatively poor reproducibility of local depth values.[37, 90] To improve the reproducibility of depth values produced by the Rodenstock system, depth values were calculated for 25 × 25 matrices of 100 × 100-μ regions, a "retinal reference plane" was defined for each depth map using three points outside the immediate peripapillary area, and each depth map was rotated to define this retinal reference plan as zero elevation.[91] In keeping with the typical pattern of glaucomatous atrophy, these three points or regions were chosen outside the immediate peripapillary area along the horizontal temporally and 30 degrees above the horizontal nasally, rather than superiorly or inferiorly.[92] Using this approach in repeated measurements in patients with glaucoma, the average standard deviation of depth values was 38 μ in the peripapillary area and 61 μ inside the optic disc margin.[93]

Several studies have examined the effect of IOP on ONH topography. Acute increases of IOP caused posterior ONH displacement in a study of glaucomatous monkeys[94] but did not produce significant change in normal human subjects.[95] When spontaneous fluctuations of IOP were followed over a matter of weeks in glaucomatous patients, IOP increases or decreases produced significant corresponding increases or decreases in cup:disc ratio and cup volume, in a reproducible fashion.[96–98] These changes were sufficient to reject the null hypothesis, even though the magnitude of change in an individual case was often well within the 95 percent confidence limits of analyzer variability.[99]

Although many studies have evaluated the capabilities of stereoscopic ONH analyzers, at this point few studies have sought to use these new capabilities to better characterize glaucomatous atrophy. Cross-sectional studies of normal subjects and ocular hypertension and patients with glaucoma have demonstrated significant differences in cup volume, rim area, and cup:disc ratio. However, there is a broad range and considerable overlap of these values, preventing useful distinction of these clinical subpopulations.[100] One longitudinal study of ocular hypertension detected significant changes in cup volume before changes in other calculated ONH statistics.[101] Patients with low-tension glaucoma were noted to have shallower cup depth and less cup volume than did patients with open-angle glaucoma.[102, 103]

Laser Tomographic Scanning. The familiar principles of an optical microscope apply to ONH imaging with indirect ophthalmoscopy, 90-diopter lens-slit lamp biomicroscopy, and fundus photography. With each technique, bright-field imaging uniformly illuminates a broad area of ONH tissue, a real, inverted image of this tissue is formed with an objective lens, and eyepiece lenses focus an image of this tissue on a broad area of film or the examiner's macula.

With the introduction of the laser and recent advances in computer capabilities for digital imaging, a new approach to ONH imaging has been developed using the confocal scanning optical microscope.[104–109] In various types of confocal scanning optical microscopy, the tissue of interest is illuminated and imaged one point at a time through a pinhole, rather than a broad area all

at once.[109–113] When the illumination and imaging light paths are superimposed using a beam splitter, illumination from a pinhole is focused to a point by the objective lens, and reflected light from this point passing back through the same optical system is focused through a pinhole onto the photodetector (Fig. 114–9A). This optical system is "confocal," because the illumination pinhole and imaging pinhole correspond to the same focal point on the object. By varying the x, y, and z coordinates of the point imaged by the optical system under microprocessor control, a three-dimensional object can be imaged.

While scanning this focal point of illumination across a given plane of focus, only reflectance from near this focal point is focused back through the imaging pinhole to the photodetector. Detection of other reflected light is markedly attenuated, because this imaging pinhole almost totally blocks other reflected light (see Fig. 114–9B), causing parts of the ONH surface that do not lie close to the plane of focus to disappear rather than to blur as with a conventional optical microscope. Perhaps the best known confocal scanning optical microscope is the compact disc player, in which the disappearance of a defocused surface is used to optically detect the binary presence or absence of surface pits while scanning the laser beam across the spinning compact disc.

In general terms, for each plane of focus selected by advancing the objective lens under steeper motor control, the illuminated and imaged focal point can be scanned rapidly horizontally and vertically across this plane of focus by steering the superimposed illumination and imaging light paths with a pair of galvanometer-controlled mirrors.[113] Superimposing the illumination

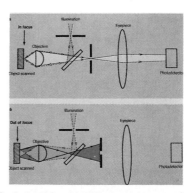

Figure 114–9. *A,* In this simplified confocal optical system, the illumination pinhole and imaging pinhole correspond to the same focal point on the object. Because the surface of the object is in focus, reflected light is focused through the imaging pinhole. Various optical elements are not shown, including mirrors used to horizontally and vertically steer the superimposed illumination and imaging light paths while scanning this focal point across each selected focal plane. Superimposing these light paths facilitates maintaining precise confocal imaging while scanning the beam across the object. *B,* As a reflective surface is moved from the plane of focus, more and more reflected light is blocked by the imaging pinhole. By advancing the focal plane depth through a particular reflecting surface location, optical section thickness can be described in terms of the depth range within which the peak reflectance will be less than 50 per cent attenuated. (From Kino GS, Corle TR: Confocal scanning optical microscopy. Physics Today 42:55, 1989.)

and imaging light paths facilitates maintaining precise confocal imaging while scanning the beam across the object. However, several technical modifications have been needed to facilitate tomographically scanning the sharply focused laser beam over the ONH at high speed through a small part of the patient's pupil. For example, separate optical elements are used to correct beam convergence for the patient's refractive error, serially adjust the plane of focus, and converge the imaging beam through the imaging pinhole. Interestingly, the high scanning rate required for the horizontal deflection mirror has required mechanically spinning a polygonal mirror at thousands of revolutions/min.[108, 109, 114–118]

Because laser tomographic scanning occurs one point at a time rather than in a brief snapshot, the finite time required for image acquisition must be limited to prevent problematic movement artifact during image acquisition. Since a laser tomographic scanner (LTS) will not image parts of the ONH surface that do not lie close to a given plane of focus, this confocal scanning optical microscope creates a "composite" ONH image much like a contour map by scanning across the ONH surface one focal plane at a time and then bringing the series of two-dimensional digitized focal plane images into registration. This registration process has been used to correct for microsaccades during image acquisition.[104, 118]

The vertical resolution of depth values obtained at each pixel in this composite ONH image is related to the number of spacing of these focal plane images, as well as other resolution-limiting features of the optical system like imaging pinhole diameter and objective lens power.[110–113] Because the measured reflectance from a given tissue interface at a given x-y location actually decreases in an approximately gaussian fashion from its peak value as the depth of the plane of focus is moved away from this tissue interface,[108, 109] these focal plane images can be thought of as optical sections with a half-width "thickness" within which reflectance from nearby tissue interfaces is attenuated to less than 50 percent of their peak value. Attempts to reduce optical section half-width thickness are limited in part by the beam-convergence restrictions imposed by passing the illuminating and imaging beam through a small pupillary aperture at a given distance from the ONH surface.[109] Despite this problem, depth values can be interpolated for a given x-y location by evaluating the "depth transfer function" of reflectance measurements sampled for that location in serial focal plane images. In theory, when several translucent tissue interfaces at a given x-y location create reflectance at several depth levels, the depth transfer function could be evaluated to separately determine their depth values.[119]

Because laser tomographic scanning evaluates ONH topography by comparing serial focal plane images rather than stereoscopic images, the wide pupillary dilatation needed for stereoscopic imaging is unnecessary. In addition, because the superimposed laser beam illumination and imaging light paths are projected through a small portion of the pupillary aperture, "pivoting" about the entrance pupil while scanning over the fundus without changing its location at the pupil, adequate imaging can be performed readily without pupillary dilatation.[105, 120] Several other features of LTS should compare favorably with conventional digital ONH imaging. The composite ONH image from the LTS should not be obscured by glare from cataracts, because reflected light from out-of-focus tissues is almost totally blocked by the imaging pinhole. This composite image forms an extended focus image without blurring due to conventional depth-of-field limitations, because the composite image is formed from a series of in-focus optical sections. Lower levels of illumination can be used, because the composite image is created one point at a time with a coherent spot of laser light rather than all at once using conventional bright-field illumination. This approach also should improve composite image sharpness by reducing diffraction-related effects[110–113] and should be less sensitive to the quality of the imaging optics.[109] Because the scanned laser beam has orders of magnitude (100 to 5000 times) and less thermal effect on the retina than the bright-field illumination levels used for conventional ophthalmoscopy or fundus photography,[121] LTSs should be safe for about an hour's continuous viewing, depending on the field of view and the laser wavelength selected[109] and should permit steady illumination with greater subject comfort. Scattered background illumination outside this focused or defocused spot is relatively low,[121] perhaps helping to produce less reflexive pupillary constriction.

The first confocal scanning optical microscope developed for ophthalmology was the Rodenstock confocal scanning laser ophthalmoscope.[108, 109, 114–117] This instrument obtains each focal plane image in 1/30th sec as a 525 horizontal line analog video signal with a field of view of 20 degrees or 40 degrees and has a focal plane section half-width thickness of about 300 μ.[108, 109] When using this videocompatible scan timing, a laser beam with a power level under 0.1 mW illuminates each small spot of imaged retina with an energy of about 10 J during an interval of about 100 nsec at a repetition rate of 30 Hz.[109] This scanner has permitted documentation of continuous fundoscopy or angiography on videotape at a rate of 30 frames/sec,[109, 122] uses a helium-neon or argon laser, and has been used for a variety of applications including NFL imaging and assessment of macular function (by modulating the intensity of the scanned laser beam to project a video image directly on the macula, just as modulating the intensity of a scanned electron beam can project a video image on a TV screen).[108, 109, 114, 115, 117, 123] Although this scanner can create ONH focal plane images at various depths,[108] its design has not been modified to automatically obtain an evenly spaced series of optical sections for LTS.

In preliminary studies with the Heidelberg LTS (Heidelberg Instruments, Heidelberg Germany) (see Fig. 114–5B), automatically completing an ONH tomographic scan of 32 consecutive focal plane sections required about 4 sec, and correction for movement artifact required registration of successive focal plane images.[105] Each two-dimensional focal plane image covering a field of view of about 15 degrees was obtained with a lateral resolution of 256 × 256 pixels, correspond-

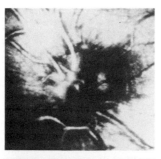
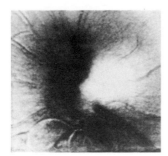
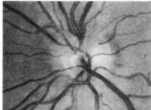

Figure 114–10. In this example from the Heidelberg Laser Tomographic Scanner, a focal plan image is shown at top left, and a corresponding fundus photograph is shown below. After evaluating a series of 32 evenly spaced focal plane images, the resultant topographic map is shown at top right, using a grayscale representation of depth values. (From Dreher AW, Tso PC, Weinreb RN: Reproducibility of topographic measurements of the normal and glaucomatous optic nerve head with the laser tomographic scanner. Am J Ophthalmol 111:221, 1991. Published with permission from The American Journal of Ophthalmology. Copyright by The Ophthalmic Publishing Company.)

ing to over 65,000 pixels with dimensions of about 15 × 15 μ. These 32 focal plane sections can be obtained with a half-width thickness of about 60 μ or less (limited in part by the beam-convergence restrictions imposed by a small pupil size),[109] while selecting an even spacing typically in the range of about 20 to 60 μ between focal plane images (Fig. 114–10).[105, 118]

In preliminary studies with the Zeiss LTS (Zeiss Instruments, Thornwood, NJ), automatically completing an ONH tomographic scan of nine consecutive focal plane sections required 0.32 sec, and depth maps were calculated without needing correction for movement artifact to adequately register successive focal plane images.[107] Each two-dimensional focal plane image covering a field of view of about 20 degrees was obtained with a lateral resolution of 578 × 672 pixels, corresponding to over 388,000 pixels with dimensions of about 10 × 10 μ. These nine focal plane sections had a "thickness" of about 300 μ and were evenly spaced with a distance of about 200 μ between focal plane images. Both the Heidelberg and Zeiss LTSs use a red helium-neon laser for illumination. Other LTSs are in the final stages of development at this time and should be commercially available soon.

To evaluate the reproducibility of depth values for the composite ONH image produced by these two systems, a standardized retinal reference plane was defined for each composite ONH image using a technique comparable to that established for the Rodenstock stereoscopic ONH analyzer.[92] After bringing repeated composite ONH images of the same subject into registration and rotating them to share a common retinal reference plane, the standard deviation of depth values was determined with the Heidelberg[105] and the Zeiss LTSs.[107] The former had an average standard deviation of less than 50 μ for each 15 × 15 μ pixel of its composite ONH image, both for normal patients without dilatation and patients with glaucoma with dilatation. This average standard deviation was independent of pupil size, cup:disc ratio, or gross fundus location. Depth value reproducibility was locally worse near vessel margins, although it was unclear whether this occurred because the reproducibility of depth values in steeply sloping regions was more sensitive to slight image misalignment, or perhaps because of spontaneous vessel pulsations. When the 10 × 10-μ pixels of the composite ONH image of the Zeiss LTS were averaged in 100 × 100-μ regions of 10 × 10 pixels, an average standard deviation of less than 28 μ was obtained for 52 percent of these regions. Pupillary dilatation was again of no benefit,[120] and depth value reproducibility was locally worse in steeply sloping regions.

Although the depth value reproducibility of LTS systems is comparable with that obtained with current stereoscopic approaches, the lateral resolution of depth maps produced by LTS systems can be much higher than for current stereoscopic approaches, when providing reliable data for each pixel.[105] Manual photogrammetry is practically limited to depth value determination at a much smaller number of points,[68] and depth value reproducibility with automated stereoscopic approaches has been reported using larger evaluation regions of perhaps 100 × 100 μ corresponding to several pixels.[37, 93] LTS depth value reproducibility could be improved by obtaining several composite ONH images in one session and bringing these images into exact three-dimensional registration (Fig. 114–11).[124] Alternatively, LTS regional depth value reproducibility could be improved at the expense of decreased lateral resolution, either by averaging depth values over areas larger than 1 pixel[107] or by using an appropriate topographic smoothing function.

NFL Evaluation

Conventional photographic documentation of NFL striations, using high-resolution, black-and-white film with a red-free filter, can be evaluated clinically to detect glaucomatous atrophy before the onset of visual field loss.[125] Diffuse or localized NFL loss has been documented in animal models of glaucoma[126] and correlates with decreased neuroretinal rim area.[127] The development of NFL defects may be a more sensitive marker for glaucomatous atrophy than changes of cup size in eyes with small ONHs and misleadingly small optic cups,[128] and in highly myopic eyes with atypical optic disc shape.[129]

However, a study of sources of variance in digitized NFL photographs found that reliable quantitative documentation required pupil dilatation to at least 6 mm, reliable optic disc positioning, and strict control of some factors in photography, film processing, and image digitization.[130] Because the short wavelength end of the visible spectrum has higher NFL reflectance,[131] a blue

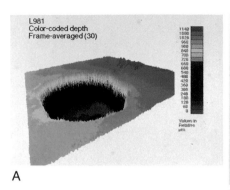

L981
Color-coded depth
Frame-averaged (30)

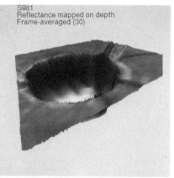

S981
Reflectance mapped on depth
Frame-averaged (30)

A

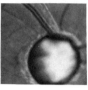

B

Figure 114–11. In this example, the Zeiss Confocal Laser Scanning Ophthalmoscope obtained 30 complete laser tomographic scans of nine focal plane images of the optic nerve head in one extended session. After the composite reflectance image and topographic map from each of these 30 scans were registered in three dimensions and cropped to the central two thirds of the image, average reflectance and average depth were calculated. The resulting topographic map is shown on the left using a false color representation of average depth values, and the gray scale image on the right shows average reflectance superimposed on this topographic map as a shaded surface. (From Cioffi GA, Eastman RD, Robin AL, et al: Confocal laser scanning ophthalmoscope. Automated registration and reproducibility. Invest Ophthalmol Vis Sci 32[Suppl]:719, 1991.)

rather than green exciting filter is preferable.[132, 133] The relative direction of subject fixation can be made more reliable using a camera modification for targeting the corneal reflex at the time of photography, following the approach developed for stereochronoscopy.[15, 16] Once digitized, digital filter can enhance the visibility of NFL striations.[31]

Possible benefits of these and other approaches[134] on the sensitivity and reliability of NFL striation evaluation require future studies. One study found that photographic image quality was often inadequate for conventional photographic NFL evaluation in normal elderly patients, particularly those over 70 yr of age.[135] Confocal scanning optical microscopy can image NFL striations with high contrast and high lateral resolution at an appropriately short wavelength but should be less dependent than photographic methods on pupil dilatation and clear media.[105, 109, 110, 115, 117, 120] NFL striations have been enhanced in this approach using digital filtering and polarization differential contrast imaging, in which changes in NFL appearance due to NFL birefringence are evaluated using two images obtained simultaneously with orthogonal polarization.[115, 117]

Local NFL thickness measurements can be obtained by direct evaluation of NFL birefringence, without inferring NFL thickness from measurements of retinal thickness or retinal surface contour. Because back-and-forth travel of light through a birefringent NFL should cause a change of polarization known as retardance, NFL thickness can be evaluated by locally measuring polarization retardance using Fourier ellipsometry.[136] In this approach, an LTS is modified to measure the polarization retardance of reflected light from each imaged point. This is performed by evaluating the effect of illuminating beam polarizer orientation on the intensity of reflected light from each imaged point passing through a second polarizer to the photodetector. Preliminary in vitro studies have demonstrated a positive correlation between polarization retardance and NFL thickness using this approach.[136] In these studies, the small standard deviation of polarization retardance

measurements corresponded with an estimated NFL thickness of 1.6 μ,[137] and retardation measurements were obtained every degree or two along a circle around the ONH.[138] An applanation-style contact lens could be used clinically to avoid significant polarization changes at the anterior corneal surface.

Topographic data have been used to assess glaucomatous atrophy by inferring NFL thickness in terms of retinal thickness or retinal surface contour in the peripapillary region.[72, 134, 139] These approaches determine depth values for the peripapillary "anterior retinal surface" using reflectance from the inner limiting membrane or NFL (or occasionally the anterior surface of retinal vessels). When depth values for the peripapillary "posterior retinal surface" are also determined using reflectance from the retinal pigment epithelium (or occasionally the surface of the choriocapillaris when necessary), peripapillary retinal thickness can be determined. When photogrammetry was used to measure peripapillary retinal thickness for 72 locations at 5-degree intervals along the optic disc margin, excluding retinal vessel sites, average retinal thickness for the entire disc margin was determined with a standard deviation that was about 5 per cent of its mean value, independent of the presence of a peripapillary halo or scleral crescent.[134] In normal patients, retinal thickness for the entire disc margin averaged 520 μ, with a standard deviation of 100 μ, and was decreased in patients with increased cup volume, cup depth, or disc area.[140]

Although the anterior and posterior retinal surfaces could be stereoscopically distinguished automatically, in theory, by computer algorithms that use measured points on each surface to cooperatively generate discrete surfaces,[44] this would require extremely accurate matching of corresponding points in stereoimages at high resolution. LTS also could distinguish the depth of the anterior and posterior retinal surfaces, in theory, by evaluating the "depth transfer function" of local retinal reflectance measurements in closely spaced series of focal plane images for each x-y location.[119] Local reflectance from particular retinal tissue interfaces could also be evaluated in a tomographic fashion using optical coherence domain interferometry.[141] In this technique, an illumination light path is focused to a point on a retinal tissue interface, and light reflected back from this point is imaged on a photodetector. However, before this "object beam" enters the eye, a beam splitter separates off a "reference beam," and a mirror reflects this reference beam back to the beam splitter to rejoin the object beam reflected from the eye. This modified Michaelson interferometer[142] creates an interference pattern over time, only if the reflected reference beam maintains a constant phase relationship with a component of the reflected object beam over time. However, the reference beam remains coherent with a component of the reflected object beam only when the difference in their round-trip path length is less than the coherence path length of the illumination source.

In preliminary in vitro studies of optical coherence domain interferometry using a broad bandwidth diode laser with a short coherence path length of 10 μ, an interference pattern was created over time only when a component of the objective beam reflected from various tissue interfaces had the same round-trip path length as the reference beam to within an "optical coherence domain" of 10 μ. This condition was detected by observing an appropriate time-dependent component of the photodetector signal while moving the reference beam mirror about a particular location with small-amplitude, high-frequency longitudinal oscillations. Even a weak, time-dependent component of the photodetector signal could be detected when superimposed on a baseline reflectance from other surfaces that was about 10 orders of magnitude larger.[141] Because this approach creates an interference pattern by matching round-trip path length for the reference beam to that for an object beam component within the 10-μ optical coherence domain, reflectance from the anterior and posterior retinal surfaces could be evaluated to precisely determine retinal thickness with known axial magnification. When using a safe level of beam intensity in a living, moving eye, practical clinical application of optical coherence domain interferometry requires adapting this mirror oscillation technique to determine depth values at a sufficiently high sampling rate.

The retinal thickness at the edge of the optic disc has also to be measured by finely focusing a laser slit beam on the anterior retinal surface at an oblique angle. Because this slit beam is also reflected from the out-of-focus posterior retinal surface as a broader, laterally shifted parallel line, retinal thickness can be sensitively determined by accurately measuring the spacing between these two parallel lines in a digitized photographic image.[143] This approach measured retinal thickness in normal eyes with a standard deviation that was about 7 percent of its mean value.[144] When the image of the two parallel lines was scanned rapidly across a high-speed photodetector, the sensitivity of retinal thickness measurements for a given pupil size was improved, corresponding with the theoretical limit due to diffraction. These thickness measurements were obtained with a standard deviation of 9 μ for thicknesses between 150 and 500 μ, using a model eye with a 6-mm pupil.[143]

When evaluating peripapillary retinal surface contour rather than retinal thickness, reproducible definition of a "retinal reference plane" has been required for good reproducibility of regional depth values for the anterior retinal surface.[91, 92] This has permitted regional depth value reproducibility in the peripapillary region of about 50 μ standard deviation or less, using either stereoscopic approaches[93] or laser tomographic scanning.[105, 107] Although current approaches define a relatively stable retinal reference plane using depth measurements outside the immediate peripapillary area that are presumably for the anterior retinal surface,[91, 92] depth values for the posterior retinal surface could be used to define a stable retinal reference plane that would not change with glaucomatous atrophy or other diseases affecting only retinal thickness.[7]

Although little is known at this point about changes in ONH imaging of peripapillary retinal thickness or NFL thickness over time, initial studies of peripapillary retinal surface contour, or "NFL height," have been quite promising. NFL height was found in cross-sectional studies to have high sensitivity and high specificity in discriminating glaucomatous eyes from normal eyes when measured around a circumferential contour 100 μ from the optic disc edge, particularly in superior and inferior quadrants.[139] Plots of NFL height along this contour had sensitivity and specificity comparable with NFL striation photography in discriminating between glaucomatous and normal eyes.[145] When averaging NFL height measurements around this contour, the average difference between patients with glaucoma and normal people was 70 μ, and the average difference between glaucoma suspects and normal people was 30 μ.[146] When averaging NFL height measurements along this contour within a 45-degree arc at 12:00 and 6:00, this polar NFL height was superior to cup volume, rim area, or cup:disc ratio in terms of correlation with visual field indices or combined sensitivity/specificity for discrimination between glaucomatous and normal eyes.[72] NFL height has also been combined with various structural and functional parameters to devise multivariable discriminant functions for improved sorting of glaucomatous and normal eyes in a population of glaucoma suspects.[147, 148]

Vascular Supply

Fluorescein angiography has demonstrated an increased incidence of ONH fluorescein filling defects in open-angle glaucoma (OAG) compared with normals.[149] These filling defects typically are located peripherally near the superior and inferior poles of the disc[150] and are most specific for glaucoma when located in the cup wall.[151] These defects generally are not seen in nonglaucomatous optic atrophy, with the exception of anterior ischemic optic neuropathy.[152] The size of these filling defects correlates with the severity of glaucomatous field loss,[153] and their location corresponds with predictions based on focal visual field abnormalities.[149, 150] Filling defects also have been noted to have larger areas in OHTN than in an age-matched normal population.[154] Among patients with low-tension glaucoma, inferotemporal filling defects are almost universal.[149, 155] The significance and role of vascular insufficiency in these types of glaucoma have been unclear, although various evidence supports a more prominent role for vascular insufficiency in low-tension glaucoma[156] than in OAG.[157]

Successive images in a conventional fluorescein angiogram[158] can be digitized and automatically brought into precise registration, allowing fluorescence to be plotted against time at multiple intravascular and extravascular points of interest, and automatic determination of the boundaries and size of filling defects.[38] The Rodenstock confocal scanning laser ophthalmoscope has also been used to perform fluorescein angiography, using a blue-green argon laser for illumination and a conventional barrier filter for imaging.[122] Because the scanned laser beam has orders of magnitude (perhaps 100 to 5000 times) less thermal effect on the retina than the bright-field illumination levels used for conventional ophthalmoscopy or fundus photography,[109, 120] angiographic imaging can be continuously performed safely every 1/30th sec for extended periods. In this fashion, a videotape angiogram can be created without discomfort to the subject, using a very low dose of fluorescein (permitting repeat doses if necessary).[122] When these angiographic images are digitized 30 times/sec and automatically brought into precise registration, rates of change of fluorescence can be followed over time for all pixels in the image at high temporal resolution, and filling delays and arteriovenous circulation times can be calculated for intravascular pixels.[159, 160]

A longitudinal study of OHTN linked development of progressive glaucomatous atrophy with progressive change in vascular supply, associating increases in pallor area (with or without visual field loss) with delays in venous filling and increases in filling defect area.[161] The significance of these delays in venous filling is unclear, although they might be a more subtle marker for the same vascular insufficiency state that infrequently leads to optic disc hemorrhage or optic disc vein miniocclusion, both of which have been associated with a significant rate of progressive glaucomatous atrophy in longitudinal studies.[162–164] The significance of these increases in filling defect area is also unclear, although they might contribute to the increased filling defect area associated with increased age in cross-sectional studies of OHTN[154] if unrecognized glaucomatous damage were present and might continue to enlarge with progressive glaucomatous field loss.[153]

The linkage between axon loss and vascular damage was also supported by a cross-sectional study evaluating NFL defects and fluorescein filling defects in OAG and OHTN. Both defects were present in all eyes with OAG and in 14 percent of eyes with OHTN, and increased NFL defect severity was associated with increased filling defect area in both groups.[165] However, NFL defects developed before fluorescein filling defects in a small longitudinal study of OAG and low-tension glaucoma.[166] Studies have evaluated arterial caliber in OAG com-

pared with normals using manual techniques,[167, 168] and automated measurements have achieved good reliability using boundary-tracking techniques.[169] Infratemporal and supratemporal arterial calibers were decreased in OAG, with the smallest arterial dimensions encountered in the quadrant with the most significant rim thinning or corresponding visual field defect.[168, 169] However, a study of OHTN and normal patients found an association between increased arterial caliber and increased IOP, suggesting autoregulatory increases in arterial caliber to increase blood flow with increased IOP.[170]

Because laser Doppler velocimetry can determine intravascular maximum erythrocyte velocity by evaluating the spectral broadening of reflected light,[171] this noninvasive technique can be combined with photographic measurements of vessel caliber to determine the blood flow rates of individual vessels as small as 40-μ caliber[172] or to determine total blood flow in the retinal circulation by evaluating blood flow in the major retinal veins.[173] When imaged while inducing an abrupt IOP increase of 40 mm, eyes with OAG have been noted to have a more immediate gross increase in pallor than normal eyes.[174] It is unclear whether this dynamic pallor increase reflects a lower neuroretinal rim capillary bed perfusion pressure or perhaps other features of vascular insufficiency or vulnerability in glaucoma.

FUTURE DIRECTIONS

Future Imaging Systems

When imaging work stations with display capabilities are networked using communication protocols with high data transfer rates, these computers can rapidly exchange data and images while sharing assorted input/output devices and data storage devices, thus enhancing network capabilities while reducing overall costs. In such a computer network, one work station in the photography laboratory might have specialized capabilities for image acquisition and archiving. Other work stations in the clinic with specialized capabilities for interactive image manipulation and display could be added with relatively little additional cost, consisting principally of a desktop display monitor and keyboard alongside a powerful computer the size of a bread box. In these computer networks, digital images could be accessed locally at the same work station. Alternatively, large digital image libraries could be shared centrally and accessed remotely by multiple users, replacing the slide room of the past, for example, with a computer-controlled "juke box" that archives images on magnetooptical disc or other cartridge media.

The past decade has witnessed continuing exponential growth in digital computer hardware capabilities, allowing these types of imaging systems to become practical in a variety of fields. In general terms, if one compares a computer with associated input/output devices today with its predecessor at the same level of expense about a decade ago, today's computer systems already have increased their resolution, capacity, and computational speed by at least one or two orders of magnitude. This progress has helped to transform digital imaging from a small, esoteric field to a dynamic, readily accessible field ranging from biomedical and industrial to desktop publishing and home computer applications, with a variety of products supported by competing hardware and software vendors. In this dynamic environment, a state-of-the-art computer quickly can become an outdated dinosaur. The great need for potential growth in commercial image-analysis systems has led to a trend away from inflexible "black box" systems with restricted compatibility, although this has been less than true in ophthalmology than in other fields with larger competitive markets. More flexible, modular image-analysis systems are emphasizing network expandability, upgradability, and multivendor compatibility with a variety of input/output devices.

Although some of the pioneering studies of ONH imaging were relatively impractical and expensive at the time, current and future technologies should make several of these approaches practical and cost-effective. For example, interactive evaluation of ONH imaging, which would have been absurdly impractical in a clinical setting not so long ago, may soon become a reality. Besides the advances in computer hardware described earlier, image-analysis systems in other fields have dramatically improved user-friendly software for interactive image manipulation and display. A popular user-friendly system on many imaging work stations allows multiple tasks to be performed concurrently, in a time-sharing fashion, with each task monitored on an on-screen "window," even when some tasks are running remotely on other work stations in the computer network. A manually controlled "mouse" corresponding to an on-screen pointer is used to provide streamlined point-to-what-you-want operation. An expandable list of command options is displayed in an on-screen menu. New commands then can be provided for a particular ongoing task by selecting the appropriate window and menu command with the mouse. Additional data needed for command execution also often can be provided graphically on the high-resolution screen using the mouse instead of the keyboard or another input device. For example, when images are displayed in a window, particular image coordinates can be entered directly by pointing at the appropriate location with the mouse. This facilitates a variety of interactive imaging commands, such as image cropping, resizing, translation, and three-dimensional rotation. These user-friendly, multiwindow environments have transformed befuddling or time-consuming image manipulations and comparisons, giving imaging work stations point-to-what-you-want speed and simplicity.

The user-friendly imaging work stations should help to make interactive ONH evaluation accessible to ophthalmologists with limited time and interest, allowing them to go beyond the artificial intelligence embodied in standardized ONH evaluation printouts when appropriate, using the computer instead as a powerful tool for amplifying their own impressive subjective perceptive abilities in image manipulations and comparisons.

This capability should not be underrated, since even the most sophisticated ONH descriptions, optimized for detecting characteristic forms of glaucomatous damage, would at least occasionally overlook atypical or subtle damage in a particular case. For example, after selecting a feature of interest for magnified examination, and perhaps selecting an appropriate surface perspective, direct flicker comparison could be performed immediately with stereoscopic color images to detect ONH damage over time. This analysis should be much more sensitive than current clinical evaluation, because it goes far beyond simply manual systems for interactive image comparison that have been surprisingly sensitive to ONH damage over time.[57]

Future ONH Descriptions

A fact that has been emphasized by preliminary experience with ONH imaging is that traditional methods of ONH description are rendered inadequate by the complexity of ONH structures and their variable change in the process of glaucomatous optic atrophy. Regarding ONH topography, for example, the concept of a cup and neural rim as two distinctly separate portions of the ONH is no longer valid. The complex topography of the ONH is such that defining the boundary between the cup and neural rim on the sloping cup wall is an arbitrary process with little diagnostic value.[3, 4]

Furthermore, emphasis on a cup:disc ratio or neural rim area fails to consider the subtle changes of glaucomatous atrophy that can occur in one or more locations throughout the disc. Localized loss in clinically significant optic disc notching, for example, easily can be lost in the noise of measuring cup-and-rim model parameters over a much larger area.[175] The relative insensitivity of the cup-and-rim model in tracking these subtle changes partly may explain why ONH imaging has not dramatically improved our ability to sensitively track glaucomatous atrophy, even though it already has provided much more detailed quantitative data on ONH status (whether in terms of pallor distribution, topography, NFL status, or vascular supply) than traditional clinical ophthalmoscopy.

Therefore, we must move beyond the traditional concept of a cup and neural rim and search for more sensitive descriptions of ONH status in glaucoma. These descriptions should avoid artificial boundaries between a cup and neural rim, seeking instead to describe significant features of ONH status (e.g., the transition zone between the cup and rim) with adequate complexity. Our current problem is somewhat analogous to the changes needed in visual field interpretation with the introduction of automated static perimetry. Rather than cling to the concept of visual field as a series of concentric lines, or isopters, around fixation, we learned to look at the overall three-dimensional contour of the retinal threshold, or "hill of vision," realizing that isopters were simply arbitrary contours along the hill of vision. As we replaced the isopter of manual, kinetic perimetry with numeric and gray-scale values of automated, static perimetry, we used strategies for interpreting the significance of change in visual field printouts that focused on areas that were more likely to be influenced by the early stages of glaucoma. In a similar fashion, we should use our clinical intuition of where glaucomatous damage is likely to occur in search for new ONH descriptions that will sensitively detect this damage.

Current clinical evaluation of ONH status involves qualitative assessment of various ONH features, at a conscious or unconscious level, and subjective integration of these observations to form a clinical impression, using our well-trained clinical intuition. When confronted with detailed quantitative data of ONH status in a clinical setting, it is natural to extrapolate similar qualitative assessments while perhaps making a few simple quantitative observations (e.g., cup:disc ratio). Given the complexities of ONH change in glaucomatous atrophy, more sophisticated quantitative ONH descriptions will probably prove most sensitive to subtle glaucomatous damage when integrating several types of data generated by ONH imaging, such as pallor distribution, topography, NFL thickness, or other as yet undetermined parameters.

Unfortunately, these new, complex ONH descriptions might be less intuitive, and their diagnostic value might be difficult to estimate subjectively. Because searching for ONH descriptions that are more sensitive to glaucomatous damage requires evaluating complex measurements based on multiple sampled variables, our search strategy should be guided by our clinical intuition and by various techniques of multivariate analysis that can evaluate the diagnostic value of these multivariable descriptions.[176] In this process, the reliability and lateral resolution of local measurements of depth, pallor, NFL thickness, or other parameters will limit the sensitivity and reliability of dependent multivariable measures of local ONH features. These complex multivariable descriptions could be automatically computed and displayed using the same computer facilities required for ONH imaging.

These ONH descriptions should help us address two problems—how to sensitively and accurately detect glaucomatous damage in a population of glaucoma suspects and how to sensitively detect progressive glaucomatous atrophy in patients with some degree of glaucomatous damage. The first problem is probably the more difficult, given the wide variation of underlying ONH features among glaucoma suspects.[100] In addition, limited longitudinal studies have observed great variability in the initial appearance and progression of optic disc and NFL abnormalities developing among a patient population with ocular hypertension.[177] Consequently, it may be necessary to presort a population of glaucoma suspects on the basis of certain ONH characteristics or functional data before designing useful multivariable functions for sorting glaucoma patients from normals in particular subsets of the glaucoma-suspect population. The second and easier problem, sensitive detection of progressive glaucomatous atrophy in glaucoma patients, may also require segregating patients with glaucoma into various

subsets, since the most sensitive features of change in glaucomatous atrophy may depend on the type of glaucoma and on the stage or degree of its progression.

Multivariate analysis has already been applied to the problem of the initial detection of glaucomatous damage. Discriminant analysis was used to formulate optimum multivariable discriminant functions for sorting patients with glaucomatous visual field loss from patients without field loss[178] and was then used to prospectively validate the predictive value of these discriminant functions in glaucoma suspects.[179] The value of this approach was also demonstrated using ONH features to predict subsequent development of visual field defects,[180] although the ONH features used at the time were relatively gross measurements like cup:disc ratio. More recent studies used discriminant analysis to sort patients with early glaucomatous visual field loss from normal controls on the basis of detailed quantitative ONH imaging data and other functional data, including NFL surface contour, cup volume, rim area, and visual field indices.[147, 148] After using a randomly selected subset of the study group to devise multivariable discriminant functions that would correctly distinguish between normal eyes and eyes with early glaucomatous visual field loss, the predictive value of these discriminant functions was tested in the remaining patients. When using discriminant functions combining these structural and functional parameters, 87 percent of eyes were classified correctly, whereas only 76 and 77 percent were correctly classified using only structural or functional parameters, respectively.[148]

Different strategies could be used to develop ONH descriptions for sensitively tracking progressive glaucomatous atrophy. In one search strategy, improved multivariable descriptions of ONH status could be developed using multivariate techniques that optimally represent the variance of the data set using a limited number of multivariable parameters.[45] However, this approach would require that the variances of the data set due to progressive glaucomatous atrophy be large compared with the variance due to underlying ONH differences across the population. Unfortunately, ONH features vary widely in cross-sectional studies of clinical subpopulations,[100] and the bulk of our clinical ONH imaging databases are cross-sectional data across clinical subpopulations rather than extensive longitudinal data over time in particular patients.[181]

For these reasons, developing multivariable descriptions of ONH imaging data that are optimally sensitive to progressive glaucomatous atrophy might at some point require collecting ONH imaging data in longitudinal studies of an animal model of glaucoma.[96] In other words, we should be able to devise more sensitive indices for tracking progressive glaucomatous atrophy by learning more about how detailed ONH imaging measurements change over time in glaucoma. After going back to the drawing board with our new ONH analyzers to develop improved ONH descriptions, the clinical value of these descriptions could be evaluated prospectively and further refined in various subpopulations of patients with glaucoma. After improving ONH descriptions for tracking progressive glaucomatous atrophy in this fashion, these multivariable descriptions could be used to refine discriminant functions designed to recognize glaucoma in various subpopulations of glaucoma suspects.

Future ONH Analyzers

To be clinically practical, a computerized ONH analyzer must provide reproducible, accurate data, be usable in a high percentage of patients, be reasonably priced, and provide a valuable, sensitive evaluation of ONH status for glaucoma management. Although first-generation ONH analyzers provided reasonably reproducible, accurate stereoscopic evaluation of ONH topography, they did not meet our other ONH analyzer requirements.[3, 4] First-generation LTS are already performing better in this regard, because they offer good reproducibility at higher lateral resolution and should be less influenced by pupil size or media opacity. Even though the cost of these units may limit their clinical practicality at the present time, there is good reason to believe that they will become more affordable as this technology matures. It is also possible that a new generation of ONH analyzers will provide more sensitive evaluation of glaucomatous damage by also measuring ONH status in terms other than topography or pallor, such as NFL thickness or other as yet undetermined parameters.

However, even when an ONH analyzer becomes available that measures these parameters at high resolution in a reproducible, accurate fashion, is usable in a high percentage of patients, and is reasonably priced, the major question still exists of how this information can best be interpreted and utilized in glaucoma management. Quite likely, it will be some combination of parameters that the clinician ultimately will use. The technique of multivariate analysis, in which the diagnostic value of various combinations of several parameters is evaluated, will undoubtedly be useful in establishing the optimum strategy for interpreting the data generated by ONH imaging. In addition, because even the most sophisticated ONH descriptions, optimized for detecting characteristic forms of glaucomatous damage, would at least occasionally overlook atypical or subtle damage in a particular case, user-friendly imaging systems will be needed that permit rapid interactive ONH evaluation in a clinical setting. These interactive imaging systems would increase the sensitivity of subjective evaluation by allowing ophthalmologists to use the computer as a powerful tool for amplifying their own impressive perceptive abilities.

Although the utility of current ONH analyzers is limited by current techniques of evaluating and describing the detailed measurements already available, future development of ophthalmic imaging systems and ONH descriptions promise to establish ONH imaging as a practical clinical tool in glaucoma management. Because these future ONH analyzers might use new strategies to interpret new parameters measured using new techniques, they might bear little resemblance to current ONH analyzers and require considerable investigation in their development. We should approach this difficult task with considerable optimism, realizing the tremendous progress that already has been made, and anticipating the high-paced technologic developments that should continue in the future. What can be accepted with relative certainty is that the day will eventually come when practical office ONH analyzers will dramatically enhance our ability to sensitively track progressive glaucomatous atrophy, providing a more sensitive evaluation of ONH status in glaucoma management and aiding the initial detection of glaucomatous damage.

REFERENCES

1. Quigley HA, Addicks EM, Green WR: Optic nerve damage in human glaucoma. Arch Ophthalmol 100:135, 1982.
2. Spaeth GL, Varma R: Assessment of the glaucomatous patient. Eye 1:29, 1987.
3. Caprioli J, Spaeth GL: Looking for better ways to measure the optic disc. Ophthalmic Surg 18:866, 1987.
4. Shields MB: The future of computerized image analysis in the management of glaucoma. Am J Ophthalmol 108:319, 1989.
5. Colenbrander A: Principles of ophthalmoscopy. In Tasman W, Jaeger EA (eds): Duane's Clinical Ophthalmology, vol. 1. Philadelphia, JB Lippincott, 1989, pp 1–21.
6. Schwartz B: Cupping and pallor of the optic disc. Arch Ophthalmol 89:272, 1973.
7. Airaksinen PJ, Tuulonen A, Werner EB: Clinical evaluation of the optic disc and retinal nerve fiber layer. In Ritch R, Shields MB, Krupin T (eds): The Glaucomas. St Louis, CV Mosby, 1989, pp 467–494.
8. Tate GW, Safir A: The slit lamp: History, principles, and practice. In Tasman W, Jaeger EA (eds): Duane's Clinical Ophthalmology, Vol. 1. Philadelphia, JB Lippincott, 1989, pp 1–44.
9. Wong D: The fundus camera. In Tasman W, Jaeger EA (eds): Duane's Clinical Ophthalmology, Vol. 1. Philadelphia, JB Lippincott, 1989, pp 1–14.
10. Allen L, Kirkendall WM, Snyder WB, et al: Instant positive photographs and stereograms of ocular fundus fluorescence. Arch Ophthalmol 75:192, 1966.
11. Donaldson DD: A new camera for stereoscopic fundus photography. Arch Ophthalmol 73:253, 1965.
12. Schwartz B: New techniques for the examination of the optic disc and clinical application. Trans Am Acad Ophthalmol Otolaryngol 81:227, 1976.
13. Krohn MA, Keltner JL, Johnson CA: Comparison of photographic techniques and films used in stereophotogrammetry of the optic disk. Am J Ophthalmol 88:859, 1979.
14. Nicholl JE, Katz LJ, Steinmann WC, et al: Optic disc computerized analysis comparing three photographic techniques. Invest Ophthalmol Vis Sci 30(Suppl):174, 1989.
15. Goldmann H, Lotmar W: Rapid detection of changes in the optic disc by stereochronoscopy. Graefes Arch Clin Exp Ophthalmol 202:87, 1977.
16. Nanba K, Iwata K, Shirakashi M: New stereochronoscopy and true chronoscopic stereo effects. Invest Ophthalmol Vis Sci 31(Suppl):457, 1990.
17. Repka MX, Uozato H, Guyton DH: Depth distortion during slit-lamp biomicroscopy of the fundus. Ophthalmology 27(Suppl):47, 1986.
18. Caprioli J: Quantitative measurements of the optic nerve head. In Ritch R, Shields MB, Krupin T (eds): The Glaucomas. St Louis, CV Mosby, 1989, pp 495–511.
19. Mansour AM: Measuring fundus landmarks. Invest Ophthalmol Vis Sci 31:41, 1990.
20. Bengtsson B, Krakau CE: Some essential optical features of the Zeiss fundus camera. Acta Ophthalmol 55:123, 1977.
21. Littmann H: The determination of the true size of objects in the

background of the living eye. Klin Monatsbl Augenheilkd 180:286, 1982.

22. Kennedy SJ, Schwartz B, Takamoto T, et al: Interference fringe scale for absolute ocular fundus measurement. Invest Ophthalmol Vis Sci 24:169, 1983.

23. Montgomery DM: Measurement of optic disc and neuroretinal rim areas in normal and glaucomatous eyes. Ophthalmology 98:50, 1991.

24. Cambier JL, Nelson MR, Brown SI, et al: Image acquisition and storage for ophthalmic fluorescein angiography. IEEE 2047:224, 1984.

25. Nelson MR, Cambier JL, Brown SI, et al: System for acquisition, analysis, and archiving of ophthalmic images (IS-2000). SPIE 454:72, 1984.

26. Friberg TR, Rehkopf PG, Warnicki JW, et al: Use of directly acquired digital fundus and fluorescein angiographic images in the diagnosis of retinal disease. Retina 7:246, 1987.

27. Laing RA, Danisch LA: An objective focusing method for fundus photography. Invest Ophthalmol 14:329, 1975.

28. Robinson P: Stereo 3D. Computer Graphics World 13:68, 1990.

29. Varma R, Spaeth GL: The PAR IS 2000: A new system for retinal digital image analysis. Ophthalmic Surg 19:183, 1988.

30. Nagin PA, Schwartz B: Approaches to image analysis of the optic disc. IEEE 1499:948, 1980.

31. Peli E, Hedges TR, Schwartz B: Computerized enhancement of the retinal nerve fiber layer. Acta Ophthalmol 64:113, 1986.

32. Peli E, Schwartz B: Enhancement of fundus photographs taken through cataracts. Ophthalmology 94(Suppl):10, 1987.

33. Coggins JM: A multi-scale description of image structure for segmentation of biomedical images. Proceedings of the Conference on Visualization in Biomedical Computing, Atlanta, May 22, 1990, pp 123–130.

34. Schwartz B: Changes in the optic disc in ocular hypertension and glaucoma. Jpn J Ophthalmol 30:143, 1986.

35. Sagaties MJ, Schwartz B: Computerized measurement of the three-dimensional distribution of optic disc pallor. Invest Ophthalmol Vis Sci 30(Suppl):174, 1989.

36. Caprioli J, Klingbeil U, Sears M, et al: Reproducibility of optic disc measurements with computerized analysis of stereoscopic video images. Arch Ophthalmol 104:1035, 1986.

37. Dandona L, Quigley HA, Jampel DH: Variability of depth measurements of the optic nerve head and peripapillary retina with computerized image analysis. Arch Ophthalmol 107:1786, 1989.

38. Nagin P, Schwartz B, Reynolds G: Measurement of fluorescein angiograms of the optic disc and retina using computerized image analysis. Ophthalmology 92:547, 1985.

39. Algazi VR, Keltner JL, Johnson CA: Computer analysis of the optic cup in glaucoma. Invest Ophthalmol Vis Sci 26:1759, 1985.

40. Varma R, Spaeth GL, Hanau C, et al: Positional changes in the vasculature of the optic disk in glaucoma. Am J Ophthalmol 104:457, 1987.

41. Takamoto T, Schwartz B: Stereochronometry: Quantitative measurement of optic disc cup changes. Invest Ophthalmol Vis Sci 26:1445, 1985.

42. Baumbach P, Wesemann W, Rassow B: Depth profiles of the optic nerve head measured by stereo-photogrammetric analysis of multiple-beam interference fringes. Invest Ophthalmol Vis Sci 30(Suppl):175, 1989.

43. Dandona L, Quigley HA, Jampel HD, et al: Limitations of computerized depth measurements. Arch Ophthalmol 108:779, 1990.

44. Marr D, Poggio T: Cooperative computation of stereo disparity. Science 194:283, 1976.

45. Echelman DA, Coggins JM: Principal component analysis for assessment of optic disc topography in glaucoma. Invest Opthalmol Vis Sci 30(Suppl):174, 1989.

46. Halberg GP: Charting and scoring the optic disc. Arch Ophthalmol 82:149, 1969.

47. Nagin P, Schwartz B, Nanba K: The reproducibility of computerized boundary analysis for measuring optic disc pallor in the normal optic disc. Ophthalmology 92:243, 1985.

48. Jonas JB, Gusek GC, Naumann GO: Optic disc, cup and neuroretinal rim size, configuration and correlations in normal eyes. Invest Ophthalmol Vis Sci 29:1151, 1988.

49. Shields MB: Gray crescent in the optic nerve head. Am J Ophthalmol 89:238, 1980.

50. Rosenthal AR, Falconer DG, Barrett P: Digital measurement of pallor-disc ratio. Arch Ophthalmol 98:2027, 1980.

51. Miller JM, Caprioli J: Videographic quantification of optic disc pallor. Invest Ophthalmol Vis Sci 29:320, 1980.

52. Mikelberg FS, Douglas GR, Drance SM, et al: Reproducibility of computerized pallor measurements obtained with Rodenstock Disk Analyzer. Graefes Arch Clin Exp Ophthalmol 226:269, 1988.

53. Miller KN, Shields MB, Ollie AR: Reproducibility of pallor measurements with the optic nerve head analyzer. Graefes Arch Clin Exp Ophthalmol 227:562, 1989.

54. Nagin P, Schwartz B: Detection of increased pallor over time: Computerized image analysis in untreated ocular hypertension. Ophthalmology 91:252, 1985.

55. Carassa R, Schwartz B, Takamoto T: Rate of change over time of optic disc cupping and pallor in relation to the initial amount of cupping and pallor. Invest Ophthalmol Vis Sci 31:458, 1990.

56. Tuulonen A, Airaksinen PJ, Schwartz B, et al: Correlation of optic disc pallor and neuroretinal rim area in glaucoma and ocular hypertension. Invest Ophthalmol Vis Sci 31(Suppl):566, 1990.

57. Heijl A, Bengtsson B: Diagnosis of early glaucoma with flicker comparisons of serial disc photographs. Invest Ophthalmol Vis Sci 30:2376, 1989.

58. Tielsch JM, Katz J, Quigley HA: Intraobserver and interobserver agreement in measurement of optic disc characteristics. Ophthalmology 95:350, 1988.

59. Klein BE, Magli YL, Richie KA: Quantitation of optic disc cupping. Ophthalmology 92:1654, 1985.

60. Krakau CE, Torlegard K: Comparison between stereo and slit image photogrammetric measurements of the optic disc. Acta Ophthalmol 50:863, 1972.

61. Kottler MS, Rosenthal AR, Falconer DG: Analog vs. digital photogrammetry for optic cup analysis. Invest Ophthalmol 15:651, 1976.

62. Schwartz B, Takamoto T: Biostereometrics in ophthalmology for measurement of the optic cup in glaucoma. SPIE 166:251, 1978.

63. Johnson CA, Keltner JL, Krohn MA, et al: Photogrammetry of the optic disc in glaucoma and ocular hypertension with simultaneous stereo photography. Invest Ophthalmol Vis Sci, 18:1252, 1979.

64. Rosenthal AR, Falconer DG, Piper I: Photogrammetry experiments with a model eye. Br J Ophthalmol 64:881, 1980.

65. Takamoto T, Schwartz B: Photogrammetric measurement of the optic disc in glaucoma. Int Arch Photogrammetry 23:732, 1980.

66. Takamoto T, Schwartz B: Stereo measurement of the optic disc cup shape: Volume profile method. Proc Am Soc Photogrammetry 1:352, 1984.

67. Takamoto T, Schwartz B: Biostereometrics in ophthalmology: Topographic analysis of the optic disc cup in glaucoma. SPIE 602:219, 1986.

68. Takamoto T, Schwartz B: Reproducibility of photogrammetric optic disc cup measurements. Invest Ophthalmol Vis Sci 26:814, 1985.

69. Holm O, Krakau CE: A photographic method for measuring the volume of papillary excavations. Ann Ophthalmol 1:327, 1970.

70. Warnicki JW, Rehkopf P, Cambier JL, et al: Development of an imaging system for ophthalmic photography. J Biol Photogr 53:9, 1985.

71. Rehkopf PG, Warnicki JW, Nelson MR, et al: Clinical experience with the ophthalmic image processing system (IS 2000). SPIE 535;282, 1985.

72. Caprioli J: The contour of the juxtapapillary nerve fiber layer in glaucoma. Ophthalmology 97:358, 1990.

73. Nicholl JE, Katz LJ, Steinmann WC, et al: Computerized image analysis of the optic disc using slits imaged on the fundus. Invest Ophthalmol Vis Sci 32(Suppl):812, 1991.

74. Iwaki M, Komurasaki Y, Miura M, et al: Comparison of the optic nerve head analyzer (Imagenet) in optic disc measurement with a non-stereo image analyzer. Invest Ophthalmol Vis Sci 31(Suppl):458, 1990.

75. Nanba K, Iwata K: Optic disc measurements of normal, ocular

hypertensive, and glaucomatous eyes with computerized image analysis. Invest Ophthalmol Vis Sci 30(Suppl):429, 1989.

76. Markovitz BJ, Spaeth GL, Katz LJ: Optimal cup drop value for best agreement between clinicians and an image analyzer in estimating cup-to-disc ratios. Invest Ophthalmol Vis Sci 32(Suppl):918, 1991.

77. Varma R, Steinmann WC, Spaeth GL, et al: Variability in digital analysis of optic disc topography. Graefes Arch Clin Exp Ophthalmol 226:435, 1988.

78. Bishop KI, Werner EB, Krupin T, et al: Variability and reproducibility of optic disk topographic measurements with the Rodenstock Optic Nerve Head Analyzer. Am J Ophthalmol 106:696, 1988.

79. Shields MB, Martone JF, Shelton AR, et al: Reproducibility of topographic measurements with the optic nerve head analyzer. Am J Ophthalmol 104:581, 1987.

80. Tomita G, Goto Y, Yamada T, et al: Reliability of optic disc measurement with a computerized stereoscopic video image analyzer. Act Soc Ophthalmol Jpn 90:1317, 1986.

81. Dandona L, Quigley HA, Jampel HD: Reliability of optic nerve head topographic measurements with computerized image analysis. Am J Ophthalmol 108:414, 1989.

82. Mikelberg FS, Douglas GR, Schulzer M, et al: The correlation between cup-disk ratio, neuroretinal rim area, optic disk area measured by the video-ophthalmograph (Rodenstock Analyzer) and clinical measurement. Am J Ophthalmol 101:7, 1986.

83. Shields MB, Tiedeman JS, Miller KN, et al: Accuracy of topographic measurements with the optic nerve head analyzer. Am J Ophthalmol 107:273, 1989.

84. Yamauchi K, Matsubara K, Funahashi M: The accuracy of optic disc measurements with the optic nerve head analyzer: In vivo and in vitro study. Invest Ophthalmol Vis Sci 30(Suppl):430, 1989.

85. Kim C, Juzych MS, Shin DH, et al: Correlation of axial length and optic disc area. Invest Ophthalmol Vis Sci 31(Suppl):459, 1990.

86. Quigley HA, Brown AE, Morrison JD, et al: The size and shape of the optic disc in normal human eyes. Arch Ophthalmol 108:51, 1990.

87. Caprioli J, Miller JM: Optic disc rim area is related to disc size in normal subjects. Arch Ophthalmol 105:1683, 1987.

88. Phillips CA, Gerber SL, Cantor LB: Effect of stereo base on computerized image analysis. Invest Ophthalmol Vis Sci 31(Suppl):458, 1990.

89. Gerber SI, Cantor LB: Variability due to image presentation in computerized optic disc analysis. Invest Ophthalmol Vis Sci 31(Suppl):458, 1990.

90. Orlando F, Nicholl JE, Steinmann WC, et al: Inherent variability of Imagenet optic disc analysis. Invest Ophthalmol Vis Sci 31(Suppl):459, 1990.

91. Caprioli J, Miller JM: Measurement of relative nerve fiber layer surface height in glaucoma. Ophthalmology 96:633, 1989.

92. Miller JM, Caprioli J: An optimal retinal reference plane for measurement of peripapillary surface contour. Invest Ophthalmol Vis Sci 31(Suppl):566, 1990.

93. Miller E, Miller JM, Hoffman D, et al: Spatial and temporal variation of fundus depth measurements. Invest Ophthalmol Vis Sci 31(Suppl):459, 1990.

94. Coleman AL, Quigley HA, Vitale S, et al: Displacement of the optic nerve head by acute changes in intraocular pressure in monkeys eyes. Ophthalmology 98:35, 1991.

95. Mehta NJ, Mitsch M, Zloty P, et al: Optic nerve head compliance during artificially-induced ocular hypertension. Invest Ophthalmol Vis Sci 31(Suppl):456, 1990.

96. Shirakashi M, Nanba K, Iwata K, et al: Quantitative analysis of reversal of cupping in primate glaucoma. Invest Ophthalmol Vis Sci 31(Suppl):457, 1990.

97. Briggs K, Shin D, Rho S, et al: Reversal of optic nerve cup depth following intraocular pressure reduction in chronic open-angle glaucoma and ocular hypertension patients. Invest Ophthalmol Vis Sci 30(Suppl):429, 1989.

98. Parrow KA, Shin DH, Tsai CS, et al: IOP-dependent dynamic changes of optic disc cupping in adult glaucoma patient. Invest Ophthalmol Vis Sci 31(Suppl):456, 1990.

99. Dandona L, Quigley HA: Changes in glaucomatous optic disc cupping or variability of computerized topographic measurements? Arch Ophthalmol 108:635, 1990.

100. Caprioli J, Miller JM: Videographic measurements of optic nerve topography in glaucoma. Invest Ophthalmol Vis Sci 29:1294, 1988.

101. Carre D, Feitl ME, Krupin T: Rodenstock optic disc topography: Long-term follow-up in ocular hypertension. Invest Ophthalmol Vis Sci 30(Suppl):173, 1989.

102. O'Brien C, Schwartz B, Takamoto T: Decreased cup depth in low tension glaucoma compared with high tension glaucoma as measured by photogrammetry. Invest Ophthalmol Vis Sci 31(Suppl):502, 1990.

103. Fazio P, Krupin T, Feitl ME, et al: Optic disc topography in patients with low-tension and primary open angle glaucoma. Arch Ophthalmol 108:705, 1990.

104. Kruse FE, Burk RO, Volcker HE, et al: Reproducibility of topographic measurements of the optic nerve head with laser tomographic scanning. Ophthalmology 96:1320, 1989.

105. Dreher AW, Tso PC, Weinreb RN: Reproducibility of topographic measurements of the normal and glaucomatous optic nerve head with the laser tomographic scanner. Am J Ophthalmol 111:221, 1991.

106. Stodmeister R, Pillunat L: Reproducibility of optic nerve head topographic measurements with a new laser scanning system. Invest Ophthalmol Vis Sci 30(Suppl):429, 1989.

107. Cioffi GA, Eastman RD, Robin AL, et al: Confocal laser scanning ophthalmoscope: Automatic registration and reproducibility. Invest Ophthalmol Vis Sci 32(Suppl):719, 1991.

108. Plesch A, Klingbeil U: Optical characteristics of a scanning laser ophthalmoscopy. San Diego, CA, SPIE Ophthalmic Imaging, 1989.

109. Webb RH: Scanning laser ophthalmoscope. In Masters BR (ed): Noninvasive Diagnostic Techniques in Ophthalmology. New York, Springer-Verlag, 1990, pp 438–450.

110. Kino GS, Corle TR: Confocal scanning optical microscopy. Physics Today 42:55, 1989.

111. Shuman H, Murray JM, DiLullo C: Confocal microscopy: An overview. Bio Techniques 7:154, 1989.

112. Wilson T: Trends in confocal microscopy. Trends Neurosci 12:486, 1989.

113. Fine A, Amos WB, Durbin RM, et al: Confocal microscopy: Applications in neurobiology. Trends Neurosci 11:346, 1988.

114. Webb RH, Hughes GW, Delori FC: Confocal scanning laser ophthalmoscope. Applied Optics 26:1492, 1987.

115. Plesch A, Klingbeil U, Bille J: Digital laser scanning fundus camera. Applied Optics 26:1480, 1987.

116. Klingbeil U, Plesch A, Rappl W, et al: Ophthalmic image analysis acquisition and analysis system. SPIE 1001:310, 1988.

117. Peli E: Electro-optic fundus imaging. Surv Ophthalmol 34:113, 1989.

118. Bartsch DU, Intaglietta M, Bille JF, et al: Confocal laser tomographic analysis of the retina in eyes with macular hole formation and other focal macular diseases. Am J Ophthalmol 108:277, 1989.

119. Bartsch DU, Bille JF, Intaglietta M, et al: Analysis of transfer functions obtained with the laser tomographic scanner in patients with macular diseases. Invest Ophthalmol Vis Sci 31(Suppl):129, 1990.

120. Sarfarazi FA, Eastman RD, Derick R, et al: Computerized optic nerve image analysis through undilated and dilated pupils with the confocal laser scanning ophthalmoscopes. Health Physics 51:81, 1986.

121. Klingbeil U: Safety aspects of laser scanning ophthalmoscopies. Health Physics 51:81–93, 1986.

122. Gabel VP, Birngruber R, Nasemann J: Fluorescein angiography with the laser scanning ophthalmoscope (SLO). Lasers Light Ophthalmol 2:35, 1988.

123. Timberlake GT, Van De Velde FJ, Jalkh AE: Clinical use of scanning laser ophthalmoscope retinal function maps in macular disease. Lasers Light Ophthalmol 2:211, 1989.

124. Cioffi GA, Sarafarazi F, Perell HF: Computerized optic nerve image analysis with the confocal laser scanning ophthalmoscope. Ophthalmology 97(Suppl):144, 1990.

125. Sommer A, Katz J, Quigley HA, et al: Clinically detectable nerve fiber atrophy preceded the onset of glaucomatous field loss. Arch Ophthalmol 109:77, 1991.
126. Iwata K, Kurosawa A, Sawaguchi S: Wedge-shaped retinal nerve fiber layer defects in experimental glaucoma: Preliminary report. Graefes Arch Clin Exp Ophthalmol 223:184, 1985.
127. Airaksinen PJ, Drance SM: Neuroretinal rim area and retinal nerve fiber layer in glaucoma. Arch Ophthalmol 103:203, 1985.
128. Jonas JB, Fernandez MC, Naumann GO: Glaucomatous optic nerve atrophy in small discs with low cup-to-disc ratios. Ophthalmology 97:1211, 1990.
129. Chihara E, Sawada A: Atypical nerve fiber layer defects in high myopes with high-tension glaucoma. Arch Ophthalmol 108:228, 1990.
130. Eikelboom RH, Cooper RL, Barry CJ: A study of variance in densitometry of retinal nerve fiber layer photographs in normals and glaucoma suspects. Invest Ophthalmol Vis Sci 31:2373, 1990.
131. Knighton RW, Jacobson SG, Kemp CM: The spectral reflectance of the nerve fiber layer of the macaque retina. Invest Ophthalmol Vis Sci 30:2393, 1989.
132. Airaksinen PJ, Nieminen H: Retinal nerve fiber layer photography in glaucoma. Ophthalmology 92:877, 1985.
133. Peli E, Hedges TR, McInnes T: Nerve fiber layer photography: A comparative study. Acta Ophthalmol 65:71, 1987.
134. Takamota T, Schwartz B: Photogrammetric measurement of nerve fiber layer thickness. Ophthalmology 96:1315, 1989.
135. Moreno J, Grazioso C, Hedges TR: Age-related issues in photographic evaluation of the retinal nerve fiber layer. Invest Ophthalmol Vis Sci 32(Suppl):918, 1991.
136. Weinreb RN, Dreher AW, Coleman A, et al: Histopathologic validation of Fourier-ellipsometry measurements of retinal nerve fiber layer thickness. Arch Ophthalmol 108:557, 1990.
137. Reiter K, Dreher AW, Weinreb RN: Accuracy and reproducibility of a retinal laser ellipsometer. Invest Ophthalmol Vis Sci 32(Suppl):812, 1991.
138. Dreher AW, Reiter K, Weinreb RN: Measurement of the circumpapillary nerve fiber layer thickness distribution by polarimetry. Invest Ophthalmol Vis Sci 32(Suppl):811, 1991.
139. Caprioli J, Ortiz-Colberg R, Miller JM, et al: Measurements of peripapillary nerve fiber layer contour in glaucoma. Am J Ophthalmol 108:404, 1989.
140. Takamoto T, Preston D, Schwartz B: Decreased retinal nerve fiber layer thickness with increased disc area, neural rim area, cup volume, and cup depth in normals measured by photogrammetry. Invest Ophthalmol Vis Sci 31(Suppl):565, 1990.
141. Huang D, Stinson WG, Schuman JS, et al: High-resolution measurement of retinal thickness using optical coherence domain reflectometry. Invest Ophthalmol Vis Sci 32(Suppl):1019, 1991.
142. Hecht E, Zajac A: Optics. London, Addison-Wesley, 1974, pp 275–301.
143. Zeimer RC, Mori MT, Khoobehi B: Feasibility test of a new method to measure retinal thickness noninvasively. Invest Ophthalmol Vis Sci 30:2099, 1989.
144. Mori MT, Shahidi M, Zeimer RC: New noninvasive method to measure changes in the nerve fiber layer thickness: Methodology and reproducibility in normal subjects. Invest Ophthalmol Vis Sci 30(Suppl):175, 1989.
145. Miller JM, Tressler C, Caprioli J: Nerve fiber layer photography and quantitative measurements of peripapillary topography in normal and glaucomatous eyes. Invest Ophthalmol Vis Sci 30(Suppl):430, 1989.
146. Caprioli J, Miller JM, Ortiz-Colberg R, et al: Profiles of the peripapillary nerve fiber layer in glaucoma. Invest Ophthalmol Vis Sci 30(Suppl):430, 1989.
147. Caprioli J, Miller E: Combined use of structural and functional measurements improves discrimination between normal and glaucomatous eyes. Invest Ophthalmol Vis Sci 31(Suppl):503, 1990.
148. Caprioli J: Discrimination between normal and glaucomatous eyes. (in preparation)
149. Spaeth GL: The Pathogenesis of Nerve Damage in Glaucoma: Contributions of Fluorescein Angiography. New York, Grune & Stratton, 1977.
150. Fishbein SL, Schwartz B: Optic disc in glaucoma. Arch Opthalmol 95:1975, 1977.
151. Adam G, Schwartz B: Increased fluorescein filling defects in the wall of the optic disc cup in glaucoma. Arch Ophthalmol 98:1590, 1980.
152. Talusan E, Schwartz B: Specificity of fluorescein angiographic defects of the optic disc in glaucoma. Arch Ophthalmol 95:2166, 1977.
153. Nanba K, Schwartz B: Fluorescein angiographic defects of the optic disc in glaucomatous visual field loss. In Greve EL, Heijl A (eds): Fifth International Visual Field Symposium. Boston, Junk, 1983, pp 67–73.
154. Loebl M, Schwartz B: Fluorescein angiographic defects of the optic disc in ocular hypertension. Arch Ophthalmol 95:1980, 1977.
155. Hitchings RA, Spaeth GL: Fluorescein angiography in chronic simple and low-tension glaucoma. Br J Ophthalmol 61:126, 1977.
156. Carter CJ, Brooks DE, Doyle DL, et al: Investigations into a vascular etiology for low-tension glaucoma. Ophthalmology 97:49, 1990.
157. Radius RL: Anatomy of the optic nerve head and glaucomatous optic neuropathy. Surv Ophthalmol 32:35, 1987.
158. Federman JL, Maguire JI: Intravenous fluorescein angiography. In Tasman W, Jaeger EA (eds): Duane's Clinical Ophthalmology, Vol. 3. Philadelphia, JB Lippincott, 1989, pp 1–39.
159. Rehkopf P, Warnicki J, Friberg T, et al: Quantification of retinal circulation time in man. Invest Ophthalmol Vis Sci 30 (Suppl):369, 1989.
160. Toonen H, Wolf S, Kaupp A, et al: Digital video fluorescein angiography and visualization of regional hemodynamics. Invest Ophthalmol Vis Sci 32(Suppl):865, 1991.
161. Tuulonen A, Nagin P, Schwartz B, et al: Increase of pallor and fluorescein-filling defects of the optic disc in the follow-up of ocular hypertensives measured by computerized image analysis. Ophthalmology 94:558, 1987.
162. Diehl DL, Quigley HA, Miller NR, et al: Prevalence and significance of optic disc hemorrhage in a longitudinal study of glaucoma. Arch Ophthalmol 108:545, 1990.
163. Tuulonen A, Takamoto T, Wu DC, et al: Optic disc cupping and pallor measurements of patients with a disk hemorrhage. Am J Ophthalmol 103:505, 1987.
164. Tuulonen A: Asymptomatic miniocclusions of the optic disc veins in glaucoma. Arch Ophthalmol 107:1475, 1989.
165. Nanba K, Schwartz B: Nerve fiber layer and optic disc fluorescein defects in glaucoma and ocular hypertension. Ophthalmology 95:1227, 1988.
166. Iwata K, Shirakashi M, Fukuchi T, et al: The glaucoma optic disc loses its capillary networks after disappearance of axons at the same location. Invest Ophthalmol Vis Sci 32(Suppl):1016, 1991.
167. Laatikainen L: Fluorescein angiographic studies of the peripapillary and perilimbal regions in simple, capsular and low-tension glaucoma. Acta Ophthalmol 111(Suppl):5, 1971.
168. Jonas JB, Nguyen XN, Gusek GC, et al: Peripapillary retinal vessel diameter in normal and glaucoma eyes. Invest Ophthalmol Vis Sci 30(Suppl):429, 1989.
169. Schwoerer J, Wu DC, Schwartz B, et al: Relative changes in vessel caliber with visual field loss in glaucoma patients measured by computerized image analysis. Invest Ophthalmol Vis Sci 30(Suppl):429, 1989.
170. Schwoerer J, Schwartz B, Banwatt R, et al: Differences in retinal vessel width between normal, ocular hypertensive and glaucoma patients. Invest Ophthalmol Vis Sci 31(Suppl):380, 1990.
171. Bonner R, Nossal R: Model for laser Doppler measurements of blood flow in tissue. Applied Optics 20:2097, 1981.
172. Milbocker MT, Feke GT, Goger DG, et al: Study of retinal arterial flow dynamics using stabilized laser doppler velocimetry. Invest Ophthalmol Vis Sci 32(Suppl):784, 1991.
173. Grunwald JE: Effect of two weeks of timolol maleate treatment on the normal retinal circulation. Invest Ophthalmol Vis Sci 32:39, 1991.
174. Robert Y, Steiner D, Hendrickson P: Papillary circulation dynamics in glaucoma. Graefes Arch Clin Exp Ophthalmol 227:436, 1989.
175. Nicholl JE, Katz LJ, Steinmann WC, et al: Localization of optic disc notching with computerized image analysis. Invest Ophthalmol Vis Sci 31(Suppl):458, 1990.

176. Kleinbaum DG, Kupper LL, Muller KE: Applied Regression Analysis and Other Multivariable Methods. 2nd ed. Boston, PWS-Kent, 1988.
177. Tuulonen A, Airaksinen PJ: Initial glaucomatous optic disk and retinal nerve fiber layer abnormalities and their progression. Am J Ophthalmol 111:485, 1991.
178. Drance SM, Schulzer M, Douglas GR, et al: Use of discriminant analysis. II: Identification of persons with glaucomatous visual field defects. Arch Ophthalmol 96:1571, 1978.
179. Drance SM, Schulzer M, Thomas B, et al: Multivariate analysis in glaucoma: Use of discriminant analysis in predicting glaucomatous visual field damage. Arch Ophthalmol 99:1019, 1981.
180. Susanna R, Drance SM: Use of discriminant analysis. I: Prediction of visual field defects from features of the glaucomatous disc. Arch Ophthalmol 96:1568, 1978.
181. Schwartz B, Takamoto T, Wu DC: Changes of optic disc cupping and pallor over time. In Krieglstein GK (ed): Glaucoma Update III. New York, Springer-Verlag, 1987, pp 84–96.

Chapter 115

■

Tonometry and Tonography

JOHN A. McDERMOTT

Schiotz developed the first device that allowed for quantification of intraocular pressure (IOP), relative reproducibility of results, combined with a simplicity and economy of design that allowed for its use in the primary physician's office. A second major step was the application of the principle of applanation by Goldmann, which improved on Schiotz's device, both simplifying further the examination and improving on the validity and reproducibility of Schiotz's instrument. As opposed to a manometer, which directly measures pressure and is impossible in an intact eye, both methods measure the pressure indirectly by deforming to some degree the surface of the globe and by "converting" this deformation into the IOP.

INDENTATION TONOMETRY

With the Schiotz tonometer a series of known, standard weights are applied to the cornea via a plunger (Fig. 115–1). The plunger indents the cornea, and a scale records the deformation of the globe. These two values are then used to determine the IOP. The plunger moves in a vertical fashion in the center of the instrument and passes through a curved footplate that sits on top of the cornea with the patient in the supine position. A "holder" fixes the footplate on the cornea but allows free movement of the plunger and the attached weights in the vertical direction. When held properly, the only force acting on the plunger and weights is the opposing force of the IOP (except for a negligible force of friction between the shaft of the holder and the plunger). A movement of the plunger from its "0" position into the cornea can be correlated with the deformation of the cornea. Since the excursion of the plunger is relatively small and would be difficult to read, a lever magnifies the excursion along a more readable calibrated scale. The greater the scale reading with a given weight, the greater will be the excursion of the plunger and the deformation of the globe. The IOP will therefore be lower.

Theoretical Basis

Unfortunately, by applying a weight to the globe one is not measuring the true "steady state" IOP. When the plunger indents the cornea, deforming the globe, the steady state IOP (P_o) is raised to a higher pressure that is the pressure induced by the tonometer (P_t). Schiotz performed experiments using a manometer to accurately measure the IOP of enucleated eyes. The experimental design allowed manipulation of the IOP in the eye. Thus P_o and P_t could be correlated with a given weight and a given scale reading. By changing the weight on the

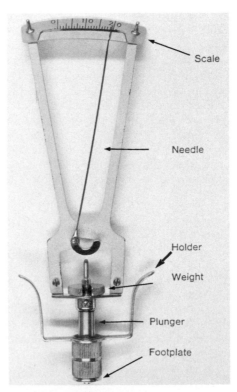

Figure 115–1. Schiotz tonometer.

tonometer and by repeating the experiment, a chart could be constructed that would indicate the P_o for any given weight and scale reading. From these data, and by repeating Schiotz's technique in his own experiments, Friedenwald derived a formula that more accurately determined the IOP.[1]

When the tonometer is placed on the eye, the indentation of the cornea results in distention of the globe. Thus the scale reading, along with indicating the indentation of the cornea, also reflects this same distention. Friedenwald's formula relates this distention to the IOP. The formula required a constant "K" or the "coefficient of ocular rigidity," which is a measure of the resistance of the eye to the distending forces of the tonometer. Friedenwald's formula allowed more accurate tables to be established. Friedenwald first published his tables in 1948, and an updated version, which Friedenwald thought to be more accurate, is known as the 1955 tables. Comparison with applanation tonometry suggests that the 1948 tables are more precise. Unfortunately, not all eyes behave in the same fashion to external pressure, and the tables established by Friedenwald are based on a single K value (0.0245 for the 1948 tables, and 0.0215 for the 1955 tables). Friedenwald determined that the value of K for an individual eye could be calculated from two tonometric scale readings using different weights. Friedenwald's "nomogram" allows one to graphically determine K from these two values. Presently, simplified tables exist that obviate the need for calculation and provide both the P_o and K values from the paired scale readings on the involved eye.

Clinical Technique

The patient is supine with the cornea anesthetized. The fingers of the examiner spread the lids carefully to avoid putting pressure on the globe. The patient is asked to fixate while the tonometer footplate is applied to the cornea, and the handle is positioned to keep the tonometer vertical and to allow free movement of the plunger to indent the cornea. The needle will oscillate with the ocular pulse, and the midpoint of the excursion is used as the scale reading. If the value is not greater than 4 units, an additional weight is added. In recording the measurement, the scale reading, the weight used, and the IOP (as read from the appropriate tables) are noted.

Limitations

The commonly available conversion tables use an average K value to calculate the IOP. If the true K of the eye is higher than the average K, the table will overestimate the true IOP. Similarly, a false-low IOP will result if the true K is less than the average K. High ocular rigidity has been reported in patients with high hyperopia,[2] extreme myopia,[3] chronic glaucoma,[3] and vasoconstrictor therapy.[3]

Low ocular rigidity may occur with high myopia,[2] miotic therapy (especially cholinesterase inhibitors)[2]

after retinal detachment surgery,[4] intravitreal injection of gas,[5] and vasodilator therapy.[3]

False-high IOP readings may be obtained with thick corneas or very steep corneas.[6] With significant corneal pathology, and on an irregular surface, Schiotz's measurements are unreliable.[7]

Since tables exist to overcome the rigidity problem, this alone has not resulted in a decline of Schiotz tonometry; rather, the ease and accuracy of applanation tonometry, without the need for a supine patient, multiple readings, and reference to tables, has allowed applanation tonometry to replace Schiotz tonometry with few exceptions. The Schiotz tonometer, however, is still the basic ingredient in tonography and is described later in this chapter.

APPLANATION TONOMETRY

Theoretical Basis

Applanation tonometry is based on the Inbert-Fick principle, which states that for an ideal sphere the pressure (P) inside the sphere is equal to the force (F) required to applanate (flatten) its surface, divided by the area (A) of flattening:

$$P = F/A$$

or

$$F = PA$$

The ideal sphere is dry, thin-walled, and readily flexible. The cornea, which is not even a true sphere, is none of these three. Because of this, there are two other significant forces at work. The force of capillary attraction (T) between the tonometer head and the tear film is additive to the external force. In addition, a force (C), independent of IOP, is required to flatten the relatively inflexible cornea. Thus,

$$F = PA$$

becomes

$$F + T = PA + C$$

or

$$P = \frac{F + T - C}{A}$$

The A, with which we are concerned, is actually on the interior surface of the cornea. The Goldmann applanator is designed so that A is equal to 7.35 mm.[2] To achieve this, the diameter of flattening of the cornea is 3.06 mm. With this value for A, the opposing forces of capillary attraction and corneal inflexibility cancel out.

$$P = \frac{F}{7.35 \text{ mm}^2}$$

In addition, with this value for A the IOP in millimeters of mercury (mmHg) is equal to ten times the force applied to the cornea in grams, which is a convenient conversion. Since only 0.5 μl is displaced from the eye and the additional increase in pressure induced in the eye from its steady state by the tonometer tip is negligible, applanation tonometery is not significantly affected by ocular rigidity.

Goldmann Applanator

The tonometer "tip," a tapered plastic cylinder containing a biprism, is the contact point with the cornea. The tip is connected via a rod to the body of the tonometer which contains an adjustable spring that provides the appropriate applanating force (Fig. 115–2). The force is adjusted manually via a knob that contains a scale indicating the force applied in grams. When the end-point is reached, the reading in grams is multiplied by 10 to convert to millimeters of mercury (Fig. 115–3).

The biprism splits the image of the circle of contact into two semicircles. When the inner margin of these semicircles just touch (see Fig. 115–2), a 3.06-mm diameter circle of cornea is applanated. The instrument is attached to the slit lamp, aligning the axis of the tip with the ocular and allowing visualization of the semicircles or mires.

Clinical Measurement

The patient is positioned at the slit lamp in the usual fashion after instilling topical anesthetic and sodium fluorescein into the tear film. The patient is instructed to fixate in the distance, to relax, and to breathe normally. If necessary, the lids are separated (without pressure). As the tip is advanced toward the cornea, gross horizontal and vertical adjustments are made by the examiner without using the oculars as the instrument approximates the cornea. The cobalt-blue filter is inserted into the slit-lamp illuminator, and maximal illumination is used. When contact is imminent, the examiner uses the ocular to observe the mires, which will

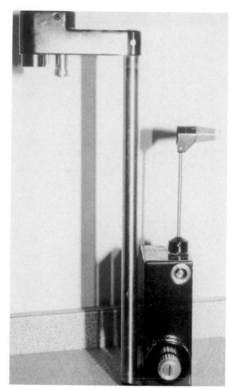

Figure 115–3. Goldmann applanation tonometer.

appear green against a blue background. If the mires are of unequal size, vertical adjustment is made. The tonometer knob is rotated until the end-point is achieved (Fig. 115–4). Ocular pulsations are noted, and the midpoint of the excursion of the internal margin of each semicircle is aligned. For accurate readings, certain precautions must be met. Valsalva maneuvers, or breath holding by the patient, must be avoided. The semicircles should be clear with distinct margins. Wider, blurred semicircles result in false-high readings as does vertical misalignment.[8] Measurements without the use of fluorescein underestimate the true IOP.[9]

Corneal astigmatism may result in false pressure readings. The error has been calculated at 1 mm for every 4 diopters (underestimated for with-the-rule; overestimates for against-the-rule). The biprism should be rotated in its housing so that the axis of least corneal curvature aligns with the red line on the prism holder; alternatively, an average of the pressure obtained with semicircles aligned horizontally and then vertically may be used.[10] Corneal curvature appears to influence applanation tonometry readings. In 200 patients examined for "routine eye examination," whose vital statistics and mean IOP demonstrated the group to be a representative sample of the general population, there was a positive correlation between corneal curvature and tonometer readings. For each 3-diopter increase in corneal power in this sample, the average intraocular pressure increased 1 mmHg.[11] Thin corneas produce false-low readings, as does a thick cornea secondary to edema.[12] A thick cornea secondary to increased collagen results in a false-high reading.[12]

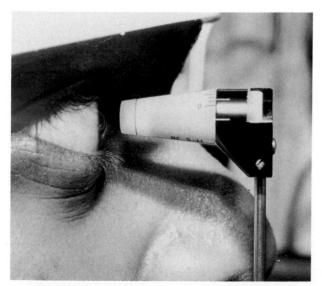

Figure 115–2. Tonometer tip approaches eye.

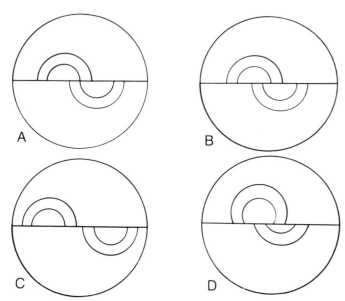

Figure 115–4. Optical endpoint of applanation. *A*, Correct endpoint. *B*, Overestimate of IOP. *C*, Underestimate of IOP. *D*, Vertical misalignment.

Prolonged contact of the applanator to the cornea should be avoided. Damage to the cornea may occur with fluorescein staining and distortion of the mires.[13] One may also observe a gradual decrease in the tonometer reading as contact is maintained on the cornea.[14]

Contaminated tonometers are well-established vectors of infection. Along with the more common bacteria and viruses that cause ocular infection, hepatitis-B surface antigen can be isolated from the tonometer tip after applanation of infected patients. Human immunodeficiency virus (HIV) (AIDS) has been isolated from human tears, although no cases of transmission from contaminated tonometers has been reported. Meticulous sterilization may reduce the risk of these pathogens. The Centers for Disease Control suggests a 5- to 10-min soaking in 3 percent hydrogen peroxide or 70 percent ethanol or isopropanol. The tip should then be washed under running water and dried thoroughly before reuse.[15]

Other Applanation Tonometers

The Perkins' applanation tonometer uses the same biprism as the Goldmann applanator. The light source is powered by battery, and a counter balance enables the instrument to be used in both the vertical and horizontal positions (Fig. 115–5). The readings are consistent and compare quite well with the Goldmann applanator. It is especially useful in the operating room for examinations under anesthesia and for invalid patients, infants, or children who cannot sit at the slit lamp.[16]

The MacKay-Marg tonometer applanates the cornea via a plunger that moves within a sleeve, similar in fashion to a Schiotz tonometer. The excursion of the plunger is electronically coupled to a transducer and graphically records the movement of the plunger on a moving strip of paper. The plunger first indents the cornea recording on the graph paper, the sum of the force required to flatten the cornea and the IOP. As the tonometer advances, the sleeve abuts the cornea, transferring the force required to flatten the cornea to the sleeve. The pressure tracing then decreases to a level that represents the IOP. Because the tonometer records instantaneously, multiple readings should be averaged in order to adjust for fluctuation in pressure due to the ocular pulsation.[17] It is especially useful in edematous or irregular corneas.[18]

The principle of the Pneumatonometer is similar to that of the MacKay-Marg tonometer. Corneal contact of the pencil-like tip records both the IOP and the force required to bend the cornea. Further advancement of the tip transfers the latter force to the surrounding "collar." In this case, the "plunger" is replaced by a column of air and the contact surface is a Silastic membrane. The air column is continually vented via a port. Changes in pressure in the column resulting from the applanation via a transducer records the measurement on a moving strip of paper. Similar to the MacKay-Marg unit, this instrument is especially useful with edematous and irregular corneas.[19]

The Tono-Pen, which is a miniature, hand-held tonometer, works on a similar principle as the MacKay-Marg tonometer. The instrument is 18 cm in length and weighs only 60 g. The MacKay-Marg wave form is internally analyzed by a microprocessor. Three to six estimations of the pressure are then averaged, and a digital readout displays the IOP with the range of the coefficient of variance. For pressures from 6 to 24 mmHg, the Tono-Pen measured an average of 1.7 mm higher than the Goldmann tonometer. Above 24 mmHg, the readings were similar. Large discrepancies (greater than 6 mmHg) were found in only 18 of 270 eyes tested. In all except 5, obvious causes such as astigmatism or corneal disease could explain the discrepancy.[20]

The noncontact tonometer applanates the cornea by means of a jet of air. Once the instrument is properly aligned with the patient's eye, a fixed distance separates the cornea from the instrument. An optical system measures the time that it takes for the air puff to flatten the cornea. This can be correlated with the IOP.[21] Mean IOP readings compare favorably with Goldmann tonometry, although relatively large discrepancies could be found in some patients. The instrument is beneficial in mass glaucoma screenings because it does not require topical anesthetic and, with proper use, there is no risk of injuring the cornea.

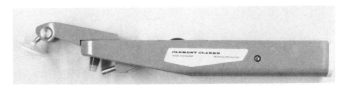

Figure 115–5. Perkins' applanation tonometer.

TONOGRAPHY

Schiotz noted that repeated tonography within a relatively short period resulted in a lowered IOP measurement. The rate at which IOP decreased seemed to be slower in eyes with glaucoma than in normal eyes.

When external pressure is applied to the eye, aqueous humor is expressed through the outflow channels resulting in this lowering of IOP. Because of its deranged outflow function, this occurred more slowly in the glaucomatous eye. In 1950, Grant described *tonography*, a technique to measure the decrease in IOP that occurs when an external weight is applied to the eye. The formulas thus derived would allow quantification of the rate at which aqueous humor could be forced through the outflow channels by the weight of the tonometer. Grant called this newly derived characteristic of the eye "the facility of aqueous outflow."[22]

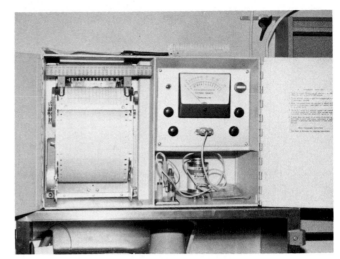

Figure 115–6. Tonography unit.

Theoretical Basis

Grant ingeniously used a paper strip recorder (such as that found in an electrocardiograph) connected to an electronic tonometer to record a continuous tracing of the changes in scale units that occurred once the tonometer was resting on the eye (Fig. 115–6).[22]

In the normal eye there is a gradual decrease in the IOP, resulting in a tracing with a gentle downward slope. In the glaucomatous eye, which has an increased resistance to expression of fluid through the outflow channels, there is less of a change in the IOP (indicated by a smaller change in the Schiotz scale units) with the resultant tracing having a flatter slope (Fig. 115–7). From the tracing, the value of the facility of aqueous outflow can be determined from Grant's equations.

The softening of the globe is due to the expression of a certain volume of fluid from the eye (ΔV). The greater the pressure applied to the eye, and the longer the time interval that the pressure is applied (T), the greater will be the value of ΔV.

$$\Delta V \propto \Delta P \times T$$

This proportion becomes a mathematical equation by the addition of a "proportionality constant," which Grant calls "C" or the *facility of aqueous outflow.*

$$\text{Solving for} \quad C = \frac{\Delta V}{\Delta P \times T}$$

The derivation of ΔV and ΔP from the tracing requires an understanding of the mechanics by which IOP is measured with the Schiotz tonometer. When the tonometer is placed on the eye, the plunger indents the cornea and the weight of the instrument distends the globe. The IOP is elevated from its "steady state" pre-tonometer value, P_o, to a higher pressure—that is, the pressure induced by the tonometer (P_t). For each scale reading, Friedenwald measured not only the volume of the corneal indentation and the volume of the distention of the globe but also the P_o and P_t (see indentation tonometry).[23, 24] As the tonometer rests on the eye, the IOP

decreases, the corneal indentation increases, and the distention of the ocular coat decreases. The value of ΔV, which is the amount of fluid expressed from the eye at the end of time T, would be the difference between the volume of corneal indentation and the volume of ocular distention at time T. Using Friedenwald's data, Grant devised tables that provide the value of ΔV, based on the initial and final Schiotz scale readings during the tracing.

Since P_o and P_t for any scale reading could be determined from Friedenwald's tables, ΔP, the pressure induced by the tonometer above the steady state is equal to $P_t - P_o$. But since the IOP decreases during the tracing, ΔP is constantly changing. Grant calculated that this changing ΔP could be represented with minimal error by averaging the values of ΔP (i.e., $P_t - P_o$) at each half-minute of the tracing. In the standard tracing, T = 4 min. With the values for ΔP, ΔV, and T, the facility of outflow C can therefore be determined in $\mu l/min/mmHg$. In clinical practice, Grant's formula is incorporated into standard tonography tables, thus the value of C may be determined by recording the initial and final Schiotz scale readings and the tonometer weight applied during the 4-min tracing.

As with Schiotz tonometry, the calculation of outflow facility is affected by ocular rigidity (see indentation tonometry). Tonography tables are based on a normal coefficient of ocular rigidity of 0.0215. With low ocular rigidity (e.g., high myopia), Schiotz tonometry underestimates the true IOP, and the resultant C value is falsely low. Routinely, however, applanation tonometry is performed just before the application of the Schiotz tonometer during tonography. A discrepancy between the two values allows an accurate calculation of C via the Friedenwald nomogram.

Test Performance

After applanation tonometry has been performed, the patient lies supine in a quiet setting. Both eyes are

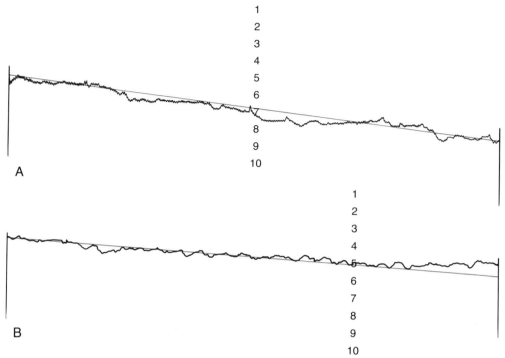

Figure 115–7. Tonography tracings. *A*, Typical tracing, "normal" C value. *B*, "Flat" tracing in an eye with a glaucomatous C value.

anesthetized and the electronic Schiotz tonometer, which is previously calibrated, is applied to the eye while the patient fixates on a ceiling target with the uninvolved eye. The proper Schiotz weight used during tonography is determined by the initial applanation, and the standard tracing of 4 min is obtained. Proper tonography requires attention to detail, and several excellent manuals have been written to help one eliminate the numerous sources of error that can occur during the performance of the test.[25, 26]

An acceptable tracing has a smooth gradual slope, with small oscillations indicating the ocular pulse and somewhat less apparent cycles of longer duration due to respirations. Any Valsalva maneuver, such as coughing or sneezing, will invalidate the tracing. When an appropriate tracing is obtained, the technician draws a line through the tracing, approximating the slope that allows one to read the scale units at time 0 and at 4 min. These are then used to determine C from the tonography tables or the Friedenwald nomogram.

Clinical Implications

Grant's initial paper, involving repeated examinations on normal eyes, determined C values with a range of 0.15 to 0.34 μl/min/mmHg, with a mean of 0.243. Subsequent studies confirmed this normal C value.[27, 28] In a given eye, outflow facility is fairly consistent and compares favorably with those obtained by perfusion experiments in enucleated eyes.[29, 30] No sex differences have been detected. C values appear to decrease gradually with aging. After initially describing the technique of tonography, Grant reported his results in over 1000 tonograms on 600 normal and glaucomatous eyes.[31] His

findings resolve the issue of whether the elevated pressure in glaucoma was caused by increased aqueous production or by decreased aqueous outflow. Without exception, reduced outflow facility could account for the elevation of IOP in the glaucomatous eyes. Lower C values, some of which were 0.0, occurred during attacks of angle-closure glaucoma. In chronic angle-closure, C values would decrease proportional to the degree of closure of the angle. Administration of topical miotics increased outflow facility, thus establishing the mechanism of these drugs.

In the initial studies, tonography appeared to demonstrate a clear demarcation between normal and glaucomatous eyes. The C value in normal eyes ranges from 0.11 to 0.44 μl/min/mmHg. In the glaucomatous eyes, C values did not exceed 0.11 μl/min/mmHg. It was anticipated that in the glaucoma suspect (i.e., patients with normal optic nerves and visual fields), patients with C values in the glaucomatous range would be especially likely to develop optic nerve damage and thus be candidates for early intervention. Subsequent studies, however, did not demonstrate such a clear-cut distinction between glaucomatous and normal eyes. There is a broad overlap in these two groups between C values of 0.10 and 0.20.[32] In another study involving more than 1300 eyes, fully 35 percent of the glaucomatous eyes had values above 0.18.[29]

To better separate normal from glaucomatous eyes, Leydecker and Becker suggested a ratio of the IOP to the C value.[33, 34] The higher the IOP and the smaller the C value, the greater will be the P_o/C ratio. Although there was still a considerable overlap, this approach seemed to enhance the separation of the two groups compared with using the C value alone. Using a P_o/C of 100 as the demarcation, 71 percent of glaucoma patients exceeded this value, whereas only 2 percent of normal people fell into this range.[33] P_o/C ratios are usually included in the standard tonographic report.

Several longitudinal studies investigated tonography and its prognostic value in predicting glaucomatous optic nerve damage in populations of glaucoma suspects. The results of these studies were equivocal.[34–38] In known glaucoma patients, attempts were made to use tonography as a prognosticator for progression of the disease. Most of these indicated that tonography added no additional information over tonometry in predicting which patients would progress.

Interest in tonography waned as it became apparent that it would offer no easy solution in predicting which glaucoma suspect would develop visual field defects. It is apparent that at any given pressure, different eyes have different susceptibilities to optic nerve damage. Advances in ocular imaging have diverted attention toward the posterior segment in determining guidelines for the initiation of treatment and documentation of stability. Although the clinical use of tonography has decreased, it is still a key research tool, especially in determining the mechanism of action of new therapeutic agents in the treatment of glaucoma.

REFERENCES

1. Friedenwald JS: Contribution to the theory and practice of tonometry. Am J Ophthalmol 20:985, 1937.
2. Drance SM: The coefficient of scleral rigidity in normal and glaucomatous eyes. Arch Ophthalmol 63:668, 1960.
3. Friedenwald JS: Contribution to the theory and practice of tonometry. Am J Ophthalmol 20:985, 1937.
4. Pemberton JW: Schiotz-applanation disparity following retinal detachment surgery. Arch Ophthalmol 81:534, 1969.
5. Aronowitz JD, Brubaker RF: Effect of intraocular gas on intraocular pressure. Arch Ophthalmol 94:1191, 1976.
6. Friedenwald JS: Some problems in the calibration of tonometers. Am J Ophthalmol 31:935, 1948.
7. Kaufman HE: Pressure measurement: Which tonometer? Invest Ophthalmol Vis Sci 11:80, 1972.
8. Goldmann H, Schmidt T: Uber Applanationstonometrie. Ophthalmologica 134:221, 1957.
9. Roper DL: Applanation tonometry with and without fluorescein. Am J Ophthalmol 90:668, 1980.
10. Moses RA: The Goldmann applanation tonometer. Am J Ophthalmol 46:865, 1958.
11. Mark HH: Corneal curvature in applanation tonometry. Am J Ophthalmol 76:223, 1973.
12. Ehlers N, Bramsen T, Sperling S: Applanation tonometry and central corneal thickness. Acta Ophthalmol 53:34, 1975.
13. Moses RA: The Goldmann applanation tonometer. Am J Ophthalmol 46:865, 1958.
14. Moses RA, Liu CH: Repeated applanation tonometry. Am J Ophthalmol 66:89, 1968.
15. Centers for Disease Control: Recommendations for preventing possible transmission of human T-lymphotropic virus type III/lymphadenopathy-associated virus in tars. MMWR 34:553, 1985.
16. Dunn JS, Brubaker RF: Perkins applanation tonometer clinical and laboratory evaluation. Arch Ophthalmol 89:149, 1973.
17. Marg E, MacKay RS, Oschsli R: Trough height, pressure and flattening in tonometry. Vis Res 1:379, 1962.
18. Kaufman HE, Wind CA, Waltman SR: Validity of MacKay-Marg electronic applanation tonometer in patients with scarred irregular corneas. Am J Ophthalmol 69:1103, 1970.
19. West CE, Capella JA, Kaufman HE: Measurement of intraocular pressure with a pneumatic applanation tonometer. Am J Ophthalmol 74:505, 1972.
20. Minckler DS, et al: Clinical evaluation of the Oculab Tono-Pen. Am J Ophthalmol 104:168, 1987.
21. Shields MB: The non-contact tonometer: Its value and limitations. Surv Ophthalmol 24:211, 1980.
22. Grant WM: Tonographic method for measuring the facility and rate of outflow in human eyes. Arch Ophthalmol 44:204, 1950.
23. Friedenwald JS: Contribution to the theory and practice of tonometry. Am J Ophthalmol 20:985, 1937.
24. Friedenwald JS: Tonometer calibration: An attempt to remove discrepancies found in the 1954 calibration scale for Schiotz tonometers. Trans Am Acad Ophthalmol Otol 61:108, 1957.
25. Drews RW: Manual of Tonography. St Louis, CV Mosby, 1971.
26. Garner LL: Tonography and the glaucomas. Springfield, IL, Charles C Thomas, 1965.
27. Becker B, Christensen RE: Water-drinking and tonography in the diagnosis of glaucoma. Arch Ophthalmol 56:321, 1956.
28. DeRoetth A, Knighton US: Clinical evaluation of the aqueous flow test: A preliminary report. Arch Ophthalmol 48:148, 1952.
29. Becker B, Constant MA: The facility of aqueous outflow: A comparison of tonography and perfusion measurements in vivo and in vitro. Arch Ophthalmol 55:305, 1956.
30. Grant WM, Trotter RR: Tonographic measurements in enucleated eyes. Arch Ophthalmol 53:191, 1955.
31. Grant WM: Clinical measurements of aqueous outflow. Arch Ophthalmol 46:113, 1951.
32. Kronfeld PC: Tonography. Arch Ophthalmol 48:393, 1952.
33. Becker B: Tonography in the diagnosis of simple (open-angle) glaucoma. Trans Am Acad Ophthalmol Otol 65:156, 1961.
34. DeRoetth A: Clinical evaluation of tonography. Am J Ophthalmol 59:169, 1965.
35. Armaly MF: Ocular pressure and visual fields: A ten-year follow-up study. Arch Ophthalmol 81:25, 1969.
36. Pohjanpelto PEJ: Tonography and glaucomatous optic nerve damage. Acta Ophthalmol 52:817, 1974.
37. Wilensky JT, Podos SM, Becker B: Prognostic indicators in ocular hypertension. Arch Ophthalmol 91:200, 1974.
38. Kass MA, Kolker AE, Becker B: Prognostic factors in glaucomatous visual field loss. Arch Ophthalmol 94:1274, 1976.

Chapter 116

∎

Diagnostic Evaluation

STANLEY J. BERKE

PROVOCATIVE TESTS FOR NARROW-ANGLE GLAUCOMA

It is estimated that 2 to 6 percent of eyes have suspiciously narrow angles (grade II or less) and 0.6 to 1.1 percent have critical narrow angles (grade I or less).[1-11] In patients older than 60 yr of age, 4.5 percent have occludable angles. In a survey of 947 eyes of patients of all ages, Spaeth[10] found that 6 percent of angles were capable of occlusion. However, most individuals with narrow angles do not develop angle-closure glaucoma, the prevalence of which is probably less than 0.2 percent of the population. This suggests that a maximum of only one of 10 people with anatomically narrow angles develops angle-closure glaucoma in his or her lifetime.

The anterior chamber depth can be estimated with a hand-held illuminator or by slit-lamp examination. If the peripheral anterior chamber depth is less than one fourth of the corneal thickness, the angles are likely to be shallow.[11] Technicians who screen patients can readily identify eyes with narrow angles by this technique. These angles must be examined carefully by gonioscopy. Some authorities prefer the Koeppe gonioscopy system to the more popular Zeiss or Goldmann lenses. However, the Koeppe gonioscopy system may give the impression of a wider angle due to posterior lens movement with the patient supine. Gonioscopy lenses capable of indentation gonioscopy (e.g., Zeiss, Posner, and Sussman) can make a narrow angle appear open if the cornea is inadvertently indented.[12-14] Even glaucomatologists have disagreed about whether or not a particular angle is occludable when judged gonioscopically with these lenses.[15]

If one could predict which patients would develop angle-closure glaucoma, prophylactic laser peripheral iridotomies would be the treatment of choice because optic nerve damage can occur soon after intraocular pressure (IOP) rises[16] and continues until the pressure decreases.[17, 18] Second, because of edema and even shallower anterior chamber, laser iridotomy technically may be more difficult to perform after the onset of an acute angle-closure attack. Furthermore, laser iridotomy may not be available if a patient travels to remote areas or if other extenuating circumstances exist.

The advent of laser iridotomy has liberalized the criteria for performing prophylactic iridotomy in eyes with normal vision and asymptomatic narrow angles. Complications of surgical iridectomy (e.g., infection, hemorrhage, hypotony, and cataract formation) are negligible when the laser is used. However, to perform laser iridotomy on all eyes with narrow angles would be an overapplication of the procedure.

Since it is usually impossible to predict which patients with narrow angles will develop angle-closure glaucoma, various adjunctive and provocative tests are available to offer additional information. Other concerns (e.g., medicolegal) may either validate or mandate performing some of these tests.

The prognostic value of provocative tests remains unknown, and both presumed false-positive and false-negative findings occur. Some ophthalmologists believe that occludability under any reasonable circumstances warrants laser iridotomy and that pharmacologic tests are justified. However, intensive provocative testing using periodic multiple tests has become less routine since the advent of laser iridotomy.

A provocative test should be as physiologic as possible to mimic a situation that might occur under natural circumstances. It is more advisable to provoke an attack of angle-closure glaucoma in the physician's office, where it can be diagnosed and treated promptly, than to allow it to occur in a place where it might not be recognized or where medical attention might not be readily available.

Mydriatic Provocative Tests

After a weak, short-acting, topical mydriatic, such as hydroxyamphetamine 1 percent (Paredrine) is instilled in one eye, IOP is measured in 1 hr or when the pupil has reached 4 mm (the point of maximum iridolenticular apposition). An IOP increase of 8 mmHg or more is indicative of a positive result. It is essential to perform gonioscopy before and after mydriasis to confirm angle-closure. Some authorities also include tonography as part of the provocative test and consider a positive finding to be one in which a 30 percent decrease in outflow facility associated with gonioscopic evidence of angle-closure occurs.[19] Patients with very narrow anterior chamber angles bilaterally should have mydriatic provocative testing performed in only one eye at a time to avoid simultaneous bilateral acute angle-closure glaucoma.

Mild cycloplegic agents such as tropicamide 0.5 percent can also be used, but with confusing results, since these agents can elevate IOP without causing angle-closure, even in the absence of pigment liberation.[20-24] Weak cycloplegic agents are used for this test; thus their effects can be reversed easily if angle-closure occurs. Pilocarpine can be administered to reverse the

1336

effects of tropicamide 0.5 percent.[25, 26] Alpha-adrenergic agonists, especially 10 percent phenylephrine, carry greater risks than other mydriatics, which paralyze the sphincter. Phenylephrine can overcome the action of miotics, and pharmacologic pupil constriction with miotics after dilatation with phenylephrine enhances the forces leading to pupillary block.[26, 27] The mydriatic test, when combined with gonioscopy, has a sensitivity of 75 percent, but its specificity is unknown.

Phenylephrine-Pilocarpine Test

After initial IOP measurement, 2 percent pilocarpine and 10 percent phenylephrine are instilled simultaneously every minute for three applications to achieve a middilated pupil.[26–30] Mapstone proposed that this provocative test maximizes pupillary block by creating a middilated pupil with full sphincter tone. Treatment with phenylephrine is repeated every 30 min, unless the IOP rises 8 mmHg. If no rise occurs after 2.5 hr, the test is terminated with an application of 0.5 percent thymoxamine. Positive results, which are indicated by an IOP increase of 8 mmHg or more, are terminated with thymoxamine and intravenous acetazolamide, 500 mg. This powerful pupillary blocking test can be difficult to control, and acute angle-closure glaucoma may be precipitated. Decreased aqueous humor outflow has been documented during positive tests.[30]

Kirsch proposed a triple test, which is an even more strenuous provocative test in which the pupil is dilated with a weak cycloplegic agent, such as tropicamide or cyclopentolate. If the result of the test is negative, the patient is given 1 liter of water orally. If the test remains negative, 4 percent pilocarpine is administered. Kirsch considers that the test has a positive result if the IOP rises 10 mmHg or more and if the angle appears closed by gonioscopy.[31]

Thymoxamine Test

Topical thymoxamine 0.5 percent, an α-adrenergic antagonist that is currently available in Europe but not in the United States, causes the radial muscle fibers of the iris to relax and allows the pupillary sphincter muscle to act unopposed in constricting the pupil and pulling the iris away from the angle wall. Unlike miotic agents, thymoxamine does not affect the trabecular meshwork or ciliary muscle. A decrease in IOP after its administration suggests that miosis has pulled the iris away from the trabecular meshwork. Thymoxamine does not affect IOP and facility of outflow if the angle is already open, thus effectively distinguishing the angle-closure component from the open-angle component.[32–37] A pure miotic agent (parasympathomimetic) lowers IOP either by reversing angle-closure or by increasing trabecular outflow. Thymoxamine also has been proposed to treat pigmentary glaucoma (see Chap. 138). The bright light and thymoxamine test is discussed later in this chapter.

Dapiprazole 0.5 percent (Rev-Eyes), another α-adrenergic antagonist, is available in the United States and is approved for reversal of routine mydriasis. Like thymoxamine, dapiprazole causes miosis and opens the angle without affecting facility of outflow, IOP, or lens-iris diaphragm. It has been shown to be safe and effective in reversing mydriasis after instillation of tropicamide 1 percent and phenylephrine 2.5 percent.[38–42] Attempting to reverse mydriasis with pilocarpine increases the pupillary-blocking forces, according to studies by Mapstone.[43] Theoretically, dapiprazole should be as effective as thymoxamine, and, therefore, useful for other diagnostic and therapeutic purposes beyond the reversal of routine mydriasis. Further clinical studies need to determine the scope of this drug's usefulness.

Dark Room Provocative Test

Some authors consider that the dark room test is the most physiologic provocative test,[44, 45] the rationale being that patients are likely to be in dim illumination during their normal lives. After gonioscopy and baseline measurement of the IOP, mydriasis is induced by placing the patient in a dark room for 1 to 2 hr. The patient is instructed to remain awake to prevent sleep-induced miosis. A radio or a companion in the room is useful for preventing sleep or a panic attack.

A rise in IOP of 8 to 10 mmHg is considered to be a positive finding when angle-closure is verified by gonioscopy. Exposure to light should be minimal during the post–dark room studies to avoid reversing the pressure-inducing mechanism.[46] Gonioscopy should be performed with minimum light and the shortest possible vertical height of the slit-lamp beam. Some clinicians have performed gonioscopy under dim illumination with infrared light.[47]

The dark room test correctly identifies only about 50 percent of patients with true angle-closure glaucoma.[48] The false-positive rate is unknown. Positive findings on dark room tests are accompanied by a tonographically decreased outflow facility. Use of a 30 percent decrease in tonographic outflow facility as an additional parameter has been reported to increase the positive yield from 30 to 67 percent in one study.[49]

As an addendum to a positive dark room test, the bright-light test (during which the patient is exposed to bright light for 15 min following a positive dark room test) can confirm angle-closure, as opposed to diurnal fluctuation in the IOP. Gonioscopy and measurement of IOP are repeated. If the elevation in IOP was caused by angle-closure, then it should return to normal within this time period.

The thymoxamine–bright-light test (the opposite of the dark room test) should be used when the bright-light test does not clearly open the angle. The aim is to induce maximal constriction of the pupillary sphincter without constricting the ciliary muscle, thus avoiding alteration of the lens and trabecular meshwork by the ciliary muscle.[33]

Prone Provocative Test

Following baseline measurement of IOP and gonioscopy,[50] the patient lies face down for 60 min without sleeping. Direct global or orbital pressure should be avoided. An IOP rise of 8 mmHg with gonioscopic confirmation of angle-closure is considered to be a positive result.[48, 50–52] It is possible to measure the IOP while the patient is still in the prone position by using a Perkins tonometer or Tonopen.

The mechanism of angle-closure with this test, which is apparently unrelated to mydriasis,[48] is uncertain, but investigators postulate that angle-closure occurs due to pupillary block associated with a slight forward shift of the lens. However one study showed no significant anterior chamber shallowing.[52] Other studies found that dark room and prone tests were more likely to yield positive results than the mydriatic test.[48, 52]

After peripheral iridectomy, about 7.5 percent of prone tests still have positive results, suggesting that the lens plays a role in these patients.[51, 53] Similarly, the results in a small number of mydriatic and dark room tests remain positive following peripheral iridectomy, presumably due to pigment dispersion into the anterior chamber or plateau iris syndrome (see Chap. 120). In one study, the number of patients with positive provocative test results was approximately 50 percent with either the prone or the dark room test alone. However, if both tests are performed separately on the same patient, the yield is almost 90 percent positive.[48]

Prone Dark Room Provocative Test

This test is the most popular of the nonpharmacologic provocative tests. Performing the prone provocative test in a dark room significantly increases the number of positive tests.[48] A survey of patients with narrow angles at the Massachusetts Eye and Ear Infirmary indicated that after a negative result on a dark room test, a patient was unlikely to develop acute angle-closure glaucoma within the next 6 mo. Therefore, some believe that suspicious patients should have this test repeated every 6 mo, as long as the result is negative.[54]

Adjunctive Tests

Another provocative test for angle-closure glaucoma uses annular compression with a 16-mm suction cup to produce a forward shift of the iris-lens diaphragm.[55] Ultrasonography for measuring anterior chamber depth has been suggested as another method of identifying angle-closure glaucoma suspects.[56] No correlation with HLA antigens was found in a study of 35 patients with angle-closure glaucoma.[57]

Conclusion

Unfortunately, provocative tests for angle-closure glaucoma are only diagnostic adjuncts.[54, 58, 59] Prospective studies have never verified their sensitivity and specificity or the predictive value. Studies have found that 10 to 30 percent of eyes with well-documented histories of angle-closure have negative provocative test results.[48, 50, 52] Many authorities believe that provocative tests are not helpful in predicting the future development of angle-closure glaucoma. Instead, careful histories and physical examinations, particularly gonioscopy, remain the hallmark of clinical decision making. In addition, the ease and efficacy of prophylactic laser iridotomy have reduced the need to perform provocative testing in eyes with very narrow angles. Ultimately, the decision to treat the asymptomatic patient with a normal IOP and a narrow angle rests on the clinical judgment of the ophthalmologist and the desire of a fully informed patient.

Any patient with narrow angles, regardless of the results of provocative testing, should be advised of the symptoms of angle-closure glaucoma and the need for immediate ophthalmologic evaluation if the symptoms occur.

PROVOCATIVE TESTS FOR OPEN-ANGLE GLAUCOMA

The aim of these tests is to determine which glaucoma-suspect patients subsequently will develop glaucoma with optic nerve damage and visual field loss. Many provocative and adjunctive tests have been studied with varied and conflicting results.

Water Provocative Tests

A 1975 report by Vucicevic and associates stated that "the water drinking test and tonography are at the present time the most popular tests for the early detection of open-angle glaucoma."[60] Many patients develop increased IOP after drinking a large quantity of water in a short time. Glaucomatous eyes may have a greater increased pressure response to water drinking than do nonglaucomatous eyes.

The test is usually performed early in the morning after an 8-hr fast. Baseline applanation tonometry is performed. The patient then promptly drinks 1 liter of water, and applanation tonometry is performed every 15 min for 1 hr.[61] Indentation tonometry by Shiotz should be avoided, because water drinking reduces ocular rigidity, independent of age and refractive error.[60, 62]

The maximum IOP is usually detected within 15 to 30 min, with the level returning to the initial IOP after 60 min in both normal and glaucomatous eyes.[60, 63, 64] An 8 mmHg increase generally is considered to be a positive response, although some investigators use 6 mmHg.[65] Spaeth found that the frequency of false-negative results on provocative tests could be reduced by considering a rise in IOP in terms of percentages rather than millimeters of mercury. A rise of more than 20 percent after water drinking was considered to be suggestive of open-angle glaucoma; an increase of greater than 30 percent made the diagnosis more likely. Several studies found that performing tonography in conjunction with a water drinking test provides additional diagnostic information.[60, 63, 64] Tonographic studies in human eyes have shown reduced aqueous outflow facility, as opposed to hypersecretion.[66–68]

Another theory suggested that reduced serum osmolality might cause increased aqueous inflow, but Spaeth[61] found that changes in IOP did not correlate closely with serum osmolality.

Roth[69] and Rasmussen and Jorgensen[70] concluded that the water provocative test had no diagnostic value due to unacceptably high rates of false-positive and false-negative results. Others, such as Leydhecker,[71] Kronfeld,[72] Drance,[73] Vucicevic and associates,[60] and Becker and Christensen[63] found that the test provided useful information, either alone or in conjunction with tonography.

We conducted a retrospective study of glaucoma-suspect patients who underwent standard water provocative testing. Of the 115 eyes followed for an average of 8 yr, we found that 86 percent with a positive result on a water drinking test subsequently developed glaucomatous optic disc changes or visual field defects. In addition, 81 percent of eyes with a negative result on a water drinking test did not develop glaucomatous optic disc changes or visual field defects. These results were found to be statistically significant by chi square analysis and were not related to age, sex, or refractive error.[74]

We believe that the water provocative test should not be completely abandoned as an adjunctive test in glaucoma suspects. Since useful information can be gained by applanation alone following water drinking, without tonography, the test can be performed easily in a general ophthalmologist's office. It can also provide specific information regarding the effect of fluid consumption on IOP. However, a prospective randomized study will be necessary to pursue the value of this historical diagnostic test.

Dilatation Provocative Tests

Although dilatation provocative tests are used primarily in narrow-angle glaucoma suspects, patients with open angles may also be affected. Strong cycloplegics have been shown to cause a significant increase in IOP (greater than 6 mmHg) in many eyes with primary open-angle glaucoma.[21] Eyes being treated with miotics are even more likely to experience this rise in pressure, which is believed to be due to inhibition of the miotic effect.[20, 75, 76] Harris and associates have demonstrated a similar response in eyes following iridectomy for angle-closure glaucoma and in nonglaucomatous eyes after several weeks of topical dexamethasone.[23, 77]

Anterior chamber pigment dispersion associated with dilatation may also elevate IOP in eyes with open angles. This occurs predominantly in eyes with pigmentary glaucoma or exfoliation syndrome.[24, 78, 79]

The fluorescein angiography provocative test, reported by Spaeth and Vacharat,[65] combines repeated instillations of a strong cycloplegic agent with water drinking to study perfusion of the optic nerve head by fluorescein angiography before and during periods of induced ocular hypertension.

Steroid Provocative Test

Francois[80] and Goldmann[81] noted that patients who received long-term treatment with corticosteroid eye drops could develop symptoms resembling open-angle glaucoma, including increased IOP, optic nerve head cupping, and visual field loss. Subsequently, hundreds of reports have linked topical, systemic, and periocular corticosteroid administration with elevated IOP and secondary open-angle glaucoma (see Chap. 129).

It was hoped that investigations of the phenomenon of ocular hypertension induced by topical steroids could identify individuals with a genetic predisposition for glaucoma. Numerous studies were performed in the 1960s and 1970s in which patients underwent topical corticosteroid testing,[82–90] usually involving application of dexamethasone 0.1 percent eye drops three to four times daily for 3 to 6 wk. These studies showed that marked ocular hypertensive responses occurred more frequently in patients with primary open-angle glaucoma and their first-degree relatives than in normal individuals. Armaly[85] and Becker[91] classified individuals according to their IOP responses to topical corticosteroid administration as low, intermediate, and high responders. Some authors concluded that the steroid response was genetic, but others disputed this finding. Some studies found that ocular hypertensives had a greater incidence of high responders, some with reversible glaucomatous field defects.[87, 89] Other studies found that the pressure response among glaucoma suspects was not significantly different from that found in a normal population.[84, 90, 92] Consequently, over the past decade, steroid provocative testing has lost favor since it did not improve the accuracy of predicting which glaucoma suspects would develop glaucomatous visual field loss.

Regardless of the predictability of the corticosteroid response, ophthalmologists should remain vigilant in reminding physicians who prescribe corticosteroids of this potentially blinding side effect.

Therapeutic Trials

Several tests have been developed based on the theory that eyes with primary open-angle glaucoma show a greater response to antiglaucoma drugs than do normal eyes.

Patients with primary open-angle glaucoma may be particularly sensitive to epinephrine, exhibiting a greater drop in IOP than normal.[93–97] The epinephrine test consists of applying 1 to 2 percent epinephrine twice daily for up to 7 days. A decrease in IOP of more than 5 mmHg is considered to be a positive response. The pressure drop 4 hr after an initial dose can also be used as an indicator of response. Becker found that the test results could be useful in predicting which ocular hypertensives would develop visual field loss.[93, 97] However, a study by Drance and associates did not confirm significant prognostic value.[98]

Hollwich[99] suggested a pilocarpine test in which an IOP drop of more than 4 mm at the peak of the diurnal curve is suggestive of glaucoma. In the acetazolamide test, the drug is given intravenously, and applanation IOP measurements are used to estimate the coefficient of aqueous outflow facility.[100] Neither of these tests has confirmed clinical value.

A uniocular therapeutic trial of a topical antiglaucoma drug is useful for determining its efficacy in individual patients.[101] A pilocarpine therapeutic test can be performed using a 2 percent concentration during a 4-hr office trial.[102]

Conclusion

The aim of provocative tests is to establish the diagnosis before damage gives rise to manifest symptoms. The physician caring for the person suspected of having open-angle glaucoma is faced with the dilemma of deciding whether or not to provide treatment, with the knowledge that a misjudgment may cause the patient a great disservice. Unfortunately, no provocative or adjunctive tests can predict with certainty which glaucoma suspects will develop glaucoma. However, some of these tests may provide useful information in evaluating patients suspected of having open-angle glaucoma.

REFERENCES

1. Gorin G: Shortening of the angle of the anterior chamber in angle-closure glaucoma. Am J Ophthalmol 49:141, 1960.
2. Scheie HG: Width and pigmentation of the angle of the anterior chamber: A system of grading by gonioscopy. Arch Ophthalmol 58:510, 1957.
3. Shaffer RN: Symposium: Primary glaucoma, III: Gonioscopy, ophthalmoscopy and perimetry. Trans Am Acad Ophthalmol Otolaryngol 62:112, 1969.
4. Becker S: Clinical Gonioscopy—A Text and Stereoscopic Atlas. St Louis, CV Mosby, 1972.
5. Jacobs IH: Anterior chamber depth measurement using the slit-lamp microscope. Am J Ophthalmol 88:236, 1979.
6. Vargas E, Drance SM: Anterior chamber depth in angle-closure glaucoma: Clinical methods of depth determination in people with and without the disease. Arch Ophthalmol 90:438, 1973.
7. Smith RJH: A new method of estimating the depth of the anterior chamber. Br J Ophthalmol 63:215, 1979.
8. Fontana ST, Brubaker RF: Volume and depth of the anterior chamber in the normal aging human eye. Arch Ophthalmol 98:1803, 1980.
9. Spaeth GL: Distinguishing between the normal narrow, the suspiciously shallow, and the particularly pathological, anterior chamber angle. Perspect Ophthalmol 1:205, 1977.
10. Spaeth GL: The normal development of the human anterior chamber angle: A new system of descriptive grading. Trans Ophthalmol Soc UK 91:709, 1971.
11. van Herick W, Shaffer RN, Schwartz A: Estimation of width of angle of anterior chamber: Incidence and significance of the narrow angle. Am J Ophthalmol 68:626, 1969.
12. Forbes M: Indentation gonioscopy and efficacy of iridectomy in angle-closure glaucoma. Trans Am Ophthalmol Soc 72:488, 1974.
13. Forbes M: Gonioscopy with corneal indentation: A method for distinguishing between appositional closure and synechial closure. Arch Ophthalmol 76:488, 1966.
14. Iwata K: A new indentation gonioscopy and evaluation of peripheral iridectomy in angle-closure glaucoma. Glaucoma 3:546, 1980.
15. Wilensky J, Herschler J, Kass M, et al: Gonioscopy. Invest Ophthalmol Vis Sci 17 (Suppl):144, 1978.
16. Hillman JS: Acute closed-angle glaucoma: An investigation into the effect of delay in treatment. Br J Ophthalmol 63:817, 1979.
17. Chandler PA: Narrow-angle glaucoma. Arch Ophthalmol 47:695, 1952.
18. Banziger T: The mechanism of acute glaucoma and the explanation for the effectiveness of iridectomy for the same. Ber Deutsch Ophthalmol Ges 43:43, 1922.
19. Becker B, Thompson HE: Tonography and angle-closure glaucoma: Diagnosis and therapy. Am J Ophthalmol 46:305, 1958.
20. Barany E, Christensen RE: Cycloplegia and outflow resistance in normal human and monkey eyes and in primary open-angle glaucoma. Arch Ophthalmol 77:757, 1967.
21. Harris LS: Cycloplegic-induced intraocular pressure elevations: A study of normal and open-angle glaucomatous eyes. Arch Ophthalmol 79:242, 1968.
22. Harris, LS, Galin MA: Cycloplegic provocative testing. Arch Ophthalmol 81:356, 1969 .
23. Harris LS, Galin MA, Mittag TW: Cycloplegic provocative testing. Arch Ophthalmol 81:356, 1969.
24. Valle O: The cyclopentolate provocative test in suspected or untreated open-angle glaucoma. III: The significance of pigment for the result of the cyclopentolate provocative test in suspected or untreated open-angle glaucoma. Acta Ophthalmol 54:654 1976.
25. Brooks AMV, West RH, Gillies WE: The risk of precipitating acute angle-closure glaucoma with the clinical use of mydriatic agents. Med J Aust 145:36, 1986.
26. Mapstone R: Normal response to pilocarpine and phenylephrine. Br J Ophthalmol 61:510, 1977.
27. Mapstone R: Dilating dangerous pupils. Br J Ophthalmol 61:510, 1977.
28. Mapstone R: Provocative tests in closed-angle glaucoma. Br J Ophthalmol 60:115, 1976.
29. Mapstone R: Partial angle closure. Br J Ophthalmol 61:525, 1977.
30. Mapstone R: Outflow changes in positive provocative tests. Br J Ophthalmol 61:634, 1977.
31. Kirsch RE: A study of provocative tests for angle-closure glaucoma. Arch Ophthalmol 74:770, 1965.
32. Wand M, Grant WM: Thymoxamine test: Differentiating angle-closure glaucoma from open-angle glaucoma with narrow angles. Arch Ophthalmol 96:1009, 1978.
33. Wand M, Grant WM: Thymoxamine hydrochloride: Effects on the facility of outflow and intraocular pressure. Invest Ophthalmol 15:400, 1976.
34. Wand M, Grant WM: Thymoxamine hydrochloride: An alpha-adrenergic blocker. Surv Ophthalmol 25:75, 1980.
35. Rutkowski PC, Fernandez JL, Galin MA, Halasa AH: Alpha-adrenergic receptor blockade in the treatment of angle-closure glaucoma. Trans Am Acad Ophthalmol Otolaryngol 77:137, 1973.
36. Halasa AH, Rutkowski PC: Thymoxamine therapy for angle-closure glaucoma. Arch Ophthalmol 90:177, 1973.
37. Ganias F, Mapstone R: Miotics in closed-angle glaucoma. Br J Ophthalmol 59:205, 1975.
38. Relf S, Gharagozzloo NA, Skuta GL, et al: Thymoxamine reverses phenylephrine-induced mydriasis. Am J Ophthalmol 106:251, 1988.
39. Allinson RW, Gerber DS, Bieber S, Hodes BL: Reversal of mydriasis by dapiprazole. Ann Ophthalmol 22:131, 1990.
40. Bucci M, D'Andrea D, Bettini A, et al: Dapiprazole for the reversal of mydriasis due to tropicamide. Glaucoma 9:94, 1987.
41. Bonomi L, Marchini G, De Gregoria M: Ultrasonographic study of the ocular effects of topical dapiprazole. Glaucoma 8:30, 1986.
42. Matsuda K, Ikuo A, Takehisa K, Konurasaki Y: Alteration of pupil-blocking force by topical dapiprazole administration. Glaucoma 13:72, 1991.
43. Mapstone, R: Mechanics of pupil block. Br J Ophthalmol 52:19, 1968.

44. Higgit AC: The dark-room test. Br J Ophthalmol 38:242, 1954.
45. Tornquist R: Dark-room test on eyes with a shallow anterior chamber. Acta Ophthalmol 19, 36:664, 1958.
46. Gloster J, Poinoosawmy D: Changes in intraocular pressure during and after the dark-room test. Br J Ophthalmol 57:170, 1973.
47. Epstein DL: Chandler and Grant's Glaucoma, 3rd ed. Philadelphia, Lea & Febiger, 1986, p 246.
48. Harris LS, Galin MA: Prone provocative testing for narrow angle glaucoma. Arch Ophthalmol 87:493, 1972.
49. Foulds WS: Observations on the facility of aqueous outflow in closed-angle glaucoma. Br J Ophthalmol 43:613, 1959.
50. Hyams SW, Friedman BZ, Neumann E: Elevated intraocular pressure in the prone position: A new provocative test for angle-closure glaucoma. Am J Ophthalmol 66:661, 1968.
51. Friedman Z, Neumann E: Comparison of prone-position, dark-room, and mydriatic tests for angle-closure glaucoma before and after peripheral iridectomy. Am J Ophthalmol 74:24, 1972.
52. Neumann E, Hyams SW: Gonioscopy and anterior chamber depth in the prone-position provocative test for angle-closure glaucoma. Ophthalmologica 167:9, 1973.
53. Hung PT, Chou LH: Provocation and mechanism of angle-closure glaucoma after iridectomy. Arch Ophthalmol 97:1862, 1979.
54. Wand M: Provocative tests in angle-closure glaucoma: A brief review with commentary. Ophthalmic Surg 5:32, 1974.
55. Nesterov AP, Kiselev GA, Devlikamova ER: New compression tests in glaucoma. II: Posterior annular compression test. Acta Ophthalmol 51:749, 1973.
56. Bellows JG: Ultrasonic diagnostic techniques in glaucoma. Ann Ophthalmol 10:91, 1978.
57. Gieser DK, Wilensky JT: HLA antigens and acute angle-closure glaucoma. Am J Ophthalmol 88:232, 1979.
58. Lowe RF: Primary angle-closure glaucoma: A review of provocative tests. Br J Ophthalmol 51:727, 1967.
59. Campbell DG: A comparison of diagnostic techniques in angle-closure glaucoma. Am J Ophthalmol 88:197, 1979.
60. Vucicevic ZM, Scheie HG, Berry A, et al: The importance and accuracy of the water drinking test and tonography. Ann Ophthalmol 7:39, 1975.
61. Spaeth GL: The water drinking test: Indications that factors other than osmotic considerations are involved. Arch Ophthalmol 77:50, 1967.
62. Vucicevic ZM, Ralston J, Burns WP, Gaffney HP: Influence of the water drinking test on scleral rigidity. Arch Ophthalmol 82:761, 1969.
63. Becker B, Christensen RE: Water-drinking and tonography in the diagnosis of glaucoma. Arch Ophthalmol 56:321, 1956.
64. Becker B: Tonography in the diagnosis of simple (open angle) glaucoma. Trans Am Acad Ophthalmol Otolaryngol 65:156, 1961.
65. Spaeth GL, Vacharat N: Provocative tests and chronic simple glaucoma. I: Effect of atropine on the water-drinking test: Intimations of central regulatory control. II: Fluorescein angiography provocative test: A new approach to separation of the normal from the pathological. Br J Ophthalmol 56:205, 1972.
66. Kimura R: Clinical studies on glaucoma. Report III. The diagnostic significance of the water-drinking test. Acta Soc Ophthalmol Jpn 71:2133, 1967.
67. Ballin N, Becker B: Provocative testing for primary open-angle glaucoma in "senior citizens." Invest Ophthalmol 6:126, 1967.
68. Armaly MF, Sayegh RE: Water-drinking test. II: The effect of age on tonometric and tonographic measures. Arch Ophthalmol 83:176, 1970.
69. Roth JA, Inadequate diagnostic value of the water-drinking test. Br J Ophthalmol 58:55, 1974.
70. Rasmussen KE, Jorgensen HA: Diagnostic value of the water-drinking test in early detection of simple glaucoma. Acta Ophthalmol 54:160, 1976.
71. Leydhecker W: The water drinking test. Br J Ophthalmol 34:457, 1950.
72. Kronfeld PC: Water drinking and outflow facility. Invest Ophthalmol 14:49, 1975.
73. Drance SM: Studies with applanation water tests. Arch Ophthalmol 69:39, 1963.
74. Gyurgyik L, Berke SJ, Weintraub J, Rahn E: Water provocative testing—Another look. (Publication pending)
75. Harris LS, Galin MA: Cycloplegic provocative testing: Effect of miotic therapy. Arch Ophthalmol 81:544, 1969.
76. Portney GL, Purcell TW: Influence of tropicamide on intraocular pressure. Ann Ophthalmol 7:31, 1975.
77. Harris LS, Galin MA, Mittage TW: Cycloplegic provocative testing after topical administration of steroids. Arch Ophthalmol 86:12, 1971.
78. Kristensen P: Mydriasis-induced pigment liberation in the anterior chamber associated with acute rise in intraocular pressure in open-angle glaucoma. Acta Ophthalmol 43:714, 1965.
79. Kristensen P: Pigment liberation test in open-angle glaucoma. Acta Ophthalmol 46:586, 1968.
80. Francois J: Cortisone et tension oculaire. Ann Ocul 187:805, 1954.
81. Goldmann H: Cortisone glaucoma. Arch Ophthalmol 68:621, 1962.
82. Becker B, Hahn KA: Topical corticosteroids and heredity in primary open-angle glaucoma. Am J Ophthalmol 57:543, 1964.
83. Francois J, Heintz-De Bree C, Tripathi RC: The cortisone test and the heredity of primary open-angle glaucoma. Am J Ophthalmol 62:844, 1966.
84. Levene R, Wigdor A, Edelstein A, Baum J: Topical corticosteroid in normal patients and glaucoma suspects. Arch Ophthalmol 77:593, 1967.
85. Armaly MF: Inheritance of dexamethasone hypertension and glaucoma. Arch Ophthalmol 77:747, 1967.
86. Kitazawa Y: Primary angle-closure glaucoma: Corticosteroid responsiveness. Arch Ophthalmol 9:946, 1970.
87. LeBlanc RP, Stewart RH, Becker B: Corticosteroid provocative testing. Invest Ophthalmol 9:946, 1970.
88. Schwartz JT, Reuling FH, Feinleib M, et al: Twin study on ocular pressure after topical dexamethasone. I: Frequency distribution of pressure response. Am J Ophthalmol 76:126, 1973.
89. Dean GO Jr, Deutsch AR, Hiatt RL: The effect of dexamethasone on borderline ocular hypertension. Ann Ophthalmol 7:193, 1975.
90. Palmberg PF, Mandell A, Wilensky JT, et al: The reproducibility of the intraocular pressure response to dexamethasone. Am J Ophthalmol 80:844, 1975.
91. Becker B: Intraocular pressure response to topical corticosteroids. Invest Ophthalmol Vis Sci 4:198, 1965.
92. Wilensky JT, Podos SM, Becker B: Prognostic indicators in ocular hypertension. Arch Ophthalmol 91:200, 1974.
93. Becker B, Shin DH: Response to topical epinephrine: A practical prognostic test in patients with ocular hypertension. Arch Ophthalmol 94:2057, 1976.
94. Palmberg PF, Hajek S, Cooper D, Becker B: Increased cellular responsiveness to epinephrine in primary open-angle glaucoma. Arch Ophthalmol 95:855, 1977.
95. Becker B, Montgomery SW, Kass MA, Shin DH: Increased ocular and systemic responsiveness to epinephrine in primary open-angle glaucoma. Arch Ophthalmol 95:789, 1977.
96. Shin DH, Kass MA, Becker B: Intraocular pressure response to topical epinephrine and HLA-B12. Arch Ophthalmol 96:1012, 1978.
97. Kass MA, Becker B: A simplified test of epinephrine responsiveness. Arch Ophthalmol 96:999, 1978.
98. Drance SM, Saheb NE, Schulzer M: Response to topical epinephrine in chronic open-angle glaucoma. Arch Ophthalmol 96:1001, 1978.
99. Hollwich F: The pilocarpine-test for the early diagnosis of glaucoma. Klin Monatsbl Augenheilkd 163:115, 1973.
100. Nissen OI, Kjer P, Olsen L: A comparison between an acetazolamide test and weight tonography in pathological and apathological circulation of the aqueous humor. Invest Ophthalmol 15:844, 1976.
101. Drance SM: The uniocular therapeutic trial in the management of elevated intraocular pressure. Surv Ophthalmol 25:203, 1980.
102. Rothkoff L, Biedner B, Biger Y, Blumenthal M: A proposed pilocarpine therapeutic test. Arch Ophthalmol 96:1380, 1978.

Chapter 117

∎

Primary Open-Angle Glaucoma

JOHN V. THOMAS

Primary open-angle glaucoma (POAG) is the most common variety of glaucoma and is thought to occur due to a hereditary predisposition. It is generally a bilateral disease, although its severity may be asymmetric in the two eyes. It has an adult onset, open and normal-appearing angles with gonioscopy, absence of secondary causes of open-angle glaucoma, and evidence of glaucomatous optic nerve damage. This optic nerve damage may take the form of changes in the appearance of the optic disc or nerve fiber layer or the presence of abnormalities in the visual field.

The term "glaucoma suspect" refers to patients with findings suggestive of POAG and to those with ocular hypertension. A patient may be called a glaucoma suspect when the following findings are noted: (1) intraocular pressure (IOP) repeatedly above 21 mmHg by applanation tonometry; (2) the optic disc or nerve fiber layer may be normal or may demonstrate changes that are suspicious for glaucomatous optic nerve damage (e.g., large cup:disc ratio; narrow disc rim; asymmetry of disc cupping between the two eyes; focal abnormalities of the disc rim such as notching or hemorrhage; localized or diffuse defects of the nerve fiber layer; and acquired peripapillary atrophy, even in the absence of elevated IOP); (3) normal visual fields; (4) onset after 30 yr of age; and (5) open, normal-appearing angles by gonioscopy.

CLINICAL MANIFESTATIONS

Epidemiology

Although there is variation in the prevalence of ocular hypertension and POAG, the data that follow are representative epidemiologic estimates. If ocular hypertension is defined as having an IOP equal to or more than 23 mmHg, its prevalence is 1.6 percent in the population older than 30 yr of age and 10.5 percent in the 70- to 79-yr age group.[1] In a normotensive population older than 30 yr of age, the incidence of developing POAG within a 5-yr interval varies from 0.5 to 1.25 percent, whereas in an ocular hypertensive population older than 30 yr of age it varies from 3 to 5 percent.[2]

In the United States, glaucoma is the second most frequent cause of blindness among whites. Among African-Americans, it is the most frequent cause of blindness, with the latter group being four to five times more likely to develop glaucoma and up to six times more likely to be blinded by this disease. Two million Americans have glaucoma, and about one half are unaware of their condition. Currently, approximately 80,000 people are blind from POAG. Each year, an additional 5000 patients go blind, and 95,000 patients lose some degree of sight. In other parts of the world such as Africa and the Carribean, a much higher proportion of patients with glaucoma are blind. While 4 percent of patients with glaucoma in the United States are blind; in Nigeria, 34 percent of patients with glaucoma are bilaterally blind and 91 percent are monocularly blind.[3] This difference in the prevalence of blindness is probably largely due to earlier detection and treatment in the United States.

Inheritance

There is a definite hereditary predisposition to the development of POAG that appears to be multifactorial and not according to simple mendelian predictions. In siblings and children of patients with glaucoma,[4] the prevalence of ocular hypertension is more than twice that of the general population. The prevalence of glaucoma is about six times that of the general population,[5] and the incidence of new cases of glaucoma is about 2.5 times greater than that found in the general population.[6] If siblings and children older than 40 yr of age are considered, the incidence of glaucoma is five times that of the general population.[7]

Risk Factors

Several ocular conditions have been implicated as risk factors in the development of glaucomatous optic nerve damage. These conditions include elevated IOP, myopia, and changes in the appearance of the optic nerve, such as a large cup:disc ratio; asymmetry of cupping; disc margin hemorrhage, especially at the superior and inferior poles of the disc; narrowing or notching of the neural rim; and acquired peripapillary atrophy.[8–13] In addition, localized or diffuse nerve fiber layer defects may indicate glaucomatous optic nerve damage.[14–16] Systemic conditions that have been implicated as risk factors in the development of glaucomatous optic nerve damage are a family history of glaucoma, increasing age, black race, diabetes mellitus, and cardiovascular disease.[17, 18]

Patients considered to be glaucoma suspects—those with a high risk of developing glaucoma—have one or more of the following characteristics: (1) elevated IOP repeatedly measured in the high 20s or above, (2) suspicious optic nerve or nerve fiber layer findings consistent with early glaucomatous optic nerve damage, and (3) the presence of ocular or systemic risk factors.

Risk factors that appear to be most significant are elevated IOP, increasing age, a family history of glaucoma, and black race.

Although the risk of developing glaucomatous optic nerve damage increases with increased IOP, the mere presence of elevated pressure correlates weakly with the presence of glaucomatous nerve damage. In one study, 28 to 36 percent of patients with a presenting IOP greater than 30 mmHg and 57 percent of patients with pressures of 40 mmHg or more presented with optic nerve damage, whereas only 6 percent of patients with moderately elevated IOP presented with nerve damage.[18] It is important to note that although IOP levels are positively correlated with the risk of developing optic nerve damage, at least one sixth of all patients with glaucoma have not had a documented IOP greater than 21 mmHg.[19]

Clinical Course

In most cases, glaucoma develops in mid-life or later, and the onset is usually gradual and asymptomatic. The IOP may be only slightly elevated in the early stages, but it generally becomes higher when the disease is more advanced. The disease tends to progress, and the facility of aqueous outflow becomes reduced with time.

Glaucomatous optic nerve damage is generally progressive, although the rate at which it occurs varies with the patient. The evidence that glaucomatous damage is progressive is seen in patients who have been treated suboptimally or in patients who failed to seek help until late in the course of the disease. Without treatment, a large proportion of patients have total optic nerve atrophy and blindness.

The likelihood that optic nerve damage will occur varies from one individual to the next, depending on the level of IOP and on the presence of other risk factors. It is estimated that approximately 1 percent of all individuals with elevated IOP will develop glaucomatous damage each year. The rate is higher if risk factors, in addition to high IOP, are present.

Clinical Findings

In POAG, findings on slit-lamp examination and the gonioscopic appearance of the angle of the anterior chamber are no different from those found in normal eyes. An extremely important part of the clinical examination in glaucoma is the evaluation of the appearance of the optic nerve head. Findings that have significance include an asymmetry of the optic cups, thinning or notching of the neural rim of the disc, an optic cup that reaches the disc margin below, a slight bending of all vessels at the margin, saucerization of the disc, a disc margin hemorrhage, and a documented progressive change in the appearance of the disc. It should be noted that in high myopia, it can be difficult to distinguish early glaucomatous disc changes from a normal disc. Nerve fiber layer defects may also be present.

Visual field abnormalities in glaucoma may include arcuate defects, nasal steps, paracentral scotomas, or a generalized depression of the field.

The IOP may vary in the course of a day from normal to significantly elevated levels. The mean value of IOP in a large normal population is approximately 16 mmHg, with a standard deviation of about 3 mmHg. Although abnormally increased IOP has been defined arbitrarily as two standard deviations above the mean, so that pressures of 21.7 mmHg or greater are considered abnormal, the clinical relevance of this number to glaucomatous damage is not clear-cut. As noted earlier, at least 16 percent of patients with glaucoma have not had demonstrable or repeated elevations of IOP above 21 mmHg, whereas many individuals with IOP repeatedly above 21 mmHg do not have and may never develop optic nerve damage during their lifetimes.

Tonography studies, although rarely done today, indicate a reduced facility of aqueous outflow from the anterior chamber. This decreased facility of outflow persists throughout the patient's life and tends to worsen with increasing age.

PATHOGENESIS

The pathogenesis of POAG is unclear. Although it is known that there is increased resistance to outflow of aqueous humor in POAG, there is much debate over the site of resistance and the morphologic changes that are responsible for reduced aqueous outflow.[20–23] The weight of the evidence appears to indicate that the primary increase in outflow resistance lies in the cribriform layer of the trabecular meshwork, consisting of the outermost part of the trabecular meshwork adjacent to the inner wall endothelium of Schlemm's canal.[24]

A decrease in vacuolization of the inner wall of Schlemm's canal in glaucomatous eyes has been postulated as the cause of increased outflow resistance.[25, 26] However, there is evidence that there is no difference in the number and size of vacuoles between normal and glaucomatous eyes.[27]

Clusters of extracellular materials called "plaques" have been found deposited within the cribrifrom layer of the trabecular meshwork and underneath the endothelial lining of Schlemm's canal.[28] The amount of this plaque material appears to be significantly greater in glaucomatous eyes than in normal eyes.[29] It is possible that these plaques could block part of the filtering area of the inner wall of Schlemm's canal and produce increased outflow resistance in glaucoma.

It has also been suggested that a loss of trabecular cells results in a fusion of the innermost trabecular sheets and partial loss of patent aqueous channels.[30, 31] It has been claimed that this appears in advanced stages of POAG and that, in most cases, the primary increase in outflow resistance lies in the cribriform layer of the meshwork.

DIFFERENTIAL DIAGNOSIS

The differential diagnosis of POAG includes chronic angle-closure glaucoma, combined-mechanism glaucoma, and secondary glaucomas such as angle recession glaucoma, pseudoexfoliation glaucoma, pigmentary glaucoma, and steroid-induced glaucoma. An accurate history and careful slit-lamp and gonioscopic examinations are required to distinguish between these conditions. Gonioscopy is done ideally when no glaucoma medications are being used, because some medications may affect angle width. Findings on gonioscopy that help to determine the type of glaucoma present include peripheral anterior synechias, abnormal vessels, abnormal pigmentation, angle recession, exudates or keratic precipitates on the trabecular meshwork, and tumors in the angle.

MANAGEMENT

Most glaucoma suspects and ocular hypertensive patients are managed by observation alone, and an assessment of the IOP, visual field, and optic disc is made at regular intervals. If a patient is a high-risk glaucoma suspect, consideration is given to treatment after carefully weighing the risk factors that contribute to optic nerve damage against the risks of treatment. This decision is individualized, taking into account the risks and rate at which glaucomatous optic nerve damage and visual impairment that are likely to occur, the patient's expected life span, and his or her tolerance of effective treatment.

In the management of glaucoma, it is helpful to select a "target pressure" in each patient. This is a level of IOP that, if achieved, will presumably prevent future optic nerve damage, It is selected by taking into account the severity of existing optic nerve damage, the level of IOP at which nerve damage occurred, the current height of the IOP, and, if known, the rapidity with which the damage occurred. It is obviously impossible to know precisely the "target pressure" for any individual, and the pressure level selected is to some extent arbitrary. However, the concept of "target pressure" is a useful one, because it provides a means of achieving the real goal of protecting the optic nerve. The adequacy and validity of the "target pressure" have to be reassessed periodically by evaluating the appearance of the optic nerve and visual field data.

In patients with advanced glaucoma or normal-tension glaucoma, the need for especially low pressures should be recognized. Obtaining pressures in the normal range is no guarantee of optic nerve stability. It is necessary to monitor optic nerve status with static perimetry, and stereo photographs of the optic disc enable detection of small deteriorations. This is essential in determining whether glaucoma is getting worse.

Treatment modalities for glaucoma consist of topical and systemic medication, laser treatment, and conventional surgical procedures. Traditionally, maximum-tolerated medical therapy has been used before laser trabeculoplasty, and laser treatment has preceded conventional surgery. This approach was designed primarily to reduce the risks of therapy for the patient. However, results from the Glaucoma Laser Trial.[32] indicate that laser trabeculoplasty is a safe and effective form of treatment when used as initial therapy for glaucoma and that after a follow-up of 2 yr, fewer patients treated initially with trabeculoplasty require the addition of glaucoma medications compared with patients initially treated with timolol. Only after a thorough analysis of the long-term results of the Glaucoma Laser Trial will it be possible to evaluate whether trabeculoplasty should become the initial treatment of open-angle glaucoma in the future.

Since glaucoma is currently a chronic, incurable disease, a patient who is a glaucoma suspect or has POAG requires life-long follow-up. On follow-up visits the clinical parameters that should be monitored regularly include a measurement of the IOP, a record of the optic disc appearance, tests of the visual fields, and occasionally tests such as diurnal IOP curves and gonioscopy.

If the optic nerve and IOP status are stable, an untreated glaucoma suspect should be evaluated every 6 to 18 mo. If the optic nerve and IOP status are stable and the patient is an untreated, high-risk glaucoma suspect, a follow-up evaluation should be performed every 3 to 6 mo. If the patient is a high-risk glaucoma suspect who is being treated and who has had newly established control of IOP, follow-up visits are made every 3 to 6 mo.

In patients with POAG who have minimal optic nerve damage and stable controlled IOP and optic nerve status, a follow-up evaluation takes place every 3 to 12 mo. Visual field examination and a record of the appearance of the optic nerve are done once or twice each year. In a patient with POAG who has moderate-to-severe optic nerve damage and stable controlled IOP and optic nerve status, a follow-up evaluation takes place every 2 to 6 mo. A visual field examination and a record of the appearance of the optic nerve are made one to three times each year.

If in a patient with POAG, IOP control has been recently established and the optic nerve status has been stabilized, follow-up visits may be every 1 to 4 mo, decreasing in frequency as stability continues to be demonstrated. It the IOP is uncontrolled and if the optic nerve status is deteriorating, it may be necessary to see a patient daily or weekly until appropriate control is achieved.

In an effort to detect glaucoma in previously undiagnosed individuals, IOP screenings have been suggested. However, performing IOP screening in the general population appears to have questionable value. One half of all patients with glaucoma will have pressures below 22 mmHg at the time of screening and will, therefore, be missed.[33, 34] In addition, a sixth or more of all patients with POAG may have IOP levels consistently below 22 mmHg. Furthermore, many individuals with elevated pressures (greater than 21 mmHg) do not have and may never develop optic nerve damage, although such a risk increases with the level of IOP.[35] If the appearance of the optic nerve and status of the visual field were evaluated in addition to IOP measurement as part of a population-based screening program, the screening, although more complex, may be more cost effective.

REFERENCES

1. Armaly MF: On the distribution of applanation pressure. I: Statistical features with the effect of age, sex and family history of glaucoma. Arch Ophthalmol 73:11, 1965.
2. Hart WM: The epidemiology of primary open angle glaucoma and ocular hypertension. *In* Ritch R, Shields MB, Krupin T (eds): The Glaucomas. St Louis, CV Mosby, 1989.
3. Amoni SS: Pattern of presentation of glaucoma in Kaduna, Nigeria. Glaucoma 2:445, 1980.
4. Becker B, Kolker AE, Roth FD: Glaucoma family study. Am J Ophthalmol 50:557, 1960.
5. Davis TG: Tonographic survey of the close relatives of patients with chronic simple glaucoma. Br J Ophthalmol 52:32, 1968.
6. Paterson G: A 9-year follow-up of studies on first degree relatives of patients with glaucoma simplex. Trans Ophth Soc UK 90:515, 1971.
7. Miller SJH: Genetics of glaucoma and family studies. Trans Ophth Soc UK 98:290, 1970.
8. Milton RC, Ganley JP: Risk of glaucoma in myopia: A population study. Invest Ophthalmol Vis Sci 16:85, 1977.
9. Perkins ES, Phelps CD: Open angle glaucoma, ocular hypertension, low tension glaucoma and refraction. Arch Ophthalmol 100:1464, 1982.
10. Drance SM, Fairclough M, Butler DM, et al: The importance of disc hemorrhage in the prognosis of chronic open angle glaucoma. Arch Ophthalmol 95:226, 1977.
11. Susanna R, Drance SM, Douglas GR: Disc hemorrhage in patients with elevated intraocular pressure: Occurrence with and without field changes. Arch Ophthalmol 97:284, 1979.
12. Primrose J: The incidence of the peripapillary halo glaucomatosus. Trans Ophth Soc UK 89:585, 1969.
13. Hitchings RA, Spaeth GL: The optic disc in glaucoma. I: Classification. Br J Ophthalmol 60:778, 1976.
14. Sommer A, Miller NR, Pollack I, et al: The nerve fiber layer in the diagnosis of glaucoma. Arch Ophthalmol 95:2149, 1977.
15. Sommer A, Pollack I, Maumenee AE: Optic disc parameters and onset of glaucomatous field loss. II: Static screening criteria. Arch Ophthalmol 97:1449, 1979.
16. Quigley HA, Miller NR, George T: Clinical evaluation of nerve fiber layer atrophy as an indicator of glaucomatous optic nerve damage. Arch Ophthalmol 98:1564, 1980.
17. Hiller R, Kahn HA: Blindness from glaucoma. Am J Ophthalmol 80:62, 1975.
18. Anderson DR: The management of elevated intraocular pressure with normal optic discs and visual fields. I: Therapeutic approach based on high risk factors. Surv Ophthalmol 21:479, 1977.
19. Sommer A, Tielsch JM, Katz J, et al: Relationship between intraocular pressure and primary open angle glaucoma among white and black Americans: The Baltimore Eye Survey. Arch Ophthalmol 109:1090, 1991.
20. Nesterov AP, Batmanov YE: Study on morphology and function of the drainage area of the eye of man. Acta Ophthalmol 50:337, 1972.
21. Nesterov AP, Batmanov YE: Trabecular wall of Schlemm's canal in the early stage of primary open angle glaucoma. Am J Ophthalmol 79:639, 1974.
22. Segawa K: Electron microscopic changes of the trabecular tissue in primary open angle glaucoma. Ann Ophthalmol 11:49, 1979.
23. Shabo AL, Reese TS, Gaasterland D: Post-mortem formation of giant endothelial vacuoles in Schlemm's canal of a monkey. Am J Ophthalmol 76:896, 1973.
24. Rohen JW, Lutjen-Drecoll E: Morphology of aqueous outflow pathways in normal and glaucomatous eyes. *In* Ritch R, Shields MB, Krupin T (eds): The Glaucomas, vol. 1. St Louis, CV Mosby, 1989.
25. Tripathi RC: Mechanism of the aqueous outflow across the trabecular wall of Schlemm's canal. Exp Eye Res 11:116, 1971.
26. Tripathi RC: Pathological anatomy of the outflow pathways of aqueous humor in chronic simple glaucoma. Exp Eye Res 25(Suppl):403, 1977.
27. Fink A, Felix MD, Fletcher RC: The electron microscopy of Schlemm's canal and adjacent structures in patients with glaucoma. Trans Am Ophthalmol Soc 70:82, 1972.
28. Rohen JW, Futa R, Lutjen-Drecoll E: The fine structure of the cribriform meshwork in normal and glaucomatous eyes as seen in tangential sections. Invest Ophthalmol Vis Sci 21:574, 1981.
29. Lutjen-Drecoll E, Shimuzu T, Rohrbach M, et al: Quantitative analysis of "plaque material" in the inner and outer wall of Schlemm's canal in normal and glaucomatous eyes. Exp Eye Res 42:443, 1986.
30. Alvarado J, Murphy C, Juster R: Trabecular meshwork cellularity in POAG and non-glaucomatous normals. Ophthalmology 91:564, 1984.
31. Fine BS, Yanoff M, Stone RA: A clinicopathologic study of four cases of POAG compared to normal eyes. Am J Ophthalmol 91:88, 1981.
32. Glaucoma Laser Trial Research Group: The Glaucoma Laser Trial (GLT). 2: Results of argon laser trabeculoplasty versus topical medicines. Ophthalmology 97:1403, 1990.
33. Kahn HA, Milton RC: Alternative definitions of open angle glaucoma: Effect on prevalence and associations in the Framingham Eye Study. Arch Ophthalmol 98:2172, 1980.
34. Leske MC: The epidemiology of open angle glaucoma: A review. Am J Epidemiol 118:166, 1983.
35. Sommer A: Intraocular pressure and glaucoma. Am J Ophthalmol 107:186, 1989.

Chapter 118

▪

Juvenile-Onset Open-Angle Glaucoma

SHLOMO MELAMED and ISAAC ASHKENAZI

DEFINITION

Some confusion still remains in the literature regarding the exact definition of juvenile-onset open-angle glaucoma (JOAG). There is still an overlap of this entity with other diagnoses such as primary open-angle glaucoma, pigmentary dispersion syndrome, congenital glaucoma, and childhood glaucomas associated with other ocular anomalies such as Sturge-Weber syndrome and aniridia.[1-5] This confusion is outdated, and more well-delineated parameters should be applied for the accurate diagnosis of this disease.

Several studies have confirmed the need for a more detailed and accurate definition of JOAG. JOAG is a distinct entity associated with special clinical signs and symptoms. The practicing ophthalmologist should be aware of these features differentiating juvenile glaucoma from all other subtypes of the disease.

Descriptive terms such as primary open-angle glaucoma of adolescents and young adults, late congenital glaucoma[1-3, 5] or developmental glaucoma[2] have failed to distinguish this disorder from other glaucomas. Ellis suggested that JOAG resulted from a congenital remnant of the pectinate ligament.[4] Scheie defined JOAG as primary open-angle glaucoma found in older children and in young adults up to 30 yr of age.[5, 6] Gorin characterized gonioscopic features related to this disease such as abnormal width and prominence of the trabecular meshwork, absence of angle recess, and mesodermal remnants in the angle.[2] Melamed and associates described open angles with various gonioscopic findings such as thickened, membrane-like trabecular meshwork, prominent iris processes that may cover the ciliary body band and scleral spur, and a high iris insertion.[7] These findings suggest that maldevelopment of the angle structures is an important component of the pathology in this disorder.

Interestingly, many patients with JOAG have a strong family history of glaucoma. This hereditary aspect of JOAG has been described by several investigators.[8-11] In our experience, the hereditary form is generally associated with various degrees of structural changes in the angle.[7] The subgroup of patients with no family history of glaucoma may have normal-looking angles or very subtle structural characteristics such as occasional prominent iris processes or "grayish" thickening of the trabecular meshwork. Additionally, a 2:1 preponderance of male patients and an association with myopia has been reported.[1] Table 118–1 summarizes the general features of JOAG.

PATHOPHYSIOLOGY

The strong family history of glaucoma in many of these patients, along with the gonioscopic findings of thickened trabecular meshwork, high iris insertion, and prominent iris processes, are strongly suggestive of angle maldevelopment as the basic pathophysiologic mechanism in JOAG. Tawara and Inomata confirmed the possible role of an abnormal, compact trabecular meshwork in a histopathologic study of specimens from patients with JOAG.[12] The compact trabecular meshwork contained cells with fine processes and an abnormal accumulation of extracellular material in the trabecular spaces. These investigations suggested that this tissue might represent an immature development of the aqueous drainage system and account for the increased

Table 118–1. GENERAL FEATURES OF JOAG

1. Age of diagnosis from 5 to 30 yr old
2. Positive family history
3. Male:female ratio 2:1
4. Myopia

Table 118–2. GONIOSCOPIC FEATURES OF JOAG

1. Open angle
2. High insertion of the iris
3. Prominent iris processes
4. Thickening of the trabecular meshwork
5. Grayish-pale color of the trabecular meshwork

resistance to aqueous outflow. Decreased outflow facility values have been reported in patients with JOAG,[7] confirming the important role of trabecular pathology in this disease.

CLINICAL SIGNS AND SYMPTOMS

Frequently, the diagnosis of JOAG is made either by chance or relatively late in the process of the disease. Similar to primary open-angle glaucoma, there are no alarming signs such as pain, ocular irritation, or visual loss that might prompt early detection. Occasionally, however, some patients have ocular pain and discomfort associated with an elevation of intraocular pressure (IOP). Colored haloes have been described by some patients.

As discussed earlier, a family history of glaucoma is an important factor in the diagnosis of JOAG. Coexistence of myopia is also common and has been described in up to 50 percent of these patients.[7]

IOP is usually elevated in both eyes. Interestingly, despite very high levels of IOP, corneal edema, ciliary congestion, and uveitis are rarely seen. Typically, pressures as high as 50 mmHg may be measured, and IOP pattern may be brittle, with marked elevations and reductions of IOP over time. Slit-lamp examination is usually unremarkable. As mentioned earlier, gonioscopic findings of wide open angles with thickened trabecular meshwork, high insertion of the iris, and prominent iris processes are very important in making the proper diagnosis (Table 118–2). However, normal-looking angles do not preclude the diagnosis of JOAG.

The optic discs vary from being entirely normal to having advanced glaucomatous cupping. Similarly, the visual fields may be full or display typical glaucomatous changes (Table 118–3).

DIFFERENTIAL DIAGNOSIS

All young patients diagnosed with glaucoma who are aged 5 to 30 yr may have JOAG. One should make the diagnosis of JOAG only when all other subtypes of

Table 118–3. DIAGNOSTIC CLUES FOR JOAG

1. Family history
2. Associated myopia
3. Elevated IOP*
4. Glaucomatous cupping
5. Visual field defects
6. Characteristic features of the angle

*IOP, intraocular pressure.

Table 118–4. DIFFERENTIAL DIAGNOSIS OF JOAG WITH ASSOCIATED OCULAR AND EXTRAOCULAR ANOMALIES

| | Associated Ocular Anomalies | | | | | |
| | Prominent Schwalbe's Ring | Chamber Angle Anomalies | Abnormalities of the | | | Extraocular Abnormalities |
			Iris	Lens	Retina	
Late congenital glaucoma	–	+	–	–	–	–
Other developmental glaucomas:						
Sturge-Weber	–	–	–	–	–	+
Aniridia	–	+	+	–	+	±
Axenfeld's anomaly	+	+	–	–	–	–
Rieger's anomaly	+	+	+	–	–	–
Rieger's syndrome	+	+	+	–	–	+
Peter's anomaly	–	+	+	+	–	–
Pigmentary glaucoma	–	–	–	–	–	–
Posttraumatic glaucoma	–	–	±	±	+	–
Early onset POAG*	–	–	–	–	–	–

*POAG, primary open-angle glaucoma.

glaucoma associated with other anomalies or related findings have been excluded. The list of differential diagnoses is summarized in Table 118–4.

Late Congenital Glaucoma

This type of glaucoma is typically associated with other signs, such as megalocornea and Haab's striae.

Other Developmental Glaucomas

Secondary glaucomas such as the Sturge-Weber syndrome, aniridia, Axenfeld's anomaly, Rieger's anomaly, and Peter's anomaly are usually distinguishable from JOAG due to their unique characteristics associated with specific ocular and extraocular abnormalities.

1. Sturge-Weber syndrome is characterized by a unilateral port wine hemangioma that presents in the distribution of the trigeminal nerve and is associated with an ipsilateral leptomeningeal angioma. Glaucoma is present in approximately half of the cases.
2. Aniridia is a congenital disorder, characterized by bilateral "absence" of the normal iris, associated with multiple ocular defects. In addition, some cases of aniridia may be associated with systemic abnormalities (e.g., Wilms' tumor).
3. Axenfeld's anomaly is a condition in which strands of iris traverse the anterior chamber angle from peripheral iris to a prominent Schwalbe's ring. Approximately half of the cases will have glaucoma.
4. Rieger's anomaly may be considered as Axenfeld's anomaly associated with corectopia, ectropion uvea, and stromal hypoplasia with hole formation of the iris. More than half of the cases have glaucoma.
5. Rieger's syndrome describes the anomaly listed earlier associated with facial, dental, and cervical anomalies.
6. Peter's anomaly is a bilateral central defect in Descemet's membrane and corneal endothelium with thinning and opacification of the corresponding area of corneal stroma, which is present at birth. Adhesions extend from the borders of this defect to the central iris. Approximately half of the patients develop glaucoma.

Pigmentary Glaucoma

Although more prevalent in young adults and associated with myopia as in the JOAG group, this entity is easily diagnosed due to well-delineated, acceptable clinical signs. These signs include a Krukenberg spindle on the corneal endothelium, posterior bowing of the peripheral iris, typical transillumination defects of the iris periphery, pigment dusting over the iris surface and heavy pigmentation of the trabecular meshwork.

Posttraumatic Glaucoma

Posttraumatic glaucoma is typically unilateral. A history of trauma to the affected eye may be present. Other signs of ocular trauma may be found, such as corneal scars, distorted pupil, dislocated lens, vitreous in the anterior chamber, or retinal pathology. Gonioscopy may reveal various degrees of angle recession or peripheral anterior synechiae.

Early Onset of Primary Open-Angle Glaucoma

As discussed previously, this descriptive entity is indistinguishable from JOAG.

Other Secondary Glaucomas

Other types of secondary glaucomas may be distinguished from JOAG on the basis of medical history and clinical findings. Examples include steroid-induced glaucoma or glaucoma secondary to uveitis.

TREATMENT OF JOAG

Medical Therapy

Medical therapy is often insufficient to control IOP in patients with JOAG.[13] In addition to poor responsiveness to medical therapy, patients with JOAG are often noncompliant due to side effects of medications and to the general youth in this patient population.

Topical drops of pilocarpine are poorly tolerated by this group of patients because of severe induced myopia and pain associated with spasm of the ciliary muscle. Recent use of slow-release drug delivery systems like the Ocusert have helped ameliorate these problems, but some patients find the Ocusert irritating and are unable to use it on a long-term basis. Topical β-blockers and epinephrine are better tolerated by the young patient. Although carbonic anhydrase inhibitors may be well tolerated in young patients, their chronic use is often problematic due to systemic side effects.

LASER THERAPY

Argon Laser Trabeculoplasty

Argon laser trabeculoplasty is generally believed to have little value in this disease.[14] Apparently, the thick and compact trabecular tissue is less affected by the laser energy. Consequently, mechanical and biologic mechanisms usually triggered by trabecular meshwork-laser interaction[15] may be less effective. This treatment modality should be tried before traditional surgical interventions in patients in whom the trabecular band is more pigmented, or in the older patient.

Nd.YAG Laser Trabeculotomy (YLT)

The role of the maldeveloped, compact trabecular meshwork in the pathophysiology of JOAG has been confirmed by a histopathologic study.[12] Cutting through such an abnormal trabecular tissue has become an attractive concept in treating these patients either surgically, by goniotomy or trabeculotomy,[1, 2, 5, 6, 16] or with the neodymium-yttrium-aluminum-garnet (Nd.YAG) laser.[7, 17]

Melamed and associates found out that a confluent Nd.YAG laser trabeculotomy extending for at least 1 clock hr was superior to focal trabeculopuncture in four quadrants.[7] Apparently, the success of this procedure is related directly to the extent of exposure of the outer wall of Schlemm's canal and its collector channels. In 75 percent of eyes treated with YLT, the procedure was initially successful in controlling IOP. Success of the treatment appeared to be related to perforation of Schlemm's canal, creating a communication with the collector channel system. The occurrence of blood reflux into the anterior chamber was seen in all successfully treated eyes.

In many of the eyes treated, outflow facility was found to be substantially increased following the procedure. Although, in some cases, a patent trabeculotomy could explain the increased outflow and IOP reduction, gonioscopy did not always contribute to our understanding of the mechanism of action of YLT. Retrodisplacement of the iris was seen in some patients and might suggest a cyclodialysis effect. Unlike patients with primary open-angle glaucoma,[18] patients with JOAG seem to respond favorably to YLT, as they do to other trabeculotomy-type procedures.[1, 5, 6, 16] It is speculated that the immaturity of the trabecular cells in these patients may interfere with the healing capacity of the injured tissue, thus permitting communication through the trabecular holes into Schlemm's canal to remain open on a long-term basis.

It is remarkable, therefore, that the JOAG group appears to respond uniquely in such a favorable way to YLT. Because no major complications were encountered with this procedure, it is suggested that patients with JOAG whose IOP levels are uncontrolled by medical treatment, should have YLT performed before more traditional surgical intervention.

SURGICAL TREATMENT

Trabeculotomy

Surgical trabeculotomy, whether performed internally from the anterior chamber[1, 5, 6] or externally from the sclera,[16] has shown relatively good results. Whereas goniotomy is the procedure of choice in infants or children with congenital glaucoma in whom the cornea is sufficiently clear to visualize the anterior chamber angle, trabeculotomy is a satisfactory second choice, and it is the preferred procedure when the cornea is hazy. Trabeculotomy has a documented higher success rate compared with goniotomy. The latter controls IOP in approximately 74 to 85 percent of eyes with congenital glaucoma.[19, 20] Trabeculotomy, on the other hand, controls IOP in more than 90 percent[21–23] of eyes with glaucoma. Although technically successful, the trabeculotomies have a tendency to close, requiring repeated procedures.

Filtration Surgery

Filtration surgery (trabeculectomy or full thickness filter) is usually less successful in the JOAG group. The main reason for the high failure rate appears to be the excessive wound healing response in younger patients, resulting in subconjunctival fibrosis. Beauchamp and Parks[24] reported a 50 percent success rate in cases of congenital glaucoma and in patients with JOAG, and quite a few of these procedures were associated with significant complications such as vitreous loss, scleral ectasia, and retinal detachment. Gressel and associates reported a success rate of 74 percent of trabeculectomies performed in patients with primary glaucomas under the

Table 118–5. TREATMENT OPTIONS OF JOAG

1. Medical treatment
2. Laser therapy
   a. Argon laser trabeculoplasty
   b. Nd.YAG* laser trabeculotomy
3. Surgical treatment
   a. Trabeculotomy
   b. Filtering surgery
   c. Setons

*Nd.YAG, neodymium-yttrium-aluminum-garnet.

age of 50 yr.[25] However, when comparing the surgical results in patients with primary glaucoma 30 to 49 yr of age to those below age 30, the former group had a considerably higher success rate (83 percent) compared with the latter group (only 44 percent). This report may suggest that, in the absence of additional confounding factors, the vigor of the healing process in young patients may be less important after a particular age. Thus, it may be important to make every effort, when possible, to control IOP in patients with JOAG using medical or laser treatment and postpone surgery for a later date.

Implantation of Setons

In an attempt to overcome the problem of scarring conjunctiva, Molteno and associates suggested the use of an aqueous drainage device for IOP control in refractory cases of what he described as JOAG.[26] The concept of bypassing the scarred anterior conjunctiva by inserting the silicone tube into the anterior chamber and placing the collecting plate at the equator has proved to be superior to repeated standard filtration surgery in these patients. However, even with the Molteno implant, a thick fibrous tissue or a tenon's cyst may form around the plate and result in IOP elevation, requiring additional surgery. In addition, one should bear in mind that the population of patients reported had an array of diagnoses and only a few of them had JOAG with no associated ocular anomalies. The success rate of the Molteno implant may be better evaluated in patients with JOAG using a more well-defined patient population (Table 118–5).

REFERENCES

1. Goldwyn R, Waltman SR, Becker B: Primary open angle glaucoma in adolescents and young adults. Arch Ophthalmol 84:579–582, 1970.
2. Gorin G: Developmental glaucoma—A concept based on correlation of gonioscopic findings with clinical manifestations. Am J Ophthalmol 58:572–580, 1964.
3. Quitko ML: Glaucoma in infants and children. New York, Appleton-Century-Crofts, 1973, pp 186–202.
4. Ellis OH: The etiology, symptomatology and treatment of juvenile glaucoma. Am J Ophthalmol 31:1589–1596, 1948.
5. Scheie HG: Infantile and juvenile glaucoma. Trans Am Acad Ophthalmol Otolaryngol 67:458–466, 1963.
6. Scheie HG: Goniopuncture: An evaluation after eleven years. Arch Ophthalmol 65:38–48, 1961.
7. Melamed S, Latina MA, Epstein DL: Neodymium-YAG laser trabeculopuncture in juvenile open angle glaucoma. Ophthalmology 94:163–170, 1987.
8. Inowe Y, Ohnishi Y: Congenital glaucoma of late onset and intraocular pressure. Jpn J Clin Ophthalmol 23:366–378, 1969.
9. Jerndal T: Dominant goniodysgenesis with late congenital glaucoma. Am J Ophthalmol 74:28–32, 1972.
10. Martin JP, Zorab EC: Familial glaucoma in nine generations of a South Hampshire family. Br J Ophthalmol 58:536–542, 1974.
11. Razemon P, Capier MJ, Couter P: Le glaucoma juvenile heredo-familial. Bull Soc Ophthalmol France 74:471–474, 1974.
12. Tawara A, Inomata H: Developmental immaturity of the trabecular meshwork in juvenile glaucoma. Am J Ophthalmol 98:82–97, 1984.
13. Walton DS: Juvenile open angle glaucoma. In Chandler PA, Grant WM (eds): Glaucoma, 2nd ed. Philadelphia, Lea & Febiger, 1979, pp 269–270.
14. Thomas JV, Simmons RJ, Belcher DL: Argon laser trabeculoplasty in the pre-surgical glaucoma patient. Ophthalmology 89:187–197, 1982.
15. Melamed S, Pei J, Epstein DL: Short term effect of argon laser trabeculoplasty in monkeys. Arch Ophthalmol 103:1546–1552, 1985.
16. Mcpherson SD Jr, Berry DP: Goniotomy vs external trabeculotomy for developmental glaucoma. Am J Ophthalmol 95:427–431, 1983.
17. Kitazawa Y, Yumita A, Shirato S, et al: Q-switched Nd-YAG laser for developmental glaucoma. Ophthalmic Surg 16:99–100, 1985.
18. Epstein DL, Melamed S, Puliafito CA, et al: Neodymium-YAG laser trabeculopuncture in open angle glaucoma. Ophthalmology 92:931–937, 1985.
19. Kwitko ML: Glaucoma in Infants and Children. New York, Appleton-Century-Crofts, 1973.
20. Shields MB: Textbook of Glaucoma, 2nd ed. Baltimore, Williams & Wilkins, 1986.
21. Gregersen E, Kessing SVV: Congenital glaucoma before and after the introduction of microsurgery: Results of "macrosurgery" 1943–1963 and of microsurgery (trabeculotomy/ectomy) 1970–1974. Acta Ophthalmol 55:422, 1977.
22. Luntz MH: Primary buphthalmos (infantile glaucoma) treated by trabeculotomy ab extreme. S Afr Arch Ophthalmol 2:219, 1974.
23. McPherson SD Jr: Results of external trabeculotomy. Am J Ophthalmol 76:918, 1973.
24. Beauchamp GR, Parks MM: Filtering surgery in children: Barriers to success. Ophthalmology 86:170–180, 1986.
25. Gressel MG, Heuer DK, Parrish RK: Trabeculectomy in young patients. Ophthalmology 91:1242–1246, 1984.
26. Molteno ACB, Ancker E, Van Biljon G: Surgical technique for advanced juvenile glaucoma. Arch Ophthalmol 102:51–57, 1984.

Chapter 119

∎

Normal-Tension Glaucoma (Low-Tension Glaucoma)

DAVID P. WELLINGTON and MURRAY A. JOHNSTONE

Historical Background

In 1857 von Graefe[1,2] astutely described "amaurosis and nerve head excavation" without a palpable elevation of pressure. Since this unorthodox description of glaucoma did not conform with current beliefs, it encountered strong opposition at the time. A half-century later, however, with the advent of the Schiotz tonometer, others began to report cases of glaucoma with normal intraocular pressure. Many terms for the condition subsequently arose and have included glaucoma-like cupping of the optic nerve head, pseudoglaucoma, posterior glaucoma, paraglaucoma posterior, and low-tension glaucoma.

At first the condition was thought to be relatively rare, and experts considered that many cases represented ischemic optic neuropathy that had been incorrectly diagnosed.[4] Attitudes changed, however, when population studies on glaucoma, which began in the 1960s, revealed that low-tension glaucoma is more prevalent than was earlier recognized.[5–15]

The concept embodied in the phrase, low-tension glaucoma, challenges traditional theories regarding the causal relationship between elevated intraocular pressure and optic nerve damage. Since its initial description, the disease process has confused and baffled ophthalmologists, and a complete understanding of its pathogenesis continues to elude investigators. Even the term "low-tension glaucoma," which has been so widely popularized, is a misnomer. Intraocular pressure is typically in the normal or high-normal range rather than in the low range in this condition, and Drance's[16] suggestion that it should be called "glaucoma with normal pressure" seems reasonable. "Normal-tension glaucoma" is a term gaining increased acceptance in recent literature,[17,18] and this name is used throughout this chapter.

Definitions

A variety of definitions for normal-tension glaucoma have been proposed. Some are purely descriptive, whereas others allude to the cause or course of the disease. In addition to cupping and visual field loss, Duke-Elder and Jay[4] included reduced aqueous outflow facility in their definition. Chandler and Grant[19] and Hoskins[20] believed that progression of visual field loss or cupping was an integral part of the definition. Spaeth[21] and Kolker and Hetherington[22] defined the condition as

optic nerve damage induced by intraocular pressure, even though the pressure was always within the normal range.

Although there may be merit to all of these definitions, it appears premature at our present state of knowledge to include causal statements in the definition of normal-tension glaucoma. Until a more thorough understanding of the pathogenesis is acquired, it would seem prudent to define the disease in a strictly descriptive manner as has been done by Levene and others.[11,23,24]

Thus, normal-tension glaucoma may be simply defined as an optic neuropathy with the classic findings of glaucomatous cupping of the optic nerve head and corresponding visual field defects in the presence of open angles, intraocular pressure consistently recorded below 21 mmHg, and the absence of any contributing ocular or systemic disorders.

CLINICAL MANIFESTATIONS

Epidemiology

INCIDENCE

The incidence of any disease depends on the criteria used to define the disease. The incidence of normal-tension glaucoma is affected by the upper limit of the intraocular pressure used, the frequency of the intraocular pressure measurements, and the degree of thoroughness used to rule out other conditions masquerading as normal-tension glaucoma.

Obviously, the higher the pressure used to separate normal-tension glaucoma from open-angle glaucoma, the higher will be the incidence of the former. There has not been collective agreement in the past regarding the exact pressure value that divides normal-tension glaucoma from high-tension glaucoma. Values have varied between 21 mmHg and 25 mmHg, depending on the author's personal preference and historical precedent. Surveys of normal distributions of intraocular pressure indicate that the mean in the normal Caucasian population is 15.6 mmHg and that 97 percent have a pressure less than 24 mmHg. Our concepts of "normal" and "abnormal" intraocular pressure are derived from statistics such as these.

The frequency of intraocular pressure measurements is a key factor in determining the incidence of normal-tension glaucoma. As the frequency of tonometric recordings increases, the likelihood of discovering an abnormally high pressure in any particular patient also increases.

Estimates of the prevalence of normal-tension glaucoma in the general community vary from 7 to 68 percent of all those found to have primary glaucomatous disc and field changes. These figures are based on a number of population surveys that have been published since 1966 (Fig. 119–1).[6, 9, 10, 13, 14, 25–28] The inconsistency of the percentages obtained by different authors may be anticipated, since many of the studies did not measure diurnal pressure fluctuations and the upper limit of "normal" intraocular pressure ranged from 20.5 to 23 mmHg. However, even with their shortcomings, it is clear from these independent population studies that normal-tension glaucoma is a common condition and may represent from one sixth to one half of all open-angle glaucoma cases.

HEREDITY

The genetic or familial component that sometimes has a role in primary open-angle glaucoma may well exert a similar influence in normal-tension glaucoma. The occurrence of cases of both types of glaucoma within the same family has often been reported.[3, 11, 29–34] There is also an isolated report of a family with a distinct type of progressive normal-tension glaucoma that presented as an autosomal dominant condition in 12 individuals spanning five generations.[35] The true significance of heredity and its influence on normal-tension glaucoma is unknown.

AGE, SEX, AND RACE

Although normal-tension glaucoma has been reported in younger individuals, it is most often seen in people over 60 yr of age.[3, 11, 29–31] Some studies indicate that the disease is more common in women,[3, 11, 29] but this may be due to the fact that women outnumber men in the older age group. There is no information to indicate a racial predilection for normal-tension glaucoma.

Typical Presentation

Clinical practices typically do not reflect a prevalence of normal-tension glaucoma like that found in clinical studies, which is probably due to a lack of detection. Most cases of primary open-angle glaucoma are first detected by an elevated intraocular pressure. Detection of normal-tension glaucoma does not occur until abnormal disc cupping or visual field defects are identified. Subtle disc changes may not be recognized without elevated intraocular pressure. This is probably the reason why most patients with normal-tension glaucoma are diagnosed at a later stage in the disease.

A typical patient with normal-tension glaucoma may present with visual symptoms relative to an extensive visual field loss, but more commonly the patient has no complaints and the index of suspicion is raised only through careful optic nerve head evaluation.

There is disagreement among authors with regard to whether the disc cupping in normal-tension glaucoma differs significantly from primary open-angle glaucoma. In a comprehensive review by Levene,[11] optic disc cupping appeared the same in both patients with normal-tension glaucoma and high-tension glaucoma. His impression, however, was that the amount of cupping was disproportionately greater than the amount of visual field loss in the normal-tension group.

Greve and Geijssen[36] have reported that optic nerve head excavations tend to be larger with steeper margins in patients with high intraocular pressure compared with the cups of patients with normal-tension glaucoma with more sloping margins. Caprioli and Spaeth[37] found that the neural rims of the patients with normal-tension glaucoma tend to be thinner in the temporal and inferior portions of the disc compared with the patients who have high-pressure glaucoma. They also agreed with Levene's observation that for a given amount of cupping the degree of glaucomatous visual field loss appeared to be less in normal-tension glaucoma.

Using stereoscopic photographs Lewis and coworkers[38] and Miller and Quigley[39] were unable to detect differences in the optic nerve heads in patients with normal-tension glaucoma and high-tension glaucoma. King and associates[40] used computed tomography and Fazio and coworkers[41] utilized quantitative optic disc topography to evaluate glaucomatous alterations of the optic nerve. Their results also failed to show any significant differences in cup:disc ratio and neuroretinal rim loss between eyes with normal-tension and high-tension glaucoma. Fazio and coworkers[41] reported, however,

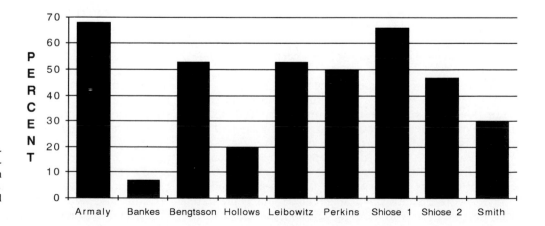

Figure 119–1. Prevalence of normal tension among newly identified glaucomas. Population studies are from references 25, 6, 26, 9, 10, 13, 14, 27, and 28, respectively.

that the volume of the optic cup did not correlate with the cup:disc ratio and neuroretinal rim area in normal-tension glaucoma. In other words, the disc volume did not increase proportionately with increases in the cup:disc ratio and decreases in the neuroretinal rim, as it did in primary open-angle glaucoma. Computed tomography techniques indicated that in normal-tension glaucoma the cupping is broadly sloping, which results in less volume change to the disc as the neuroretinal rim tissue is lost.

Javitt and coworkers[42] have observed that focal loss of neural rim tissue is sometimes associated with pronounced excavation and also with loss of lamina cribrosa. The authors found that pitlike localized cupping was present in 74 percent of their patients with normal-tension glaucoma but only in 15 percent of those with high-tension glaucoma. They suggest that the acquired pits may signal a primary structural or vascular weakness of the optic nerve that makes it abnormally susceptible to the damaging effects of intraocular pressure.

Rivaling the controversial nature of optic nerve cupping in normal-tension glaucoma is the issue of visual field loss. Levene[11] noted that a larger proportion of patients with normal-tension glaucoma have visual field defects closer to fixation. Greve and Geijssen[43] and Caprioli and Spaeth[44] report that the defects are denser, steeper, closer to fixation, and more often located in the superior half of the visual field in normal-tension glaucoma. Other investigators who have compared the field defects of normal-tension glaucoma and high-tension glaucoma at approximately the same stage of disc damage have failed to show any differences in the pattern of the defects.[14, 45, 46]

One of the problems in the past has been that many studies have not compared the same stage of the glaucomatous process. As already mentioned, open-angle glaucoma is often detected earlier because of elevated pressure even without a major optic nerve head abnormality. Normal-tension glaucoma is often recognized only after considerable tissue damage at the optic nerve has occured. When investigators specifically compare the two conditions at the same stage of the disease, differences in nerve head appearance seem to be less pronounced. King and coworkers[47] reported that when eyes with normal-tension glaucoma and high-tension glaucoma are matched for the degree of cupping, the pattern of visual field loss is identical. Similarly when eyes with normal-tension and high-tension glaucoma are matched for the degree of visual field loss, cupping is identical.

As the technology of automated perimetry has become more sophisticated, articles dealing with the statistical analysis of visual field sensitivity have yielded some interesting findings. By utilizing indices such as mean deviation and corrected pattern standard deviation, quantitative information regarding diffuse and localized visual field damage can be obtained.[48, 49] Drance and associates[50] showed that in patients with arcuate defects limited to one hemifield, there was twice as much diffuse loss of sensitivity in the spared hemifield in eyes with chronic open-angle glaucoma compared with the patients with normal-tension glaucoma. In a

subsequent article,[51] patients with normal-tension glaucoma and high-tension glaucoma who were matched closely for extent of field damage were studied. The undisturbed areas of the visual fields in both groups were tested, and the results showed that the group with normal-tension glaucoma had greater areas with normal light sensitivity. These studies and the work of others[52, 53] support the hypothesis that patients who have glaucoma and lower intraocular pressure have more localized damage, whereas patients who have higher intraocular pressure have more diffuse damage.

Research in the field of chromatic sensitivity has led to some findings that further support the idea that the visual damage of high-tension glaucoma differs from that of normal-tension glaucoma. Drance's group compared the chromatic thresholds at various wavelengths of patients with high-tension glaucoma and normal-tension glaucoma who had similar visual field defects.[54] They discovered that the patients who had high-tension glaucoma revealed statistically significantly greater sensitivity losses, especially in the blue color range, compared with the patients with normal-tension glaucoma. It is known that blue chromatic signals travel in larger diameter axons than do red-green signals in the primate visual system. In experimental animal glaucoma models it has been shown that larger diameter axons are more susceptible to increased pressure than are small axons. More study in this area needs to be done, but preliminary findings seem to suggest that the mechanism of damage in high-tension glaucoma involves larger axons and more diffuse damage, whereas in normal-tension glaucoma the damage is more localized and is confined to the small axonal fibers.

Risk Factors

It is important for the ophthalmologist to realize that certain factors may affect the incidence and severity of normal-tension glaucoma. Although these factors may not be causal, the frequency with which they are seen leads many authorities to believe that their presence significantly increases the risk for developing normal-tension glaucoma. Age and family history represent general risk factors. Both ocular and systemic risk factors may also be identified (Fig. 119–2).

OCULAR RISK FACTORS

Intraocular Pressure. In most cases of normal-tension glaucoma the intraocular pressures cluster at the upper end of the so-called normal range. Many people consider that intraocular pressure may be an important risk factor for patients with normal-tension glaucoma just as it is in high-tension glaucoma. Cartwright and Anderson[55] studied a group of patients with normal-tension glaucoma with asymmetric intraocular pressures. In a statistically significant number the cupping and field loss were greater in the eye with the higher pressure. In a more recent study of unequal mean intraocular pressures and asymmetric visual field defects in patients with normal-tension glaucoma, Critchton and coworkers[56] confirmed that visual field damage was usually greater on the side

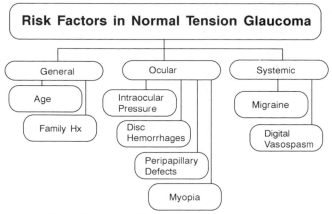

Risk Factors in Normal Tension Glaucoma

- General
  - Age
  - Family Hx
- Ocular
  - Intraocular Pressure
  - Disc Hemorrhages
  - Peripapillary Defects
  - Myopia
- Systemic
  - Migraine
  - Digital Vasospasm

Figure 119–2. Flow chart illustrating risk factors to consider in normal-tension glaucoma. (Hx, history.)

with the higher mean intraocular pressure. These findings suggest that the level of pressure is a factor in producing optic nerve cupping and visual field defects in normal-tension glaucoma. The authors of both of these studies point out, however, that many patients with asymmetric visual field loss do not have appropriately unequal mean intraocular pressures. Thus, there must be factors other than intraocular pressure that contribute to the field loss in such patients.

In a retrospective study by Sugiura and associates,[57] cases of progressive and nonprogressive normal-tension glaucoma were reviewed. Both the mean and maximum intraocular pressures were significantly higher in the group that showed progression of optic disc changes and visual field defects. Yamagami and associates[58] compared intraocular pressure and field defects between pairs of eyes in 46 patients with normal-tension glaucoma. By using discriminant analysis with the Humphrey (30-2) STATPAC program they determined that in eyes in which the more advanced field defects were associated with the higher intraocular pressure, the mean pressure level was 15 mmHg or higher. Below this cut-off level, intraocular pressure showed no significant correlation to visual field damage. The authors concluded that intraocular pressure can be an aggravating factor in normal-tension glaucoma, especially if the mean follow-up pressure is 15 mmHg or above.

Optic Disc Hemorrhage. Bjerrum is reported to have been the first person to describe optic disc hemorrhage and its relationship to glaucoma in 1889.[59] Since then, many articles have described the prevalence of optic disc hemorrhage in glaucoma and its importance as a prognostic sign of future progressive optic nerve damage.[26, 60–67] Several authors[11, 29, 30, 68] have studied the incidence of optic disc hemorrhage in normal-tension glaucoma, and the prevailing evidence indicates that there is a higher frequency of such hemorrhages in patients with normal-tension glaucoma compared with their chronic open-angle glaucoma counterparts.

In 1986 Kitazawa and colleagues[69] reported on a retrospective study in which they found optic disc hemorrhage in 20.5 percent of their patients with normal-tension glaucoma (Fig. 119–3). A prospective study was also conducted in which patients with normal-tension glaucoma were followed monthly for 6 mo. In this group the overall incidence of hemorrhage was 24.8 percent (28 of 113 eyes). When compared with patients with primary open-angle glaucoma in their study, the prevalence of disc hemorrhage in normal-tension glaucoma was five times greater. Other results from their investigation indicated that eyes with normal-tension glaucoma seem to consist of two different groups: one group that develops recurrent disc hemorrhage and another group that is very unlikely to bleed through the entire course of the disease.

Shiose[70] reported that the type of cupping affects the frequency of optic disc hemorrhage. He found that eyes with unidirectional cupping showed over twice as many hemorrhages as did those with expansive cupping. The true significance of splinter or flame-shaped hemorrhage, which is usually located at the inferotemporal or superotemporal neuroretinal rim of the optic disc, is unclear. Many authorities have presumed that it represented a chronic ischemic process in the optic nerve head.[23] Others[71] consider that it is a consequence of structural changes of the nerve rather than of local infarction or vascular insufficiency. They suggest that as the lamina cribrosa becomes distorted, the shearing of laminar plates could damage blood vessels and cause bleeding. Is optic disc hemorrhage a sign of progressive disease and does it have prognostic importance when it occurs in normal-tension glaucoma? Certainly more investigation needs to be done before this question can be

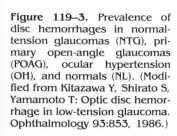

Figure 119–3. Prevalence of disc hemorrhages in normal-tension glaucomas (NTG), primary open-angle glaucomas (POAG), ocular hypertension (OH), and normals (NL). (Modified from Kitazawa Y, Shirato S, Yamamoto T: Optic disc hemorrhage in low-tension glaucoma. Ophthalmology 93:853, 1986.)

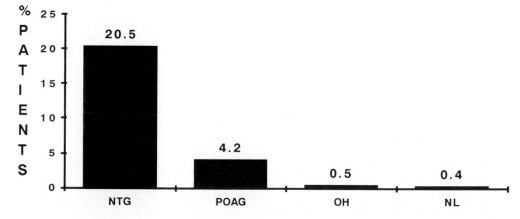

answered with certainty. At our present state of knowledge it seems reasonable to consider the finding of optic disc hemorrhage in normal-tension glaucoma as cause for concern and to include this finding in the list of probable risk factors.

Peripapillary Defects. The absence of retinal pigment epithelium around or adjacent to an optic disc is often described as a chorioscleral halo or crescent. Several authors[72, 73] have found a high prevalence of such peripapillary abnormalities in patients with glaucoma. Rockwood and Anderson[74] reported that the crescents or halos were especially common in patients with disc damage at normal or only mildly elevated intraocular pressure. In a more recent study, Buus and Anderson[75] compared the incidence and size of peripapillary changes in patients with normal-tension glaucoma with cupped discs with a group of patients with ocular hypertension and healthy discs. The frequency and average area of bared peripapillary choroid and sclera were significantly higher in the normal-tension group. It has also been shown that the location of the chorioscleral crescent usually corresponds to the sector of greatest disc damage.[76, 77]

The term senile sclerotic glaucoma[78] has been used to describe cases of cupping that are prominently associated with peripapillary changes. This implies that vascular sclerosis is a factor in the pathogenesis, but this supposition has not been proved. In some cases, peripapillary atrophy of the retinal pigment epithelium may progressively occur along with the gradually increasing disc cupping and may simply be part of the overall glaucomatous process.[74] In other cases, preexisting congenital peripapillary defects may exist that predispose certain eyes to glaucomatous change.[79, 80] In other patients the peripapillary defects may be age-related but may precede the glaucoma and may somehow cause the disc to become more vulnerable to subsequent damage.[81, 82]

At the present time the evidence seems to indicate that there is a correlation between disc damage and peripapillary crescents and halos. Because of their increased incidence in normal-tension glaucoma they may be considered an anatomic risk factor, but further research is needed to determine their causal relationship, if any, to the glaucomatous process.

Myopia. It is generally believed that myopic eyes are more sensitive to pressure than are nonmyopic eyes. Perkins and Phelps[83, 84] have looked at the distribution of refractive error in glaucoma and have determined that myopia occurs more frequently among patients with open-angle glaucoma, ocular hypertension, and normal-tension glaucoma than would be expected in the normal population. It is theorized that the congenital misalignment of the peripapillary tissue layers in myopia may contribute in some way to an increased vulnerability to pressures even in the normal range. Leighton and Tomlinson[85] reported a higher incidence of axial myopia in patients with normal-tension glaucoma compared with patients who have chronic open-angle glaucoma. Although some authors[30, 86] could not confirm this observation, there is suggestive evidence that myopia should be considered a risk factor in normal-tension glaucoma.

SYSTEMIC RISK FACTORS

Vascular Disease. The relationship between systemic blood pressure and normal-tension glaucoma has always been a controversial issue. Early observations by Sjogren[3] indicated that low blood pressure was a frequent finding in individuals with normal-tension glaucoma. Other authors[31, 87–89] later agreed with the impression that blood pressures were lower in patients with normal-tension glaucoma compared with those in patients with high-tension glaucoma. In 1972, Drance[23] reported the high prevalence of hemodynamic crises including myocardial infarction and perioperative hypotension among his patients with normal-tension glaucoma. He also showed that such patients were less likely to develop progressive visual field loss.[30, 90] Subsequently, some authors[29] have confirmed these findings whereas others have not.[11, 31, 89, 91]

Another area of disagreement involves the association of normal-tension glaucoma with systemic vascular disease. There is a popular belief that generalized vascular disease is common in normal-tension glaucoma. Articles can be found in the literature that both support[31] and refute this impression.[26, 30, 88, 89] In an investigation by Drance and coworkers[92] a thorough search for vascular etiologic factors was conducted on 162 subjects comprised of individuals with normal-tension glaucoma, open-angle high-tension glaucoma, and nonglaucomatous age-matched controls. Extensive noninvasive vascular and rheologic profiles were performed on all three groups. These included biochemical, coagulation, and hematology tests and multiple blood pressure recordings taken before and after exercise. When the test results of the three groups were compared, no statistically significant differences were detected. Because of the lack of diagnostic abnormalities, the authors concluded that there is no evidence to support a generalized organic vascular pathology for normal-tension glaucoma. They suggest that if vascular factors are important in the cause of normal-tension glaucoma then they must be localized or vasospastic.

The role of vasospasm in normal-tension glaucoma was first reported by Corbett and associates.[93] In 1985, this group studied patients with normal-tension glaucoma for evidence of central nervous system involvement. Their neurologic evaluation included a detailed history and physical examination, electroencephalography, computed tomography scan, and neurobehavioral tests. Although no correlation between normal-tension glaucoma and central nervous system disease could be detected, the authors were surprised to find that 48 percent of their patients with normal-tension glaucoma gave a positive history of classic migraine. In a followup study[94] the frequency of headache with migrainous symptomatology was compared in normal-tension glaucoma, open-angle glaucoma, and ocular hypertension and also in the normal eye. In age-matched groups the frequency of migraine headache was highest in patients with normal-tension glaucoma. Although a more recent survey of the prevalence of migraine in Japan failed to confirm these findings,[95] many authors theorize that vasospastic events may play a significant role in the pathogenesis of normal-tension glaucoma.[96]

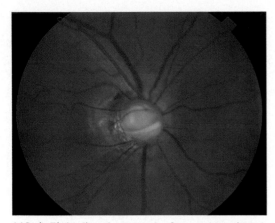

Figure 119–4. Right disc photograph of normal-tension glaucoma in a 45-year-old woman. The excavated disc shows pitlike focal loss of lamina cribrosa centrally. Risk factors exhibited by this patient include (1) positive family history: mother with primary open-angle glaucoma, sister with normal-tension glaucoma; (2) myopia; (3) peripapillary crescent; (4) migraine; (5) digital vasospasm; and (6) disc hemorrhage noted during the initial examination.

Inspired by Phelps' observations and the work of others such as Gasser and associates[97] and Flammer and associates,[98] Drance and coworkers[99] studied the occurrence of vasospasm in nonglaucomatous subjects and in patients with normal-tension glaucoma. Doppler measurements of capillary blood flow in the finger were compared in the two groups. Both the mean baseline digital blood flow and the blood flow after exposure to cold water were significantly lower in the patients with normal-tension glaucoma compared with the individuals with normal eyes. It was also noted that subjects with a history of migraine had a greater vasospastic response after exposure to cold than did those without migraine. Nail fold capillaroscopy studies by Gasser and Flammer[100] compared the blood-flow velocity in high-tension glaucoma, normal-tension glaucoma, and control groups. There were no measurable differences in the morphologic findings, but the patients with normal-tension glaucoma showed a statistically significant de-

crease in capillary blood-cell velocity when compared with the high-tension and control subjects. This difference became even more pronounced after cold provocation.

It is obvious that the whole subject of vascular disease as it relates to the cause of normal-tension glaucoma is still poorly understood. There appears to be strong evidence that vasospasm may be a key factor. Migraine and other conditions that reflect vasomotor instability may constitute a significant risk factor for the development of normal-tension glaucoma. Figures 119–4 and 119–5 document disc and field findings in a patient who illustrates many of the risk factors seen in normal-tension glaucoma.

PATHOGENESIS

The true nature of normal-tension glaucoma and its relationship to chronic open-angle glaucoma remains controversial. Are normal-tension glaucoma and high-tension glaucoma two separate disease entities with different etiologies or is the underlying pathologic process the same in both? Some investigators believe that normal-tension glaucoma should be classified as a primary open-angle glaucoma in which the optic nerve is more susceptible to the effects of lower intraocular pressure.[30] Other investigators believe that normal-tension glaucoma and primary open-angle glaucoma may have different causes.[29, 37, 44]

What factors other than intraocular pressure cause the optic nerves of patients with normal-tension glaucoma to be vulnerable to an acceleration of neuronal loss? The "mechanical theory" of glaucomatous nerve damage implies that increased intraocular pressure distorts the lamina cribosa and causes compression damage to the axons and interference with axoplasmic flow. Proponents of this theory believe that in normal-tension glaucoma there may be local weaknesses of the structural components of the nerve itself. A connective tissue defect at the lamina or in the glial support tissue could increase the nerve's susceptibility to damage, even in the presence of normal pressure.

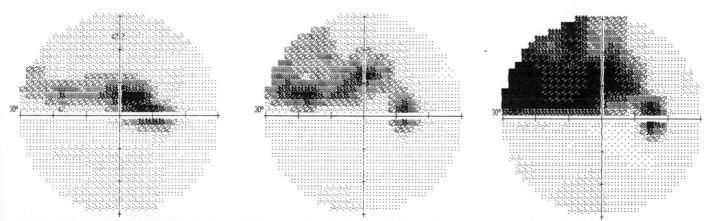

Figure 119–5. Right visual fields of same patient as in Figure 119–4, showing progressive deterioration over an 18-mo period. After institution of maximally tolerated medical therapy and laser trabeculoplasty, pressures have been reduced to the range of 7 to 11 mmHg. Visual fields have remained stable since November, 1988.

The "ischemic theory" of glaucomatous damage proposes that elevated intraocular pressure causes a relative ischemia of the optic nerve head that eventually destroys axons. Many authorities have long considered that hypoperfusion of the optic nerve head also has a primary role in the development of normal-tension glaucoma. In 1972 Drance observed that patients with normal-tension glaucoma often had a history of a previous acute hypotensive episode.[90, 101] Hayreh[102] believed that normal-tension glaucoma differed from anterior ischemic optic neuropathy only in the fact that the latter was a more acute process. The literature contains many reports of an increased incidence of cardiovascular and hematologic abnormalities associated with normal-tension glaucoma. Hypercoagulability,[30] hypercholesterolemia, increased blood viscosity,[103, 104] abnormal ophthalmodynamometry,[30, 31, 105, 106] carotid artery disease,[107, 108] hemodynamic crises,[90, 101] hypertension, hypotension,[3, 30] and migraine,[93] have all been implicated in normal-tension glaucoma. Other studies,[31, 87, 103, 104, 109–111] however, have failed to show a higher prevalence of vascular disease in normal-tension glaucoma when compared with high-tension glaucoma. From the bulk of evidence to date it does seem that hypoperfusion of the optic nerve head is an important consideration, but its precise role in the pathogenesis of normal-tension glaucoma remains uncertain. It is possible that all glaucomatous damage is pressure-induced but that there are many factors that reduce optic nerve resistance to any given pressure, vascular disease being only one of them.

It is becoming increasingly clear that an arbitrary separation of normal-tension glaucoma and high-tension glaucoma into two distinct groups on the basis of pressure is untenable. Because of the obvious overlap, it appears more appropriate to consider normal-tension glaucoma and primary open-angle glaucoma as different ends of the same spectrum. At the high-pressure end of the spectrum, glaucomatous damage results from susceptibility factors that are strongly pressure dependent. At the low-pressure end, the mechanisms of damage are only slightly pressure dependent or are possibly pressure independent. As knowledge of mechanisms and susceptibility factors increases, a more accurate classification of normal-tension glaucoma and primary open-angle glaucoma based on pathophysiologic differences may be developed.

DIFFERENTIAL DIAGNOSIS

The diagnosis of normal-tension glaucoma is a diagnosis of exclusion. Entities in the differential diagnosis that must be excluded are shown in Figure 119–6.

Undetected Intraocular Pressure Elevation

TRANSIENT ELEVATIONS OF INTRAOCULAR PRESSURE

Ruling out undetected chronic open-angle high-tension glaucoma should be a primary initial objective. Diurnal variations in intraocular pressure are commonly seen in both the normal population and in the glaucoma population. It is therefore helpful to record the intraocular pressure of a normal-tension glaucoma suspect at frequent intervals throughout the day. Even a diurnal

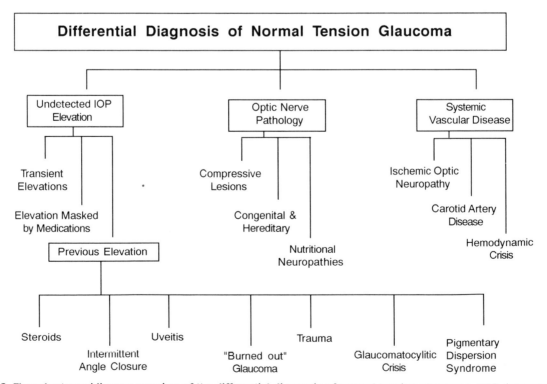

Figure 119–6. Flow chart providing an overview of the differential diagnosis of normal-tension glaucoma. (IOP, intraocular pressure.)

pressure curve determination in the office may not detect transient spikes in pressure that occur late in the day or night. Such spikes may occur at the same time every day or may occur in an irregular pattern. In addition to daily fluctuations some individuals show fluctuation of intraocular pressure over several days, weeks, or months—the so-called "phasic variation."[112] Wilensky and Geiser[113] and others suspect that many patients who have been diagnosed as having normal-tension glaucoma are, in fact, experiencing abnormal phasic pressure variations. Their intraocular pressures may be normal for weeks, but then for several days the pressure rises to abnormal levels at which time glaucomatous damage occurs. It is thought by some that spikes of high pressure often occur in patients with abnormally low outflow facility who, for unknown reasons, at times secrete a greater amount of aqueous. On such occasions a sporadic rise in intraocular pressure is thus produced.

There is considerable evidence that altering body position affects intraocular pressure. Many authors[114–117] have documented that intraocular pressure increases when an individual changes from a sitting position to a supine position. Intraocular pressure increases in a position-dependent manner when the head is below the heart.[118] This mechanism has been reported as a cause of "pseudo-low-tension glaucoma" by Rice and Allen.[119] In this case, a patient with optic nerve cupping and visual field loss had repeatedly normal intraocular pressure during the office visit. When it was learned that the patient practiced yoga exercises daily by doing full headstands, the authors measured the pressure during this inverted position and found that it rose to 37 mmHg. It is possible that postural changes of intraocular pressure play a more significant role in normal-tension glaucoma than is presently realized.

Eliminating transient elevations of intraocular pressure from the differential diagnosis of normal-tension glaucoma is not an easy task. Home tonometry has been advocated and is gaining in popularity.[120, 121] As newer advances occur in this area it is hoped that more patients will be able to accurately monitor their own intraocular pressures in a nonoffice setting. This would significantly reduce the practical difficulties that the ophthalmologist now faces in diagnosing normal-tension glaucoma.

PREVIOUS ELEVATION OF INTRAOCULAR PRESSURE

When considering the differential diagnosis of normal-tension glaucoma the clinician must be careful to exclude patients whose history indicates that they have experienced elevated intraocular pressure in the past that subsequently became normalized. Such an example is the individual who develops secondary glaucoma from the use of corticosteroids. Upon cessation of the steroid therapy the intraocular pressure returns to normal but the patient is left with permanent, albeit nonprogressive, disc cupping and visual field loss. Other conditions that could produce a temporary but damaging elevation of intraocular pressure include uveitis, trauma, glaucomatocyclitic crisis, pigmentary dispersion syndrome, and intermittent angle-closure. At the time of initial pres-

entation these secondary glaucomas may be in remission, and it is only through a careful history and examination that their prior existence can be suspected.

One entity that has been frequently mentioned in the literature is "burned-out glaucoma." Patients with this condition are described as having had chronic open-angle glaucoma in the past with high tension and the resultant sequelae. Late in the course of the disease the untreated intraocular pressure drops as the result of ciliary body atrophy and aqueous hyposecretion. When first seen, such patients have normal intraocular pressure, very low outflow facility, and are usually elderly with end-stage glaucomatous disease. Some authors feel that burned-out glaucoma exists as a distinct entity[113] whereas others think that the progression of chronic open-angle glaucoma to a burned-out state is uncommon.[122, 123]

ELEVATION MASKED BY MEDICATION

The clinician must always keep in mind that certain systemic medications may mask the existence of chronic open-angle glaucoma. Aqueous secretion requires the presence of specific enzyme systems that are inhibited by the digitalis glycosides. A single daily dose of digoxin in the digitalized patient is sufficient to maintain the secretory inhibition of aqueous and to significantly lower intraocular pressure. In one study[124] digoxin suppressed aqueous formation by 45 percent; acetazolamide suppressed aqueous formation by 50 percent; and a combination of these two inhibitors reduced aqueous formation by 65 percent.

Beta-blockers constitute another category of systemic drugs that can lower intraocular pressure. Several studies have shown that patients with uncontrolled glaucoma have had their intraocular pressure normalized with 10 to 40 mg of propranolol (Inderal) administered orally three times a day.[125, 126] Similarly, systemic nadolol (Corgard) is effective in lowering intraocular pressure.[127] Timolol (Blocadren, Timolide) may also be expected to produce an ocular hypotensive effect when taken orally.

In the differential diagnosis of normal-tension glaucoma the clinician must consider the dampening effect that certain systemic medications may have on intraocular pressure. A careful history of the current systemic medications is important. In some cases short-term discontinuance of a systemic drug may be useful to detect the presence of a hidden high-tension glaucoma.

Optic Nerve Pathology

COMPRESSIVE LESIONS

Nonglaucomatous optic nerve disease must always be considered in the differential diagnosis of normal-tension glaucoma. Because of their treatable nature, compressive lesions of the visual pathway should be foremost on the list of important entities to be considered. Optic atrophy caused by tumors of the optic nerve or chiasm have been mistaken for glaucomatous cupping.[128, 129] In one study, 8 of 141 (5.7 percent) of subjects suspected of having glaucoma by optic disc screening were found to have intracranial lesions.[27] Visual field defects that mimic those of glaucoma can also result from tumors as reported by Hupp and associates.[130]

CONGENITAL AND HEREDODEGENERATIVE ABNORMALITIES

Anomalies of the optic nerve head that may simulate glaucomatous cupping need to be recognized. These anomalies include congenitally large physiologic cups, hypoplastic discs, myopic discs, oblique insertion of the optic nerve, colobomas, pits, and drusen of the nerve head. Since many of these conditions may also be associated with visual field defects, the clinician must be vigilant to properly identify these entities.

Hereditary disorders such as Leber's disease and Behr's syndrome should be included in the list of conditions that cause optic neuropathy. The optic atrophy associated with these conditions usually poses no diagnostic problem since cupping is not part of the clinical picture. Mention should be made, however, of a dominant form of juvenile optic atrophy that is characterized by temporal disc pallor and temporal sectoral excavation.[131] In such cases the visual field generally shows cecocentral defects with mild reduction of central acuity. At times, however, progressive glaucomatous-like field defects and deeply excavated discs have been reported.[35, 132]

NUTRITIONAL NEUROPATHIES

Nutritional amblyopia, pernicious anemia, and vitamin B deficiency are often included in the differential diagnosis of normal-tension glaucoma. In most cases the optic neuropathy produced by these entities should not pose a diagnostic problem, since the field defects are usually central or cecocentral and the discs are not cupped. One should always keep in mind, however, that at times atypical glaucoma field deficits may have a cecocentral appearance.[133] In such cases it is conceivable that the ocular findings of a patient with atypical normal-tension glaucoma may mimic a toxic or nutritional optic atrophy.

Systemic Vascular Disease

ISCHEMIC OPTIC NEUROPATHY AND CRANIAL ARTERITIS

A number of systemic vascular conditions can produce optic nerve and visual field changes that may masquerade as normal-tension glaucoma. Altitudinal and arcuate scotomata have frequently been associated with ischemic optic neuropathy, cranial arteritis, and emboli. In all of these conditions infarction of the optic nerve is believed to play a dominant role. Disc edema may be present initially, but as the swelling resolves optic atrophy ensues and temporal disc pallor appears. In some cases cupping develops and resembles that seen in normal-tension glaucoma.[11, 129, 134–138]

In the early literature some authors classified normal-tension glaucoma as a chronic form of ischemic optic neuropathy.[24, 102, 139] Indeed, in an atypical case without a history of sudden visual loss and in the presence of a glaucomatous appearing disc, it may be very difficult to exclude ischemic optic neuropathy from the differential diagnosis.

HEMODYNAMIC CRISES

Acute hypotensive episodes due to events such as myocardial infarction, cardiac arrest, massive hemorrhage, or shock have been thought by some investigators to play a role in the production of cupping and visual field loss. Decreased perfusion may lead to optic nerve damage in patients who experience a hemodynamic crisis. Drance and coworkers[90] reported that a history of an acute hypotensive episode was significantly more prevalent among patients who showed disc cupping and field loss with normal intraocular pressure than in ocular hypertensive controls. They also pointed out that the visual field defects in these patients were usually nonprogressive.[30, 140]

Although a subsequent study[91] has not confirmed Drance's observations, it is still important for the clinician to inquire about the possibility of past hemodynamic crises when the differential diagnosis of normal-tension glaucoma is being considered.

CAROTID ARTERY DISEASE

Carotid artery disease has been thought by some authors to cause or be associated with optic disc ischemia,[141–144] but whether there is any relationship between normal-tension glaucoma and carotid artery disease remains controversial.[11, 89, 145] Because isolated case reports of cupping and carotid disease have been reported,[146] it should be listed in the differential diagnosis. In elderly patients sclerotic vessels can cause temporal compression effects on the optic nerve in the sella.[139, 142, 143, 147–149] In such cases progressive visual field loss and optic atrophy may ensue. Some cases of arteriosclerotic chiasmal syndrome cause nasal depressions in the field that could be mistaken for glaucomatous damage.

DIAGNOSTIC EXAMINATION

History

A thorough history is important in the diagnostic work-up of patients with normal-tension glaucoma. Many entities can be excluded from the differential diagnosis simply by asking the appropriate questions. The ocular history should include inquiries about previously elevated intraocular pressures, past episodes of visual loss, ocular inflammation and trauma, and the use of corticosteroid eye medications. Attempts to elicit a family history of glaucoma and other ocular disease should be made.

The medical history should be evaluated for hypotensive episodes associated with severe blood loss, trauma, shock, and myocardial infarction. Information should also be included about past illnesses, especially atherosclerotic and cardiovascular disease, that might be sources of embolization.

A history suggestive of temporal arteritis, such as weight loss and cranial tenderness, should be sought, and a review of possible nutritional inadequacies or abuses should be made. A detailed history of the administration of past and present systemic medications is essential, including digitalis drugs, β-blocking agents, and corticosteroid preparations. The clinician should also inquire about the occurrence of migraine headache and other vasomotor disturbances.

Ocular Examination

In the patient suspected of having normal-tension glaucoma, several aspects of the ocular examination deserve special emphasis. During the external ocular evaluation the pupillary reflexes should always be carefully assessed. An afferent pupillary defect (Marcus Gunn pupil) indicates optic nerve disease. Although a positive test does not differentiate between glaucomatous neuropathy and other forms of optic atrophy, it might help to rule out a congenital disc anomaly.

In the office the intraocular pressure should be measured by an accurate tonometric technique, such as applanation. The Schiotz tonometer can yield false low readings, especially in patients with reduced scleral rigidity. In order to evaluate the diurnal variations of intraocular pressure, diurnal tension curves are very useful. Although not routinely practical, the ideal curve would include applanation pressure recordings every other hour throughout a 24-hr period. A valuable alternative is office tonometry performed every 1 to 2 hr during the day, beginning as early in the morning and continuing as late in the evening as is feasible. To enhance the tonometric study, certain patients and cooperative family members can be successfully trained to use a tonometer at home. In such cases valuable information regarding pressure levels during nonoffice hours can be obtained. In the past the Schiotz tonometer has been most frequently utilized for this purpose. The clinician must remember to correlate Schiotz values with those obtained by applanation tonometry before interpreting such results. The ideal tonometer for home use would be an applanation instrument that would allow the patient to record his or her own intraocular pressure without assistance. Such instruments are presently being developed, and with improved technology the self-tonometer may become a valuable addition to the clinician's armamentarium.[120, 121]

In addition to diurnal variations of intraocular pressure, it should be remembered that episodic and phasic elevations may occur over periods of several weeks to months. Such elevations must always be suspected in patients with the diagnosis of normal-tension glaucoma. Repeated diurnal tension curves and home tonometry represent options to identify these intermittent elevations, although there is a limit to feasibility and resources available for such endeavors in a clinical setting.

Gonioscopy must be included in the ocular examination in order to rule out secondary and narrow-angle glaucoma. The anterior chamber angle in normal-tension glaucoma has a normal open appearance since there are no specific characteristics to differentiate it from primary open-angle glaucoma.

Examination of the optic nerve should be accomplished with both the direct ophthalmoscope and slit-lamp biomicroscopy. Obtaining a high magnification stereoscopic view of the disc by means of a Hruby or hand-held 90-diopter lens is extremely helpful in the accurate assessment of cupping. The contours of the optic disc surface can be studied in significant detail by this technique.

A permanent record of the optic disc appearance is an essential part of the examination. Stereophotography, when available, is an excellent way to document optic disc pathology. Alternatively, sketches of the discs may be included in the patient's chart and updated on subsequent visits as needed. Both drawings and photos are invaluable in monitoring the progression of glaucomatous defects when following a patient over several years.

Through careful optic nerve examination, the list of conditions that may resemble glaucomatous optic neuropathy can be shortened. Congenital disc anomalies can usually be correctly diagnosed by observation alone. In nonglaucomatous optic atrophy, pallor of the neuroretinal rim and only a modest excavation of the disc are common findings. In contrast, glaucomatous atrophy is typically characterized by marked excavation of the disc, often with undermining of the disc rim. Pallor of neuroretinal rim tissue uninvolved in the excavation is less frequent. At times, however, it is not possible to ophthalmoscopically distinguish glaucomatous from nonglaucomatous disc cupping. In these cases, the history and other diagnostic studies must serve to make the distinction.

Measurement of the visual field is another aspect of the ocular examination that deserves emphasis. Either kinetic or static perimetric techniques may be employed, but for the sake of consistency the same method should be used on subsequent testing of any given individual. If visual field defects do not correlate well with the appearance of the disc, the results should be interpreted with caution.

Tonography has been used to study the aqueous humor dynamics in normal-tension glaucoma, and a wide range of results have been reported. Some patients with normal-tension glaucoma have reduced outflow facilities whereas others do not. For research purposes tonography is valuable, but it currently is not commonly used in the clinical work-up of the patient with normal-tension glaucoma.

Because reduced optic nerve perfusion may play a significant role in normal-tension glaucoma, many have thought that opthalmodynamometry would be a useful diagnostic test. A number of studies have been done in which the ophthalmic artery pressure was measured and compared among patients with normal-tension glaucoma, patients with primary open-angle glaucoma, and normal subjects. After reviewing the literature Levene[11] concluded that there is no evidence for a lowered ophthalmic artery perfusion gradient in normal-tension glaucoma. He thought that the results of both ophthalmodynamometry and ophthalmodynamography were inconsistent. This continues to be the prevailing belief of clinicians.

Medical Examination

A thorough physical examination by a general physician is valuable in patients suspected of having normal-tension glaucoma. A search for vascular disease includes measuring the blood pressure, listening for carotid bruits, identifying cardiac valvular disease, and feeling for temporal artery tenderness.

Laboratory tests include a complete blood count to rule out anemia and a sedimentation rate if history or findings suggest temporal arteritis. Biochemical, coagulation, and hematologic testing may be considered, but one study did not find them to be of benefit.[92] If there is a suspicion of neurologic disease, skull and orbital x-rays may be obtained. Additionally computed tomography or magnetic resonance imaging may be considered.

In some cases part of the medical evaluation might include the short-term discontinuation of certain systemic medications, such as β-blocking agents or digitalis, in order to assess their possible masking of an otherwise elevated intraocular pressure. Such action should be undertaken in conjunction with the attending medical physician.

MANAGEMENT

Just as the pathogenesis of normal-tension glaucoma is controversial, so too is the management. Since the specific causative factors in the development of normal-tension glaucoma are unclear, the decisions of whether, when, and how to treat the disorder are based on incomplete information. If one believes that intraocular pressure participates in the production of the damage, then lowering the pressure should logically be a primary therapeutic goal. Some, however, question the benefits of pressure reduction in patients with normal-tension glaucoma.

Recognizing our inadequate knowledge related to management, the Foundation for Glaucoma Research has organized "The Collaborative Low-Tension Glaucoma Study." The purpose of this multicentric international study that began in 1986 is two-fold: (1) to determine whether aggressive lowering of intraocular pressure halts visual field and/or optic nerve damage in patients with normal-tension glaucoma and (2) to assess the risks and side effects of the aggressive treatment required to reduce the pressure to low-normal levels.

Hopefully, this study will help to answer some of the troublesome questions about normal-tension glaucoma. These questions include: (1) To what extent is intraocular pressure involved in the mechanism of nerve damage?; (2) Are other factors involved in the process of nerve damage?; (3) Is it clinically feasible and worthwhile to aggressively lower the intraocular pressure?; and (4) What is the risk-benefit ratio of the aggressive treatment required to substantially reduce the intraocular pressure from its spontaneous normal level? While awaiting the results of "The Collaborative Low-Tension Glaucoma Study," the therapeutic approach advocated by most authorities is to lower intraocular pressure as much as possible by using medications, laser techniques, or surgery (Fig. 119–7).

When the diagnosis of normal-tension glaucoma has been established, baseline office diurnal curves are very helpful in defining the pretreatment pressure range. Before treatment one must consider what a reasonable target pressure will be. For example, if the patient has advanced damage with pressures documented to be consistently in the mid teens, pressure reduction to the very low teens or the 8 to 10 range would be appropriate. On the other hand, if pressure prior to treatment was consistently in the 18 to 20 range, a reduction to the mid to low teens might be adequate. Many patients with normal-tension glaucoma are diagnosed late in their disease when small increments of change are difficult to identify in an extensively cupped disc. Progression of field loss may also be difficult to identify in eyes that already have advanced field loss. There is typically a correspondingly large component of short- and long-term fluctuation that makes real progression difficult to identify. Despite its limitations, perimetry usually remains the most useful means of detecting progressive disease.

Some authors[113] believe that the reduction in baseline pressure may not always be a necessary goal of treatment. Patients with normal-tension glaucoma may experience damage only during transient or phasic pressure elevations. In such cases the reduction or elimination of these pressure spikes may be an appropriate therapeutic goal that is not easily assessed with random office pressure measurements. To evaluate the effectiveness of treatment, repeated diurnal pressure measurements may be useful.

Medical treatment is usually started with miotics. If a significant pressure reduction is not achieved, carbonic anhydrase inhibitors can be utilized. The question of whether to use β-blockers and adrenergic agonists in normal-tension glaucoma has not been answered. Some authorities believe that these drugs may exert a deleterious autonomic effect on circulation. It has been shown in rabbits that the topical administration of timolol, betaxolol, and phenylephrine causes substantial constriction of the arterioles supplying the ciliary processes.[150] If a comparable vasoconstriction occurs in the optic nerve, glaucomatous optic disc damage may be increased. Because of their possible adverse influences on optic nerve perfusion pressure, some clinicians have postulated that such vasoactive drugs may be more injurious than beneficial to patients with normal-tension glaucoma.[151, 152]

Others advocate their use as long as the drugs are well tolerated and effective in reducing the intraocular pressure.[113, 153] Grunwald has shown that retinal artery blood flow[154] and perfusion pressure[155] increase following

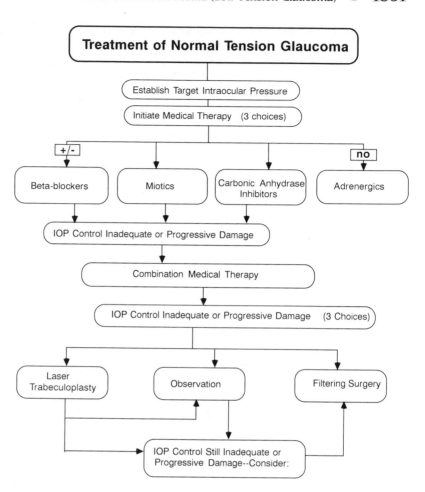

Figure 119–7. A flow chart illustrating one therapeutic approach for the management of normal-tension glaucoma. (IOP, intraocular pressure.)

treatment with timolol, but the issue of what may happen at the level of the arterioles in the optic nerve remains to be answered.

If medical therapy fails to lower pressure to the predetermined target level, laser trabeculoplasty may be justified. Some clinicians claim successful reduction of pressure with argon laser therapy,[156, 157] whereas others do not. Demailly and associates[158] reported on a randomized study of patients with normal-tension glaucoma in which eyes treated with early laser trabeculoplasty were compared with eyes managed only with antiglaucomatous drugs. He found no difference between the two groups with respect to intraocular pressure or to visual status after a 7-yr follow-up.

Wilensky and Gieser[113] utilized tonography as a therapeutic tool to aid in the selection of candidates for argon laser trabeculoplasty. They believe that patients with normal-tension glaucoma with a reduced outflow facility show the best response to laser therapy. After the procedure the facility of outflow is often improved, which may allow the treated eye to handle periodic increases in aqueous production with less fluctuation in pressure.

Despite medical and laser therapy some patients with normal-tension glaucoma fail to have a significant reduction in pressure and continue to show progression of optic nerve and visual field damage. Filtering surgery is often utilized in these cases in an effort to achieve low

or even "subnormal" pressures. Successful results using full-thickness filtration procedures have been reported by Chandler and others.[113, 156, 159–161] These reports provide suggestive evidence that progressive deterioration can be arrested by surgically reducing intraocular pressure below 12 mmHg.

Unfortunately, patients with normal-tension glaucoma may continue a relentless downhill course regardless of therapy. A retrospective study of all patients with normal-tension glaucoma treated at Wills Eye Hospital in Philadelphia over a 5-yr period revealed that 62 percent continued to show progressive visual field damage as measured by Octopus computerized perimetry.[162] All of the patients were treated medically, and 65 percent underwent at least one surgical procedure. This rate of progressive field loss was significantly greater than that seen in a group of patients with primary open-angle glaucoma similarly studied at the same institution.

The search for better treatment modalities continues. Reduction of intraocular pressure has been the common therapeutic goal in the past. With increasing evidence that optic nerve head ischemia may play a role in normal-tension glaucoma, some authorities believe that treatment should also be aimed at enhancing optic nerve perfusion. Gasser and colleagues[97, 163] have studied patients with normal-tension glaucoma who also have digital vasospasm. They discovered that visual field impairment can be temporarily aggravated or provoked by cooling one hand in cold water. They assume this temporary reduction of mean sensitivity as measured by Octopus perimetry is due to ocular vasospasm.[164] Further studies showed that treatment of these patients with an oral calcium channel blocker, nifedipine, produced a statistically significant improvement of visual field mean sensitivity. Unfortunately, not all reports on nifedipine therapy are encouraging. Lumme and coworkers[165] could show no change in the rate of progression of optic disc cupping in the patients with normal-tension glaucoma who were treated with nifedipine compared with patients treated with acetazolamide and those who received no treatment at all.

Kitazawa and associates[166] conducted a prospective study on randomly selected patients with normal-tension glaucoma treated with nifedipine for 6 mo and found that visual field mean sensitivity improvement occurred in some cases. Those who responded favorably to the calcium channel blocker tended to be younger, showed a greater recovery rate from digital vasospasm induced by cold exposure, and had less marked pretreatment visual field defects. The authors postulate that patients who showed visual field improvement may have retained the reactivity of peripheral vessels to the calcium channel blockers and that the resultant vasodilatation then improved the blood supply to the optic nerve.

The antiserotonin agent, nastidrofuryl (Praxilen), is another drug that may show future promise in the treatment of normal-tension glaucoma. This drug, which dilatates the peripheral vessels and capillaries without decreasing the systolic blood pressure, has been used successfully in patients with peripheral arteriography, Raynaud's phenomenon, and stroke. Mermoud and associates[167, 168] report that patients with normal-tension glaucoma who received oral nastidrofuryl for up to 11 mo showed a significant improvement in visual acuity and an increase in the visual field mean sensitivity when compared to a nontreated control group. More research is needed to determine whether medications that alter vasospasm, such as calcium channel blockers or antiserotonin agents, will be able to significantly modify the disease process in normal-tension glaucoma.

REFERENCES

1. von Graefe A: Amaurose mit Sehnervenexcavation. Archiv f Ophthalmol 3(II):484, 1857.
2. von Graefe A: Die iridectomie bei amauros mit sehnervenexcation. Archiv f Ophthalmol 3(II):546, 1857.
3. Sjogren H: A study of pseudoglaucoma. Acta Ophthalmol 24:239, 1946.
4. Duke-Elder S, Jay B: System of Ophthalmology. Vol II: Diseases of the Lens and Vitreous: Glaucoma and Hypotony. St Louis, CV Mosby, 1969.
5. Armaly MF: Ocular pressure and visual fields: A ten year follow-up study. Arch Ophthalmol 81:25, 1969.
6. Bankes JLK, Perkins ES, Tsolakis S, et al: Bedford glaucoma survey. Br Med J 1:791, 1968.
7. Bengtsson B: Manifest glaucoma in the aged. II: Cases detected by ophthalmoscopy. Acta Ophthalmol 57:929, 1979.
8. Bengtsson B, Krakau CET: Automatic perimetry in a population survey. Acta Ophthalmol 57:929, 1979.
9. Hollows FC, Graham PA: Intraocular pressure, glaucoma and glaucoma suspects in a defined population. Br J Ophthalmol 50:570, 1966.
10. Leibowitz HM, Krueger DE, Maunder LR, et al: The Framingham eye study monograph. Surv Ophthalmol 24 (Suppl):335, 1980.
11. Levene RZ: Low-tension glaucoma: A critical review and new material. Surv Ophthalmol 24:621, 1980.
12. Perkins ES: The Bedford glaucoma survey. I: Long-term follow-up of borderline cases. Br J Ophthalmol 57:179, 1973.
13. Perkins ES: The Bedford glaucoma survey. II: Rescreening the normal population. Br J Ophthalmol 57:186, 1973.
14. Shiose Y: Prevalence and clinical aspects of low tension glaucoma. In Henkind P (ed): Acta 24th International Congress of Ophthalmology. Philadelphia, JB Lippincott, 1983.
15. Wallace J, Lovell HG: Glaucoma and intraocular pressure in Jamaica. Am J Ophthalmol 67:93, 1969.
16. Drance SM: Low-tension glaucoma, enigma and opportunity. Arch Ophthalmol 103:1131, 1985.
17. American Academy of Ophthalmology: Primary Open-Angle Glaucoma: Preferred Practice Pattern. San Francisco, American Academy of Ophthalmology, 1989.
18. Hoskins HD Jr, Kass MA: Becker-Shaffer's Diagnosis and Therapy of the Glaucomas, 6th ed. St Louis, CV Mosby, 1989.
19. Chandler PA, Grant WM: Glaucoma, 2nd ed. Philadelphia, Lea & Febiger, 1979.
20. Hoskins HD: Definition, classification and management of the glaucoma suspect. In Transactions of the New Orleans Academy of Ophthalmology: Symposium on glaucoma. St Louis, CV Mosby, 1981.
21. Spaeth GL: Low-tension glaucoma: Its diagnosis and management. Doc Ophthalmol Proc Ser 22:263, 1980.
22. Kolker AE, Hetherington J Jr: Becker-Shaffer's Diagnosis and Therapy of the Glaucomas, 5th ed. St Louis, CV Mosby, 1983.
23. Drance SM: Some factors involved in the production of low tension glaucoma. Br J Ophthalmol 56:229, 1972.
24. Hayreh SS: Pathogenesis of optic nerve damage and visual field defects. In Heilmann K, Richardson KT (eds): Glaucoma: Conceptions of a Disease: Pathogenesis, Diagnosis, Therapy. Philadelphia, WB Saunders, 1978.
25. Armaly MF: On the distribution of applanation pressure and arcuate scotoma. In Paterson G, Miller SJH, Paterson GD (eds): Drug Mechanisms in Glaucoma. Boston, Little, Brown, 1966.
26. Bengtsson B: Aspects of the epidemiology of chronic glaucoma. Acta Ophthalmol Suppl 146:1, 1981.
27. Shiose Y, Komuro K, Itoh T, et al: New system for mass screening of glaucoma, as part of automated multiphasic health testing services. Jpn J Ophthalmol 25:160, 1981.
28. Smith J: Diurnal intraocular pressure correlation to automated perimetry. Ophthalmology 92:858, 1985.
29. Chumbley LC, Brubaker RF: Low-tension glaucoma. Am J Ophthalmol 81:761, 1976.
30. Drance SM, Sweeney VP, Morgan RW, et al: Studies of factors involved in the production of low-tension glaucoma. Arch Ophthalmol 89:457, 1973.
31. Goldberg I, Hollows FC, Kass MA, et al: Systemic factors in patients with low-tension glaucoma. Br J Ophthalmol 65:56, 1981.
32. Maumenee AE: Visual loss in glaucoma. In Transactions of the New Orleans Academy of Ophthalmology: Symposium on Glaucoma. St Louis, CV Mosby, 1981.
33. Paterson G: A nine-year follow-up on first-degree relatives of patients with glaucoma simplex. Trans Ophthalmol Soc UK 90:515, 1970.
34. Perkins ES: Family studies in glaucoma. Br J Ophthalmol 58:529, 1974.
35. Bennett SR, Alward WLM, Folberg R: An autosomal dominant form of low-tension glaucoma. Am J Ophthalmol 108:238, 1989.
36. Greve EL, Geijssen HC: The relationship between excavation and visual field in patients with high and low intraocular pressures. Doc Ophthalmol Proc Ser 35:35, 1983.
37. Caprioli J, Spaeth GL: Comparison of the optic nerve head in high- and low-tension glaucoma. Arch Ophthalmol 103:1145, 1985.
38. Lewis RA, Hayreh SS, Phelps CD: Optic disc and visual field correlations in primary open-angle and low-tension glaucoma. Am J Ophthalmol 96:148, 1983.
39. Miller KM, Quigley HA: Comparison of optic disc features in low tension and typical open angle glaucoma. Ophthalmol Surg 18:882, 1987.

40. King D, Douglas GR, Drance SM, et al: Optic nerve analysis in low-tension glaucoma versus high pressure glaucoma. Invest Ophthalmol Vis Sci 27 (Suppl):41, 1986.
41. Fazio P, Krupin T, Feitl M, et al: Optic disc tomography in patients with low-tension and primary open angle glaucoma. Arch Ophthalmol 108:705, 1990.
42. Javitt JC, Spaeth GL, Katz JL, et al: Acquired pits of the optic nerve. Ophthalmology 97:1038, 1990.
43. Greve EL, Geijssen HC: Comparison of visual fields in patients with high and with low intraocular pressures. Doc Ophthalmol Proc Ser 35:101, 1983.
44. Caprioli J, Spaeth GL: Comparison of visual field defects in the low-tension glaucomas with those in the high-tension glaucomas. Am J Ophthalmol 97:730, 1984.
45. Motolko M, Drance SM, Douglas GR: The visual field defects of low-tension glaucoma. Arch Ophthalmol 100:1074, 1982.
46. Phelps CD, Hayreh SS, Montague PR: Visual fields in low-tension glaucoma, primary open-angle glaucoma and anterior ischemic optic neuropathy. Doc Ophthalmol Proc Ser 35:113, 1983.
47. King D, Drance SM, Douglas G, et al: Comparison of visual field defects in normal-tension glaucoma and high-tension glaucoma. Am J Ophthalmol 101:204, 1986.
48. Flammer J, Drance SM, Augustiny L, et al: Quanitification of glaucomatous visual field defects with automated perimetry. Invest Ophthalmol Vis Sci 26:176, 1985.
49. Heijl A, Lindgren G, Olsson J: A package for the statistical analysis of visual fields. Doc Ophthalmol Proc Ser 49:153, 1987.
50. Drance SM, Douglas GR, Airaksinen PJ, et al: Diffuse visual field loss in chronic open-angle glaucoma and low-tension glaucoma. Am J Ophthalmol 104:577, 1987.
51. Chauhan BC, Drance SM, Douglas GR, et al: Visual field damage in normal-tension and high-tension glaucoma. Am J Ophthalmol 108:636, 1989.
52. Caprioli J, Sears M, Miller, JM: Patterns of early visual field loss in open-angle glaucoma. Am J Ophthalmol 103:512, 1987.
53. Glowazki A, Flammer J: Is there a difference between glaucoma patients with rather localized visual field damage and patients with more diffuse visual field damage? Doc Ophthalmol Proc Ser 49:317, 1987.
54. Yamazaki Y, Lakowski R, Drance, SM: A comparison of the blue color mechanism in high- and low-tension glaucoma. Ophthalmology 96:12, 1989.
55. Cartwright MJ, Anderson DR: Correlation of asymmetric damage with asymmetric intraocular pressure in normal-tension glaucoma (low-tension glaucoma). Arch Ophthalmol 106:898, 1988.
56. Critchton A, Drance SM, Douglas GR, et al: Unequal intraocular pressure and its relation to asymmetric visual field defects in low-tension glaucoma. Ophthalmology 96:1312, 1989.
57. Sugiura T, Ito M, Mizokami K: A comparative study of optic disc appearances in progressive and non-progressive low-tension glaucoma. Acta Soc Ophthalmol Jpn 95:343, 1991.
58. Yamagami J, Shirato S, Araie M: The influence of the intraocular pressure on the visual field of low-tension glaucoma. Acta Soc Ophthalmol Jpn 94:514, 1990.
59. Bjerrum J: Om en tilfojelse til den saedvanlige synsfelfundersøgelse samt om synsfeltet ved glaukom. Nord Ophthalmol Tskr (Kbh) 2:141, 1889.
60. Begg IS, Drance SM, Sweeney, VP: Ischemic optic neuropathy in chronic simple glaucoma. Br J Ophthalmol 55:73, 1971.
61. Drance SM, Fairclough M, Butler DM, et al: The importance of disc hemorrhage in the prognosis of chronic open-angle glaucoma. Arch Ophthalmol 95:226, 1977.
62. Kottler MS, Drance SM: Studies of hemorrhage on the optic disc. Can J Ophthalmol 11:102, 1976.
63. Susanna R, Drance SM: Use of discriminant analysis. I: Prediction of visual field defects from features of the optic disc. Arch Ophthalmol 96:1568, 1978.
64. Susanna R, Drance SM, Douglas GR: Disc hemorrhages in patients with elevated intraocular pressure, occurrence with and without field changes. Arch Ophthalmol 97:284, 1979.
65. Airaksinen, PJ: Are optic disc hemorrhages a common finding in all glaucoma patients? Acta Ophthalmol 62:193, 1984.
66. Airaksinen PJ, Tuulonen A: Early glaucoma changes in patients with and without an optic disc hemorrhage. Acta Ophthalmol 62:197, 1984.
67. Richler M, Werner EB, Thomas D: Risk factors for progression of visual field defects in medically treated patients with glaucoma. Can J Ophthalmol 17:245, 1982.
68. Gloster J: Incidence of optic disc hemorrhages in chronic open-angle glaucoma and ocular hypertension. Br J Ophthalmol 65:452, 1981.
69. Kitazawa Y, Shirato S, Yamamoto T: Optic disc hemorrhage in low-tension glaucoma. Ophthalmology 93:853, 1986.
70. Shiose Y: Quantitative disc pattern as a new parameter for glaucoma screening. Glaucoma 1:41, 1979.
71. Quigley HA, Addicks EM, Green, WR: Optic nerve damage in human glaucoma. Arch Ophthalmol 100:135, 1982.
72. Primrose J: The incidence of the peripapillary halo glaucomatosus. Trans Ophthalmol Soc UK 89:585, 1969.
73. Wilensky JT, Kolker AE. Peripapillary changes in glaucoma. Am J Ophthalmol 81:341, 1976.
74. Rockwood EJ, Anderson DR: Acquired peripapillary changes and progression in glaucoma. Graefes Arch Clin Exp Ophthalmol 226:510, 1988.
75. Buus DR, Anderson DR: Peripapillary crescents and halos in normal-tension glaucoma and ocular hypertension. Ophthalmology 96:16, 1989.
76. Anderson DR: Correlation of the peripapillary anatomy with the disc damage and field abnormalities in glaucoma. Doc Ophthalmol Proc Ser 35:1, 1983.
77. Heijl A, Samander C: Peripapillary atrophy and glaucomatous visual field defects. Doc Ophthalmol Proc Ser 42:403, 1985.
78. Geijssen HC, Greve EL: The spectrum of primary open angle glaucoma. I: Senile sclerotic glaucoma versus high tension glaucoma. Ophthal Surg 18:207, 1987.
79. Fantes FE, Anderson DR: Clinical histologic correlation of human peripapillary anatomy. Ophthalmology 96:20, 1989.
80. Anderson, DR: The mechanisms of damage of the optic nerve. In Krieglstein GK, Leydhecker W (eds): Glaucoma Update, II. Berlin, Springer-Verlag, 1983.
81. Kasner O, Feuer WJ, Anderson DR: Possibly reduced prevalence of peripapillary crescents in ocular hypertension. Can J Ophthalmol 24:221, 1989.
82. Anderson DR: Glaucoma: The damage caused by pressure. XLVI Edward Jackson Memorial Lecture. Am J Ophthalmol 108:489, 1989.
83. Perkins ES, Phelps CD: Open-angle glaucoma, ocular hypertension, low-tension glaucoma and refraction. Arch Ophthalmol 100:1464, 1982.
84. Phelps CD: Effect of myopia on prognosis in treated primary open-angle glaucoma. Am J Ophthalmol 93:622, 1982.
85. Leighton DA, Tomlinson A: Ocular tension and axial length of the eyeball in open-angle glaucoma and low-tension glaucoma. Br J Ophthalmol 57:499, 1973.
86. Bengtsson B: Findings associated with glaucomatous visual field defects. Acta Ophthalmol 58:20, 1980.
87. Leighton DA, Phillips GI: Systemic blood pressure in open-angle glaucoma, low-tension glaucoma and the normal eye. Br J Ophthalmol 56:447, 1972.
88. Gramer E, Leydhecker W: Glaukom ohne hochdruck: Eine klinische studie. Klin Monatsb Augenheilkd 186:262, 1985.
89. Demailly P, Cambien F, Plovin PF, et al: Do patients with low-tension glaucoma have particular cardiovascular characteristics? Ophthalmologica 188:65, 1984.
90. Drance SM, Morgan RW, Sweeney VP: Shock-induced optic neuropathy: A cause of non-progressive glaucoma. N Engl J Med 288:392, 1973.
91. Jampol LM, Board RJ, Maumenee AE: Systemic hypotension and glaucomatous changes. Am J Ophthalmol 85:154, 1978.
92. Carter CJ, Brooks DE, Doyle DL, et al: Investigations into a vascular etiology for low-tension glaucoma. Ophthalmology 97:49, 1990.
93. Corbett JJ, Phelps CD, Eslinger P, et al: The neurologic evaluation of patients with low-tension glaucoma. Invest Ophthalmol Vis Sci 26:1101, 1985.
94. Phelps CD, Corbett JJ: Migraine and low-tension glaucoma. Invest Ophthalmol Vis Sci 26:1105, 1985.
95. Usui T, Iwata K, Shirakashi M, et al: Prevalence of migraine in low-tension glaucoma and primary open-angle glaucoma in Japanese. Br J Ophthalmol 75:224, 1991.

96. Drance SM: The neurologic evaluation of patients with low-tension glaucoma. Surv Ophthalmol 31:74, 1986.

97. Gasser P, Flammer J, Guthauser U, et al: Bedeutung des vasospastischen syndroms in der augenheilkunde. Klin Monatsbl Augenheilkd 183:503, 1986.

98. Flammer J, Guthauser U, Mahler F: Does ocular vasospasm help cause low tension glaucoma? Doc Ophthalmol Proc Ser 49:397, 1987.

99. Drance SM, Douglas MD, Wijsman K, et al: Response of blood flow to warm and cold in normal and low-tension glaucoma patients. Am J Ophthalmol 105:35, 1988.

100. Gasser P, Flammer J: Blood-cell velocity in the nailfold capillaries of patients with normal-tension and high-tension glaucoma. Am J Ophthalmol 111:585, 1991.

101. Drance SM: The visual field of low tension glaucoma and shock-induced optic neuropathy. Arch Ophthalmol 95:1359, 1977.

102. Hayreh SS: Anterior Ischemic Optic Neuropathy. New York, Springer-Verlag, 1975.

103. Winder AF: Circulatory lipoprotein and blood glucose levels in association with low-tension and chronic simple glaucoma. Br J Ophthalmol 61:641, 1977.

104. Winder A, Patterson G, Miller SJH: Biochemical abnormalities associated with ocular hypertension and low tension glaucoma. Trans Ophthalmol Soc UK 94:518, 1974.

105. Francois J, Neetens A: The deterioration of the visual field in glaucoma and the blood pressure. Doc Ophthalmol 28:70, 1970.

106. Gafner F, Goldmann H: Experimentelle untersuchungen uber den zusammenhang von augendrucksteigerung und gesichtfeld schadigung. Ophthalmologica 130:357, 1955.

107. Morax V: Glaucome simple au atrophie avec excavation. Ann Ocul (Paris) 153:25, 1916.

108. Thiel R: Glaukom ohne hochdruck. Ber Dtsch Opthalmol Gessell 48:133, 1930.

109. Duke-Elder S: Fundamental concepts in glaucoma. Arch Ophthalmol 42:538, 1949.

110. Hatsuda TA: Low-tension glaucoma. Folia Ophthalmol Jpn 28:244, 1977.

111. Joist JH, Lichtenfeld P, Mandell AI, et al: Platelet function, blood coagulability and fibrinolysis in patients with low tension glaucoma. Arch Ophthalmol 94:1893, 1976.

112. Duke-Elder S: The phasic variations in the intraocular tension in primary glaucoma. Am J Ophthalmol 35:1, 1952.

113. Wilensky JT, Gieser DK: Low-tension glaucoma. In Weinstein GW (ed): Contemporary Issues in Ophthalmology: Open-Angle Glaucoma, Vol. 3. New York, Churchill Livingstone, 1986.

114. Kriegelstein GK, Langham ME: Influence of body position on the intraocular pressure of normal and glaucomatous eyes. Ophthalmologica 171:132, 1975.

115. Hyams SW, Frankel A, Keroub C, et al: Postural changes in intraocular pressure with particular reference to low tension glaucoma. Glaucoma 6:178, 1984.

116. Linder BJ, Trick GL, Wolf ML: Altering body position affects intraocular pressure and visual function. Invest Ophthalmol Vis Sci 29:1492, 1988.

117. Tsukahara S, Sasaki T: Postural changes of IOP in normal persons and in patients with primary wide open-angle glaucoma and low-tension glaucoma. Br J Ophthalmol 68:389, 1984.

118. Friberg TR, Sanborn G, Weinreb RN: Intraocular and episcleral venous pressure increase during inverted posture. Am J Ophthalmol 103:523, 1987.

119. Rice R, Allen RC: Yoga in glaucoma. Am J Ophthalmol 100:738, 1985.

120. Alpar JJ: The use of home tonometry in the diagnosis and treatment of glaucoma. Glaucoma 5:130, 1983.

121. Zeimer RC, Wilensky JT, Gieser DK, et al: Application of a self-tonometer to home tonometry. Arch Ophthalmol 104:49, 1986.

122. Grant WM, Burke JF: Why do some people go blind from glaucoma? Ophthalmology 89:991, 1982.

123. Kolker AE: Visual prognosis in advanced glaucoma: A comparison of medical and surgical therapy for retention of vision in 101 eyes with advanced glaucoma. Trans Am Ophthalmol Soc 75:539, 1977.

124. Simon K, Bonting SL: Possible usefulness of cardiac glycosides in treatment of glaucoma. Arch Ophthalmol 68:227, 1962.

125. Reynolds PM, Crick RP: A clinical trial of oral propranolol (Inderal) in patients with medically uncontrolled chronic simple glaucoma. Glaucoma 3:539, 1980.

126. Ohrstrom A, Pandolfi M: Long-term treatment of glaucoma with systemic propranolol. Am J Ophthalmol 86:340, 1978.

127. Duff GR: The effect of twice daily nadolol on intraocular pressure. Am J Ophthalmol 104:343, 1987.

128. Trobe JD, Glaser JS, Cassady JC: Optic atrophy differential diagnosis by fundus observation alone. Arch Ophthalmol 98:1041, 1980.

129. Trobe JD, Glaser JS, Cassady JC, et al: Nonglaucomatous excavation of the optic disc. Arch Ophthalmol 98:1046, 1980.

130. Hupp SL, Savino PJ, Schatz NJ, et al: Nerve fiber bundle visual field defects and intracranial mass lesions. Can J Ophthalmol 21:231, 1986.

131. Smith DP: Diagnostic criteria in dominantly inherited juvenile optic atrophy: A report of 3 new families. Am J Optom Physiol Opt 49:183, 1972.

132. Sandvig K: Pseudoglaucoma of autosomal dominant inheritance: A report on three families. Acta Opthalmol (Kbh) 39:33, 1961.

133. Pickett JE, Terry SA, O'Connor PS, et al: Early loss of central visual acuity in glaucoma. Ophthalmology 92:891, 1985.

134. Sebag J, Thomas JV, Epstein DL, et al: Optic disc cupping in arteritic anterior ischemic optic neuropathy resembles glaucomatous cupping. Ophthalmology 93:357, 1986.

135. Quigley H, Anderson DR: Cupping of the optic disc in ischemic optic atrophy. Trans Am Acad Ophthalmol Otolaryngol 83:755, 1977.

136. Lichter PR, Henderson JW: Optic nerve infarction. Am J Ophthalmol 85:302, 1978.

137. Beck RW, Savino PJ, Repka MX, et al: Optic disc structure in anterior ischemic optic neuropathy. Ophthalmology 91:1334, 1984.

138. Doro S, Lessel S: Cup-disc ratio and ischemic optic neuropathy. Arch Ophthalmol 103:1143, 1985.

139. Duke-Elder S, Scott GI: System of Ophthalmology. Vol. 12: Neuroophthalmology. St Louis, CV Mosby, 1971.

140. Drance SM, Sweeney VP, Morgan RW, et al: Studies of factors involved in the production of low-tension glaucoma. Arch Ophthalmol 89:457, 1973.

141. Harrington DO: Some unusual and difficult visual field defects. Trans Ophthalmol Soc UK 92:15, 1972.

142. Lyle DJ: Arteriosclerotic optic atrophy. Proc Soc Med 50:937, 1957.

143. Magnus JA: A case of pseudo-glaucoma. Br J Ophthalmol 31:692, 1947.

144. Etzikson LY: Calcification of basal arteries and so-called pseudo-glaucoma. Vest Oftal 31:7, 1952.

145. Jampol LM, Miller NR: Carotid artery disease and glaucoma. Br J Ophthalmol 62:324, 1978.

146. Gittinger JW, Miller NR, Keltner JL, et al: Glaucomatous cupping—sine glaucoma. Surv Ophthalmol 25:383, 1981.

147. Knapp A: Association of sclerosis of cerebral basal vessels with optic atrophy and cupping. Arch Ophthalmol 8:637, 1932.

148. McLean JM, Ray BS: Soft glaucoma and calcification of the internal carotid arteries. Arch Ophthalmol 38:154, 1947.

149. Knapp A: Course in certain cases of atrophy of the optic nerve with cupping and low tension. Arch Ophthalmol 23:41, 1940.

150. Van Buskirk EM, Bacon DR, Fahrenbach WH: Ciliary vasoconstriction after topical adrenergic drugs. Am J Ophthalmol 109:511, 1990.

151. Flammer J, Drance SM: The effect of a number of glaucoma medications on the differential light threshold. Doc Ophthalmol Proc Ser 35:145, 1983.

152. Flammer M, Robert Y, Gloor B: Influence of pindolol and timolol treatment on the visual fields of glaucoma patients. J Ocul Pharmacol 2:30, 1986.

153. Werner EB: Low-tension glaucoma. In Ritch R, Shields MB, Krupin T (eds): The Glaucomas, 1st ed. St Louis, CV Mosby, 1989.

154. Grunwald J: Effect of timolol maleate on the retinal circulation of human eyes with ocular hypertension. Invest Ophthalmol Vis Sci 31:521, 1990.

155. Grunwald E, Furubayashi C: Effect of topical timolol maleate on the ophthalmic artery blood pressure. Invest Ophthalmol Vis Sci 30:1095, 1989.

156. Abedin S, Simmons RJ, Grant W: Progressive low-tension glau-

coma: Treatment to stop glaucomatous cupping and field loss when these progress despite normal intraocular pressure. Ophthalmology 89:1, 1982.

157. Schwartz AL, Perman KI, Whitten M: Argon laser trabeculoplasty in progressive low-tension glaucoma. Ann Ophthalmol 16:560, 1984.

158. Demailly P, Lehrer M, Kretz G: Argon laser trabeculoplasty in low-tension glaucoma: A prospective study of tonometric and perimetric results. J Francais d'Ophthalmol 3:183, 1989.

159. Epstein DL: Progressive low-tension glaucoma. In Epstein DL (ed): Chandler and Grant's Glaucoma, 3rd ed. Philadelphia, Lea & Febiger, 1986.

160. Mellin KB: Filtering surgery in low tension glaucoma. Dev Ophthalmol 18:138, 1989.

161. DeJong N, Greve EL, Hoyng PFJ, et al: Results of a filtering procedure in low tension glaucoma. Int Ophthalmol 13:131, 1989.

162. Gliklich RE, Steinmann WC, Spaeth GL: Visual field change in low-tension glaucoma over a five-year follow-up. Ophthalmology 96:316, 1989.

163. Gasser P, Flammer J, Guthauser U, et al: Do vasospasms provoke ocular diseases? Angiology 41:213, 1990.

164. Gasser P, Flammer J: Influence of vasospasm on visual function. Doc Ophthalmol 66:3, 1987.

165. Lumme P, Tuulonen A, Airaksinen PJ, et al: Neuroretinal rim area in low tension glaucoma: Effect of nifedipine and acetazolamide compared to no treatment. Acta Ophthalmol 69:293, 1991.

166. Kitazawa, Y, Shirai H, Go FJ: The effect of Ca²⁺-antagonist on visual field in low-tension glaucoma. Graefes Arch Clin Exp Ophthalmol 227:408, 1989.

167. Mermoud A, Faggioni R: Treatment of normal pressure glaucoma with a serotonin S2 receptor antagonist, nastidrofuryl. Klin Monatsb Augenheilkd 198:332, 1991.

168. Mermoud A, Faggioni R, VanMelle GD: Double-blind study in the treatment of normal tension glaucoma with naftidrofuryl. Ophthalmologica 201:145, 1990.

Chapter 120

▪

Primary Angle-Closure Glaucoma

DAVID G. CAMPBELL

Closure of the iridocorneal angle constitutes an intriguing and multifactorial phenomenon. It can occur silently or can present suddenly with the fury and rage of a hurricane. Either way, untreated, it can rob a person of vision, either slowly and clandestinely or quickly and painfully.

This chapter on primary angle-closure glaucoma (ACG) begins with definitions and general concepts in the field of angle-closure, and is followed by discussions of the specific primary ACGs.

HISTORICAL COMMENT

Before the discovery and use of gonioscopy, ophthalmologists did not fully distinguish between open-angle glaucoma and ACG. They did recognize a glaucoma that could be sudden and another that was slow in development. Von Graefe[1] discovered in 1857 that a surgical peripheral iridectomy could cure some glaucomas, but it was not until the 1920s that the reason for this cure in some cases was understood—that is, that iridectomy relieved the forces of relative pupillary block.[2, 3]

DEFINITIONS

ACG can be classified in a number of different ways. Four different classifications are in common use. The first classification divides these glaucomas by the type of mechanism of closure—primary versus secondary angle-closure. A second classification divides these glaucomas by the location of the mechanism causing the closure—

anterior ACG versus the posterior ACG, with the iris as the reference point. The third classification involves the timing and the course of the closure process—acute, intermittent (subacute), and chronic angle-closure. Finally, an important and fourth classification involves the nature of the trabecular meshwork coverage—appositional angle closure versus synechial angle-closure.

Angle closure occurs when the peripheral iris comes to rest against the trabecular meshwork and covers it. Angle-closure glaucoma occurs when enough of the trabecular meshwork is occluded to produce elevated intraocular pressure (IOP) greater than 22 mmHg.

Primary Versus Secondary ACG

Primary ACG may be defined as glaucoma caused by predisposing anatomic factors that, associated with physiologic factors (aqueous production and flow, lens enlargement with age) and with pupillary movement (generally dilatation), lead to angle closure. There is no precipitating or initiating known primary pathologic process that leads to a secondary closure in this group other than the anatomic and physiologic factors just mentioned. Primary ACG will presently be further subdivided.

Secondary ACG, by contrast, includes those glaucomas caused by a preceding pathologic process within the eye that causes the angle to close as a secondary response to the primary pathologic process. An example of secondary ACG is closure due to the prior development of peripheral iris and ciliary body cysts that enlarge and push the peripheral iris forward, closing the angle.

Anterior Versus Posterior ACG

Anterior ACG can be defined as glaucoma caused by pathologic processes that contract and pull the iris anteriorly to cover the trabecular meshwork.[4] These pathologic processes all cause initial synechial closure. Examples include angle-closure caused by a proliferating fibrovascular membrane (neovascular glaucoma), by a proliferating endothelial membrane (iridocorneoendothelial syndrome), by contracting inflammatory keratic precipitates making contact with the iris from the surface of the trabecular meshwork (sarcoidosis), and by other processes. In contrast, posterior ACG is considered to include those glaucomas that are caused by forces posterior to the iris surface that push the peripheral iris against the trabecular meshwork. These processes at first cause appositional, and then, later, if uninterrupted, synechial closure. There are many examples of this type of closure, including all of the primary ACGs and many of the secondary posterior ACGs, such as the angle closure caused by uveochoroidal effusion or by growth of a tumor posterior to the iris.

Acute Versus Chronic ACG

ACGs can be divided according to the timing or suddenness of onset, into acute or sudden ACG and chronic or nonsudden ACG. In acute ACG, the iris quickly covers the entire or almost the entire trabecular meshwork, leading to sudden, severe, often painful elevation of IOP.

By contrast, in chronic ACG, the iris slowly comes to rest against the trabecular meshwork and to cover it, initially covering only small portions, leading to slow and gradual elevation of IOP. This process can often be painless and asymptomatic.

Acute ACG can be further subclassified according to whether or not spontaneous resolution of the attack occurs. If it does not remit spontaneously, the attack is generally called an acute or fully developed attack of angle-closure. If spontaneous resolution of the attack occurs (to be discussed later), the attack is called an intermittent (or subacute) attack of ACG.

Appositional Versus Synechial ACG

A final classification and an important distinction to make in ACG involves divides the closure clinically and pathologically into appositional versus synechial closure.

In appositional angle-closure, the iris rests against the trabecular meshwork and covers it, preventing aqueous outflow in the areas covered, in the absence of synechia formation. In this situation, with or without treatment, the iris may spontaneously fall away from the trabecular meshwork, permitting normal aqueous escape once again and lowering IOP. Synechial ACG exists when the iris has become permanently adherent to the trabecular meshwork, chronically obstructing aqueous outflow.

The permanent adherence is caused by fibrosis that develops between the anterior surface of the iris and the surface of the trabecular meshwork. In this situation, neither natural causes, pharmacologic treatment, nor iridectomy or iridotomy causes the iris to fall away from the trabecular meshwork. Surgical therapy, goniosynechialysis, and laser therapy in some early cases can separate these adhesions.

Further Classification of Primary ACG Into Four Types

1. Relative pupillary block ACG (RPB ACG)
2. Plateau iris configuration ACG (PIC ACG)
3. Nanophthalmic ACG
4. Mobile lens ACG

Primary ACG, defined earlier as glaucoma that develops as a result of preexisting anatomic and physiologic factors, without a preceding primary pathologic event, can be classified into four categories according to the mechanism of closure: (1) RPB ACG (most common), (2) PIC ACG, (3) nanophthalmic (tiny eye) ACG, and (4) mobile lens (forward lens) ACG.

An old term, *acute congestive glaucoma*, is generally no longer used to describe acute ACG. The term arose because it was once believed that congestion of the cilliary body caused acute primary ACG. This is no longer considered to be the case.

GENERAL PRINCIPLES CONCERNING PRIMARY ACG

Primary ACG Versus Primary Open-Angle Glaucoma

In primary ACG, before coverage of the angle and closure, the trabecular meshwork is normal and is functioning normally, and the facility of outflow and the IOP thus are normal. After the meshwork becomes covered by the iris, the facility of outflow decreases and the IOP rises.[5] Once the meshwork is uncovered again, at least in the initial stages of the disease process, both the meshwork and pressure are normal. In chronic open-angle glaucoma, the angle is open and is not covered by the peripheral iris at any time. The associated elevation of IOP is due to a different pathology, an obstruction to flow deeper within the trabecular meshwork and outflow channels.

Impermeability of the Iris to Fluid Flow

In ACG, the pressure elevates when the iris covers the trabecular meshwork because fluid cannot freely flow through the iris. If fluid could pass with almost no resistance through the iris, then coverage of the trabecular meshwork by the iris would do little harm, theoretically. The portion of the iris that is most impermeable to aqueous flow is the posterior pigmented epithelium of the iris. These cells have tight junctions and resist fluid flow. Proof for this can be seen clinically when a surgeon, in an attempt to perform a surgical iridectomy to treat ACG, excises only the anterior stroma, leaving the posterior pigment layer intact. When this happens and RPB is therefore unrelieved, the posterior pigment layer bulges forward into the anterior chamber, even farther forward than the surrounding stroma of the iris, demonstrating that this layer is indeed both impermeable to fluid flow and sensitive to the greater pressure in the posterior chamber.

Importance of the Small Eye and the Small Anterior Chamber

The development of angle-closure associated with primary ACG is in general a multifactorial phenomenon. A number of different anatomic factors usually combine, each contributing to angle-closure in differing degrees.

Eyes that generally become involved with primary ACG are usually smaller than normal. Investigators have shown that they are on the average 1 mm shorter than normal in their anterior-posterior dimension.[6, 7] Studies have also shown that the corneas[7, 9] and the anterior chambers are smaller, both centrally,[8, 10] peripherally,[11] and by volume,[12] in these eyes. These anatomic factors often decrease the space between the anterior surface of the peripheral iris and the surface of the trabecular meshwork, causing the angle to be described as "narrow" and to be predisposed to angle-closure.

Importance of the Lens; Lens-Eye Disproportion

The presence of the lens in the eye is an indispensable factor in the causation of primary ACG. In small eyes, the lens may be relatively normal in size but the relationship between a lens size and eye size is disproportionate. This disproportion increases as patients age and the lens enlarges and displaces the iris into a more forward position. This contributes to the development of an increasingly more narrow angle—that is, an angle in which there is little space between the peripheral iris and the trabecular meshwork.[6, 13]

In early life, the lens is relatively small and does not anatomically push the iris forward out of its natural or resting position of flatness and perpendicularity to the optical axis within the eye. In adulthood and senescence, the presence of the lens, now enlarged and enlarging further, pushes the iris forward slightly, causing the iris to lose its flatness and to become anteriorly bowed. The gradual and natural enlargement of the lens throughout life is a major factor in closure. If the lens enlarges more than normal, the angle can be further narrowed, predisposing to closure.[6, 7, 14]

If the lens is removed, the iris reassumes an anatomic position that is flat and posterior, causing the angle to widen considerably and the iris to reside in a position

that makes the development of primary ACG impossible. *In other words, if there is no lens, there can be no primary ACG.*

In addition to lens enlargement, slight forward movement of the lens has been measured as an eye becomes older, and this movement also causes the angle to narrow.[6]

Development of RPB

A factor in the development of primary ACG is RPB.[2, 3, 15] This is the precipitating factor in the most common type of primary RPB ACG. In a normal human adult eye, the pupil and the central region of the posterior surface of the iris make appositional contact with the anterior surface of the lens. The area of the apposition probably increases with age as the lens enlarges and the pupil becomes smaller. Because of this apposition and because the aqueous is generated in the posterior chamber, a slight difference in pressure develops between the posterior and the anterior chambers, with the greater pressure in the posterior chamber (Fig. 120–1). This slight difference is due to resistance caused by the apposition described.[16] The resistance or blockage is described as relative because the blockage is not absolute and permanent. If the pupillary margin of the iris becomes synechially adherent to the lens in its entirety (i.e., for 360 degrees), as can occur after inflammation, then the blockage becomes absolute, the iris bows forward in a characteristic rounded or ballooned form, and the angle closes, resulting in a secondary type of angle-closure called iris bombé ACG.

RPB, as stated, causes a slight buildup of pressure in the posterior chamber, thus causing the peripheral iris to bulge forward slightly more than it would if the pressure differential were not there. If the angle is spacious, this slight forward bulge is of no consequence within the eye, and this is the case in most normal-sized or large eyes. If, however, for anatomic reasons, there is little room in the angle, this peripheral bulge can lead to angle-closure, either suddenly or gradually.

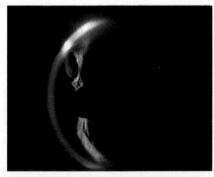

Figure 120–1. Slit-lamp photograph illustrating an incomplete surgical peripheral iridectomy with an intact posterior pigment layer. The layer can be seen to bulge forward into the anterior chamber owing to relative pupillary block and higher pressure in the posterior chamber. (From Campbell DG: A comparison of diagnostic techniques in angle-closure glaucoma. Am J Ophthalmol 88:199, 1979. Published with permission from The American Journal of Ophthalmology. Copyright by The Ophthalmic Publishing Company.)

Multifactorial Nature of ACG

As discussed earlier, there are many causes of angle closure in primary ACG. Of chief importance are a relatively small eye, a normal-sized or enlarged lens, and the presence of relative pupillary block. In some cases, closure is due to all three in equal proportion; in others, lens enlargement may be the dominant factor; and in others, the smallness of the eye may predominate.

Proportionality Principle: The Direct Relationship Between the Degree of Closure and the Elevation of the IOP

An important concept, established by Chandler and Grant,[5] states that in general the degree of elevation of IOP in angle-closure is directly proportional to the degree of closure. Goldmann's equation states that the perfusion pressure in the eye (perfusion pressure can be defined as the IOP minus the episcleral venous pressure and is the pressure that therefore drives fluid across the trabecular meshwork and out of the eye) is directly proportional to the resistance to flow in the eye if aqueous production remains constant, as it generally does over the short term. Hence, if resistance increases as it does in angle-closure and if aqueous production remains normal or nearly normal (as it does except in very high-pressure situations like acute ACG), the IOP increases proportionately.

For example, if half of the trabecular meshwork becomes covered by the iris, the resistance to outflow doubles, as does perfusion pressure. If the initial perfusion pressure was a normal 7 mmHg and hence the initial IOP was a normal 16 mmHg (the normal perfusion pressure of 7 is obtained by subtracting 9, the normal episcleral venous pressure, from the normal IOP of 16), the perfusion pressure would be doubled to 14 and the IOP would elevate to 23 (14 plus 9). Thus a normal eye has some reserve, and it can withstand closure of as much as one-half of the angle without a severe rise in pressure and fortunately without a rise in pressure that would damage most optic nerve heads. If, however, this eye then has half of the remaining angle closed (i.e., an additional 90 degrees), the resistance will double once again and so again will the perfusion pressure. The perfusion pressure (now 14) will double to 28, and the IOP will elevate to 37 (28 plus 9). Thus, with three-fourths of the angle closed, the pressure has elevated to a worrisome level. Further closure causes rapidly escalating IOP.

Unfortunately, there seems to be no compensatory mechanism to keep IOP normal within the eye and therefore to protect it by lowering aqueous production whenever resistance increases in the outflow channels, whether it be due to angle closure or some other mechanism. Inflow generally remains unchanged, and the eye pressure responds accordingly.

The proportionality concept, more fully stated, holds that the elevation of IOP following angle closure depends on the degree of closure and the status of the underlying trabecular meshwork. If the meshwork is normal, as in the previous example, the pressures do not initially elevate to high levels. If the meshwork is abnormal, as in early chronic open-angle glaucoma, the baseline IOP will be higher initially and hence closure of half of the angle will have a more profound effect. For example, if the initial perfusion pressure is 14 and hence the initial IOP is 23 (i.e., 14 plus 9), closure of half of this angle and hence a doubling of the resistance will double the perfusion pressure to 28 and raise the IOP to approximately 37 (28 plus 9). This is a much greater IOP effect than in a normal eye. This explains why a patient with early primary open-angle glaucoma poorly tolerates closure of portions of the angle, even a degree of closure that may be well tolerated in a normal eye. This relationship also offers one explanation for previously stable and well-controlled chronic open-angle glaucoma that becomes difficult to control. Silent, chronic angle closure should be searched for if the angle is narrow.

In the human eye, one cannot expect exact mathematical correlation as outlined earlier, but these general concepts are useful in thinking about ACG. For instance, if a patient presents with an initial IOP of 37 mmHg and gonioscopy reveals 60 degrees (or 2 hr) of angle closure, one knows that in a normal eye this degree of closure alone cannot cause this elevation and therefore assumes with surety that the trabecular meshwork must be abnormal as well.

These concepts, elucidated by Grant, permit correlation between gonioscopy and IOP as well as tonography determinations. A fact that may be taken for granted is also true—that the trabecular meshwork appears to function equally in its entire circumference of 360 degrees. If this were not the case and, for instance, if all of the outflow in a given eye exited through only 180 degrees, then coverage of this 180 degrees would cause marked elevation of IOP and coverage of the opposite 180 degrees would have no effect at all. This does not appear to be the case in humans.

For further expostulation on this concept, refer to Chandler and Grant's discussion and table in their text on glaucoma.[5]

MECHANISMS OF CLOSURE AND REVERSAL IN PRIMARY ACG

As stated earlier, primary ACG can be thought of as falling into four categories, the first being by far the most common and the remaining three relatively uncommon: (1) RPB ACG, (2) PIC ACG, (3) nanophthalmic ACG, and (4) mobile lens ACG.

RPB ACG and Its Reversal

MECHANISM OF CLOSURE

RPB, with its secondary peripheral bulging of the iris (Fig. 120–2), has a major role in the most common type

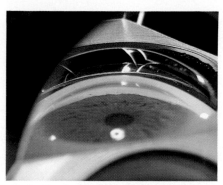

Figure 120–2. Gonioscopic photograph of a patient with relative pupillary block, angle-closure glaucoma. The fully distributed convexity of the iris characteristic of this type of closure is seen.

of angle-closure, at least in the closure that is the most common in the United States. The mechanism of the closure was described earlier. RPB ACG is usually found in the context of a slightly small eye and a slightly small anterior segment, in an adult or elderly patient, and in association with a lens that has slowly enlarged as a result of its normal growth throughout life. The lens enlarges at the expense of the central and peripheral depth and volume of the anterior chamber. As the lens enlarges, it is likely that more and more of the central posterior iris makes contact with the anterior surface of the lens, increasing the relative block to anterior chamber fluid flow and slightly increasing the pressure differential between the posterior chamber and the anterior chamber. The slightly increased pressure in the posterior chamber causes the peripheral iris not in contact with the lens to bulge anteriorly.

The peripheral bulging of the iris may be maximal when the pupil is in the middilatated position, between 3 and 6 mm in diameter.[17] In this position, RPB exists owing to iris-lens apposition, and at the same time the peripheral iris is relaxed slightly, allowing for more forward bulge and for possible closure. The posterior vector forces of the iris musculature, holding the iris to the lens, may be maximal with this degree of dilatation.[16]

Three different causes have been identified for the pupil to reside in middilatation for a long enough period of time for an acute attack of angle closure to occur: prolonged awake exposure to dim lighting or darkness with relaxation of the sphincter muscle, prolonged severe emotional stress with secondary dilation due to adrenergic stimulation of the dilator muscle, and topical or systemic pharmacologic therapy capable of dilating the pupil.

The level of aqueous production may also be a factor in the degree of peripheral iris bulging created by RPB. It is known that a normal eye can vary its production during different times by perhaps 100 percent—that is, it may secrete approximately 1.5 μL/min during the night[18] and 3.0 during the day. If a person with observable iris bulging is given acetazolamide, which can decrease aqueous production by 50 percent, the peripheral iris in some cases can be seen to fall back slightly. It is also possible, but not proved, that the reduction of

aqueous inflow at night may help explain, along with miosis, the spontaneous resolution of some evening attacks of subacute ACG. This variation may also explain why a person might develop closure at one time during middilatation and not during another. It is also possible that increased aqueous production, stimulated by adrenergic mediators, may have a role in stress-induced acute ACG.

Thus, relative pupillary block ACG can be defined in the following manner. We can recognize that smallness of the anterior chamber and relative lens-eye disproportion[19] or actual increase in lens size to a size slightly larger than normal all may play a part in narrowing the angle. However, if these factors do not close the angle themselves and the additional factor of peripheral iris bulging due to RPB does, then the glaucoma can be named after this last factor. In addition, reversal of the bulging, if it opens the angle, constitutes further proof that it was this last factor that was the final precipitant.

REVERSAL OF RPB ACG BY IRIDECTOMY OR IRIDOTOMY

The peripheral bulge of the iris and the angle closure caused by this bulge can generally be reversed by creating a hole in the peripheral iris by either a surgical peripheral iridectomy or a surgical laser iridotomy. A hole in the periphery of the iris almost immediately equalizes the pressure in the anterior and posterior chambers. With the pressure no longer greater in the posterior chamber, the peripheral iris tends to move slightly posteriorly, toward its more normal anatomic position. This can be seen at the time of laser iridotomy if one observes the configuration and position of the peripheral iris and its change within minutes after the hole has been created. The depth of the peripheral angle increases. Posterior iris pigment, released at the time of iridotomy, can be seen to flow within a gush of aqueous into the anterior chamber, demonstrating in another way that the pressure was higher in the posterior chamber and that it is now being equalized.

REVERSAL OF PERIPHERAL IRIS BULGE: PHARMACOLOGIC MIOSIS AND LASER PERIPHERAL IRIDOPLASTIC TECHNIQUES

The peripheral bulge of the iris, although not the disparity of pressure between the two chambers, can be reversed pharmacologically by drugs that constrict the pupil. The miosis causes the peripheral iris to flatten slightly, producing a generally beneficial effect of opening an angle closed by this mechanism or of widening an angle made narrow by this mechanism. One might ask if miosis does not increase iris lens contact and therefore does not make the RPB effect greater. Clinical observation suggests that tautening of the peripheral iris creates a stronger force than that created by possible slight increase in the pressure differential between the two chambers. Hence the parasympathomimetic drugs exert their beneficial effects not by decreasing RPB but by decreasing the peripheral convexity.

Peripheral bulging can also be reduced somewhat by laser peripheral iridoplasty, a technique to be described later, to be used only primarily for RPB ACG if an iridotomy cannot be performed.

In some eyes, RPB can be reversed by maximal pupillary dilation, which results in a pupil dilated to a point where it has visibly pulled away from the lens surface. This tends to occur more in young eyes that can dilate more fully. This approach should not be used in the therapy of ACG because the dilation is impractical on a long-term basis owing to increased light sensitivity and is impractical on a short-term basis, as perhaps in a case of acute ACG, because the pupil often does not dilate well, because partial dilation might make the closure worse, and because partial dilation might make subsequent and more beneficial miosis difficult. See the later discussion on Mobile Lens ACG and Its Reversal for an exception to this statement.

PIC ACG and Its Reversal

MECHANISM FOR CLOSURE

PIC ACG, which is rare, has an anatomic factor for closure in addition to the general factors (small eye, lens-eye disproportion, and RPB) mentioned earlier.[20–22] In this type of angle closure, the lens is situated slightly more posteriorly than in RPB ACG, so that the central depth of the anterior chamber is greater than in RPB ACG. The peripheral depth remains narrow, however, and the configuration of the iris suggests to the gonioscopist a peripheral plateau (i.e., a relatively flat central iris that falls off rather steeply in the periphery as if off a plateau into a narrow angle) (Fig. 120–3). Because it has been shown that iridotomy does not always prevent subsequent attacks of ACG in these eyes, particularly when they dilate, it is believed that with dilation, peripheral pleating of the iris in the narrow peripheral angle space mechanically causes the peripheral iris to close the angle and cover the trabecular meshwork directly without a major role for RPB.

REVERSAL OF PIC ACG

The treatment for PIC ACG is iridotomy to relieve RPB, although it may be contributing only in a minor way, and then to prevent the peripheral pleating or bunching of the iris in the angle when the iris is dilated by either chronic miotic therapy, which pulls the peripheral iris away from the trabecular meshwork, or by treating the peripheral iris by laser iridoplasty, causing the peripheral iris to contract permanently away from the trabecular meshwork.

Nanophthalmic ACG and Its Reversal

Although it is not the purpose of this chapter to discuss nanophthalmos and the angle-closure associated with this disease, for the purpose of completeness in

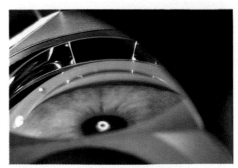

Figure 120–3. Gonioscopic photograph of a patient with plateau iris configuration, angle-closure glaucoma. The centrally flat iris falls off abruptly at the periphery. (From Campbell DG: A comparison of diagnostic techniques in angle-closure glaucoma. Am J Ophthalmol 88:201, 1979. Published with permission from The American Journal of Ophthalmology. Copyright by The Ophthalmic Publishing Company.)

regard to mechanisms of closure, a paragraph is included. Here, in these very small eyes, generally 20 mm or less in axial length, it appears that the mere presence of the lens, with aging and its increase in size, pushes the peripheral iris forward against the trabecular meshwork. Though RPB undoubtedly has a role, as perhaps does dilation, as in PIC angle closure, neither of these factors seems to play a major part because both iridotomy and maximum iridoplasty treatment can often fail and the angle may inexorably continue to close. The mechanism of closure seems to be slow enlargement of the lens itself and its relative size compared with the small eye and its anterior chamber. In some cases, it seems that the only way to prevent inexorable angle closure is to remove the lens, although surgery in these eyes is extremely hazardous and should not be considered without full knowledge of the special complications that can occur.

The fact that a lens can become too large for an eye and can cause closure merely by its large relative size can be illustrated by another secondary ACG, phacomorphic angle closure glaucoma. Here a very large or mature cataract can push the peripheral iris forward and close the angle. In this condition, iridectomy and peripheral iridoplasty can be ineffective. This closure is reversed by removing the enlarged cataractous lens.

Mobile Lens ACG and Its Reversal

The concept of another primary ACG is introduced in this chapter because, over the years, another type of ACG has been found to present in a seemingly primary fashion—that is, with no known underlying primary pathologic cause of the angle-closure. This type of angle-closure resembles that noted by Levene[23] and is described in more detail later. In this form of angle-closure, the lens moves forward excessively into the anterior chamber, beyond its usual position in RPB and in PIC. It is possible that zonule laxity or positive pressure in the vitreous space accounts for the forward movement. In contrast to RPB and to PIC ACG, this

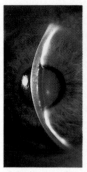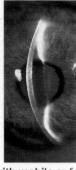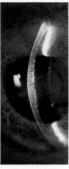

Figure 120–4. A patient with mobile or forward lens angle-closure glaucoma, with the lens one corneal thickness behind the iris (left picture). The middle and right photos show increasing deepening of the anterior chamber with mydriatic-cycloplegic therapy. (From Campbell DG: A comparison of diagnostic techniques in angle-closure glaucoma. Am J Ophthalmol 88:203, 1979. Published with permission from The American Journal of Ophthalmology. Copyright by The Ophthalmic Publishing Company.)

glaucoma is exacerbated by miotic therapy and can be improved by mydriadic-cycloplegic therapy (Fig. 120–4), which may worsen the previously mentioned forms of angle closure. Here, the mydriatic-cycloplegic therapy tightens the ciliary body-zonular ring and moves the lens posteriorly. Iridotomy is often of little value. The mechanism appears to be excessive forward movement of the lens with secondary closure of the angle.

Mechanism of Acute ACG Attack in RPB ACG

MECHANISM OF AN ACUTE ATTACK

As stated earlier, closure can be gradual or sudden (i.e., chronic or acute). The mechanisms discussed generally pertain to chronic or gradual closure. One can then ask, in a patient with a narrow angle, why does that patient go for months or years without a problem and then, over a period of hours, develop an acute attack? In general, in an acute angle-closure attack, the entire trabecular meshwork is covered abruptly, preventing almost all flow of aqueous out of the eye. In this situation, the IOP rises rapidly, as aqueous continues to be produced. The IOP can rise 1 mmHg/min following total closure. Therefore, severe pressure elevations can be seen within 45 min to 1 hr of onset.

The major factor that seems to predispose to an acute attack of angle closure is prolonged, stationary middilation of the pupil, generally between 3 and 6 mm. With the iris in this configuration, RPB continues to exist, causing the pressure in the posterior chamber to be greater than in the anterior chamber. At the same time, the peripheral iris has become slightly lax and is therefore free to bulge slightly more forward, more so than in a more constricted pupillary configuration. It seems that these two factors, combined with a narrow angle, lead to an acute attack.

Attacks frequently occur after a period of time in dim light, supposedly as a result of constant middilation of the pupil. This is the basis for the provocative dark room test, a test used to determine if a narrow angle is capable of actual closure. Attacks also occur after periods of severe stress,[24–26] periods that can also cause dilatation of the pupil due to adrenergic stimulation. Medications, either topical or systemic, that are capable of dilating the pupil can also lead to an acute attack.

OTHER POSSIBLE FACTORS

The thinness or the thickness of the iris could be a hypothetical additional factor in RPB ACG, with a thinner iris perhaps more likely to bulge forward.

It is also possible that the level of aqueous production at the time of the acute attack may be a factor. It is known that aqueous production can vary in the human eye by a factor of 2, and it is possible that episodes of acute ACG occur at times of peak or maximum aqueous production, which would be expected to lead to enhanced peripheral iris bulging. It is also possible that in acute ACG associated with stress, adrenergic stimulation may increase aqueous production, which may be an additional factor in sudden closure.

In regard to the maximum pressure that can be reached in an acute attack, IOP can rise to 60 to 80 mmHg and then does not rise higher. It seems that when the pressure exceeds arterial ciliary process pressure, the production of aqueous stops or slows and the pressure stabilizes. At this point, the pressure within the radial vessels of the iris may be exceeded, explaining the sectoral iris infarction with later atrophy that can occur.

MECHANISM OF SPONTANEOUS RESOLUTION OF INTERMITTENT (SUBACUTE) ATTACKS

Attacks of acute angle-closure occasionally resolve spontaneously. In many cases, they resolve when a patient lies down and rests or sleeps. It is possible that the resolution occurs because relative miosis occurs during sleep, with the miosis pulling the peripheral iris away from the trabecular meshwork. It is also possible that the known reduction in aqueous production during sleep could play a part, reducing peripheral iris bulge,[18] or that relaxation with decreased adrenergic stimulation may have a role.

Miotic-Induced ACG

Angle closure can occasionally be induced by topical pharmacologic miosis, such as high concentrations of direct- or indirect-acting parasympathomimetic agents. In eyes thus affected, the lens may move forward more than the small amount usually produced by these agents, contributing to closure.[27–29] Treatment includes discontinuation of the offending medication and peripheral iridotomy to relieve existent RPB to create slightly more space in the angle.

Accommodative Effort-Induced ACG

Acute or subacute angle-closure glaucoma can occasionally be induced by prolonged reading (i.e., by accommodative effort). The mechanism is unknown but may involve forward movement of the lens. The possible part played by the slightly forward rotation of the ciliary body that occurs in accommodation in these rare cases is unknown. The treatment is to perform iridotomy and to reverse any RPB component and then to perform iridoplasty if necessary.

CLINICAL AND PATHOLOGIC CHANGES FOLLOWING THE DEVELOPMENT OF PRIMARY ACG

The pathologic changes that occur within the eye after the development of primary ACG can be discerned clinically and in the pathology laboratory. Unfortunately, the mechanisms *causing* primary ACG cannot be well appreciated in the pathology laboratory. This is because artifactual changes occur within the eye after death or enucleation. The lens can artifactually become displaced posteriorly, along with the iris, totally obscuring the anatomic configurations that led to the angle closure. Without aqueous production, the physiologic configurational changes caused by RPB disappear as well.

The changes that occur in the trabecular meshwork in association with primary ACG are poorly understood, primarily because the meshwork is not well visualized in routine thick-section light microscopy. In the future, it is hoped that thin-section, 1-μm light microscopy, and transmission and scanning electron microscopy may help delineate the specific pathologic changes that occur in ACG.

The pathologic changes that occur *after* the development of primary ACG can be divided into those following the development of acute or subacute attacks, associated with sudden marked elevation of IOP, and those that are due to chronic gradual elevation of IOP.

Pathologic Changes Following Sudden, Severe Elevation of IOP

The pathologic findings that can occur in the eye after an acute attack of angle-closure glaucoma and severe elevation of IOP can be seen in the cornea, in the iris, in the lens, perhaps in the trabecular meshwork, in the ciliary body, and in the disc.

CORNEA: EDEMA AND ENDOTHELIAL CELL COUNT REDUCTION

Acute, severe elevation of IOP can cause an excessive amount of fluid to pass into the cornea from the anterior chamber. This initially manifests as a collection of fluid in and between the epithelial cells and is seen clinically as bedewing of the cornea, microcystic edema formation, and laking of fluid within and under the epithelium. Edema can at times be seen within the stroma of the cornea as well, particularly after an acute attack. Specular microscopy studies have shown that the number of endothelial cells can be reduced after an acute attack, suggesting damage to and loss of these cells.[30–33]

IRIS: NECROSIS AND SYNECHIA FORMATION

During an acute attack of ACG, it appears that once IOP elevates to between approximately 50 and 70 mmHg, blood flow through the iris or through portions of it can be severely compromised. Ischemia of the iris tissue results, with the posterior pigment layer being the most resistant. Least resistant seem to be the iris stroma and the sphincter and dilator muscles, which are damaged by the ischemic process.[34–36] The loss of iris stroma is manifested by the development of sectorial iris atrophy with thinning and loss of stromal tissue, often resulting in sectors that appear thin, distorted, and gray on clinical examination. Grayish loss of tissue in a circumferential manner can often be seen at the pupillary margin. Necrosis of both the sphincter and the dilator muscle often leaves the pupil in a permanently fixed, irregular middilated configuration. Loss and breakdown of cells from the posterior pigmented layer of the iris with dispersion of a moderate amount of pigment can occasionally be observed.

During attacks of acute IOP elevation, both anterior and posterior synechia formation can occur. The most harmful process is peripheral anterior synechia formation of iris to the trabecular meshwork, leading to synechial closure and loss of trabecular outflow in the sections involved. The exact nature of the fibrosis leading to the closure is unknown. If the IOP is high and the eye is inflamed, significant synechial closure can be seen within approximately 2 to 7 days. Posterior synechiae to the surface of the lens at the pupillary margin also occur under the same circumstances.

LENS: GLAUKOMFLECKEN AND GENERALIZED CATARACT FORMATION

Acute elevation of IOP can damage the central lenticular epithelial cells and the subepithelial cortex.[37–39] After an attack of acute angle closure, whitish subepithelial changes can be seen in the pupillary space in association with the development of a film or mat that may represent a fibrin layer on the surface of the exposed lens in the pupillary region. The glaukomflecken develop only in the exposed pupillary region (Fig. 120–5). Pathologic sections reveal damage to the overlying epithelial cells and coagulation changes in the anterior subepithelial fibers. Although the exact cause of these whitish, milky, sometimes dotlike and sometimes larger star-shaped changes is unknown, they are pathognomonic of an episode of previous severe and acute elevation of IOP, although the cause does not

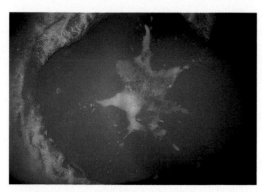

Figure 120–5. Glaukomflecken of the lens and an irregularly fixed and middilated pupil following an attack of acute angle-closure glaucoma.

necessarily have to be a primary ACG attack. In addition to glaukomflecken, generalized cataract formation often occurs gradually after acute attacks.

CILIARY BODY: CILIARY BODY HYPOSECRETION

Clinical observations suggest that the ciliary body is physiologically damaged by a prolonged acute ACG attack with high IOP when the pressure is lowered suddenly. Clinicians have long noted that if severe elevation of IOP is reduced suddenly, either by sudden opening of the angle (either by medical therapy or by iridotomy with reduction of RPB) or, more interestingly, if the IOP is suddenly reduced by the use of medical treatment that markedly decreases aqueous production (topical β-blocker therapy, systemic carbonic anhydrase therapy), or reduced fluid content in the eye (osmotic therapy), or if the pressure is reduced by surgically opening the eye (as in iridectomy or following paracentesis), the IOP can remain low and in the normal range for days even though the angle remains totally closed. Closure may be due to the development of peripheral anterior synechiae or persistence of appositional closure. This temporary reduction in aqueous inflow can be termed *temporary ciliary body hyposecretion*. Aqueous production generally does return to normal or toward normal, and if the angle remains closed, the IOP will generally elevate to high levels once again. Later, we will see that we can occasionally take advantage of this hyposecretion in the treatment of some resistant acute ACG attacks.

The high IOP and its diminution can also lead to the development of inflammation in the eye. Cell and flare can be seen owing to breakdown of the blood-aqueous barrier. If cell and flare are noted within the eye after an attack of pain and if IOP is normal, one should consider the possibility of a preceding attack of intermittent or subacute ACG. Keratic precipitates do not form with the inflammation associated with primary ACG. If keratic precipitates are seen in association with high IOP and angle-closure, one should suspect a secondary mechanism for the closure, such as the development of iris bombé or synechial closure due to inflammatory debris.

OPTIC NERVE: SWELLING AND ATROPHY WITHOUT INCREASED CUPPING; LOSS OF VISION

Acute IOP rise leads to acute congestion of the nerve, with blockage of axonal flow at the level of the lamina cribrosa.[34] Acute swelling of the nerve can be seen clinically during or after an acute attack.[40] Later, the disc can develop increased pallor and atrophy with visual loss but without significant cupping. These acute changes due to high IOP can lead to drastic reduction in vision on a temporary or a permanent basis. Visual field testing during or after acute attacks can show generalized constriction of the peripheral isopters, nerve fiber bundle defects, or central reduction in sensitivity.[41, 42]

Pathologic Changes After Chronic ACG

OPTIC NERVE: TYPICAL GLAUCOMATOUS CUPPING AND VISUAL FIELD LOSS

In chronic ACG, IOP generally elevates in a slow and often silent manner much as it does in chronic open-angle glaucoma. Instead of acute swelling of the disc with subsequent development of pallor and atrophy, without significant cupping, as occurs after an attack of severe acute ACG, the findings in chronic angle closure are those of gradual enlargement of the optic cup often associated with loss of neuroretinal rim tissue, as in chronic open-angle glaucoma. The pathologic consequences are similar to those of chronic open-angle glaucoma, with the gradual development of typical glaucomatous visual field defects. In either case, the end result can be total blindness due to optic nerve damage.

Pathologic Changes in the Trabecular Meshwork in Primary ACG

The trabecular meshwork changes associated with primary ACG are poorly understood and can be divided into three categories: (1) the changes that occur in association with and underneath the development of synechial angle closure, (2) the changes that occur underneath chronic appositional angle closure, and (3) the changes that occur after severe or repeated attacks of acute appositional angle closure.

UNDERNEATH SYNECHIAL ANGLE-CLOSURE

Pathologic studies of the trabecular meshwork underneath chronic synechial ACG reveal degeneration, fibrosis, and sclerosis of the trabecular meshwork. These findings have led clinicians to believe that long-standing synechial closure does severely damage and compromise the function of the trabecular meshwork in this situation. Clinical and perfusion studies also demonstrate that the underlying trabecular meshwork is permanently damaged and nonfunctional, particularly if the meshwork has resided under the synechial closure for more than 1 yr.[43]

UNDERNEATH CHRONIC APPOSITIONAL ANGLE-CLOSURE

The changes that can occur in the trabecular meshwork after chronic appositional closure and hypoperfusion of the meshwork are poorly understood. I have seen one case in which long-standing chronic appositional angle-closure led to permanent damage to the trabecular meshwork, as evidenced by persistent clinical elevation of IOP after opening of the angle and by the histologic appearance of loss of intertrabecular spaces, associated with severe fibrosis of the intertrabecular spaces. This suggests that a secondary open-angle glaucoma may follow chronic appositional ACG.

FOLLOWING SEVERE ACUTE ATTACKS OF APPOSITIONAL CLOSURE THAT REVERSE

The changes that occur—if indeed they exist—in the trabecular meshwork after acute repeated appositional attacks of glaucoma have not been documented pathologically. It is not known if intermittent acute ACG causes permanent damage to the trabecular meshwork, but this has been suggested by some clinicians. In general, if the acute attacks are interrupted, the trabecular meshwork will initially function normally.

DIAGNOSTIC EVALUATION AND DIAGNOSTIC TECHNIQUES IN PRIMARY ACG

Refractive Error

As previously stated, eyes predisposed to ACG are, in general, small.[6-8, 44, 45] Affected eyes are usually hyperopic, and determination of a patient's refractive error can be one of the first clues that an eye may be predisposed to angle closure.[13]

Corneal Size

Many patients with ACG have smaller anterior chambers and slightly smaller corneas than normal.[7, 8, 46] Clinicians in training should routinely measure the horizontal corneal diameter of patients for a while. This promotes perspective and shows that the corneas of patients with ACG tend to be slightly smaller. The normal horizontal corneal diameter, from white to white, is approximately 11.5 to 12.0 mm in adults, and corneas that measure 11.0 mm or less are considered small.

Eye Length: Ultrasound Measurement

Eyes predisposed to ACG are often shorter than normal. Ultrasound measuring units are becoming more widely available, making it easier to obtain this measurement. A normal eye, from the front of the cornea to the front of the retina, measures approximately 23.5 mm. Eyes that are predisposed to ACG average 1 mm shorter than normal.[47]

Central Anterior Chamber Depth

The depth of the central anterior chamber is, in general, decreased in primary ACG.[8, 12, 44, 45, 47–50] The depth of the central anterior chamber should be assessed and estimated in corneal thicknesses at slit-lamp biomicroscopy, because this measurement too can alert a clinician to the possibility of ACG. In this way, the central corneal depth can be considered to be shallow, moderate, or deep. In general, if the central corneal depth is six corneal thicknesses or greater, it can be considered to be deep. If it is four to five corneal thicknesses, it can be considered to be moderate in depth. If it is three corneal thicknesses, it can be considered to be quite shallow. The central thickness of the cornea is approximately 0.5 mm, and hence a shallow anterior chamber (three corneal thicknesses) is approximately 1.5 mm in depth. A moderate anterior chamber (four to five corneal thicknesses) is 2.0 to 2.5 mm in depth, and deep anterior chambers (six corneal thicknesses or greater) are 3.0 mm or greater. In general, in RPB ACG, the central corneal depth will be found to be three to four corneal thicknesses or 1.5 to 2.0 mm.[51, 52] In PIC ACG, the central corneal depth may be deeper, approximately five corneal thicknesses, or 2.5 mm centrally. In the rare mobile lens or forward lens angle closure, the central corneal depth will be found to be abnormally shallow or "too shallow," and the lens will be found to reside one to two corneal thicknesses, or 0.5 to 1.0 mm, behind the central endothelium, demonstrating its abnormal forward position.

Accurate measurement of the central anterior chamber depth, to 0.1 mm, may be obtained by measurement with the Haag-Streit AC pachymeter, that fits easily onto the same manufacturer's slit lamp. This instrument, similar to the corneal pachymeter, is essential for accurate measurement of subtle changes in lens position or anterior chamber depth.

Peripheral Anterior Chamber Depth: van Herick's Test

The peripheral anterior chamber is shallow in all primary ACG.[11, 17, 44, 53–55] Clinical assessment of the peripheral anterior chamber depth at slit-lamp biomicroscopic examination is one of the most important assessments in regard to anterior chamber examination. Van Herick and colleagues introduced the concept of the examination of the peripheral depth many years ago, and this clinical test has proved to be invaluable (Fig. 120–6).[55] If one is asking the question, does the patient have an angle that may have closed, or may close spontaneously, or may be capable of closing with

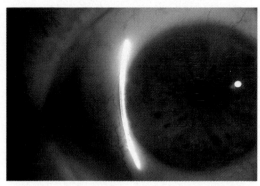

Figure 120–6. Positioning of the slit beam for clinical evaluation of the peripheral depth of the anterior chamber, right eye, van Herick's test.

dilation?—this test is almost as valuable as gonioscopic evaluation. The test is performed by evaluating the depth of the temporal anterior chamber as far temporally as can be seen. As originally shown by van Herick and Shaffer, if the peripheral depth in this region is one-fourth corneal thickness or less, the possibility of angle closure exists. If the depth is slitlike, angle-closure is even more likely.

Gonioscopy

Gonioscopy constitutes the most important clinical examination in ACG.[20, 56-60] Accurate gonioscopy is essential to intelligent understanding, diagnosis, and therapy of these glaucomas.

Gonioscopy of the narrow angle and accurate determination of the closure status are difficult and require skill that is acquired with patience and time. It is relatively easy to evaluate a wide-open angle, and it makes little difference which gonioscopic lens is used, but it is considerably more difficult to evaluate some closed angles, some partially closed angles, or some angles that are open but extremely narrow. The first problem encountered in gonioscopy of a narrow angle derives from the fact that the iris is convex and hence difficult to see over, so that the first difficulty to overcome is to view over the anteriorly bowed iris down into the narrow angle. Once this view has been obtained, the next task is to determine the status of the angle—that is, if the angle is narrow but open or if actual closure exists.

GONIOSCOPIC LENSES

Direct (Koeppe's Lens) Gonioscopy

Initially, all gonioscopy was performed with a Koeppe lens or a similar lens using a direct view of the angle with a hand-held magnification system and hand-held light. This was the method used by Saltzman, the father of gonioscopy, and the one used until the introduction of indirect mirror lenses. One of the advantages of this system was the ability to move up over the convex iris with the equipment and look easily down into the narrow angle. This is still an excellent system and is perhaps the best way to evaluate a narrow angle.[58] The system is cumbersome, however, requiring a supine patient in a relatively large room and costly equipment that is difficult to purchase today. This form of gonioscopy is also more time-consuming and has been largely abandoned by most American ophthalmologists.

Indirect Gonioscopy, Mirror Lens Gonioscopy

Direct gonioscopy has been largely supplanted by indirect gonioscopy performed at the slit lamp. This type of gonioscopy permits visualization of the angle off a mirror with slit-lamp illumination and biomicroscopic magnification. This is the type of gonioscopy used by most ophthalmologists today because it is less expensive, requires less space because patients are examined sitting at the slit lamp, and takes advantage of the superior lighting, the superior magnification if necessary, and the superior optical clarity of the modern slit lamp.

Indirect Gonioscopy: Vaulting Versus Direct-Contact Lenses

The indirect gonioscopy system uses two basic types of lenses: lenses that vault the cornea and require a fluid or gel to fill the space between the lens and the eye and lenses that make direct contact with the cornea and require no additional fluid.

Two basic types of lenses vault the cornea: lenses with a low mirror placement and less angulation with the plane of the iris (which give a lower or flatter view across the anterior chamber and do not generally allow a view into the apex of a narrow angle unless the patient looks toward the lens and the mirror is tilted toward the angle being viewed; generally three-mirror lenses) and lenses with mirrors that are mounted higher and with a greater angulation to the horizontal and generally allow a view into the apex of a narrow angle without requiring the patient to move the eye (generally one- or two-mirror lenses). Each lens allows evaluation of and a view into the narrow angle that is almost as good as direct gonioscopy, and each is considerably easier to use.

In patients with small eyes and small palpebral fissures, the smaller base diameter of a one-mirror lens may be easier to insert than the larger-based three-mirror lens. A practical point to remember about gonioscopy is that some patients may be considerably more comfortable if the anesthetic drop is repeated once for more complete anesthesia. Also, patients tolerate a lengthy examination more comfortably if the lens is not held in place with excessive pressure, which can cause considerable ache in the eye.

Lenses that make direct contact with the cornea (the Zeiss and Sussman four-mirror lenses are currently the most popular) require anesthesia, as do all lenses, but do not require a fluid or gel between the lens and the eye. The examination is thus simpler and easier to perform. Corneal wrinkling, caused by pressure, may slightly obscure the view, however, particularly if a patient must move the eye for the examiner to see into the depth of the angle. Increasingly more ophthalmologists are switching to these lenses because of their simplicity, speed, greater acceptance by patients, and ability to permit indentation evaluation.

GONIOSCOPY IN ANGLE CLOSURE

Two important questions must be answered in the gonioscopic evaluation of a narrow angle: First, is the angle open or closed?; second, if the angle is closed, is the closure appositional or synechial?

NORMAL OPEN ANGLE VERSUS CLOSED ANGLE

Once a lens has been chosen and a view over the convex iris has been obtained, the first task is to determine if the angle is open or closed. If the angle is found to be closed, the examiner may then want to determine if the closure is appositional or synechial. The first evaluation requires familiarity with the normal appearance of the open angle. Only then can it be determined if the structures normally seen are not being seen (i.e., are covered by the peripheral iris).

Schwalbe's Line

Clinicians should be familiar with the appearance of Schwalbe's line and should know that although this line may not be discernible in many eyes, two features of the line, when present, are pathognomonic: First, protuberance or a slight shelflike quality of the line into the anterior chamber is occasionally noted. Second, inferiorly, pigment may collect on it and delineate it in a circumferential but nonwavy manner (a wavy inferior line can exist more anteriorly in the periphery of the inferior cornea and is known as *Sampaolesi's line*). If the gonioscopist can definitely identify this line in one area or another, a useful landmark has been discovered.

Trabecular Meshwork

The observer should be familiar with three pathognomonic aspects of the trabecular meshwork itself: first, the very important change in texture and color between the periphery of the cornea, which appears white owing to the sclera seen in its background, and the meshwork itself, which has a slightly porous or textured appearance and is less white; second, the characteristic pigmentation pattern of the trabecular meshwork itself, of dispersed pigment within the meshwork that darkens the posterior portion of the trabecular meshwork, that portion overlying Schlemm's canal. By adulthood, most but not all patients have dispersed enough pigment to make this finding helpful. This pigment is especially prominent inferiorly and nasally. This pigment band is wider than the pigment line that may delineate Schwalbe's line. Third, the blush of blood in Schlemm's canal that can be occasionally seen also identifies the posterior trabecular meshwork. This blush is more commonly seen in supine patients undergoing Koeppe gonioscopy than it is in upright patients at slit-lamp gonioscopy.

Scleral Spur

Perhaps the most definite and important landmark is the scleral spur, the white band of connective tissue making up the posterior aspect of the trabecular groove and lying posterior to the trabecular meshwork. When the meshwork or the spur is seen, either in its entirety, the angle is open in that region.

Iris Contour

In addition to determination of the status of the angle in regard to closure, other assessments should be made. First, the contour of the iris should be observed and recorded, Is the iris convex and, if so, to what degree? Is the iris evenly convex, as is characteristic of RPB ACG, or is the iris flat centrally and does it then drop into a narrow angle peripherally, as in PIC ACG?

One occasionally sees an angle that appears to be closed and wonders if the angle is open and nonpigmented or truly closed and therefore not observed. As an aid, part of the angle often is open somewhere (it is usually not entirely closed except in an acute attack). If the examiner is not sure whether an area is open or closed but suspects closure, it is advisable to rotate around the circumference of the angle until a definitely open or partially open area with landmarks can be found. These landmarks may be a shelved Schwalbe's line, or the typical trabecular pigmentation found in most elderly eyes, or the whitish line of the scleral spur, the most reliable landmark. If one of these can be found, then it is possible to rotate to the area in question and usually make an accurate determination by comparison. Difficulty can be encountered when Schwalbe's line is flat and the trabecular meshwork has no pigmentation. Here, I rely on the texture change of the meshwork previously described.

Although indentation gonioscopy has not yet been described, it can be helpful at this point, when one is not sure if the trabecular meshwork is covered. Posterior deformation of the peripheral iris may now reveal a trabecular meshwork that was obviously appositionally covered, confirming the impression of closure.

Shaffer's Classification of the Angle

After the iris has been observed, the narrowness of the angle, if open, should be ascertained. I prefer Shaffer's classification of the narrow angle, dividing it into slitlike inlets of 10, 20, 30, and 40 degrees, noting that inlets 20 degrees or greater generally do not close and that those of 10 degrees or less are at considerable risk and also noting that this classification is subjective and probably subject to considerable interpersonal variation.[20]

A Drawing of the Findings

Once the examination is complete—and it may have taken more than one rotation of 360 degrees to be certain of the result—the findings should be accurately drawn in a double circle diagram. In general, if the posterior two-thirds of the trabecular meshwork is covered, that area is probably almost completely blocked and nonfunctional. A general assessment should be made of what percentage of the angle is closed and where. It is convenient to divide the circumference into 30-degree segments or clock hours.

INDENTATION GONIOSCOPY: THE DIFFERENTIATION BETWEEN APPOSITIONAL AND SYNECHIAL CLOSURE

Once the initial evaluation of the angle has been determined, if portions of the angle have been found to be closed, the angle needs to be reexamined to determine if the closure is appositional or synechial. Indentation gonioscopy, introduced by Forbes (Fig. 120–7), can answer this question.[61–63] For this gonioscopic examination, only one of the lenses described, the contact four-mirror lens, is practical. The other lenses, which vault the cornea, are not capable of the central corneal indentation necessary for the examination. With central compression of the four-mirror contact lens on the cornea, aqueous can be forced from the central anterior chamber out into the angle, pushing the peripheral iris posteriorly and opening the closed angle if the closure is appositional.

This is not an easy technique to learn but can be mastered with patience and practice. If I am going to perform this test, I use gonioscopy gel of some kind on the lens to try and reduce epithelial cell damage. Corneal wrinkling with indentation can to a degree obscure the view of the angle. If straightforward central indentation of the lens does not cause sufficient peripheral posterior deformation of the iris, tilting the lens with impression of the mirror away from the observed angle (i.e., tilting inward the mirror that is being looked into) and even sliding the lens toward the angle being viewed may be necessary for complete examination.

It is not always possible to perform an accurate or complete examination. The lower the initial pressure, the easier the examination, and if the pressure is extremely high, indentation may be very difficult. The patient may not be able to cooperate fully. In some cases of closure due to iris bombé, the technique may be inadequate in that indentation cannot overcome the extreme bowing in this condition.

Ophthalmologists today almost routinely use indirect gonioscopy for initial evaluation of a narrow angle. Many use a vaulting mirror, and others use a direct four-mirror contact lens. If one chooses to use the contact lens for all examinations, and especially if one is a beginner, one must be careful not to cause undetected indentation and unwanted opening of an apposi-

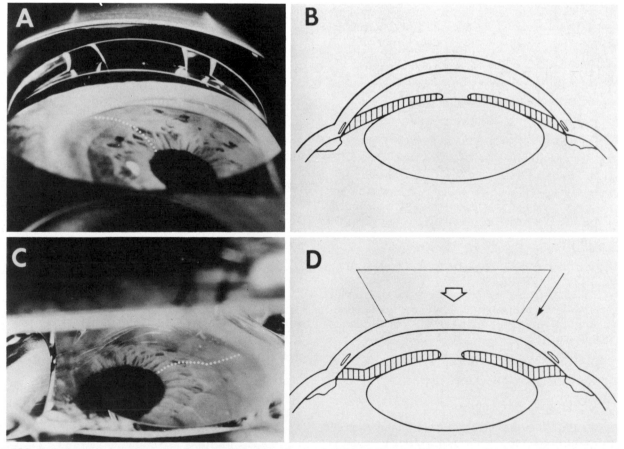

Figure 120–7. Indentation gonioscopy. Gonioscopic view of a convex iris and appositionally closed angle before indentation. *B,* Drawing of same. *C,* Goniophotograph during indentation, revealing flattening of the peripheral iris and opening of the appositionally closed angle. *D,* Drawing of same.

tionally closed angle in the initial angle evaluation, leading to the erroneous diagnosis of an open angle.

Use of Topical Glycerin for an Edematous Cornea

When the cornea is cloudy as a result of edema due to severe elevation of the IOP, gonioscopy can be extremely difficult and sometimes impossible. The almost instant partial clearing of the cornea with a drop of topical glycerin produced by corneal dehydration can improve the visibility of the angle substantially. One can be disappointed, however, in that although the central view of the anterior chamber at slit-lamp examination can be markedly improved, the oblique gonioscopic view may be only marginally improved.

An enhanced view of the central anterior chamber is extremely important, however, in evaluation and accurate assessment of the differential diagnostic possibilities in a patient who presents with acute or seemingly acute IOP elevation. A diagnosis of acute ACG may be entertained, but other causes of acute or seemingly acute IOP rise must be ruled out. A clearer view through the central cornea may allow visualization of previously unappreciated fine neovascular tufts at the pupillary margin and an open and neovascularized or a closed angle (compatible with neovascular glaucoma). It may also allow observations such as a hypermature lens with heavy flare and some cells in the anterior chamber (compatible with phacolytic glaucoma), a hypermature swollen lens and a closed angle (phacomorphic ACG), khaki-colored ghost cells in the aqueous and an open angle (ghost cell glaucoma), or mutton-fat keratic precipitates and cell and flare in the anterior chamber (compatible with uveitic glaucoma).

Examination of the Contralateral Eye

If a patient presents with an acute IOP elevation and the cornea is so edematous that an adequate diagnostic view of the anterior chamber and angle is not possible, examination of the contralateral eye can be extremely valuable. If the diagnosis is acute RPB ACG, the fellow eye will generally be found to have a very narrow angle as well. If the fellow eye has a deep anterior chamber (and rare anisometropia has been ruled out by examining the patient's refraction), one should consider sudden open-angle glaucoma and unilateral ACG in the differential diagnosis.

Surgical Chamber-Deepening Procedure

Simmons and Chandler introduced the chamber-deepening procedure as a modification of Shaffer's technique to answer the question, if an angle is seen to be entirely closed in association with an acute attack, is that closure appositional or synechial?[64] If a patient with neglected or long-standing acute ACG was seen and was taken to the operating room, the question whether to perform a peripheral iridectomy or a filtration procedure arose. If the angle was synechially closed 360 degrees, an iridectomy was useless and a filtration procedure was indicated. On the other hand, if the angle is appositionally closed for 360 degrees, then an iridectomy to open the angle is all that is indicated. To answer the question about the type of closure and the appropriate surgical therapy, Shaffer suggested performing an iridectomy and then closing the eye and performing gonioscopy to determine how much of the angle had opened after relief of RPB.[65] It was then possible to determine whether further surgery, a filtration procedure, was indicated.

Chandler and Simmons altered the procedure by initially performing paracentesis, artificially deepening the chamber with saline through the paracentesis site (today this is done with a viscoelastic substance), and performed gonioscopy in the operating room before choosing a surgical procedure (Figs. 120–8 and 120–9). If the eye was found to be synechially closed for 360 degrees, a filtration procedure was performed. If the eye was open 360 degrees, an iridectomy was indicated. If the angle was partially synechially closed, the surgeon would perform an iridectomy unless the closure was very extensive (generally 9 hr or more [270 degrees or more]), and then a filtration procedure would generally be done. Today, one would consider goniosynechialysis as well (discussed later).

It is important to be aware of a small technical point when performing a chamber-deepening procedure. After paracentesis is performed and a small amount of aqueous is allowed to escape the anterior chamber, the limbus of the cornea should be gently indented for 360 degrees. This important step forces fluid from the posterior chamber into the anterior and allows the peripheral iris to move more posteriorly when the anterior chamber is refilled and deepened.

In the chamber-deepened configuration, the lens is pushed slightly posteriorly and the peripheral iris drastically so. Gonioscopic evaluation of the angle is thus facilitated, because synechial closure, if it exists, becomes quite obvious. In addition, the angle becomes wide enough to accept surgical instruments safely, advantageous in performing goniosynechialysis (described later).

Laser Iridotomy as a Diagnostic as Well as Therapeutic Technique in ACG

Today, the development of indentation gonioscopy allows differentiation between appositional and synechial closure in the office most but not all of the time. More importantly, the development of laser iridotomy has made iridotomy so simple and so safe that it can be used to avoid operating room surgery, and laser iridotomy can be used as a diagnostic as well as a therapeutic

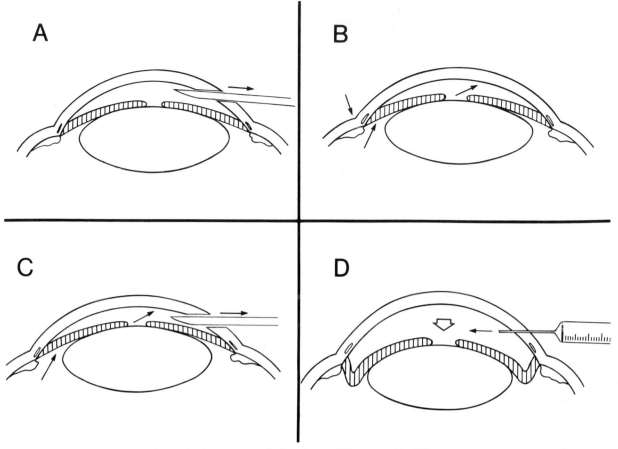

Figure 120–8. *A* to *D*, The chamber deepening procedure of Chandler and Simmons. Fluid is evacuated from the anterior and posterior chambers, and fluid is then reintroduced to deepen the anterior chamber artifically.

technique. If an angle is completely closed and indentation gonioscopy is not possible or is not diagnostic, iridotomy can be performed. If the closure was due to RPB, as it usually is, then the appositional portions of the closure will open and the synechial portions will not. One can then reexamine the patient with gonioscopy to make the determination.

Tonography in ACG

Using tonography, Grant originally showed that in ACG, the trabecular meshwork, the pressure, and the tonographic facility of outflow are normal when the angle is open and that these are abnormal when the angle is closed.

Diagnostic Mistakes To Avoid

Acute or intermittent (subacute) ACG can occasionally masquerade as other diseases and be misdiagnosed. The headaches and eye aches associated with subacute attacks can be mistaken for migraine headaches or other types of headaches. If this might be the case and narrow angles are found, a patient must be observed during an attack and have the IOP measured and the angle examined at that time. An acute attack of ACG can cause nausea and vomiting. If the patient or the physician does not pay attention to the eye, an unnecessary and unrewarding gastrointestinal work-up may be performed. Cells and flare may be seen in an eye after spontaneous resolution of a subacute attack. The history of sudden pain, dilatation rather than constriction of the pupil, an absence of keratic precipitates, and a narrow or partially closed angle should lead to the correct diagnosis of subacute ACG and away from the incorrect diagnosis of spontaneous uveitis or iritis. Again, after spontaneous resolution of an acute attack, the associated disc swelling and venous swelling should not be misinterpreted as either papillitis or vein occlusion. In addition, if a patient with known (or more likely unknown) narrow angles develops ocular pain after surgery with general anesthesia, one should not automatically assume this is due to corneal irritation or abrasion. Acute ACG should be ruled out, because anticholinergic medications are frequently used by anesthesiologists, and they can lead to pupillary dilation and closure in individuals at risk. Severe ocular damage can ensue if days are allowed to pass with a mistaken diagnosis of corneal abrasion.

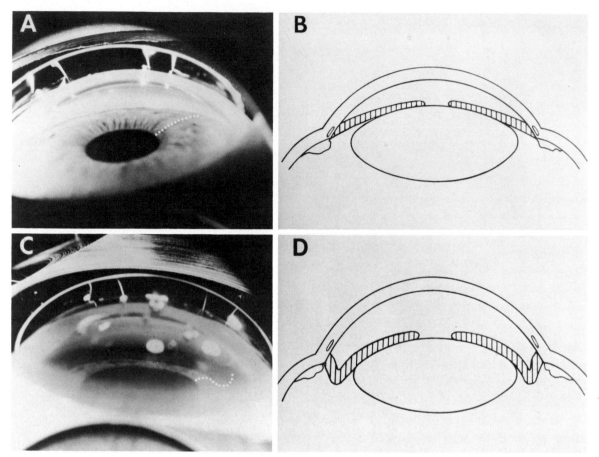

Figure 120–9. The chamber deepening procedure. *A,* gonioscopic photo in the operating room showing closed angle. *B,* Drawing of same. *C,* Deep peripheral chamber following chamber deepening. *D,* Drawing of same. The deepened configuration, reliably held with viscoelastic substance, makes goniosynechialysis possible.

THERAPEUTIC MODALITIES IN PRIMARY ACG

Pharmacologic Therapy

MIOTIC THERAPY: PARASYMPATHOMIMETIC AGENTS

Pilocarpine, a direct-acting parasympathomimetic drug, is an important and frequently used drug in ACG. It is the main drug to be used pharmacologically to reverse the angle closure of RPB, PIC, and nanophthalmic ACG. In these cases, if the closure is appositional, the strong miosis pulls peripheral iris tissue out of the angle and flattens the peripheral iris tissue as well. If the forces causing the angle closure are not too strong, this may open the angle and reduce the elevated IOP. If the closure has been chronic, medical therapy may control the IOP and prevent further closure, either appositional or synechial. In general, however, medical therapy should only be used until more definitive surgical therapy can be applied (i.e., peripheral iridotomy for RPB and peripheral iridoplasty for PIC ACG).

Using pilocarpine or other parasympathomimetic therapy alone in the treatment of chronic ACG can be dangerous: The forces causing closure may initially be overcome, but as years go by this may no longer be the case, and chronic closure may develop despite therapy. This closure may also be masked by the open-angle pressure-lowering effect of the pilocarpine, and the treating doctor therefore may not suspect that this harmful effect is occurring. If a patient refuses laser or surgical therapy, the angle should be examined gonioscopically once a year while parasympathomimetic therapy continues.

Pilocarpine is also the drug of choice to treat acute ACG of the types described earlier. If an acute attack has just begun and is only minutes or an hour or two old, pilocarpine 2 to 4 percent alone may suffice to abort the attack.

In an acute attack of ACG, one wants to constrict the sphincter muscle maximally. As stated earlier, this maximal constriction may increase RPB, and although this effect theoretically might worsen the ACG, the beneficial effect of flattening the peripheral iris usually far outweighs any increase in RPB.

In an acute attack of ACG, the pupillary sphincter, the iris muscle that responds to the pilocarpine, may be in one of three conditions: (1) perfused and therefore responsive to immediate pharmacologic therapy; (2)

nonperfused because of high and prolonged IOP elevation and therefore reversibly nonresponsive to pharmacologic therapy, in which case the muscle would be expected to respond when the pressure is lowered by other medical means; and (3) nonperfused and perhaps necrotic and therefore rendered permanently nonresponsive to miotic therapy. Because there is no way to determine accurately the status of the sphincter, pilocarpine should be administered immediately so that if and when the sphincter can react, pilocarpine will be in the anterior chamber and on the receptors to cause it to do so.

One must take care not to place too much pilocarpine on the eye needlessly by exceeding the maximum dose necessary for saturation of the receptors and thus unnecessarily increase the likelihood of unwanted systemic toxicity and poisoning. Signs of this toxicity include diaphoresis, salivation, nausea and vomiting, defecation, hypotension, bradycardia, and respiratory bronchospasm and distress. Some of these symptoms might be falsely attributed to the acute glaucoma attack and be neglected.

The initial treatment of an acute attack should start with one drop of 2 percent pilocarpine placed in the eye every 5 min times three. One drop of 2 percent pilocarpine is equivalent to 1 mg. In a normal eye, a maximum aqueous concentration is achieved within 5 min. The two additional drops further increase the intraocular concentration. If the pupil does not immediately respond, one drop should be placed in the eye every 30 min times three, then perhaps one drop every 2 hr until miosis is achieved, keeping in mind that the diaphoretic subcutaneous dose of pilocarpine is 5 mg and a dangerous toxic systemic dose is 100 mg.

If the pupil cannot respond because the IOP is too high and arterial perfusion to the sphincter has been interrupted, one should reduce the frequency of administered pilocarpine drops until other medications administered to lower the IOP have had time to take effect.[66, 67]

If the ACG attack has been continuing for days and the sphincter is not only fixed but is irregular in shape, permanent necrosis may be present.

If the contralateral eye is extremely narrow but uninvolved in an acute attack, a drop of 1 percent pilocarpine is indicated for this eye because the adrenergic response of the stress of the acute attack in the other eye might precipitate a second attack that should be avoided by this precaution.

REDUCTION OF AQUEOUS FORMATION

Standard pressure-lowering medications that decrease aqueous formation can be used to treat chronic ACG but should be used only after appropriate surgical therapy. These agents too could mask the slow pressure rise of further chronic closure if the precipitating mechanism has not been reversed, as stated earlier.

In an acute ACG attack, these medications have a strong role in initial therapy. If the pupil does not immediately respond to pilocarpine therapy within 5 to 10 min or if it is not expected to respond initially (the attack is many hours old and IOP is greater than 50 to 60 mmHg), then medications to lower IOP by means other than opening the angle should be administered. A topical β-blocker and acetazolamide should be given immediately if not contraindicated. One drop of timolol maleate 0.5 percent should be placed on the eye, perhaps repeated in 30 min. If the attack is not broken, it should be repeated at 4 and 8 hr, then every 12 hr.

Diamox, 500 mg/PO, should be given immediately if the patient is not nauseated or vomiting and can tolerate oral medication. If not, 500 mg IV should be given.

It is hoped that these medications will rapidly lower IOP to less than 40 to 50 mmHg and will allow reperfusion of the sphincter for it to respond to pilocarpine.

OSMOTIC REDUCTION OF OCULAR PRESSURE

In an attack of acute ACG, the pressure can be reduced pharmacologically in three ways: first, by opening the closed angle with miotic therapy; second, by reducing aqueous formation; and third, by osmotically reducing the aqueous volume within the eye. Oral osmotic agents are generally tried first, and if these fail, then a systemic intravenous agent can be used. These agents work by drawing fluid osmotically out of the eye across the blood-eye barrier into the vascular space.

If a patient is not nauseous and can tolerate oral agents, glycerol (glycerin) can be given, 1.0 to 1.5 g/kg in a 50 percent solution. It is usually mixed in refrigerated orange juice for palatability. IOP begins to fall quickly and has usually reached its maximum within 45 to 60 min. It is hoped that this reduction will allow the miotic to constrict the pupil and open the angle. If the pupil remains nonreactive, the lower IOP may allow the cornea to clear of edema, permitting emergency laser peripheral iridotomy or iridoplasty (perhaps in conjunction with the use of topical glycerin as well). The pressure may remain low for 5 to 6 hr but generally rises again if the angle has not been opened. The treatment can be repeated if necessary at that time.

Glycerol can cause hyperglycemia in diabetic patients and may therefore be contraindicated in this group. Dehydration occurs not only in the eye but also the brain and can lead to headache and possible disorientation and coma. Caution should be used in elderly patients with renal, cardiovascular, or diabetic disease. Nausea and vomiting can be precipitated by this agent. Diuresis must be expected, and acute retention can occur.

Isosorbide can be safely used in diabetic persons because it causes no hyperglycemia. It is given orally at a dose of 1.5 to 2.0 g/kg. It may cause less nausea as well.

If the oral agents cannot be used, then intravenous mannitol, if not contraindicated, can be extremely effective in helping to lower IOP. Mannitol is given in a 20 percent solution 2 g/kg IV, during ½ hr. IOP diminishes soon thereafter, generally reaching its maximum decrease at 1 hr. With all osmotic agents, patients cannot be allowed to drink water and reverse the osmotic effect. Urea, formerly used, should not be given because tissue extravasation around the needle can cause severe sloughing of the skin and tissue. Again, extreme care should be used with these strong osmotic agents, and all the previously listed complications with oral agents can occur with mannitol. Diuresis might require catheterization.

REDUCTION OF PAIN AND ANXIETY

In acute ACG attacks, especially if prolonged, the pain can be severe and unrelenting. Intramuscular morphine may provide some relief. In addition, if indicated, a retrobulbar block can also afford immediate relief. It may also allow easier gonioscopic examination and laser therapy.

MYDRIATIC-CYCLOPLEGIC THERAPY

Mydriatic-cycloplegic therapy can, in some conditions, by dilatation of the ciliary body ring with secondary tightening of the zonular ring, pull the lens posteriorly. This treatment, first described as a therapy for malignant or posterior aqueous diversion glaucoma, is contraindicated in all cases of primary ACG except mobile or forward lens ACG. It is indicated in this form. In the others, dilatation can only be expected to make things worse (discussed earlier).

With extreme dilatation of the iris, especially in young patients, who can dilate fully, the iris can lift off the lens and RPB can be relieved. Theoretically, this could break an attack of RPB ACG. An iris suffering an acute attack would not be expected to dilate well, however, and if dilatation failed, the medication would make the necessary constriction more difficult.

Laser Therapy

PERIPHERAL IRIDOTOMY

The technique of peripheral iridotomy is discussed later. I prefer Nd.YAG to argon laser iridotomy because of its speed, relative ease, and the decreased dispersion of melanin particles. During an acute ACG attack, however, the procedure can be difficult, can be associated with hemorrhage, and can be impossible in some eyes with cloudy corneas.

PERIPHERAL IRIDOPLASTY

The peripheral iris is treated with surface argon laser burns that are of large size (500 μm), long duration (0.5 sec), and low power (approximately 250 mW for brown irides and 400 mW for blue), working up to a point where visible surface reaction and contraction occur. Approximately six applications per quadrant should be used, leaving space in between the applications for perfusion of the iris and avoiding possible neovascularization. Slight ocular discomfort may be felt by the patient at this point. The power setting should be as low as possible. Only topical anesthesia is required. Patients should be warned that one treatment may not suffice

and that a second treatment may be necessary to obtain a permanent effect (i.e., posterior positioning of the peripheral iris). The applications are performed with a contact lens with straight-on applications. I prefer to use a gonioscopy lens so that as the peripheral iris treatments are applied straight on, rapid visualization of the effect in the angle can be seen through the gonioscopy mirror.

Patients should be told ahead of time that the treatment might cause slight permanent dilatation of the pupil and that it will cause delayed discoloration of the peripheral iris.

PERIPHERAL LASER SYNECHIALYSIS

In early synechial closure, peripheral laser synechialysis may be an effective means of opening a synechially closed angle and should be attempted before surgical goniosynechialysis. If the synechiae are firm, however, laser therapy may not be effective.

PUPILLOPLASTY: LASER THERAPY FOR ACUTE ACG

In acute RPB ACG, if laser attempts at iridotomy and peripheral iridoplasty have failed or are not feasible because of corneal clouding, distortion of the pupil by pupilloplasty might pull a middilated pupil away from the lens and break the pupillary block.[68, 69]

Surgical Therapy

PERIPHERAL IRIDECTOMY

If all medical and laser attempts have failed to break an attack of RPB ACG, surgical iridectomy may be indicated. This might be combined with the chamber-deepening procedure to determine the degree of synechial closure (discussed earlier).

CHAMBER-DEEPENING PROCEDURE

This procedure was described earlier. It is theoretically possible that this procedure could be therapeutic as well as diagnostic—that is, that the deepening could cause early synechiae to fall away from the trabecular meshwork. In reality, however, the deepening and posterior displacement of the peripheral iris are often not strong enough to dislodge synechial closure.

GONIOSYNECHIALYSIS

If the angle becomes synechially completely closed or almost completely closed (270 degrees or more), a goniosynechialysis procedure can be considered.[70, 71] This relatively new operation takes advantage of the development of viscoelastic substances for surgery and the fact that the meshwork will function well if reopened if it has not been closed and covered for too long a time, perhaps 6 mo or less (Fig. 120–10).

Candidates for this procedure are patients who have

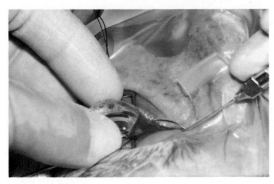

Figure 120–10. An eye about to undergo goniosynechialysis, with a surgical Barkan's lens on the eye and a curved spatula prepared to enter the eye.

had significant synechial closure for 6 months or less. Included are patients who have developed closure after an attack of acute ACG, patients with closure secondary to recent iris bombé, and patients with an angle that has closed after complicated surgery or trauma.

The technique involves the use of the chamber-deepening procedure as described. With the angle held reliably widened and the lens pressed posteriorly by a viscoelastic substance, the peripheral iris can be teased from the trabecular meshwork with a spatula.

One often may not know if the underlying meshwork was normal before closure or how long the closure has existed. If a patient has had an attack of acute closure and the other eye has normal pressure, indicating no chronic open-angle glaucoma, and if the disc in the involved eye is normal, suggesting the absence of long-term preexisting chronic ACG, one can assume the patient may be a good candidate. Results have generally been favorable in synechial closure cases of less than 6 mo duration.

PARACENTESIS

Before the introduction of laser iridotomy, an acute attack of ACG that could not be broken medically required an emergent trip to the operating room for at least a surgical iridectomy. Now that this is most often not necessary (i.e., because most acute attacks are treated with laser iridotomy), there may be a place for paracentesis in some cases of resistant acute ACG. If a patient is suffering from an acute attack that cannot be broken medically and if this attack has been continuing for some days, the cornea may be too edematous or cloudy to perform laser iridotomy. Osmotic therapy may often be contraindicated in an elderly patient, or its use may pose considerable risk, perhaps contributing to the failure of medical therapy. Perhaps it will take many hours or will be almost impossible to obtain an operating room for a surgical iridectomy procedure. One may wonder if there is anything one can do to relieve a patient's pain and high IOP and allow a controlled and comfortable laser iridotomy at a later time.

A simple solution to this problem involves paracentesis. The eye is treated with topical antibiotics, and a retrobulbar injection is given. A patient who has been in severe pain for hours to days feels immediate relief. The paracentesis procedure can be performed sterilely in the office with the patient supine, using an office operating microscope or loupes, or can be performed at the slit lamp, perhaps with more difficulty. A lid speculum is used, as well as toothed forceps to hold the eye absolutely still. A very sharp disposable blade is slipped through the peripheral cornea temporally into the shallow anterior chamber. This should only be performed by someone skilled in the maneuver of paracentesis and should be done with maximum control. The IOP is reduced, and the patient can then be admitted to the hospital for a night of rest. The next morning, the IOP is usually still low because of the ciliary body shock phenomenon (discussed earlier), the pupil may have been constricted by pilocarpine, the cornea has cleared, and the candidate can have laser iridotomy with relative ease.

Gonioscopy will be enhanced by the clear cornea, and a determination of appositional versus synechial closure can often be made. All this can be done in a much more controlled environment than the one that exists in an acute situation.

Although risks are involved with this approach, including intraocular infection, intraocular hemorrhage, and lens damage, these risks are present for a surgical iridectomy as well. The use of mannitol in the elderly can also pose considerable risks, which can even be life-threatening.

FILTRATION SURGERY

Filtration surgery may become necessary in ACG if extensive, permanent synechial angle-closure has developed.

LENS EXTRACTION

If ACG occurs with a coincident cataract that causes enough visual loss to require removal, removing the lens will halt the angle closure process. Hence it can be the treatment of choice in this situation.

CORNEAL INDENTATION

Just as indentation gonioscopy can open an appositionally closed angle, so can it or other forms of indentation of the cornea open the angle in acute ACG. This therapy, introduced by Anderson, should be tried if other simple means have failed to break an attack of acute ACG.[72]

RPB ACG

Epidemiology

Prevalence. ACG in general is much rarer than chronic open-angle glaucoma, being one fourth to one tenth less common in the United States and Europe.[73–75] In the general population, less than 1 percent of people are likely to develop ACG.

Age. ACG due to RPB is generally a disease of advanced adulthood and senescence, with some cases occurring in midadulthood but most cases in the sixth and seventh decades of life.[76, 77] This pattern is due to gradual lens enlargement and increasing miosis with advanced age.

Sex. ACG occurs more frequently in females than in males,[78–83] possibly because a woman's eye is smaller than a man's eye and is therefore more prone to closure.

Race. ACG occurs relatively commonly in the white race, more so perhaps in Northern than in Mediterranean Europeans. A high rate of ACG is noted in Eskimos,[80–82, 84] and perhaps a lower rate in blacks.[44, 79, 85, 86] Blacks reportedly develop less acute ACG but develop chronic angle closure relatively more frequently.[79, 87–89] This may be due to the thicker iris in the black population, apparent at laser iridotomy. The thicker iris may be less prone to the peripheral bulging seen in eyes with thinner irides with RPB.

Heredity. It is generally believed that ACG can be inherited but, because of the many factors that contribute to ACG, that the inheritance may be multifactorial and polygenic and that in general the family history may or may not be contributory.[57, 90, 91]

Symptoms

ACUTE ACG

Signs and Symptoms

In an acute attack of ACG, after the development of very high IOP, a patient develops redness of the eye with ciliary flush, visual blurring and halo formation due to corneal edema formation, mild to severe pain, a fixed and middilated pupil, and perhaps nausea and vomiting.

In an acute attack of ACG, middilatation of the pupil, often induced by stress, a darkened environment, or pharmacologic dilatation, can lead to closure of the angle for reasons described earlier. In this situation, the closure is entire and the IOP rapidly elevates over a period of hours to approximately 60 to 70 mmHg. When the IOP reaches approximately the 50 to 60 mmHg range, fluid is forced into the normal cornea and epithelial edema begins to occur. The result is blurring of vision and the development of colored halos around lights. These halos are persistent and cannot be blinked away as halos can when they are due to mucus or dryness, other causes of blurring. At about the same or perhaps slightly higher IOP, severe aching pain develops in the eye as well. This pain can be centered in the eye or can radiate adjacent to the eye in the distribution of the trigeminal nerve.

If prolonged, the attack can lead to a vagal response with nausea and vomiting. As the IOP exceeds that of the arteries in the iris, the pupil becomes fixed in middilatation, usually 3 to 6 mm, and does not react to light and sometimes not to pharmacologic agents. As corneal edema increases, the visual acuity can continue to diminish.

The optic nerve head can begin to have its blood supply interrupted by the high IOP, and the retinal artery may pulsate, signifying that the IOP has exceeded retinal diastolic pressure and should be lowered as quickly as possible.

The correct diagnosis of acute ACG is made primarily by finding severe elevation of IOP in association with a closed angle determined gonioscopically. Central visual acuity is often markedly reduced owing to corneal edema and later because of optic nerve damage as well. The eye may be found to be hyperopic and small, with a shallow peripheral and central anterior chamber. The cornea may be mildly to extremely edematous. The pupil may be fixed, middilated, and irregular. Flare and cell may be found in the anterior chamber. The disc may be swollen, and the visual field reduced.

In making the diagnosis, topical glycerin may be used, and the other possible causes of acute or seemingly acute pressure elevation, mentioned earlier, should be ruled out.

One should look for the telltale signs of previous acute attacks listed earlier (e.g., sector iris atrophy, glaukomflecken). The contralateral eye should be examined for the presence of a similarly narrow angle.

If the contralateral eye is not shallow peripherally (and the rare anisometropia is not the cause), then other causes of sudden unilateral elevation of IOP must be sought because the two eyes are usually quite similar in anatomic make-up.

Differential Diagnosis of Sudden Elevation of IOP

In addition to acute ACG, other pathologic conditions that can raise the pressure rather suddenly or seemingly so should be ruled out. These conditions include (1) phacolytic glaucoma with its open angle, mature lens, and cell and flare with macrophages in the anterior chamber, (2) inflammatory glaucoma with some cell and flare and perhaps keratic precipitates, which do not occur in ACG, with again an open angle, (3) ghost cell glaucoma with a history of vitreous hemorrhage, trauma to the anterior hyaloid face, an open angle, and pathognomonic khaki-colored cells in the anterior chamber and on the trabecular meshwork, and (4) neovascular glaucoma with its often closed angle, dilated pupil with ectropion uveae, and pathognomonic neovascularization of the pupillary border, perhaps with a known history of diabetes mellitus or a prior central retinal vein occlusion. The causes of unilateral angle closure glaucoma must also be ruled out, such as central retinal vein occlusion with anterior chamber shallowing, the rare peripheral uveal effusion with closure, the extremely rare sudden massive subretinal hemorrhage due to macular degeneration, forward movement of the lens secondary to a choroidal melanoma, lens dislocation in Marfan's syndrome and Weil-Marchesani syndrome, iris bombé ACG secondary to inflammation, and other rare forms of unilateral ACG.[94]

INTERMITTENT, SPONTANEOUSLY RESOLVING (SUBACUTE) ACG

Spontaneous resolution of an ACG attack usually results from miosis due to entering a lighted area or sleeping (perhaps the miosis of sleep resolves the problem) or possibly from relaxing and decreasing adrenergic stimulation. These attacks are marked by development of halos and perhaps some ocular discomfort and can forewarn of a full-blown attack that does not resolve spontaneously. When a patient with narrow angles presents with such a past history, an iridotomy is indicated if any closure is seen; if not, a provocative test is indicated. If the provocative test results in closure, an iridotomy is indicated. These subacute attacks can occur during the development of chronic angle closure as well.[93, 94]

CHRONIC ACG

Chronic ACG glaucoma,[95–98] which can be caused by any of the primary mechanisms of closure, can present silently. At first only a few hours of angle become appositionally closed. More hours are slowly added until the pressure begins to rise silently, without halos or pain. The condition can therefore be unnoticed, and typical glaucomatous cupping and field loss can occur as in the chronic open-angle glaucomas. Appositional closure can gradually convert to synechial, although little is known about the time sequence of this pathologic change.

Patients may occasionally have subacute attacks or even a full-blown acute attack of ACG after years of slow development of chronic ACG.

The treatment of all RPB ACG is to interrupt the closure process and restore normal IOP and thus halt disc damage and field loss.

Treatment

ACUTE ACG

In acute ACG, if the pressure is not reduced promptly, permanent visual loss can ensue as a result of optic nerve damage. Permanent damage to the nerve can perhaps occur within 24 to 48 hr. Once the appropriate diagnosis of RPB ACG has been made, treatment should promptly be instituted. Pilocarpine, a β-blocker, and acetazolamide should be administered. If prompt lowering of the IOP does not ensue, osmotic agents should be considered. If medical therapy reduces the IOP to a safe level and the angle opens, vigilance can be relaxed. The patient can be treated with 1 percent pilocarpine therapy every 6 hr, and iridotomy/iridectomy can either be performed immediately or can be delayed until the cornea clears of edema and the iris becomes less hyperemic. Definitive treatment, peripheral iridotomy, can then be performed. If the pressure decreases to a safe level (about 30 mmHg or lower) but the angle remains closed, signifying that the reduction was due only to decreased aqueous formation and osmotic fluid removal, monitoring cannot be relaxed because the IOP

can be expected to elevate once again. Laser therapy should immediately be attempted, including iridotomy as first choice or possibly peripheral iridoplasty if iridotomy cannot be performed. Laser pupillary distortion might be considered in an attempt to break the RPB. Indentation of the cornea should be considered as well. If all these attempts fail and the IOP reelevates, surgical iridectomy might be considered at this time. If an operating room is not available, retrobulbar block and paracentesis might be considered as an alternative (discussed earlier under Paracentesis), with the idea that the cornea may be clear within hours thereafter, allowing laser iridotomy. If a patient is taken to the operating room, a chamber-deepening procedure might be considered, and if the angle opens almost entirely, an iridectomy should be performed. If the angle is totally synechially closed, operative goniosynechialysis should be considered. If goniosynechialysis is not feasible owing to poor visibility or inexperience with the procedure, then a filtration procedure should be performed.

In acute ACG, the first line of medical therapy is the use of a parasympathomimetic agent to try to cause miosis and pull the peripheral iris taut and away from the trabecular meshwork. Pilocarpine 2 percent can be used, one drop every 5 min times three, then one drop every 15 min times three then every 1 hr times four. If the attack has been prolonged and the pupillary sphincter muscle is paralyzed, pilocarpine may be ineffective in constricting the pupil. If this is anticipated, other measures to lower the IOP should be tried as well to try to lower the IOP to 40 mmHg or below, permitting the pupillary sphincter to function. This would include the use of topical β-blocker drops, the use of oral or intravenous acetazolamide (500 mg either PO or IV), and the possible use of an osmotic agent such as isosorbide or intravenous mannitol. If the medications do not work within 1 hr or so and a laser is accessible, laser iridotomy should be performed to try to open the angle.

One must be alert for pilocarpine toxicity and avoid systemic absorption with canalicular compression or lid closure. One should not use a nonselective β-blocker in patients with asthma or bradycardia and should consider a selective blocker or none at all. Diamox should be avoided in patients with an allergy to sulfa medications, although cross-reaction is rare, and the adverse cardiac effects of osmotic agents should be considered.

SUBACUTE ACG

If the diagnosis of subacute attacks of ACG has been established through history or by ocular examination, which might reveal signs of previous attacks such as sector iris atrophy or glaukomflecken, or if small portions of synechial closure are seen in a narrow angle, then iridotomy is indicated.

CHRONIC ACG

When the diagnosis of chronic angle-closure is made, iridotomy is indicated.

PLATEAU IRIS CONFIGURATION ACG

Epidemiology

A second primary ACG called *plateau iris configuration ACG* is increasingly being recognized. In this rare syndrome, the anatomic configuration of the iris is such that the angle closes despite the creation of a patent iridotomy following dilation of the pupil owing to crowding of peripheral iris tissue in the angle. This occurs despite the absence of peripheral bulging due to RPB, although the only sure way to be certain that this is the case is to perform an iridotomy and see if the angle closes either immediately thereafter after or even years later.

The distribution of this type of ACG is unknown. This form of glaucoma is rare in the United States but may in the future be found to be relatively more common in areas of the world where brown irides are prevalent.

Symptoms and Signs

Patients with PIC ACG tend to present with either acute, intermittent, or chronic ACG. The central anterior chambers are generally deeper than in RPB ACG, usually being four to six corneal thicknesses centrally. The peripheral chamber is shallow, however, and van Herick's test is positive, warning the examiner to be careful with dilation of the pupil. The contour of the iris is different from that in RPB, offering a main differentiating feature. The iris is flatter centrally and then drops off at the periphery somewhat precipitously, as if off a plateau. The appearance sometimes is that of a peripheral roll. Indentation gonioscopy may help in the differential diagnosis. In RPB ACG, following indentation, the peripheral iris usually hugs the lens and is flattened in the periphery without a peripheral iris roll. In PIC ACG, indentation gonioscopy may demonstrate a peripheral roll. If closure exists, it can be at first appositional and then later synechial.

Treatment

Despite the fact that RPB may not be the major factor in the cause of the glaucoma, iridotomy should be performed first. This is because we are often not sufficiently knowledgeable in determining the difference between these two syndromes (and some cases appear to overlap), and therefore, the pupillary block component should be removed with an iridotomy. If the angle continues to close after this procedure, the diagnosis of PIC ACG has been confirmed and further treatment may be necessary. This treatment could be either permanent pharmacologic miotic therapy or peripheral iridoplasty. I prefer the latter.

NANOPHTHALMIC ACG

Nanophthalmic ACG is the subject of another chapter.

MOBILE LENS (FORWARD LENS) ACG

An extremely rare type of angle closure can present primarily and can perhaps be called *mobile lens* or *forward lens syndrome ACG*. In this glaucoma, the lens moves excessively forward in the eye for an unknown reason, and this forward movement closes the angle primarily. This glaucoma was described by Levene.[23] The lens behaves as if the zonules were lax or as if posterior aqueous diversion existed, pushing the lens forward. The lens can excessively shallow the anterior chamber to a depth of perhaps one to three corneal thicknesses, and if this excessive shallowing is seen, this rare syndrome should be suspected. Examination of the other eye may reveal a deep chamber centrally and peripherally and an angle that could not possibly close with dilation, and this finding as well should alert the examiner to the possibility of this rare syndrome.

It is important to suspect this syndrome because the treatment is opposite to the three primary ACGs mentioned above (i.e., the treatment is mydriatic-cycloplegic therapy). Parasympathomimetic treatment, which benefits RPB and PIC ACG, exacerbates this glaucoma. In other words, this glaucoma behaves in some respects like postoperative malignant glaucoma.

If the examiner suspects this type of angle closure but cannot be certain, it is advisable to treat the patient conventionally and then reverse therapy if pilocarpine shallows the central anterior chamber. Careful attention to the depth of the central anterior chamber and its measurement is essential.

If mydriatic-cycloplegic therapy fails, combined with an iridotomy, which should be performed in all primary ACG, peripheral iridoplasty can be tried but is often unsuccessful. In this case, one can consider either lens extraction with intraocular lens replacement or a possible vitrectomy, or suffer the consequences of synechial angle closure and the probable need for a filtration procedure.

ASYMPTOMATIC PATIENTS WITH NARROW ANGLES

If a patient has a narrow but entirely open angle and has been asymptomatic in the past and the examiner wants to know if that patient is at risk for an attack of acute ACG in the future or if the patient should be protected by an iridotomy, it is reasonable to think that an iridotomy is indicated if closure can be precipitated by either physiologic or pharmacologic means.

Iridotomy cures RPB ACG and should be performed on all patients who have this disease or who can be induced to develop closure by any of the provocative tests. I recommend that patients who have angle closure (documented gonioscopically) or who can be induced to develop angle-closure (documented gonioscopically) should have an iridotomy. Patients who have anatomically similar eyes with closure in one eye should have iridotomy of the other eye because studies show high risk for closure in the uninvolved eye in the future. Studies have shown that the other eye has an approximate 50 percent chance of developing an acute attack within 5 years.

An examiner may perform gonioscopy on a patient and believe that the angle is extremely narrow and potentially occulable and that the patient thus is at risk for an acute attack. I believe that if actual closure is found or can be induced, then an iridotomy is indicated but should not be performed only for a narrow angle when the IOP is normal and it cannot be induced to close. A possible exception to this rule might be made for a patient who will travel to or live in a remote area where modern medical care may be unavailable.

FUTURE CONSIDERATIONS

Many advances have been made in our understanding of the field of primary ACG. It would be advantageous to be able to predict more accurately which eye with a narrow angle will close and which will not. Perhaps further anatomic studies of angle anatomy in small eyes, combined with a more complete knowledge of closing physiologic events, will provide insight. It may be possible to devise a better provocative test than we now have. The safety of laser peripheral iridotomy needs to be established. If this is done, perhaps the use of laser iridotomy will be liberalized to all patients with asymptomatic but extremely narrow angles.

REFERENCES

1. von Graefe A: Uber die iridectomie bei glaukom und uber den glaucomatosen process. 3:456, 1857.
2. Banziger T: The mechanism of acute glaucoma and the explanation for the effectiveness of iridectomy for the same. 43:43, 1922.
3. Curran E: A new operation for glaucoma involving a new principle in the aetiology and treatment of chronic primary glaucoma. Arch Ophthalmol 49:131, 1920.
4. Shields M, Ritch R: Classification and mechanisms. In Ritch R, Shields M (eds): The Secondary Glaucomas. St. Louis, CV Mosby, 1982.
5. Chandler P, Grant W: Lectures on Glaucoma. Philadelphia, Lea & Febiger, 1965.
6. Lowe R: Causes of shallow anterior chamber in primary angle-closure glaucoma: Ultrasonic biometry of normal and angle-closure glaucoma eyes. Am J Ophthalmol 67:87, 1969.
7. Storey J, Phillips CI: Ocular dimensions in angle-closure glaucoma. Br J Physiol Opt 26:228, 1971.
8. Tomlinson A, Leighton D: Ocular dimensions in the heredity of angle-closure glaucoma. Br J Ophthalmol 57:475, 1973.
9. Alsbirk P: Limbal and axial chamber depth variations: A population study in Eskimos. Acta Ophthalmol 64:593, 1987.
10. Weekers R, Grieten J, Lavergne G, et al: Etude des dimensions de la chambre anterieure de l'oeil humain I partie: Considerations biometriques. Ophthalmologica 142:650, 1961.
11. Tornquist R: Peripheral chamber depth in shallow anterior chamber. Br J Ophthalmol 43:169, 1959.
12. Lee DA, Brubaker RF, Ilstrup DM: Anterior chamber dimensions in patients with narrow angles and angle-closure glaucoma. Arch Ophthalmol 102:46, 1984.
13. Fontana S, Brubaker R: Volume and depth of the anterior chamber in the normal aging human eye. Arch Ophthalmol 98:1803, 1980.
14. Lowe R, Clark B: Radius of curvature of the anterior lens surface: Correlations in normal eyes and eyes involved with primary angle-closure glaucoma. Br J Ophthalmol 57:471, 1973.
15. Raeder J: Untersuchungen uber die Lage und Dicke der Linse im menschlichen Augen bei physiologischen und pathologischen Zustanden nach einer neuen Methode gemessen. Arch Ophthalmol cx:73–108, 1922.
16. Mapstone R: Mechanics of pupil block. Br J Ophthalmol 52:19, 1968.
17. Chandler P: Narrow-angle glaucoma. Arch Ophthalmol 47:695, 1952.
18. Reiss GR, Lee DR, Topper JE, et al: Aqueous humor flow during sleep. Invest Ophthal Vis Sci 25:776, 1984.
19. Panek WC, et al: Biometric variables in patients with occludable anterior chamber angles. Am J Ophthalmol 110:185, 1990.
20. Shaffer R: Gonioscopy, ophthalmoscopy, and perimetry. JT Trans Am Acad Ophthalmol Otolaryngol 64:112, 1960.
21. Tornquist R: Angle-closure glaucoma in an eye with a plateau type of iris. JT Trans Am Acad Ophthalmol Otolaryngol 36:413, 1958.
22. Wand M, Lee DR, Topper JE, et al: Plateau iris syndrome. JT Trans Am Acad Ophthalmol Otolaryngol 83:122, 1977.
23. Levene R: A new concept of malignant glaucoma. Arch Ophthalmol 87:197–506, 1972.
24. Inman W: Emotion and acute glaucoma. Lancet 2:1188, 1929.
25. Egan J: Shock glaucoma. Am J Ophthalmol 40:227, 1955.
26. Cross M, Croll L: Emotional glaucoma. Am J Ophthalmol 49:297, 1960.
27. Rieser J, Schwartz B: Miotic induced malignant glaucoma. Arch Ophthalmol 87:706, 1972.
28. Merritt J: Malignant glaucoma induced by miotics postoperatively in open-angle glaucoma. Arch Ophthalmol 95:1988, 1977.
29. Gorin G: Angle-closure glaucoma induced by miotics. Am J Ophthalmol 62:1063, 1966.
30. Bigar F, Witmer R: Corneal endothelial changes in primary acute angle-closure glaucoma. Ophthalmology 89:596, 1982.
31. Markowitz S, Morin J: The endothelium in primary angle-closure glaucoma. Am J Ophthalmol 98:103, 1984.
32. Olsen T: The endothelial cell damage in acute glaucoma: On the corneal thickness response to intraocular pressure. Acta Ophthalmol 58:257, 1980.
33. Setala K: Corneal endothelial cell density after an attack of acute glaucoma. Acta Ophthalmol 57:1004, 1979.
34. Anderson D, Davis E: Sensitivities of ocular tissues to acute pressure-induced ischemia. Arch Ophthalmol 93:267, 1975.
35. Charles S, Hamasaki D: The effect of intraocular pressure on the pupil size. Arch Ophthalmol 83:729, 1970.
36. Rutkowski P, Thompson H: Mydriasis and increased intraocular pressure. I: Pupillographic studies. Arch Ophthalmol 87:21, 1972.
37. Lowe R: Primary acute angle-closure glaucoma: Damage to cornea and lens. Br J Ophthalmol 49:460, 1965.
38. Jones B: Cataracta glaucomatosa and its role in the diagnosis of the acute glaucomas. 59:753, 1959.
39. Sugar H: Cataracta glaucomatosa acuta. Am J Ophthalmol 29:1396, 1946.
40. Zimmerman LE, de Venecia G, Hamasaki D: Pathology of the optic nerve in experimental acute glaucoma. 6:109, 1967.
41. Douglas G, Drance S, Shulzer M: The visual field and nerve head in angle-closure glaucoma. A comparison of the effects of acute and chronic angle closure. Arch Ophthalmol 93:409, 1975.
42. Lowe R: Primary angle-closure glaucoma: A review 5 years after bilateral surgery. Br J Ophthalmol 57:457, 1973.
43. Campbell DG, Vela A: Modern goniosynechialysis for the treatment of synechial angle-closure glaucoma. Ophthalmology 91:1052, 1984.
44. Clemmesen V, Luntz M: Lens thickness and angle-closure glaucoma: A comparative oculometric study in South African Negroes and Danes. Acta Ophthalmol 54:193, 1976.
45. Delmarcelle Y, Francois J, Gols F, et al: Biometrie oculaire clinique (oculometrie). 172:1, 1976.

46. Alsbirk P: Corneal diameter in Greenland Eskimos. Acta Ophthalmol 53:635, 1975.
47. Lowe R: Primary angle-closure glaucoma: A review of ocular biometry. 5:9, 1977.
48. Tornquist R: Chamber depth in primary acute glaucoma. Br J Ophthalmol 40:421, 1956.
49. Smith R: A new method of estimating the depth of the anterior chamber. Br J Ophthalmol 63:215, 1979.
50. Jacobs I, Krohn D: Central anterior chamber depth after laser iridectomy. Am J Ophthalmol 89:865, 1980.
51. Lowe R: Aetiology of the anatomical basis for primary angle-closure glaucoma: Biometrical comparisons between normal eyes and eyes with primary angle-closure glaucoma. Br J Ophthalmol 54:161, 1970.
52. Alsbirk P: Anterior chamber depth and primary angle-closure glaucoma. I: An epidemiologic study in Greenland Eskimos. Acta Ophthalmol 53:89, 1975.
53. Aizawa K: Studies on the depth of the anterior chamber. Jpn J Ophthalmol 4:272, 1960.
54. Chan R, Smith J, Richardson K: Anterior segment configuration correlated with Shaffer's grading of anterior chamber angle. Arch Ophthalmol 99:104, 1981.
55. van Herick W, Shaffer R, Schwartz A: Estimation of width of angle of anterior chamber: Incidence and significance of the narrow angle. Am J Ophthalmol 68:626, 1969.
56. Spaeth G: The normal development of the human anterior chamber angle: A new system of descriptive grading. Trans Ophthalmol Soc UK 91:709, 1971.
57. Spaeth G: Gonioscopy: Uses old and new. The inheritance of occludable angles. Ophthalmology 85:222, 1978.
58. Campbell D: A comparison of diagnostic techniques in angle-closure glaucoma. Am J Ophthalmol 88:197, 1979.
59. Gorin G: The value of gonioscopy in the diagnosis and treatment of angle closure glaucoma. Bibl Ophthalmol 47:125, 1957.
60. Scheie H: Width and pigmentation of the angle of the anterior chamber: A system of grading by gonioscopy. Arch Ophthalmology 58:510, 1957.
61. Forbes M: Gonioscopy with corneal indentation: A method for distinguishing between appositional closure and synechial closure. Arch Ophthalmol 76:488, 1966.
62. Forbes M: Indentation gonioscopy and efficacy of iridectomy in angle-closure glaucoma. Trans Am Ophthalmol Soc 72:488, 1974.
63. Gorin G: Re-evaluation of gonioscopic findings in angle-closure glaucoma: Static versus manipulative gonioscopy. Am J Ophthalmol 71:894, 1971.
64. Chandler P, Simmons R: Anterior chamber deepening for gonioscopy at time of surgery. Arch Ophthalmol 74:177, 1965.
65. Shaffer R: Operating room gonioscopy in angle closure glaucoma surgery. Trans Am Ophthalmol Soc 55:59, 1957.
66. Airaksinen P, Airaksinen PJ, Saari KM, et al: Management of acute closed-angle glaucoma with miotics and timolol. Br J Ophthalmol 63:822, 1979.
67. Ganias F, Mapstone R: Miotics in closed-angle glaucoma. Br J Ophthalmol 59:205, 1975.
68. Ritch R: Argon laser treatment for medically unresponsive attacks of angle-closure glaucoma. Am J Ophthalmol 94:197, 1982.
69. Shin DH: Argon laser iris photocoagulation to relieve acute angle-closure glaucoma. Am J Ophthalmol 93:348, 1982.
70. Campbell D, Vela A: Modern goniosynechialysis for the treatment of synechial angle-closure glaucoma. Ophthalmology 91:1052, 1984.
71. Shingleton BJ, Chang MA, Bellows AR, et al: Surgical goniosynechialysis for angle-closure glaucoma. Ophthalmology 97:551, 1990.
72. Anderson D: Corneal indentation to relieve acute angle-closure glaucoma. Am J Ophthalmol 88:1091, 1979.
73. Barkan O: Iridectomy in narrow angle glaucoma. Am J Ophthalmol 37:504, 1954.
74. Hollows F, Graham P: Intraocular pressure, glaucoma, and glaucoma suspects in a defined population. Br J Ophthalmol 50:570, 1966.
75. Bankes J, Tsolakis S, Wright J: Bedford glaucoma survey. Br Med J 1:791, 1968.
76. Lowe R: Angle-closure glaucoma. The second eye: An analysis of 200 cases. 21:65, 1961.
77. Lehrfeld L, Reber J: Glaucoma at the Wills Hospital. Arch Ophthalmol 18:712, 1937.
78. Lowe R: Comparative incidence of angle-closure glaucoma among different national groups in Victoria, Australia. Br J Ophthalmol 47:721, 1963.
79. Alper M, Laubach J: Primary angle-closure glaucoma in the American Negro. Arch Ophthalmol 79:663, 1968.
80. Arkell S, Lightman DA, Sonner A, Taylor HR, et al: The prevalence of glaucoma among Eskimos of northwest Alaska. Arch Ophthalmol 105:482, 1987.
81. Clemmesen V, Alsbirk P: Primary angle-closure glaucoma (a.c.g.) in Greenland. Acta Ophthalmol 49:47, 1971.
82. Drance S: Angle closure glaucoma among Canadian Eskimos. Can J Ophthalmol 8:252, 1973.
83. Smith R: The incidence of the primary glaucomas. 78:215, 1958.
84. Alsbirk P: Angle-closure glaucoma surveys in Greenland Eskimos. Can J Ophthalmol 8:260, 1973.
85. Luntz M: Primary angle-closure glaucoma in urbanized South African Caucasoid and Negroid communities. Br J Ophthalmol 57:445, 1973.
86. Wilensky J: Racial influences in glaucoma. Ann Ophthalmol 9:1545, 1977.
87. Neumann I, Zauberman H: Glaucoma survey in Liberia. Am J Ophthalmol 59:8, 1965.
88. Roger F: Eye diseases in the African continent. Am J Ophthalmol 45:343, 1958.
89. Venable H: Glaucoma in the Negro. JAMA 44:7, 1952.
90. Lowe R: Primary angle-closure glaucoma: Inheritance and environment. Br J Ophthalmol 56:13, 1972.
91. Francois J: Multifactorial or polygenic inheritance in ophthalmology. Acta Intl Cong Ophthalmol 10:1–39, 1985.
92. Chandler P, Trotter R: Angle-closure glaucoma: Subacute types. Arch Ophthalmol 53:305, 1955.
93. Bhargava S, Leighton D, Phillips C: Early angle-closure glaucoma: Distribution of iridotrabecular contact and response to pilocarpine. Arch Ophthalmol 89:369, 1973.
94. Playfair T, Watson P: Management of chronic or intermittent primary angle-closure glaucoma: A long-term follow-up of the results of peripheral iridectomy used as an initial procedure. Br J Ophthalmol 63:23, 1979.
95. Pollack I: Chronic angle-closure glaucoma: Diagnosis and treatment in patients with angles that appear open. Arch Ophthalmol 85:676, 1971.
96. Foulds W, Phillips C: Some observations on chronic closed-angle glaucoma. Br J Ophthalmol 41:208, 1957.
97. Gorin G: Shortening of the angle of the anterior chamber in angle-closure glaucoma. Am J Ophthalmol 49:141, 1960.
98. Lowe R: Primary creeping angle-closure glaucoma. Br J Ophthalmol 48:544, 1964.

Chapter 121

∎

Combined-Mechanism Glaucoma

KATHLEEN A. LAMPING

Since the early 1900s, classification of the glaucomas has been based on anterior chamber depth and the status of the angle, as observed with a gonioscope. In 1938, Barkan observed that increased tension could result from permanent adhesions in the angle caused by contact between the peripheral iris and the trabecular meshwork; this observation marked a great step forward.[1] At the American Academy of Ophthalmology and Otolaryngology Symposium on Glaucoma in 1949, the division of primary glaucoma into wide-angle versus narrow-angle was advised.[2]

Chandler and Grant were instrumental in increasing our understanding of narrow-angle glaucoma. Through careful clinical observations correlated with the experimental findings of Grant's work with tonography, it became apparent that almost all glaucomas were secondary to obstruction to the outflow system, rather than aqueous hypersecretion.[3, 4] In 1952, Chandler observed that mixed forms of glaucoma occur—that is, the narrow-angle mechanism is superimposed on a type caused by a defective filtration apparatus.[5]

The final proof of the fundamental difference in the mechanism of wide- and narrow-angle glaucoma was Chandler's discovery of obstruction to outflow from the anterior chamber in cases of untreated wide-angle glaucoma at all stages of the disease, whether the tension was normal or elevated. In cases of primary wide-angle glaucoma in which the diagnosis could be established in one eye by the usual clinical methods, obstruction to flow was also present in the fellow eye, which to date had shown no clinical evidence of the disease. During a phase of elevated tension in narrow-angle glaucoma when the angle was closed, as observed gonioscopically, obstruction to outflow was proportionate to the height of the tension and to the degree of angle-closure. These investigations led to our present understanding of angle-closure glaucoma.[5, 6]

The concept of pupillary block also evolved through the efforts of early investigators, including Chandler, Grant, Barkan, Sugar, and Mapstone. Both Barkan and Chandler considered that pupillary block was the product of contact between the iris and the lens. Sugar[7] stated that the posteriorly directed vector of force exerted by the iris sphincter was responsible. Mapstone[8] provided rigorous mathematical analysis to explain the pupillary block mechanism. We are now fully aware that the primary angle-closure glaucomas develop in the presence of pupillary block, restricting the passage of aqueous humor from the posterior to the anterior chamber. This pressure differential balloons the peripheral iris forward into contact with the trabecular meshwork.

Primary angle-closure glaucoma has been further sub-divided into acute, subacute, and chronic angle-closure. Subacute primary angle-closure with pupillary block can be considered prodromal, intermittent, and subclinical; its symptoms are often minimal and relieved without treatment. Chronic primary angle-closure with pupillary block has also been referred to as "creeping angle-closure"[9] and "shortening of the angle."[10] This situation involves relative pupillary block that causes a gradual angle-closure with no symptoms. The resultant optic nerve damage and visual field loss are identical to those seen in primary open-angle glaucoma. By definition, a combined-mechanism glaucoma exists when a patent iridectomy relieves the pupillary block but fails to lower the intraocular pressure to a level that prevents optic nerve damage and visual field loss. Since this condition can be easily mistaken for primary open-angle glaucoma, it is essential that we learn from our predecessors and perform regular and careful gonioscopy. An iridectomy early in the course of the disease may save the patient from chronic medication usage or filtration surgery.

CLINICAL MANIFESTATIONS

Combined angle-closure glaucoma may occur when an increased obstruction to aqueous outflow, caused by a ballooning of the peripheral iris against the trabecular meshwork, results in permanent synechial closure. In this situation, pupillary block is usually the initial cause of the bowing of the peripheral iris (Fig. 121–1). After pupillary block has been relieved by a patent iridectomy, however, permanent synechial closure causes an increase in intraocular pressure. Because repeated attacks of acute or subacute angle-closure may permanently damage the trabecular meshwork, combined mechanism glaucoma may also exist in the absence of visible peripheral anterior synechiae. After a peripheral iridectomy for presumed angle-closure glaucoma, intraocular pressures remained elevated, despite an open and normal-appearing angle, in six of 267 (2.2 percent) eyes in one study.[11] After acute attacks of angle-closure glaucoma, an abnormal amount of pigment has also been observed in the trabecular meshwork, which may cause an obstruction of outflow and an associated increase in intraocular pressure.

Occasionally, a patient may have evidence of both primary open-angle glaucoma and an associated angle-closure component within the same eye. There is a low prevalence of each of these entities in the general population. It seems reasonable to conclude that patients with narrow angles are more likely to have chronic angle-closure glaucoma as opposed to the simultaneous occurrence of these two forms of primary glaucoma.

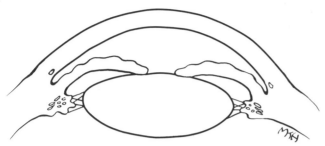

Figure 121–1. Pupillary block leading to angle-closure.

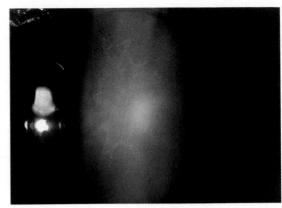

Figure 121–2. Subcapsular lens opacities (glaukomflecken of Vogt); a sequela of prior angle-closure.

CLINICAL COURSE AND FINDINGS

Primary chronic angle-closure glaucoma is not really a distinct disease entity; it includes a spectrum of angle-closure types, including acute, subacute, and chronic forms. Each of these forms is characterized by an insidious onset secondary to relative pupillary block that initially creates appositional closure that may progress to permanent synechial closure.

Primary chronic angle-closure glaucoma is totally asymptomatic and closely resembles primary angle-closure glaucoma. The use of miotics or epinephrine derivatives may aggravate this condition. Miotics cause forward displacement of the lens-iris diaphragm, and epinephrine derivatives may cause pupillary dilatation that further crowds angle structures. As optic nerve and associated visual field changes are identical, gonioscopy is the key to the correct diagnosis. In the initial stages, medication may temporarily control intraocular pressure. With progressive development of peripheral anterior synechiae, however, all medical treatment eventually fails to lower the intraocular pressure. The need for regular, careful gonioscopy cannot be overemphasized. Progressive chronic angle-closure may be prevented after a peripheral laser iridectomy is performed, thus saving the patient from either a lifetime of medical treatment or filtering surgery.

Individuals may also have intermittent episodes of angle-closure (prodromal, subacute, subclinical). These patients may present with the classic symptoms of an acute angle-closure glaucoma—that is, ocular pain, headaches, blurred vision, or halos; their symptoms may be mild and are self-limited. In some instances, these patients may be treated for "atypical" migraine, sinusitis, or anxiety attacks. A careful history, combined with a thorough ocular examination and a strong index of suspicion, may lead to a diagnosis of angle-closure glaucoma. In addition to narrow angles, these patients may show the classic signs of acute angle-closure glaucoma, including segmental iris atrophy, a fixed nonreactive pupil, and glaukomflecken (Fig. 121–2). Patients who have experienced angle-closure attacks in one eye are at high risk for an attack in the fellow eye; similarly, the fellow eye may develop chronic or creeping angle-closure.

Optic nerve changes may differ in patients experiencing acute or subacute glaucoma attacks, compared with patients with chronic angle-closure glaucoma.[12] Due to chronic elevation of intraocular pressure, the optic nerve and visual field changes seen in chronic angle-closure glaucoma appear to be identical to changes observed in patients with primary chronic open-angle glaucoma. Few of these patients retain a normal optic nerve head. They exhibit asymmetry of the optic cup and abnormalities of the neuroretinal rim. Following an acute attack of glaucoma or a sudden, dramatic rise in pressure, the neuroretinal rim may appear pale with a normal cup:disc ratio (Fig. 121–3).

Patients who have had an acute angle-closure glaucoma attack may develop a chronic angle-closure glaucoma, especially if the attack was not treated promptly. Although the first intracular pressure spike after an episode of angle-closure may be broken by laser iridectomy, either in an acute or subacute attack, successfully performing this procedure has little value in predicting the future course of the intraocular pressure. Postsurgical gonioscopy can help to establish the prognosis. If much of the angle is closed by peripheral anterior synechiae in the early postsurgical period, the intraocular pressure may still be low because of anterior segment inflammation. Once the inflammation subsides, the intraocular pressure may rise. Because this rise may not occur for months, the patient should be warned and followed regularly. The roles of laser iridoplasty and surgical goniosynechialysis in this situation are discussed under Management.

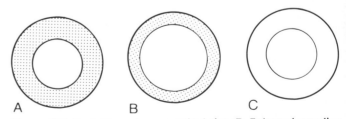

Figure 121–3. A, Normal neuroretinal rim. B, Enlarged cup:disc ratio typical of primary chronic open-angle glaucoma or primary chronic angle-closure glaucoma. C, A pale neuroretinal rim with preservation of the cup:disc ratio as seen after an acute attack of angle-closure glaucoma.

From the previous discussion, it should be apparent that an evaluation of the anterior chamber depth and gonioscopy of the anterior chamber angle are the keys to accurate diagnosis. Evaluation of anterior chamber depth can be performed with the oblique flash light test, which is a useful screening mechanism. When a pen light is placed near the temporal iris, the entire iris is illuminated in a wide open angle. In the presence of peripheral iris shallowing, only the distal nasal iris will be illuminated.

Slit-lamp examination of the anterior chamber angle has more diagnostic value and should be performed with every initial ocular examination. Van Herick[13] and co-workers developed this technique for comparing the peripheral anterior chamber depth with corneal thickness. If the width of the slit-lamp beam from corneal endothelium to anterior iris stroma (peripheral anterior chamber depth) is less than one quarter of the corneal thickness, the angle is considered capable of occlusion (Fig. 121–4); there is a risk of chronic peripheral anterior synechia or an acute glaucoma attack. All patients should, of course, be gonioscoped; however, a high index of suspicion for chronic angle-closure glaucoma should exist if slit-lamp examination reveals a shallow anterior chamber. The risk of developing angle-closure can also be assessed by various other methods. Patients with less than or equal to 2.5 mm of central anterior chamber depth may be at risk for developing angle-closure glaucoma.[14] Using photogrametric measurements, Lee[15] and associates noted that anterior chamber volume was at least 50 percent lower in eyes with various forms of angle-closure than in normal eyes. Unfortunately, no sophisticated method or biometric factor alone can allow the ophthalmologist to diagnose chronic angle-closure glaucoma without slit-lamp evaluation and gonioscopy.

Gonioscopy remains the principle method for determining the cause of aqueous obstruction. A conscious effort must be applied to learn accurate gonioscopy. Chronic angle-closure glaucoma is frequently not appreciated, making an inaccurate assessment of the angle in this condition common.

There are various methods of correlating angle structure with potential for angle-closure. Scheie[16] proposed that anterior chamber angle structures be classified as they are visualized. Shaffer[17] devised a classification system based on angular width. Many clinicians prefer to describe and draw the angle; this is probably the most useful method, because different portions of the angle have different depths. A general principle to remember is that angles in which portions of posterior trabeculum are obscured are at risk of developing angle-closure glaucoma. If peripheral anterior synechiae are present with no other cause than an anatomically narrow angle, chronic angle-closure glaucoma exists.

Three instruments are available for gonioscopy: Koeppe, Goldmann, and Zeiss. The Koeppe lens allows direct visualization of the angle and causes less distortion of the anterior chamber angle (Fig. 121–5). It does not, however, magnify the angle enough to identify subtle changes. The Goldmann lens is the prototype of the gonioprism, which uses indirect gonioscopy (Fig. 121–6). The Zeiss lens, which uses compression to open the angle, is essential for the correct diagnosis and treatment of chronic angle-closure glaucoma. The Zeiss four-mirror lens, also a gonioprism, has a diameter of 7.7 mm and is smaller than the corneal diameter (Fig. 121–7A). When compression is applied, it will, therefore, artifactually open the angle (see Fig. 121–7B). When compression is applied with the Goldmann lens, the angle may appear artifactually more narrow.

The importance of gonioscopy with corneal indentation using a four-mirror gonioprism cannot be overemphasized. It is necessary to gonioscope hundreds of eyes in order to become comfortable with this procedure. Begin with a cooperative patient with open angles. Using the superior mirror, verify angle structures and then observe the peripheral iris, which normally has a slightly convex appearance. The same routine should be performed with the Goldmann lens, which allows for a more detailed examination of specific structures; compare the results of the examination with each lens.

If an angle appears narrow or your index of suspicion is high for a narrow angle component, Zeiss compression

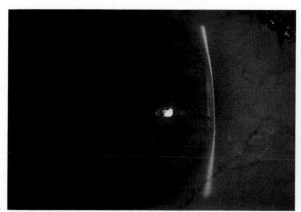
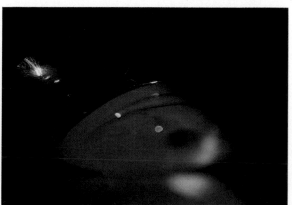

A   B

Figure 121–4. A, Narrow width of slit-lamp beam from corneal endothelium to anterior iris stroma indicates that angle may be occludable. B, Gonioscopy confirms appositional closure.

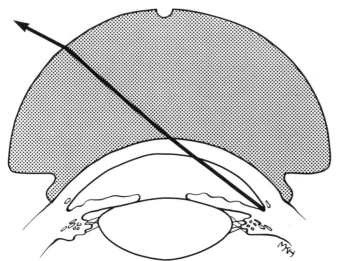

Figure 121–5. Koeppe's lens enables direct visualization of the angle.

is mandatory. Although the extent of occlusion can be determined using a Goldmann lens alone, appositional closure cannot be distinguished accurately from synechial closure. Identification of synechial closure is the key to accurately diagnosing chronic angle-closure glaucoma. This distinction is considerable; if peripheral anterior synechiae are present, the treatment is a laser iridectomy. Medical treatment alone will only temporize the situation and may even aggravate it. The technique for gonioscopy with indentation, as described by Forbes,[18] will now be explained in detail.

A single drop of local anesthetic is applied prior to

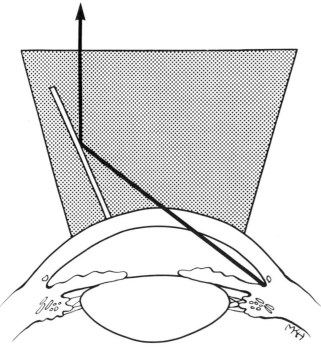

Figure 121–6. The Goldmann lens is used for indirect gonioscopy.

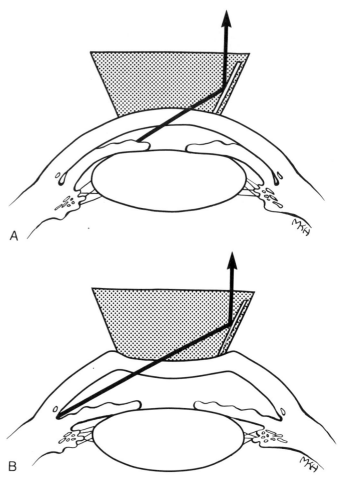

Figure 121–7. *A,* The diameter of the Zeiss lens is narrower than the diameter of the cornea. *B,* When compression is applied, the angle opens.

insertion. No methylcellulose is required. With the Zeiss lens centered on the cornea, the angle structures can be seen through all four mirrors. After carefully determining the status of the undisturbed angle, the lens is pressed against the corneal apex. This produces an indentation of the central cornea and displacement of aqueous humor to the periphery of the anterior chamber, with consequent posterior displacement of the peripheral iris and deepening of the chamber angle. This pressure may cause a slight retrodisplacement of the globe in the orbit, requiring a forward movement of the slit lamp toward the eye to keep the angle structures in focus. A few folds in Descemet's membrane may appear, but generally will not obstruct the view. After the angle has been widened, the pressure of the lens is gradually released until the folds in Descemet's membrane disappear. At this point, the angle has been restored to its undisturbed configuration. This procedure may be repeated several times until the examiner is comfortable with the findings.

Although all chamber angles may be observed in this fashion, the technique is especially useful when some degree of closure is suspected. Areas of appositional closure are readily opened by this procedure, and adhesions are clearly exposed (Figs. 121–8 and 121–9).

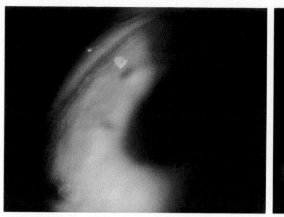
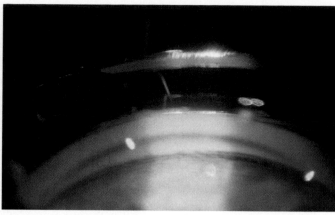

A
B

Figure 121–8. *A,* No angle structures are identified with Zeiss' gonioscopy. *B,* With Zeiss' compression, angle structures are readily visible; no peripheral anterior synechiae are seen and appositional closure exists.

The technique may be refined in order to produce a maximum displacement of aqueous humor into a particular portion of the angle being studied. The lens may be decentered 2 to 3 mm away from the area under visualization. The cornea is then indented from this eccentric position, forcing most of the displaced aqueous toward the opposite half of the chamber angle. A simple rule is to move the goniolens in the direction of the mirror being used. This refinement is extremely effective and, with more experience, the examiner will tend to use it automatically. It must be emphasized that meaningful results are obtained when the angle is examined thoroughly both with and without corneal identation.

Careful attention to the focal lines reflected from the posterior surface of the cornea and the anterior surface of the iris may also help to determine the existence of appositional closure or synechial closure.[19] It may be presumed that an open space exists between the iris periphery and the anterior wall of the angle from the displacement of the focal lines reflected from the posterior cornea and the anterior iris surface (Fig. 121–10). When synechial closure exists, the focal lines are not displaced; instead, they are continuous and form a geometric angle, the apex of which corresponds to the point of contact between the anterior and posterior walls of the chamber angle. The absence of displacement of

the focal lines indicates that there is fusion between the root of the iris and the trabecular meshwork (Fig. 121–11).

DIFFERENTIAL DIAGNOSIS

Some eyes may exhibit sequelae of previous attacks of angle-closure glaucoma, including posterior synechiae, glaukomflecken, iris atrophy, and optic nerve pallor. Peripheral anterior synechiae are also seen and are usually scattered, peaked, and broad (Fig. 121–12).

A reported 24 to 72 percent of patients will develop an elevated pressure in the postoperative period following an iridectomy for an acute angle-closure attack.[20, 21] Since this elevation can occur months to years after the attack, patients should be warned of the need for lifelong care. Although an elevation in pressure is seen more commonly in patients with extensive peripheral anterior synechiae, it may also occur in eyes without any evidence of synechia closure.

Patients with chronic primary angle-closure with pupillary block have no symptoms or clinical manifestations of previous glaucoma attacks. Intraocular pressure is moderately elevated and often does not respond to treatment. On gonioscopy, apposition is seen between the iris and the trabecular meshwork over most of the circumference of the angle (see Fig. 121–12). The ap-

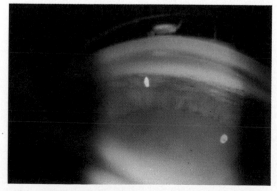

Figure 121–9. With compression, the angle opens and peripheral anterior synechiae are identified.

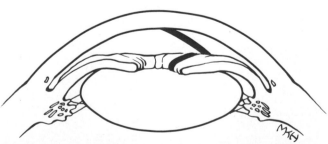

Figure 121–10. Displacement of focal lines indicates that an open space exists between the iris periphery and the chamber angle wall.

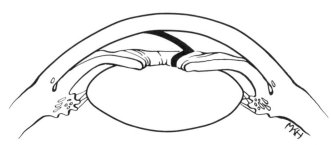

Figure 121–11. Focal lines are not displaced but form an angle, the apex corresponding to the point of contact between the anterior and the posterior walls of the chamber angle. Synechial closure exists.

position usually begins in the superior angle and progresses in both directions toward 6 o'clock. When approximately 60 percent of the angle is occluded, the intraocular pressure rises. If peripheral anterior synechiae are present, they are usually continuous—rather than scattered, as seen after an angle-closure attack. It is speculated that the lack of inflammation and vascular congestion explain the difference in character of the synechiae.

In primary chronic angle-closure glaucoma, the optic nerve generally begins to show signs of glaucomatous cupping, as observed in patients with primary chronic open-angle glaucoma. It is important, however, to realize that there may be no cupping and the optic nerve may be pale and atrophic if a patient has previously experienced either an acute or subacute attack of angle-closure glaucoma. This optic nerve atrophy is similar to the changes in the optic nerve that are seen with either a compressive lesion or secondary to an ischemic optic neuritis. In these conditions, however, the visual acuity is often markedly diminished. Primary chronic angle-closure glaucoma is rarely associated with a diminished visual acuity until the final stage of the disease. A diagnosis of angle-closure glaucoma should, therefore, be considered in the face of a pale optic nerve with no glaucomatous cupping and a preserved central acuity.

Provocative tests, such as the darkroom test and mydriatic test, may be useful in distinguishing primary open-angle glaucoma from primary chronic angle-closure glaucoma. Problems with these tests may arise, however, if a positive darkroom test is based solely on a rise in intraocular pressure, which could occur when a diurnal intraocular pressure rise coincides with the test. It is only when the rise is associated with a change in angle configuration—that is, when the angle has become more narrow with an associated rise in intraocular pressure—that the diagnosis of chronic angle-closure should be considered.

The thymoxamine test may also be useful, but it is not available in the United States. Thymoxamine, an adrenergic-blocking agent, causes relaxation of the radial muscle fibers of the iris, thus allowing the pupillary sphincter muscle to act unapposed in constricting the pupil and pulling the iris away from the angle. It does not act on the ciliary muscle. Thymoxamine can reverse elevated intraocular pressure that is secondary to appositional closure.

Intraocular pressure is not always helpful in establishing the diagnosis of chronic angle-closure glaucoma. In the early stages of primary chronic angle-closure glaucoma, appositional closure can exist with no peripheral anterior synechiae and intraocular pressures are often normal (Fig. 121–13). It is only when a significant portion of the angle (usually greater than two thirds) becomes closed with permanent synechiae that we begin to note an increase in intraocular pressure. By this time, of course, the damage is irreversible.

Tonography may occasionally play a role in the diagnosis and management of chronic angle-closure glaucoma. For example, there may be wide fluctuations in intraocular pressure in the immediate postoperative phase after laser iridectomy. If the facility of outflow is subnormal by tonography, a low intraocular pressure may be expected to rise once the postoperative phase stabilizes. This may be especially true after an acute angle-closure attack, as the intraocular pressure during the early post-attack phase may not reflect the true outflow status.

The most helpful techniques in making a correct diagnosis of combined-mechanism glaucoma include a careful history, a thorough understanding of and ability

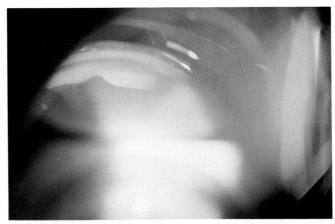

Figure 121–12. Broad and extensive synechial formation after acute angle-closure.

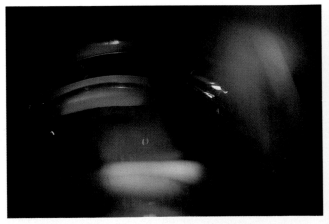

Figure 121–13. Appositional closure; no angle structures are identified.

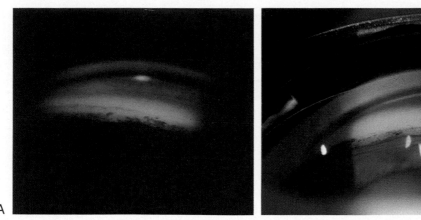

Figure 121–14. *A,* Prominent uveal meshwork; fine branching twiglike endings with lacy, open character may be confused with peripheral anterior synechiae. *B,* Peripheral anterior synechiae, which are solid and uniform.

to perform gonioscopy, and an index of suspicion for this entity.

Combined-mechanism glaucoma or primary chronic angle-closure glaucoma is most frequently mistaken for primary open-angle glaucoma. The previous discussion has emphasized the importance of gonioscopy in distinguishing between these two entities. If the posterior trabeculum is observed, the examiner should suspect that a narrow angle is contributing to the decrease in outflow facility. If synechiae are noted and are not secondary to another disease or previous surgical procedure, primary chronic angle-closure glaucoma exists.

In many patients, a prominent uveal meshwork may possibly be confused with peripheral anterior synechiae (Fig. 121–14*A*). Uveal meshwork may be more prominent in the nasal angle. In blue-eyed patients, this meshwork lines the angle overlying the ciliary body band, scleral spur, and trabecular meshwork. It appears as a delicate gray or colorless structure that interferes with the visibility of the angle. It is more conspicuous in brown eyes due to increased pigmentation. Typically, the anterior edge of the uveal meshwork is on the trabecular meshwork and has many fine branching twiglike endings. The feature that seems to be the most consistent in distinguishing normal tissue from peripheral anterior synechiae is a difference in the apparent solidity of tissue. The uveal meshwork in adult eyes regularly has the lacy, open character of a meshwork made up of many interconnected strands. Angle structure can be identified between the strands. Conversely, peripheral anterior synechiae have more uniform and solid characteristics of iris stroma and block the view of angle structures (see Fig. 121–14*B*).

Peripheral anterior synechiae may occur in other conditions and may mimic primary chronic angle-closure glaucoma. In primary angle-closure glaucoma, the synechiae are generally low, diffuse, and not bridging (Fig. 121–15).

It must also be remembered that any condition that secondarily causes shallowing of the anterior chamber may cause permanent synechial closure. These conditions include both inflammatory and postsurgical conditions in which adhesions may develop between the

iris, vitreous face, or intraocular lens. Pupillary block occurs most often after a complicated cataract extraction but may also be noted in a quiet eye with an intact posterior capsule and a well-positioned posterior chamber intraocular lens. Unfortunately, we are all too familiar with shallow anterior chambers secondary to filtering surgery. Peripheral anterior synechiae that occur after prolonged absence of the anterior chamber following surgery are usually broad bands of adhesions to the iris at various levels. Some may appear as tentlike synechiae. Bridging synechiae may also exist. Peripheral anterior synechiae secondary to chronic iridocyclitis generally are tentlike or found in broad columns. The remainder of the angle is wide open.

In all of these patients, we must maintain a high index of suspicion so that proper treatment is instituted and permanent synechial angle-closure is not allowed to occur.

The fact that permanent synechial closure may occur after argon laser trabeculoplasty emphasizes the importance of treating the anterior trabecular meshwork. To avoid this complication of an otherwise relatively low-risk procedure, one must have a thorough appreciation of all angle structures and avoid postoperative inflammation. If the angle is inaccessible to treatment, either

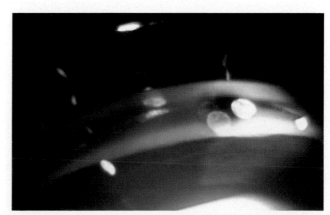

Figure 121–15. Low, diffuse synechial closure, typical of primary chronic angle-closure glaucoma.

iridoplasty or iridectomy should be performed to open the angle, enabling proper treatment of the trabecular meshwork and avoiding peripheral anterior synechiae. These synechiae are typically small and irregular and may occasionally extend to the posterior trabecular meshwork (Fig. 121–16).

Permanent synechial closure may also occur after scleral buckling procedures. Closure of the angle may develop from two different mechanisms. One mechanism is forward displacement of vitreous humor and lens by the combination of scleral indentation and suprachoroidal fluid. Another mechanism is an anterior rotation of the ciliary processes caused by an effusion that separates the ciliary body from the sclera. In this condition, pupillary block is not the mechanism. An iridectomy alone will not prevent posterior synechiae, and a laser iridoplasty or surgical goniosynechialysis may be necessary to pull the peripheral iris from the trabecular meshwork.

Permanent angle-closure may occur after central retinal vein occlusion or after panretinal photocoagulation. Again, the proposed mechanism is a forward shift of the ciliary body caused by a suprachoroidal effusion.

Other entities that may secondarily cause angle-closure include subluxation or dislocation of the lens, either after trauma or as an isolated congenital anomaly. Several syndromes, such as Ehlers-Danlos, Weill-Marchesani, and Marfan's, may include permanent synechial closure secondary to pupillary block induced by ectopia lentis. These conditions and others are discussed in the chapter on lens-induced glaucomas.

Ciliary body cysts and tumors may also cause permanent synechial closures. This diagnosis may be suspected when there is a considerable difference in the width of the chamber angle in various portions of the circumference. As previously discussed, plateau iris may cause a closed angle in the absence of pupillary block.

In neovascular glaucoma, a fibrovascular membrane develops; peripheral anterior synechiae form when this membrane contracts. These synechiae are broad, extensive, and associated with new vessels on the anterior iris stroma (Fig. 121–17). When broad synechiae exist in

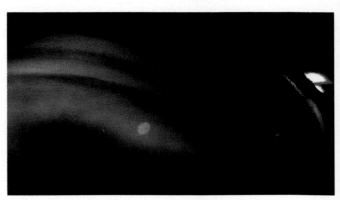

Figure 121–17. Broad, extensive synechial closure associated with contraction of a fibrovascular membrane in neovascular glaucoma.

end-stage neovascular glaucoma, the new vessels may not always be prominent and it may be confused with angle-closure glaucoma. If the patient is at risk for development of neovascular glaucoma, a careful search for new vessels must be made under high slit-lamp magnification. Gonioscopy of the fellow eye may be beneficial as well. If the fellow eye has a wide-open angle, the condition is less likely to be primary angle-closure glaucoma.

Essential iris atrophy is characterized by special peripheral anterior synechiae that are gross, extend anterior to Schwalbe's line, and may be directly visible with the slit lamp. This syndrome is unilateral and is associated with ectopia uveae and corectopia, as well as holes in the iris.

Attachments between the peripheral iris and Schwalbe's line that bridge the angle are also seen with posterior embryotoxin, Axenfeld's anomaly, and Reiger's anomaly. These attachments from an abnormally thick and prominent uveal meshwork (iris processes); they are not peripheral anterior synechiae.

Epithelial downgrowth may also be associated with broad-based synechiae. This condition develops in an aphakic or pseudophakic patient, usually after a wound leak. The eye is usually infected and photophobic. One may also see a typical scalloped membrane on the corneal endothelial surface.

In primary chronic angle-closure glaucoma, peripheral anterior synechiae will develop due to appositional closure, as opposed to secondary disease or prior surgery. The diagnosis can be made if peripheral anterior synechiae are identified (Fig. 121–18). It should be emphasized, however, that the absence of peripheral anterior synechiae under indentation gonioscopy does not rule out chronic appositional angle-closure glaucoma.

EPIDEMIOLOGY

Patients who are at risk for primary chronic angle-closure glaucoma are similar to those who are susceptible to acute angle-closure attacks. Primary angle-closure glaucoma is considerably less common than primary open-angle glaucoma, although a precise ratio between

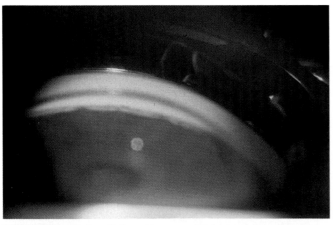

Figure 121–16. Small, irregular synechiae seen after argon laser trabeculoplasty.

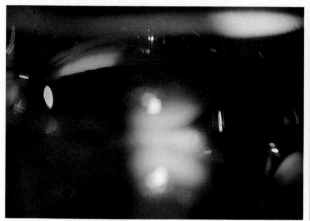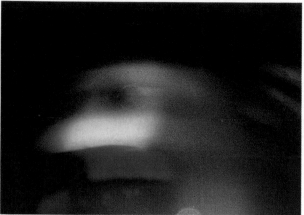

Figure 121–18. Various forms of primary chronic angle-closure glaucoma. *A,* Complete synechial closure (with Zeiss' compression). *B,* Appositional closure; anterior trabecular meshwork is the only structure identified.

the two conditions has not been established. Studies of the anterior chamber angle within a large population have shown that between 5 and 6 percent of individuals had suspiciously narrow angles; between 0.64 and 1.1 percent had angles that were considered critically narrow.[13, 22] The incidence and prevalence of pupillary block in a population are influenced by age, race, heredity, and refraction.

Age. The depth and volume of the anterior chamber diminish with age. Other changes associated with aging that increase the relative risk of pupillary block include an increased thickness of the lens, more anterior displacement of the lens secondary to an increased zonular laxity, and an increase in miosis. All of these factors increase the contact between the iris and lens, thus inducing pupillary block.

Pseudoexfoliation of the lens capsule, which occurs more frequently in the older population, increases the incidence of angle-closure secondary to weak zonular attachments. It is important to recognize, however, that primary chronic angle-closure glaucoma may develop in younger patients as well.

Race. Blacks are more susceptible to primary chronic angle-closure glaucoma than to acute angle-closure glaucoma. There is no complete explanation for this phenomenon.

Sex. Females have a more shallow anterior chamber depth, making them more susceptible to acute angle-closure glaucoma. A correlation between sex and primary chronic angle-closure glaucoma, however, has not been ascertained.

Refractive Error. Hyperopes maintain a smaller depth and volume of the anterior chamber and should be considered to be at higher risk for developing primary chronic angle-closure glaucoma.

PATHOPHYSIOLOGY

Relative pupillary block and chronic angle-closure glaucoma trypically occur in eyes with small anterior segments. Using photogeometric images, Lee and coworkers[15] found that anterior chamber volume was reduced in patients with chronic angle-closure glaucoma compared with normal individuals. Decreased corneal diameter[23] and central anterior chamber depth[24] have also been noted in eyes susceptible to angle-closure glaucoma.

Lens size and position also contribute to pupillary block. An anterior position of the lens with respect to the ciliary body (Fig. 121–19), increased lens thickness, and increased anterior lens curvature have been identified in patients with angle-closure glaucoma.

Each factor listed is associated with increased contact between the iris and the lens, accentuating pupillary block. Three trends associated with aging predispose an eye to angle-closure glaucoma: the lens thickens with age and assumes a more anterior position and the pupil becomes more miotic.

Patients with pseudoexfoliation of the lens capsule have a high incidence of angle-closure glaucoma. This is thought to be secondary to laxity of the zonules, causing a forward displacement of the lens-iris diaphragm.

Resistance to flow or relative pupillary block causes the pressure in the posterior chamber to be slightly higher than in the anterior chamber. Usually this pressure differential is of little importance. The process of

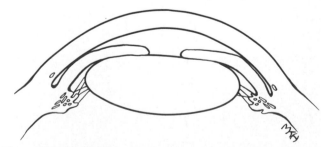

Figure 121–19. Pupillary block caused by the forward shift of the lens-iris diaphragm secondary to laxity of the zonules.

angle-closure is initiated if the pupillary block sufficiently increases and pushes the peripheral iris forward into contact with the trabecular meshwork. In chronic angle-closure glaucoma, the condition begins as appositional closure and progresses gradually toward synechial formation. This closure consists of a permanent, progressive fusion between the root of the iris and the trabecular meshwork—thus accounting for the terms "shortening of the angle" and "creeping angle-closure."

MANAGEMENT

Since laser iridectomy has been shown to be safe and effective, the treatment and management of primary angle-closure glaucoma has been simplified. A dilemma arises, however, in determining which patients are candidates for a laser iridectomy. A laser iridectomy is easy to perform, but it should not be used for all cases of narrow angles. Although laser iridectomy is safer than a surgical iridectomy, there are complications—that is, decreased visual acuity, corneal and lenticular burns, inflammation, transient or permanent pressure elevation, hypopyon, and hyphema (Fig. 121–20). The relative risks and benefits must be carefully weighed for each patient.

Laser iridectomy is unequivocally indicated in an eye that has had a documented acute or subacute angle-closure glaucoma attack. A peripheal iridectomy is recommended for a patient with narrow angles who gives a classic history of angle-closure attacks. Prophylactic laser iridectomy should be performed on the fellow eye, because these eyes are at high risk for acute or chronic angle-closure; an exception to this rule is made if anisometropia exists and the fellow eye has a wide-open angle.

In asymptomatic patients, the indications for performing a laser iridectomy are less clear cut. If an elevation in intraocular pressure exists and appositional closure is seen on gonioscopy, a laser iridectomy should be performed. If peripheral anterior synechiae are identified and there is no secondary cause for their existence, a laser iridectomy must be performed regardless of the

intraocular pressure level. Chronic appositional angle-closure alone should be a strong indicator for performing a laser iridectomy.

By definition, combined-mechanism glaucoma exists when the intraocular pressure is uncontrolled after a peripheral iridectomy is performed. Once patency of the iridectomy is achieved, the intraocular pressure should be managed as a chronic open-angle glaucoma, initially using either β-blockers or epinephrine derivatives. Miotics can be used safely after an iridectomy is performed. Gonioscopy should still be regularly performed, however, since miotics may occasionally cause a forward shift of the lens (even in the presence of a patent peripheral iridectomy) and further angle-closure. Miotics will not be effective in the presence of a total 360 degrees of synechial closure. Carbonic anhydrase inhibitors are useful, but obviously have a number of well-known systemic side effects. Argon laser trabeculoplasty was found effective in primary chronic angle-closure glaucoma in 53 percent of patients who did not respond to medication.[25] In the successfully treated eyes, 6.5 clock hours of open angle were available for treatment. Other investigators, however, have concluded that argon laser trabeculoplasty is unlikely to benefit eyes with narrow-angle glaucoma, even after pupillary block has been relieved.[26] Even with a patent iridectomy, the approach to the angle may be difficult. In this situation, iridoplasty is a useful adjunct and can be performed at the same time as trabeculoplasty. It should be emphasized that iridoplasty is not a replacement for iridectomy as treatment for chronic angle-closure glaucoma. Iridoplasty may be used to widen the angle and allow a clear view of the angle structures, enabling precise placement of the laser beam during trabeculoplasty. Despite these innovations in technique, argon laser trabeculoplasty is not as successful in narrow-angle glaucoma as it is in primary open-angle glaucoma.

Iridoplasty may also be beneficial after an acute or subacute glaucoma attack. Again, this procedure does not replace iridectomy; it is indicated if peripheral synechiae remain after iridectomy eliminates pupillary block. When performed in the immediate postoperative period, burns placed in the peripheral iris will cause contraction of the surrounding iris stroma between the site of the burn and angle wall. Successful performance of this procedure will produce widening of the angle. This technique is discussed elsewhere in this section. The author's personal technique is to pretreat with 4 percent pilocarpine to place the iris on stretch. Using an Abraham iridectomy lens at the most peripheral portion of the iris, three to four burns are placed per clock hour using a 500-μm spot size at 0.5 sec and 200 to 400 mW. The areas closed with peripheral anterior synechiae are treated. This procedure is useful only in the immediate postoperative period; once the angle is open, the prognosis for trabecular function improves with a shorter duration of synechial closure.

The anterior chamber deepening technique introduced by Chandler and Simmons[27] may be indicated along with intraoperative goniosynechialysis in a select group of patients. A paracentesis is first performed

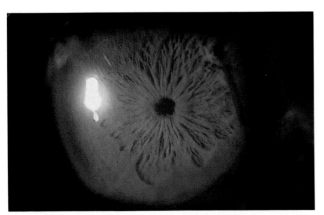

Figure 121–20. Hyphema associated with neodymium:yttrium-aluminum-garnet (Nd.YAG) laser iridectomy.

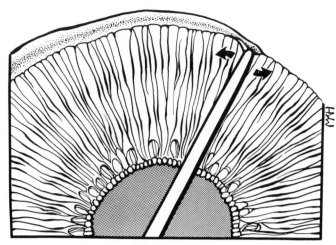

Figure 121–21. Peripheral anterior synechiae may be lysed with a spatula.

compression on the posterior lip of this incision allows aqueous to egress and the anterior chamber to shallow. A muscle hook is then used to force posterior chamber fluid through the pupil into the anterior chamber. This allows the angle to deepen easily, as there is now no resistance in the posterior chamber. The anterior chamber can be deepened with a viscoelastic material to a depth that can depress the lens posteriorly and force the peripheral iris backward. The angle can then be easily assessed intraoperatively with a Koeppe lens. If peripheral anterior synechiae are identified, they may be separated from the trabecular meshwork using a smooth-tipped irrigating cyclodialysis spatula, as described by Campbell and Vella (Fig. 121–21).[28] This technique is useful after an acute or subacute glaucoma attack and may save a patient from filtration surgery. It is not recommended unless there are 270 degrees or more of synechial closure and outflow facility is compromised. A filtering operation would be favored over synechialysis if significant cupping and visual field loss exist.

If optic nerve damage and visual field loss progress despite maximum tolerated medication and argon laser trabeculoplasty, the next alternative is filtration surgery. It should be remembered that patients with narrow preoperative angles are at risk for postoperative malignant glaucoma (aqueous diversion syndrome). This should be suspected in a patient who develops a flat anterior chamber with elevated intraocular pressure. Postoperative cycloplegic agents should be used routinely in this patient population.

Patients with combined-mechanism glaucoma are more difficult to manage surgically than patients with primary open-angle glaucoma. The success rate of trabeculoplasty is not as favorable as with primary open-angle glaucoma. More complications develop after filtering surgery in this population, such as a flat anterior chamber and malignant glaucoma. For these reasons, it is obviously advantageous to make the diagnosis early, thus preventing these complications.

REFERENCES

1. Barkan O: Glaucoma: Classification, causes and surgical control: Results of microgonioscopic research. Am J Ophthalmol 21:1099, 1938.
2. Friedenwald JS: Symposium on primary glaucoma. I: Terminology, pathology, and physiological mechanisms. Trans Am Acad Ophthalmol Otolaryngol 53:169, 1949.
3. Grant WM: A tonographic method for measuring the facility and rate of aqueous flow in human eyes. Arch Ophthalmol 44:204, 1950.
4. Grant WM: Clinical measurements of aqueous outflow. Arch Ophthalmol 46:113, 1951.
5. Chandler PA: Narrow angle glaucoma. Arch Ophthalmol 47:695, 1952.
6. Chandler PA, Trotter RR: Angle-closure glaucoma, subacute types. Arch Ophthalmol 53:305, 1955.
7. Sugar HS: Newer conceptions in the classification of glaucomas. Am J Ophthalmol 32:425, 1949.
8. Mapstone R: Mechanics of pupil block. Br J Ophthalmol 52:19, 1968.
9. Lowe RF: Primary creeping angle-closure glaucoma. Br J Ophthalmol 48:544, 1964.
10. Gorin G: Shortening of the angle of the anterior chamber in angle-closure glaucoma. Am J Ophthalmol 49:141, 1960.
11. Hyams SW, Keroub C, Pokotilo E: Mixed glaucoma. Br J Ophthalmol 61:105, 1977.
12. Douglas GR, Drance SM, Schulzer M: The visual field and nerve head in angle-closure glaucoma: A comparison of the effects of acute and chronic angle closure. Arch Ophthalmol 93:409, 1975.
13. Van Herick W, Shaffer RN, Schwartz A: Estimation of width of angle of anterior chamber: Incidence and significance of the narrow angle. Am J Ophthalmol 68:626, 1969.
14. Alsbirk PH: Anterior chamber depth and primary angle-closure glaucoma. I: An epidemiologic study in Greenland Eskimos. Acta Ophthalmol (Copenh) 53:89, 1975.
15. Lee DA, Brubaker RF, Ilstrup DM: Anterior chamber dimensions in patients with narrow angles and angle-closure glaucoma. Arch Ophthalmol 102:46, 1984.
16. Scheie HG: Width and pigmentation of the angle of the anterior chamber: A system of grading by gonioscopy. Arch Ophthalmol 58:510, 1957.
17. Shaffer RN: Symposium: Primary glaucoma III, gonioscopy, ophthalmoscopy, and perimetry. Trans Am Acad Ophthalmol Otolaryngol 62:112, 1960.
18. Forbes M: Indentation gonioscopy and efficacy of iridectomy in angle-closure glaucoma. Trans Am Ophthalmol Soc 72:488, 1974.
19. Gorin G: Shortening of the angle of the anterior chamber in angle-closure glaucoma. Am J Ophthalmol 49:141, 1960.
20. Krupin T, Mitchel KB, Johnson M, et al: The long-term effects of iridectomy for primary acute angle-closure glaucoma. Am J Ophthalmol 89:875, 1982.
21. Bobrow JC, Drews RC: Long-term results of peripheral iridectomy. Glaucoma 3:319, 1981.
22. Spaeth GL: The normal development of the human anterior chamber angle: A new system of descriptive grading. Trans Ophthalmol Soc UK 91:707, 1971.
23. Alsbirk PH: Corneal diameter in Greenland Eskimos: Anthropometric and genetic studies with special reference to primary angle-closure glaucoma. Acta Ophthalmol (Copenh) 53:635, 1975.
24. Aizawa K: Studies on the depth of the anterior chamber. Jpn J Ophthalmol 4:272, 1960.
25. Belcher CD, Thomas JV, Simmons RJ: Photocoagulation in Glaucoma and Anterior Segment Disease. Baltimore, Williams & Wilkins, 1984, p 83.
26. Wishart PK, Nagasubramaniaw S, Hitchings RA: Argon laser trabeculoplasty in narrow angle glaucoma. EYE 1:567, 1987.
27. Chandler PA, Simmons RJ: Anterior chamber deepening for gonioscopy at time of surgery. Arch Ophthalmol 74:177, 1965.
28. Campbell DG, Vella A: Modern goniosynechialysis for the treatment of synechial angle-closure glaucoma. Ophthalmology 91:1052, 1984.

Chapter 122

■

The Exfoliation Syndrome— A Continuing Challenge

DOUGLAS H. JOHNSON

The exfoliation syndrome has been recognized for over half a century and has come to be respected for the aggressive glaucoma that may often accompany it. Glaucoma develops in up to 50 percent of patients with exfoliation syndrome and tends to be more difficult to control, with higher intraocular pressures and a poorer response to medication than primary open-angle glaucoma. Despite longstanding recognition of the exfoliation syndrome, its worldwide distribution, and a multitude of studies, the reason why exfoliation syndrome develops is unknown. Also unknown is why only certain patients with the condition develop glaucoma, and how to predict which of these patients will develop glaucoma. Thus, the exfoliation syndrome continues to present a series of challenges: to understand the pathogenesis of the condition, to be wary of the glaucoma that may develop, and to predict which patients will develop glaucoma with time.

Exfoliation syndrome has been associated with glaucoma since first reported by Lindberg, in 1917.[1] He found the characteristic white dandruff-like flakes on the lens and pupillary margin in 50 percent of his patients with glaucoma. Later authors have confirmed and expanded on Lindberg's report. Vogt (1925) attributed the material to a true exfoliation or delamination of the lens capsule, while Busacca (1927) and years later Dvorak-Theobald (1954) attributed the material to an abnormal precipitation on the lens capsule.[2-4] Dvorak-Theobald called it "*pseudo*exfoliation" to distinguish it from true exfoliation and delamination of the lens capsule as seen in glass blowers. More recent studies have again pointed to the lens capsule as a partial source of the material and have given rise to the term "exfoliation syndrome."[5-9] Other synonyms have included senile exfoliation of the lens capsule,[2, 5] senile uveal exfoliation,[10] fibrillopathia epitheliocapsularis,[6] the basement membrane exfoliation syndrome,[11] and glaucoma capsulare.[6, 10, 11]

CLINICAL MANIFESTATIONS

Diagnosis Based on Slit-Lamp Examination

The hallmark of exfoliation syndrome is the appearance of whitish granular deposits and dandruff-like flakes on the anterior capsule of the crystalline lens (Fig. 122–1). Characteristically this presents as a central, homogeneous appearing disc of gray granular material, of the approximate size of the pupil at its smallest diameter. A clear intermediate zone, lacking exfoliative material, surrounds this in a concentric ring. This in turn is surrounded by an outer peripheral zone of exfoliative material. It is thought that the intermediate clear zone is caused by movement of the iris and pupillary border, rubbing exfoliative material off the lens. The exfoliative material may sometimes appear as a partially detached sheet, resembling a delamination of the anterior capsule. Exfoliative material also characteristically appears as fine white flakes on the pupillary border of the iris (Fig. 122–2). Several variations of these presentations can occur, including lack of the central disc of exfoliative material, streaks of exfoliative material in the intermediate clear zone, or a very subtle, delicate appearance of the granular material in portions of the central disc area with no other clinically apparent manifestations in the intermediate or peripheral zones (see Fig. 122–1C and D).

Dilatation of the pupil is often helpful in diagnosing exfoliation syndrome, as the intermediate clear zone and peripheral exfoliative zone become readily apparent. An undilatated pupil will constrict under the light of the slit lamp during examination and will become small enough to hide the intermediate clear zone and the obvious demarcation with the central disc. Without these visible transitions the homogeneous nature of the exfoliative material in the central disc can make a diagnosis difficult. Reports indicate that up to 20 percent of exfoliative cases are missed if examined with undilatated pupils.[12]

Exfoliative material may also be seen in other locations. Flakes and granular globs may appear in the drainage angle on the trabecular meshwork, on the corneal endothelium, on the zonular fibers, on the ciliary processes, or on the anterior vitreous face (see Fig. 122–2).

Pigment may also be a clue to exfoliation syndrome. Gonioscopy often reveals a moderate to dense degree of pigmentation, frequently in a discontinuous segmental fashion in the trabecular meshwork (Fig. 122–3). The pigmentation is characteristically black, but never as dense or as homogeneous as the continuous "mascara line" seen on the meshwork in pigmentary glaucoma. Pigment is also present on Schwalbe's line in the inferior portions of the eye. The pigment probably arises from the iris, where atrophy of the pupillary ruff of pigment and scattered transillumination defects occur. These defects are much more central and in a different pattern

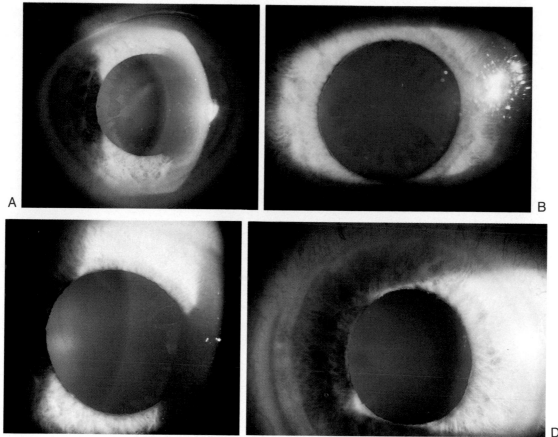

Figure 122–1. *A*, Slit-lamp photograph of typical anterior lens capsule findings in exfoliation syndrome. Note the central disc of exfoliative material, the intermediate clear zone where most of the material has been rubbed off by the iris, and the peripheral granular zone. The pupil has been dilatated. *B*, Exfoliation syndrome. The intermediate zone is not as well defined because of bridging strands of exfoliative material. *C*, Exfoliation syndrome, with no central disc of exfoliative material. The peripheral granular zone is readily seen, but only after pupil dilatation. *D*, Exfoliation syndrome, subtle. The central disc and strands bridging the intermediate zone are visible through careful observation.

than the midperipheral radial spokes of transillumination of pigment dispersion syndrome.

Exfoliative material has also been described in the conjunctiva, iris, and skin, although this is only seen microscopically on biopsy specimens.[13–18]

Epidemiology

A DISEASE FROM SCANDINAVIA?

Lindberg's first description of the exfoliation syndrome was in a series of patients in Finland, and high prevalence rates and a plethora of studies continue to be reported from the Nordic countries. It is not unique to Scandinavia, however, as the syndrome has been described in most other peoples of the world.[12] Exfoliation syndrome has been reported in Japanese, Indians, Australian aborigines, blacks from the Bantu tribe in South Africa, American Navajo Indians, Peruvian Indians, and in many European countries (Table 122–1). Prevalence rates vary, however. Not only do true differences in the prevalence rates exist, but also differ-ences in examination techniques among studies exist. Dilatation of the pupil by the examiner, age of population studied, and prospective versus retrospective data collection can all affect results. Prevalence rates appear highest and most accurate in prospective studies using pupil dilatation. One such series of prospective screenings in retirement homes for the elderly indicates prevalence rates of 6.3 percent in Norway, 4.7 percent in England, and 4 percent in Germany.[23] Rates in other populations tend to be similar or lower: 0.2 percent in Japanese, 2 percent in Indians, 4.4 percent in Peruvian Indians,[12] and 1.8 percent in the Framingham, Massachusetts study.[19] Exfoliation syndrome is more common with age (see later).

No specific dominant nor recessive inheritance pattern has been described in exfoliation syndrome, yet a genetic or ethnic predisposition seems to play a role. The condition is common in Norway and Finland (up to 20 percent prevalence reported in Finland)[12, 22] but less common in Denmark (2 percent),[25] Austria, and Switzerland (2 percent).[12] It has been reported in 10 percent of blacks in South Africa[28] yet in only 0.4 percent of blacks with glaucoma in Louisiana,[32] whose ancestral homes were mainly West Africa. It is rare in Eskimos.

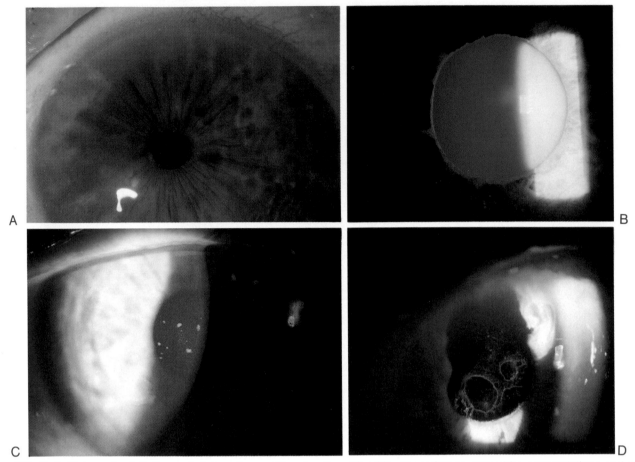

Figure 122–2. *A,* Flakes of exfoliative material on the pupillary border of the iris, appearing as gray-white accumulations and small clumps of material. *B,* Peripupillary iris transillumination in exfoliation syndrome. The pupillary ruff of the pigment is missing, and scattered patchy transillumination defects with a moth-eaten appearance occur in the nearby iris. The edge of the central disc of exfoliative material appears as a whitish ring in this photograph. *C,* Flakes of exfoliative material adherent to central corneal endothelium. *D,* Whitish exfoliative material coating strands of vitreous on the anterior hyaloid face years after intracapsular cataract extraction.

INFLUENCED BY CLIMATE?

The frequency of reports and high prevalence rates in the Nordic countries lead to the idea that northern latitudes, cold air, hours of sunlight, or some other climate-related factor is involved in producing exfoliation syndrome. Evidence for this is mixed, however. Exfoliation syndrome is common in Laplanders but is rare in Eskimos, both groups living at similar latitudes.[12] It is also prevalent in Saudi Arabia (13.2 percent),[26] which has a radically different climate than that found in the northern latitudes.

Ultraviolet light exposure has also been suggested as influencing exfoliation syndrome. Evidence to support this theory is mixed, also. One study found more exfoliation syndrome in people from the mountainous areas of Pakistan than in those living on the plains,[12, 33] yet other studies of people living at high altitudes (e.g., Himalayas, Andes mountains) report a low prevalence of exfoliation.[12] Attempts to correlate exfoliation with other signs associated with ultraviolet exposure, such as pterygia, climatic keratopathy, or cataract, have failed to reveal significant correlations.[12]

A DISEASE OF AGE

Exfoliation syndrome is more common with age (see Table 122–1). It is rare before age 50 but becomes increasingly common thereafter, nearly doubling in incidence every decade.[12] Forsius reported a prevalence of 10 percent among Finns 50 to 69 yr of age and a prevalence of 25.3 percent among Finns over 70 yr of age.[12] The Framingham study reported a prevalence of 0.6 percent for people who are 52 to 64 yr of age, rising to 5.0 percent by 75 to 85 yr of age.[19] Similar age-dependent increases have been reported in North Carolina,[20] France,[21] and Saudi Arabia.[26]

A UNILATERAL DISEASE?

Exfoliation syndrome often occurs unilaterally. Reports indicate from 48 to 76 percent of cases appear to be unilateral at the time of diagnosis.[19, 34–38] The reason is unknown. Most theories of pathogenesis point toward a metabolic or degenerative process, which would be expected to be present bilaterally. The condition may actually be bilateral, however, with asymmetric appear-

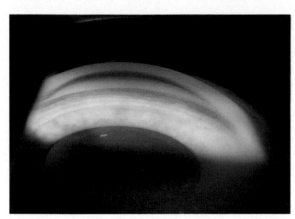

Figure 122–3. Gonioscopic view of the angle in exfoliation syndrome. Moderate to heavy degree of pigmentation is evident in trabecular meshwork. The peripheral granular zone of exfoliative material is evident on the anterior lens surface.

ance between the eyes. Along this line, Mizuno studied unilateral exfoliation patients and found exfoliative material on the ciliary processes in 76 percent of the presumably uninvolved fellow eyes of these patients.[39] In addition, studies indicate that from 13 to 43 percent of patients with unilateral exfoliation syndrome will develop it in the fellow eye after 5 to 10 yr.[36, 38, 40, 41]

Risk of Glaucoma

AT TIME OF INITIAL DISCOVERY OF EXFOLIATION

About 20 percent of patients with newly discovered exfoliation syndrome also have glaucoma or elevated intraocular pressure found at the same examination. (Studies vary, with the incidence of actual glaucoma ranging from 6 to 24 percent).[26, 27, 37, 38, 42] This indicates that careful attention should be focused on the optic disc examination as well as on intraocular pressure in a patient newly found to have exfoliation syndrome. Overall, about 50 percent of patients with exfoliation syndrome are ultimately diagnosed with glaucoma, whether found at the time of the initial examination or at a later time (figures vary from 20 to 85 percent).[21, 34, 36–38, 41]

Even in the absence of overt glaucoma, higher intraocular pressure is often found in an eye with exfoliation.[19, 26, 37, 38, 43, 44] The examiner should be aware of this and should schedule a reexamination after a reasonable period of time. Thus, because of the frequency of glaucoma that may be present or may develop in exfoliation syndrome, visual field examination, optic disc photographs, and tonography should be obtained if the disc or pressure is suspicious.

RISK OF GLAUCOMA WITH TIME

Five percent of patients with exfoliation syndrome and no glaucoma at the initial examination develop an elevated intraocular pressure or glaucoma after 5 yr, and 15 percent overall develop elevated pressure after 10 yr.[38] (Figures vary with different studies, ranging from 5 to 34 percent at 5 yr.[38, 43–46]) These figures again indicate that exfoliation syndrome can be considered a warning sign that glaucoma may develop. Patients with exfoliation syndrome must be followed faithfully at regular intervals, and an accurate observation of the disc should be made at each examination. Suspicious discs or pressures may entail reexamination after several months, whereas a patient with exfoliation syndrome and normal discs and pressures should be observed annually or at 2-yr intervals.

PREVALENCE OF EXFOLIATION SYNDROME IN OPEN-ANGLE GLAUCOMA

The reverse side of the coin regarding exfoliation syndrome and glaucoma indicates that, overall, many patients with open-angle glaucoma actually have exfoliation syndrome with glaucoma. Surveys of patients with established open-angle glaucoma indicate that between 3 and 47 percent of these open-angle glaucoma cases are exfoliative glaucoma, and figures in the United States range from 3 to 28 percent.[20, 31, 35, 36, 41, 47–50] This is also age-dependent, with an increasing proportion of exfoliative glaucoma in the older patients with open-angle glaucoma. The distinction of exfoliative glaucoma versus primary open-angle glaucoma has direct clinical importance, because intraocular pressures in eyes with exfoliation syndrome and glaucoma tend to go out of control more often and at shorter intervals than in primary open-angle glaucoma. Eyes with exfoliative glaucoma should thus be watched frequently and faithfully (i.e., three or four times each year rather than two or three times each year).

Clinical Course of Exfoliation Syndrome

GLAUCOMA: AN AGGRESSIVE GLAUCOMA THAT MAY REQUIRE LASER OR TRADITIONAL SURGERY

As mentioned earlier, glaucoma may develop at some point in up to 50 percent of patients with exfoliation syndrome, and the glaucoma that develops may be more difficult to control. One study found that 61 percent of patients with exfoliative glaucoma had either laser trabeculoplasty (35 percent) or glaucoma surgery (26 percent) by the time they had died.[51] This study also reported that 25 percent of patients with exfoliative glaucoma were blind in at least one eye, and 8 percent of patients were blind in both eyes (comprising some 15 percent of the patients with bilateral exfoliative glaucoma in that study). Numerous studies have commented on the failure of long-term medical treatment and late failures of laser trabeculoplasty.[35, 36, 44, 45, 50–56]

Table 122–1. PREVALENCE OF EXFOLIATION SYNDROME IN GENERAL POPULATION (PROSPECTIVE STUDIES, PATIENTS 50+ YEARS, DILATATED PUPIL EXAMINATION)

Country	Age (Yr)	No. of Patients Studied	% with Exfoliation
United States			
Framingham, MA[19]	52–85	1906	1.8
	52–64	1060	0.6
	65–74	585	2.6
	75–85	261	5.0
North Carolina[20]	60–89	2121	3.2
	60–69	522	1.7
	70–79	345	3.8
	80–89	122	7.8
Scandinavia/Nordic Countries			
Finland			
Forsius[12]	50+	443	20.5
	50–69	152	11.8
	70+	291	25.1
Krause*[22]	60+	795	22.4
	60–69	239	14.2
	70–79	383	21.9
	80+	173	34.7
Norway[23]	60+	766	6.3
Sweden[24]	65–74	760	18.0
Denmark[25]	60+	209	1.9
	70+	84	4.8
Iceland[12]	50–69	155	11.0
	70+	324	31.5
England[23]	60+	801	4.0
Germany[23]	60+	491	4.9
France[21]	50+	4042	5.5
	50–60		0.7
	61–65		2.7
	66–70		4.0
	71–75		6.5
	76–80		8.2
	80+		12.8
India[12]	50+	100	2.0
Tunisia[12]	50+	126	9.5
Saudi Arabia[26]	50+	250	13.2
	50–59	103	7.8
	60–69	79	8.9
	70+	68	26.5
Peru (Indians)[12]	50+	159	4.4
American Navajo Indians[27]	60+	50	38.0
South Africa[28]	60+	854	10.0
Australia (Aborigines)[29]	61+	184	16.3
Japan			
Nanba[30]	60+		5.1
Shimizu[31]*	50+	23,645	0.2

*Not dilatated.

CATARACT SURGERY: WEAK ZONULES, LENS DISLOCATION, AND VITREOUS LOSS

Subluxation of the crystalline lens is a rare but definite complication of exfoliation syndrome.[57] The attachment of the zonular fibers to the ciliary body is thought to be weakened, perhaps by accumulation of exfoliative material between the zonular fiber and its insertion.[57] This can not only cause the rare lens subluxation but may also predispose the eye to surgical complications in this era of extracapsular cataract surgery. Several studies have reported significantly higher rates of zonular breaks, capsular dialysis, or vitreous loss (5 to 10 times normal) in eyes with exfoliation syndrome.[58–60] This has been due mainly to zonular rupture causing displacement of the posterior capsule and may occur despite the most gentle and atraumatic surgery possible.

Surgeons should anticipate weakened zonules during cataract surgery. Preoperative signs may be obvious, as lens dislocation, or may be subtle, as iridodinesis or phacodinesis. These more subtle signs are best seen during slit-lamp examination while asking the patient to move the eye briefly and should be checked routinely on all patients with exfoliative syndrome who are con-sidering cataract surgery. Problems with the posterior capsule or vitreous encountered during surgery are also an obvious warning of potential problems in the unop-erated fellow eye. Surgical technique should be adjusted accordingly, including consideration of performing the intracapsular technique rather than a repeat of a prob-lem-filled extracapsular attempt. If extracapsular surgery is to be performed, several caveats should be considered: gentle anterior capsulotomy, longer corneoscleral inci-sion, hydrodissection of nucleus, gentle nucleus expres-sion, and gentle irrigation-aspiration of the remaining cortex.

PATHOGENESIS

Exfoliative Material— Characteristic Filaments and Fibrils, Yet of Unknown Origin

Exfoliative material appears to be a homogeneous, eosinophilic, periodic acid-Schiff (PAS)-positive staining substance under light microscopy (Fig. 122–4).[4, 6, 61–63] PAS staining indicates a material rich in polysaccharides.

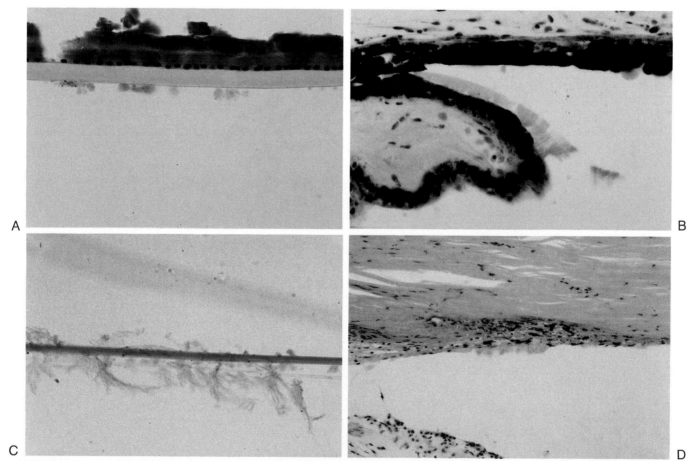

Figure 122–4. *A,* Light microscopic view of anterior lens capsule in exfoliation syndrome. Eosinophilic bushlike clumps of exfoliative material are lined up on anterior capsule. H&E, ×400. *B,* Ciliary process in exfoliation syndrome. The pale pink homogeneous coating of exfoliative material has been artifactually separated from ciliary process in some portions. H&E, ×400. *C,* Zonular fiber coated with exfoliative material. H&E, ×400. *D,* Trabecular meshwork in exfoliation syndrome. Clumps of material coat the uveal meshwork. H&E, ×200.

Transmission electron microscopy shows exfoliative material to be a randomly arranged tangle of filaments and fibrils embedded in an amorphous ground substance (Fig. 122–5). The filaments are small, threadlike rods about 10 nm in diameter, whereas the larger fibrils have a diameter of about 50 nm. The fibrils show a characteristic banding.[6–9, 61–63] The amorphous ground substance is thought to consist of glycosaminoglycans, consistent with the PAS staining, whereas the filaments and fibrils are protein.[64]

Scanning electron microscopy demonstrates exfoliative material to be a rough-appearing coating that, under higher power, is a fine net of fibrillar material and bushlike excrescences of coarser fibers (Figs. 122–6 and 122–7).[62] The distribution and appearance vary, resembling a precipitate in some areas of the lens and a more homogeneous, matted group of fibers in other areas.

A variety of enzymatic, histochemical, and immunologic tests have been performed on exfoliative material.[61, 63, 64, 67–69] These tests indicate that the fibrils and filaments consist of noncollagenous protein, because they are insoluble in enzymes and do not contain hydroxyproline. Amino acid analysis of exfoliative material is compatible with three possibilities: microfibrils of elastin, basement membrane, or amyloid.[70]

Elastin. A close association between zonular fibers and exfoliative material has long been recognized.[71, 72] Zonular fibers consist of oxytalan, a type of elastic filament. Elastic tissue consists of two major components: elastin, an amorphous-appearing, insoluble protein, and elastic filaments, of which there are several variations including oxytalan. The elastic filaments themselves consist of glycoproteins. Ultrastructural, histochemical, and antigenic similarities exist between elastic filaments and exfoliative material.[73, 74] Elastic tissue also occurs in other areas of the eye besides zonules,

and studies of exfoliative material in the conjunctiva have found that exfoliative material is frequently associated with the normal elastic system of that tissue.[75] Increased amounts of exfoliative material also occur near areas of elastosis, leading one group of researchers to propose that exfoliative fibers are a type of elastosis.[18, 75]

Basement Membrane. Numerous studies have described exfoliative material in association with basement membranes, which often appear duplicated, disrupted, or degenerated. These changes are present in the lens capsule and have also been noted in the iris, ciliary processes, and conjunctiva.[6–8, 13–18, 76, 77] Basement membrane is a conglomeration of material secreted by epithelial cells and is present in structures throughout the eye. It consists of collagen filaments intermixed with glycoproteins (laminin and fibronectin) and proteoglycans. The diffuse locations of exfoliative material in accompaniment with abnormal-appearing basement membrane has led some investigators to call the condition the "basement membrane exfoliation syndrome."[11] Whether basement membranes throughout the body are affected is unclear, because reports are contradictory with regard to the presence of the material in the skin in sites distant to the eye.[18, 78]

Amyloid. Several studies have found that exfoliative material reacts with stains suggestive of amyloid: Congo red, thioflavin T, and thioflavin S.[79, 80] Both amyloid and exfoliative material also stain with ruthenium red and react positively for tyrosine and tryptophan on histochemical tests.[63, 66, 69, 81] Several patients with amyloidosis (primary systemic nonfamilial and also systemic familial) have been reported to have deposits on the equator of the lens capsule and on the surfaces of the iris, reminiscent of exfoliative deposits.[82, 83] Although these cross-reactivities and similarities are alluring, they are not

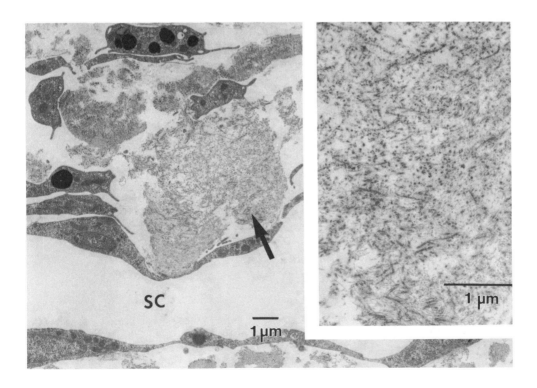

Figure 122–5. Exfoliative material, accumulation near Schlemm's canal (SC). The material is a randomly arranged tangle of filaments and fibrils embedded in an amorphous ground substance. Filaments are small, threadlike rods with a 10-nm diameter. Fibrils are larger rods with a 50-nm diameter. Transmission electron micrograph, ×7500. *Inset:* Magnified view of exfoliative material, ×25,000.

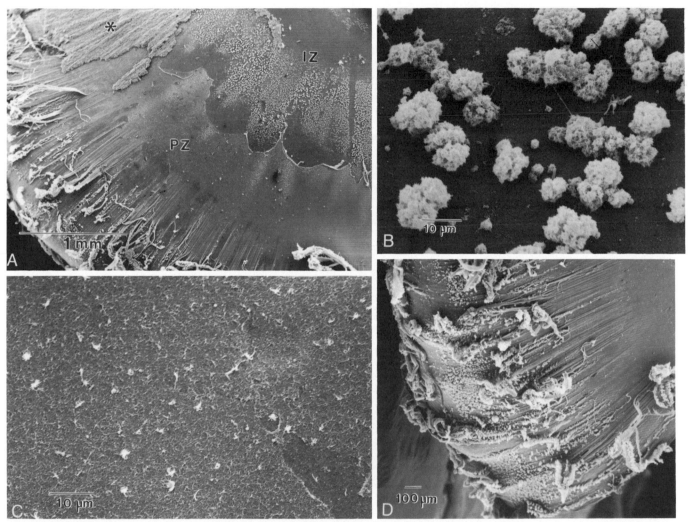

Figure 122–6. *A,* The anterior lens surface in exfoliation syndrome. Portions of the intermediate zone (IZ) contain granular accumulations of exfoliative material. A sharp demarcation line is evident between the intermediate zone and the peripheral zone (PZ). Zonular fibers appear as broken strands, some encrusted with exfoliative material. The iris pigment epithelium is artifactually adherent to lens surface in the upper portion of photograph *(asterisk).* Scanning electron micrograph, ×27. *B,* Intermediate zone with rounded, bushlike accumulations of exfoliative material. Underlying lens capsule is relatively smooth and free of material. Scanning electron micrograph, ×1000. *C,* Peripheral zone. Dense feltlike mat of exfoliative material lies directly on the lens capsule. Note the lack of bushlike accumulations in contrast to the intermediate zone as shown in *B.* Scanning electron micrograph, ×1000. *D,* The equatorial zone of the lens surface in exfoliation syndrome. Granular accumulations of exfoliative material are prominent on the anterior edge of the equator, near insertion of zonular fibers. Under higher magnification, these granules of material consist of numerous fine threads (see *E*). Scanning electron micrograph, ×40.

Illustration continued on following page

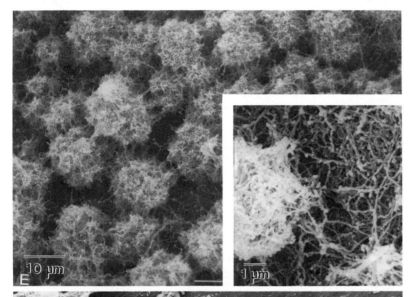

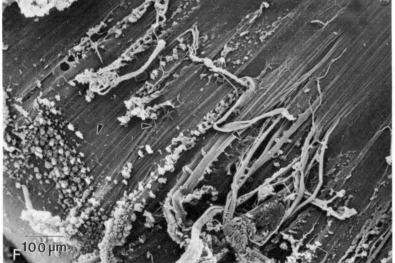

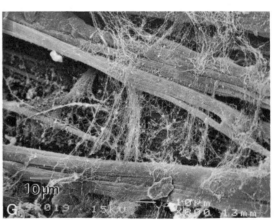

Figure 122–6. *Continued E,* Higher power views of granular accumulations of exfoliative material seen in *D.* Note that each "granule" consists of a tangle of threadlike fibrils and filaments. ×1000. *Inset:* ×9000. *F,* The anterior equatorial zone of lens surface, exfoliation syndrome. Broken zonular fibers, some encrusted with barnacle-like exfoliative material, are evident, along with granular accumulations as seen in *D.* This higher power view also shows cobweb-like bundles of exfoliative fiber *(arrowheads).* Scanning electron micrograph, ×100. *G,* Higher power view of cobwebs of exfoliative fibers covering zonular fiber insertions, as shown in *F,* ×800.

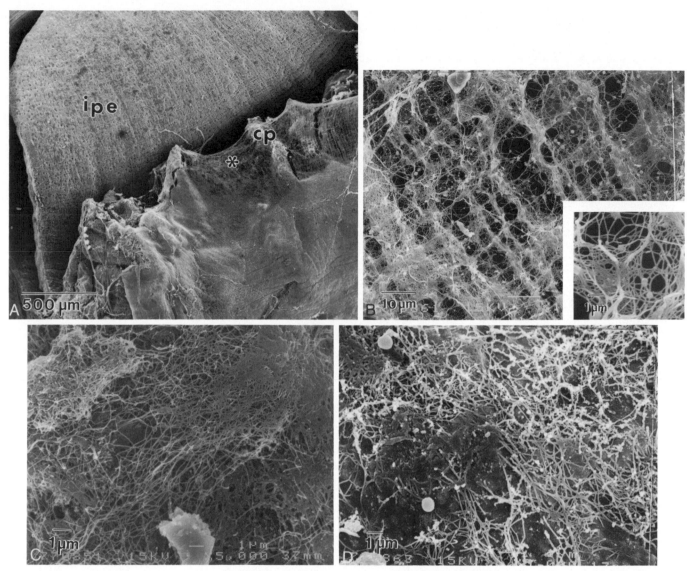

Figure 122–7. *A,* Posterior iris surface and ciliary processes in exfoliation syndrome. Note the dense mat of exfoliative material stretching between ciliary processes *(asterisk).* (ipe, iris pigment epithelium; cp, ciliary processes.) Scanning electron micrograph, ×35. *B,* Higher power views of mat of exfoliative material shown in part *A.* Note tangle of fibrils forming the mat, with entrapped pigment granules scattered throughout, ×1000. *Inset:* ×5000. *C,* Exfoliative material covering ciliary process in denser tangles than in *B,* ×5000. *D,* Exfoliative material covering the posterior iris surface. Note the similarity to the material on the posterior iris surface as shown in *C,* ×5000.

pathognomonic. Amyloid is usually thought to consist of immunoglobin light chains, and antibody cross-reactivity has not been demonstrated between κ and λ light chains and exfoliative material.[84] In addition, other studies have failed to find exfoliation to stain with Congo red and also comment on the nonspecificity of the thioflavin reaction.[61, 63, 69]

Source of Exfoliative Material

INTRAOCULAR SITES

Lens. The hallmark of exfoliation syndrome is its appearance on the lens. Histologically, five regions of the lens are described, compromising not only the three clinically observed regions (central disc, intermediate clear zone, peripheral granular zone) but also anterior and posterior equatorial regions.[63, 85] The posterior capsule does not appear to be involved in the exfoliation syndrome. Surprisingly, the clinically obvious appearance of exfoliative material in the central and peripheral regions may be the result of aqueous-borne deposition and polymerization, because the underlying lens capsule remains intact and does not show evidence of production of the material.[6–9, 63] Intrinsic capsular changes are present in the equatorial zones, however, leading to the conclusion that the material is produced in these areas.[6–9, 63] An amorphous layer of material has been described within the capsule or underlying the capsule and resting on the epithelial cells, in the equatorial zones. The amorphous layer itself is discontinuous and appears as multiple discoid plaques scattered throughout the area. In addition, vertical striations of bundles of exfoliative fibers are present, appearing to originate in pits in the lens epithelium and traverse both the amorphous layer of the capsule and the capsule itself.[6-9, 63]

Ciliary Processes. Exfoliative material often coats the ciliary processes and appears intermixed with a multilaminar basement membrane on electron microscopy.[4, 9, 13, 62, 63, 77] Clinically, exfoliative material has been seen on the ciliary processes of exfoliative eyes and also in the fellow eyes of a number of cases of "unilateral" exfoliation syndrome.[39] The presence and presumed production of exfoliative material in the ciliary processes, as well as in the iris pigment epithelium, may explain the clinical observation of its appearance on the pupil margin years after intracapsular cataract extraction.[86]

Iris. Exfoliative material has been found in the iris pigment epithelium, blood vessel walls, and on the anterior stroma.[16, 17, 63] Accumulations of the material are seen on the pigment epithelial layer, both posteriorly and at the pupillary margin. Microscopically, exfoliative material is intermixed with a duplicated and disorganized basement membrane of the iris pigment epithelial cells, which also have degenerative and disruptive changes. Iris vasculature may contain subendothelial accumulations of the material, often in conjunction with disrupted basement membranes.[16, 17, 63] These changes may occlude the lumen in some areas and may explain the clinical observation of dropout and leakage of iris vessels and the occasional areas of vasoproliferation seen with fluorescein angiography.[87-89]

Trabecular Meshwork. It is uncertain if exfoliative material is produced locally by the trabecular meshwork. Most studies agree on its presence in the aqueous channels of the uveal meshwork, the intertrabecular spaces, juxtacanalicular tissue, and Schlemm's canal,[4, 61, 90, 91] all consistent with a washing in and deposit of aqueous-borne material. Studies do not agree on the presence of exfoliative material within the trabecular lamellae, which would be the evidence needed to indicate local production by the trabecular cells. Some studies have described exfoliative material to be present in the subcellular regions of the trabecular lamellae and also within trabecular cell vacuoles, suggesting local production,[90] whereas others have reported that these structures are normal.[61, 91] Exfoliation syndrome is also associated with increased pigmentation of the meshwork. This pigment is undoubtedly washed in from the aqueous and appears as granules within trabecular cells as well as in the intertrabecular spaces.

Zonules. Although exfoliative material frequently coats the zonular fibers and has structural and histochemical similarities with them, the zonular fibers themselves are usually intact and unaffected.[4, 7] The zonular ruptures and lens dislocations described clinically may result from exfoliative material accumulating at the insertion of the zonular fibers into the ciliary body, weakening this attachment.[92]

EXTRAOCULAR SITES

Conjunctiva. Exfoliative material has been demonstrated in both the bulbar and palpebral conjunctiva.[14, 15, 35, 75, 78, 93, 94] Although conceivable that its presence in the bulbar conjunctiva could be due to washout from within the eye through scleral channels, its presence in the palpebral conjunctiva makes this less likely. In addition, it is present in the conjunctival stroma, associated with the endogenous elastic fibers of this tissue, and is not necessarily in intimate association with vessels or lymphatics.[75, 93, 94] Streeten and associates commented on the association of exfoliative fibrils with elastosis, finding an intermingling of the fibrils with elastic fibrils and suggested that exfoliation syndrome may be a type of elastosis, resulting from an abnormal aggregation of components related to elastic microfibrils.[75]

Skin. Although an early study did not find exfoliative material in the eyelid skin or oral mucosa of patients with exfoliation syndrome,[78] a later study found it in several skin sites distant from the eye.[18] Areas with exfoliative fibrils were retroauricular skin, buttock skin, and eyelid skin. The exfoliation material was found primarily along elastic fibers and appeared to be influenced by an accompanying dermal elastosis.[18]

Cause of the Glaucoma

Opinions on the nature of the glaucoma have varied through the years, and four major theories have been proposed. Vogt believed that the glaucoma was secondary, owing to blockage of trabecular spaces by exfoliative material.[2] Others have thought that the glaucoma was primary and that exfoliation was only an additional factor.[34, 35] Additional theories have proposed that exfoliation and glaucoma were both due to degeneration of the uvea,[10, 34] or that the glaucoma was caused by pigment blockage.[34] Most researchers now believe the glaucoma is a secondary process, distinct from primary open-angle glaucoma.[36, 90, 91, 94] Several clinical observations support this idea. First, exfoliative glaucoma has a more aggressive clinical course, with higher intraocular pressures and a poorer response to medication.[35, 45, 51, 53, 54] Second, steroid challenge tests, looking for intraocular elevation after topical steroid treatment, revealed no increased incidences of "high responders." This is in contrast to the increased number of "high responders" found in primary open-angle glaucoma.[95, 96] Finally, elevated intraocular pressure occurs much more commonly in patients with exfoliation syndrome than in an otherwise matched control population. This is particularly noticeable in unilateral exfoliation syndrome in which the affected eye develops glaucoma and the unaffected eye only rarely does.[34, 37, 38, 44, 46, 55]

Histologic observation also indicates that exfoliative glaucoma is distinct from primary open-angle glaucoma. First, exfoliative material can be found throughout the aqueous channels of the trabecular meshwork, accumulating especially heavily in the finely porous juxtacanalicular area.[90, 91, 97] Exfoliative material is not present in primary open-angle glaucoma. The exfoliative material may well obstruct the porosity of this tissue, decreasing the net area available to aqueous outflow, and may also serve as a nidus for the accumulation of pigment, cellular debris, and extracellular matrix components and further decrease the porosity of this critical portion of the aqueous outflow channels. The second difference between exfoliative glaucoma and primary open-angle glaucoma is the occurrence of "plaques" of material seen in primary glaucoma.[97] These plaques are actually fibrillar tendons with their surrounding collagen sheaths, running through the juxtacanalicular tissue. When histologic sections are cut in the usual radial orientation (sagittal sections), the tendons and sheaths appear as discontinuous plaques, whereas in tangential sections they appear as tendons. The tendon sheaths become thicker with age and are especially thick in primary glaucoma, appearing as an increase in "plaque material" when viewed with the standard sagittal histologic sections.[97] Exfoliative glaucoma eyes do not have this excess tendon sheath/plaque material but rather have amounts similar to control eyes.[97] This indicates a fundamental difference in the nature of exfoliative glaucoma and of primary glaucoma.

Pigment may be a contributing factor in the pathogenesis of exfoliative glaucoma. Some authors believe that pigment may be the primary cause of the glaucoma, whereas others consider that it is a contributing factor.[34, 36, 94] A relationship between the amount of pigment seen with gonioscopy and the incidence of glaucoma has been suggested.[36, 94] Histologically, pigment is present within trabecular cells and occasionally within the intertrabecular spaces, although the outflow spaces do not appear narrowed enough because of this to produce elevated pressure.[91]

A vexing question remains: Why do only some eyes with exfoliation syndrome develop glaucoma? One factor may be simply the amount of exfoliative material present. Eyes with larger amounts might be expected to develop glaucoma, and eyes with small amounts of exfoliative material may not. This relationship is not always borne out clinically, however, because glaucoma can develop in eyes with even subtle findings of exfoliation syndrome. An additional explanation probably lies in the innate differences among individual patients. The cells in the trabecular meshwork are metabolically active, containing a variety of synthetic and digestive enzymes, and are thought responsible for cleaning the meshwork of debris. These metabolic activities and capabilities may vary among patients, with some meshworks less able to handle the continuing burden of exfoliative material. The final portion of the trabecular meshwork, the juxtacanalicular tissue, is an area rich in collagen and extracellular matrix, through which aqueous humor must diffuse. The composition and porosity of this region are determined in part by the trabecular cells and thus may also vary between eyes. Exfoliative material probably passes through this tissue more easily in some eyes than others. With time, the cellular and extracellular capacities of almost any eye to deal with chronic, repetitive, or large amounts of exfoliative material may become inadequate, causing obstruction of aqueous channels and glaucoma.

DIFFERENTIAL DIAGNOSIS

Few things are easily confused with exfoliation syndrome. The heavy pigmentation of the trabecular mesh-

work seen on gonioscopy in exfoliation syndrome tends to be segmental, unlike the diffuse, darker brown or black pigmentation of pigmentary glaucoma. Iris transillumination also differs, because pigmentary glaucoma has elongated radial spokes in the periphery of the iris whereas exfoliation syndrome has moth-eaten patchy peripupillary transillumination defects, often with some loss of the pupillary ruff.[94]

Synechiae, fibrin, or cyclitic membranes may involve the anterior lens capsule with white debris but may lack the homogeneous granular appearance and characteristic flakes of exfoliative material. True delamination or exfoliation of the anterior lens capsule presents as a clear diaphanous membrane with a free edge floating in the aqueous.[98] This condition is rare and differs from the occasional sheet of gray-white material that may peel off the lens capsule in exfoliation syndrome (pseudoexfoliation).

Systemic amyloidosis may produce ocular changes, including deposition of white, flaky material in the anterior segment.[82, 83] Glaucoma may accompany this condition. It differs from exfoliation syndrome in being much less common and also in having systemic manifestations.

TREATMENT

The frequent occurrence of glaucoma in exfoliation syndrome and its aggressive nature require that the clinician be wary of the condition. Regular periodic examinations (annually or every other year) should be performed on patients with exfoliation syndrome, with initial baseline optic disc drawings or photographs. Tonography may give an indication of the function of the outflow channels, with borderline or abnormal values indicating more frequent follow-up.

Once glaucoma is diagnosed, standard medical treatment is used. Regular examinations are again important (at least every 6 mo), because intraocular pressure will become more difficult to control with time. Laser trabeculoplasty is especially successful in exfoliation syndrome, and studies report average initial success rates up to 80 percent in lowering intraocular pressure.[54, 99] The increased success rate is thought to be due to the higher starting intraocular pressures and the generally increased trabecular pigmentation. As in primary open-angle glaucoma, success rates decrease with time, averaging 50 percent or less by 5 yr. Reports on the success of retreatment with laser therapy are mixed, and most indicate less successful results.[99] If medications and laser therapy are unsuccessful in controlling the glaucoma, routine filtration surgery can be performed with success rates similar to that of surgery in primary open-angle glaucoma.[54]

REFERENCES

1. Lindberg JG: Clinical studies of depigmentation of the pupillary margin and transillumination of the iris in cases of senile cataract and also in normal eyes of the aged. [Original in German] M.D. Thesis, Diss Helsingfors, Finland, 1917.
2. Vogt A: A new slit lamp finding of the pupillary area: Light blue peripupillary membranous formations originating from the ante-

rior lens capsule. [Original in German] Klin Monatsabl Augenheilkd 75:1, 1925.

3. Busacca A: Structure and importance of the membranous precipitates in the anterior and posterior eye chambers. [Original in German] Graefes Arch Klin Exp Ophthalmol 119:135, 1927.

4. Dvorak-Theobald G: Pseudo-exfoliation of the lens capsule. Am J Ophthalmol 37:1, 1954.

5. Sunde OA: Senile exfoliation of the anterior lens capsule. Acta Ophthalmol 45(Suppl):1, 1956.

6. Bertelsen TI, Drablös PA, Flood PR: The socalled senile exfoliation (pseudoexfoliation) of the anterior lens capsule, a product of the lens epithelium: Fibrillopathia epitheliocapsularis. Acta Ophthalmolgica 42:1096, 1964.

7. Ashton N, Shakib M, Collyer R, Blach R: Electron microscopic study of pseudo-exfoliation of the lens capsule. I: Lens capsule and zonular fibers. Invest Ophthalmol 4:141, 1965.

8. Dark AJ, Streeten BW, Jones D: Accumulation of fibrillar protein in the aging human lens capsule. Arch Ophthalmol 82:815, 1969.

9. Seland JH: The ultrastructural changes in the exfoliation syndrome. Acta Ophthalmologica 66(Suppl 184):28, 1988.

10. Weekers L, Weekers R, Dednjoid J: Pathogenesis of glaucoma capsulare. Doc Ophthalmol 5/6:555, 1951.

11. Eagle RC Jr, Font RL, Fine BS: The basement membrane exfoliation syndrome. Arch Ophthalmol 97:510, 1979.

12. Forsius H: Exfoliation syndrome in various ethnic populations. Acta Ophthalmologica 66(Suppl 184):71, 1988.

13. Shakib M, Ashton N, Blach R: Electron microscopic study of pseudo-exfoliation of the lens capsule. II: Iris and ciliary body. Invest Ophthalmol 4:154, 1965.

14. Ringvold A: Electron microscopy of the limbal conjunctiva in eyes with pseudo-exfoliation syndrome (PE syndrome). Virchows Arch Abt A Path Anat 355:275, 1972.

15. Speakman JS, Ghosh M: The conjunctiva in senile lens exfoliation. Ophthalmology 94:1757, 1976.

16. Ringvold A: Electron microscopy of the wall of iris vessels in eyes with and without exfoliation syndrome (pseudoexfoliation of the lens capsule). Virchows Arch Abt A Path Anat 348:328, 1969.

17. Ghosh M, Speakman JS: The iris in senile exfoliation of the lens. Can J Ophthalmol 9:289, 1974.

18. Streeten BW, Dark AJ, Wallace RN, et al: Pseudoexfoliative fibrillopathy in the skin of patients with ocular pseudoexfoliation. Am J Ophthalmol 110:490, 1990.

19. Hiller R, Sperduto RD, Krueger DE: Pseudoexfoliation, intraocular pressure, and senile lens changes in a population-based survey. Arch Ophthalmol 100:1080, 1982.

20. Cashwell LF Jr, Shields MB: Exfoliation syndrome: Prevalence in a southeastern United States population. Arch Ophthalmol 106:335, 1988.

21. Colin J, Le Gall G, Le Jeune B, Cambrai MD: The prevalence of exfoliation syndrome in different areas of France. Acta Ophthalmologica 66(Suppl 184):86, 1988.

22. Krause U, Alanko HI, Kärnä J, et al: Prevalence of exfoliation syndrome in Finland. Acta Ophthalmologica 66(Suppl 184):120, 1988.

23. Aasved H: The geographical distribution of fibrillopathia epitheliocapsularis, so-called senile exfoliation or pseudoexfoliation of the anterior lens capsule. Acta Ophthalmologica 47:792, 1969.

24. Ekström C: Prevalence of pseudoexfoliation in a population of 65–74 years of age. Acta Ophthalmol 65(Suppl 182):9, 1987.

25. Backhaus B, Lorentzen SE: Prevalence of pseudoexfoliation in non-glaucomatous eyes in Denmark. Acta Ophthalmol 44:1, 1966.

26. Summanen P, Tönjum AM: Exfoliation syndrome among Saudis. Acta Ophthalmologica 66(Suppl 184):107, 1988.

27. Faulkner HW: Pseudo-exfoliation of the lens among the Navajo Indians. Am J Ophthalmol 72:206, 1971.

28. Bartholomew RS: Pseudo-capsular exfoliation in the Bantu of South Africa. Br J Ophthalmol 55:693, 1971.

29. Taylor HR, Hollows FC, Moran D: Pseudoexfoliation of the lens in Australian Aborigines. Br J Ophthalmol 61:473, 1977.

30. Nanba K, Sabre K, Imai A, Sakurai I: Clinical evaluation of pseudoexfoliation and capsular glaucoma. Folia Ophthalmol Jpn 29:1567, 1978.

31. Shimizu K, Kimura Y, Aoki K: Prevalence of exfoliation syndrome in the Japanese. Acta Ophthalmologica 66(Suppl 184):112, 1988.

32. Ball SF: Exfoliation syndrome prevalence in the glaucoma popu-

lation of south Louisiana. Acta Ophthalmologica 66(Suppl 184):93, 1988.

33. Mohammad S, Kazmi N: Subluxation of the lens and ocular hypertension in exfoliation syndrome. Pakistan J Ophthalmol 22:77, 1986.

34. Tarkkanen A: Pseudoexfoliation of the lens capsule. Acta Ophthalmologica (Suppl 71):9, 1962.

35. Layden WE, Shaffer RN: Exfoliation syndrome. Am J Ophthalmol 78:835, 1974.

36. Roth M, Epstein DL: Exfoliation syndrome. Am J Ophthlamol 89:477, 1980.

37. Kozart DM, Yanoff M: Intraocular pressure status in 100 consecutive patients with exfoliation syndrome. Ophthalmology 89:214, 1982.

38. Henry CJ, Krupin T, Schmitt M, et al: Long-term follow-up of pseudoexfoliation and the development of elevated intraocular pressure. Ophthalmology 94:545, 1987.

39. Mizuno K, Muroi S: Cycloscopy of pseudoexfoliation. Am J Ophthalmol 87:513, 1979.

40. Hansen E, Sellevold OJ: Pseudoexfoliation of the lens capsule. II: Development of the exfoliation syndrome. Acta Ophthalmologica 47:161, 1969.

41. Aasved H: The frequency of fibrillopathia epitheliocapsularis (so-called senile exfoliation or pseudoexfoliation) in patients with open angle glaucoma. Acta Ophthalmologica 49:194, 1971.

42. Aminlari A: Glaucoma capsulare. Glaucoma 5:134, 1983.

43. Aasved H: Intraocular pressure in eyes with and without fibrillopathia epitheliocapsularis (so-called senile exfoliation or pseudoexfoliation). Acta Ophthalmologica 49:601, 1971.

44. Brooks AMV, Gillies WE: The presentation and prognosis of glaucoma in pseudoexfoliation of the lens capsule. Ophthalmology 95:271, 1988.

45. Crittendon JJ, Shields MB: Exfoliation syndrome in the southeastern United States. II: Characteristics of patient population and clinical course. Acta Ophthalmologica 66(Suppl 184):103, 1988.

46. Klemetti A: Intraocular pressure in exfoliation syndrome. Acta Ophthalmologica 66(Suppl 184):54, 1988.

47. Sziklai P, Süveges I: Glaucoma capsulare in patients with open-angle glaucoma in Hungary. Acta Ophthalmologica 66(Suppl 184):90, 1988.

48. Valle O: Prevalence of simple and capsular glaucoma in the central hospital district of Kotka. Acta Ophthalmologica 66(Suppl 184):116, 1988.

49. Cashwell LF Jr, Shields MB: Exfoliation syndrome in the southeastern United States. I: Prevalence in open-angle glaucoma and non-glaucoma populations. Acta Ophthalmologica 66(Suppl 184):99, 1988.

50. Horven I: Exfoliation syndrome: Incidences and prognosis of glaucoma capsulare in Massachusetts. Arch Ophthalmol 76:505, 1966.

51. Thorburn W: The outcome of visual function in capsular glaucoma. Acta Ophthalmologica 66(Suppl 184):132, 1988.

52. Smith RJH: Nature of glaucoma in the pseudoexfoliation syndrome. Trans Ophthalmol Soc UK 99:308, 1979.

53. Tarkkanen A: Exfoliative glaucoma. Glaucoma 6:266, 1984.

54. Hetherington J Jr: Capsular glaucoma: Management philosophy. Acta Ophthalmologica 66(Suppl 184):138, 1988.

55. Pohjanpelto P: Influence of exfoliation syndrome on prognosis in ocular hypertension ≧25 mm: A long-term follow-up. Acta Ophthalmologica 64:39, 1986.

56. Olivius E, Thorburn W: Prognosis of glaucoma simplex and glaucoma capsulare: A comparative study. Acta Ophthalmol 56:921, 1978.

57. Bartholomew RS: Lens displacement associated with pseudocapsular exfoliation. Br J Ophthalmol 54:744, 1970.

58. Guzek JP, Holm M, Cotter JB, et al: Risk factors for intraoperative complications in 1000 extracapsular cataract cases. Ophthalmology 94:461, 1987.

59. Skuta GL, Parrish RK, Hodapp E, et al: Zonular dialysis during extracapsular cataract extraction in pseudoexfoliation syndrome. Arch Ophthalmol 105:632, 1987.

60. Naumann GOH, Erlanger Augenblätter-Group: Exfoliation syndrome as a risk factor for vitreous loss in extracapsular cataract surgery: Preliminary report. Acta Ophthalmologica 66(Suppl 184):129, 1988.

61. Horven I: Exfoliation syndrome: A histological and histochemical study. Acta Ophthalmologica 44:790, 1966.
62. Dickson DH, Ramsay MS: Fibrillopathia epitheliocapsularis (pseudoexfoliation): A clinical and electron microscope study. Can J Ophthalmol 10:148, 1975.
63. Morrison JC, Green WR: Light microscopy of the light exfoliation syndrome. Acta Ophthalmologica 66(Suppl 184):5, 1988.
64. Davanger M: On the molecular composition and physico-chemical properties of the pseudo-exfoliation material. Acta Ophthalmologica 55:621, 1977.
65. Davanger M: The pseudo-exfoliation syndrome: A scanning electron microscopic study. I: The anterior lens surface. Acta Ophthalmologica 53:809, 1975.
66. Dickson DH, Ramsey MS: Symposium on pseudocapsular exfoliation and glaucoma: Fibrillopathia epitheliocapsularis: Review of the nature and origin of pseudoexfoliative deposits. Trans Ophthalmol Soc UK 99:284, 1979.
67. Ringvold A: Ultrastructure of exfoliation material (Busacca deposits). Virchows Arch Abt A Path Anat 350:95, 1970.
68. Streeten BW, Gibson SA, Li Z-Y: Lectin binding to pseudoexfoliative material and the ocular zonules. Invest Ophthalmol Vis Sci 27:1516, 1986.
69. Ringvold A: Exfoliation syndrome: Immunological aspects. Acta Ophthalmologica 66(Suppl 184):35, 1988.
70. Ringvold A: A preliminary report on the amino acid composition of the pseudo-exfoliative material (PE material). Exp Eye Res 15:37, 1973.
71. Gifford H Jr: A clinical and pathologic study of exfoliation of the lens capsule. Trans Am Ophthalmol Soc 55:189, 1957.
72. Streeten BW, Dark AJ, Barnes CW: Pseudoexfoliative material and oxytalan fibers. Exp Eye Res 38:523, 1984.
73. Streeten BW, Gibson SA, Dark AJ: Pseudoexfoliative material contains an elastic microfibrillar-associated glycoprotein. Trans Am Ophthalmol Soc 84:304, 1986.
74. Li Z-Y, Streeten BW, Wallace RN, Gibson SA: Immunolocalization of fibrillin on pseudoexfoliative material and the ocular zonules. Invest Ophthalmol Vis Sci 28(Suppl):32, 1987.
75. Streeten BW, Bookman L, Ritch R, et al: Pseudoexfoliative fibrillopathy in the conjunctiva: A relation to elastic fibers and elastosis. Ophthalmology 94:1439, 1987.
76. Ringvold A: The distribution of the exfoliation material in the iris from eyes with exfoliation syndrome (pseudoexfoliation of the lens capsule). Virchows Arch [A] 351:168, 1971.
77. Ghosh M, Speakman JS: The ciliary body in senile exfoliation of the lens. Can J Ophthalmol 8:394, 1973.
78. Ringvold A: On the occurrence of pseudo-exfoliation material in extrabulbar tissue from patients with pseudo-exfoliation syndrome of the eye. Acta Ophthalmologica 51:411, 1973.
79. Ringvold A, Husby G: Pseudo-exfoliation material: An amyloid-like substance. Exp Eye Res 17:289, 1973.
80. Meretoja J, Tarkkanen A: Occurrence of amyloid in eyes with pseudo-exfoliation. Ophthalmol Res 9:80, 1977.
81. Davanger M, Pedersen OO: Pseudo-exfoliation material on the anterior lens surface: Demonstration and examination of an interfibrillar ground substance. Acta Ophthalmologica 53:3, 1975.
82. Meretoja J, Tarkkanen A: Pseudoexfoliation syndrome in familial systemic amyloidosis with lattice corneal dystrophy. Ophthalmol Res 7:194, 1975.
83. Schwartz MF, Green WR, Michels RG, et al: An unusual case of ocular involvement in primary systemic nonfamilial amyloidosis. Ophthalmology 89:394, 1982.
84. Dark AJ, Streeten BW, Cornwall CC: Pseudoexfoliative disease of the lens: A study in electron microscopy and histochemistry. Br J Ophthalmol 61:462, 1977.
85. Gradle HS, Sugar HS: Concerning the chamber angle. II: Exfoliation of the zonular lamella and glaucoma capsulare. Am J Ophthalmol 23:982, 1940.
86. Sugar HS: Onset of the exfoliation syndrome after intracapsular lens extraction. Am J Ophthalmol 89:601, 1980.
87. Vannas A: Pseudoexfoliation of the lens capsule and capsular glaucoma. Acta Ophthalmol 105:29, 1969.
88. Vannas A: Vascular changes in pseudoexfoliation of the lens capsule in capsular glaucoma: A fluorescein angiographic and electron microscopic study. Graefes Arch Klin Exp Ophthal 184:248, 1972.
89. Friedburg D, Bischof G: Fluorescein angiographic features of the pseudoexfoliation syndrome. Glaucoma 4:13, 1982.
90. Ringvold A, Vegge T: Electron microscopy of the trabecular meshwork in eyes with exfoliation syndrome (pseudoexfoliation of the lens capsule). Virchows Arch [A] 353:127, 1971.
91. Richardson TM, Epstein DL: Exfoliation glaucoma: A quantitative perfusion and ultrastructural study. Ophthalmology 88:968, 1981.
92. Takei Y, Mizuno K: Electron-microscopic study of pseudo-exfoliation of the lens capsule. Graefes Arch Klin Exp Ophthalmol 205:213, 1978.
93. Roh YB, Ishibashi T, Ito N, Inomata H: Alteration of microfibrils in the conjunctiva of patients with exfoliation syndrome. Arch Ophthalmol 105:978, 1987.
94. Prince AM, Streeten BW, Ritch R, et al: Preclinical diagnosis of pseudoexfoliation syndrome. Arch Ophthalmol 105:1076, 1987.
95. Tarkkanen A, Horsmanheimo A: Topical steroids and non-glaucomatous pseudoexfoliation. Acta Ophthalmol 44:323, 1966.
96. Pohjola S, Horsmanheimo A: Topically applied corticosteroids in glaucoma capsulare. Arch Ophthalmol 85:150, 1971.
97. Lutjen-Drecoll E, Tamm E: Differences in the amount of 'plaque-material' in the outflow system of eyes with chronic simple and exfoliation glaucoma. In Krieglstein GK (ed): Glaucoma Update III. Berlin, Springer-Verlag, 1987, p 17.
98. Cashwell LF Jr, Holleman IL, Weaver RG, van Rens GH: Idiopathic true exfoliation of the lens capsule. Ophthalmology 96:348, 1989.
99. Svedbergh B: Argon laser trabeculoplasty in capsular glaucoma. Acta Ophthalmol (Copenh) 66(Suppl 184):141, 1988.

Chapter 123

Pigmentary Dispersion Syndrome and Glaucoma

THOMAS M. RICHARDSON

Glaucoma, in the presence of an anatomically open-drainage angle of the eye, is usually due to an increased resistance to the flow of aqueous humor from the eye because of an abnormality that resides within the aqueous drainage system. In the absence of trauma, but in the presence of particulate substances in the aqueous outflow system, the glaucoma is considered a secondary open-angle glaucoma. One of the most easily recognized particulate substances in the drainage angle often associated with glaucoma is pigment.

Around the turn of the 20th century von Hippel[1] first brought attention to the relationship of glaucoma and pigment. A few years later Levinsohn[2] suggested that the pigment that caused the glaucoma probably came from the pigmented epithelium of the iris. Over the next few decades several investigators took positions both in support of[3, 4] and against[5–7] the likelihood that pigment was a major factor in the cause of glaucoma.

The modern concept of what has come to be known as pigmentary glaucoma originated from the work of Sugar,[8] who in 1940 described a 29-year-old man with glaucoma who also had degeneration of the pigment epithelium of the iris with deposits of pigment on the anterior segment surfaces. The term pigmentary glaucoma was applied to this entity by Sugar and Barbour[9] in 1949 when they delineated the clinical features that have come to be recognized as the hallmarks of this unusual type of glaucoma. The origin of the pigment particles observed in this condition is now generally recognized to be the pigmented neuroepithelium of the iris and perhaps the ciliary body.[10–12]

Subsequent to this early work, many cases of pigmentary glaucoma were reported, and in 1966 a review of 147 cases by Sugar[12] highlighted additional features of this disease. In 1981 Scheie and Cameron[13] presented data from a large number of patients studied between 1946 and 1977 that essentially confirmed the work of Sugar.

CLINICAL MANIFESTATIONS

Ocular Findings

Pigmentary glaucoma is a bilateral disorder that occurs with greater incidence in men than in women. It is commonly associated with myopia and has a younger age of onset than primary open-angle glaucoma. It is distinguished by a loss of pigment from the pigmented epithelium of the iris, particularly in the midperipheral

region (Fig. 123–1). This results in radial transillumination defects in the iris and in dispersion of melanin pigment into the aqueous humor. The displaced pigment is deposited on several surfaces in the anterior segment, including the lens, zonules, iris, cornea, and trabecular meshwork (Fig. 123–2). Accumulation of pigment particles in the aqueous outflow system is believed to be the cause of the associated glaucoma.

On the corneal endothelium, pigment is generally deposited as a central, vertically oriented, brown band known as Krukenberg's spindle. The spindle can vary from 1 to 6 mm in length and can be up to 3 mm in width. Its vertical form probably results from the vertical meeting of aqueous convection currents. Pigment deposition on the cornea occasionally occurs as more diffusely distributed punctate deposits. Endothelial cell function is not known to be compromised by the presence of the pigment deposits, and there is no significant difference in central endothelial cell density and corneal thickness in patients with pigmentary dispersion syndrome when compared with control eyes that are matched for age, sex, and refractive error.[14]

Regions of pigment loss in the iris appear as radial, slitlike, midperipheral transillumination defects detected by careful retroillumination (see Fig. 123–1). These are

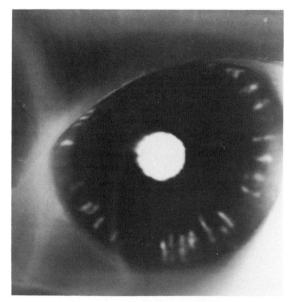

Figure 123–1. Iris transillumination in a patient with pigmentary glaucoma; spokelike, midperipheral, radial defects result from loss of pigment from the pigment epithelium.

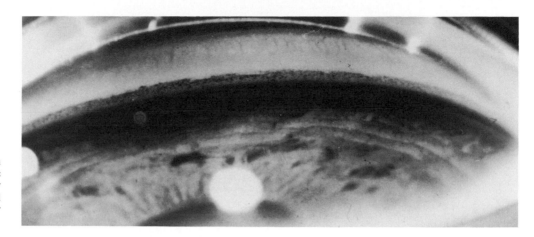

Figure 123–2. Goniophotograph of the anterior chamber angle from a patient with pigmentary glaucoma shows a dense band of pigment in the trabecular meshwork.

best observed by a dark-adapted examiner positioning the probe of a fiberoptic transilluminator over the sclera to achieve a bright red reflex through the pupil. The radial pattern of iris defects should be present if the diagnosis of pigmentary glaucoma is to be made reliably. Pigment deposition on the anterior surface of the iris may also be detected.

The anterior chamber in pigmentary glaucoma is characteristically deep, whereas the iris assumes a concave configuration that is most marked in the midperiphery (Fig. 123–3). Upon gonioscopic examination, the angles are open; a characteristic and dense band of hyperpigmentation is situated on the trabecular meshwork; and a ring of pigment is located along Schwalbe's line and anteriorly (Sampaolesi line) (see Fig. 123–2).

Other sites of pigment deposition are the zonular fibers and the surface of the lens. Pigment on the lens is usually located at the insertion of the zonular fibers on the posterior capsule.

Age of Onset

The age of onset of pigmentary dispersion syndrome is unknown. In the series of Scheie and Cameron,[13] the

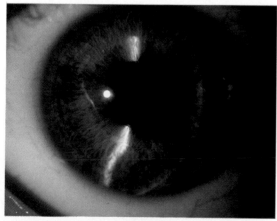

Figure 123–3. Slit lamp photograph of the anterior segment shows a deep anterior chamber with peripheral sagging of the iris.

youngest patient was 14 yr old. The age at diagnosis for men is about 35 to 45 yr of age and for women is 40 to 50 yr of age. As would be expected, the mean age of patients with pigmentary dispersion syndrome at the time of diagnosis is younger than those with primary open-angle glaucoma.

Risk Factors

Males outnumber females in most pigmentary glaucoma series. Most patients with pigmentary dispersion syndrome, both with and without glaucoma, are myopic. In a study correlating age, refraction, and intraocular pressure status, Berger and associates found that the higher the myopia, the younger will be the age at which glaucomatous damage tends to develop.[15]

Patients with pigmentary dispersion syndrome appear to have a deeper anterior chamber than do control subjects.[16] In a study reported by Kaiser-Kupfer and associates,[17] three of four related patients with pigmentary dispersion syndrome with markedly asymmetric pigment dispersion and normal intraocular pressures in both eyes were found to have an anterior chamber depth 0.2 mm greater in the most affected eye.

Most patients with pigmentary dispersion syndrome are white. The disease is rare in blacks and Asians. In the series of Scheie and Cameron,[13] five patients were described as mulatto. Pigmentary glaucoma has been reported in a black albino.[18] Krukenberg's spindles were reported to develop during pregnancy in four black women, only one of whom was slightly myopic.[19] However, whether these cases represented true pigmentary dispersion syndrome is uncertain.

Clinical Course and Progression

Pigmentary dispersion syndrome can occur in the absence of elevated intraocular pressure. Except for the elevated pressures and signs of glaucomatous damage, these eyes appear clinically like those with pigmentary glaucoma. The true prevalence of pigmentary dispersion syndrome in the population is unknown, and the frequency with which glaucoma develops is difficult to estimate. Considerable variation occurs in the time between the diagnosis of pigment dispersion and the onset of glaucoma. In some cases it can take up to 12 to 20 yr.[12, 20, 21] Even after 20 yr of follow-up, some patients with diffuse pigment dispersion have not developed abnormal pressures.[22] A long-term retrospective study of 65 patients with pigmentary dispersion revealed glaucoma in 36 percent of males and in 33 percent of females after a mean follow-up time of 17 yr.[20] Apparently, both sexes had an equal chance of developing glaucoma once a patient was identified as having pigmentary dispersion syndrome, even though the ratio of male to female patients with the syndrome in the study was found to be 1.6 : 1.0.

In a retrospective study of 111 patients with pigmentary dispersion syndrome or pigmentary glaucoma, Farrar and associates identified several risk factors for the development of glaucoma and the severity of glaucoma in patients with pigmentary dispersion syndrome.[23] These included male gender, black race, severe myopia, and Krukenberg's spindles. Thus, although pigmentary dispersion syndrome is rare in blacks, those with the dispersion might be more likely to develop glaucoma. The discrepancy between this study and that of Migliazzo and associates with respect to the frequency with which male and female patients with pigmentary dispersion syndrome might develop glaucoma has not been explained.[20]

The progressive nature of pigmentary glaucoma was documented in a prospective study by Richter and associates[24] describing 110 eyes of 55 patients with pigmentary dispersion syndrome or pigmentary glaucoma, followed for a mean of 27 mo (6 to 43 mo). Of these eyes, 62 percent remained stable, 34 percent had worsening of their glaucoma, and 5 percent improved. During the course of the study, 45 eyes (41 percent) had clinically detectable dispersion of pigment. There was a significant association between progression of glaucoma and active pigment dispersion, which was more commonly associated with an elevated intraocular pressure than with increased optic nerve cupping or visual field loss at stable intraocular pressures. Interestingly, there were no differences in the frequency of active pigment dispersion and worsening of glaucoma when patients in various age groups (less than 44 yr; 45 to 64 yr; greater than 65 yr) were compared. This study suggested that risk factors for increasing intraocular pressure, in patients with pigmentary glaucoma or pigment dispersion syndrome, could include increasing iris transillumination defects, increasing corneal pigmentation, and the presence of pigment granules on the anterior lens capsule in the undilatated pupillary zone.

Pigmentary glaucoma is usually a progressive disease that requires medical or surgical management to prevent damage to the optic disc and glaucomatous field loss. Sometimes, however, it has a mild course or becomes less severe, particularly with increasing age. Ten percent of 102 patients in a study by Lichter and Shaffer[25] had a definite decrease in the amount of pigment in the trabecular meshwork, suggesting that pigment could pass out of the meshwork as the patient aged. Transilluminating areas of the iris have also been observed to disappear on occasion,[22, 26] suggesting resurfacing of these areas by pigment epithelium or pigment-containing cells. It has also been possible to discontinue treatment for glaucoma in a few patients whose intraocular pressure returned to normal after several years of treatment.[22, 27, 28]

Hereditary Factors

There have been scattered reports of families with multiple members having pigmentary dispersion syndrome. Krukenberg's spindles were reported in mother and daughter in three familes,[29-31] and in twin brothers in another.[32] Stankovic[33] described a family in which pigmentary glaucoma was observed through four generations and considered these cases to show autosomal recessive inheritance. Pigmentary dispersion syndrome was reported by Kaiser-Kupfer and associates in two brothers, their father, and a paternal uncle.[17]

More recent studies have pointed to an autosomal dominant mode of inheritance. These studies include that of Mandelkorn and associates, who reported on four families in whom 6 of 19 relatives of probands had pigmentary dispersion syndrome.[34] McDermott and associates[35] detected pigmentary dispersion syndrome in 25 percent of 48 immediate relatives of 21 probands and 47 percent of immediate adult relatives. In this study, phenotypic expression usually appeared after the second decade.

Piccolino and associates[36] reported on two brothers with pigmentary glaucoma who also had widespread symmetric degeneration of the retinal pigment epithelium. Their observations support the hypothesis that an early defect can affect the pigment epithelium in both the anterior and posterior segments of the eye.

PATHOGENESIS

Loss of Pigment From the Iris

Loss of pigment from the iris in pigmentary glaucoma has been suggested to result from congenital atrophy or degeneration of the iris neuroepithelium.[37, 38] In 1979 Campbell[26] proposed a pathogenetic mechanism that accounts for many of the features of this pigment release (Fig. 123–4; see also Fig. 123–3). Pigment granules may be dislodged mechanically from the pigmented epithelium of the iris by a back-and-forth rubbing of the posterior peripheral iris surface against packets of zonules that insert anteriorly on the lens surface (see Fig. 123–4). The midperipheral radial pattern of iris transillumination defects (see Fig. 123–1) corresponds well to the location of the zonules. Scanning electron microscopic studies have confirmed that the iris defects consistently follow the course of the zonular fibers.[39] Loss of pigment, however, can progress to involve the entire neuroepithelial layer (Fig. 123–5).

The aforementioned theory can also account for the observation that pigmentary glaucoma predominantly affects younger males with mild to moderate myopia.

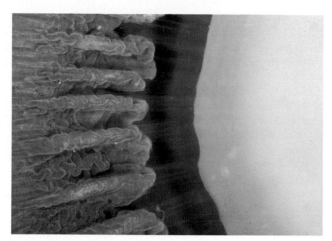

Figure 123–4. Photograph of the posterior view of the anterior segment. Zonular fibers that arise from the pars plicata and insert into the lens periphery are seen contrasted against the surface of the iris pigment epithelium.

The young myopic eye can continue to enlarge into the patient's 20s or early 30s. This increase in the diameter of the globe could be associated with an enlargement of the ciliary body ring relative to the lens, resulting in sagging of the peripheral iris such that it establishes contact with the zonular fibers. During normal physiologic movement, rubbing of the concave iris against the zonules could result in pigment liberation. Because of the larger size of the eye in men, there is a greater chance in males that the peripheral iris is sufficiently concave to permit iridozonular rubbing.

Campbell's[26] theory may also explain why the severity and incidence of pigmentary glaucoma decrease with increasing age. Except in the young myope, the eye generally stops enlarging when maturity is reached. The lens, however, continues to grow slowly until late in life. On the other hand, the average size of the pupil decreases with age. These two factors can create a relative pupillary block that causes the peripheral iris to shift anteriorly away from the zonules.[26] This phenomenon could explain the decreased severity and incidence of pigmentary glaucoma with age.

An unexplained feature of pigmentary glaucoma is its relative rarity in blacks and Asians, even though their uveae are heavily pigmented and it is not uncommon to find pigment in the angle. In normotensive eyes of black and white patients, no differences can be detected in intraocular pressure, facility of outflow, or rate of aqueous humor production.[40] One relevant difference between the two groups could be the degree of iris pigmentation and compactness of the stroma.

In darkly pigmented individuals, the iris is heavily laden with pigment and its anterior surface usually appears velvety smooth and uniformly compact. In lightly pigmented persons, the iris is not only lighter in color but also has a more lacy texture, with deep crypts and easily visualized stromal blood vessels. Although no differences in iris thickness have been documented histologically, darker irides do appear to be more compact with a larger number of melanocytes within the stroma.[41]

Increased stromal density in darkly pigmented irides is also suggested by studies that demonstrate a slower responsiveness of dark irides to various topically applied drugs, including miotics and mydriatics, when compared with light irides.[42] Such differences are thought to be caused by a slower penetration of the drugs through a denser stroma. Stromal characteristics such as heavy pigmentation and compactness might prevent peripheral iris sagging, which is believed to be essential for the development of the pigmentary dispersion syndrome.[26]

Fluorescein angiographic studies of 10 patients with pigmentary dispersion syndrome or pigmentary glaucoma have provided evidence that deficiencies in the vasculature of the iris could contribute to the cause of pigmentary glaucoma.[43] In these patients, the iris tissue was hypoperfused, radial vessels were decreased in number, and dye leaked from the pupillary margin and into the peripupillary tissue. In cases in which the fellow eye was essentially unaffected by the pigment dispersion, vascular changes were present but less marked, suggesting that they precede the degenerative changes in the pigment epithelium.

Development of Glaucoma

Despite our detailed knowledge of the clinical features of pigmentary glaucoma, the pathogenesis of the glaucoma remains a topic of debate. Currently, there is no animal model in which to test various hypotheses concerning the pathophysiology of the disease. Furthermore, few specimens have been made available for histopathologic studies. Hypotheses that have been advanced to explain the elevation of intraocular pressure in pigmentary glaucoma include those that suggest that the pressure elevation is caused by the presence of

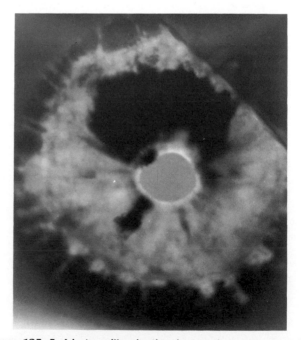

Figure 123–5. Iris transillumination in a patient with extensive pigment loss from the iris neuroepithelium.

pigment in the anterior segment and those that suggest that the two features are not causally related.

Among the second group is the hypothesis that pigmentary glaucoma is simply a variant of primary open-angle glaucoma. This opinion is supported by a study indicating that patients with the pigmentary dispersion syndrome, who develop an elevated intraocular pressure after the administration of topical corticosteroids, belong to a class of individuals genetically predisposed to open-angle glaucoma.[44] However, another study of pressure responses to corticosteroids suggested that pigmentary glaucoma is, in fact, a separate and distinct entity from primary open-angle glaucoma.[45]

Another hypothesis relates pigmentary glaucoma to the presence of a developmental defect in the anterior chamber angle structures.[25, 46, 47] In addition to interfering with the outflow of aqueous humor through the aqueous outflow system, this defect gives rise to mesodermal angle anomalies such as abnormal iris processes and is responsible for the presence of pigment in the trabecular meshwork. However, prominent iris processes seem to occur with equal frequency in myopic eyes, whether or not they have open angles or excessive pigment in the trabecular meshwork.[22] Other iris abnormalities, such as hyperplasia of the iris dilator muscle and degeneration of iris nerve fibers, have been observed in patients with pigmentary dispersion syndrome,[48, 49] but the significance of these findings to the development of glaucoma remains obscure.

Hypotheses that suggest that elevation of intraocular pressure in pigmentary glaucoma is caused, at least initially, by an accumulation of melanin pigment in the trabecular meshwork have gained the most support (Fig. 123–6). The pigment is thought to block the flow of aqueous humor through the outflow channels.[8] An increase in the resistance to fluid flow through the aqueous outflow system has been demonstrated in enucleated human and primate eyes following perfusion with pigment particles isolated from the iris pigment epithelium.[50, 51]

Clinical evidence for this hypothesis has been obtained from patients with pigmentary dispersion syndrome who develop a shower of pigment into the anterior chamber either spontaneously or after vigorous exercise.[52, 53] Tonography on one such patient revealed an acute rise in intraocular pressure accompanied by a decrease in the facility of outflow.[52] In a more recent study of the effects

of exercise on intraocular pressure, Smith and associates[54] found an acute pressure rise in 2 of 19 eyes in 10 patients with pigmentary glaucoma. Although pressure decreased in the remaining eyes, the average decrease was significantly less than the pressure fall normally expected from exercise and which in fact occurred in their normal volunteers. The observations suggested that the pigment showers observed in 84 percent of the pigmentary glaucoma eyes following exercise had a marked dampening effect on the pressure fall that normally occurs after exercise.

Transient rises in intraocular pressure have also been observed after the release of pigment into the anterior chamber following dilatation of the pupil.[55] Topical administration of mydriatics, especially sympathomimetics such as phenylephrine, often result in the liberation of pigment into the aqueous humor.[56, 57] However, phenylephrine either reduces or has no effect on intraocular pressure in normal individuals or on those with primary open-angle glaucoma.[58] In patients with either pigmentary or exfoliative glaucoma, mydriasis can induce an acute rise in intraocular pressure associated with pigment release, suggesting increased susceptibility of these eyes to temporary obstruction of the aqueous outflow system by pigment particles.[55]

The prognostic value of intraocular pressure responses to phenylephrine was investigated by Epstein and associates.[52] After topical administration of phenylephrine to a group of patients who had bilateral pigmentary dispersion syndrome with or without glaucoma, 15 percent of the patients developed an elevation of intraocular pressure greater than 2 mmHg, whereas only 2.5 percent developed a 4 + pigment reaction in the anterior chamber. As in an earlier study by Kristensen,[55] most patients who developed a rise in intraocular pressure already had either pigmentary or exfoliative glaucoma.

Of interest in Epstein's[52] study is the finding that pigment liberation in response to phenylephrine tended to be greatest in the older patient with pigment dispersion, who already had glaucoma and had been treated with topical antiglaucoma medication. This is unexpected since the incidence of pigmentary glaucoma decreases with increasing age. Another interesting finding in Kristensen's[55] study is that repeated mydriasis results in smaller and smaller showers of pigment into the anterior chamber. However, after a 2-wk recovery pe-

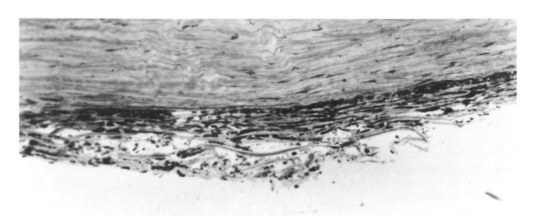

Figure 123–6. Light microscopic view of a section through the trabecular meshwork in pigmentary glaucoma. Heavy melanin deposits extend through the entire depth of the meshwork.

riod from mydriatics, induction of mydriasis produces pigment liberation almost as intense as the initial response. This latter finding suggests that pigment or pigment-containing cells might regenerate at the sites of previously liberated pigment.[26] In neither study was there any correlation between the extent of iris transillumination and the grade of phenylephrine-induced pigment liberation.

Although the aforementioned studies show that aqueous outflow can be obstructed temporarily by pigment particles, it is evident that the mere presence of pigment particles in the trabecular meshwork is not sufficient to account for glaucoma. In some individuals with pigment dispersion and dense pigmentation of the trabecular meshwork, elevated intraocular pressure or abnormal outflow facility may not develop even after 20 yr of observation.[22]

Important questions that arise then are what factors determine the fate of pigment particles in the aqueous outflow system and how are these factors related to the elevation of intraocular pressure. An examination of the tissue responses of the aqueous outflow system to the presence of pigment particles has provided valuable insight into why some patients with pigment dispersion develop glaucoma and others do not. In persons with the pigmentary dispersion syndrome, it is common on gonioscopy to find a dense band of pigment in the trabecular meshwork (see Fig. 123–2). Histopathologic studies have shown that the pigment particles are situated both within and outside the cells that line the trabecular beams (Figs. 123–7 and 123–8).[24, 38, 48, 58, 59] The intertrabecular spaces occasionally contain large pigment-laden cells that could be either phagocytes or cells derived from the iris stroma (Fig. 123–9). Frequently, the amount of pigment contained both within and outside the cells of the trabecular meshwork appears sufficient to obstruct the intertrabecular spaces. Such

restriction of the aqueous outflow channels is probably sufficient to impede the flow of aqueous humor and cause elevation of intraocular pressure.

Electron microscopic studies of the aqueous outflow system obtained from patients with pigmentary glaucoma who do not respond to medical therapy reveal that there may be another stage in the obstructive process. In these patients, endothelial cells of the trabecular meshwork degenerate, cell debris and pigment particles occlude the intertrabecular spaces, and trabecular beams appear sclerotic[60] (Figs. 123–10 and 123–11). Trabecular endothelial cells have a selective capacity to phagocytize materials that can potentially obstruct the outflow channels.[61, 62] Excessive phagocytosis, however, can apparently lead to detachment of cells from the trabecular beams[29, 38] (Fig. 123–12), or disruption of the cells in situ (see Fig. 123–8).[60] As it occurs in pigmentary glaucoma, apparently this process produces the cell debris that fills the intertrabecular spaces and leaves the trabeculas denuded of cells and unprotected from the aqueous humor and its contents. As a result, the trabecular beams degenerate and sclerose and the intertrabecular spaces collapse (see Figs. 123–10 and 123–11).

As a result of these observations, we have postulated that the obstruction of the aqueous outflow system and the development of glaucoma in the pigmentary dispersion syndrome probably occur in two stages as shown schematically in Figure 123–13. In the first stage, pigment liberated from the iris neuroepithelium enters the intertrabecular spaces and is accumulated in the trabecular endothelial cells as a result of phagocytosis. Accumulation of small amounts of pigment over a short period can cause acute obstruction of the intertrabecular space, with a transient elevation of intraocular pressure. Excessive phagocytosis of pigment leads to detachment of trabecular cells from the beams and migration of cells into the intertrabecular spaces. Some trabecular cells

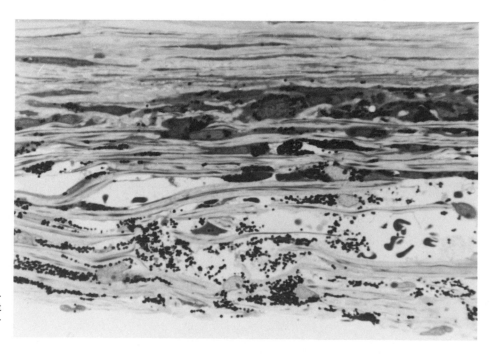

Figure 123–7. Section through trabecular meshwork shows melanin pigment within and outside of trabecular meshwork cells.

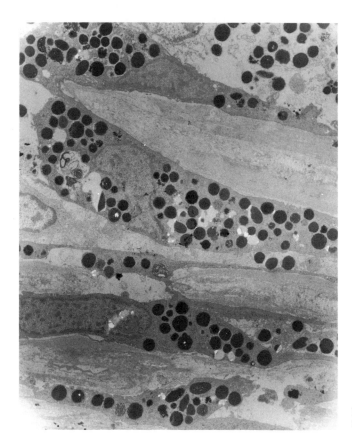

Figure 123–8. The trabecular meshwork with phagocytized pigment. Minimal intertrabecular space is available.

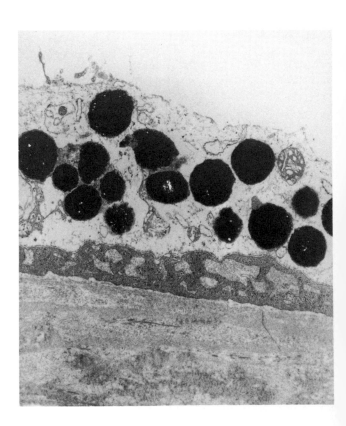

Figure 123–9. A healthy trabecular meshwork cell interposed between a degenerating cell and the trabecular beam.

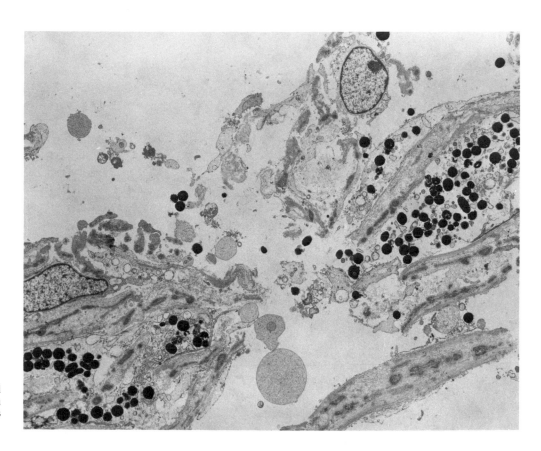

Figure 123–10. Fragmented trabecular cells and beams with denudation and cellular debris in the intertrabecular spaces.

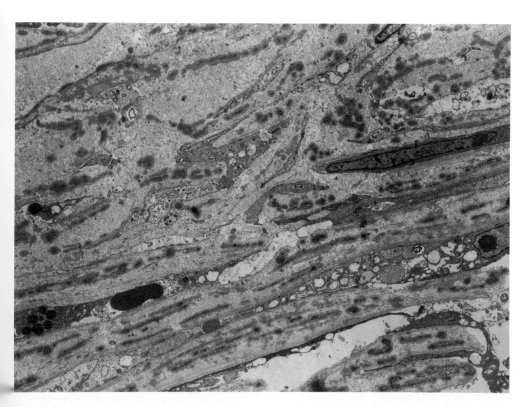

Figure 123–11. Collapse and fusion of the trabecular mesh-work in a patient with advanced pigmentary glaucoma.

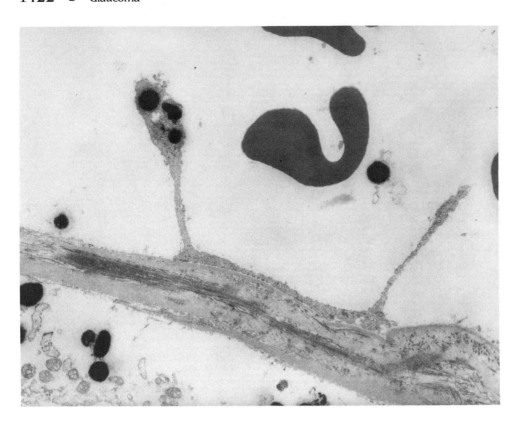

Figure 123–12. Trabecular beam that is denuded except for a small region of attachment of a migrating trabecular cell.

undergo cytolysis, resulting in further accumulation of pigment and cell debris in the intertrabecular spaces. There is evidence that the remaining attached trabecular cells attempt to spread over the denuded portions of the trabeculas (Fig. 123–14).

During this first stage, a level of homeostasis is probably achieved, with only an occasional or low-grade elevation of intraocular pressure. This stage is probably clinically reversible, provided that the trabecular meshwork retains the capacity for self-repair. If it loses this capacity, the second stage of the process is entered in which denuded trabecular beams disintegrate and undergo sclerosis. This second stage is probably irreversible because of irreparable damage to the trabecular tissues (see Fig. 123–11).

This scheme helps to explain the great variation in the clinical course of this disease among individuals. Transient increases in pressure after a mydriasis-induced pigment shower and the acute obstruction of outflow resulting from injection of iris pigment into the anterior chamber of human and animal eyes are consistent with events in stage 1 of the disease. In this clinically revers-

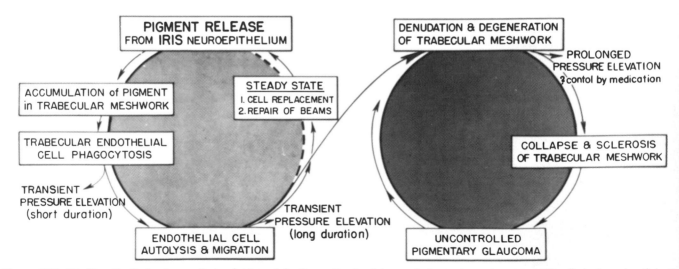

Figure 123–13. Hypothetical scheme that might explain the pathophysiology of pigmentary glaucoma. The first stage is clinically reversible and is characterized by transient rises in intraocular pressure. The second stage, marked by irreparable damage to trabecular tissues, is irreversible and is usually accompanied by uncontrolled glaucoma.

ible stage, obstruction by pigment particles is transient, producing only a temporary rise in intraocular pressure. The key to reversibility appears to reside in several responses of trabecular endothelial cells including phagocytosis of pigment particles, detachment and migration of pigment-laden cells away from the beams, and resurfacing of denuded beams by new or healthier trabecular cells (see Fig. 123–14) that can repair mildly damaged trabecular sheets before they undergo degeneration and collapse. The inability of the trabecular meshwork to carry out any of these functions could reflect a primary defect in the trabecular endothelial cells. Such defects could explain why some individuals with pigmentary dispersion syndrome develop severe glaucoma, whereas others with an identical clinical picture have a normal intraocular pressure. Individuals who have a mild to moderate pressure elevation and who appear to recover from the disease can be thought of as having a less severe endothelial cell defect.

DIFFERENTIAL DIAGNOSIS

Other abnormalities in which pigment is disseminated in the anterior chamber include uveitis, cysts of the iris and ciliary body, dispersion of melanoma cells, postoperative conditions, and aging changes. Pigmentary dispersion, with or without elevation of intraocular pressure, can usually be easily distinguished from these entities because most occur unilaterally and present characteristic features on history and examination. Also, in these conditions trabecular pigmentation is less dense and is usually unevenly distributed throughout the circumference of the trabecular meshwork.

Exfoliation syndrome with glaucoma is the disease most similar to pigmentary glaucoma. Like pigmentary glaucoma, it is characterized by a loss of pigment from the iris neuroepithelium, iris transillumination defects, pigment dispersion in the anterior segment (including Krukenberg's spindle), trabecular pigmentation, and elevation of intraocular pressure. However, careful history, examination, and biomicroscopy easily distinguish the two diseases. The age of onset for exfoliative glaucoma is later than pigmentary glaucoma and usually occurs over the age of 60 and rarely under the age of 40. Exfoliation shows no sexual or racial preference, although some reports suggest a higher prevalence of the disease in Scandinavians. The incidence of the disease appears to be independent of the size and shape of the eye (myopia). Pigmentation of the trabecular meshwork is less intense than in pigmentary glaucoma, and iris transillumination characteristically begins at the pupillary border and not the midperiphery. Approximately 50 percent of patients with exfoliation syndrome appear clinically affected in only one eye, compared with pigmentary dispersion, which is usually bilateral. The most apparent distinguishing characteristic is the presence of white flakes of exfoliation material at the pupillary border on the anterior lens surface that is the hallmark of the exfoliation syndrome.

A secondary form of pigmentary glaucoma apparently can occur after the implantation of a posterior chamber

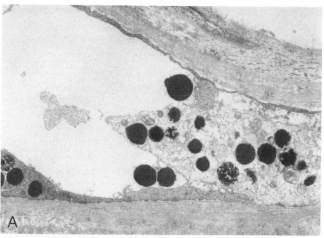
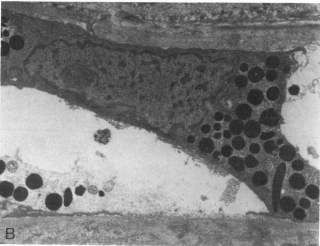

Figure 123–14. A and B, Attenuated processes of healthy trabecular cells spread to cover denuded portions of beams or to replace damaged or degenerating cells. The mere presence of melanin within the cells does not determine whether such cells remain attached to the beams.

intraocular lens.[63–65] Excessive trauma to the iris at the time of lens implantation or continued contact of the intraocular lens with the iris postoperatively are thought to be responsible for the pigment liberation. This condition can be distinguished from pigment dispersion syndrome by its monocular occurrence in the operated eye, a history of posterior chamber lens implantation, and mild to marked atrophy of the iris pigment epithelium in areas adjacent to the lens. Intraocular pressure elevation is usually transient or easily controlled with topical medication, although in some cases laser trabeculoplasty may be required.

MANAGEMENT

Medical Therapy

There is often a rather insidious rise in intraocular pressure in pigmentary glaucoma, with tensions commonly rising to 60 mmHg or more. Patients with pigmentary dispersion syndrome are also susceptible to rather wide fluctuations in intraocular pressure. Because of the early age of onset and the wide fluctuations of intraocular pressure, patients with pigmentary glaucoma require a somewhat different approach to management than do those with other forms of open-angle glaucoma. In patients who remain in stage 1 of the disease, that is, the trabecular meshwork retains the capacity to undergo self-repair, only the occasional "crisis" of pressure elevation requires therapy and the condition can eventually go into remission. However, if the trabecular meshwork has limited or no capacity to recover and the disease enters stage 2, the management is determined by the effectiveness of the medication and the residual functional capacity of the meshwork.

Once long-term medical management is required in pigmentary glaucoma, the approach is basically the same as for primary open-angle glaucoma. In theory, drugs that constrict the pupil and make the peripheral iris more taut might decrease iridozonular rubbing and consequent liberation of pigment. However, miotics are poorly tolerated by young individuals because of the associated spasm of accommodation and blurring of vision. Miotics should be used cautiously in young myopic patients with pigmentary glaucoma, because of the reported association with retinal detachment in patients with associated chorioretinal degeneration. All patients with pigmentary glaucoma who are being considered for miotic therapy should have a careful peripheral retinal examination.

Epinephrine compounds alone, or in combination with other agents, have proved to be effective in reducing intraocular pressure in pigmentary glaucoma.[22] In a clinical study reported by Scheie and Cameron,[13] epinephrine alone or combined with pilocarpine appeared to be more effective in this regard in patients with pigmentary glaucoma than in those with primary open-angle glaucoma. Beta-adrenergic blocking agents are also effective and have a relatively low incidence of undesirable side effects. Carbonic anhydrase inhibitors can be used on a short-term basis to reduce the severity of an acute pressure rise or on a long-term basis when indicated and tolerated by the patient.

Surgical Therapy

Laser trabeculoplasty is useful as an interim treatment in the management of advanced pigmentary glaucoma. Although the initial result is good, a larger proportion of patients with pigmentary glaucoma treated with laser trabeculoplasty lose control of intraocular pressure over time when compared with similarly treated patients with primary open-angle glaucoma.[66, 67] Also, this loss of control can occur in less time (9 mo compared with 2 to 3 yr). Lunde[66] found that the loss of control tended to occur in patients who were older and who had glaucoma for a longer period. In a series of 50 eyes with pigmentary glaucoma that had undergone laser trabeculoplasty, Hagadus and associates[67] found an inverse correlation between the age of the patient and the duration of successful control. Because laser trabeculoplasty can

result in worsening of glaucoma, these patients must be watched carefully following treatment.

Surgical management of patients with pigmentary glaucoma follows the same principles and considerations used in the management of primary open-angle glaucoma. The appearance and change in the optic nerve along with visual field defects should be the principal guidelines used in deciding whether surgery is needed. Most patients respond well to standard filtration operations.

REFERENCES

1. von Hippel E: Zur pathologischen Anatomie des Glaucoma. Arch Ophthalmol 52:498, 1901.
2. Levinsohn G: Beitrag zur pathologische Anatomie und Pathologie des Glaukoms. Arch Augenheilkd 62:131, 1909.
3. Koeppe L: Die Rolle der Irispigment beim Glaukom. Ber Dtsch Ophthalmol Ges 40:478, 1916.
4. Jess A: Zur Frage des Pigmentglaukoms. Klin Monatsbl Augenheilkd 71:175, 1923.
5. Vogt A: Atlas der Spaltlampenmikroskopie. Klin Monatsbl Augenheilkd 81:711, 1928.
6. Birch-Hirschfeld A: Menschlichen Auges durch Röntgenstrahlen. Z Augenheilkd 45:199, 1921.
7. Evans WH, Odom RE, Wenass EJ: Krukenberg's spindle: A study of 202 collected cases. Arch Ophthalmol 26:1023, 1941.
8. Sugar HS: Concerning the chamber angle. I: Gonioscopy. Am J Ophthalmol 23:853, 1940.
9. Sugar HS, Barbour FA: Pigmentary glaucoma: A rare clinical entity. Am J Ophthalmol 32:90, 1949.
10. Bick MW: Pigmentary glaucoma in females. Arch Ophthalmol 58:483, 1957.
11. Scheie HG, Fleischauer HW: Idiopathic atrophy of the epithelial layers of the iris and ciliary body. Arch Ophthalmol 59:216, 1958.
12. Sugar HS: Pigmentary glaucoma: A 25-year review. Am J Ophthalmol 62:499, 1966.
13. Scheie HG, Cameron JD: Pigment dispersion syndrome: A clinical study. Br J Ophthalmol 65:264, 1981.
14. Shihab Z, Murrell WJ, Lamberts DW, Avera B: The corneal endothelium and central corneal thickness in pigmentary dispersion syndrome. Arch Ophthalmol 104:845, 1986.
15. Berger A, Ritch R, McDermott JA, Wang RF: Pigmentary dispersion, refraction and glaucoma. Invest Ophthalmol Vis Sci Suppl 28:114, 1987.
16. Davidson JA, Brubaker RF, Ilstrup DM: Dimensions of the anterior chamber in pigment dispersion syndrome. Arch Ophthalmol 101:81, 1983.
17. Kaiser-Kupfer MI, Kupfer C, McCain L: Asymmetric pigment dispersion syndrome. Trans Am Ophthalmol Soc 81:310, 1983.
18. Wever PA, Dingle JB: Pigmentary glaucoma in a black albino. Ann Ophthalmol 15:454, 1983.
19. Duncan TE: Krukenberg spindles in pregnancy. Arch Ophthalmol 91:355, 1974.
20. Migliazzo CV, Shaffer RN, Nykin R, Magee S: Long-term analysis of pigmentary dispersion syndrome and pigmentary glaucoma. Ophthalmology 93:1528, 1986.
21. Sugar HS: Symposium: glaucoma—Discussion of the three preceding papers. Trans Am Acad Ophthalmol Otolaryngol 78:328, 1974.
22. Epstein DL: Pigment dispersion and pigmentary glaucoma. In Chandler PA, Grant WM (eds): Glaucoma. Philadelphia, Lea & Febiger, 1979.
23. Farrar SM, Shields MB, Miller KN, Stoup CM: Risk factors for the development and severity of glaucoma in the pigment dispersion syndrome. Am J Ophthalmol 108:223, 1989.
24. Richter CU, Richardson TM, Grant WM: Pigmentary dispersion syndrome and pigmentary glaucoma: A prospective study of the natural history. Arch Ophthalmol 104:211, 1986.
25. Lichter PR, Shaffer RM: Diagnostic and prognostic signs in pigmentary glaucoma. Trans Am Acad Ophthalmol Otolaryngol 74:984, 1970.

26. Campbell DG: Pigmentary dispersion and glaucoma: A new theory. Arch Ophthalmol 97:1667, 1979.
27. Grant WM: Personal communication, 1981.
28. Speakman JS: Pigmentary dispersion. Br J Ophthalmol 65:249, 1981.
29. Seissinger J: Weitere Beiträge zur Kenntnis der Axenfeld-Krukenberg'schen Pigmentspindel. Klin Monatsbl Augenheilkd 77:37, 1926.
30. Strebel J, Steiger O: Korrelation der Vererbung von Augenleiden (Ectopia lentium cong, Ectopia pupillae, Myopie) und sog nicht angeborenen Herzfehlern. Arch Augenheilkd 78:208, 1915.
31. Vogt A: Weitere Ergebnisse der Spaltlampenmikroskopie des vorderen Bulbaschnittes (Cornea, vorderer Glaskörper, Conjunctiva, Lidrander). I: Abschnitt, Hornhaut. Arch Ophthalmol 106:63, 1921.
32. Mauksch H: Zerfall des retinalen Pigmentblattes der Iris bei zwei Brüdern. Z Augenheilkd 57:262, 1925.
33. Stankovic J: Den Beitrag zur Kenntnis der Vererbung des Pigmentglaukom. Klin Monatsbl Augenheilkd 139:165, 1961.
34. Mandelkorn RM, Hoffman ME, Olander KW, et al: Inheritance and the pigmentary dispersion syndrome. Ann Ophthalmol 15:577, 1983.
35. McDermott JA, Rich R, Berger A, Wang RF: Inheritance of pigmentary dispersion syndrome. Invest Ophthalmol Vis Sci Suppl 28:153, 1987.
36. Piccolino FC, Calalria G, Polizzi A, Fioretto M: Pigmentary retinal dystrophy associated with pigmentary glaucoma. Graefes Arch Clin Exp Ophthalmol 227:335, 1989.
37. Brini A, Porte A, Roth A: Atrophie des couches epitheliales de l'iris: Étude d'un cas de glaucome pigmentaire au microscope optique et au microscope electronique. Doc Ophthalmol 26:403, 1969.
38. Rodrigues MM, Spaeth GL, Weinreb S, Sivalingam E: Spectrum of trabecular pigmentation in open-angle glaucoma: A clinicopathologic study. Trans Am Acad Ophthalmol Otolaryngol 81:258, 1976.
39. Kampik A, Green WR, Quigley HA, Pierce LH: Scanning and transmission electron microscopic studies of two cases of pigment dispersion syndrome. Am J Ophthalmol 91:573, 1981.
40. Boles-Carenini B, Buten RE, Spurgeon WM, Ascher KW: Comparative topographic study of normotensive eyes of white and Negro persons. Am J Ophthalmol 40:224, 1955.
41. Yanoff M, Fine BS: Ocular Pathology: A Text and Atlas. New York, Harper & Row, 1975.
42. Chen KK, Poth EJ: Racial difference as illustrated by the mydriatic action of cocaine, euphthalmine, and ephedrine. J Pharm Exp Ther 36:429, 1929.
43. Gillies WE: Pigmentary glaucoma: A clinical review of anterior segment pigment dispersal syndrome. Aust N Z J Ophthalmol 13:325, 1985.
44. Becker B, Podos SM: Krukenberg's spindles and primary open-angle glaucoma. Arch Ophthalmol 76:635, 1966.
45. Becker B, Shin DDH, Cooper DG, Kass MA: The pigment dispersion syndrome. Am J Ophthalmol 83:161, 1977.
46. Calhoun FP Jr: Pigmentary glaucoma and its relation to Krukenberg's spindles. Am J Ophthalmol 36:1398, 1953.
47. Lichter PR: Pigmentary glaucoma: Current concepts. Trans Am Acad Ophthalmol Otolaryngol 78:309, 1974.
48. Fine BS, Yanoff M, Scheie HG: Pigmentary "glaucoma": A histologic study. Trans Am Acad Ophthalmol Otolaryngol 78:314, 1974.
49. Kupfer C, Kuwabara T, Kaiser-Kupfer M: The histopathology of pigmentary dispersion syndrome with glaucoma. Am J Ophthalmol 80:857, 1975.
50. Bellows AR, Jocson VL, Sears ML: Iris pigment granule obstruction of the aqueous outflow channels in enucleated monkey eyes. Paper presented at the Association for Research in Vision and Ophthalmology, 1974.
51. Grant WM: Experimental aqueous perfusion in enucleated human eyes. Arch Ophthalmol 69:783, 1963.
52. Epstein DL, Boger WP III, Grant WM: Phenylephrine provocative testing in the pigmentary dispersion syndrome. Am J Ophthalmol 85:43, 1978.
53. Schenker HI, Luntz MH, Kels B, et al: Exercise-induced increase of intraocular pressure in the pigmentary dispersion syndrome. Am J Ophthalmol 89:598, 1980.
54. Smith DL, Kae SF, Robbani BS, et al: The effects of exercise on intraocular pressure in pigmentary glaucoma patients. Ophthalmol Surg 20:561, 1989.
55. Kristensen P: Mydriasis-induced pigment liberation in the anterior chamber associated with acute rise in intraocular pressure in open-angle glaucoma. Acta Ophthalmol 43:714, 1965.
56. Havener VH: Ocular Pharmacology, 4th ed. St Louis, CV Mosby, 1978.
57. Mapstone R: Pigment release. Br J Ophthalmol 65:258, 1981.
58. Hoffmann F, Kumitrescu L, Hager H: Pigment-glaukom. Klin Monatsbl Augenheilkd 166:609, 1975.
59. Iwamoto T, Witmer R, Landolt E: Light and electron microscopy in absolute glaucoma with pigment dispersion phenomena and contusion angle deformity. Am J Ophthalmol 72:420, 1971.
60. Richardson TM, Hutchinson BT, Grant WM: The outflow tract in pigmentary glaucoma: A light and electron microscopic study. Arch Ophthalmol 195:1015, 1977.
61. Rohen JW, van der Zypen E: The phagocytic activity of the trabecular meshwork endothelium: An electron microscopic study of the vervet (cercopithecus aethiops). Graefes Arch Clin Exp Ophthalmol 175:143, 1968.
62. Sherwood M, Richardson TM: Evidence for in vivo phagocytosis by trabecular endothelial cells. Invest Ophthalmol Vis Sci Suppl 21:66, 1980.
63. Huber C: The gray iris syndrome: An iatrogenic form of pigmentary glaucoma. Arch Ophthalmol 102:397, 1984.
64. Smith JP: Pigmentary open-angle glaucoma secondary to posterior chamber intraocular lens implantation and erosion of the iris pigment epithelium. J Am Intraocul Implant Soc 11:174, 1985.
65. Woodhams JT, Lester JC: Pigmentary dispersion glaucoma secondary to posterior chamber intraocular lenses. Ann Ophthalmol 16:852, 1984.
66. Lunde MW: Argon laser trabeculoplasty in pigmentary dispersion syndrome with glaucoma. Am J Ophthalmol 96:721, 1983.
67. Hagadus J, Ritch R, Pollack I, et al: Argon laser trabeculoplasty in pigmentary glaucoma. Invest Ophthalmol Vis Sci Suppl 25:94, 1984.

Chapter 124

■

Inflammatory Glaucoma

PHILIP M. FIORE

Inflammatory glaucoma comprises a group of heterogeneous disorders that have elevated intraocular pressure in common. There are many presentations of ocular inflammation resulting from various causes including acute trauma, infectious agents, immunologic processes, biologic conditions, or idiopathic conditions (Table 124–1). When present for a sufficient time or of sufficient severity, ocular inflammation can produce a number of damaging side effects such as retinal scarring, cataract formation, corneal edema, and glaucoma. Inflammatory glaucoma is a difficult and challenging condition to manage both because many of the inflammatory diseases are chronic and because the damage that they produce is often permanent.

GENERAL SIGNS AND SYMPTOMS

Acute ocular inflammation characteristically produces pain, photophobia, lacrimation, and blurred vision. The eye is often injected from vascular congestion with ciliary flush and can be tender to palpation. Examination of the anterior chamber reveals cells and increased protein (flare) in the aqueous fluid. The aqueous cells can collect on the endothelium, forming fine keratic precipitates or a hypopyon (Fig. 124–1). Cells may also be present in the anterior vitreous, where they appear much larger from the magnification of the lens. Inflammation of a granulomatous nature is more often seen in a quiet eye with little or no pain and mild, if any, ciliary injection. Granulomatous inflammation produces characteristic "mutton-fat" keratic precipitates on the endothelium. Ocular inflammation can also cause posterior and peripheral anterior synechia, cataract formation, band keratopathy, and glaucoma.

SECONDARY GLAUCOMA

Patients with iritis can have a low, normal, or elevated intraocular pressure. The variation in pressure depends

on the effect that inflammation has on both the aqueous outflow and the rate of aqueous secretion (Table 124–2). Iritis can affect the trabecular meshwork with increased resistance to aqueous outflow while decreasing the rate of production from hyposecretion. The actual pressure depends on the balance of inflow and outflow, because each is affected by inflammation.

Several factors may affect aqueous outflow (Table 124–3). Swelling and dysfunction of the endothelial cells or infiltration and obstruction of the trabecular meshwork by inflammatory material such as white blood cell aggregates, macrophages, lymphocytes, and fibrin may cause diminished outflow with subsequent increased intraocular pressure.[1] Normal serum components have also been reported to cause obstruction to outflow pathways.[2] This obstruction to outflow cannot be observed by gonioscopy. However, on occasion, inflammatory material can accumulate on the meshwork forming precipitates similar to keratic precipitates. These can be seen by gonioscopy and are a sign of trabecular inflammation and possible dysfunction.

Prostaglandins are mediators of acute inflammation and can cause many of the signs of ocular inflammation including vasodilation, increased vascular permeability, and miosis.[3] Topical administration of prostaglandins have caused increased intraocular pressure.[4, 5] Agents that can inhibit their synthesis or function can be of potential benefit in ocular inflammatory disease.

Ocular inflammation, acute, recurrent, or chronic, can cause structural changes in an eye leading to the development of permanent secondary glaucoma. Posterior synechia, if complete, leads to iris bombé and angle-

Table 124–1. MAJOR INFLAMMATORY DISORDERS ASSOCIATED WITH GLAUCOMA

1. Idiopathic anterior uveitis
2. Fuchs' heterochromic iridocyclitis
3. Sarcoidosis
4. Glaucomatocyclitis crisis
5. Herpetic keratouveitis
6. Idiopathic inflammatory precipitates in angle
7. Syphilitic interstitial keratitis
8. Juvenile rheumatoid arthritis
9. Scleritis and episcleritis

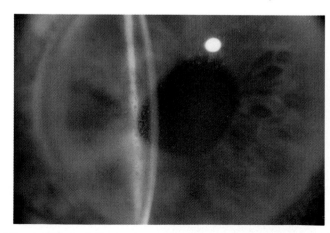

Figure 124–1. Inflammatory glaucoma with prominent keratic precipitates.

Table 124–2. INFLAMMATION AND INTRAOCULAR PRESSURE

Aqueous Secretion	Aqueous Outflow	Intraocular Pressure
Hyposecretion	Normal	Low
Hyposecretion	Outflow obstruction	Normal
Normal	Outflow obstruction	High

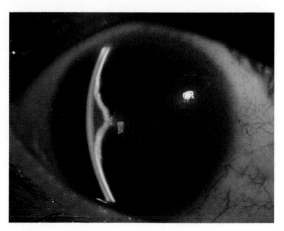

Figure 124–2. Iris bombé complicating uveitis.

closure (Fig. 124–2). Peripheral anterior synechia, if broad or extensive enough, causes progressive angle-closure and glaucoma. Even without extensive posterior or peripheral anterior synechia, an angle can have a "dirty" appearance after many episodes of iritis.

TREATMENT

The management of patients with uveitis and elevated intraocular pressure must be directed both at reducing the acute inflammation and controlling the intraocular pressure. Every attempt should be made to prevent any permanent structural damage from prolonged inflammation because that could cause permanent glaucoma or visual loss.

The initial treatment of uveitis has been with cycloplegia and corticosteroids. Cyclopentolate, homatropine, or atropine are used to dilate the pupil and break any posterior synechia. They also reduce ciliary spasm, decreasing the patient's pain and photophobia. Corticosteroids have a nonspecific antiinflammatory effect, quieting the intraocular inflammation without changing the underlying physiologic or biologic cause of the inflammation. Almost all causes of ocular inflammation can be nonselectively suppressed with corticosteroids.

The antiinflammatory effects of corticosteroids have been ascribed to decreasing capillary permeability,[6, 7] suppression of inflammatory mediators,[6] and inhibiting the formation of granulation tissue.[8] Corticosteroids stabilize intracellular lysozomes[9] and suppress the release of prostaglandins in the inflammatory response.[10] Corticosteroids can be used topically, subconjunctivally, or systemically. Ocular penetration after topical administration is increased in the inflamed eye. Most cases of anterior segment inflammation can be controlled with frequent instillation of prednisolone 1 percent or dexamethasone 0.1 percent. As the inflammation subsides, the frequency of use is slowly tapered.

Although effective in reducing inflammation, corticosteroids cause elevated intraocular pressure in 20 to

Table 124–3. MECHANISMS OF OUTFLOW OBSTRUCTION

1. Infiltration and obstruction of the trabecular meshwork
2. Swelling and dysfunction of the trabecular cells
3. Abnormal aqueous fluid
4. Release of prostaglandins
5. Posterior synechia with iris bombé and angle-closure
6. Peripheral anterior synechia
7. Formation of an inflammatory or hyaline membrane over the trabecular meshwork

30 percent of the population after prolonged use.[11] Certain topical corticosteroids (e.g., medrysone and fluorometholone) have a decreased tendency to elevate intraocular pressure[12–14] but also to have less antiinflammatory effect. In treating inflammatory glaucoma it can be very difficult to determine whether increasing intraocular pressure is induced by steroids or is secondary to increased aqueous production after reduced inflammation. Corticosteroids are often quickly tapered, resulting in the return of inflammation, hyposecretion, and decreased intraocular pressure. This setting only prolongs the inflammation with increased opportunity for permanent ocular damage. Inflammation that does not respond to topical steroids may require subconjunctival or systemic treatment. Long-acting periocular steroids should be avoided because they may result in a delayed and often irreversible increase in intraocular pressure.[15] The long-term use of either topical[16] or systemic[17] corticosteroids may also cause posterior subcapsular cataracts.

Flurbiprofen, a topical nonsteroidal antiinflammatory agent, has been introduced to prevent pupillary miosis during cataract surgery.[18] This agent inhibits the production of inflammatory mediators such as prostacyclin, thromboxane, prostaglandin E_2, and leukotrienes by inhibiting the cyclooxygenase pathway and to a lesser extent the lipoxygenase pathway in the degradation of arachidonic acid.[19, 20] The antiinflammatory and antiprostaglandin activities have been used with some success to prevent the breakdown of the blood-aqueous barrier[21] and reduce inflammation after cataract extraction.[22] Although topical nonsteroidal antiinflammatory agents do not appear to be as effective in suppressing inflammation as corticosteroids are, their use should be considered in patients with uveitis and in patients with steroid-induced ocular hypertension requiring further antiinflammatory therapy.

Some severe inflammatory conditions may not respond to corticosteroid therapy, and immunosuppressive therapy should be considered. Methotrexate[23] and low-dose prednisone with azathioprine or chlorambucil[24] have resulted in response rates of 60 to 70 percent.

Treatment of secondary glaucoma from inflammatory disease is directed at controlling the inflammation as described. Elevated intraocular pressure should be initially treated medically with topical epinephrine, β-adrenergic antagonists, and carbonic anhydrase inhibitors. Miotics are generally avoided because they may exacerbate inflammation and may lead to formation of posterior synechia. Patients developing posterior synechia should be dilated frequently to prevent the formation of a secluded pupil. Eyes with posterior synechia and iris bombé need emergent laser iridectomy to prevent secondary angle-closure.

Laser trabeculoplasty has a limited and uncertain role in the control of intraocular pressure. In one series only one of five eyes with uveitis had a response to laser trabeculoplasty.[25] Another investigator reported no reduction in intraocular pressure in three patients with nongranulomatous uveitis.[26] Furthermore, two of the patients sustained pressure elevations and significant flare-up of their inflammation requiring surgery in the first 4 wk after laser therapy. Finally, one investigator did report reduced intraocular pressure in three of four eyes with glaucoma secondary to uveitis.[27] The possibility of further exacerbation of inflammation with peripheral anterior synechia formation must be considered before attempting laser trabeculoplasty.

The surgical treatment of inflammatory glaucoma is difficult and often yields poor results. Failure of filtration surgery from conjunctival scarring is accelerated by recurrent or preexisting inflammation. Full-thickness filtration procedures have been shown to be more effective than trabeculectomy.[28] The use of postoperative 5-fluorouracil has improved the success rate of filtration and should be considered in all cases.[29] The Molteno implant has been used with success in refractory cases of glaucoma and should be considered in inflammatory glaucoma, especially after previous surgical failure.[30] Cyclocryotherapy and cyclophotocoagulation are reserved for end-stage disease.

FUCHS' HETEROCHROMIC IRIDOCYCLITIS

Fuchs' heterochromic iridocyclitis syndrome, first described by Fuchs in 1906, consists of chronic, low-grade iritis with secondary posterior subcapsular cataract and glaucoma.[31] The condition is rare, occurs unilaterally in 90 percent of cases, and is associated with a change in iris color.[32] The disease is insidious, slowly progressive, and usually first detected in the third and fourth decades of life.[33] Men and women appear equally affected.[32]

Patients with Fuchs' heterochromic iridocyclitis typically have quiet, white eyes with no pain, photophobia, or discomfort. They usually seek medical attention for decreased vision as the cataract progresses. The inflammation consists of low-grade flare and cells with stellate keratic precipitates and fine filaments scattered over the entire endothelium.[32, 33] The inflammation is chronic and nongranulomatous, characterized by a predominance of lymphocytes and plasma cells.[34] There are also anterior vitreous opacities and small white nodules on the anterior iris.[32]

Heterochromia is a classic feature of this disease with hypochromia most often seen in affected eyes with dark irides caused by stromal atrophy (Fig. 124–3).[35, 36] In light irides, the affected eye may be darker because the stromal atrophy can reveal the dark posterior pigment epithelium.[32] The iris atrophy may cause loss of normal iris architecture and a moth-eaten appearance with small hole formation seen on retroillumination.[33] Another characteristic finding is neovascularization of the iris and angle with fine fragile vessels. These vessels can bleed with minor trauma, but intraoperative hemorrhage is rare.[37–40] Angle neovascularization does not lead to peripheral anterior synechia and is not associated with the development of glaucoma. Fluorescein angiography demonstrates leakage from iris vessels in all affected eyes.[41]

Posterior subcapsular cataract formation, a late finding of the disease, develops in all affected eyes if followed long enough.[42] Cataract extraction is generally uncomplicated and well tolerated with good visual results and little exacerbation of inflammation.[32, 33, 39, 40] Chorioretinal lesions have been reported in greater frequency in patients with Fuchs' heterochromic iridocyclitis.[31, 43, 44]

The major late complication of heterochromic iridocyclitis is secondary glaucoma. An early study reported secondary glaucoma in only a small proportion of uni-

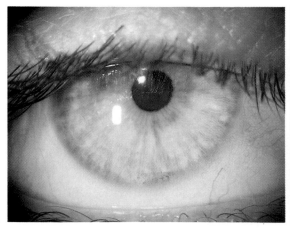
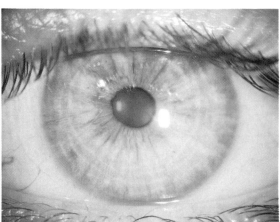

Figure 124–3. A (right) and B (left), Eyes of a patient with Fuchs' heterochromic iridocyclitis in the *right* eye.

lateral cases.[45] A more recent long-term study reported 15 percent of patients with secondary glaucoma at the time of diagnosis and another 44 percent developing glaucoma during an average follow-up of 12 yr.[42] There is a higher incidence of glaucoma in patients with bilateral disease, 25 to 33 percent than in those with unilateral disease, 5 to 13 percent.[32, 46, 47] Glaucoma also appears to be more common in black patients (38 percent) compared with white patients (11 percent) with heterochromic iridocyclitis.[48] Increased intraocular pressure is believed to be caused by decreased aqueous outflow secondary to trabecular meshwork obstruction by plasma cells and lymphocytes and, by the formation of an inflammatory or hyaline membrane over the trabecular meshwork.[34, 49]

The inflammation of Fuchs' iridocyclitis is benign and does not require aggressive treatment with corticosteroids. In fact, steroids have little effect in controlling the chronic inflammation and can cause steroid-induced glaucoma and accelerated cataract formation.[35] Elevated intraocular pressure initially responds to β-adrenergic antagonists, miotics, and carbonic anhydrase inhibitors. With time the glaucoma becomes refractory to medical treatment.[42] Argon laser trabeculoplasty, which should be used cautiously, is not very effective because of the formation of a hyaline membrane over the trabecular meshwork. Filtration surgery may eventually be necessary to control refractory intraocular pressure.

SARCOIDOSIS

Sarcoidosis is a noncaseating granulomatous disease of unknown cause affecting a number of systemic organs including the lung, liver, spleen, central nervous system, skin (Fig. 124–4), and eye. Granulomas consist of small islands of macrophages, epitheloid cells, giant cells, and a surrounding rim of lymphocytes. Although the initial stimulus for the development of sarcoidosis is unknown, an alteration in T lymphocytes and cell-mediated activity is involved.[50] The condition occurs more frequently in blacks and women and first occurs in young adults under the age of 40.

The ocular manifestations of sarcoidosis occur in 10 to 38 percent of patients with systemic disease.[51–54] Sarcoidosis most commonly affects the anterior segment but can also involve the posterior segment and the orbit. The ocular inflammation of sarcoidosis is a chronic granulomatous uveitis having mutton-fat keratic precipitates, with iris (Busacca) and pupil (Koeppe) nodules. Frequently, patients present with noninjected and painless eyes with bilateral involvement, although the disease can present acutely in one eye. Chronic inflammation can lead to the formation of a pupillary membrane, posterior synechia, peripheral anterior synechia, cataract, and band keratopathy.

Posterior segment involvement consisting of chorioretinopathy, periphlebitis, and retinopathy has been reported in 25 percent of cases of sarcoidosis.[52, 53, 55] Posterior segment involvement usually also signifies anterior segment involvement. Vitreous opacities are present in 30 percent of eyes with chorioretinal sarcoi-

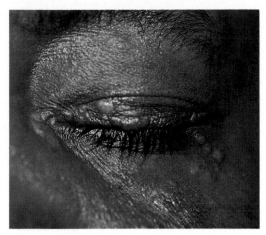

Figure 124–4. Skin granulomas in a 42-year-old black man with sarcoidosis.

dosis.[55] Lacrimal gland involvement also occurs in a large number of cases.

Secondary glaucoma occurs in 11 percent of patients with anterior segment inflammation.[53] Persistent inflammation leads to trabecular meshwork damage with scarring, occlusion, or obstruction of the meshwork.[56] Angle-closure glaucoma can develop from progressive peripheral anterior synechia or iris bombé caused by posterior synechia or a pupillary membrane.

Sarcoidosis is a chronic disease with many exacerbations and remissions. Ocular inflammation can present only rarely, or the disease can have a chronic relapsing course with greater ocular damage.[57] Corticosteroids and cycloplegia are the mainstay of treatment in controlling the anterior inflammation. With posterior, orbital, or systemic involvement, systemic steroids should be considered. Low-dose cyclosporine therapy has been reported to be helpful in patients with sarcoidosis who do not respond to corticosteroids.[58]

Glaucoma should be treated medically for as long as possible. Beta-adrenergic antagonists and carbonic anhydrase inhibitors are used to decrease aqueous production. Miotics are avoided because they can exacerbate the effects of inflammation. Laser trabeculoplasty can be tried but is frequently ineffective in these cases. Refractory glaucoma on maximal medications requires glaucoma surgery. Surgical success is improved if all inflammation is allowed to subside, if possible, before filtration surgery is attempted. Full-thickness surgery is frequently preferred in inflammatory glaucoma due to sarcoidosis, especially if the patients are young or black.

GLAUCOMATOCYCLITIS CRISIS

Glaucomatocyclitis crisis was first recognized as a syndrome by Posner and Schlossman in 1942.[59, 60] It is an unusual and important type of acute recurrent uveitis and secondary glaucoma. The syndrome consists of recurrent attacks of very mild inflammation and elevated intraocular pressure. The inflammation characteristically is out of proportion to the glaucoma when compared with hypertensive uveitis, which presents with severe uveitis and mildly elevated intraocular pressure.

Glaucomatocyclitis crisis often occurs in patients between the ages of 20 and 50 yr. The condition is generally unilateral and recurrent, however bilateral cases have been reported.[61] Patients present with only mild ocular discomfort, some blurring of vision, and halos if corneal edema is present. The eye is white and quiet; the pupil is often slightly dilated; and the anterior chamber is deep with an open angle.[59, 62] Intraocular pressure is found to be very elevated, above 30 mmHg and often in the 40 to 50 mmHg range.[60] Signs of anterior inflammation are characteristically minimal with some aqueous flare, rare cells, and only a few keratic precipitates that are small, flat, nonpigmented, and concentrated over the inferior endothelium.[60] Posterior synechia or peripheral anterior synechia do not form. The inflammatory reaction can be seen with elevated intraocular pressure but often occurs several days after the intraocular pressure rises with the degree of elevated intraocular pressure not proportional to the amount of inflammation.[63] The attacks last from several days and may take as long as 2 wk to resolve. Recurrences tend to occur at intervals of a few months to several years.

The cause of glaucomatocyclitic crisis is unclear. The increased intraocular pressure, however, results from an acute drop in the facility of outflow during the attack with an increased outflow after the attack.[64] Increased aqueous production has also been reported.[65, 66] There have been many suggestions with regard to possible factors in the development of glaucomatocyclitis crisis such as an abnormal vascular process,[67] an autonomic defect,[59] an allergic condition,[62] a variant of developmental glaucoma,[63] or a cytomegalovirus infection.[68]

Prostaglandins have been found to play a role in the disease. Elevated levels of prostaglandins in the aqueous humor have been found during an acute attack and the concentration correlated with the level of intraocular pressure.[69] Treatment with oral indomethacin, an inhibitor of prostaglandin synthesis, or subconjunctival polyphloretin phosphate, a prostaglandin antagonist, decreased the intraocular pressure.[69] Increased levels of prostaglandins in the anterior chamber may also be responsible for both the decreased facility of outflow and the breakdown of the blood-aqueous barrier allowing for leakage of protein and cells into the anterior chamber.[70] The vascular effects of prostaglandins may explain the tortuous iris vessels and leakage of fluorescence seen by iris angiography.[67]

Eyes with glaucomatocyclitic crisis were long believed to maintain normal visual fields and optic nerves between attacks.[59, 60] It is now clear that some patients with glaucomatocyclitic crisis have abnormal aqueous humor dynamics between episodes, and some patients have underlying primary open-angle glaucoma.[71] Also, patients can develop optic nerve cupping and visual field loss because of frequent repeated attacks or because of underlying primary open-angle glaucoma.[71] In one study patients were followed long-term after an attack and were found to have a greater incidence of elevated intraocular pressure, steroid responsiveness, decreased facility of outflow, and cupping and field loss in both the affected and nonaffected eye.[71]

Glaucomatocyclitic crisis is treated initially with topical corticosteroids to control the inflammation,[62] and antiglaucoma medications, β-adrenergic antagonists, epinephrine, or carbonic anhydrase inhibitors to lower intraocular pressure. Mydriatics are seldom used and have little effect because there is little ciliary muscle spasm. Miotics are also seldom used to control pressure because of their limited effect. Oral indomethacin may be effective since prostaglandins have been implicated in the disease.[69] Although little clinical data exist, flurbiprofen may be tried to control the inflammation and prostaglandin levels. Most attacks of glaucomatocyclitic crisis are self-limited, and moderate episodes of increased intraocular pressure are well tolerated. Laser trabeculoplasty is generally not effective in controlling the elevations of intraocular pressure. An occasional patient may require filtering surgery because of progressive cupping and field loss.[71] Successful filtering surgery prevents the elevations in intraocular pressure but does not prevent the recurrent episodes of inflammation.[72, 73]

HERPETIC KERATOUVEITIS

There are four major viruses within the herpesvirus family that are human pathogens, herpes simplex virus, varicella zoster virus, cytomegalovirus, and Epstein-Barr virus. The herpes simplex virus and the varicella zoster virus are the two most important pathogens that affect the human eye.

Herpes Simplex

Herpes simplex virus occurs in humans in two forms, types 1 and 2. Herpes simplex type 1 most commonly causes the oral and ocular infections, whereas type 2 is associated with genital infections. The majority of the adult population have circulating antibodies to herpes simplex type 1 from prior exposure to the virus and carry the virus in an inactive state. Primary ocular infection with the herpes simplex virus causes an acute follicular conjunctivitis with regional lymphadenopathy and often a vesicular, ulcerative blepharitis. Most patients also present with the typical herpetic epithelial keratitis. Recurrent episodes affect principally the cornea and are more troublesome, causing epithelial keratitis, stromal keratitis, and uveitis. Repeated episodes of herpes simplex keratouveitis can lead to secondary glaucoma.

Herpes simplex keratouveitis is often associated with increased intraocular pressure. The increased pressure is seen more frequently in patients with uveitis than with only keratitis (Fig. 124–5). In one report 28 percent of patients with herpes simplex keratouveitis had increased intraocular pressure and of these 94 percent had either disciform or stromal keratitis.[74] The periods of elevated intraocular pressure from herpetic keratouveitis may be intermittent and have a mean duration of 2 mo. The

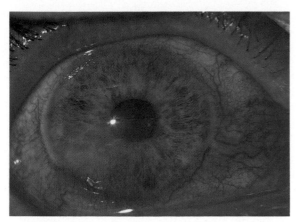

Figure 124–5. Herpes simplex keratouveitis and glaucoma in a 56-year-old man.

increased intraocular pressure is presumed to be due to increased aqueous viscosity, trabecular blockade with inflammatory cells and fibrin, or trabeculitis with edema of the meshwork.[74–76] Virus particles have been identified in the iris.[77]

Treatment of herpes simplex is directed toward preventing or reducing viral replication. A variety of topical antiviral agents such as idoxuridine, vidarabine, and trifluridine are presently available to treat herpes simplex (see Chap. 6). Although topical corticosteroids are useful and often necessary for suppressing uveitis, they may increase viral replication and may cause reactivation of epithelial herpes and should be used with an antiviral agent. Prolonged corticosteroid use may also lead to steroid-induced glaucoma.[78]

Increased intraocular pressure from active herpes keratouveitis should be controlled initially with β-adrenergic antagonists, carbonic anhydrase inhibitors, or epinephrine. As ocular inflammation subsides, the intraocular pressure usually returns to normal. However, approximately 12 percent of patients will have a persistent elevated intraocular pressure requiring continued antiglaucoma therapy.[74] Filtration surgery may be required occasionally and should be avoided or postponed until the inflammation has subsided,[74] if possible. Adjunctive therapy with 5-fluorouracil may improve the results of filtration surgery in an acutely inflamed eye.

Varicella Zoster

Varicella (chickenpox) infection and herpes zoster infection represent different clinical manifestations of the same virus. The initial infection is varicella, whereas the recurrent infection is known as herpes zoster, occurring in individuals with partial immunity resulting from a prior varicella infection. Zoster is caused by the reactivation of latent varicella virus. Ophthalmic herpes zoster is a disease that primarily affects the elderly during the sixth and seventh decades of life. Ocular complications occur in 50 percent of cases and include blepharitis, conjunctivitis, keratitis, scleritis, iridocyclitis, retinitis, and optic neuritis.[79–81] When herpes zoster

involves the ophthalmic division of the trigeminal nerve, especially the nasociliary branch, there is very often an associated keratitis, iridocyclitis, and secondary open-angle glaucoma.[82]

Herpes zoster ophthalmicus presents with the typical vesicular rash affecting the periorbital, nasal, and forehead of one side. Pain may precede the appearance of the rash by 24 to 48 hr. The cornea can have a dendritic pattern and, with the presence of stromal keratitis, sensation is affected and may not recover, leading to trophic ulcers. Anterior uveitis presents with blurred vision, photophobia, ciliary injection, iris edema, and miosis.[83] The associated iridocyclitis is usually chronic and can be either granulomatous or nongranulomatous with pigmented keratic precipitates and possible hypopyon formation.[84] Posterior synechia often develop, but peripheral anterior synechia are uncommon.[85]

Secondary glaucoma occurs commonly in association with herpes zoster keratouveitis in 16 percent of affected eyes (Fig. 124–6).[82] The increased intraocular pressure results from the inflammatory obstruction to outflow or from repeated inflammatory damage to the trabecular meshwork.[86, 87] Intraocular pressure can increase transiently during an exacerbation of the disease and, with persistent recurrences, may become chronically elevated. In some cases hypotony develops, presumably from hyposecretion of the ciliary body from ischemia.

Treatment of herpes zoster ophthalmicus begins with corticosteroids to control the inflammation and cycloplegia to reduce ciliary spasm and prevent posterior synechia. Steroids are reserved for patients with stromal keratitis or keratouveitis and intact epithelium. Oral acyclovir has been used successfully to shorten the duration and reduce the severity of dendritic keratopathy, stromal keratitis, and uveitis.[88, 89] Elevated intraocular pressure is controlled initially with β-adrenergic antagonists, carbonic anhydrase inhibitors, and epinephrine. Miotics should be avoided because they exacerbate the condition. Laser trabeculoplasty is not considered to be effective as in other inflammatory glaucomas. Filtration surgery may occasionally be required.

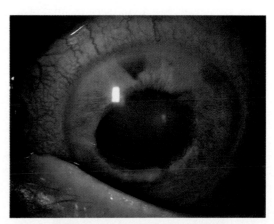

Figure 124–6. Herpes zoster uveitis and glaucoma in a 52-year-old woman. Note the irregular pupil and iris atrophy. Patient had undergone iridectomies for angle-closure glaucoma before development of herpes zoster.

IDIOPATHIC INFLAMMATORY PRECIPITATES IN ANGLE

Chandler and Grant[85] described idiopathic inflammatory precipitates on the trabecular meshwork as a relatively rare cause of secondary glaucoma often mistaken for primary open-angle glaucoma. These patients with elevated intraocular pressure have no ocular complaints and typically present with white, quiet eyes. There may be some cells in the aqueous and rarely some precipitates on the back of the cornea. Gonioscopy reveals inflammatory precipitates confined to the surface of the trabecular meshwork. Sometimes only an irregularity in the attachment of the iris root may be an indication that trabecular precipitates are or have been present.[85] The magnitude of the increase in intraocular pressure does not correlate with the amount of precipitates seen on the trabecular meshwork. The condition is bilateral in 86 percent of patients and usually occurs after the fifth decade.[90] Several other ocular conditions have been found to cause trabecular precipitates.

Sarcoidosis is a possible cause of inflammatory precipitates on the trabecular meshwork that should be ruled out. Often the patient will have other manifestations of the disease such as corneal endothelial deposits, Busacca or Koeppe nodules, inflammation in the vitreous or retina, and systemic involvement. Isolated precipitates on the trabecular meshwork with no other findings should always raise the possibility of sarcoid disease.[85]

Glaucomatocyclitic crisis has been reported to occasionally demonstrate a few tiny precipitates in the angle.[85] These eyes also present unilaterally with minimal pain and the absence of injection. They can, however, manifest several small keratic precipitates on the corneal endothelium with trace cells in the aqueous humor associated with the episode of intraocular pressure elevation.

Trabecular inflammatory deposits have also been reported occurring after argon laser trabeculoplasty (Fig. 124–7).[91] This syndrome should be recognized, and patients undergoing argon laser trabeculoplasty should be followed closely in the immediate and intermediate postoperative periods. An increase in the intraocular pressure above baseline following trabeculoplasty warrants careful gonioscopic examination to rule out inflammatory precipitates.

The detection of even solitary, subtle inflammatory precipitates on the trabecular meshwork usually indicates a diffuse process of trabecular inflammation.[85] The intraocular pressure elevation is probably caused by an accumulation of inflammatory cells and debris in the trabecular meshwork. Organization of the precipitate may lead to peripheral anterior synechiae formation with a characteristic uneven insertion into the angle.

Treatment of idiopathic trabecular precipitates consists of initial frequent topical corticosteroids along with β-blockers, carbonic anhydrase inhibitors, and epinephrine to control intraocular pressure. With continued steroid use the precipitates gradually disappear in 1 to 2 wk with the return of intraocular pressure to normal levels. It is important to make a correct diagnosis of idiopathic trabecular precipitates so that proper treatment is instituted. If the condition is not recognized and the eye is treated for primary open-angle glaucoma, the precipitates may increase and gradually lead to peripheral anterior synechia with closure of the angle and permanent glaucoma. Argon laser trabeculoplasty treatment is not indicated because it may exacerbate the condition.

SYPHILITIC INTERSTITIAL KERATITIS

Syphilitic interstitial keratitis is associated with secondary glaucoma in both congenital disease or adult acquired disease. The glaucoma can occur during the acute phase of interstitial keratitis or many years later after the cornea has healed and the inflammation has subsided.

Congenital syphilis is caused by the in utero transmission of the *Treponema pallidum* organism from a syphilitic mother to her fetus.[92] The manifestations of the disease affect approximately 70 percent of infected newborn infants. Congenital syphilis can present with a variety of ocular findings, including acute and chronic iritis, interstitial keratitis, scleritis, chorioretinitis, retinal periphlebitis, optic neuritis, and secondary cataracts.[93]

Interstitial keratitis is the most characteristic ocular finding in congenital syphilis and commonly appears between the sixth and twelfth years. Corneal edema and infiltrates present with lacrimation and photophobia. Vascularization of the corneal stroma is characteristic and may be so pronounced as to give the cornea a pink "salmon patch" appearance. Iridocyclitis is virtually always present and is often associated with elevated intraocular pressure. The condition generally begins in one eye and becomes bilateral in 90 percent of cases. With the advent of antibiotics and better diagnosis, treatment, and prophylaxis, early acute interstitial keratitis and secondary glaucoma have become rare.

Interstitial keratitis from congenital syphilis is associated with adult secondary glaucoma in 15 to 20 percent of patients.[94] The glaucoma develops an average of

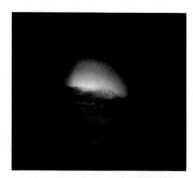

Figure 124–7. Goniophotograph demonstrating keratitic precipitates in the angle following argon laser trabeculoplasty.

27 yr after the initial episode of interstitial keratitis has subsided.[95] The majority of these patients do not have a reactivation of their inflammation. Clinical evidence has shown two different forms of late glaucoma, a deep-chamber, open-angle type,[96] and a shallow-chamber, narrow-angle type.[97] Both types occur with equal frequency and present with characteristic changes of congenital syphilis, such as corneal scarring with ghost vessels and chorioretinal atrophy.

Patients having the open-angle variety of secondary glaucoma present with a normal anterior chamber depth and a flat iris insertion. Gonioscopy reveals open angles with a "dirty appearance" having varying amounts of old, postinflammatory synechias that do not correlate with the amount of outflow obstruction.[98] There are no signs of active inflammation, and the glaucoma may present in one or both eyes. The appearance of the angle remains stable as the glaucoma becomes worse. The pathology of the condition appears to be endothelialization of the open portions of the angle with formation of a hyaline membrane.[95, 96, 98, 99] Secondary open-angle glaucoma from syphilitic interstitial keratitis responds poorly to antiglaucoma medications.[95, 98] Argon laser trabeculoplasty is likely to be of little benefit because of the angle endothelialization. Filtering surgery is often required for intraocular pressure control.

The narrow-angle type of secondary glaucoma in congenital syphilis presents with a shallow anterior chamber and a convex iris. The interstitial keratitis in childhood may affect the development of these eyes resulting in a small anterior segment.[100] These eyes also have no signs of active inflammation, unless an acute attack of angle-closure glaucoma has occurred and caused varying amounts of old peripheral anterior synechia. Peripheral iridectomy is curative in eyes without permanent synechial angle-closure.[98] In other eyes with permanent peripheral anterior synechia, medical therapy, surgical goniosynechialysis, or filtering surgery may be necessary.

Adult acquired syphilis can affect the eye with iritis, interstitial keratitis, chorioretinitis, and optic neuritis. Interstitial keratitis resembles the congenital variety but is usually uniocular, milder, and limited to a sector of the cornea.

JUVENILE RHEUMATOID ARTHRITIS

Juvenile rheumatoid arthritis is a chronic disease occurring in children before they reach puberty. The disease clinically takes three different forms: acute systemic, oligoarticular, and polyarticular, based on the degree of articular and systemic involvement at the time of onset.[101] The acute systemic form, characterized by Still, consists of an evanescent salmon-pink macular rash, fever, polyarthritis, hepatosplenomegaly, leukocytosis, and polyserositis seen commonly in boys under 4 yr of age.[102] Uveitis is not associated with this disease. The oligoarticular and polyarticular forms occur mostly in girls and lack the systemic features. Iritis occurs in 10 percent of these patients and is more common in the oligoarticular form (19 to 29 percent) than in the polyarticular disease (2 to 5 percent).[103, 104] Iritis is also more frequently associated with patients having negative rheumatoid factor and positive antinuclear antibodies.[104, 105]

The iritis associated with juvenile rheumatoid iritis is usually asymptomatic but occasionally presents with pain, redness, tearing, and photophobia.[103, 106] The uveitis is clinically chronic and nongranulomatous, having occasional small keratic precipitates and frequent posterior synechia formation. Histopathologic study of these eyes has revealed a granulomatous inflammation of the uveal tract.[107] The iritis develops after the appearance of the arthritis in 90 percent of patients with no temporal association between the activity of ocular disease and joint disease. Common late sequela of rheumatoid iritis are band keratopathy, cataract formation, and glaucoma.[106, 108–110]

Secondary glaucoma is seen in approximately 19 percent of patients with longstanding iritis in juvenile rheumatoid arthritis.[108] The glaucoma occurs from progressive peripheral anterior synechia and inflammatory damage to the trabecular meshwork or may be steroid-induced. Angle-closure can occur from posterior synechia and iris bombé. Additionally, systemic steroid therapy for the control of juvenile rheumatoid arthritis or topical steroid therapy for ocular inflammation may cause steroid-induced glaucoma.

Ocular inflammation in juvenile rheumatoid arthritis is managed with topical and occasionally periorbital steroids. Cycloplegic agents are necessary to prevent posterior synechia formation. The surgical treatment of cataracts and glaucoma is difficult.[106, 109] Elevated intraocular pressure is initially treated medically with β-adrenergic antagonists and carbonic anhydrase inhibitors. Iridectomy may be necessary to relieve pupillary block caused by posterior synechia. Surgical control of elevated intraocular pressure not responsive to medical therapy is difficult. A modified goniotomy technique has been reported to have been effective in 7 of 15 eyes for up to 2 yr.[111] These results are similar to those seen with conventional glaucoma filtration procedures.[109] The use of 5-fluorouracil may improve the results of filtration surgery in these young patients. Alternatively, the use of setons may provide successful surgical glaucoma control.

SCLERITIS AND EPISCLERITIS

Secondary glaucoma is frequently associated with inflammation of the sclera and episclera and should be remembered in dealing with these conditions. Intraocular pressure should be measured during every examination of patients with scleritis or episcleritis.

Episcleritis is a benign, frequently recurring inflammatory disease of the episclera. The onset is acute, producing a nodular or diffuse red congestion of the episclera with occasional ocular discomfort. Scleral vessels, although sometimes congested, appear normal in configuration and there is no scleral edema. A small number of patients with episcleritis can present with uveitis or glaucoma.

Elevated intraocular pressure in episcleritis can be due to primary open-angle glaucoma, steroid-induced glaucoma, or acute open-angle glaucoma.[112] In the secondary open-angle glaucoma due to episcleritis, the episclera is markedly edematous and the eyelids are swollen. These patients have extremely painful eyes, which is uncommon in typical episcleritis. The intraocular pressure is markedly elevated; the cornea is edematous; the pupil is miotic; and the angle is open.[113] The elevated intraocular pressure is thought to be due to edema of the trabecular meshwork.[114] The episcleral venous pressure may be elevated, but venous congestion is absent. The condition responds well to cycloplegia and topical steroids. Elevated intraocular pressure is controlled with β-adrenergic antagonists and carbonic anhydrase inhibitors.

Scleritis is a more painful and destructive inflammatory disease of the sclera with 46 percent of patients having an associated systemic condition, usually a connective tissue disorder.[115, 116] Scleritis is more common in the fourth to sixth decades of life and occurs more frequently in women. Patients present with severe ocular pain, often localized to the involved area. The affected scleral area is very injected, edematous, and elevated with a loss of the normal radial vascular pattern. The area is always tender to palpation. Several distinct types of scleritis can be identified clinically.

Glaucoma is a frequent complication of scleritis, occurring in 12 percent of patients in a series of 310 patients.[112] In a histopathologic study of 92 eyes enucleated because of scleral disease, 49 percent had glaucoma.[114] Increased intraocular pressure in scleritis can result from primary open-angle glaucoma, glaucoma due to uveitis, glaucoma with active limbal uveitis and trabecular meshwork inflammation, steroid-induced glaucoma, vasculitis of the episcleral vessels, primary angle-closure glaucoma, pupillary block glaucoma caused by posterior synechia, angle-closure caused by choroidal effusion, angle-closure due to peripheral anterior synechia, and neovascular glaucoma.[112, 117, 118]

Appropriate therapy for elevated intraocular pressure in the presence of scleritis depends on accurate diagnosis of the cause of glaucoma. Active scleritis should be treated with nonsteroidal antiinflammatory agents, topical or systemic steroids, and immunosuppressive agents as necessary.[119] Antiglaucoma medical therapy with β-adrenergic antagonists and carbonic anhydrase inhibitors are used to lower intraocular pressure. Angle-closure caused by primary or secondary pupillary block is treated with laser iridotomy. Residual synechial closure may be treated with laser gonioplasty or surgical goniosynechialysis. Angle-closure due to choroidal effusion is treated with intensive cycloplegics. Persistently elevated intraocular pressure can be treated with filtering surgery in an area of uninvolved conjunctiva.[120] Cyclocryotherapy or cyclophotocoagulation can exacerbate an already inflamed eye, and setons should be used cautiously because the presence of foreign material may stimulate further inflammation.

REFERENCES

1. Freddo TF, Patterson MM, Scott DR, Epstein DL: Influence of mercurial sulfhydryl agents on aqueous humor outflow pathways in enucleated eyes. Invest Ophthalmol Vis Sci 25:278, 1984.
2. Epstein DL, Hashimoto J, Grant WM: Serum obstruction of aqueous outflow in enucleated human eyes. Am J Ophthalmol 86:101, 1978.
3. Beitch BR, Eakins KE: The effects of prostaglandins on the intraocular pressure of the rabbit. Br J Pharmacol 37:158, 1969.
4. Kass MA, Podos SM, Moses RA, Becker B: Prostaglandin E1 and aqueous humor dynamics. Invest Ophthalmol 11:1022, 1972.
5. Bethel RA, Eakins KE: The mechanism of the antagonism of experimentally induced ocular hypertension by polyphloretin phosphate. Exp Eye Res 13:83, 1972.
6. Ebert RH, Barclay WR: Changes in connective tissue reaction induced by cortisone. Ann Intern Med 37:506, 1952.
7. Leopold IH, Purnell JE, Cannon EJ, et al: Local and systemic cortisone in ocular disease. Am J Ophthalmol 34:361, 1951.
8. Leopold IH: Treatment of eye disorders with anti-inflammatory steroids. Ann N Y Acad Sci 82:939, 1959.
9. Thomas L: The role of lysozomes in tissue injury. In Zeifach BW, Grant L, McCluskey RT (eds): The Inflammatory Process. New York, Academic Press, 1965, p 449.
10. Floman Y, Floman N, Zor U: Inhibition of prostaglandin E release by anti-inflammatory steroids. Prostaglandins 11:591, 1976.
11. Becker B: Intraocular pressure response to topical corticosteroids. Invest Ophthalmol 4:198, 1965.
12. Podos SM, Krupin T, Asseff C, Becker B: Topically administered corticosteroids preparations: Comparison of intraocular pressure effects. Arch Ophthalmol 86:251, 1971.
13. Stewart RH, Kimbrough RL: Intraocular pressure response to topically administered fluorometholone. Arch Ophthalmol 97:2139, 1979.
14. Kass M, Cheetham J, Duzman E, Burke PJ: The ocular hypertensive effect of 0.25% fluorometholone in corticosteroid responders. Am J Ophthalmol 102:159, 1986.
15. Herschler J: Intractable intraocular hypertension induced by repository triamcinolone acetonide. Am J Ophthalmol 74:501, 1972.
16. Becker B: Cataracts and topical corticosteroids. Am J Ophthalmol 58:872, 1964.
17. Oglesby RB, Black RL, von Sallmann L, Bunim JL: Cataracts in patients with rheumatic diseases treated with corticosteroids. Arch Ophthalmol 66:625, 1961.
18. Keats RH, McGowan KA: Clinical trial of flurbiprofen to maintain pupillary dilation during cataract surgery. Ann Ophthalmol 16:919, 1984.
19. Brogden RN, Heel RC, Speight TM, Avery GS: Flurbiprofen: A review of its pharmacological properties and therapeutic use in rheumatoid arthritis. Drugs 18:417, 1979.
20. Kantor TG: Physiology and treatment of pain and inflammation: Analgesic effects of flurbiprofen. Am J Med 80(Suppl 3A):3, 1986.
21. Araie M, Sawa M, Takase M: Topical flurbiprofen and diclofenac suppress blood-aqueous barrier breakdown in cataract surgery: A fluorophotometric study. Jpn J Ophthalmol 27:535, 1983.
22. Sabiston D, Tessler H, Sumers K: Reduction of inflammation following cataract surgery by the nonsteroidal anti-inflammatory drug, flurbiprofen. Ophthal Surg 18:873, 1987.
23. Wong VG, Hersch EM: Methotrexate in the therapy of cyclitis. Trans Am Acad Ophthalmol Otolaryngol 69:279, 1965.
24. Andrasch RH, Pirofski B, Burns RP: Immunosuppressive therapy for severe chronic uveitis. Arch Ophthalmol 96:247, 1978.
25. Tuulonen A, Airaksinen PJ: Laser trabeculoplasty II in secondary glaucoma and after failed trabeculectomy in primary open angle glaucoma. Acta Ophthalmol 61:1016, 1983.
26. Lieberman MF, Hoskins HD Jr, Hetherington J Jr: Laser trabeculoplasty and the glaucomas. Ophthalmology 90:790, 1983.
27. Thomas JV, Simmons RJ, Belcher CD III: Argon laser trabeculoplasty in the presurgical glaucoma patient. Ophthalmology 89:187, 1982.
28. Hoskins HD: Secondary glaucomas. In Heilmann K, Richardson

KT (eds): Glaucoma: Concepts of a Disease. Stuttgart, Germany, Georg Thieme, 1978, p 377.

29. Jampel HD, Jabs DA, Quigley HA: Trabeculoplasty with 5-fluorouracil for adult inflammatory glaucoma. Am J Ophthalmol 109:168, 1990.

30. Melamed S, Fiore PM: Molteno implant surgery in refractory glaucoma. Surv Ophthalmol 34:441, 1990.

31. Fuchs E: Ueber Komplikatintionen der Heterochromie. Z Augenheilkd 15:191, 1906.

32. Franceschetti A: Heterochromic cyclitis (Fuchs' syndrome). Am J Ophthalmol 39:50, 1955.

33. Kimura SJ, Hogan MJ, Thygeson P: Fuchs' syndrome of heterochromic cyclitis. Arch Ophthalmol 100:1622, 1982.

34. Perry HD, Yanoff M, Scheie HG: Rubeosis in Fuchs' heterochromic iridocyclitis. Arch Ophthalmol 93:337, 1975.

35. Kimura SJ: Fuchs' syndrome of heterochromia cyclitis in brown-eyed patients. Trans Am Ophthalmol Soc 76:76, 1978.

36. O'Conner GR: Heterochromic iridocyclitis. Trans Ophthalmol Soc UK 104:219, 1985.

37. Ward DM, Hart CT: Complicated cataract extraction in Fuchs' heterochromic uveitis. Br J Ophthalmol 51:530, 1967.

38. Feldman ST, Deutch TA: Hyphema following Honan balloon use in Fuchs' heterochromic iridocyclitis. Arch Ophthalmol 104:967, 1986.

39. Smith RE, O'Conner GR: Cataract extraction in Fuchs' syndrome. Arch Ophthalmol 91:39, 1974.

40. Gee SS, Tabbara KF: Extracapsular cataract extraction in Fuchs' heterochromic iridocyclitis. Am J Ophthalmol 108:310, 1989.

41. Saari M, Vuorre I, Nieminen H: Fuchs' heterochromic cyclitis: A simultaneous bilateral fluorescein angiography study of the iris. Br J Ophthalmol 62:715, 1978.

42. Liesigang TJ: Clinical features and prognosis in Fuchs' uveitis syndrome. Arch Ophthalmol 100:1622, 1982.

43. Arffa RC, Schlaegel TF: Chorioretinal scars in Fuchs' heterochromic iridocyclitis. Arch Ophthalmol 102:1153, 1984.

44. De Abreu MT, Belfort R Jr, Hirata PS: Fuchs' heterochromic cyclitis and ocular toxoplasmosis. Am J Ophthalmol 93:739, 1982.

45. Francois J: Nouvelle contribution à l'heterochromie de Fuchs. Bull Soc Belge Ophthalmol 102:607, 1952.

46. Huber A: Glaucoma as a complication in heterochromia of Fuchs. Ophthalmologica 142:66, 1961.

47. Francois J, Beheyt J: Heterochromie de Fuchs bilaterale. Ann Ocul (Paris) 188:55, 1955.

48. Tabbut BR, Tessler HH, Williams D: Fuchs' heterochromic iridocyclitis in blacks. Arch Ophthalmol 106:1688, 1988.

49. Melamed S, Lahav M, Sandbank U, et al: Fuchs' heterochromia iridocyclitis: An electron microscopic study of the iris. Invest Ophthalmol Vis Sci 17:1193, 1978.

50. James DG, Neville E, Walker A: Immunology of sarcoidosis. Am J Med 59:388, 1975.

51. Johns CJ, Schonfeld SA, Scott PP, et al: Longitudinal study of chronic sarcoidosis with low-dose maintenance corticosteroid therapy. Ann N Y Acad Sci 465:702, 1986.

52. James DG, Anderson R, Langley D, Ainslie D: Ocular sarcoidosis. Br J Ophthalmol 48:461, 1964.

53. Obenauf CD, Shaw HE, Sydnor CF, Klintworth GK: Sarcoidosis and its ophthalmic manifestations. Am J Ophthalmol 86:648, 1978.

54. Siltzbach LE, James DG, Neville E, et al: Course and prognosis of sarcoidosis around the world. Am J Med 57:847, 1974.

55. Gould H, Kaufman HE: Sarcoid of the fundus. Arch Ophthalmol 65:453, 1961.

56. Iwata K, Nanba K, Sobue K, Abe H: Ocular sarcoidosis: Evaluation of intraocular findings. Ann N Y Acad Sci 278:445, 1976.

57. Karma A, Huti E, Poukkula A: Course and outcome of ocular sarcoidosis. Am J Ophthalmol 106:467, 1988.

58. Bielory L, Holland C, Gascon P, Frohman L: Uveitis, cutaneous and neurosarcoid: Treatment with low dose cyclosporine. Transplant Proc 20(Suppl 4):144, 1988.

59. Posner A, Schlossman A: Syndrome of recurrent attacks of glaucoma with cyclitis symptoms. Arch Ophthalmol 39:517, 1948.

60. Posner A, Schlossman A: Further observation on the syndrome of glaucomatocyclitis crisis. Trans Am Acad Ophthalmol Otolaryngol 57:531, 1953.

61. Levatin P: Glaucomatocyclitis crisis occurring in both eyes. Am J Ophthalmol 41:1056, 1956.

62. Theodore FH: Observations on glaucomatocyclitis crisis. Br J Ophthalmol 36:207, 1952.

63. Hart CT, Weatherill JR: Gonioscopy and tonography in glaucomatocyclitis crisis. Br J Ophthalmol 52:682, 1968.

64. Grant WM: Clinical measurements of aqueous outflow. Arch Ophthalmol 46:113, 1951.

65. Nagataki S, Mishima S: Aqueous humor dynamics in glaucomatocyclitis crisis. Invest Ophthalmol 15:365, 1976.

66. Spivey BE, Armaly MF: Tonographic findings in glaucomatocyclitis crisis. Am J Ophthalmol 55:47, 1963.

67. Raitta C, Vannas A: Glaucomatocyclitis crisis. Arch Ophthalmol 95:608, 1977.

68. Bloch-Michel E, Dussaix E, Cerqueti P, Patarin D: Possible role of cytomegalovirus in the etiology of the Posner-Schlossman syndrome. Int Ophthalmol 11:95, 1987.

69. Masuda K, Izawa Y, Mishima S: Prostaglandins and glaucomatocyclitis crisis. Jpn J Ophthalmol 19:368, 1975.

70. Eakins KE: Increased intraocular pressure produced by prostaglandins E1 and E2 in the cat eye. Exp Eye Res 10:87, 1970.

71. Kass MA, Becker B, Kolker AE: Glaucomatocyclitis crisis and primary open-angle glaucoma. Am J Ophthalmol 75:668, 1973.

72. Hung PT, Chang JM: Treatment of glaucomatocyclitis crisis. Am J Ophthalmol 77:169, 1974.

73. Varma R, Katz LJ, Spaeth GL: Surgical treatment of acute glaucomatocyclitis crisis in a patient with primary open angle glaucoma. Am J Ophthalmol 105:99, 1988.

74. Falcon MG, Williams HP: Herpes simplex kerato-uveitis and glaucoma. Trans Ophthalmol Soc UK 98:101, 1978.

75. Townsend WM, Kaufman HE: Pathogenisis of glaucoma and endothelial changes in herpetic kerato-uveitis in rabbits. Am J Ophthalmol 71:904, 1971.

76. Hogan MJ, Kimura SJ, Thygeson P: Pathology of herpes simplex keratitis. Trans Am Ophthalmol Soc 61:75, 1963.

77. Witmer R, Iwamoto J: Electron microscope observation of herpes-like particles. Arch Ophthalmol 79:331, 1968.

78. Thygeson P: Chronic herpetic kerato-uveitis. Trans Am Ophthalmol Soc 65:211, 1967.

79. Liesegang TJ: Ocular complication from herpes zoster ophthalmicus. Ophthalmology 92:316, 1985.

80. Pavan-Langston DR: Ocular viral diseases. In Galasso GJ, Merigan TC, Buchanan RA (eds): Antiviral Agents and Viral Diseases of Man. New York, Raven Press, 1979, pp 253–303.

81. Haynes RE: Varicella zoster infection in normal and compromised hosts. In Galasso GJ, Merigan TC, Buchanan RA (eds): Antiviral Agents and Viral Diseases of Man. New York, Raven Press, 1979, pp 647–679.

82. Womack LW, Liesegang TJ: Complication of herpes zoster ophthalmicus. Arch Ophthalmol 101:42, 1983.

83. Raber I, Laibson PR: Herpes zoster ophthalmicus. In Liebowitz H (ed): Corneal Disorders: Clinical Diagnosis and Management. Philadelphia, WB Saunders, 1984, p 404.

84. Sears ML, Fenton RH: Unusual corneal lesion following herpes ophthalmicus. Br J Ophthalmol 51:775, 1967.

85. Epstein DL: Chandler and Grant's Glaucoma, 3rd ed. Philadelphia, Lea & Febiger, 1986.

86. Naumann G, Gass JDM, Font RL: Histopathology of herpes zoster ophthalmicus. Am J Ophthalmol 65:533, 1968.

87. Hedges DR, Albert DM: The progression of the ocular abnormalities of herpes zoster: Histopathologic observations of nine cases. Ophthalmology 89:165, 1982.

88. Cobo LM, Foulks JN, Liesegang T, et al: Oral acyclovir in the therapy of acute herpes zoster ophthalmicus: An interim report. Ophthalmology 92:1574, 1985.

89. Cobo LM, Foulks JN, Liesegang T, et al: Oral acyclovir in the therapy of acute herpes zoster ophthalmicus. Ophthalmology 93:763, 1986.

90. Roth M, Simmons RJ: Glaucoma associated with precipitates on the trabecular meshwork. Ophthalmology 86:1613, 1979.

91. Fiore PM, Melamed S, Epstein DL: Trabecular precipitates and elevated intraocular pressure following argon-laser trabeculoplasty. Ophthalmic Surg 20:697, 1989.

92. Fiumara NJ: Syphilis in newborn children. Clin Obstet Gynecol 18:183, 1975.
93. Wilhelmus KR, Yokoyama CM: Syphilitic episcleritis and scleritis. Am J Ophthalmol 104:595, 1987.
94. Lichter PR, Shaffer RN: Interstitial keratitis and glaucoma. Am J Ophthalmol 68:241, 1969.
95. Tsukahara S: Secondary glaucoma due to inactive congenital syphilitic interstitial keratitis. Ophthalmologica 174:188, 1977.
96. Knox DL: Glaucoma following syphilitic interstitial keratitis. Arch Ophthalmol 66:44, 1961.
97. Sugar HS: Late glaucoma associated with inactive syphilitic interstitial keratitis. Am J Ophthalmol 53:602, 1962.
98. Grant WM: Late glaucoma after interstitial keratitis. Am J Ophthalmol 79:87, 1975.
99. VanHorn DI, Schultz RE: Electron microscopy of syphilitic interstitial keratitis. Invest Ophthalmol 10:469, 1971.
100. Luyckx-Bacus J, Delmarcelle Y: Recherches biométriques sur des yeaux presentant une microcornée ou une megalocornée. Bull Soc Belge Ophthalmol 149:433, 1968.
101. Calabro JJ, Mareschano JM: The early natural history of juvenile rheumatoid arthritis. Med Clin North Am 52:567, 1968.
102. Still GF: On a form of chronic disease in children. Med Chir Trans 80:47, 1897.
103. Calabro JJ, Parrino GR, Atchoo PP, et al: Chronic iridocyclitis in juvenile arthritis. Arthritis Rheum 13:406, 1970.
104. Schaller J, Kupfer C, Wedgwood RJ: Iridocyclitis in juvenile rheumatoid arthritis. Pediatrics 44:92, 1969.
105. Smiley WK: Ocular involvement in juvenile rheumatoid arthritis (Still's disease). Proc R Soc Med 66:1163, 1973.
106. Chylack LT, Bierfang DC, Bellows AR, Stillman JS: Ocular manifestations of juvenile rheumatoid arthritis. Am J Ophthalmol 79:1026, 1975.
107. Hinzpeter EN, Naumann G, Bartelheimer HK: Ocular histopathology in Still's disease. Ophthalmol Res 2:16, 1971.
108. Kanski JJ: Anterior uveitis in juvenile rheumatoid arthritis. Arch Ophthalmol 95:1794, 1977.
109. Key SN III, Kimura SJ: Iridocyclitis associated with juvenile rheumatoid arthritis. Am J Ophthalmol 80:425, 1975.
110. Wolf MD, Lichter PR, Ragsdale CG: Prognostic factors in the uveitis of juvenile rheumatoid arthritis. Ophthalmology 94:1242, 1987.
111. Hass JS: Surgical treatment of open angle glaucoma. In Symposium on Glaucoma: Transactions of the New Orleans Academy of Ophthalmology. St. Louis, CV Mosby, 1967.
112. Watson PG, Hayreh SS: Scleritis and episcleritis. Br J Ophthalmol 60:163, 1976.
113. Harbin T, Pollack J: Glaucoma in episcleritis. Arch Ophthalmol 93:948, 1795.
114. Wilhelmus K, Grierson I, Watson PG: Histopathologic and clinical associations of scleritis and glaucoma. Am J Ophthalmol 91:679, 1981.
115. McGavin DD, Williamson J, Forrester JV, et al: Episcleritis and scleritis: A study of the clinical manifestation and associations with rheumatoid arthritis. Br J Ophthalmol 60:192, 1976.
116. Watson PG, Hazleman BL: The Sclera and Systemic Disorders. London, WB Saunders, 1976, pp 155–201.
117. Quinlan MP, Hitchings RA: Angle closure glaucoma secondary to posterior scleritis. Br J Ophthalmol 62:330, 1978.
118. Philips CD: Angle closure glaucoma secondary to ciliary body swelling. Arch Ophthalmol 92:287, 1974.
119. Watson PG: The management of scleritis. In Bellows JD (ed): Contemporary Ophthalmology Honoring Sir Stewart Duck-Elder. Baltimore, Williams & Wilkins, 1972, pp 77–78.
120. Watson PG, Grierson I: The place of trabeculectomy in the treatment of glaucoma. Ophthalmology 88:175, 1981.

Chapter 125

■

Glaucoma Associated With Ocular Trauma

DAVID P. TINGEY and BRADFORD J. SHINGLETON

Long after the immediate problems of ocular trauma have been resolved, glaucoma may persist or reappear even years or decades later. Awareness of the various forms and pathogenesis of glaucoma in traumatized eyes is important in early detection and treatment as well as recognizing which eyes might be at future risk for the development of late-onset glaucoma.

Following an ocular injury, the intraocular pressure may be found initially to be high or low. Several mechanisms exist to explain a low pressure. These mechanisms include aqueous hyposecretion on the basis of ciliary contusion and inflammation, increased egress of aqueous through a cyclodialysis cleft, or loss of integrity of the wall of the globe. Elevated intraocular pressure has multiple causes as well, all of which tend to reflect a reduced facility of outflow of aqueous humor.

It is useful to categorize the types of glaucoma in trauma as either immediate onset or delayed onset (Table 125–1). The type of trauma is also important to consider and is conventionally divided into blunt and penetrating trauma. A broader classification would include chemicals, electromagnetic radiation, and surgery as additional causes of trauma that might induce glaucoma.

IMMEDIATE EARLY-ONSET GLAUCOMA AFTER TRAUMA

Contusion

Occasionally, intraocular pressure elevation in the setting of blunt trauma is noted in the absence of any obvious intraocular damage. The angle is typically open, and there is no evidence of angle recession, trabecular disruption, or hyphema. Inflammation in the form of flare and cells in the anterior chamber may be present. The presumed mechanism of this pressure rise is acute inflammation of the trabecular meshwork with a corresponding reduction in the facility of outflow. This pres-

Table 125–1. IMMEDIATE AND DELAYED CAUSES OF TRAUMATIC GLAUCOMA

Immediate	Delayed
Contusion	Angle recession
Trabecular disruption	Peripheral anterior synechiae
Hyphema	Lens induced
Massive choroidal hemorrhage	Phacolytic
Chemical (alkali)	Phacomorphic
	Lens particle
	Lens subluxation
	Ghost cells
	Closure of cyclodialysis cleft
	Fibrous/epithelial downgrowth
	Retained intraocular foreign body
	Rhegmatogenous retinal detachment

sure rise is typically self-limited, and improvement may be hastened by a short course of topical antiinflammatory agents.

Trabecular Disruption

Careful gonioscopy within 48 hr of injury in patients with hyphema has documented evidence of trauma-related changes in the trabecular zone.[1] These abnormalities vary from sharply demarcated hemorrhage into Schlemm's canal and possibly the outer trabecular sheets to full-thickness rupture of the trabecular meshwork for part of its circumference. A trabecular flap may be created with a point of rupture at or just below the insertion of the trabecular sheets at Schwalbe's line. Hinging of the flap occurs at the region of the scleral spur. These lesions may or may not be associated with increased intraocular pressure at the time of injury. There are often other factors such as inflammation that could also account for the increase in intraocular pressure. Trabecular lesions tend to scar with time and become more difficult to recognize. It has been hypothesized by some that angle recession is only a marker for significant injury and that the late development of glaucoma may correlate better with the amount of trabecular disruption observed acutely.[1]

Hyphema

The presence of a hyphema following ocular trauma is an indicator of significant intraocular injury. There are several possible mechanisms for the occurrence of glaucoma in the setting of acute hyphema. These include contusion of the outflow apparatus, physical disruption of the meshwork, and plugging of the meshwork with red blood cells.

Acute pressure elevation may pose a threat to vision as a result of optic nerve damage or corneal staining. Intraocular pressure can be elevated in as many as 27 percent of patients acutely; however, this pressure elevation is often mild and self-limited.[2]

The level and duration of intraocular pressure elevation that is safe for the optic nerve is difficult to quantitate. Susceptibility varies among patients. Goldberg[2] found in a prospective study of 137 patients with traumatic hyphema that optic atrophy tended to occur with pressures at or greater than 35 mmHg and durations varying from 5 to 14 days. Optic atrophy as a direct result of trauma may be a confounding factor.

The level and duration of intraocular pressure elevation required to produce corneal blood staining is also difficult to quantitate. Blood staining occurs more readily in the presence of a total hyphema that is allowed to remain for at least 6 days with intraocular pressures elevated above 25 mmHg.[2] Corneas with endothelial damage secondary to trauma or preexisting disease are more susceptible to blood staining with only marginal pressure elevation.

Severely elevated intraocular pressure may be found in patients with sickle cell hemoglobinopathy following accumulation of even small amounts of blood in the anterior chamber.[3] The presumed mechanism is obstruction of trabecular outflow by sickled erythrocytes. Optic atrophy at only slightly elevated intraocular pressures has also been reported in these patients.[3, 4] Suboptimal blood flow to the optic nerve on the basis of sickling has been proposed as a mechanism for this sensitivity. Patients with either sickle cell disease or trait are susceptible to these complications. Several of the conventional pharmacologic agents used for lowering intraocular pressure may be potentially harmful in the patient with sickle cell hemoglobinopathy. Carbonic anhydrase inhibitors may increase sickling as a result of systemic acidosis. Since methazolamide theoretically causes less systemic acidosis than acetazolamide, methazolamide may be a safer choice in this clinical situation. Carbonic anhydrase inhibitors or osmotic agents may increase hemoconcentration and viscosity in an already compromised ocular microvasculature. Acetazolamide can increase ascorbate in the aqueous, and this may worsen the sickling process. Epinephrine agents may further compromise blood flow as a result of vasoconstriction. The presence of hyphema in the sickling patient calls for the judicious use of pharmacologic agents to control even mild pressure elevations and a lower threshold on the part of the clinician for performing a washout of sickled erythrocytes from the anterior chamber.

Rebleeding into the anterior chamber after an initial hyphema can be a potentially devastating complication. This typically occurs between days 2 and 6 after the initial injury. The reported incidence of rebleeding varies between 6 and 33 percent.[2, 4–6] Rebleeding is of particular concern because it may be accompanied by markedly elevated intraocular pressure and its attendant complications. Aminocaproic acid has been shown to decrease the rate of rebleeding in some patients.[4, 6] Some authors have advocated the use of systemic steroids for reducing the incidence of secondary hemorrhage[7, 8]; however, Spoor and associates showed no benefit from oral corticosteroids in a prospective study.[9] Dieste and associates have described an unusual intraocular pressure complication of the use of aminocaproic acid. In patients with larger hyphemas (more than one third of the anterior chamber), exaggerated clot lysis occasionally develops 1 to 2 days after cessation of aminocaproic acid.[10] The lysed cells and debris obstruct the trabecular outflow of aqueous humor. Intraocular pressure may be refractory to medical treatment and may require surgery.

The treatment of acute pressure elevation as a result of hyphema entails the use of conventional pharmacologic agents to control pressure elevation with the exception of miotic agents. Cycloplegic agents and topical steroids are often used as well for the associated traumatic iritis. If topical or systemic steroids are used for the treatment of hyphema, the physician must be aware of the potential effect of intraocular pressure elevation with chronic steroid use in some patients.

Surgical intervention is reserved for cases in which the intraocular pressure cannot be controlled by conventional medicines and the pressure is potentially threatening the optic nerve or cornea. Many surgical procedures have been reported, including anterior chamber washout,[11] clot expression,[12] delivery of the clot with a cryoprobe,[13] automated hyphemectomy,[14] and ultrasonic emulsification and aspiration.[15] Adjunctive procedures have included peripheral iridectomy in the setting of pupillary block resulting from the clot.[16] Trabeculectomy for short-term pressure control has been utilized.[17] Cyclodiathermy to control recurrent bleeding has also been described.[18]

Paracentesis and anterior chamber washout is the simplest and safest procedure. Evacuation of suspended anterior chamber cells and debris is effective in lowering intraocular pressure and can be performed by simple irrigation or by manual coaxial irrigation or aspiration. Removal of the entire clot is not required. In addition to being relatively easy to perform, this technique spares the conjunctiva for future filtration surgery if required (Fig. 125–1 A and B).

Glaucoma may also occur several years after the initial hyphema. This glaucoma may be on the basis of any of several mechanisms that are dealt with later in this chapter.

Massive Choroidal Hemorrhage

The occurrence of massive hemorrhage into the choroidal space is a rare cause of acute pressure elevation following ocular trauma. Typically, the anterior chamber is shallow both axially and peripherally. The red reflex is poor, and indirect ophthalmoscopy reveals choroidal elevation. The lens-iris diaphragm is pushed forward, resulting in obstruction of the trabecular meshwork. The intraocular pressure may be markedly elevated as a result of this secondary angle-closure.

Initial treatment consists of a topical β-blocker as well as oral carbonic anhydrase inhibitors and a systemic hyperosmotic agent, if needed. Miotics should be avoided because they may cause further shallowing of the anterior chamber. Cycloplegics may be effective in tightening the lens-zonule diaphragm and deepening the

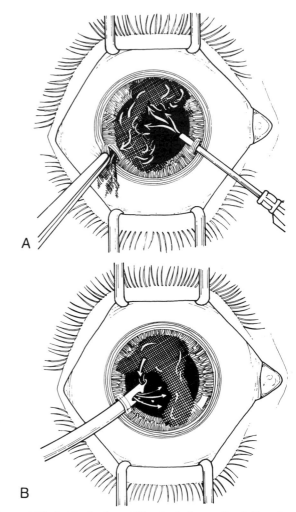

Figure 125–1. Illustration of the technique of anterior chamber washout for hyphema with the use of direct irrigation (A) and the Simcoe coaxial irrigation/aspiration cannula (B).

anterior chamber. High-dose oral steroids are recommended by some people who believe that steroids will stabilize the choroidal vessels.

Surgical intervention is required occasionally. Drainage of blood from the suprachoroidal space may be warranted in certain situations. Indications include persistent elevation of intraocular pressure that has not responded to medical therapy, lens-cornea apposition, and so-called "kissing choroidals" with retina-to-retina apposition. Generally it is advisable to wait for several days if possible before draining the blood, because this allows time for the blood to be fully sequestered in the suprachoroidal space.

Chronic synechial closure of the angle may be a long-term sequela of massive suprachoroidal hemorrhage. This may require later intervention in the form of medical therapy, laser iridoplasty (gonioplasty), surgical goniosynechialysis, conventional filtration surgery, or a cycloablative procedure depending on the individual circumstances.

In the setting of age-related macular degeneration, trauma may rarely lead to massive choroidal detachment with intraretinal dissection. This results in a "Y-suture" apposition of posterior segment tissues pushing the lens-iris diaphragm forward and leading to angle-closure.[19] Intraocular pressure rises dramatically, and vision is often reduced to no light perception. Medical or surgical therapy rarely restores vision.

Chemical Trauma

Alkali burns are well known for their ability to cause severe damage to the ocular structures as a result of tissue saponification. This is in contrast to acids that more often produce an injury that is self-limited as a result of tissue coagulation. Glaucoma is more often associated with alkali burns, and thus this section is restricted to alkali burns.

Glaucoma may be an immediate or late complication of an alkali burn. Hughes[20] in 1946 documented several cases of elevated intraocular pressure that occurred late after an alkali burn. It was not until the 1960s that pressure elevation was documented acutely following an alkali burn.[21, 22] This pressure rise occurred in the setting of a gonioscopically open angle.

The nature of the acute pressure rise was studied in rabbits by Chiang and associates who demonstrated a dicrotic pressure rise following the application of sodium hydroxide.[23] There was an immediate pressure rise of 40 mmHg followed by a gradual decline in pressure to 20 mmHg above normal in 10 min. A second, gradual pressure rise then occurred, reaching 40 mmHg above normal at 1 hr. At 3 hr after application, the pressure was 20 mmHg above normal.

Paterson and Pfister[24] set out to determine the exact mechanisms of these pressure rises in rabbits. They believed that shrinkage of the outer coats of the eye was the major cause of the initial pressure spike. Lid contraction and extraocular muscle spasm were not significant factors in raising the pressure. Prostaglandin release with inflammation was implicated as the major factor in the second hypertensive phase. They also postulated that blockage of the trabecular meshwork with inflammatory debris might play a later role in the rise in intraocular pressure.

Intraocular pressure may be overlooked in the initial evaluation and treatment of the patient with a severe alkali burn. In addition to the conventional therapies directed at the anterior segment consequences of an alkali burn, treatment of any pressure elevation is important. This includes topical β-blocker therapy, oral carbonic anhydrase inhibitors, and systemic hyperosmotic agents as needed. Miotics should be avoided in the setting of intense inflammation. Topical epinephrine has been effective in blunting the second hypertensive phase in experimental animal models. Antiinflammatory medications and adequate cycloplegia are also important. Anterior chamber paracentesis and aspiration of aqueous fluid may be required if the intraocular pressure is extremely high during the initial hypertensive phase. This reduces the intraocular pressure and removes debris and alkali directly from the anterior chamber.

Glaucoma may appear or reappear years after the initial alkali burn. This is generally considered to be a result of ongoing inflammation with secondary peripheral anterior synechiae. The treatment of this late-onset glaucoma would include conventional medical and surgical therapies addressed at this underlying mechanism of chronic angle-closure.

LATE-ONSET GLAUCOMA AFTER OCULAR TRAUMA
Angle Recession

Collins[25] gave the first pathologic description of angle recession resulting from blunt trauma to the eye in 1892. In 1949 D'Ombrain[26] commented on his observations of a chronic traumatic glaucoma that he believed was the result of a proliferative lesion scarring the trabecular meshwork. He made no observation of pathologic deepening of the anterior chamber angle. In 1962 Wolff and Zimmerman[27] tied together the pathologic entity of angle recession with the clinical phenomenon of unilateral chronic glaucoma following trauma.

Angle recession is common following blunt ocular trauma. In patients with traumatic hyphema, angle recession occurs in 71 to 100 percent of eyes.[28–31] Despite this high incidence of angle recession, glaucoma is uncommon, occurring in approximately 7 to 9 percent of eyes.[28, 30, 32] Some authors have attempted to correlate the degree of angle recession with the development of glaucoma. Alper[33] believed that the risk of glaucoma developing was highest if more than 240 degrees of angle appeared recessed.

Elevated intraocular pressure may occur months or decades following the initial injury. Blanton[28] observed a bimodal pattern with glaucoma occurring either within the first year or after 10 yr. The earlier onset group often had less angle recession, and the intraocular pressure rise was transient in some patients. Other authors have found that extensive angle recession equal to or more than 270 degrees was usually present in the early-onset group.[1]

Pathologically, recession of the anterior chamber angle appears as a separation between the longitudinal and circular fibers of the ciliary body muscle.[27] The longitudinal muscles characteristically remain attached to the scleral spur. There is retrodisplacement of the iris root. Iridodialysis or cyclodialysis may also be observed. The lens may display changes such as cataract, subluxation, or dislocation. In the acute setting, frank hyphema may also be observed. Late evaluation shows the effects of healing. The inner circular muscle of the ciliary muscle may be atrophied, giving the ciliary body band a broad and more fusiform appearance. The trabecular meshwork displays variable degrees of fibrosis and hyalinization.

A newly formed hyaline membrane may be observed. This hyaline change is continuous with Descemet's membrane and extends over the trabecular meshwork for variable distances. Peripheral anterior synechiae may also be present.

The clinical presentation of glaucoma secondary to angle recession is variable and depends somewhat on the time of presentation relative to the initial injury. Elevated intraocular pressure immediately after injury may be due to extensive angle recession, although it may also be due to other causes as cited earlier in this chapter. More often angle-recession glaucoma presents years after the initial event as a chronic unilateral glaucoma. In a pathologic review of 100 eyes enucleated for unilateral glaucoma, Miles and Boniuk[34] found 11 eyes with angle deformity as the principal cause for their glaucoma. None of these deformities had been recognized clinically. Eight of these 11 patients gave a history of previous trauma to the eye ranging from 6 mo to 24 yr prior to the onset of glaucoma.

It is important to attempt to elicit a history of previous ocular trauma when confronted with a case of unilateral glaucoma. Examination can often reveal asymmetry of anterior chamber depth between the two eyes with the involved eye having a greater chamber depth. There are often associated findings of ocular trauma, such as tears in the iris sphincter or root. The iris stroma may be thinned with pigmentation occurring in clumps. There may be a difference in pigmentation between the two irides as a result of blood or pigment having been dispersed into the chamber at the time of injury. Tonjum[35] evaluated injured eyes acutely and found that the pupillary sphincter was often paretic or paralyzed in the same sector as the chamber angle deformity. This pupillary change often, but not always, recovered with time. The lens may demonstrate subluxation with iridophacodonesis, or it may be frankly dislocated. Cataractous changes may also be present. The posterior segment can also display signs of previous trauma such as pigment in the vitreous, macular edema, retinal pigment epithelial hyperplasia, choroidal or retinal scars, retinal tearing, or frank retinal detachment.

Gonioscopy reveals a deepening of the angle in which the exposed face of the ciliary body appears wider than is usual and the iris root appears posteriorly displaced (Fig. 125–2). Uveal processes are disrupted, and the scleral spur may appear abnormally white. Bilateral, simultaneous Koeppe gonioscopy is an effective technique for detecting subtle recession. A gray-white membrane is often observed covering the angle recess many years after the initial injury.[33] The optic nerve may display typical glaucomatous cupping that may be far advanced as the late and insidious onset of this glaucoma occasionally avoids early detection.

The mechanism of intraocular pressure elevation in this secondary open-angle glaucoma appears to be a decrease in aqueous filtration. Herschler[1] emphasized that the tear into the ciliary body is more of a marker for significant injury and that the glaucoma itself is related to accompanying scarring of the trabecular meshwork. He was able to document a high incidence of visible damage to the trabecular meshwork and Schlemm's canal in eyes gonioscoped within 48 hr of injury. These trabecular lesions became less apparent over time as opposed to the ciliary body tears. The facility of outflow, as measured by tonography, is re-

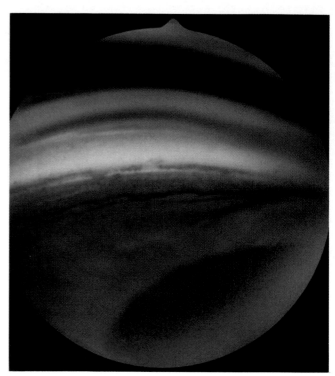

Figure 125–2. Gonioscopic view of traumatic angle recession.

duced and correlates with the degree of angle recession and glaucoma.[29] Tesluk and Spaeth studied 13 patients who had developed unilateral angle recession glaucoma and found that approximately 50 percent of these patients had evidence of frank or probable glaucoma in their fellow eye on the basis of intraocular pressure, disc appearance, or visual field changes.[36] This has raised the question of a possible underlying predisposition to the development of glaucoma in some injured patients.

The treatment of angle-recession glaucoma falls along conventional medical therapeutic routes. Failure of medicines to control the pressure requires further intervention. Argon laser trabeculoplasty may be helpful in some patients provided that the initial intraocular pressure is not too high.[37, 38] Filtration surgery is often effective in controlling the pressure if the conjunctiva has not been previously scarred by the injury itself or previous surgical interventions resulting from related ocular injuries such as cataract or retinal detachment. Failure of conventional filtration techniques may lead to the subsequent placement of a seton or to a cyclodestructive procedure depending on the individual circumstances.

Peripheral Anterior Synechiae

Attachment of peripheral iris to the cornea or chamber angle has many causes. The essential elements required for peripheral anterior synechia formation are apposition and inflammation. Both of these may occur in the setting of ocular trauma. Organization of blood and inflammatory debris in the angle can occur following hyphema. Penetrating trauma may shallow the chamber for extended periods, resulting in extensive synechial closure of the angle. Endothelialization of the angle has been observed following blunt trauma with resultant angle-closure. Penetrating trauma may result in epithelial or fibrous downgrowth into the anterior chamber causing synechial closure. Massive choroidal hemorrhage leads to apposition, which may remain after the hemorrhage has resolved. The occurrence of synechial closure following trauma necessitates careful and repeated gonioscopy following a traumatic event.

Treatment of synechial closure can often be directed at attempting to reopen the angle, particularly if the intervention occurs early rather than late. Iridogonioplasty with the argon laser may be sufficient to pull the iris away from the angle. Failing this, surgical goniosynechialysis may be effective in reopening the angle for filtration. If the angle is permanently closed with ensuing high intraocular pressure, therapy is directed at lowering the pressure with more conventional medical and surgical methods.

Ghost Cell Glaucoma

Ghost cell glaucoma was initially described by Campbell, Simmons, and Grant.[39] They showed that following vitreous hemorrhage, fresh red blood cells degenerated into ghost cells in the vitreous usually within 1 or 2 wk (Fig. 125–3). In the event of anterior hyaloid face disruption, these cells gain access to the anterior chamber. The normal red blood cell is pliable and passes through the trabecular meshwork, whereas the ghost cells are rigid and do not pass through the meshwork easily. These cells produce an obstruction to aqueous outflow with a resultant rise in intraocular pressure. Ghost cell glaucoma has been reported to occur after cataract extraction, vitrectomy, or trauma.

Campbell reviewed the clinical characteristics of 14 patients with traumatic ghost cell glaucoma.[40] He found that all patients shared a common clinical course: severe trauma to the eye causing anterior chamber and vitreous hemorrhages. The anterior chamber hemorrhages gradually cleared. In the vitreous, the fresh red blood cells slowly converted to ghost cells that were then able to

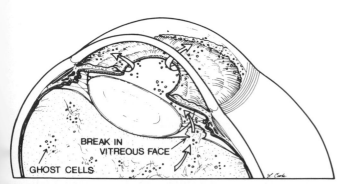

Figure 125–3. Illustration of ghost cell glaucoma, demonstrating hemorrhage within the vitreous cavity and escape of ghost cells through a break in the anterior hyaloid face into the anterior chamber.

pass forward through a disrupted hyaloid face. The ghost cells had a characteristic ochre color that distinguished them from fresh red blood cells. Occasionally, they would layer out in the anterior chamber and create a "pseudohypopyon." The glaucoma occurred anywhere from 2 wk to 3 mo following the trauma but was most common 1 mo after the injury. The intraocular pressure was usually in the range of 30 to 50 mmHg.

Histopathologic examination of one eye revealed a relatively normal-looking angle with ghost cells in the anterior chamber. The vitreous cavity demonstrated degenerated macrophages laden with red blood cell debris along the hyaloid face. Ghost cells were present in the vitreous cavity. The anterior hyaloid face appeared disrupted. Ghost cells had a characteristic crenated shrunken appearance by phase contrast microscopy. Heinz bodies representing denatured hemoglobin was appreciated in the cytoplasm of some ghost cells.[40]

The treatment of ghost cell glaucoma includes conventional medical therapy followed by surgery in cases that do not respond. Campbell found that less than half of his cases responded to medical therapy alone.[40] The surgery of choice is anterior chamber irrigation, which is often effective. If this should fail, a pars plana vitrectomy may be necessary to ensure complete removal of all blood components trapped in the vitreous body.

Lens-Induced Glaucoma

The lens-induced glaucomas are a group of secondary glaucomas that share the lens as a common pathogenic cause (Fig. 125–4). The angle in this category of glaucomas may be open or closed. The major categories of lens-induced glaucoma are lens dislocation, lens swelling, phacolytic glaucoma, and lens particle glaucoma.[41] All of these glaucomas may be associated with previous trauma to the eye.

Lens Dislocation. The lens may be dislocated or subluxed as a direct result of trauma that disrupts the zonules. Once mobilized the lens may advance forward, producing pupillary block with angle-closure. With a complete dislocation of the lens posteriorly, the pupil may become blocked with vitreous that can also produce a pupillary block angle-closure glaucoma.

Clinically, such patients may present with an acutely painful red eye and decreased vision. A previous history of trauma is helpful in making a diagnosis because the presentation may mimic primary acute angle-closure glaucoma. The cornea is edematous. The chamber is shallowed both axially and peripherally with iris convexity. The angle appears closed gonioscopically. Comparison of refractive error, chamber depth, and angle depth of both eyes may help to rule out primary angle-closure glaucoma if the unaffected eye does not have a shallow configuration. If vitreous is blocking the pupil, this may be appreciated at slit-lamp examination. The posteriorly dislocated lens may also be seen by ophthalmoscopy in these cases.

Treatment of this form of glaucoma is directed at relieving the pupillary block. Generally, this is achieved

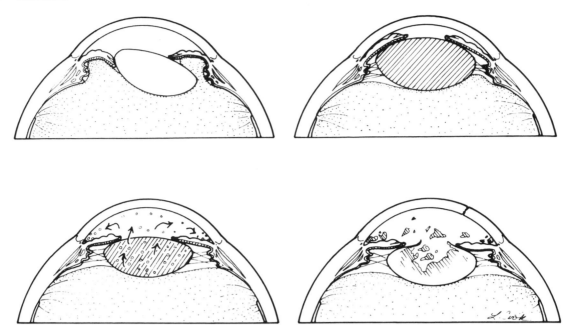

Figure 125–4. Illustration of the four types of lens-induced glaucoma. Clockwise from upper left: lens subluxation, phacomorphic, lens particle, and phacolytic.

with laser iridotomy or surgical iridectomy. Lensectomy may be undertaken only when other methods of visual rehabilitation prove unsuccessful or if pupillary block recurs. Lensectomy may be performed by using an intracapsular technique with anterior vitrectomy as needed, or the lens may be removed via a pars plana lensectomy/vitrectomy approach.

Lens Swelling. A cataract may develop as a result of trauma. Occasionally a cataractous lens becomes intumescent. Such swollen lenses can subsequently cause angle-closure glaucoma as a result of pupillary block or direct angle compromise by mass effect.

A previous history of trauma and asymmetry of anterior chamber depth on clinical examination are vital in establishing a reason for this type of glaucoma.

Cataract surgery relieves the pupillary block and angle compromise and restores vision. Peripheral anterior synechiae may contribute to an elevated intraocular pressure as a result of chronic pupillary block, and each patient should be evaluated carefully for this. Iridogonioplasty or goniosynechiolysis may be required. In cases in which any potential for vision is negligible, iridotomy or iridectomy may be performed without cataract extraction, although cataract removal is still the treatment of choice.

Phacolytic Glaucoma. Phacolytic glaucoma is seen in the setting of a hypermature cataract. An open-angle glaucoma occurs as a result of leakage of high molecular weight proteins through an intact lens capsule. For diagnosis and management, see Chapter 126.

Lens-Particle Glaucoma. Lens-particle glaucoma is characterized by the presence of frankly disrupted lens capsule with obvious fragments of lens material in the anterior chamber. For clinical presentation, diagnosis, and management, see Chapter 126.

Delayed Closure of a Cyclodialysis Cleft

The occurrence of a cyclodialysis cleft following trauma is associated with hypotony as a result of suppression of aqueous production and increased aqueous outflow via the uveoscleral pathway. Goldmann[42] postulated that a reduction in the normal flow of aqueous across the trabecular meshwork resulted in a reduced permeability of the meshwork to aqueous outflow. This is believed to account for the marked acute pressure elevation that can be seen to occur following closure of an existing cyclodialysis cleft.

Delayed closure of a cyclodialysis cleft can be a difficult diagnosis to make. The patient presents with an acutely elevated pressure, corneal edema, a formed anterior chamber, and a gonioscopically open angle. A previous history of trauma should raise the suspicion of the examiner. When closure of a cleft is suspected, treatment with miotics and phenylephrine may be effective in reopening the cleft and in lowering the pressure. A repeat gonioscopy then often provides the diagnosis.

Epithelial Downgrowth

The downgrowth of epithelium into the eye may occur in the presence of a patent fistula from the external surface of the eye to its internal surface or following the implantation of epithelial cells within the eye. This is a rare occurrence that has a poor prognosis when it occurs. The common clinical settings include previous cataract surgery, filtration surgery, and penetrating trauma. See Chapter 138 for a discussion of the clinical findings, diagnosis, and management.

Retained Intraocular Foreign Body

As a form of trauma and penetrating injury, a retained foreign body may be associated with several types of glaucoma. A flat anterior chamber combined with inflammation can result in secondary angle-closure glaucoma following the formation of extensive peripheral anterior synechiae. Prolonged leakage and fistulization at the site of penetration can produce an epithelial downgrowth situation as discussed previously. Frank disruption of the lens capsule may result in lens particle glaucoma, phacomorphic glaucoma, or phacolytic glaucoma. A late manifestation of iron-containing foreign bodies is siderotic glaucoma with its associated heterochromia, mydriasis, and rustlike discoloration of the anterior subcapsular surface of the lens and the posterior corneal surface.

Patients may present immediately with a clear history and evidence of an intraocular foreign body, or they may appear months or years after the initial event in a more subtle fashion with unilateral cataract, chronic inflammation, glaucoma, or reduced retinal function. Ocular examination is directed at looking for evidence of penetration such as a discrete area of iris transillumination, a small lenticular capsular rupture, or a corneal or scleral wound.

A dilated ocular examination may allow direct visualization of a foreign body. Occasionally, a foreign body is located in the anterior chamber angle and is evident on gonioscopy only. Some patients may have signs of chalcosis or siderosis as outlined previously.

Appropriate studies including plain film x-rays, computed tomography scans, and ultrasound are helpful in confirming the diagnosis.

Rhegmatogenous Retinal Detachment

Rhegmatogenous retinal detachment is most commonly associated with ocular hypotension due to a decrease in aqueous production.[43] As many as 5 or 10 percent of patients with rhegmatogenous retinal detachment demonstrate ocular hypertension.[44] This may be the result of preexisting open-angle glaucoma or inflammation secondary to a long-standing detachment. However, there exists a small group of patients with no preexisting glaucoma who develop a secondary open-angle glaucoma that resolves when the retinal detachment is repaired. This was well described by Schwartz[45] who collected 11 such cases. Interestingly, 5 of the 11 cases were associated with previous ocular trauma.

The original proposed mechanism was inflammation of the trabecular meshwork with a resultant decrease in outflow facility. Others[46] hypothesized that pigment was being released and obstructed the trabecular meshwork. Matsuo demonstrated photoreceptors in the aqueous humor by transmission electron microscopy in seven patients with this syndrome. He first proposed that the photoreceptors could be obstructing aqueous outflow.[47]

Unilateral glaucoma in the presence of a rhegmatogenous retinal detachment is an unusual presentation and emphasizes the importance of careful funduscopic examination in all cases of unilateral glaucoma.

Treatment consists of repairing the retinal detachment. This promptly and permanently returns the intraocular pressure to normal, provided that there are no associated ocular abnormalities such as angle recession that could contribute to chronic elevation of intraocular pressure.

REFERENCES

1. Herschler J: Trabecular damage due to blunt anterior segment injury and its relationship to traumatic glaucoma. Trans Am Acad Ophthalmol Otolaryngol 83:239, 1977.
2. Read J, Goldberg MF: Comparison of medical treatment for traumatic hyphema. Trans Am Acad Ophthalmol Otolaryngol 78:799, 1974.
3. Goldberg MF: The diagnosis and treatment of sickled erythrocytes in human hyphemas. Trans Am Ophthalmol Soc 76:481, 1978.
4. Crouch ER, Frenkel M: Aminocaproic acid in the treatment of traumatic hyphema. Am J Ophthalmol 81:355, 1976.
5. Edwards WC, Layden WE: Traumatic hyphema: A report of 184 consecutive cases. Am J Ophthalmol 75:110, 1973.
6. McGetrick JJ, Jampol LM, Goldberg MF, et al: Aminocaproic acid decreases secondary hemorrhage after traumatic hyphema. Arch Ophthalmol 101:1031, 1983.
7. Yasuna E: Management of traumatic hyphema. Arch Ophthalmol 91:190, 1974.
8. Rynne MV, Romano PE: Systemic corticosteroids in the treatment of traumatic hyphema. J Pediatr Ophthalmol Strabismus 17:141, 1980.
9. Spoor TC, Hammer M, Belloso H: Traumatic hyphema: Failure of steroids to alter its course: A double-blind prospective study. Arch Ophthalmol 98:116, 1980.
10. Dieste MC, Hersh PS, Kylstra JA, et al: Intraocular pressure increase associated with epsilon-aminocaproic acid therapy for traumatic hyphema. Am J Ophthalmol 106:383, 1988.
11. Belcher CD, Brown SVL, Simmons RJ: Anterior chamber washout for traumatic hyphema. Ophthalmic Surg 16:475, 1985.
12. Sears ML: Surgical management of black ball hyphema. Trans Acad Ophthalmol Otolaryngol 74:820, 1970.
13. Hill K: Cryoextraction of total hyphema. Arch Ophthalmol 80:368, 1968.
14. McCuen BW, Fung WE: The role of vitrectomy instrumentation in the treatment of severe traumatic hyphema. Am J Ophthalmol 88:930, 1979.
15. Kelman CD, Brooks DL: Ultrasonic emulsification and aspiration of traumatic hyphema: A preliminary report. Am J Ophthalmol 71:1289, 1971.
16. Parrish RK, Bernardino V: Iridectomy in the surgical management of eight ball hyphema. Arch Ophthalmol 100:435, 1982.
17. Weiss JS, Parrish RK, Anderson DR: Surgical therapy of traumatic hyphema. Ophthalmic Surg 14:343, 1983.
18. Gilbert HD, Smith RE: Traumatic hyphema: Treatment of secondary hemorrhage with cyclodiathermy. Ophthalmic Surg 7(3):31, 1975.
19. Pesin SR, Katz LJ, Augsburger JJ, et al: Acute angle closure glaucoma from spontaneous massive hemorrhagic retinal or choroidal detachment. Ophthalmology 97:76, 1990.
20. Hughes WF: Alkali burns of the eye. 1: Review of the literature and summary of present knowledge. Arch Ophthalmol 35:423, 1946.
21. Grant WM: Toxicology of the Eye. Springfield, IL, Charles C Thomas Publisher, 1965, p 35.
22. Highman VN: Early rise in intraocular pressure after ammonia burns. Br Med J 1:359, 1969.
23. Chiang TS, Moorman LR, Thomas RP: Ocular hypertensive response following acid and alkali burns in rabbits. Invest Ophthalmol 10:270, 1971.

24. Paterson CA, Pfister RR: Intraocular pressure changes after alkali burns. Arch Ophthalmol 91:211, 1974.
25. Collins ET: On the pathological examination of three eyes lost from concussion. Trans Ophthalmol Soc UK 12:180, 1892.
26. D'Ombrain A: Traumatic monocular chronic glaucoma. Trans Ophthalmol Soc Aust 5:116, 1986.
27. Wolff SM, Zimmerman LE: Chronic secondary glaucoma: Associated with retrodisplacement of iris root and deepening of the anterior chamber angle secondary to contusion. Am J Ophthalmol 54:547, 1962.
28. Blanton FM: Anterior chamber angle recession and secondary glaucoma: A study of the aftereffects of traumatic hyphemas. Arch Ophthalmol 72:39, 1964.
29. Tonjum AM: Intraocular pressure and facility of outflow late after ocular contusion. Acta Ophthalmol 46:886, 1968.
30. Monney D: Angle recession and secondary glaucoma. Br J Ophthalmol 57:608, 1973.
31. Canavan YM, Archer DB: Anterior segment consequences of blunt ocular injury. Br J Ophthalmol 66:549, 1982.
32. Kaufman JH, Tolpin DW: Glaucoma after traumatic angle recession: A ten year prospective study. Am J Ophthalmol 78:648, 1974.
33. Alper MG: Contusion angle deformity and glaucoma: Gonioscopic observations and clinical course. Arch Ophthalmol 69:455, 1963.
34. Miles DR, Boniuk M: Pathogenesis of unilateral glaucoma: A review of 100 cases. Am J Ophthalmol 62:493, 1962.
35. Tonjum AM: Gonioscopy in traumatic hyphema. Acta Ophthalmol 44:650, 1968.
36. Tesluk GC, Spaeth GL: The occurrence of primary open angle glaucoma in the fellow eye of patients with unilateral angle cleavage glaucoma. Ophthalmology 92:904, 1985.
37. Robin AL, Pollack IP: Argon laser trabeculoplasty in secondary forms of open angle glaucoma. Arch Ophthalmol 101:382, 1983.
38. Thomas JV, Simmons RJ, Belcher CD: Argon laser trabeculoplasty in the pre-surgical glaucoma patient. Ophthalmology 89:187, 1982.
39. Campbell DG, Simmons RJ, Grant WM: Ghost cells as a cause of glaucoma. Am J Ophthalmol 97:2141, 1973.
40. Campbell DG: Ghost cell glaucoma following trauma. Ophthalmology 88:1151, 1981.
41. Epstein DL: Diagnosis and management of lens-induced glaucoma. Ophthalmology 89:227, 1982.
42. Goldmann H: Klinische Studien zum Glaucomproblem. Ophthalmologica 125:16, 1953.
43. Dobbie JG: A study of the intraocular fluid dynamics in retinal detachment. Arch Ophthalmol 69:159, 1963.
44. Linner E: Intraocular pressure in retinal detachment. Acta Ophthalmol 84:101, 1966.
45. Schwartz A: Chronic open angle glaucoma secondary to rhegmatogenous retinal detachment. Am J Ophthalmol 75:205, 1973.
46. Baruch E, Bracha R, Godel V, et al: Glaucoma due to rhegmatogenous retinal detachment; Schwartz's syndrome. Glaucoma 3:229, 1981.
47. Matsuo N, Takabatake M, Ueno H, et al: Photoreceptor outer segments in the aqueous humor in rhegmatogenous retinal detachment. Am J Ophthalmol 101:673, 1986.

Chapter 126

■

Lens-Induced Glaucoma

DAVID M. CHACKO and ROBERT C. ROSENQUIST

Glaucomas in which the lens plays a role, either by size or by position or by causing inflammation, have been classified as lens-induced glaucomas. In the past, significant confusion existed about the terminology and mechanisms causing the glaucoma. Terms such as phacotoxic reaction, phacogenetic glaucoma, phacotopic glaucoma, lens-induced uveitis, and endophthalmitis phacoanaphylactica were used.[1–7]

Some standardization of terminology has occurred in recent years. Phacolytic glaucoma and lens particle glaucoma are secondary open-angle glaucomas. The iridocorneal angle is open, and there is blockage of the trabecular meshwork by lens proteins. Phacomorphic glaucoma and lens displacement glaucoma are secondary angle-closure glaucomas. Phacoanaphylactic uveitis, now termed lens-induced uveitis, is not truly an anaphylactic reaction but is a granulomatous reaction that can result in glaucoma with either open-angle, angle-closure, or combined open-angle and angle-closure glaucoma.

PHACOLYTIC GLAUCOMA
(Fig. 126–1)

The syndrome of glaucoma secondary to hypermature cataracts (Fig. 126–2) was first described by Gifford in

1900. Glaucoma of this type was characterized as having open angles and the presence of large histiocytes in the anterior chamber. Flocks and coworkers hypothesized that the rise in intraocular pressure was due to the blockage of the trabecular meshwork by solubilized protein leaking through intact lens capsules from morgagnian cataracts.[8]

The patients are generally older and have long-standing cataracts and decreased vision. A rapid onset of pain and redness as well as a further decrease in vision are typical. Clinical examination reveals elevated intraocular pressures, usually in excess of 35 mmHg. Perilimbal injection and corneal edema are usually present. The iridocorneal angle is usually open with essentially no peripheral anterior synechiae, but gonioscopic evaluation is not always possible due to corneal edema. The anterior chamber is deep with dense flare and minimal to moderate cells. Occasionally, iridescent particles have been reported in the aqueous.[9] White flocculent material can often be seen attached to the lens capsule and floating in the anterior chamber, occasionally forming a pseudohypopyon. No true keratic precipitates are seen.[10–12]

Histopathologic studies of enucleated eyes with phacolytic glaucoma have indicated that the lens capsule is usually intact, although the posterior capsule is fre-

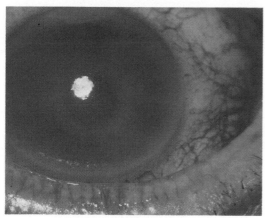

Figure 126–1. Phacolytic glaucoma. (Courtesy of David D. Donaldson, M.D.)

quently attenuated. The lens protein has liquified and leaks through an intact capsule.[8] Lens protein induces chemotactic migration of macrophages, the principal inflammatory cell in phacolytic glaucoma.[13] These large cells have small nuclei and foamy cytoplasm due to the ingested lens proteins.[14] The iridescent particles seen in the aqueous correspond to calcium oxalate and cholesterol crystals.[15, 16]

Significant ambiguity has existed in the literature regarding the exact mechanism of increased intraocular pressure in phacolytic glaucoma. Initially, it was suggested that both bloated macrophages and lens debris were blocking the trabecular meshwork.[8] Gradually the emphasis shifted to the macrophages, because it was shown histologically that macrophages were present in the trabecular meshwork of eyes with phacolytic glaucoma.[14] However, Epstein and coworkers noted that the cellular response in the anterior chamber did not correlate with degree of blockage of the trabecular meshwork. They suggested that soluble high molecular weight lens protein was most likely causing the decreased outflow of aqueous humor.[10, 17, 18] Furthermore, Yanoff and Scheie noted that macrophages in the anterior chamber do not result in glaucoma in children.[7]

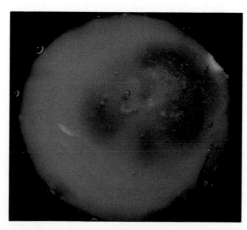

Figure 126–2. Hypermature cataract that caused phacolytic glaucoma. (Courtesy of David D. Donaldson, M.D.)

Diagnosis of phacolytic glaucoma can usually be made on clinical grounds alone. Characteristic features of uveitis, high intraocular pressure, and a hypermature cataract give the clinician reasonable confidence in making the diagnosis. If the diagnosis is uncertain, an anterior chamber paracentesis showing the presence of bloated macrophages should confirm the diagnosis.[10] Millipore filtration of aqueous humor can aid in diagnosis.[19]

Cataract extraction is the definitive treatment. Prior to surgery, medical therapy should be used to reduce the intraocular pressure and inflammation. Surgery may be delayed for several days in cases with severe uveitis to allow for intensive topical and possible subconjunctival steroid therapy. Patients should be evaluated daily. Suppression of the uveitis and control of the intraocular pressure before surgery are beneficial, although not always possible. Intracapsular cataract extraction has been recommended in the past over extracapsular cataract extraction because of the possibility of precipitating phacoanaphylaxis.[20] Extracapsular surgery has been used successfully for phacolytic glaucoma.[21] Extracapsular cataract extraction, which is more familiar to current surgeons than is intracapsular cataract extraction, is the preferred surgical technique providing that the zonules are intact.

LENS-INDUCED UVEITIS

This type is an intractable uveitis due to lens protein liberated by lens capsule disruption. It is a rare event that is precipitated by extracapsular cataract surgery or by traumatic rupture of the lens capsule. It develops after a latent period during which the immune system is sensitized to the lens protein and results in a chronic granulomatous inflammation in the involved eye. Rarely the fellow eye also develops a "sympathetic" reaction, resulting in bilateral phacoanaphylaxis.[22]

The onset of uveitis is variable, ranging from hours to months, but typically occurs from 1 to 14 days.[23] A latent period of 1 yr has been reported.[24] Clinical examination reveals large mutton-fat keratic precipitates on the corneal endothelium, a severe cellular response in the anterior chamber, and occasionally a hypopyon. The onset of lens-induced uveitis is usually associated hypotony, but the development of posterior synechiae or peripheral anterior synechiae can cause a secondary glaucoma. Lens debris and cellular elements may also obstruct outflow. The inflammation can progress to the formation of cyclitic membranes and phthisis bulbi.[11]

The inflammation in lens-induced uveitis has been described as a well localized abscess with lens material at the center.[25] The inflammatory cells form a zonal granuloma around the lens material with polymorphonuclear cells in the zone adjacent to the lens. Concentric layers of epithelioid cells, giant cells, lymphocytes, and plasma cells are next.[7, 9, 11] Extensive infiltration of the uveal tract can occur, and the entire mass can become encased in granulation tissue.[9] Large foamy macrophages are also present in the aqueous fluid.[26]

In embryogenesis, isolation of lens proteins from the immune system occurs early. When the lens capsule is disrupted and the lens proteins are exposed, they presumably act as foreign antigens and incite an inflammatory response. Experimental studies in rabbits have provided support for this hypothesis, but no demonstrable increase in antibodies to lens protein in humans has been shown.[23, 27]

Lens-induced uveitis requires more than just exposure of lens proteins. Actual sensitization of the immune system must occur during the latent period. Otherwise, a significantly greater percentage of patients with extracapsular cataract extraction would be at risk for lens-induced uveitis. It has been suggested that a genetic predisposition for lens-induced uveitis must exist and that rupture of the lens capsule is the triggering event.[7] The precise sequence of events from the lens protein exposure to granulomatous uveitis is unknown, but once sensitization occurs the fellow eye is at increased risk for lens-induced uveitis as a "sympathetic" event or after extracapsular cataract surgery.[24, 25]

Correct diagnosis of lens-induced uveitis is frequently not made until a histopathologic specimen can be obtained. A granulomatous uveitis presenting with a history of cataract surgery or trauma to the lens should raise the index of suspicion for lens-induced uveitis. The differential diagnosis includes *Propionibacterium acne* endophthalmitis and sympathetic ophthalmitis.[11, 28] Surgical retrieval of lens material for histologic analysis confirms the diagnosis.[24]

Surgery to remove residual lens material is curative, but to prevent progression of the inflammation all lens remnants must removed. Although intraocular lenses do not cause the uveitis, some sources suggest that any intraocular lens should be removed to facilitate complete retrieval of lens residue.[9, 24] Cataracts in the fellow eye should be extracted by using the intracapsular cataract technique, because of the increased risk of lens-induced uveitis.[4, 29]

LENS PARTICLE GLAUCOMA

Lens material in the anterior chamber is capable of inducing a spectrum of inflammatory responses in the eye depending on the amount of liberated lens protein and immunologic differences (Fig. 126–3). Like lens-induced uveitis, lens particle glaucoma requires surgical or traumatic disruption of the lens capsule with the release of cortical material into the aqueous.[24] However, lens particle glaucoma is a limited response that consists mainly of bloated macrophages and lens debris and is not the severe granulomatous uveitis seen in lens-induced uveitis. The severity of the glaucoma is proportional to the amount of free cortical material in the aqueous humor.[24]

The precipitating event for lens particle glaucoma is usually extracapsular cataract surgery, traumatic injury to the capsule, or neodymium:yttrium-aluminum-garnet (Nd.YAG) laser posterior capsulotomy in which cortical material is freed. Onset of glaucoma is usually delayed

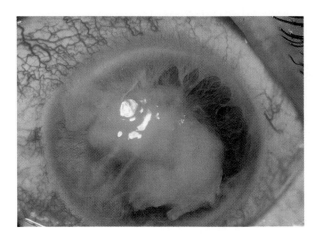

Figure 126–3. Lens-particle glaucoma. (Courtesy of David D. Donaldson, M.D.)

after the precipitating event by a few days to weeks. However, glaucomatous uveitis has been reported years after surgical cataract extraction.[29] The patient may present with pain, redness, or decreased vision or may be asymptomatic. Slit-lamp examination reveals dense flare and cells with white particles in the aqueous corresponding to lens cortex. If treatment is significantly delayed, peripheral anterior synechiae and posterior synechiae can form.[12]

The lens protein is the major component that causes obstruction of outflow facility in lens particle glaucoma, such as in phacolytic glaucoma.[10] The cellular contribution to outflow obstruction is minimal. The macrophages remove lens debris and accelerate the return to normal intraocular pressures. Most proteins in the normal lens are low molecular weight proteins, although high molecular weight proteins are present and possibly contribute to the blockage.[17, 18, 30] Eyes with preexisting decreased outflow facility are more likely to develop increased intraocular pressure with lens protein in the aqueous.[31]

An appropriate history and clinical examination are frequently sufficient to make the diagnosis.[10] If signs and symptoms are minimal, an anterior chamber paracentesis may reveal the presence of large eosinophilic staining macrophages and lens material that would aid in confirming the diagnosis.[24] The differential diagnosis includes primary open-angle glaucoma and other secondary open-angle glaucomas.

Medical therapy is useful for eyes with minimal to moderate amounts of free cortical material. Treatment with aqueous suppressants, cycloplegics, and topical steroids often suffice until residual lens material is absorbed.[11, 20] Intensive topical steroid therapy can delay absorption of lens protein and should be avoided. Surgical removal of lens debris is recommended if the intraocular pressure cannot be controlled by a reasonable trial of medical therapy. Prolonged inflammation may cause persistent glaucoma due to posterior synechiae and pupillary membranes.[20]

PHACOMORPHIC GLAUCOMA

Secondary angle-closure glaucoma due to lens intumescence is called phacomorphic glaucoma.[1] Rapid swelling of the lens can occur in eyes with advanced senile cataracts and in eyes with cataracts caused by trauma and inflammation. Rapid lens swelling may result in pupillary block or forward displacement of the lens-iris diaphragm.[11]

Phacomorphic glaucoma should be differentiated from primary angle-closure in which normal lens growth, short axial length, preexisting differences in the anatomy of the iridocorneal angle, zonular relaxation, and pupillary block can cause acute intraocular pressure elevations.[11] Phacomorphic glaucoma may be conceptualized as persistent appositional closure despite elimination of the pupillary block.

Asymmetric central shallowing of the anterior chamber in the presence of a unilateral mature intumescent cataract and elevated intraocular pressure should alert the examiner to the possibility of phacomorphic glaucoma.[32] Initial management includes reduction of the intraocular pressure with topical β-adrenergic antagonists, carbonic anhydrase inhibitors, and osmotic agents. Lens extraction is the treatment of choice. One may consider a trial of laser iridotomy and possibly gonioplasty if a visual need for cataract extraction does not exist. If the angle remains appositionally closed despite laser intervention, cataract extraction should be done.

LENS DISPLACEMENT GLAUCOMA (Fig. 126–4)

Displacement of the lens (ectopia lentis) with either partial or complete disruption of the zonules (dislocation) can cause angle-closure glaucoma (Fig. 126–5). Anterior movement of the lens or prolapse of vitreous may result in a pupillary block. Traumatic disruption of the zonules is the most common cause, but the list of syndromes and isolated disorders associated with ectopia lentis is extensive.[32]

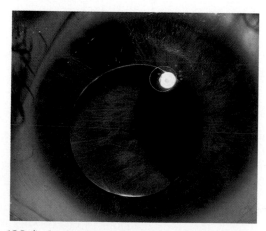

Figure 126–4. Angle-closure glaucoma caused by congenitally dislocated lens. (Courtesy of David D. Donaldson, M.D.)

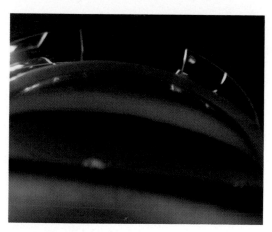

Figure 126–5. Dislocated lens in Marfan's syndrome that caused pupillary block angle-closure glaucoma. A surgical iridectomy was performed. (Courtesy of David D. Donaldson, M.D.)

Patients with ectopia lentis have symptoms of decreased visual acuity, although minimally subluxed lenses may be asymptomatic. On examination, phacodonesis and iridodonesis can be seen. Medical therapy is initiated with topical β-adrenergic antagonists, osmotic agents, and carbonic anhydrase inhibitors. Miotics may exacerbate a pupillary block and should be avoided. Lens removal is not indicated unless the lens is in the anterior chamber, there is evidence of lens-induced uveitis, or for improvement of vision.[11, 32] Pars plana lensectomy is preferable if posterior lens displacement is present.

REFERENCES

1. Appleton B, Lowrey A Jr: Phacogenic glaucoma. Am J Ophthalmol 47:682, 1959.
2. Irvine SR, Irvine AR Jr: Lens-induced uveitis and glaucoma. I: Endophthalmitis phacoanaphylactica. Am J Ophthalmol 35:177, 1952.
3. Irvine SR, Irvine AR Jr: Lens-induced uveitis and glaucoma. II: The phacotoxic reaction. Am J Ophthalmol 35:370, 1952.
4. Irvine SR, Irvine AR Jr: Lens-induced uveitis and glaucoma. III: "Phacogenetic glaucoma": Lens-induced glaucoma; mature or hypermature cataract; open iridocorneal angle. Am J Ophthalmol 35:489, 1952.
5. Riise P: Endophthalmitis phacoanaphylactica. Am J Ophthalmol 60:911, 1965.
6. Smith ME, Zimmerman LE: Contusive angle recession in phacolytic glaucoma. Arch Ophthalmol 5:737, 1922.
7. Yanoff M, Scheie HG: Cytology of human lens aspirate: Its relationship to phacolytic glaucoma and phacoanaphylactic endoophthalmitis. Arch Ophthalmol 80:160, 1968.
8. Flocks M, Littwin CS, Zimmerman LE: Phacolytic glaucoma. Arch Ophthalmol 54:37, 1955.
9. Apple DJ, Mamalis N, Steinmetz RL, et al: Phacoanaphylactic endophthalmitis associated extracapsular cataract extraction and posterior chamber intraocular lens. Arch Ophthalmol 102:1528, 1984.
10. Epstein DL: Diagnosis and management of lens-induced glaucoma. Ophthalmology 89:227, 1982.
11. Gressel MG: Lens-induced glaucoma. *In* Duane T, Jaeger EA (eds): Clinical Ophthalmology. Philadelphia, JB Lippincott, 1988.
12. Hoskins HD Jr, Kass MA: Becker-Shaffer's Diagnosis and Therapy of the Glaucomas, 6th ed. St Louis, CV Mosby, 1989.
13. Rosenbaum JT, Samples JR, Seymour B, et al: Chemotactic activity of lens proteins and the pathogenesis of phacolytic glaucoma. Arch Ophthalmol 105:1582, 1987.

14. Apple DJ, Rabb MF: Clinical Applications of Ocular Pathology, 3rd ed. St Louis, CV Mosby, 1985.
15. Bartholomew RS, Rebello PF: Calcium oxalate crystals in aqueous. Am J Ophthalmol 88:1026, 1979.
16. Brooks AMV, Grant G, Gillies WE: Comparison of specular microscopy and examination of aspirate in phacolytic glaucoma. Ophthalmology 97:85, 1990.
17. Epstein DL, Jedziniak JA, Grant WM: Obstruction of aqueous outflow by lens particles and by heavy-molecular-weight soluble lens proteins. Invest Ophthalmol Vis Sci 17:272, 1978.
18. Epstein DL, Jedziniak JA, Grant WM: Identification of heavy-molecular-weight soluble protein in aqueous humor in human phacolytic glaucoma. Invest Ophthalmol Vis Sci 17:398, 1978.
19. Goldberg MF: Cytological diagnosis of phacolytic glaucoma utilizing millipore filtration of the aqueous. Br J Ophthalmol 51:847, 1967.
20. Epstein DL: Lens-induced glaucoma. In Epstein D (ed): Chandler and Grant's Glaucoma, 3rd ed. Philadelphia, Lea & Febiger, 1986.
21. Lane SS, Kopietz LA, Lindquist TD, et al: Treatment of phacolytic glaucoma with extracapsular cataract extraction. Ophthalmology 95:749, 1988.
22. deVeer JA: Bilateral endophthalmitis phacoanaphylacta. Arch Ophthalmol 49:607, 1953.
23. Rahi AHS, Misra RN, Morgan G: Immunopathology of the lens. III: Humoral and cellular immune responses to autologous lens antigens and their roles in ocular inflammation. Br J Ophthalmol 61:371, 1977.
24. Richter C, Epstein DL: Lens-induced open-angle glaucoma. In Ritch R, Shields MB, Krupin T (eds): The Glaucomas, 1st ed. St Louis, CV Mosby, 1989.
25. Duke-Elder S: Diseases of the lens and vitreous, glaucoma and hypotony. In Duke-Elder S (ed): System of Ophthalmology. London, H. Kimpton, 1984.
26. Perlman EM, Albert DM: Clinically unsuspected phacoanaphylaxis after ocular trauma. Arch Ophthalmol 95:244, 1977.
27. Nissen SH, Anderson P, Anderson HMK: Antibodies to lens antigen in cataracts after cataract surgery. Br J Ophthalmol 65:63, 1981.
28. Meisler KM, Palestine AG, Vastine DW, et al: Chronic proprionibacterium endophthalmitis after extracapsular cataract extraction and intraocular lens implantation. Am J Ophthalmol 102:733, 1986.
29. Forstot SL, Price PK, Hovland DR, et al: Phacolytic glaucoma after extracapsular cataract extraction. Glaucoma 5:206, 1983.
30. Jedziniak JA, Nicoli DG, Baram H, et al: Quantitative verification of the existence of high molecular weight protein aggregates in the intact normal human lens by light-scattering spectroscopy. Invest Ophthalmol Vis Sci 17:51, 1978.
31. Savage FA, Thomas JV, Belcher CD, et al: Extracapsular cataract extraction and posterior chamber intraocular lens implantation in glaucomatous eyes. Ophthalmology 92:1506, 1985.
32. Liebman JM, Ritch R: Glaucoma secondary to lens intumescence and dislocation. In Ritch R, Shields MB, Krupin T (eds): The Glaucomas, 1st ed. St Louis, CV Mosby, 1989.

Chapter 127

Iridocorneal Endothelial Syndrome

M. BRUCE SHIELDS

HISTORIC BACKGROUND AND TERMINOLOGY

During the latter part of the 19th century, a number of isolated case reports appeared in the literature describing a uniocular condition that was characterized by striking abnormalities of the iris with corectopia, iris atrophy, and occasional hole formation. Some cases had additional findings that included glaucoma and corneal edema. However, it was not until a report by Harms[1] in 1903 that these disorders became recognized as a discrete entity. Because the iris abnormalities were the most striking feature, and because the pathogenesis was unknown, the condition became known as "essential iris atrophy."

Many reports of essential iris atrophy appeared in the literature during the first half of the 20th century. During the second half of this century, additional reports appeared, which suggested that essential iris atrophy might be only one variation of a broader spectrum of disorders. In 1956, Chandler[2] described patients with a similar form of uniocular glaucoma, who differed from those with essential iris atrophy by having mild or absent iris changes, but more frequent corneal edema. In 1969, Cogan and Reese[3] reported two additional patients with uniocular features that resembled those described by Harms and Chandler but that differed by the additional finding of pigmented nodules on the iris.

In 1978, Campbell and associates[4] postulated that the various clinical conditions described earlier were all linked by a common abnormality of the corneal endothelium, which was responsible for the corneal edema, as well as for the secondary iris changes and glaucoma. This theory was supported by clinical and histopathologic studies.[5, 6] The term "iridocorneal endothelial (ICE) syndrome" was proposed to encompass this spectrum of disease[6] and has become generally accepted. Within this spectrum, the following three clinical variations have been distinguished, primarily on the basis of iris changes (Table 127–1).

Progressive Iris Atrophy

This variation was originally referred to as essential iris atrophy or progressive essential iris atrophy. However, since the iris atrophy is not the essential or primary feature of the disease, the term "progressive iris atrophy" is more commonly used. As with all forms of the ICE syndrome, corneal edema and secondary glaucoma with characteristic peripheral anterior synechia may be present. The distinguishing feature, however, is the extreme atrophy of the iris with hole formation.

Table 127–1. MAJOR CLINICAL VARIATIONS

Names	Characteristic Features
1. Progressive iris atrophy	Iris features predominate, with marked corectopia, atrophy, and hole formation
2. Chandler's syndrome	Changes in the iris are mild to absent, whereas corneal edema, often at normal intraocular pressure, is typical
3. Cogan-Reese syndrome	Nodular, pigmented lesions of the iris are the hallmark and may be seen with the entire spectrum of corneal and other iris defects

Chandler's Syndrome

The variation described by Chandler in 1956 has subsequently become known as Chandler's syndrome. The corneal edema occurs somewhat more frequently in this variation, but the changes in the iris are limited to slight corectopia and mild stromal atrophy or may be absent altogether. Intermediate variations between progressive iris atrophy and Chandler's syndrome may also be seen, in which changes in the iris are more extensive than the latter condition but lack the hole formation of the former variation. In one study of 37 consecutive cases of the ICE syndrome, Chandler's syndrome was the most common clinical variation and accounted for 21 cases (56 percent), with the remaining cases being equally divided between the other two major clinical variations.[7]

Cogan-Reese Syndrome

Since the report by Cogan and Reese in 1969, it has been confirmed that pigmented nodules of the iris may occur throughout the complete spectrum of the ICE syndrome.[8, 9] This variation has become known as the Cogan-Reese syndrome. Similar cases have been described with diffuse nevi, rather than nodules, on the surface of the iris, and this has been referred to as the iris nevus syndrome.[8] There has been a tendency to group the Cogan-Reese syndrome and iris nevus syndrome together as variations of the ICE syndrome. However, the iris lesions of the two conditions are clinically and histologically different, and there is insufficient evidence to include the iris nevus syndrome as a clinical variation of the ICE syndrome.

GENERAL FEATURES OF PATIENTS

It is important to recognize that the clinical variations described earlier represent only minor differences within a common spectrum of disease. Although subtle differences with regard to the frequency and severity of corneal edema and secondary glaucoma have been recognized between the clinical variations,[7] which are discussed later, all patients with the ICE syndrome share the following general features.

The condition is almost always clinically uniocular, although subclinical abnormalities of the corneal endothelium are seen in the fellow eye of some patients. The syndrome is usually recognized in early to middle adulthood, with a predilection for women. Familial cases are rare, and there is no consistent association with any other ocular or systemic disorder.

The most common presenting manifestations are abnormalities of the iris, reduced visual acuity, or pain. Some patients may be prompted to seek medical attention because they notice a displacement of the pupil or a dark spot on the iris, which usually represents the atrophy or hole formation. Other patients may first notice reduced vision in the involved eye. This occurs typically in the morning, when the corneal edema is more severe, and subsides during the day, as exposure to air dehydrates the cornea. In more advanced cases, the patient may have chronic reduction in vision due to corneal edema or glaucomatous optic atrophy. The pain is usually due to corneal edema and much less commonly to elevated intraocular pressure.

CLINICOPATHOLOGIC FEATURES
(Table 127–2)

Cornea

A common feature throughout ICE syndrome is a corneal endothelial abnormality, which Chandler[2] described by slit-lamp examination as having a fine-hammered silver appearance of the posterior cornea, similar to that of Fuchs' dystrophy, but less coarse (Fig. 127–1). Specular microscopy of the corneal endothelium reveals a characteristic, diffuse abnormality with variable degrees of pleomorphism in size and shape, dark areas within the cells, and loss of the clear hexagonal margins (Fig. 127–2).[10] This characteristic abnormality of the corneal endothelium is present in all clinical

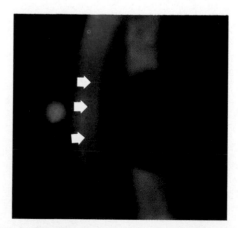

Figure 127–1. Slit-lamp view showing fine-beaten silver appearance of corneal endothelial abnormality (*arrows*) in the iridocorneal endothelial (ICE) syndrome.

Figure 127–2. Specular microscopic appearance of corneal endothelial cells in ICE syndrome, showing pleomorphism in size and shape, dark areas within the cells, and loss of clear hexagonal margins. (From Shields MB: Textbook of Glaucoma, 2nd ed, p 222. © 1987, the Williams & Wilkins Co., Baltimore.)

variations of ICE syndrome and is the strongest evidence that they represent a spectrum of disease. Whenever the diagnosis is in doubt, it can usually be confirmed by the specular microscopic findings, which are essentially pathognomonic.

In many patients with ICE syndrome, the corneal endothelial abnormality may cause no symptoms. In other cases, it may cause corneal edema with variable degrees of reduced vision and pain, as described earlier. In some patients, the corneal edema may be aggravated by elevated intraocular pressure, although other patients may have the edema with pressures that are normal or only slightly elevated. A slight reduction in endothelial cell count and mild cellular pleomorphism may be observed in the fellow eye of some patients, although this is almost always asymptomatic and never leads to the full clinical manifestations of ICE syndrome.[11]

In some patients, the persistent corneal edema may lead to marked reduction in visual acuity, frequently requiring penetrating keratoplasty. Electron microscopic studies of the posterior cornea in these cases have revealed varied and complex alterations of cells, lining multilayered collagenous tissue posterior to a normal Descemet's membrane (Fig. 127–3).[12–14] Descriptions of the cellular layer differ among reports, which may relate to the varied response of the corneal endothelium in this syndrome, even within different areas of the same eye. Some cells have evidence of metabolic activity or have undergone division. Filopodial processes and cytoplasmic actin filaments suggest that these cells are capable of migration.[13, 14] In some specimens, the endothelial cells are present in multiple layers, suggesting a loss of contact inhibition.[13] Other specimens reveal a monolayer of reduced cell density with disrupted and

Table 127–2. CLINICOPATHOLOGIC FEATURES

Structures	Clinical Appearance	Histopathology
1. Cornea	a. Fine-hammered silver appearance of posterior cornea in all cases	a. Abnormal endothelial cells lining multilayered collagenous tissue posterior to Descemet's membrane
	b. Corneal edema in some cases	b. Stroma and epithelial edema associated with marked endothelial cell abnormality
2. Anterior chamber angle	a. Secondary glaucoma with open angle	a. Single layer of endothelial cells and Descemet's-like membrane extending from the cornea across the open anterior chamber angle
	b. Secondary glaucoma with peripheral anterior synechia extending to or beyond Schwalbe's line	b. Peripheral anterior synechia created by contracture of the cellular membrane
3. Iris	a. Corectopia, ectropion uvea, and extensive iris atrophy with hole formation (progressive iris atrophy)	a. Cellular membrane extends from the angle onto the iris, with subsequent contracture producing clinical findings
	b. Normal iris or minimal corectopia and mild atrophy of the iris stroma (Chandler's syndrome)	b. Normal iris or cellular membrane producing the milder clinical findings
	c. Pigmented, pedunculated nodules on the iris surface with any degree of iris atrophy (Cogan-Reese syndrome)	c. Nodules composed of tissue resembling the underlying iris stroma, surrounded by cellular membrane

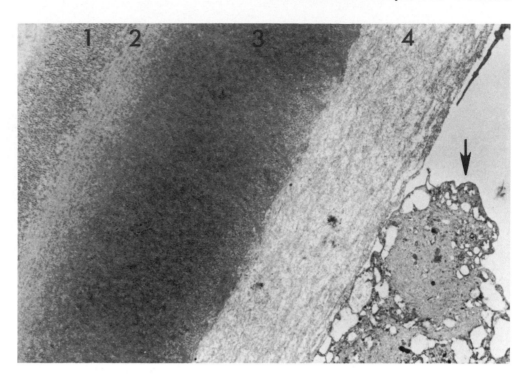

Figure 127–3. Transmission electron microscopic view of inner corneal surface in ICE syndrome, showing part of an abnormal cell (*arrow*) on a four-layered membrane composed of the anterior nonbanded (1) and posterior-banded (2) portions of Descemet's membrane with abnormal compact collagenous (3) and loose collagenous (4) layers. ×6875. (From Shields MB, McCracken JS, Klintworth KG, Campbell DG: Corneal edema in essential iris atrophy. Published courtesy of *Ophthalmology* 86: 1533–1550, 1979.)

necrotic cells and occasional acellular zones. Chronic inflammatory cells have also been observed in some cases.[13, 14] Although the corneal endothelial abnormality is found consistently in all variations of ICE syndrome, corneal edema appears to be more severe in patients with Chandler's syndrome.[7]

Anterior Chamber Angle

The typical gonioscopic appearance of patients with ICE syndrome is that of broad peripheral anterior synechia, often extending to or beyond Schwalbe's line (Fig. 127–4). This finding does not differ significantly among the clinical variations of ICE syndrome by either gonioscopic or histologic examination. Histologic studies reveal a cellular membrane, consisting of a single layer of endothelial cells and a Descemet's-like membrane, which is continuous with the cellular and collagenous layers of the posterior cornea. This membrane is usually seen in association with the peripheral anterior synechia, although it may also be seen covering an otherwise open anterior chamber angle.

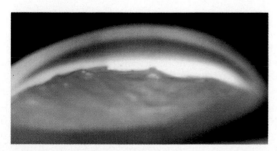

Figure 127–4. Gonioscopic appearance in ICE syndrome with broad peripheral anterior synechia extending beyond trabecular meshwork.

These changes in the anterior chamber angle are presumed to be the mechanism of the secondary glaucoma in ICE syndrome. Most patients with ICE syndrome, who develop the secondary glaucoma, have extensive peripheral anterior synechia, although this does not correlate precisely with the glaucoma, and some patients may have an anterior chamber angle that appears to be entirely open. In the latter cases, the obstruction to aqueous outflow is presumably due to the membrane covering the trabecular meshwork. Although the anterior chamber angle alterations are seen in all variations of ICE syndrome, the associated secondary glaucoma appears to be more severe with progressive iris atrophy and Cogan-Reese syndrome.[7]

Iris

Although the abnormalities of the iris are the least significant with regard to visual dysfunction, they do constitute the primary basis for distinguishing clinical variations within ICE syndrome.

Progressive iris atrophy is characterized by marked atrophy of the iris, associated with variable degrees of corectopia and ectropion uvea (Fig. 127–5). The pupil is typically displaced toward the quadrant with the most prominent area of peripheral anterior synechia. The hallmark of progressive iris atrophy is hole formation of the iris, which occurs in two forms.[5] The most common finding is a "stretch hole," in which the iris is markedly thinned in the quadrant away from the direction of the pupillary distortion, with hole formation in the area that is being stretched. Less commonly, "melting holes" develop without associated corectopia or iris thinning, and fluorescein angiographic studies suggest that this may be associated with ischemia of the iris.[9]

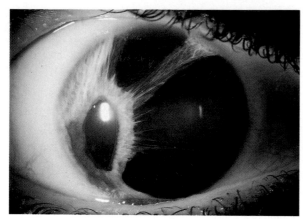

Figure 127–5. Progressive iris atrophy, a variation of ICE syndrome, with marked inferior corectopia and iris atrophy with multiple iris holes.

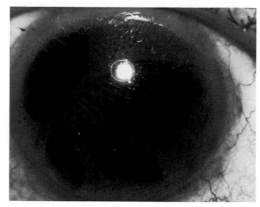

Figure 127–7. Cogan-Reese syndrome, a variation of ICE syndrome, with ectropion uvea and marked corectopia with iris atrophy, hole formation, and numerous dark nodules on the iris surface. (From Shields MB, Campbell DG, Simmons RJ, Hutchinson BT: Iris nodules in essential iris atrophy. Arch Ophthalmol 94:406–410, 1976. Copyright 1976, American Medical Association.)

Histopathology of the iris in this and in all variations of ICE syndrome includes a monolayer of cells, often with a Descemet's-like membrane, on portions of the anterior iris surface, continuous with the similar layer that was described in the anterior chamber angle. These structures are most often found in the quadrant toward which the pupil is distorted.[4]

In some cases of Chandler's syndrome, the iris may appear entirely normal. The diagnosis may be difficult in these cases, and it should be emphasized that the corneal endothelium must always be examined carefully in cases of uniocular glaucoma. In most cases, however, patients with Chandler's syndrome have slight corectopia and mild atrophy of the iris stroma (Fig. 127–6). As previously noted, there are intermediate variations between Chandler's syndrome and progressive iris atrophy, in which the degree of corectopia and stromal atrophy is more severe than that typically seen in Chandler's syndrome but is lacking the hole formation of progressive iris atrophy.

Patients with Cogan-Reese syndrome may have any degree of iris abnormality from no corectopia or stromal atrophy to marked changes with hole formation. The distinguishing feature in these patients, however, is the presence of pigmented, pedunculated nodules on the surface of the iris (Fig. 127–7). In some cases, other features of ICE syndrome may be present for many years before the nodules appear. Histologically, the nodules appear to consist of tissue similar to that in the underlying iris stroma, and they are always surrounded by the previously described cellular membrane.[4, 6]

PATHOGENESIS

Theories of Etiology

The precise cause of ICE syndrome remains unknown. The absence of a positive family history suggests that the condition is acquired, rather than inherited, and the onset in early to middle adulthood, as well as the histologic finding of a fully developed Descemet's membrane, suggest that it is acquired at some point after birth. The finding of chronic inflammatory cells in the corneal specimens has raised the possibility of a viral cause,[13] although similar cells have been found in the endothelium of corneas with inherited diseases.[14] All we can say at the present time is that ICE syndrome is apparently an acquired disorder in which the full manifestations are limited to one eye. Further study is needed to establish the precise cause.

Theories of Mechanism

Although the precise cause awaits further elucidation, the mechanism that leads to the various changes in ICE syndrome has been established with reasonable certainty. The membrane theory of Campbell[4] holds that the abnormality of the corneal endothelium is the primary defect in ICE syndrome. The endothelial defect causes the corneal edema and leads presumably to the proliferation of the previously described cellular membrane across the anterior chamber angle and onto the surface of the iris. The observation of filopodial pro-

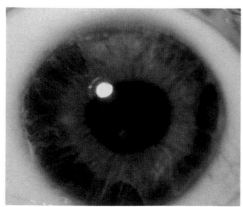

Figure 127–6. Chandler's syndrome, a variation of ICE syndrome, with irregular pupil and stromal iris atrophy.

cesses, cytoplasmic actin filaments, and apparent loss of contract inhibition are all consistent with the concept of migrating cells. Subsequent contracture of the cellular membrane is believed to cause the formation of the peripheral anterior synechia, as well as most, if not all, of the iris changes. As the membrane in one quadrant contracts to create the peripheral anterior synechia and the corectopia and ectropion uvea toward the synechia, the iris in the opposite quadrant is put on stretch, especially when it is anchored by additional peripheral anterior synechia in that quadrant. This stretching is considered to be the primary cause of the iris atrophy and hole formation, although other factors, such as ischemia, may also be involved.

The cellular membrane is also believed to be responsible for the development of the nodular lesions of the iris in Cogan-Reese syndrome. It has been postulated that the membrane, as it grows across the iris, encircles and pinches off portions of the iris stroma to create the nodules.[4, 15] As previously noted, the associated secondary glaucoma in all variations of ICE syndrome is believed to be due to an obstruction of the trabecular meshwork by the peripheral anterior synechia or, less commonly, by the cellular membrane.

Each clinical variation is believed to have the same basic mechanism described earlier. In some cases, the difference in clinical features may simply be due to the time at which the patient is seen. For example, a patient with the initial findings of Chandler's syndrome may later develop iris hole formation or nodules, changing the diagnosis to progressive iris atrophy or to Cogan-Reese syndrome, respectively. In other cases, however, patients do not progress and, as previously noted, Chandler's syndrome appears to be the most common variant of ICE syndrome.[7] It may be that the endothelial cells in these patients are more disrupted or less able to migrate, which could explain the more severe corneal edema as well as the less severe glaucoma and iris changes compared with the other variants in this spectrum of disease.[7, 13]

DIFFERENTIAL DIAGNOSIS
(Table 127–3)

There are several disorders of the cornea or iris, many of which have associated glaucoma, that could be con-

Table 127–3. DIFFERENTIAL DIAGNOSIS

Categories	Entities
1. Corneal endothelial disorders	a. Posterior polymorphous dystrophy b. Fuchs' endothelial dystrophy
2. Dissolution of the iris	a. Axenfeld-Rieger syndrome b. Aniridia c. Iridoschisis
3. Nodular iris lesions	a. Iris melanoma b. Iris nevus syndrome c. Neurofibromatosis d. Nodular inflammatory disorders

fused with the various forms of ICE syndrome. It may be helpful to think of these conditions in the following three categories: corneal endothelial disorders, dissolution of the iris, and nodular lesions of the iris.

Corneal Endothelial Disorders

Two conditions with primary endothelial abnormalities that might be confused with ICE syndrome are posterior polymorphous dystrophy and Fuchs' endothelial dystrophy. With regard to posterior polymorphous dystrophy, the differential diagnosis is further compounded by the fact that a small subset of these patients have anterior chamber angle and iris findings that resemble ICE syndrome, as well as occasional associated glaucoma. However, the condition is bilateral and familial, and the clinical appearance of the corneal endothelial abnormality is more that of blisters or vesicles. The clinical appearance of the endothelial abnormality in Fuchs' dystrophy, on the other hand, may be difficult to distinguish from that of ICE syndrome. However, this condition is also bilateral and does not have the anterior chamber angle or iris features of the latter condition.

Dissolution of the Iris

Several conditions are characterized by changes in the iris that could be confused with that of ICE syndrome. The condition with the most striking clinical and histopathologic similarities to ICE syndrome is Axenfeld-Rieger syndrome. Patients with this syndrome typically have iridocorneal adhesions of the anterior chamber angle with secondary glaucoma, as well as changes in the iris that are very difficult to distinguish from those of ICE syndrome. However, the bilateral and familial nature of Axenfeld-Rieger syndrome allows a distinction to be made between these two conditions. Some advanced cases of progressive iris atrophy might resemble aniridia, in which a rudimentary stump of iris is present. Again, however, the latter condition is bilateral and congenital. Another condition associated with dissolution of the iris is iridoschisis. The iris changes in this condition, however, differ from that of ICE syndrome by a separation of superficial layers of iris stroma, usually in elderly individuals.

Nodular Lesions of the Iris

The nodular lesions of Cogan-Reese syndrome may be confused with similar nodular iris lesions in a variety of additional conditions. Most important in this regard is the fact that the nodular lesions in Cogan-Reese syndrome have been mistaken for melanomas of the iris, leading to enucleation. It is important, therefore, to make the distinction between these two conditions in order not only to avoid enucleation in the benign condition but also to recognize the melanoma when it is present. In most cases, the melanomas are larger and more diffuse than the small, pedunculated nodules of Cogan-Reese syndrome. Other patients may have iris nevi that might cause confusion with Cogan-Reese syndrome. As previously noted, a specific condition has been described as the iris nevus syndrome, in which additional features resembling ICE syndrome might be present. Other patients may have iris melanosis, in which pedunculated nodules are difficult to distinguish from those of Cogan-Reese syndrome, although this condition is typically bilateral and may be familial. Other conditions with nodules of the iris include neurofibromatosis and nodular inflammatory disorders, such as sarcoidosis.

MANAGEMENT

In the management of patients with ICE syndrome, the primary concern has to do with the corneal edema and the secondary glaucoma.

Corneal Edema

Mild corneal edema, especially with normal intraocular pressure, can often be controlled with hypertonic saline solutions. Some patients may also find it useful to allow the warm air of a hair dryer to blow toward their face in order to accelerate the dehydration of the cornea in the morning. Soft contact lenses may also be helpful in some cases of more persistent corneal edema. When intraocular pressure elevation is present, medical reduction of the pressure may also help to reduce the corneal edema. In severe cases, however, the corneal edema persists despite low intraocular pressures, and penetrating keratoplasty is usually required.

Secondary Glaucoma

In the early stages of secondary glaucoma associated with ICE syndrome, the intraocular pressure elevation can often be controlled medically, especially with drugs that reduce aqueous production, such as the β-blockers and carbonic anhydrase inhibitors. Epinephrine may also be useful in some cases. Miotics are rarely effective, owing to the mechanical obstruction of the trabecular meshwork.

When the intraocular pressure can no longer be controlled medically, filtering surgery is usually indicated. Laser trabeculoplasty is rarely effective in these cases. Patients with ICE syndrome generally do well with glaucoma filtering surgery, although some patients have late failure due to the endothelialization of the fistula. In some cases, these can be reopened with application of a neodymium:yttrium-aluminum-garnet (Nd.YAG) laser.

REFERENCES

1. Harms C: Einseitige spontane Luckenbildung der Iris durch Atrophie Ohne mechanische Zerrung. Klin Monatsbl Augenheilkd 41:522, 1903.
2. Chandler PA: Atrophy of the stroma of the iris: Endothelial dystrophy, corneal edema, and glaucoma. Am J Ophthalmol 41:607, 1956.
3. Cogan DG, Reese AB: A syndrome of iris nodules, ectopic Descemet's membrane, and unilateral glaucoma. Doc Ophthalmol 26:424, 1969.
4. Campbell DG, Shields MB, Smith TR: The corneal endothelium and the spectrum of essential iris atrophy. Am J Ophthalmol 86:317, 1978.
5. Shields MB, Campbell DG, Simmons RJ: The essential iris atrophies. Am J Ophthalmol 85:749, 1978.
6. Eagle RC Jr, Font RL, Yanoff M, Fine BS: Proliferative endotheliopathy with iris abnormalities: The iridocorneal endothelial syndrome. Arch Ophthalmol 97:2104, 1979.
7. Wilson MC, Shields MB: A comparison of the clinical variations of the iridocorneal endothelial syndrome. Arch Ophthalmol 107:1465, 1989.
8. Scheie HG, Yanoff M: Iris nevus (Cogan-Reese) syndrome: A cause of unilateral glaucoma. Arch Ophthalmol 93:963, 1975.
9. Shields MB, Campbell DG, Simmons RJ, Hutchinson BT: Iris nodules in essential iris atrophy. Arch Ophthalmol 94:406, 1976.
10. Hirst LW, Quigley HA, Stark WJ, Shields MB: Specular microscopy of the iridocorneal endothelial syndrome. Am J Ophthalmol 89:11, 1980.
11. Kupfer C, Kaiser-Kupfer MI, Datiles M, McCain L: The contralateral eye in the iridocorneal endothelial (ICE) syndrome. Ophthalmology 90:1343, 1983.
12. Shields MB, McCracken JS, Klintworth GK, Campbell DG: Corneal edema in essential iris atrophy. Ophthalmology 86:1533, 1979.
13. Alvarado JA, Murphy CG, Maglio M, Hetherington J: Pathogenesis of Chandler's syndrome, essential iris atrophy, and the Cogan-Reese syndrome. I: Alterations of the corneal endothelium. Invest Ophthalmol Vis Sci 27:853, 1986.
14. Rodrigues MM, Stulting RD, Waring GO III: Clinical, electron microscopic, and immunohistochemical study of the corneal endothelium and Descemet's membrane in the iridocorneal endothelial syndrome. Am J Ophthalmol 101:16, 1986.
15. Eagle RC Jr, Font RL, Yanoff M, Fine BS: The iris naevus (Cogan-Reese) syndrome: Light and electron microscopic observations. Br J Ophthalmol 64:446, 1980.

Chapter 128

■

Ocular Tumors and Glaucoma

RANDALL OZMENT

The association of intraocular tumors and glaucoma has long been recognized. Von Graefe has been credited with the dictum, "the degree of tension of the eyeball is a guide to diagnosis."[1] In years past great emphasis was given to the presence or absence of glaucoma to differentiate rhegmatogenous retinal detachment or retinal detachment due to an intraocular tumor. In 1896, Marshall reported his findings of associated glaucoma and intraocular tumors from his study of 100 eyes enucleated for "malignant disease both of the choroid and also the retina."[2] His study included uveal melanoma and retinoblastoma. Marshall found elevated intraocular pressure in 53 percent of the eyes that he studied. He also reported decreased intraocular pressure in 7 percent and normal intraocular pressure in 40 percent. In his attempt to understand the mechanism of glaucoma secondary to intraocular tumors, Marshall reported a close correlation of the width of the anterior chamber angle to the development of glaucoma. Most eyes with glaucoma were found to have a closed angle or "restricted angle." Marshall states "in all cases tension bears a direct relation to the size and condition of the angle of the anterior chamber." He found a higher incidence of closed angles with tumors of the choroid versus the ciliary body.

In 1935 Terry and Johns reported a 33 percent incidence of glaucoma in eyes with uveal sarcoma.[3] Of 94 eyes, 23 were found histopathologically to have damage to the filtration angle as a result of a tumor being present within the eye.

In 1938 Dunnington published a review of 55 cases of "intraocular sarcoma" (uveal malignant melanoma).[1] He reported that glaucoma was present in 27 percent of eyes studied. When eyes were grouped according to primary location of the tumor, either choroid or ciliary body, glaucoma occurred in 29 percent and 12 percent, respectively.

Shields and coworkers presented the results of a survey of 2704 eyes with intraocular tumors.[4] One hundred twenty-six eyes or 5 percent were found to have a tumor-induced elevation of intraocular pressure. The survey included uveal melanoma, retinoblastoma, metastatic tumors, and other miscellaneous neoplasms. In their survey, metastatic tumors to the iris and ciliary body were more likely to result in elevated intraocular pressure compared with choroidal melanoma and retinoblastoma.

Most earlier studies report a higher incidence of glaucoma in eyes with intraocular tumors compared with the larger, more recent 1987 survey of Shields and coworkers. This may well represent earlier detection of intraocular tumors with modern equipment and diagnostic studies used for ophthalmic examinations. The percentage of eyes with intraocular tumors that develop glaucoma is small. The group of patients with tumor-induced glaucoma is a very small fraction of all patients with glaucoma. Nevertheless, because of the serious morbidity and mortality associated with some intraocular tumors, proper diagnosis and treatment of the tumor and any tumor-related pathology is mandatory for the overall well-being of the patient.

The systemic well-being of the patient must always be considered paramount in caring for patients with intraocular tumors. Treatment of the tumor itself to prevent a possible fatal outcome should be the primary goal of care given to any patient with an intraocular tumor. Management of ocular tumors often requires enucleation of the eye; thus, glaucoma secondary to the tumor is not a problem. However, in eyes retaining good vision with malignant tumors that do not undergo enucleation, or tumors known to be benign, management of associated glaucoma may be required. Medical management of intraocular pressure is often effective. However, in many cases surgical therapy may be a consideration. Eyes containing malignant intraocular tumors should not undergo fistulizing operations for control of their glaucoma. Fistulizing operations place the patient at risk for extraocular spread of tumor. If there is uncontrolled glaucoma in an eye with a malignant tumor, enucleation may be in the best interest of the patient. Conversely, fistulizing glaucoma operations may be appropriate for eyes with secondary glaucoma associated with a benign intraocular tumor.

To facilitate the ease of use of this chapter for the clinician caring for patients with intraocular tumors or glaucoma, it is divided into primary ocular tumors, metastatic tumors, and miscellaneous tumors with ocular involvement. Within the first two sections, there is an anatomic division of the eye starting with the iris, then moving posteriorly to the ciliary body, optic nerve, retina, and finally the choroid. Specific tumors and secondary glaucomas are discussed under each anatomic subheading.

PRIMARY OCULAR TUMORS AND GLAUCOMA

Primary Iris Tumors

Glaucoma secondary to tumors of the iris may occur with both benign and malignant neoplasms. Depending on the underlying mechanism producing the elevation of intraocular pressure, the clinical presentation of glaucoma secondary to iris tumors may be acute or chronic angle-closure glaucoma, chronic open-angle glaucoma, hemorrhagic glaucoma, or inflammatory glaucoma. The underlying mechanism of glaucoma may be direct invasion of aqueous outflow pathways by tumor cells, dispersion of pigment or melanin granules causing obstruction of aqueous outflow pathways, tumor cell dispersion into the trabecular meshwork causing obstruction of outflow, and inflammatory cells obstructing aqueous outflow.

Iris Nevus. Benign iris nevi are common clinical findings in many patients. Histologically, they consist of benign spindle-shaped cells. An iris nevus rarely results in a pathologic process in the eye. However, diffuse growth of an iris nevus within the anterior chamber and into the chamber angle involving the trabecular meshwork has been documented clinically and histopathologically.[5] A secondary open-angle glaucoma may result when a nevus grows to involve the angle and aqueous outflow pathways.

Iris Melanocytoma. Iris melanocytoma, a pigmented iris tumor composed of benign polyhedral nevus cells, is a rare clinical entity. Pigment dispersion and secondary elevation of intraocular pressure with significant reduction of outflow facility has been documented in an eye containing a necrotic iris melanocytoma.[6] Following removal of the tumor by iridocyclectomy, the intraocular pressure and outflow facility returned to normal. This occurred concurrently with resolution of heavy pigmentation of the trabecular meshwork. The obstruction of outflow was thought to be secondary to pigment collecting in the outflow pathways as it was released from the necrotic tumor. Direct involvement of the outflow pathways by an iris melanocytoma has also occurred and has resulted in increased intraocular pressure with impaired facility of outflow.[7]

Iris Pigment Epithelium Adenoma. Iris pigment epithelium adenoma is a rare benign tumor of the iris pigment epithelium. Glaucoma associated with this tumor has been attributed to pigment dispersion into the trabecular meshwork.[8] Resolution of the elevated intraocular pressure occurred following removal of the tumor by iridocyclectomy in a single case.

Iris Malignant Melanoma. Malignant melanoma of the iris may result in secondary tumor-induced glaucoma. The incidence of glaucoma associated with iris melanoma ranges from 7 to 48 percent.[4, 9, 10] Diffuse iris melanomas are more likely to result in secondary glaucoma compared with smaller circumscribed tumors.[4]

Secondary glaucoma associated with primary iris melanoma may occur from several different mechanisms. Direct growth of solid tumor into the anterior chamber angle and aqueous outflow pathways causing obstruction of aqueous outflow is the most common mechanism of glaucoma associated with iris melanoma.[4, 10] Both indirect seeding of aqueous outflow pathways by tumor cells and dispersion of pigment from iris melanomas have resulted in secondary open-angle glaucomas (Fig. 128–1).[4, 9]

Melanomalytic glaucoma is seen only in eyes with pigmented intraocular tumors and therefore may occur

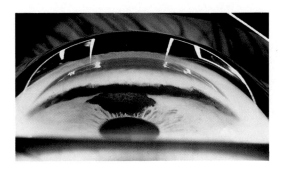

Figure 128–1. Midstromal iris melanoma with extensive tumor seeding into the angle structures.

in eyes with iris melanoma.[11–13] Melanomalytic glaucoma results from an obstruction of aqueous outflow pathways by macrophages containing melanin granules dispersed from the tumor. Melanin-filled macrophages may occupy the anterior chamber angle and mechanically obstruct aqueous outflow. Light and electron microscopy of eyes with melanomalytic glaucoma have shown the trabecular meshwork surface and intertrabecular spaces filled with melanin-laden macrophages.[12]

The differential diagnosis of glaucoma secondary to iris tumors is relatively brief. Pigmentary glaucoma, uveitic glaucoma, glaucoma secondary to metastatic tumors to the iris, and variants of the iridocorneal endothelial syndromes may be confused with glaucoma secondary to primary iris tumors. However, with a tumor present on the iris, proper diagnosis is usually made clinically. In some patients a fine-needle biopsy, aqueous aspiration, or excisional biopsy is needed to confirm the diagnosis.

Management of iris tumors in eyes with good visual acuity generally involves frequent observation of the lesion. Photographic documentation of the lesion is helpful in determining the stability or growth of the tumor. Most malignant iris tumors have relatively benign histopathologic characteristics and may be observed over long periods when the lesion is documented to be stable and nongrowing.[9, 10, 14]

Elevated intraocular pressure in eyes with iris tumors may be managed by medical means. Surgical fistulizing operations performed in eyes with malignant iris tumors carry the significant risk of promoting extraocular spread of tumor cells and is contraindicated.

Iris tumors of limited size may be removed by iridectomy or iridocyclectomy.[14] Eyes containing tumors resulting in pigmentary dispersion and glaucoma have had resolution of the pigment dispersion and glaucoma following removal of the tumor by iridectomy and iridocyclectomy.[4, 8] Uncontrollable glaucoma secondary to iris tumors may require enucleation of the eye.

Primary Ciliary Body Tumors

Benign and malignant tumors involving the ciliary body may result in increased intraocular pressure and glaucoma. However, many eyes with tumors of the ciliary body may have decreased intraocular pressure.[1, 2, 15, 16] Hypotony may occur secondary to decreased aqueous production as a result of a tumor involving the ciliary body and ciliary processes. In many patients, only a mild relative hypotony is present when comparing involved and uninvolved eyes. Eyes with glaucoma secondary to ciliary body tumors have tumor-related pathology affecting the outflow pathways to a greater extent than the tumor pathology has reduced aqueous production by involvement of the ciliary processes.

As with glaucoma related to iris tumors, the presentation of glaucoma related to ciliary body tumors may be varied. The glaucoma may present as acute or chronic angle-closure glaucoma, chronic open-angle glaucoma, hemorrhagic glaucoma, or uveitic glaucoma.[13, 15, 17] The presentation depends on the underlying mechanism producing the glaucoma.

Ciliary Body Medulloepithelioma. Medulloepithelioma is a tumor that arises most commonly from the nonpigmented ciliary epithelium. Medulloepithelioma may have a benign or malignant histopathologic appearance and clinical course. Medulloepithelioma generally occurs during childhood but may be seen in early adulthood.

In a large series of medulloepitheliomas involving the ciliary body, approximately 50 percent of the eyes had glaucoma at the time of initial examination.[17] Rubeosis iridis with resultant angle-closure was a common cause of glaucoma associated with medulloepithelioma of the ciliary body. Direct tumor growth into the chamber angle involving outflow pathways was also documented. Tumor-induced angle-closure glaucoma caused by mechanical displacement of the angle structures also resulted in glaucoma in several eyes reported. A single eye developed elevated intraocular pressure following recurrent intracameral hemorrhage and hyphema.[17]

Ciliary Body Melanocytoma. Melanocytoma, a benign pigmented tumor of the uveal tract, may occur in the ciliary body. Melanocytoma of the ciliary body has been associated with glaucoma. A single case report has demonstrated invasion of a ciliary body melanocytoma into the angle structures, resulting in an elevated intraocular pressure and glaucoma.[18]

Ciliary Body Malignant Melanoma. As many as 17 to 55 percent of eyes with ciliary body melanoma may have a tumor-induced glaucoma.[4, 15, 16] Secondary elevation of intraocular pressure in eyes with ciliary body melanoma may be produced by a variety of mechanisms. Most commonly pigment dispersion or direct invasion of the angle structures is found. In one large series of 96 eyes with ciliary body melanoma, pigment dispersion was the mechanism of pressure elevation in half of the glaucomatous eyes.[19] Thirty-one percent of eyes with elevated intraocular pressure were found to have direct tumor involvement of the angle structures by tumor growth from the ciliary body. Seeding of angle structures by tumor cells (Fig. 128–2), rubeosis iridis with neovascular glaucoma, and mechanical tumor-induced angle-closure have all been reported as mechanisms of elevation of intraocular pressure in eyes containing ciliary body melanomas.

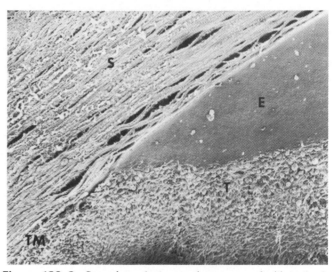

Figure 128–2. Scanning electron microscopy of ciliary body melanoma tumor cells seeding the trabecular meshwork. E, exudate; S, sclera; TM, trabecular meshwork. (From Shields MB, Klintworth GK: Anterior uveal melanomas and intraocular pressure. Ophthalmology 87:503–517, 1980.)

Melanomalytic glaucoma may occur in eyes with malignant melanoma of the ciliary body. This glaucoma caused by mechanical obstruction of outflow pathways by melanin-laden macrophages was described originally by Yanoff in 1970 in an eye with a necrotic melanoma of the ciliary body.[11] Large accumulations of macrophages engorged with melanin were seen histologically lining the anterior chamber angle and were present within the trabecular meshwork (Fig. 128–3).

The differential diagnosis of glaucoma secondary to ciliary body tumors includes open- and closed-angle glaucomas. Pigmentary dispersion glaucoma, uveitic glaucoma, hemorrhagic glaucoma, neovascular glaucoma, acute angle-closure glaucoma, and chronic angle-closure glaucoma must all be considered in the differential diagnosis.

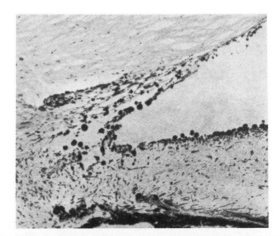

Figure 128–3. Pigment-laden macrophages lining the anterior chamber angle with involvement of the trabecular meshwork in melanomalytic glaucoma. (From Yanoff M and Scheie H: Melanocyte glaucoma: Report of a case. Arch Ophthalmol 84:471–473, 1970. Copyright 1970, American Medical Association.)

Management of glaucoma in eyes with ciliary body tumors may be done by medical means. As with iris tumors, surgical fistulizing operations are contraindicated with malignant ciliary body tumors. Fistulizing operations carry the significant risk of promoting extraocular spread of tumor cells. Enucleation often follows the discovery of eyes with glaucoma and ciliary body tumors for control of the glaucoma and histologic diagnosis of the tumor when malignancy is suspected clinically.

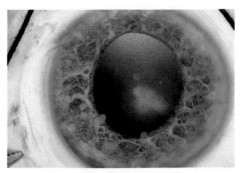

Figure 128–4. Anterior segment seeding by retinoblastoma with secondary glaucoma.

Primary Tumors of the Optic Nerve

Optic Nerve Melanocytoma. Melanocytomas most commonly arise within the intraocular portion of the optic nerve. A single case report has documented neovascular glaucoma associated with a melanocytoma of the optic nerve head.[20] Necrosis of the tumor resulted in occlusion of the central retinal artery and an ischemic retinal syndrome. Secondary neovascularization of the anterior segment occurred resulting in synechial angle-closure.

Management of glaucoma in eyes with melanocytomas of the optic nerve head should be done conservatively, with medical therapy followed by surgical therapy as needed.

Primary Retinal Tumors

Retinoblastoma. Glaucoma may occur secondarily in eyes with retinoblastoma. The incidence of glaucoma secondary to retinoblastoma ranges from 2 to 22 percent in published series.[4, 21] The clinical presentation of glaucoma may occur as acute angle-closure, uveitic glaucoma, or neovascular glaucoma.

The most common mechanism of secondary glaucoma in eyes with retinoblastoma is neovascularization of the iris and angle structures with formation of peripheral anterior synechiae. Neovascular glaucoma accounted for 73 percent of glaucoma associated with retinoblastoma in one large study.[4] Histologic studies have identified neovascularization of the anterior segment in 50 to 59 percent of eyes containing retinoblastoma.[22, 23] Most eyes with neovascularization of the anterior segment contain large tumors involving the posterior pole with involvement of the central retinal vessels or large branch retinal vessels.[4, 21] Histologically, occlusion of these large vessels has resulted in ischemic retinopathy. The ischemic retinopathy in these eyes may secondarily cause anterior segment neovascularization. Angiogenic factors from the tumor itself may also play a role in neovascularization of the anterior segment of the eye.[24]

Anterior displacement of the lens with resultant pupillary block and angle-closure is the second most common mechanism, resulting in glaucoma in eyes containing retinoblastoma.[4, 21, 22] These eyes generally contain retinal detachments secondary to intraretinal or subretinal tumor with massive subretinal exudation of fluid. The space-occupying tumor and subretinal fluid displaces the lens anteriorly, resulting in pupillary block and angle-closure. Massive tumor involvement of the posterior segment may cause anterior displacement of the lens-iris diaphragm to the extent of obliterating the anterior chamber, resulting in an angle-closure glaucoma.

A less common mechanism of glaucoma in eyes with retinoblastoma is massive tumor involvement of the entire globe with direct involvement of the anterior chamber structures by tumor cells.[21] Seeding of the trabecular meshwork by tumor cells from posterior tumors may also occur (Fig. 128–4).[4] Many eyes containing retinoblastoma have a combination of the aforementioned mechanisms, resulting in glaucoma.

The differential diagnosis of glaucoma secondary to retinoblastoma would include glaucoma associated with uveitis, persistent hyperplastic primary vitreous, retinopathy of prematurity, and other causes of neovascularization of the anterior segment. The young age of patients in which retinoblastoma occurs helps to eliminate from the differential diagnosis many of the usual and more common causes of neovascularization of the anterior segment seen in adults. Neovascularization of the anterior segment in a child should raise the suspicion of possible retinoblastoma.

The treatment of retinoblastoma often requires enucleation of the eye for treatment of the tumor. However, in bilateral cases in which it is desirable to retain at least one eye, radiation therapy or photocoagulation may be used to treat the tumor. The management of glaucoma may then require medical therapy. Fistulizing glaucoma operations are contraindicated because of the risk of extraocular spread of tumor cells.

Primary Tumors of the Choroid

Choroidal Malignant Melanoma. Two to 14 percent of eyes containing malignant melanoma of the choroid may develop secondary glaucoma.[1, 4, 19] Earlier reports of the incidence of glaucoma in eyes with choroidal melanoma are higher than those found in the past 20 yr. At the turn of the century and during the early 1900s the incidence of glaucoma in eyes with choroidal melanoma was reported to be as high as 29 to 67 percent.[1–3] This difference in incidence of glaucoma may be due to the earlier diagnosis of choroidal melanoma as a result of the routine use of the indirect ophthalmoscope that has occurred in the past several decades.

The clinical presentation of glaucoma in eyes containing malignant melanoma of the choroid may be variable. Glaucoma secondary to choroidal melanoma may present clinically as neovascular glaucoma, acute or chronic angle-closure glaucoma, hemorrhagic glaucoma, or uveitic glaucoma. The clinical presentation depends on the inducing mechanism.

The most common mechanism of glaucoma in eyes with malignant melanoma of the choroid is neovascularization of the anterior segment.[4] Neovascularization is seen primarily in eyes containing large choroidal tumors with total retinal detachment. The association of long-standing retinal detachment and anterior segment neovascularization is well recognized. The exact mechanism, however, is not completely understood.

The second most common mechanism of glaucoma associated with choroidal melanoma is anterior displacement of the lens-iris diaphragm by the tumor mass, resulting in pupillary block with development of peripheral anterior synechiae and angle-closure glaucoma.[4, 13] The angle-closure glaucoma may occur as an acute angle-closure or as a more insidious chronic angle-closure.

Hemorrhage within the eye secondary to the choroidal melanoma may cause glaucoma. Massive suprachoroidal hemorrhage secondary to choroidal melanoma with anterior displacement of the lens-iris diaphragm may result in angle-closure glaucoma.[4] Direct extension of tumor into the anterior chamber has resulted in hyphema with elevated intraocular pressure.

Anterior extension of choroidal melanoma to involve the anterior segment may result in glaucoma without hemorrhage. Direct invasion of the chamber angle by tumor cells may elevate the intraocular pressure by directly involving outflow pathways.[4]

Spontaneous necrosis of choroidal malignant melanomas is known to occur. The inflammatory response in eyes with necrosis of a malignant melanoma may result in a secondary open-angle glaucoma. The presumed mechanism is obstruction of aqueous outflow pathways by inflammatory cells.[25]

Many eyes with a choroidal malignant melanoma that have developed glaucoma contain large intraocular tumors and decreased vision. Often these eyes undergo enucleation for treatment of the tumor. Management of glaucoma is therefore not an issue. However, in eyes with coexisting glaucoma and choroidal malignant melanoma that have retained good vision, the tumor may be treated with radiation or surgical resection. The elevated intraocular pressure should be managed by medical means.

METASTATIC TUMORS TO THE EYE AND GLAUCOMA

Metastatic Tumors to the Iris

Metastatic tumors involving only the iris are relatively rare. In a large series of uveal metastasis in 256 eyes, only 11 eyes had iris metastases.[4] Seven of these eyes had elevation of intraocular pressure. In a second large series of 199 metastatic carcinomas to the eye, only six involved the iris alone.[26] Twenty of the eyes had involvement of both the iris and the ciliary body, with two involving the iris predominantly and nine involving the iris and the ciliary body equally. The most common primary tumor sites that metastasize to the iris are the lung in males and the breast in females. Cutaneous melanoma and kidney are also known primary tumor sites that may metastasize to the iris.[26, 27]

Clinical presentation of glaucoma associated with metastatic disease to the iris is generally an acute process. Most commonly, the presentation is that of an acute iridocyclitis with pain, redness, and decreased vision. Elevated intraocular pressure is then found on examination. A tumor mass is often seen on the iris surface, and the tumor may be identified in the angle structures.

The most common mechanism of glaucoma in eyes with metastatic disease to the iris is direct invasion of the aqueous outflow pathways by tumor cells.[4, 27] Squamous cell carcinomas metastatic to the iris and anterior segment may form an "epithelial-like" lining over the anterior chamber structures that is very similar to epithelialization of the anterior chamber following anterior segment surgery.[26] Less commonly, hyphema from an iris metastasis may result in a hemolytic glaucoma.[4]

The differential diagnosis of glaucoma secondary to metastatic disease to the iris includes glaucoma associated with uveitis, hyphema, iris cysts, and primary iris tumors. Medical management of glaucoma associated with iris metastasis is appropriate. Radiation to metastatic lesions may also be useful as well as chemotherapy to treat the systemic tumor. Enucleation may be necessary when there is intractable pain present secondary to glaucoma.

A unique and rare "black hypopyon" and secondary glaucoma may occur in eyes with cutaneous melanoma metastatic to the iris.[28, 29] Free-floating melanoma tumor cells and pigment laden macrophages have been documented to form the "black hypopyon." It is postulated that these tumor cells and macrophages mechanically obstruct aqueous outflow pathways.

Metastatic Tumors to the Ciliary Body

Metastatic disease isolated to the ciliary body is rare. In one series of 199 cases of metastasis to the eye, none were completely isolated within the ciliary body.[26] Twenty of the 199 involved both the ciliary body and the iris, with 9 of the 20 predominantly involving the ciliary body. A second study of 256 eyes with uveal metastases revealed three patients with metastasis to the ciliary body.[4] Two of the three eyes had secondary elevation of intraocular pressure.

The clinical presentation of glaucoma secondary to ciliary body metastasis is similar to that associated with iris metastasis. In general, an acute iritis is seen with an associated elevation of intraocular pressure and a tumor involving the anterior chamber angle. The most common primary tumor site is usually the lung or the breast, such as with iris metastasis.[26]

Direct extension of a tumor from the ciliary body into the anterior chamber and involving the angle structures is the most common mechanism of secondary glaucoma in tumors metastatic to the ciliary body.[4, 26] Hemorrhagic glaucoma, neovascularization of the anterior chamber, and mechanical angle-closure resulting from forward displacement of the iris-lens diaphragm by tumor are other mechanisms by which glaucoma may occur in eyes with metastasis to the ciliary body.[26]

Management of glaucoma secondary to metastasis to the ciliary body is similar to the glaucoma associated with iris metastasis. Medical therapy to control the intraocular pressure along with radiation therapy or chemotherapy to treat the tumor may all be beneficial. Enucleation may be done for uncontrolled glaucoma that produces pain.

Metastatic Tumors to the Choroid

The posterior choroid is the most common site within the eye to which tumors metastasize.[27] In published series, 74 to 94 percent of uveal metastasis involve the choroid.[4, 27] Breast carcinoma accounts for most metastatic disease to the choroid.[27] Lung carcinoma is the second most common primary tumor to metastasize to the choroid.[27] In male patients, a lung tumor is the most frequent tumor involving the choroid compared with breast carcinoma in females.[27] Kidney, testicle, prostate, pancreas, colon, and other gastrointestinal tumors are all known to metastasize to the choroid.[4, 27, 30] Glaucoma associated with metastasis to the choroid is rare in comparison with glaucoma associated with metastasis to the anterior uveal tract. In one large series, glaucoma associated with metastasis to the choroid occurred in only 1 percent of eyes.[4] This percentage is strikingly different compared with eyes containing metastasis to the iris or ciliary body, which have an incidence of glaucoma as high as 56 to 64 percent.[4, 26]

Angle-closure glaucoma is the most common form of glaucoma in eyes with metastasis to the choroid.[4] Angle-closure glaucoma is produced in eyes with metastasis to the choroid by anterior displacement of the iris-lens diaphragm. Serous detachment of the retina or choroidal detachment often contribute to the anterior displacement of the iris-lens diaphragm.

Glaucoma secondary to metastasis to the choroid may be managed by medical means to lower intraocular pressure. Radiation to the metastatic lesion along with chemotherapy may also be appropriate to treat the metastatic tumor. Enucleation is required for glaucoma associated with intractable pain.

MISCELLANEOUS TUMORS INVOLVING THE EYE AND GLAUCOMA

Glaucoma Secondary to Leukemia

The ocular manifestations of leukemia are well described.[31] The eyes may be involved in both acute lymphocytic leukemia and chronic lymphocytic leukemia. Leukemic involvement of the ocular tissues of both the posterior and anterior segments of the eye has been reported. The incidence of ocular involvement in leukemia ranges from 50 to 80 percent of eyes in published studies.[31, 32] Despite frequent ocular involvement by leukemia, glaucoma secondary to leukemia is relatively rare. When glaucoma is present, it is most often secondary to anterior segment involvement.

Anterior segment involvement of leukemia may present as a conjunctivitis, iris heterochromia, iritis, hyphema, and pseudohypopyon.[31] Elevated intraocular pressure may occur in eyes with leukemic involvement of the anterior segment secondary to iritis, hyphema, or pseudohypopyon consisting of leukemic cells. Leukemic infiltrates involving the trabecular meshwork and tissue surrounding Schlemm's canal has been documented histopathologically in eyes with elevated intraocular pressure.[33, 34] Epibulbar leukemic infiltrates of the bulbar conjunctiva and episcleral tissue may involve aqueous veins.[35] Epibulbar leukemic infiltrates have been implicated as a mechanism by which secondary glaucoma may occur in eyes with leukemic involvement.

Management of the glaucoma may be done by medical means to control the intraocular pressure. Radiation therapy or chemotherapy to treat the underlying tumor may also promote resolution of the glaucoma.[31, 33, 35]

Glaucoma Secondary to Multiple Myeloma

The ocular manifestations of multiple myeloma are well known.[36] One of the prominent features are cysts of the pars plana and ciliary body. The ciliary body cysts have been implicated in the dislocation of the crystalline lens with resulting lens-induced angle-closure glaucoma. Forward displacement of the iris root by ciliary body cysts has also been implicated in secondary angle-closure glaucoma associated with multiple myeloma.[37]

The presentation of glaucoma secondary to multiple myeloma may be that of acute or chronic angle-closure. If the mechanism is found to be lens induced angle-closure, removal of the lens may be curative. If the mechanism is direct forward displacement of the iris root, medical therapy to lower intraocular pressure should be used. Laser iridectomy or laser cyst puncture may be useful in managing secondary angle-closure glaucoma due to ciliary body cysts.

Glaucoma Secondary to Large Cell Lymphoma

Large cell lymphoma (reticulum cell sarcoma) may occur in the eye and masquerade as a unilateral or bilateral uveitis. The diagnosis is made by biopsy of the vitreous for cytology to document the presence of lymphoma cells. Diffuse infiltration of the uveal tract by large cell lymphoma has resulted in an acute glaucoma secondary to closure of the angle by necrotic swollen iris tissue.[38] Glaucoma secondary to chronic intraocular inflammation, with and without chronic angle-closure, has been reported to occur in eyes with large cell lymphoma.[39, 40] Intraocular lymphoma may also result in elevated intraocular pressure by tumor cells seeding the anterior chamber angle.[4] The tumor is best treated with radiation therapy. The glaucoma should be managed by medical means.

Glaucoma Secondary to Juvenile Xanthogranuloma

Juvenile xanthogranuloma is a benign histiocytic proliferation affecting the skin and eye seen in infants and young children. Typical skin lesions of the disease are yellow-orange papules found on the skin of the head and neck.

Ocular manifestations are most commonly seen in the anterior segment as an iris tumor that is lightly pigmented or salmon colored.[41] Spontaneous hyphema often occurs in the presence of iris involvement. Juvenile xanthogranuloma is the most common cause of spontaneous hyphema in children. Typical skin lesions may not be present, even with ophthalmic involvement.[41, 42] The presentation is often acute with a red and painful eye. On examination hyphema, iris tumor, and elevated intraocular pressure are found.[41, 42]

Glaucoma may occur in eyes with juvenile xanthogranuloma by several mechanisms. Direct involvement of the iris and adjacent angle structures by proliferating histiocytes may obstruct aqueous outflow.[41] Glaucoma may also develop following recurrent spontaneous hyphema.[41, 42] Resolution of glaucoma secondary to juvenile xanthogranuloma may occur following treatment of the tumor by topical or systemic steroids.[42–45] Low-dose radiation therapy to involved iris tissue has also promoted resolution of the tumor and of the associated glaucoma.[42, 44]

Glaucoma Secondary to Histiocytosis

Histiocytosis-X is a proliferation of histiocytes that typically involve multiple organ systems. A secondary open-angle glaucoma has been associated with histiocytosis-X.[46] Aqueous aspiration demonstrated that histiocytes were present in the aqueous. These histiocytes were implicated as a mechanism of obstruction of aqueous outflow.

SUMMARY

Glaucoma associated with intraocular tumors represents only a small fraction of all glaucoma; however, the proper diagnosis and management of patients with glaucoma associated with intraocular tumors is important. Proper recognition and management is mandatory because of the possible fatal outcome of some malignant ocular tumors. The systemic well-being of patients with glaucoma associated with ocular tumors is the primary consideration. Prevention of a fatal outcome due to death caused by a tumor is paramount.

The mechanisms of outflow obstruction secondary to intraocular tumors are varied. Recognition and understanding of the mechanisms involved in glaucomas associated with intraocular tumors is important in rendering proper care to affected patients.

REFERENCES

1. Dunnington JH: Intraocular tension in cases of sarcoma of the choroid and ciliary body. Arch Ophthalmol 20:359–363, 1938.
2. Marshall CD: Tension in cases of intra-ocular tumour. Trans Ophthalmol Soc UK 16:155–169, 1896.
3. Terry TL, Johns JP: Uveal sarcoma—Malignant melanoma. Am J Ophthalmol 18:903–913, 1935.
4. Shields CL, Shields JA, Shields MB, Augsburger JJ: Prevalence and mechanisms of secondary intraocular pressure elevation in eyes with intraocular tumors. Ophthalmology 94:839–846, 1987.
5. Narieman AN, Ahmed H, Zimmerman LE, Fine BS: Diffuse iris nevus manifested by unilateral open angle glaucoma. Ophthalmology 99:125–127, 1981.
6. Shields JA, Annesley WH, Spaeth GL: Necrotic melanocytoma of iris with secondary glaucoma. Am J Ophthalmol 84:826–829, 1977.
7. Thomas CI, Purnell EW: Ocular melanocytoma. Am J Ophthalmol 67:79–86, 1969.
8. Shields JA, Augsburger JJ, Sanborn GE, Klein RM: Adenoma of the iris-pigment epithelium. Ophthalmology 90:735–739, 1983.
9. Jakobiec FA, Silbert G: Are most iris "melanomas" really nevi? Arch Ophthalmol 99:2117–2132, 1981.
10. Cleasby GW: Malignant melanoma of the iris. Arch Ophthalmol 60:403–417, 1958.
11. Yanoff M, Scheie HG: Melanomalytic glaucoma. Arch Ophthalmol 84:471–473, 1970.
12. Van Buskirk EM, Leure-DuPree AE: Pathophysiology and electron microscopy of melanomalytic glaucoma. Am J Ophthalmol 85:160–166, 1978.
13. Yanoff M: Mechanisms of glaucomain eyes with uveal malignant melanomas. Int Ophthalmol Clin 12:51–62, 1972.
14. Rones B, Zimmerman LE: The prognosis of primary tumors of the iris treated by iridectomy. Arch Ophthalmol 60:193–205, 1958.
15. Shields MB, Klintworth GK: Anterior uveal melanomas and intraocular pressure. Ophthalmology 87:503–517, 1980.
16. Foos RY, Hull SN, Straatsma BR: Early diagnosis of ciliary body melanomas. Arch Ophthalmol 81:336–344, 1969.
17. Broughton WL, Zimmerman LE: A clinicopathologic study of 56 cases of intraocular medulloepitheliomas. Am J Ophthalmol 85:407–418, 1978.
18. Bowers JF: Melanocytoma of the ciliary body. Arch Ophthalmol 71:649–652, 1964.
19. Yanoff M: Glaucoma mechanisms in ocular malignant melanomas. Am J Ophthalmol 70:898–904, 1970.
20. Croxatto JO, Ebner R, Crovetto L, Morales AG: Angle closure glaucoma as initial manifestation of melanocytoma of the optic disc. Ophthalmology 90:830–834, 1983.
21. Yoshizumi MO, Thomas JV, Smith TR: Glaucoma-inducing mechanisms in eyes with retinoblastoma. Arch Ophthalmol 96:105–110, 1978.
22. Walton DS, Grant WM: Retinoblastoma and iris neovascularization. Am J Ophthalmol 65:598–599, 1968.
23. Spaulding AG: Rubeosis iridis in retinoblastoma and pseudoglioma. Trans Am Ophthalmol Soc 76:584–609, 1978.
24. Folkman J: Tumor angiogenesis factor. Cancer Res 34:2109–2113, 1974.
25. Reese AB, Archila EA, Jones IS, Cooper WC: Necrosis of malignant melanoma of the choroid. Am J Ophthalmol 69:91–104, 1970.
26. Ferry AP, Font RL: Carcinoma metastatic to the eye and orbit. Arch Ophthalmol 93:472–482, 1975.
27. Ferry AP, Font RL: Carcinoma metastatic to the eye and orbit. Arch Ophthalmol 92:276–286, 1974.

28. Char DH, Schwartz A, Miller TR, Abele JS: Ocular metastases from systemic melanoma. Am J Ophthalmol 90:702–707, 1980.
29. Harper JI, Wormald RPL: Bilateral black hypopyon in a patient with self-healing cutaneous malignant melanoma. Br J Ophthalmol 67:231–235, 1983.
30. Hart WM: Metastatic carcinoma to the eye and orbit. Int Ophthalmol Clin 2:465–482, 1962.
31. Kincaid MC, Green WR: Ocular and orbital involvement in leukemia. Surv Ophthalmol 27:211–232, 1983.
32. Allen KA, Straatsma BR: Ocular involvement in leukemia and allied diseases. Arch Ophthalmol 66:490–508, 1961.
33. Fonken HA, Ellis PP: Leukemic infiltrates in the iris. Arch Ophthalmol 76:32–36, 1966.
34. Rowan PJ, Sloan JB: Iris and anterior chamber involvement in leukemia. Ann Ophthalmol 6:1081–1085, 1976.
35. Glaser B, Smith JL: Leukaemic glaucoma. Br J Ophthalmol 50:92–94, 1966.
36. Ashton N: Ocular changes in multiple myelomatosis. Arch Ophthalmol 73:487–494, 1965.
37. Baker TR, Spencer WH: Ocular findings in multiple myeloma. Arch Ophthalmol 91:110–113, 1974.
38. Duker JS, Shields JA, Ross M: Intraocular large cell lymphoma presenting as massive thickening of uveal tract. Retina 7:41–45, 1987.
39. Collyer R: Reticulum cell sarcoma of eye and orbit. Can J Ophthalmol 7:247–249, 1972.
40. Klingele TG, Hogan MJ: Ocular reticulum cell sarcoma. Am J Ophthalmol 79:39–47, 1975.
41. Zimmerman L: Ocular lesions of juvenile xanthogranuloma. Trans Am Acad Ophthalmol Otol 69:412–442, 1965.
42. Gass JD: Management of juvenile xanthogranuloma of the iris. Arch Ophthalmol 71:344–347, 1964.
43. Schwartz LW, Rodrigues MM, Hallett JW: Juvenile xanthogranuloma diagnosed by paracentesis. Am J Ophthalmol 77:243–245, 1974.
44. Hadden OB: Bilateral juvenile xanthogranuloma of the iris. Br J Ophthalmol 59:699–702, 1975.
45. Bruner WE, Stark WJ, Green WR: Presumed juvenile xanthogranuloma of the iris and ciliary body in an adult. Arch Ophthalmol 100:457–459, 1982.
46. Epstein DL, Grant WM: Secondary open-angle glaucoma in histiocytosis X. Am J Ophthalmol 84:332–336, 1977.

Chapter 129

■

Corticosteroid-Induced Glaucoma

CLAUDIA A. ARRIGG

Over the years, clinical and experimental investigations have documented the effects of corticosteroids on the eye. It is well established that topical, systemic, or periocular steroid administration can cause an increase in intraocular pressure and a decrease in the facility of aqueous outflow.[1–5] The clinical findings typically resemble primary open-angle glaucoma. Despite their popularity as antiallergic and antiinflammatory agents,[6, 7] corticosteroids can have tragic consequences and should be used only with judicious monitoring.

In 1954, Francois published the first report of an intraocular pressure rise following long-term therapy with topical cortisone. He also noted optic nerve cupping and atrophy and visual field loss, which suggested a picture very similar to open-angle glaucoma.[8]

Other reports followed shortly thereafter. Armaly found that the topical application of dexamethasone in normal eyes resulted in increased intraocular pressure and a reduction in outflow facility and rate of aqueous formation.[1] The magnitude of the effect was greatest among older people and those with glaucomatous eyes.[1, 2] Becker and Mills also noted that chronically administered topical steroids not only produced a glaucoma-like state in otherwise healthy eyes but also exacerbated preexisting glaucoma.[3] However, unlike primary open-angle glaucoma, this condition was usually reversible on cessation of the drug.

A number of drugs have been implicated in corticosteroid-induced glaucoma, including dexamethasone,[1, 2, 6–14] betamethasone,[3, 4, 15–18] prednisolone,[3, 5, 19] medrysone,[7, 10] fluorometholone,[20, 21] hydrocortisone,[3, 5, 10, 22] cortisone,[8, 23] prednisone,[5, 23] and flurandrenolide.[24]

EPIDEMIOLOGY

Corticosteroid-induced glaucoma can occur in any age group, in either sex, or from steroid therapy for any ocular or systemic disease. Approximately one third of the normal population develops a moderate increase in intraocular pressure following topical corticosteroid use.[3, 4, 25] However, 5 to 6 percent of the normal population develops markedly increased intraocular pressure of more than 31 mmHg after 4 to 6 wk of topical corticosteroid therapy.[15, 26–28] In contrast, almost all patients with primary open-angle glaucoma or low-tension glaucoma develop some elevation of the intraocular pressure after topical steroid therapy.[2, 4, 15, 28]

A genetic basis for this finding was proposed in landmark papers in the 1960s by Armaly[26–28] and Becker.[4, 15] Using different classification criteria, both authors independently postulated a relationship between the inheritance of the intraocular pressure response to topical corticosteroids and the inheritance of primary open-angle glaucoma. Becker and Hahn also proposed that the pressure response to topical steroid testing was genetically determined by a simple monogenic autosomal mechanism. The recessive homozygote state was hypothesized to be present in patients with primary open-angle glaucoma.[4]

Although all patients on steroids have the potential of developing corticosteroid-induced glaucoma, some persons are at a higher risk. Individuals who are particularly susceptible are those with primary open-angle glaucoma or a family history of glaucoma.[2–4, 6, 15, 16, 29] In addition, highly myopic patients (>5.0 diopters) with no evidence or family history of glaucoma have a high rate (88 percent) of an elevated intraocular pressure rise in response to topical steroid testing.[30, 31] Persons with diabetes mellitus have a greater prevalence of primary open-angle glaucoma and an elevated intraocular pressure response to topical corticosteroids.[32]

Many patients with ocular complications of renal and connective-tissue disease (e.g., rheumatoid or psoriatic arthritis, systemic lupus erythematosus) are treated with topical and systemic steroids.[23, 33] Unlike the 5 to 6 percent of normal eyes found to have a marked pressure rise by Becker and Armaly, Gaston found that 15 percent of patients with connective tissue disease had a dramatic response to topical steroid testing and concluded that damage to the trabecular meshwork from their disease may be the cause of their glaucoma.[34]

Patients undergoing surgery are at risk if steroids are used either preoperatively or postoperatively. Corticosteroid-induced glaucoma has developed in patients using topical corticosteroids following cataract surgery[35] as well as filtration surgery, despite the presence of a functioning filtering bleb,[21, 36, 37] although this finding has been disputed.[38]

Recent studies have questioned the precision and reproducibility of the intraocular response to topical dexamethasone testing.[39] Furthermore, Schwartz and associates found a low concordance of pressure response in monozygotic twins to topical testing, indicating either a limited role for the genetic basis for the monogenic inheritance of the corticosteroid response or poor reproducibility to topical steroid testing.[12, 13] In addition, dexamethasone provocative testing has been found to have limited prognostic ability both for the development of glaucoma in steroid responders[9, 40] and visual field loss in glaucoma suspects.[41]

ROUTES OF ADMINISTRATION

Most corticosteroid-induced glaucoma comes from exogenous steroids, which may be given topically, periocularly, or systemically. Endogenous steroids can also cause this condition (Table 129–1).

Table 129–1. CORTICOSTEROID-INDUCED GLAUCOMA

Exogenous corticosteroids
1. Ocular (topical)
   a. Eyedrops
   b. Ocular ointments
   c. Inadvertent administration to the eye from the lids or the face
2. Periocular injection
3. Systemic
   a. Oral
   b. Topical to the skin
   c. Injection

Endogenous corticosteroids
1. Adrenal hyperplasia
2. Adrenal adenoma or carcinoma
3. Ectopic adrenocorticotropic hormone (ACTH) syndrome

Modified from Kass MA, Johnson T: Corticosteroid-induced glaucoma. *In* Ritch R, Shields MB, Krupin T (eds): The Glaucomas. St Louis, CV Mosby Company, 1989.

Topical Route

Of the various routes of steroid administration, topical therapy most commonly causes elevated intraocular pressure by having a greater effect than systemic therapy on aqueous outflow facility.[42] When administered to normal eyes, topical steroids can cause an intraocular pressure rise that correlates with the duration and frequency of drug administration.[1, 4, 26] Nevertheless, the topical application of corticosteroids is still considered safer than the systemic route because of the multiple other potentially devastating side effects of systemic steroid administration. The topical route includes ocular drops and ointment, as well as steroid lotions, creams, and ointment applied to the face or eyelids.[17, 24, 43–45]

Periocular Route

Subconjunctival,[46, 47] sub-Tenon's,[48, 49] and retrobulbar injections[50] may cause dangerous and prolonged elevations of intraocular pressure because of their long duration of action. The increased pressure from these repository steroids can be sustained for 1 yr or more after the injection.[47, 48] A patient's response to topical steroids does not predict the response to periocular steroids.[49] The advantages of periocular steroids are (1) a high local concentration; (2) a long duration of action, determined by the solubility of the steroid and the location of the injection; and (3) their effectiveness against inflammatory disorders of the posterior segment.[46–48] The inferior quadrant is the preferred injection site, in order to save the superior conjunctiva for possible future filtration surgery.

Systemic Route

Although systemic administration of corticosteroids is the least likely to cause intraocular pressure elevation, the pressure rise may occur as long as weeks to years following treatment.[19, 23, 42, 51] When systemic steroids are administered concurrently with topical corticosteroids (e.g., in patients with uveitis with underlying collagen vascular disease or patients with asthma),[38, 42, 51] the combined treatment may have an additive effect, resulting in a higher intraocular pressure than if a single route was used. Even steroids applied to the skin at remote sites can be systemically absorbed, raising the intraocular pressure in susceptible individuals.[52] This pressure effect also occurs when occlusive dressings to large parts of the body are impregnated with fluorinated glucocorticoids.[52]

Endogenous Route

The endogenous production of glucocorticoids, for example, in Cushing's syndrome, can also cause an increase in the intraocular pressure. In one report, the increased intraocular pressure and decreased outflow facility returned to normal following adrenalectomy.[53]

CLINICAL COURSE

An increase in intraocular pressure may occur as soon as a few hours[14] or as long as months to years following the administration of steroids.[3, 25, 52] The height and duration of the pressure rise depend on factors such as drug potency, penetration, dosage, and length of administration, as well as on individual susceptibility, age, and underlying ocular or systemic disease.[1, 2, 10, 24, 50]

Both chronic and acute forms of corticosteroid glaucoma respond to cessation of the corticosteroid therapy and to treatment with antiglaucoma medication, if needed. Even in patients with visual field loss and optic cupping and atrophy, the outflow facility and intraocular pressure generally return to baseline values in days to weeks after discontinuation of the medication.[3, 25, 38] Rarely, the intraocular pressure remains persistently elevated for months or years after the steroids have been discontinued, perhaps as a result of damage to the outflow channels.[52] In one report, despite cessation of therapy, increased intraocular pressure reversed in one eye but remained elevated in the other eye that had received greater and more prolonged flurandrenolide therapy.[24]

Clinical Findings

The clinical findings in corticosteroid-induced glaucoma typically resemble those of primary open-angle glaucoma in teenagers and adults: (1) open and normal-appearing angle by gonioscopy, (2) white and painless eye, (3) optic disc cupping, (4) visual field defects, (5) elevated intraocular pressure, and (6) decreased outflow facility.[3–5, 25] Patients are usually asymptomatic. However, an acute presentation can occur if the intraocular pressure is elevated enough, such as following intensive systemic steroid therapy (rarely following topical treatment). In this situation, patients may develop corneal edema, blurred vision, ciliary hyperemia, and pain, although the anterior chamber depth and angle remain normal.[25]

The age of the patient may determine the clinical form of corticosteroid-induced glaucoma. A recent report suggests that a marked elevation in intraocular pressure to 0.1% dexamethasone instillation occurs frequently in children under 10 years of age.[54] Infants develop a picture similar to congenital glaucoma. Signs include tearing, photophobia, blepharospasm, cloudy corneas with an enlarged corneal diameter, Descemet's membrane breaks, elevated intraocular pressure, and optic disc cupping. Unlike congenital glaucoma, however, the anterior chamber angle is normal.[55]

Additional ocular findings from topical steroid use include mydriasis,[56, 57] increased corneal thickness,[58] corneal ulcers,[43, 59] posterior subcapsular cataracts,[38, 43, 59] delayed wound healing, ptosis,[56, 57] and skin atrophy of eyelids.[43] Importantly, systemic steroids are known to cause cushingoid facies, truncal obesity, hirsutism, buffalo hump, cutaneous striae, easy bruisability, delayed wound healing, osteoporosis, fluid retention, peptic ulcers, diabetes, hypertension, and psychiatric disorders.[50]

PATHOGENESIS

Many mechanisms have been proposed to explain the elevated intraocular pressure and decreased outflow facility seen in corticosteroid-induced glaucoma. The most commonly held hypothesis is that glycosaminoglycans accumulate in the outflow pathways causing an increase in outflow resistance.[1, 2, 52, 60, 61] Glycosaminoglycans, normally present in the aqueous outflow channels, are depolymerized by hyaluronidase that is contained in lysosomes. Francois showed that corticosteroids protect the lysosomal membrane and thus inhibit the release of hydrolases from the lysosomes.[62] In turn, glycosaminoglycans cannot depolymerize and accumulate in the ground substance, retain water, and narrow the trabeculae. It is only when glycosaminoglycans become depolymerized from the liberation of the catabolic enzymes from lysosomes that they no longer retain water, the trabeculae widen, and aqueous outflow is facilitated.[25, 52, 62, 63]

Other investigators have postulated that in primary open-angle glaucoma, an abnormal accumulation of dihydrocortisols in trabecular cells may potentiate exogenous glucocorticoid activity. In particular, 5β-dihydrocortisol can potentiate the increased intraocular pressure caused by exogenous glucocorticoids in primary open-angle glaucoma. This theory may explain why patients with open-angle glaucoma have an increased susceptibility to pressure elevation from corticosteroids.[64–70]

An alternative explanation is that corticosteroids inhibit prostaglandin synthesis by human trabecular cells. Dexamethasone can inhibit synthesis of both prostaglandins E_2 and $F_2\alpha$, whose normal function is to lower the intraocular pressure by increasing the outflow facility.[71, 72]

Another theory involves phagocytosis. Endothelial cells lining the trabecular meshwork can act as phagocytes of debris in aqueous humor. Corticosteroids suppress phagocytic activity, causing aqueous debris accumulation in the trabecular meshwork and decreased outflow.[73]

DIFFERENTIAL DIAGNOSIS

To diagnose corticosteroid-induced glaucoma, the most important consideration is a careful history of any type of past or present use of steroids. For example, when previously stable open-angle glaucoma becomes difficult to control, the physician must consider whether systemic steroids, started to treat some other disease, could be contributing to this change or whether the underlying glaucoma is progressing. The history and examination of the patient should also include observation for symptoms and signs of endogenous corticosteroid production.

A history of steroid use may also be important in evaluating a patient with a shallow anterior chamber. In the presence of corticosteroid-induced glaucoma, a shallow anterior chamber can be mistaken for chronic angle-closure glaucoma. In presumed low-tension glaucoma, the intraocular pressure and outflow facility may be of normal range, but advanced cupping and visual field loss may be present. Since these latter findings may be sequelae of corticosteroid-induced glaucoma, a comprehensive history is crucial.[50] In patients with uveitis, it is often difficult to determine whether an elevated intraocular pressure is due to an inflammatory condition or from the steroids used to treat the disease. In unilateral cases, examination of the pressure of the uninvolved eye may be helpful in determining steroid responsiveness.

MANAGEMENT

The most effective management of corticosteroid-induced glaucoma is discontinuation of the drug.[25] The intraocular pressure generally returns to normal within a few days to weeks,[3] although it may take months or years.[52] Once the corticosteroid is discontinued, the time required to regain normal intraocular pressure does not correlate with either the height of intraocular pressure rise or the extent of decreased aqueous outflow facility.[38]

Whenever steroids must be used for a particular disease entity, it is important to choose the safest drug with the fewest side effects, lowest concentration, shortest action, lowest dosage frequency, and most effective route of administration.[10] As corticosteroid-induced glaucoma can develop at any point during therapy, the baseline intraocular pressure should be established before treatment is initiated and then followed closely every 2 to 3 wk for the entire duration of treatment. Corticosteroid-responsive individuals should be followed carefully for the development of glaucoma-like visual field defects and disc changes.[18, 40, 41] Medical management with antiglaucoma therapy may be necessary.

The treatment of choice for patients with glaucoma or a known steroid responder is medrysone or fluorometholone,[10, 20, 21] because these two agents have the least effect on intraocular pressure. Fluorometholone is less likely to increase the intraocular pressure than dexamethasone because of its chemical structure, specifically, deoxygenation at the C_{21} position.[20, 21] Nonsteroidal antiinflammatory agents have not been shown to cause a pressure elevation.[74]

In the case of uncontrolled intraocular pressure following repository steroids, the depot site of the injection may require excision.[47–49]

In some patients, glaucoma may persist even after discontinuation of steroid therapy.[52] Argon laser trabeculoplasty has variable success in treating corticosteroid-induced glaucoma but may be a viable approach prior to filtering surgery.[75–77] However, if progressive optic nerve cupping and visual field loss develop, filtering surgery is indicated.[25, 38]

In all cases, if additional systemic steroid therapy is used, it is important to watch for the development of a pressure rise in the contralateral eye.

CONCLUSION

Corticosteroid therapy remains a common cause of visual loss. All physicians should be aware of the potentially devastating and deleterious consequences of unrestricted or prolonged use of topical and systemic corticosteroids. The recognition and management of corticosteroid-induced glaucoma should be well understood by every ophthalmologist.

REFERENCES

1. Armaly MF: Effect of corticosteroids on intraocular pressure and fluid dynamics. I: The effect of dexamethasone in the normal eye. Arch Ophthalmol 70:482, 1963.
2. Armaly MF: Effect of corticosteroids on intraocular pressure and fluid dynamics. II: The effect of dexamethasone in the glaucomatous eye. Arch Ophthalmol 70:492, 1963.
3. Becker B, Mills DW: Corticosteroids and intraocular pressure. Arch Ophthalmol 70:500, 1963.
4. Becker B, Hahn KA: Topical corticosteroids and heredity in primary open-angle glaucoma. Am J Ophthalmol 57:543, 1964.
5. Goldmann H: Cortisone glaucoma. Arch Ophthalmol 68:621, 1962.
6. Jilani FA, Khan AM, Kesharwani RK: Study of topical corticosteroid response in glaucoma suspects and family members of established glaucoma patients. Indian J Ophthalmol 35(3):141, 1987.
7. Mithal S, Sood AK, Maini AK: Management of vernal conjunctivitis with steroid induced glaucoma—A comparative study. Indian J Ophthalmol 35:298, 1987.
8. Francois J: Cortisone et tension oculaire. Ann Ocul 187:805, 1954.
9. Klemetti A: The dexamethasone provocative test: A predictive tool for glaucoma? Acta Ophthalmol 68:29, 1990.
10. Podos SM, Krupin T, Asseff C, et al: Topically administered corticosteroid preparations. Arch Ophthalmol 86:251, 1971.
11. Podos SM, Becker B, Beaty C, et al: Diphenylhydantoin and cortisol metabolism in glaucoma. Am J Ophthalmol 74:498, 1972.
12. Schwartz JT, Reuling FH, Feinleib M, et al: Twin study on ocular pressure after topical dexamethasone. I: Frequency distribution of pressure response. Am J Ophthalmol 76:126, 1973.
13. Schwartz JT, Reuling FH, Feinleib M, et al: Twin study on ocular pressure following topically applied dexamethasone. II: Inheritance of variation in pressure response. Arch Ophthalmol 90:281, 1973.
14. Weinreb RN, Polansky JR, Kramer SG, et al: Acute effects of dexamethasone on intraocular pressure in glaucoma. Invest Ophthalmol Vis Sci 26:170, 1985.
15. Becker B: Intraocular pressure response to topical corticosteroids. Invest Ophthalmol Vis Sci 4(2):198, 1965.
16. Becker B, Chevrette L: Topical corticosteroid testing in glaucoma siblings. Arch Ophthalmol 76:484, 1966.
17. Eisenlohr JE: Glaucoma following the prolonged use of topical steroid medication to the eyelids. J Am Acad Dermatol 8:878, 1983.
18. Kitazawa Y, Horie T: The prognosis of corticosteroid-responsive individuals. Arch Ophthalmol 99:819, 1981.
19. McDonnell PJ, Kerr Muir MG: Glaucoma associated with systemic corticosteroid therapy (Letter). Lancet 17;2(8451):386, 1985.
20. Morrison E, Archer DB: Effect of fluorometholone (FML) on the intraocular pressure of corticosteroid responders. Br J Ophthalmol 68:581, 1984.

21. Akingbehin AO: Comparative study of the intraocular pressure effects of fluorometholone 0.1% versus dexamethasone 0.1%. Br J Ophthalmol 67:661, 1983.
22. Munjal VP, Dhir SP, Jain IS: Steroid induced glaucoma. Indian J Ophthalmol 30:379, 1982.
23. Bernstein HN, Schwartz B: Effects of long-term systemic steroids on ocular pressure and tonographic values. Arch Ophthalmol 68:742, 1962.
24. Brubaker RF, Halpin JA: Open-angle glaucoma associated with topical administration of flurandrenolide to the eye. Mayo Clin Proc 50:322, 1975.
25. Francois J: Corticosteroid glaucoma. Ann Ophthalmol 9(9):1075, 1977.
26. Armaly MF: Statistical attributes of the steroid hypertensive response in the clinically normal eye. I: The demonstration of three levels of response. Invest Ophthalmol Vis Sci 14:187, 1965.
27. Armaly MF: The heritable nature of dexamethasone-induced ocular hypertension. Arch Ophthalmol 75:32, 1966.
28. Armaly MF: Inheritance of dexamethasone hypertension and glaucoma. Arch Ophthalmol 77:747, 1967.
29. Davies TG: Tonographic survey of the close relatives of patients with chronic simple glaucoma. Br J Ophthalmol 52:32, 1968.
30. Podos SM, Becker B, Morton WR: High myopia and primary open-angle glaucoma. Am J Ophthalmol 62:1039, 1966.
31. Wang RF, Guo BK: Steroid-induced ocular hypertension in high myopia. Chin Med J 97(1):24, 1984.
32. Becker B: Diabetes mellitus and primary open-angle glaucoma. Am J Ophthalmol 71:1, 1971.
33. Wilson DM, Martin JH, Niall JF: Raised intraocular tension in renal transplant recipients. Med J Aust 1:482, 1973.
34. Gaston H, Absolon MJ, Thurtle OA, et al: Steroid responsiveness in connective tissue diseases. Br J Ophthalmol 67:487, 1983.
35. Kwitko ML: Postoperative open-angle glaucoma following topical application of steroids. Can Med Assoc J 94:966, 1966.
36. Thomas R, Jay JL: Raised intraocular pressure with topical steroids after trabeculectomy. Graefes Arch Clin Exp Ophthalmol 226:337, 1988.
37. Wilensky JT, Snyder D, Gieser D: Steroid-induced ocular hypertension in patients with filtering blebs. Ophthalmology 87:240, 1980.
38. Epstein DL: Corticosteroid glaucoma. In Epstein DL (ed): Chandler and Grant's Glaucoma, 3rd ed. Philadelphia, Lea & Febiger, 1986.
39. Palmberg PF, Mandell A, Wilensky JT, et al: The reproducibility of the intraocular pressure response to dexamethasone. Am J Ophthalmol 80:844, 1975.
40. Lewis JM, Priddy T, Judd J, et al: Intraocular pressure response to topical dexamethasone as a predictor for the development of primary open-angle glaucoma. Am J Ophthalmol 106:607, 1988.
41. Wilensky JT, Podos SM, Becker B: Prognostic indicators in ocular hypertension. Arch Ophthalmol 91:200, 1974.
42. Godel V, Regenbogen L, Stein R: On the mechanism of corticosteroid-induced ocular hypertension. Ann Ophthalmol 10(2):191, 1978.
43. Cubey RB: Glaucoma following the application of corticosteroid to the skin of the eyelids. Br J Dermatol 95:207, 1976.
44. Nielsen NV, Sorensen PN: Glaucoma induced by application of corticosteroids to the periorbital region. Arch Dermatol 114:953, 1978.
45. Zugerman C, Sauders D, Levit F: Glaucoma from topically applied steroids. Arch Dermatol 112:1326, 1976.
46. Kalina RE: Increased intraocular pressure following subconjunctival corticosteroid administration. Arch Ophthalmol 81:788, 1969.
47. Mills DW, Siebert LF, Climenhaga DB: Depot triamcinolone-induced glaucoma. Can J Ophthalmol 21(4):150, 1986.
48. Herschler J: Intractable intraocular hypertension induced by repository triamcinolone acetonide. Am J Ophthalmol 74:501, 1972.
49. Herschler J: Increased intraocular pressure induced by repository corticosteroids. Am J Ophthalmol 82:90, 1976.
50. Kass MA, Johnson T: Corticosteroid-induced glaucoma. In Ritch R, Shields MB, Krupin T (eds): The Glaucomas. St Louis, CV Mosby, 1989.
51. Godel V, Feiler-Ofry V, Stein R: Systemic steroids and ocular fluid dynamics. II: Systemic versus topical steroids. Acta Ophthalmol 50:664, 1972.
52. Spaeth GL, Rodrigues MM: Steroid-induced glaucoma. A: Persistent elevation of intraocular pressure. B: Histopathological aspects. Trans Am Ophthalmol Soc 75:353, 1977.
53. Hass JS, Nootens RH: Glaucoma secondary to benign adrenal adenoma. Am J Ophthalmol 78:497, 1974.
54. Ohji M, Kinoshita S, Ohmi E, Kuwayama Y: Marked intraocular response to instillation of corticosteroids in children. Am J Ophthalmol 112:450, 1991.
55. Alfano JE, Platt D: Steroid (ACTH)-induced glaucoma simulating congenital glaucoma. Am Ophthalmol 61:911, 1966.
56. Newsome DA, Wong VG, Cameron TP, Anderson RR: "Steroid-induced" mydriasis and ptosis. Invest Ophthalmol 10:424, 1971.
57. Spaeth GL: The effect of autonomic agents on the pupil and the intraocular pressure of eyes treated with dexamethasone. Br J Ophthalmol 64:426, 1980.
58. Baum JL, Levene RZ: Corneal thickness after topical corticosteroid therapy. Arch Ophthalmol 79:366, 1968.
59. St Clair-Roberts D: Steroids, the eye, and general practitioners. Br Med J 292:1414, 1986.
60. Sood NN, Raghu Ram AR: Histopathological and histochemical analysis of trabeculectomy specimens in open angle and steroid induced glaucoma—A clinico-pathological study. Indian J Ophthalmol 31:947, 1983.
61. Johnson D, Bradley J, Acott T: The effect of dexamethasone on glycosaminoglycans of human trabecular meshwork in perfusion organ culture. Invest Ophthalmol Vis Sci 31(12):2568, 1990.
62. Francois J: Corticosteroid glaucoma. Ophthalmologica 188:76, 1984.
63. Francois J, Benozzi G, Victoria-Troncoso V, et al: Ultrastructural and morphometric study of corticosteroid glaucoma in rabbits. Ophthalmic Res 16:168, 1984.
64. Southren AL, Gordon GG, Munnangi PR, et al: Altered cortisol metabolism in cells cultured from trabecular meshwork specimens obtained from patients with primary open-angle glaucoma. Invest Ophthalmol Vis Sci 24(10):1413, 1983.
65. Southren AL, Gordon GG, I'Hommedieu D, et al: 5β-dihydrocortisol: Possible mediator of the ocular hypertension in glaucoma. Invest Ophthalmol Vis Sci 26(3):393, 1985.
66. Southren AL, Gordon GG, Weinstein BI: Genetic defect in cortisol metabolism in primary open angle glaucoma. Trans Assoc Am Physicians 98:361, 1985.
67. Southren AL, I'Hommedieu D, Gordon GG, et al: Intraocular hypotensive effect of a topically applied cortisol metabolite: 3 alpha, 5 beta-tetrahydrocortisol. Invest Ophthalmol Vis Sci 28:901, 1987.
68. Weinstein BI, Gordon GG, Southren AL: Potentiation of glucocorticoid activity by 5β-dihydrocortisol: Its role in glaucoma. Science 222:172, 1983.
69. Weinstein BI, Munnangi P, Gordon GG, et al: Defects in cortisol-metabolizing enzymes in primary open-angle glaucoma. Invest Ophthalmol Vis Sci 26:890, 1985.
70. Weinstein B, Kandalaft N, Ritch R, et al: 5α-Dihydrocortisol in human aqueous humor and metabolism of cortisol by human lenses in vitro. Invest Ophthalmol Vis Sci 32(7):2130, 1991.
71. Weinreb RN, Mitchell MD, Polansky JR: Prostaglandin production by human trabecular cells: In vitro inhibition by dexamethasone. Invest Ophthalmol Vis Sci 24(12):1541, 1983.
72. Polansky JR, Kurtz RM, Alvarado JA, et al: Eicosanoid production and glucocorticoid regulatory mechanisms in cultured human trabecular meshwork cells. Prog Clin Biol Res 312:113, 1989.
73. Bill A: The drainage of aqueous humor. Invest Ophthalmol 14(1):1, 1975.
74. Shields MB: Steroid-induced glaucoma. In Shields MB: Textbook of Glaucoma, 2nd ed. Baltimore, Williams & Wilkins, 1987.
75. Hoskins HD Jr, Kass MA: Secondary open-angle glaucoma. In Hoskins HD Jr, Kass MA: Becker-Shaffer's Diagnosis and Therapy of the Glaucomas, 6th ed. St Louis, CV Mosby, 1989.
76. Thomas J: Laser trabeculoplasty. In Belcher CD, Thomas J, Simmons R (eds.): Photocoagulation in Glaucoma and Anterior Segment Disease. Baltimore, Williams & Wilkins, 1984.
77. Reiss G, Wilensky J, Higginbotham E: Laser trabeculoplasty. Surv Ophthalmol 35(6):407, 1991.

Chapter 130

Glaucoma Associated With Increased Episcleral Venous Pressure

EVE JULIET HIGGINBOTHAM

The diagnosis and management of open-angle glaucoma secondary to increased episcleral venous pressure (EVP) is sometimes challenging. The diagnosis can be easily missed if the clinical presentation does not show evidence of an obvious sign such as pulsatile exophthalmos. If unprepared, the unsuspecting ophthalmic surgeon may encounter unexpected intraoperative complications such as choroidal hemorrhage. Moreover, the management of some cases may involve other physicians such as a neuroradiologist, an oncologist, or a neurosurgeon. It thus behooves the clinician to be fully aware of the clinical entities associated with elevated EVP.

The importance of the role of EVP in aqueous dynamics has evolved over several decades. The aqueous veins are important contributors to EVP. The relationship between aqueous veins and aqueous outflow began to be recognized when Lauber, in the early 1900s, provided evidence histologically that the canal of Schlemm was connected to the episcleral venous network.[1] Several investigations were made with animals, and the results suggested a functional link between the anterior chamber and the aqueous veins. Lauber[1] noted in 1901 the dilution of red blood cells in the anterior ciliary veins of the dog compared with an aliquot of blood taken from the paw of the same animal. In 1923, Seidel[2] injected India ink in the anterior chamber of a rabbit and subsequently noted the appearance of the ink in the episcleral veins. As a natural extension of these observations in animals, Ascher[1, 3] noted the presence of aqueous veins in humans and described their physiologic importance to aqueous flow in 1942. These vessels, which were once thought to be empty, were described as containing clear fluid, the aqueous humor. Ascher's observations sparked great interest in aqueous veins, the pressure generated within these vessels, and the influence of EVP on intraocular pressure (IOP).

The diagnosis of glaucoma secondary to elevated EVP can be divided into three genral areas: arteriovenous anomalies, venous obstruction, and the idiopathic variety.[4] The first category, arteriovenous anomalies, can be subdivided into six entities: carotid cavernous sinus fistula, orbital varices, Sturge-Weber syndrome, orbital-meningeal shunts, carotid jugular venous shunts, and intraocular vascular shunts. Venous obstruction can present as a retrobulbar tumor, thyroid ophthalmopathy, superior vena cava syndrome, congestive heart failure, thrombosis of the cavernous sinus or orbital vein, vasculitis involving the episcleral vein or orbital vein, and jugular vein obstruction. Finally, patients may present without any apparent cause of their elevated EVP and may show evidence of either a sporadic or familial form of the disease. A brief review of the anatomy of the ocular and orbital venous system and the physiology and the various methods of measuring EVP will provide the reader with a general foundation for understanding the basic mechanism of this secondary open-angle glaucoma prior to the discussion of each of the specific disorders.

ANATOMY OF THE EPISCLERAL VENOUS SYSTEM

According to Duke-Elder and Wybar,[5] the ciliary circulation consists of the vortex system, the anterior ciliary system, and the posterior ciliary system. The vortex system drains most of the choroid, ciliary body, and iris. The venules of the choroid, arising from the choriocapillaris, converge with neighboring venules to form subsequently larger veins that pass to the outer layer of the choroid. The larger veins subsequently converge to form a single vortex vein in each quadrant. The vortex veins drain into the posterior ciliary veins, which subsequently drain into the orbital veins.[6] The venous drainage of the ciliary body consists of venous blood from the ciliary muscle and processes and subsequently passes posteriorly into the vortex vein. The iris veins drain into the ciliary body and eventually enter the vortex venous system.

The drainage of blood from the anterior and outer region of the ciliary body makes up the anterior ciliary venous system.[5] The branches of this system connect with the efferent channel of the canal of Schlemm before linking up with the episcleral venous plexus. The anterior ciliary veins form a deep and superficial plexus. The deep plexus, which consists of numerous flat and tortuous veins, directly communicates with the canal of Schlemm through collector channels. The superficial portion of the plexus drains directly into the episcleral venous plexus. Other authors have referred to these systems as indirect and direct venous drainage systems, respectively.[4] This anterior ciliary venous system communicates with the venous plexuses of the Tenon's capsule and conjunctiva and eventually drains into the ophthalmic veins. The posterior ciliary venous system is

1467

relatively unimportant.[5] This system drains primarily the posterior portion of the sclera.

There are variable anastomoses connecting the retinal and ciliary venous systems.[7] Anastomotic channels are noted between the retinal venous system and the vortex system when central venous pressure is high.[8] However, no significant connection between the vortex veins and the episcleral veins in humans has been noted.[7] For a more complete discussion of the anatomy of the retinal and vortex venous systems, the reader is referred to Principles & Practice of Ophthalmology: Basic Sciences, Chapter 14.

The three major routes of venous drainage in the orbit are the superior ophthalmic vein, inferior ophthalmic vein, and the facial veins, all of which are interconnected (Fig. 130–1).[9] The superior ophthalmic vein, located in the upper and medial aspect of the orbital margin, is formed by the supraorbital and angular veins of the face. The angular vein establishes a link between the superficial veins of the face via the anterior facial vein and the deep veins of the orbit. The superior ophthalmic vein leaves the orbit via the superior orbital fissure and then traverses downward to the cavernous sinus. Along its course there may be varicosities that may contribute to a pulsating exophthalmos.[5] The two superior vortex veins and branches of the ethmoid venous system drain into the superior ophthalmic vein. The inferior ophthalmic vein receives branches from the lower lid, the area surrounding the lacrimal sac, the inferior rectus, and inferior oblique muscles and two inferior vortex veins. Along its course, the inferior ophthalmic vein divides into two branches. The superior branch may either pass through the superior orbital fissure, beneath the annulus of Zinn, and enter the cavernous sinus or may enter into the superior ophthalmic vein. The inferior branch, if present, passes

through the inferior orbital fissure and ultimately drains into the pterygoid plexus.

There are three principal directions of blood flow through the orbital venous system. Flow may be backward via the superior and inferior ophthalmic veins to the cavernous sinus and the cranial system. Venous drainage may also be directed forward via anastomoses of the ophthalmic veins to the facial system. Moreover, flow may be downward to the pterygoid venous plexus.[5]

PHYSIOLOGY OF EVP

EVP plays a significant role in aqueous humor dynamics. Aqueous humor, which is produced primarily by a combination of ultrafiltration, diffusion, and active transport in the posterior segment, passes through the pupil and exits the eye by one of two pathways—by way of the anterior surface of the ciliary body or through the trabecular meshwork, Schlemm's canal, collector channels, and subsequently aqueous veins. These pathways have been termed alternatively unconventional and conventional pathways, respectively.[3, 10] Flow of fluid by way of the unconventional pathway is independent of pressure. Outflow via the conventional route is passive and largely depends on the difference between the pressure within the eye (IOP) and EVP. Fluid therefore naturally flows in the direction of the lower pressure, EVP. However, there is resistance (R) within the conventional outflow system, particularly across the juxta-canalicular trabecular meshwork. The relationship between these parameters thus is as follows:

$$Flow = (IOP - EVP)/R \qquad (1)$$

As EVP increases in relation to IOP, or as resistance increases, flow decreases. However, resistance does not

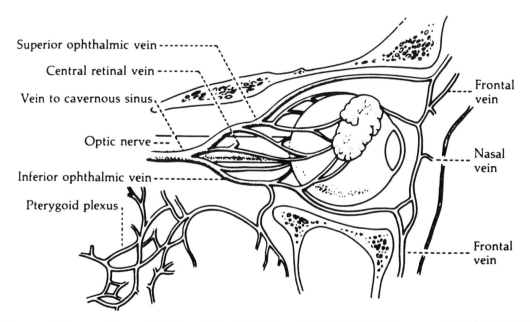

Figure 130–1. Venous drainage of the orbit. (From Weinreb RN, Jeng S, Goldstick BJ: Glaucoma secondary to elevated episcleral venous pressure. *In* Ritch R, Shields MB, Krupin T [eds]: The Glaucomas. St Louis, CV Mosby, 1989, p 1128.)

necessarily remain constant when there are changes in IOP and may actually increase as the IOP increases due to collapse of the aqueous outflow system. Equation 1 would be therefore modified as follows[11]:

$$R = R_i + R_iQ(IOP - EVP) \qquad (2)$$

in which R_i is the initial resistance measured when the IOP and EVP are equivalent and Q represents the change in resistance following an increase in the difference of IOP and EVP measuring 1 mmHg. Incorporating equation 2, equation 1 would be written as follows:

$$Flow = (IOP - EVP)/R_i + R_iQ(IOP - EVP) \qquad (3)$$

This equation suggests that EVP can influence flow within the conventional outflow pathway in two ways: the pressure gradient and resistance.

At steady state, aqueous production, F_{ap}, should be equal to flow across the conventional pathway, F_c, in addition to flow across the unconventional pathway, F_u.

$$F_{ap} = F_c + F_u \qquad (4)$$

Using equation 1 as an approximation of flow across the conventional pathway, the following equation arises:

$$F_{ap} = (IOP - EVP)/R + F_u \qquad (5)$$

Solving for IOP, equation 5 appears as follows:

$$IOP = (F_{ap} - F_u)R + EVP \qquad (6)$$

It should be noted that EVP may not be independent of IOP and aqueous production. Aqueous production may decrease when IOP increases, a concept referred to as pseudofacility. When the EVP was increased in an experimental study, the IOP was noted to increase 80 percent of the increment. The 20 percent difference was thought to be due to a decrease in aqueous production or to the egress of fluid via pathways other than the anterior chamber.[12] The existence of pseudofacility, however, has not been documented fluorophotometrically.[13]

The relationship of IOP and EVP has been studied by several investigators. Using a micropuncture technique, Maepea and Bill evaluated the correlation of IOP and EVP in cynomolgus monkeys.[14] A positive relationship linking these variables was noted and was expressed as follows by these investigators: IOP = 0.68EVP + 11. The increase in EVP induced by increasing IOP in these animals was not statistically significant. Similarly in humans, a positive correlation (+0.59) was noted by Weigelin and Lohlein[15] in 172 individuals with IOPs ranging from 7 to 24 mmHg. Moreover, when IOP and EVP were measured in individuals in both the supine and head-down vertical position, an increase in EVP of 0.83 ± 0.21 mmHg was reported for every 1 mmHg rise in IOP.[16] Kaskel and coworkers[17] noted an increase in EVP more than IOP when individuals changed from a sitting position to a recumbent position. Finally, the EVP as well as IOP were noted to be lower during the third trimester in pregnancy.[18]

In contrast, a negative correlation between IOP and EVP has been noted by others. Talusan and coworkers[19] reported on findings in normotensive eyes and in eyes with primary open-angle glaucoma. A decrease in EVP from 8.5 to 6 mmHg corresponded with an increase in IOP from 20 to 40 mmHg. Similarly, Kupfer[20] noted a lower mean EVP in normotensive eyes, 8.4 ± 0.3 mmHg versus ocular hypertensive eyes, 7.7 ± 0.2 mmHg. Differences in IOP between eyes could not be attributed to differences in EVP according to Podos and coworkers.[21]

The impact of EVP on aqueous humor dynamics is indeed complex and depends mainly on variations in the clinical circumstance as well as on methods of measurement. Certainly, equation 6 suggests a positive correlation existing between IOP and EVP. However, considering the confusion in the literature, these calculations are mere approximations. Additional clinical evaluation is needed to untangle the existing controversies.

METHODS OF MEASURING EVP

There are essentially four methods for clinically determining EVP noninvasively: torsion balance, pressure chamber, air jet, and an indirect method.

Considerable attention has been given to the proper identification of EVP and to the determination of the appropriate end-point. Unlike conjunctival veins that move when an applicator is placed on the eye, episcleral veins remain immobile. Episcleral veins are most visible between the 1 and 5 o'clock positions and the 7 and 11 o'clock positions between the equator and the limbus. The accuracy of the end-point has been investigated by both Brubaker[22] and Gaasterland and Pederson.[23] Brubaker[22] compared three methods for determining EVP: torsion balance, pressure chamber, and direct cannulation. Three different end-points were evaluated: (1) an end-point at which the vascular stream first narrows, (2) an end-point at which 50 percent of the stream narrows compared with baseline, and (3) a point at which the stream is completely obliterated. The pressure chamber method gave results that were most agreeable with direct cannulation of episcleral veins, and the second method of determining the end-point most closely resembled physiologic conditions. Gaasterland and Pederson[23] compared a pressure chamber method with direct cannulation using three different categories for the end-point: (1) slight indentation, (2) intermittent indentation, and (3) sustained collapse of the vein. Utilization of either endpoints (2) or (3) resulted in an overestimation of the EVP. Complete obliteration of the vein forces fluid into collateral pathways that may not adequately accommodate the additional volume, a circumstance that subsequently increases EVP. The accepted end-point therefore becomes either 50 percent reduction in color or 50 percent reduction in perfused vessel width.[10] Each of the methods is discussed briefly.

Torsion Balance Method

In 1949, Goldmann[24] described a technique based on the assumption that a known force applied to a known area of conjunctiva increases the pressure within the vessel by an amount equivalent to the applied force per unit area (F/A). Essentially the torsion balance device consists of a lever connected to a suspended torsion spring. The diameter of the tip that is in contact with the eye measures 0.5 mm. Increasing degrees of pressure are applied to the conjunctiva until the desired endpoint is reached. The average value for EVP obtained using this method is 10.0 ± 1 mmHg.[10]

Pressure Chamber Method

The pressure chamber method was described by Seidel[25] in 1923. This device is based on a similar principle compared with the torsion balance method. One side of a small chamber consists of a thin, distensible membrane, and the other side consists of a transparent glass through which the episcleral vein is directly viewed. The membrane is in contact with the vessel and the pressure within the chamber increases until the desired end-point is reached. The pressure within the chamber is assumed to be comparable with the pressure within the vessel. Zeimer[26] and associates developed a commercially available device that can be easily mounted on a slit lamp and requires only one observer to complete the measurement (Fig. 130–2). A mean value for EVP measuring 9.8 ± 1.8 mmHg using this pressure chamber method has been noted.[10]

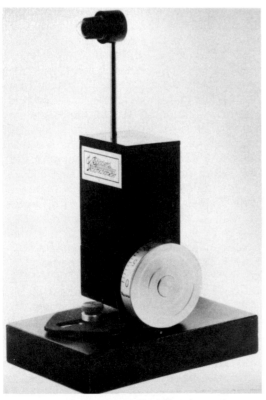

Figure 130–2. Episcleral Venomanometer based on the pressure chamber method. This instrument mounts easily on the slit-lamp microscope, the membrane is positioned in contact with the episcleral vessel, and the graduated wheel measures the episcleral venous pressure in millimeters of mercury. (Courtesy of Eyetech Ltd., Skokie, IL.)

Air Jet Method

Krakau[27] and associates described a noninvasive method of determining EVP using an air jet that requires no topical anesthetic. The force that is required to achieve the desired end-point is measured. Widakowich[28] underscored the importance of measuring EVP in a vein as close to Schlemm's canal as possible using this method. Krakau[27] reported a mean value of 10.4 ± 0.8 mmHg using an air jet device.

Indirect Method

The eye is first compressed with an impression tonometer. The IOP rapidly decreases then increases to a level equal to EVP. The average pressure measured using this method is 10.4 ± 4.1 mmHg.[10, 29]

CLINICAL ENTITIES ASSOCIATED WITH ELEVATED EVP

Arteriovenous Anomalies

CAROTID CAVERNOUS SINUS FISTULA

Carotid cavernous sinus fistula is an arteriovenous shunt between the internal or external carotid arteries and the cavernous sinus. In recent years, based on clinical and angiographic differences, this entity has been further classified into two subcategories—traumatic and spontaneous.[30] The traumatic carotid cavernous fistulas have also been called high-flow fistulas or direct fistulas (direct communication of the intracavernous trunk of the internal carotid artery and the cavernous sinus) when using descriptions related to velocity of flow or anatomy.

The "traumatic" presentation is typically a young individual who presents following a severe head injury with pulsating exophthalmos, conjunctival chemosis, engorgement of the episcleral vein, severely restricted ocular motility, bruit, and ocular ischemia. The proptosis can increase slowly for several weeks before stabilizing. Lid swelling as well as dermal cyanosis may be particularly evident if the superior ophthalmic vein is significantly enlarged. An ocular bruit can be noted in 50 to 95 percent of patients and is amplified with exercise. Diplopia may be a presenting complaint as well due to the involvement of the cranial nerves, most often the sixth cranial nerve; mechanical restriction may also be noted. Patients may have retrobulbar pain that may be associated with a constant noise and a bruit.[31] The provoking injury can be a basal skull fracture or any penetrating injury to the orbit injuring the medial or inferomedial wall of the orbit as well as the superior orbital fissure. Such trauma can account for 75 percent of the cases of carotid-cavernous fistulas.[31] These fistulas can also occur following surgery involving the internal carotid artery or following a rupture of a preexisting aneurysm of the internal carotid artery. Visual loss and papilledema have also been associated.[31]

An incidence of 50 percent loss of vision has been

reported due to damage to the optic nerve associated with the initial injury, papilledema, venous congestion of the retina, and chronic secondary glaucoma.[31] Glaucoma can occur secondary to increased EVP, orbital congestion, neovascularization following central retinal vein occlusion, or angle-closure.

The spontaneous clinical entity, otherwise described as low flow or dural (indirect), is more insidious. These fistulas involve small intracavernous dural branches of the internal carotid artery and dural branches from the ascending pharyngeal and internal maxillary arteries from the external carotid artery. This communication may involve the ipsilateral or contralateral cavernous sinus. There may be drainage either anteriorly via the superior ophthalmic vein, the deep sylvian vein, or the sphenoparietal sinus or there may be posterior drainage by way of the superior and inferior petrosal sinuses. If there is no significant anterior drainage, these fistulas may be asymptomatic.[32] Typically, a middle-aged to elderly individual presents with minimal proptosis without pulsations, arterialized episcleral veins, and usually no history of trauma (Figs. 130–3 and 130–4). Of 20 patients diagnosed as having a spontaneous carotid cavernous fistula, one patient had papilledema; four patients had choroidal detachment; two patients demonstrated exudative retinal detachment; and three patients had central venous thrombosis.[33] In elderly patients, there may be a predisposition to the development of carotid cavernous fistulas due to degenerative vascular changes within the sinus.[31] These fistulas have also been reported in association with Ehlers-Danlos syndrome[34] and pseudoxanthoma elasticum.[35] In 64 patients reported by Jorgensen and Guthoff,[36] spontaneous carotid cavernous fistulas accounted for 31 percent of the secondary glaucomas associated with elevated EVP. Other clinical entities that should be differentiated from these fistulas include the following: dysthyroid orbitopathy, pseudotumor of the orbit, orbital cellulitis, episcleritis, and any sphenoorbital mass lesion.[32]

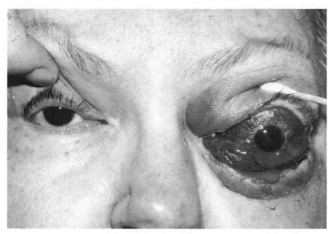

Figure 130–4. Proptosis, chemosis, and arterialization of episcleral venous vessels in a patient with a carotid cavernous fistula. (Courtesy of Dr. WT Cornblath and Dr. JD Trobe.)

The diagnosis of a carotid cavernous fistula is made clinically and angiographically. Ocular pulse amplitude as measured by pneumotonometry, has been shown to be a useful noninvasive tool to evaluate patients with carotid cavernous fistulas. In 15 patients with carotid cavernous fistulas, the difference in the ocular pulse amplitude between eyes was noted to be greater in patients with fistulas than in patients without orbital disease and patients with orbital disease without any evidence of a fistula.[37] Once there is a high level of suspicion clinically, the next step is angiography. Miller[32] points out the importance of performing not only selective internal carotid arteriography but also selective external carotid arteriography, particularly when a dural cavernous fistula is suspected. Dural fistulas have been noted to close spontaneously following angiography. Three of five patients with dural arteriovenous shunts were noted to improve spontaneously following angiography in one group of patients.[38] The symptoms and signs of some patients may worsen in the course of their disease; these findings may be an indication of spontaneous thrombosis of the superior ophthalmic vein.[39] Systemic steroids may be beneficial in these cases.[32] However, spontaneous improvement has been reported.[39]

Computed tomography, orbital ultrasound, and magnetic resonance imaging may demonstrate enlargement of the extraocular muscles, dilatation of the superior ophthalmic vein, and enlargement of the cavernous sinus (Fig. 130–5). Color Doppler imaging is a noninvasive technique that provides two-dimensional structural imaging and Doppler evaluation of blood flow. This technique has been used successfully to evaluate patients with traumatic and spontaneous carotid cavernous fistulas and may eliminate the need to perform computed tomography and magnetic resonance imaging.[40] Depending on the vessel feeding the shunt, treatment may involve ligation of the carotid artery proximal to the ophthalmic artery or embolization. Embolization using detachable balloon catheters has also been utilized successfully to close fistulas.[40–42] Hanneken and coworkers[41]

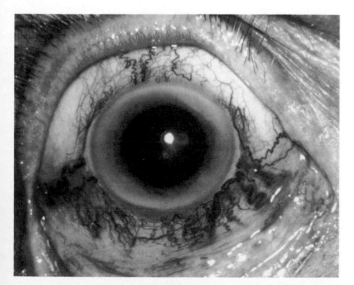

Figure 130–3. Dilatated episcleral venous vessels and proptosis in a patient with a carotid cavernous fistula. (Courtesy of Dr. WT Cornblath and Dr. JD Trobe.)

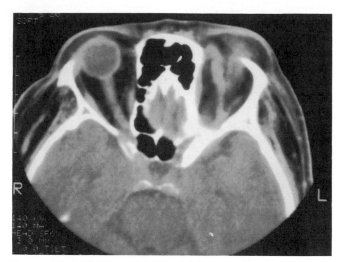

Figure 130–5. Computed tomographic scan of a dilatated superior ophthalmic vein in the patient depicted in Figure 130–4. (Courtesy of Dr. WT Cornblath and Dr. JD Trobe.)

successfully treated four patients, three of whom showed evidence of a spontaneous fistula and one who had a traumatic fistula, by advancing a detachable balloon through the superior ophthalmic vein. There were no intraoperative or postoperative complications. Nevertheless, any intervention with respect to these fistulas must be balanced by the relevant risks.[31, 43]

In cases that are complicated by secondary open-angle glaucoma, aqueous suppressants can be used initially. Miotics may increase the inflammation in an already injected eye. Since most cases of the dural arteriovenous fistula resolve spontaneously, the pressure can be controlled until the fistula resolves. Laser trabeculoplasty in these patients can result in choroidal effusion and a flat anterior chamber (Robert Ritch, M.D., Personal communication). Angle-closure glaucoma has been reported in association with dural shunts. In such cases orbital congestion plays a significant role. Choroidal effusions may be present in addition to a dilatated superior ophthalmic vein. These patients can be treated initially with aqueous suppressants as well as with hyperosmotics. Laser iridotomy can be performed to eliminate the contribution of pupillary block. Cycloplegics can be added to encourage a posterior shift of the lens-iris diaphragm. Laser gonioplasty or goniosynechialysis may be beneficial in further opening the angle. If neovascular glaucoma occurs as a result of ocular ischemia, panretinal photocoagulation is indicated.[44]

ORBITAL VARIX

A shunt between the intracranial and extracranial venous systems forms the orbital venous plexus. An orbital varix can be created when there is dilatation of the orbital veins as a result of posterior dilatation of the intracranial vessels.[31] Alternatively, an orbital varix may be congenital and occur as an abnormal, tortuous, dilatated vein.[45] Orbital varix has been associated with the Klippel-Trenaunay-Weber syndrome.[46] A common clinical sign of an orbital varix is intermittent exophthalmos, which occurs by placing the head in a dependent position, by sneezing, or by performing a Valsalva maneuver. By increasing pressure within the jugular vein, the orbital varix becomes distended, resulting in proptosis. These episodes may be associated with symptoms of blurred vision, headache, nausea, and pain. When the patient ceases the inciting maneuver, the proptosis lessens. Over a period of years these episodes may become longer and more difficult to reverse.[31] A 15 percent incidence of blindness has been noted as a result of optic nerve damage after repeated episodes of proptosis.[47] The presence of associated systemic venous abnormalities, for example, involving the buccal mucosa, extremities, and abdomen, should be investigated.[31]

Occasionally, patients may present with orbital varix thrombosis. Patients may have symptoms indicative of an acute orbital process (i.e., pain, diplopia, blurred vision, and proptosis). Bullock[48] and associates described three patients who presented with orbital varix thrombosis. All three patients had a characteristic body habitus, a "bull-neck," that may have contributed to the stagnation and subsequent thrombosis of their orbital varices. The authors point out the importance of differentiating this clinical entity from cavernous sinus thrombosis and superior ophthalmic vein thrombosis. Only one of the three patients had glaucoma.

The diagnosis of an orbital varix can be made both clinically and by utilizing orbital venography. However, cases have been reported in the absence of any evidence of proptosis[49, 50] and were not demonstrated with orbital venography.[50] The observation of a phlebolith can be demonstrated on plain roentgenogram but can be suggestive of other vascular lesions such as a venous angioma, arteriovenous fistula, and an arteriovenous malformation.[48] Computed axial tomography, particularly if combined with jugular compression or the Valsalva maneuver[51, 52] as well as magnetic resonance imaging, can assist the clinician in making the diagnosis.[49, 53] Color Doppler imaging offers a noninvasive method of evaluating orbital varices.[54]

Orbital varices can be managed conservatively[31, 48, 51, 55–57] or surgically.[45, 46, 49, 50, 58] Electrically induced thrombosis has been described as a treatment.[59] Complete surgical removal may not be possible.[31, 48] Indications for surgery include repeated or unrelenting episodes of thrombosis, intractable pain, severe proptosis, and compressive optic neuropathy.[48] The glaucoma, which is secondary to elevated EVP and decreased outflow facility, can be managed medically.[60] Since many of the varices resorb or recanalize eventually with subsequent improvement of symptoms, conservative management is suggested.

STURGE-WEBER SYNDROME (ENCEPHALOTRIGEMINAL ANGIOMATOSIS)

A hemiparetic, epileptic patient with a facial hemangioma was presented to the Clinical Society of London by Sturge in 1879. He postulated that the facial manifestations were related to the neurologic component of the presenting patient's disorder. Previously in 1860,

Schirmer had presented a patient with a facial hemangioma and buphthalmos but no evidence of involvement of the central nervous system. In 1910, Durck was the first to report the presence of cerebral calcification in association with a facial nevus. Weber characterized the radiologic appearance of a case similar to that of Sturge, and the disorder has subsequently been called the Sturge-Weber syndrome. Alternatively, the term encephalotrigeminal angiomatosis has been proposed because of the involvement of the trigeminal nerve. Others favor the label encephalofacial angiomatosis, because the facial lesion may extend beyond the distribution of the trigeminal nerve.[61]

Sturge-Weber syndrome is characterized by a cutaneous hemifacial angioma that stops at the midline and an ipsilateral angioma of the meninges and the brain (Fig. 130–6). Other characteristics that may be noted are the following: epilepsy, gyriform calcifications, glaucoma, mental retardation, hemiparesis, and a homonymous hemianopia.[32, 61] The characteristic facial hemangioma is unilateral in 90 percent of cases and can involve the lower face, scalp, and neck.[62]

Glaucoma has been reported to occur in 30 percent of cases.[9, 63] Sixty percent of patients develop glaucoma before 2 years of age, and the remaining patients develop glaucoma later in childhood or early adulthood.[63–65] Glaucoma is often present in the ipsilateral eye when the facial angioma involves the eyelid or conjunctiva.[66] In an evaluation of 106 patients with facial port-wine stains and Sturge-Weber syndrome, involvement of the first division of cranial nerve 5 was the determinant of ocular involvement.[67] An angioma of the choroid can be found in 31 percent[68] to 50 percent[69] of patients with Sturge-Weber syndrome. The choroidal hemangioma found in Sturge-Weber syndrome is flat and diffusely involves the choroidal vasculature. There is often associated diffuse angiomatosis involving the episcleral and subconjunctival perilimbal tissues.[70] Other less commonly seen ocular abnormalities include iris heterochromia and retinal vascular tortuosity.[71]

Facial nevus flammeus has been associated with an orbital vascular malformation in the absence of any leptomeningeal angiomatosis. Glaucoma, ipsilateral to the facial lesion, was also noted. These cases were not considered to be characteristic of Sturge-Weber syndrome.[72] Nevus flammeus and unilateral glaucoma have been reported in association with retinitis pigmentosa.[73] This occurrence was thought to be coincidental.

Patients with Klippel-Trenaunay-Weber syndrome can exhibit angiomas of the face and extremities and associated ocular findings similar to those of Sturge-Weber syndrome, but in addition these patients show evidence of varicosities on the affected side as well as local hypertrophy or atrophy of the bone and soft tissues in the involved areas.[32, 65, 74] Other closely related disorders include Jahnke's syndrome (facial angioma without glaucoma), Schirmer's syndrome with buphthalmos, Lawford's syndrome with late onset glaucoma, and Mille's syndrome with a choroidal hemangioma without glaucoma.[65]

There have been many theories to explain the cause of the glaucoma associated with Sturge-Weber syndrome.[61, 62, 64] The neural theory proposes a congenital modification of the sympathetic innervation to the eye resulting in dilatation of the uveal capillaries and a decrease in blood flow. This theory would suggest that heterochromia of the iris would be more commonly seen. Moreover, Horner's syndrome, which is characterized by a sympathetic abnormality, is not associated with glaucoma. The cranial theory suggests that an occult angioma of the meninges interferes with tributaries draining into the cavernous sinus. However, there are instances when patients have evidence of glaucoma without intracranial angiomas. Since choroidal hemangiomas are often noted, some investigators have proposed a hypersecretion theory—that is, transudation of fluid from the choroidal hemangioma results in glaucoma. However, unless there are specific characteristics of the choroidal hemangioma associated with Sturge-Weber syndrome that distinguish it from a hemangioma occurring alone without glaucoma, this theory does not seem valid. Other theories include the mechanical blockage of the aqueous outflow system by an angioma in the angle and angle-closure secondary to peripheral anterior synechiae.

There are two theories that deserve particular attention: A decrease in outflow facility due to either malformation of the aqueous outflow system or secondary to elevated EVP. Several investigators have noted changes in the angle similar to those found in congenital glaucoma.[9, 63, 65, 75–77] A "high" insertion of the iris and ciliary muscle and the existence of a "Barkan membrane" have been described. Cibis and coworkers[65] analyzed the trabeculectomy specimens taken from patients with Sturge-Weber syndrome noting a compact trabecular meshwork with amorphous material filling the deeper intertrabecular spaces (Fig. 130–7). The beams appeared much thicker than what might be expected for the patients' ages. These changes were rem-

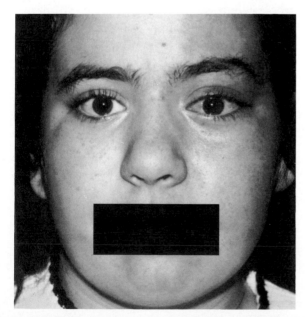

Figure 130–6. Young patient with facial angioma and ipsilateral glaucoma. No cerebral involvement has been documented. (Photograph by Frances McIver.)

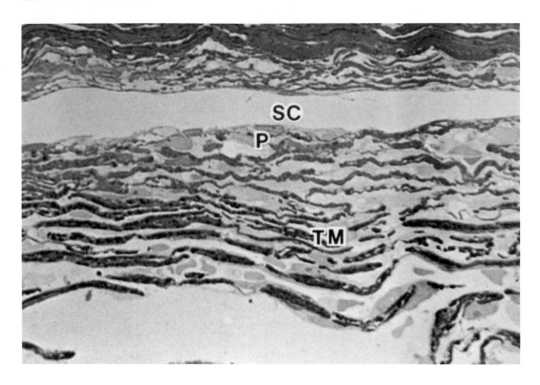

Figure 130–7. Light micrograph of a trabeculectomy specimen from a patient with Sturge-Weber syndrome. Note the compact trabecular meshwork (TM) and pericanalicular region (P). (SC, Schlemm's canal.) ×800. (From Cibis GW, Tripathi RC, Tripathi BJ: Glaucoma in Sturge-Weber syndrome. Ophthalmology 91:1064, 1984.)

iniscent of primary open-angle glaucoma. Phelps[62] raised three objections to any theory based solely on anterior chamber malformation: (1) The pathophysiology of congenital glaucoma is poorly understood. (2) The typical changes seen in infants are not seen in older cases of Sturge-Weber syndrome. (3) The vascular component of this syndrome is such an overwhelming feature of this entity, it is difficult to exclude its contribution.

In 1971, Weiss[9] proposed that the glaucoma observed in Sturge-Weber syndrome was secondary to elevated EVP. He suggested that the arteriovenous shunts within an episcleral hemangioma increased the pressure within the vessels draining Schlemm's canal. In support of his theory, Phelps[62] noted an elevation in EVP in 12 glaucomatous eyes associated with Sturge-Weber syndrome measuring 18.5 ± 5.8 mmHg compared with 9.1 ± 1.6 mmHg in the uninvolved fellow eyes. Episcleral hemangiomas[78] and elevated episcleral venous pressure[79] have been noted by others. Those who refute this theory point out the surgical success of procedures such as goniotomy and trabeculotomy in these cases as evidence that a primary abnormality in the aqueous outflow system is the primary mechanism. It is likely that the basis of the glaucoma seen in Sturge-Weber syndrome is a combination of an anomaly in the anterior chamber as well as elevated EVP.[80]

An analysis by Iwach and coworkers[66] lends insight into the management of glaucoma associated with Sturge-Weber syndrome both medically and surgically. Thirty-six eyes of 30 patients with either early- or late-onset glaucoma with a mean follow-up of 122 mo were reviewed. Primarily a surgical approach was used for infants, and a combination of medications, laser trabeculoplasty, and either goniotomy, trabeculotomy, or trabeculectomy was used in late-onset cases. Median postoperative intervals during which the patients were considered stable based on IOP or absence of disc deterioration were calculated for each of the interventions and were reported as follows: goniotomy (12 mo), trabeculotomy (21 mo), trabeculectomy (21 mo), argon laser trabeculoplasty (25 mo), and medications (57 mo). The authors favored either goniotomy or trabeculotomy because trabeculectomies were complicated by a 24 percent incidence of intraoperative choroidal effusions. Choroidal effusion[81] and expulsive hemorrhage have been noted to be a significant problem intraoperatively by others as well.[82] Bellows and associates[83] suggest performing a posterior sclerotomy prior to entering the eye when undertaking filtration surgery to allow adequate drainage of any choroidal effusion that might occur intraoperatively. Ali and coworkers avoided the occurrence of a choroidal effusion in their cases by using a releasable suture and tight suturing of the scleral flap.[84] Others favor combining procedures such as trabeculotomy-trabeculectomy[85] and trabeculectomy and cyclocryotherapy.[86] Considering the difficulty in treating these patients medically and surgically, the prognosis is fair. Keverline and Hiles[87] emphasize the importance of early intervention prior to worsening of the glaucomatous status. Of the 35 eyes evaluated by Iwach and coworkers,[66] 23 eyes showed evidence of IOP less than 25 mmHg and 13 eyes demonstrated visual acuity better than 20/40 at the patients' last visit.

MISCELLANEOUS ARTERIOVENOUS ANOMALIES

Orbital-meningeal shunts, carotid jugular venous shunts, and intraocular vascular shunts are clinical entities that are also associated with elevated EVP.[4] Michelsen[88] and associates distinguish vascular malformations from vascular neoplasms such as hemangiomas.

Vascular malformations can be further subdivided into venous malformations without an arterial component (orbital varix), true arteriovenous malformations of the orbit, and arteriovenous malformations that are primarily extraorbital but with orbital manifestations. Frequent physical findings are pulsating or nonpulsating exophthalmos, chemosis, restricted ocular motility, chemosis, visual loss, glaucoma, and a bruit.

Howard and coworkers[89] reported a case of 19-year-old patient who presented with progressive swelling of the upper lid and proptosis. Cerebral angiography documented the presence of an arteriovenous malformation that was supplied primarily by a distal branch of the internal maxillary artery as well as by the superficial temporal and middle meningeal arteries. The lesion was treated initially by embolization of a rapidly polymerizing Silastic liquid but subsequently required surgical removal following a recurrence 4 yr later. Arteriovenous malformations[90, 91] and aneurysms[92, 93] within the orbit can mimic orbital tumors. Angiography can establish the diagnosis. The associated glaucoma is due to the increased pressure within the vortex veins that is secondary to increased orbital pressure.[92, 93] The glaucoma can be treated initially with topical medications and carbonic anhydrase inhibitors; however, treatment of the underlying problem must be undertaken to achieve long-term stabilization of the glaucoma.[93]

Venous Obstruction

RETROBULBAR TUMOR

Proptosis is the most significant clinical sign seen in association with orbital tumors. Any difference of 2 mm or more of protrusion of the globes when comparing two orbits should raise suspicions of orbital disease until proven otherwise.[63] Depending on the size and consistency of the lesion, the secondary orbital congestion can lead to an increase in EVP.[93, 94] Tumors that occur commonly in the region of the superior orbital fissure and the cavernous sinus include the following: meningiomas, pituitary adenomas, and metastatic tumors. The diagnosis can be confirmed using neuroimaging studies and ultrasonography. These tumors may be treated medically, surgically, or radiotherapeutically.[44] The underlying cause must be treated to achieve long-term stabilization of the IOP.[93]

THYROID OPHTHALMOPATHY

Thyroid ophthalmopathy is characterized by proptosis, restriction in ocular motility, a decrease in obitonometry readings, conjunctival chemosis, epiphora, papilledema, refractive changes, ocular discomfort, and elevation in IOP.[95] The mechanism of the increase in IOP may occur by a variety of mechanisms: elevated EVP due to orbital congestion, contraction of the extraocular muscles, chronic exposure leading to chronic inflammation and secondary angle-closure,[4] and finally, increased mucopolysaccharide deposit within the aqueous outflow system.[96] There is no evidence of direct influence of the thyroid on IOP.[97] An incidence of glaucoma measuring 5 percent was reported in one series of patients.[96] In the same series of 74 patients, the degree of proptosis correlated with the likelihood of finding elevation in IOP. In another series of patients, 2 of 29 evidenced glaucoma and 11 demonstrated a reduced outflow facility (Po/C as measured by tonography >100).[98] Patients with glaucoma can be treated with topical medications and carbonic anhydrase inhibitors. Treatment of the thyroid disease is necessary and may involve orbital decompression or systemic steroids.[95]

SUPERIOR VENA CAVA SYNDROME

The presenting signs characterizing the superior vena cava syndrome include the following: edema of the lid, face, and conjunctiva; vascular engorgement of the fundus, episclera, and conjunctiva; proptosis; and papilledema and glaucoma. The glaucoma may be bilateral; the IOP may increase in the supine position and may decrease in the sitting position. Depending on the duration of the underlying disorder, there may not be any optic nerve deterioration.[99] Malignancy is the underlying basis for this syndrome in 97 percent of cases.[100] Aortic aneurysms, enlarged hilar nodes, thyroid disease,[4] and inflammatory jugular phlebostenosis[101] have been associated with this entity. Treatment should be aimed at the underlying cause. Miotics have been reported to be effective in lowering the IOP.[102] Aqueous suppressants should also be considered.

CONGESTIVE HEART FAILURE

Congestive heart failure was linked to glaucoma secondary to elevated EVP by Etienne.[103] However, a later report by Bettelheim did not confirm this relationship.[104] Additional clinical studies are needed to further elucidate this relationship.

THROMBOSIS OF CAVERNOUS SINUS OR ORBITAL VEIN

Patients with thrombosis of the cavernous sinus can present with the signs and symptoms of orbital disease previously mentioned: proptosis, involvement of the cranial nerves 3, 4, 5, and 6, as well as signs of obstruction of venous drainage of the cavernous sinus. In addition there may be retrobulbar pain. Septic cavernous sinus thrombosis may be accompanied by systemic symptoms such as fever, headache, nausea, vomiting, and somnolence. Tolosa-Hunt syndrome is the primary entity to differentiate. Orbital venography can assist in the diagnosis. The correct diagnosis is important because the treatment for thrombosis of the cavernous sinus is heparin therapy, and the therapy for Tolosa-Hunt syndrome is systemic steroids.[105]

VASCULITIS INVOLVING EPISCLERAL VEIN OR ORBITAL VEIN

In patients with either episcleritis or scleritis associated with a variety of systemic diseases such as rheu-

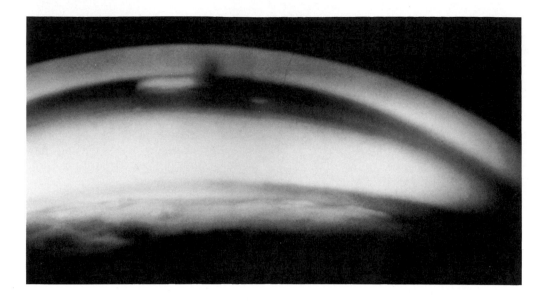

Figure 130–8. Reflux of blood in Schlemm's canal in a patient with idiopathic elevation of episcleral venous pressure. (Courtesy of G. Skuta, M.D.)

matoid arthritis, ankylosing spondylitis, erythema nodosum, and turberculosis, glaucoma was reported in 11.6 percent of patients with scleritis and in 4 percent of patients with episcleritis. The cause of glaucoma was related to either edema in the aqueous outflow system, peripheral anterior synechiae, or chronic steroids.[106] Patients with chronic inflammatory disease associated with glaucoma are best treated with aqueous suppressants. Low-dose topical steroids should be considered in place of more potent formulations. Laser trabeculoplasty may not be effective in most cases.[107] Finally, filtration surgery may need to be supplemented with utilization of antimetabolites to enhance success.[108]

JUGULAR VEIN OBSTRUCTION

The reader is referred to the discussion regarding superior vena cava syndrome.

Idiopathic Elevation of EVP

In cases that demonstrate no angiographic or radiographic evidence of an underlying cause for elevated EVP, the patient may be considered to be either familial or sporadic. Talusan[109] reported six unilateral cases and one bilateral case in patients with dilatated episcleral veins and increased EVP. No evidence of arteriovenous connections could be found angiographically. Two of the patients showed evidence of glaucomatous cupping and field changes, and five demonstrated more cupping in the eye that had the higher EVP. Evidence of idiopathic dilatated episcleral vessels and open-angle glaucoma has been documented by others.[110–113] This association should be suspected in individuals with asymmetric IOP and chronically red eye. On gonioscopic examination, as in any patient with elevated EVP, there may be a reflux of blood in Schlemm's canal (Fig. 130–8). If filtration surgery becomes necessary, a posterior sclerotomy prior to entering the eye may be beneficial.[83]

SUMMARY

The anatomy, physiology, and methods of measuring EVP were reviewed (Table 130–1). There are three general categories of clinical entities associated with elevated EVP: arteriovenous and venous anomalies, venous obstruction, and idiopathic. Topical glaucoma medication and carbonic anydrase inhibitors can be used initially to control IOP. However, the underlying cause must be resolved in order to achieve long-term stabilization of IOPs. Laser trabeculoplasty can be attempted; filtration surgery may be needed ultimately in intractable cases in order to completely bypass the resistance that occurs as a result of elevation in EVP and any primary or secondary changes within the aqueous outflow pathway.

Table 130–1. CLASSIFICATION OF ELEVATED EPISCLERAL VENOUS PRESSURE

Venous obstruction
1. Retrobulbar tumor
2. Thyroid ophthalmopathy
3. Superior vena cava syndrome (mediastinal tumor)
4. Congestive heart failure
5. Thrombosis of cavernous sinus or orbital vein
6. Vasculitis involving episcleral vein or orbital vein
7. Jugular vein obstruction
Arteriovenous anomalies
1. Carotid cavernous sinus fistula
2. Orbital varix
3. Sturge-Weber syndrome
4. Orbital-meningeal shunts
5. Carotid jugular venous shunts
6. Intraocular vascular shunts
Idiopathic elevation of episcleral venous pressure
1. Sporadic
2. Familial

From Weinreb RN, Jeng S, Goldstick BJ: Glaucoma secondary to elevated episcleral venous pressure. *In* Ritch R, Shields MB, Krupin T (eds): The Glaucomas. St Louis, CV Mosby, 1989, p 1130.

Acknowledgments

The author wishes to acknowledge Wayne Cornblatt, M.D., for reviewing the manuscript and Nancy Thomas for her secretarial assistance.

REFERENCES

1. Ascher KW: The aqueous veins: Physiologic importance of the visible elimination of intraocular fluid. Am J Ophthalmol 25:1174, 1942.
1a. Lauber H: Anat. 18:437, 1901 quoted by Ascher KW.
2. Seidel E: Weitere experimentelle Untersuchungen uber die quelle und den Verlauf der intraokularen Saftsrommung. XX: Uber die Messung des Blutdruckes in dem episcleral Venengeflecht, den vorderen ciliar, und den Wirbelvenen normaler Augen. Graefes Arch Clin Exp Ophthalmol 112:252, 1923.
3. Ascher KW: Aqueous veins: Preliminary note. Am J Ophthalmol 25:31, 1942.
4. Weinreb RN, Jeng S, Goldstick BJ: Glaucoma secondary to elevated episcleral venous pressure. In Ritch R, Shields MB, Krupin T (eds): The Glaucomas. St Louis, CV Mosby, 1989.
5. Duke-Elder S, Wybar KC: The Anatomy of the Visual System. St Louis, CV Mosby, 1961.
6. Heyreh SS, Baines JAB: Occlusion of the vortex veins: An experimental study. Br J Ophthalmol 57:217, 1973.
7. Yablonski ME, Podos SM: Glaucoma secondary to elevated episcleral venous pressure. In Ritch R, Shields MB (eds): The Secondary Glaucomas. St Louis, CV Mosby, 1982.
8. Anderson DR: Vascular supply to the optic nerve of primates. Am J Ophthalmol 70:341, 1970.
9. Weiss DL: Dual origin of glaucoma in encephalotrigeminal haemangiomatosis. Trans Ophthalmol Soc UK 93:477, 1971.
10. Zeimer RC: Episcleral venous pressure. In Ritch R, Shields MB, Krupin T (eds): The Glaucomas. St Louis, CV Mosby, 1989.
11. Brubaker RF: Computer-assisted instruction of current concepts in aqueous humor dynamics. Am J Ophthalmol 82:59, 1976.
12. Kupfer C, Sanderson P: Determination of pseudofacility in the eye of man. Arch Ophthalmol 80:194, 1968.
13. Brubaker RF: Physiology of aqueous humor formation. In Drance SM, Neufeld A (eds): Applied Pharmacology in the Medical Treatment of Glaucoma. New York, Grune & Stratton, 1984.
14. Maepea O, Bill A: The pressures in the episcleral veins, Schlemm's canal and the trabecular meshwork in monkeys: Effects of changes in intraocular pressure. Exp Eye Res 49:645, 1989.
15. Weigelin E, Lohlein H: Blutdruckmessungen an den episkleralen Gefassen des Auges bei kreislaufgesunden Personen. Graefes Arch Clin Exp Ophthalmol 153:202, 1952.
16. Friberg TR, Sanborn G, Weinreb RN: Intraocular and episcleral venous pressure increase during inverted posture. Am J Ophthalmol 103:523, 1987.
17. Kaskel D, Muller-Breitenkamp R, Williams I, et al: Augeninnendruck, episkleralvenendruck und blutdruck bei anderung der korperlage. Graefes Arch Clin Exp Ophthalmol 208:217, 1978.
18. Wilke K: Episcleral venous pressure and pregnancy. Acta Ophthalmol Suppl 125:40, 1975.
19. Talusan ED, Fishbein SL, Schwartz B: Increased pressure of dilated episcleral veins with open-angle glaucoma without eophthalmos. Ophthalmology 90:257, 1983.
20. Kupfer C: Clinical significance of pseudofacility. Am J Ophthalmol 75:193, 1973.
21. Podos SM, Minas TF, Macr FJ: A new instrument to measure episcleral venous pressure: Comparison of normal eyes and eyes with primary open angle glaucoma. Arch Ophthalmol 80:209, 1968.
22. Brubaker R: Determination of episcleral venous pressure in the eye. Arch Ophthalmol 77:110, 1967.
23. Gaasterland DE, Pederson JE: Episcleral venous pressure: A comparison of invasive and noninvasive measurements. Invest Ophthalmol Vis Sci 24:1417, 1983.
24. Goldmann H: Eid Kammerwasservenen und das Poiseuille'sche Gesetz. Ophthalmologica 118:496, 1949.
25. Seidel E: Weitere experimentelle Untersuchungen uber die quelle und den verlauf der Intraokularen Saftstromung. XX: Mitteilung uber die Messung des Blutdruckes in dem episcleralen Venengeflecht, den vorderen Ciliarund den Wirbelvenen normaler Augen. Graefes Arch Clin Exp Ophthalmol 115:112, 1923.
26. Zeimer RC, Gieser DK, Wilensky JT, et al: A practical venomanometer: Measurement of episcleral venous pressure and assessment of the normal range. Arch Ophthalmol 101:1447, 1983.
27. Krakau CET, Widakowich J, Wilke K: Measurements of the episcleral venous pressure by means of an air jet. Acta Ophthalmologica 51:185, 1973.
28. Widakowich J: Episcleral venous pressure and flow dynamics. Acta Ophthalmol 54:500, 1976.
29. Stepanik J: Neues Verfahren zur Bestimmung des extrokularen episcleralen Venendruckes. Graefes Arch Clin Exp Ophthalmol 177:116, 1969.
30. Phelps CD, Thompson HS, Ossoinig KC: The diagnosis and prognosis of atypical carotid-cavernous fistula (red-eyed shunt syndrome). Am J Ophthalmol 93:423, 1982.
31. Flanagan JC: Vascular problems of the orbit. Symposium: Tumors of the lids and orbit. Ophthalmology 86:896, 1979.
32. Miller N: Walsh and Hoyt's Clinical Neuro-Ophthalmology, 4th ed. Baltimore, Williams & Wilkins, 1988.
33. Jorgensen JS, Guthoff R: Ophthalmoscopic findings in spontaneous carotid cavernous fistula: An analysis of 20 patients. Graefes Arch Clin Exp Ophthalmol 226:34, 1988.
34. Graf CJ: Spontaneous carotid-cavernous fistula: Ehlers-Danlos syndrome and related conditions. Arch Neurol 13:662, 1965.
35. Rios-Montenegro EN, Behrens MM, Hoyt WF: Pseudoxanthoma elasticum: Association with bilateral carotid rete mirabile and unilateral carotid-cavernous sinus fistula. Arch Neurol 26:151, 1972.
36. Jorgensen JS, Guthoff R: Die Rolle des episkleralen Venendrucks bei der Entstehung von Sekundarglaukomen. Klin Mbl Augenheilk 193:471, 1988.
37. Golnik KC, Miller NR: The diagnosis of carotid-cavernous sinus fistulas by ocular pulse amplitude. Presented at the North American Neuro-ophthalmology Society Meeting, Park City, Utah, 1991.
38. Slusher MM, Lennington RB, Weaver RG, et al: Ophthalmic findings in dural arteriovenous shunts. Ophthalmology 86:720, 1979.
39. Sergott RC, Grossman RI, Savino PJ, et al: The syndrome of paradosical worsening of dural-cavernous sinus arteriovenous malformation. Ophthalmology 94:205, 1987.
40. Flaharty PM, Lief WE, Sergott RC, et al: Color Doppler imaging: A new noninvasive technique to diagnose and monitor carotid cavernous sinus fistulas. Arch Ophthalmol 109:522, 1991.
41. Hanneken AM, Miller NR, Debrun GM, et al: Treatment of carotid-cavernous fistulas using a detachable balloon catheter through the superior ophthalmic vein. Arch Ophthalmol 107:87, 1989.
42. Wu ZX, Wang ZC: Treatment of traumatic carotid-cavernous fistula with detachable balloon. Chin Med J 103:840, 1990.
43. Barrow DL, Fleisher AS, Hoffman JC: Complications of detachable balloon catheter technique in the treatment of traumatic intracranial arteriovenous fistulas. J Neurosurg 56:396, 1982.
44. Fiore PH, Latina MA, Shingleton BJ, et al: The dural shunt syndrome. I: Management of glaucoma. Ophthalmology 97:56, 1990.
45. Guoxiang S, Wenfang T, Dongfang Q: Surgical treatment of orbital varices. Chin Med J 92:723, 1979.
46. Rathbun JE, Hoyt WF, Beard C: Surgical management of orbitofrontal varix in Klippel-Trenaunay-Weber syndrome. Am J Ophthalmol 70:109, 1970.
47. Duke-Elder S, MacFaul PA: System of Ophthalmology: XIII, The Ocular Adnexa. St Louis, CV Mosby, 1974.
48. Bullock JD, Goldberg SH, Connelly PJ: Orbital varix thrombosis. Ophthalmology 97:251, 1990.
49. Kubota T, Kuroda E, Fujii T, et al: Orbital varix with a pearly phlebolith: Case report. J Neurosurg 73:291, 1990.

50. Rosenblum P, Zilkha A: Sudden visual loss secondary to an orbital varix. Surv Ophthalmol 23:49, 1978.
51. Winter J, Centeno RS, Bentson JR: Maneuver to aid diagnosis of orbital varix by computed tomography. AJNR 3:39, 1982.
52. Jorgensen JS: Ein Ungewohnlicher Fall: episklerale und orbitale Varizen. Klin Mbl Augenheilk 191:146, 1987.
53. Osborn RE, DeWitt JD, Lester PD, et al: Magnetic resonance imaging of an orbital varix with CT and ultrasound correlation. Comput Radiol 10:155, 1986.
54. Lieb WE, Merton DA, Shields JA, et al: Colour Doppler imaging in the demonstration of an orbital varix. Br J Ophthalmol 74:305, 1990.
55. McCord CD, Spitalny LA: Localized orbital varices. Arch Ophthalmol 80:455, 1968.
56. Golan A, Savir H, Matz S: Intermittent exophthalmos due to orbital varicose vein accompanied by varicose vein of the legs. Ann Ophthalmol 8(1):61, 1976.
57. Salmenson BD, Gelfand YA, Welsh NH, et al: Orbital varix: An unusual cause of proptosis: A case report. SAMT 74:529, 1988.
58. Sales MJ, Frise P, Roux FX, et al: Les Varices Orbitaires—A propos d'une observation. Bull Soc Ophtalmol Fr 11 (LXXXIX):1287, 1989.
59. Handa H, Mori K: Large varix of the superior ophthalmic vein: Demonstration by angular phlebography and removal by electrically induced thrombosis: case reports. J Neurosurg 29:202, 1968.
60. Kollarits C, Gaasterland D, DiChiro G, et al: Management of a patient with orbital varices, visual loss, and ipsilateral glaucoma, Ophthalmol Surg 8:54, 1977.
61. Alexander GL, Norman RM: The Sturge-Weber Syndrome. Bristol, John Wright & Sons, 1960.
62. Phelps CD: The pathogenesis of glaucoma in Sturge-Weber syndrome. Ophthalmology 85:276, 1978.
63. Font RL, Ferry AP: The phakomatoses. Int Ophthalmol Clin 12:1, 1972.
64. Miller SJH: Symposium: The Sturge-Weber syndrome. Proc R Soc Med 56:419, 1963.
65. Cibis GW, Tripathi RC, Tripathi B: Glaucoma in Sturge-Weber syndrome. Ophthalmology 91:1061, 1984.
66. Iwach A, Hoskins HD, Hetherington J, et al: Analysis of surgical and medical management of glaucoma in Sturge-Weber syndrome. Ophthalmology 97:904, 1990.
67. Enjolras O, Riche MC, Merland JJ: Facial port-wine stains and Sturge-Weber syndrome. Pediatrics 76:48, 1985.
68. Uram M, Zubillaga C: The cutaneous manifestations of Sturge-Weber syndrome. J Clin Neuro-Ophthalmol 2:245, 1982.
69. Danis P: Aspects ophtalmologiques des angiomatose du systeme nerveus. Acta Neurol Psychiatr Belg 50:615, 1950.
70. Witschel H, Font R: Hemangioma of the choroid: A clinicopathologic study of 71 cases and a review of the literature. Surv Ophthalmol 20:415, 1976.
71. Board RJ, Shields MB: Combined trabeculotomy-trabeculectomy for the management of glaucoma associated with Sturge-Weber syndrome. Ophthalmol Surg 12:813, 1981.
72. Hofeldt AJ, Zaret CR, Jakobiec FA, et al: Orbital angiomatosis. Arch Ophthalmol 97:484, 1979.
73. Maul ED, Kass MA: Retinitis pigmentosa associated with nevus flammeus and unilateral glaucoma. Ann Ophthalmol 9:603, 1977.
74. Kramer W: Klippel-Trenaunay syndrome. In Vinken PJ, Bruyn GW (eds): Handbook of Clinical Neurology, vol 14: The Phakomatoses. New York, Elsevier, 1972.
75. Barkan O: Goniotomy for glaucoma associated with nevus flammeus. Am J Ophthalmol 43:545, 1957.
76. O'Brien CS, Porter WC: Glaucoma and nevus flammeus. Arch Ophthalmol 9:715, 1933.
77. Dickens CJ, Hoskins HD: Developmental glaucoma. In Isenberg SJ: The Eye in Infancy. Chicago, Year Book Medical Publishers, 1989.
78. Baikoff G, Colin J, Bechetoille A, et al: Maladie de Sturge-Weber et glaucome. Bull Soc Ophtalmol Fr 4-5 (LXXX), 1980.
79. Jorgensen JS, Guthoff R: Sturge-Weber-Syndrom: Glaukom mit erhohtem episkleralen Venendruck. Klin Mbl Augenheilk 191:275, 1987.
80. Spencer WH: Glaucoma. In Spencer WH (ed): Ophthalmic Pathology: An Atlas and Textbook, 3rd ed, vol 1. Philadelphia, WB Saunders, 1985.
81. Shibab ZM, Kristan RW: Recurrent intraoperative choroidal effusion in Sturge-Weber syndrome. J Pediatr Ophthalmol Strabismus 20:250, 1983.
82. Theodossiadis G, Damanakis A, Kousandrea CH: Aderhauteffusion wahrend einer antiglaukomatosen Operation bei einem Kind mit Sturge-Weber-Syndrom. Klin Mbl Augenheilk 186:300, 1985.
83. Bellows AR, Chylack LT, Epstein DL: Choroidal effusion during glaucoma surgery in patients with prominent episcleral vessels. Arch Ophthalmol 97:493, 1979.
84. Ali MA, Fahmy IA, Spaeth GL: Trabeculectomy for glaucoma associated with Sturge-Weber syndrome. Ophthalmol Surg 21:352, 1990.
85. Board RJ, Shields MB: Combined trabeculotomy-trabeculectomy for the management of glaucoma associated with Sturge-Weber syndrome. Ophthalmol Surg 12:813, 1981.
86. Wagner RS, Caputo AR, Negro RG, et al: Trabeculectomy with cyclocryotherapy for infantile glaucoma in the Sturge-Weber syndrome. Ann Ophthalmol 20:289, 1988.
87. Keverline PO, Hiles DA: Trabeculectomy for adolescent onset glaucoma in the Sturge-Weber syndrome. J Pediatr Ophthalmol 13:144, 1976.
88. Michelsen WJ, Hilal SK, Stern J: The management of arteriovenous malformations of the orbit. In Jakobiec FA (ed): Ocular and Adnexal Tumors. Birmington, Aesculapius Publishing Co, 1978.
89. Howard GM, Jakobiec FA, Michelsen WJ: Orbital arteriovenous malformation with secondary capillary angiomatosis treated by embolization with Silastic liquid. Ophthalmology 90:1136, 1983.
90. Murali R, Berenstein A, Hirschfeld A: Intraorbital arteriovenous malformation with spontaneous thrombosis. Ann Ophthalmol 13(4):457, 1981.
91. Levy JV, Zemek L: Ophthalmic arteriovenous malformation. Am J Ophthalmol 62:971, 1966.
92. Terry TL, Fred GB: Abnormal arteriovenous communication in the orbit involving the angular vein. Arch Ophthalmol 19:90, 1938.
93. Nordmann PJ, Lobstein A, Gerhard JP: A propos de 14 cas de glaucome par hypertension veineuse d'origine extraoculaire. Ophthalmologica 142:501, 1961.
94. Bietti PGB, Vanni V: Glaucome secondaire à une obstruction veineuse extraoculaire. Ophthalmologica 142:227, 1961.
95. Cant JS, Wilson TM: The ocular and orbital circulations in dysthyroid ophthalmopathy. Trans Ophthal Soc UK 94:416, 1974.
96. Manor RS, Kurz O, Lewitus Z: Intraocular pressure in endocrinological patients with exophthalmos. Ophthalmolgica 168:241, 1974.
97. Bouzas AG: The Montgomery Lecture, 1980. Endocrine ophthalmopathy. Trans Ophthal Soc UK 100:51, 1980.
98. Haddad HM: Tonography and visual fields in endocrine exophthalmos. Am J Ophthalmol 64:63, 1967.
99. Alfano JE, Alfano PA: Glaucoma and the superior vena caval obstruction syndrome. Am J Ophthalmol 42:685, 1956.
100. Lokich JJ, Goodman R: Superior vena cava syndrome. JAMA 231:58, 1975.
101. Meyer O: Inflammatory jugular phlebostenosis as the cause of glaucoma exogenicum. Br J Ophthalmol 30:682, 1946.
102. Bedrossian EH: Increased intraocular pressure secondary to mediastinal syndrome. Arch Ophthalmol 47:641, 1952.
103. Etienne R: Chronic glaucoma and hypertension of the pulmonary artery. Bull Soc Ophtalmol Fr 70:510, 1957.
104. Bettelheim H: Der episklerale venendruck bei pulmonaler hypertension. Graefes Arch Clin Exp Ophthalmol 177:108, 1969.
105. Brismar G, Brismar J: Aseptic thrombosis of orbital veins and cavernous sinus. Acta Ophthalmologica 55:9, 1977.
106. Watson PG, Hayreh SS: Scleritis and episcleritis. Br J Ophthalmol 60:163, 1976.
107. Robin AL, Pollack IP: Argon laser trabeculoplasty in secondary forms of open-angle glaucoma. Arch Ophthalmol 101:382, 1983.
108. Weinreb RN: Adjusting the dose of 5-fluorouracil after filtration surgery to minimize side effects. Ophthalmology 94:564, 1987.

109. Talusan ED, Fishbein SL, Schwartz B: Increased pressure of dilated episcleral veins with open-angle glaucoma without exophthalmos. Ophthalmology 90:257, 1983.
110. Radius RL, Maumenee E: Dilated episcleral vessels and open-angle glaucoma. Am J Ophthalmol 86:31, 1978.
111. Jorgensen JS, Guthoff: Zur Genese der einseitig dilatierten

episkleralen Gefase und Erhohung des intraokularen Drucks. Klin Mbl Augenheilk 190:428, 1987.
112. Bigger JF: Glaucoma with elevated episcleral venous pressure. South Med J 68:1444, 1975.
113. Jorgensen JS, Payer H: Erhohter episkleraler Venendruck bei uvealer effusion. Klin Mbl Augenheilk 195:14, 1989.

Chapter 131

■

Epithelial and Fibrous Proliferation

ROBERT A. LYTLE and RICHARD J. SIMMONS

Intraocular proliferation of epithelium from the ocular surface is a rare but devastating complication of intraocular surgery or penetrating trauma. Ingrowth of fibroblasts from episcleral connective tissue or cornea may mimic epithelialization. The incidence of these dreaded sequelae has diminished with an improved understanding of their pathogenesis and also with modern microsurgical techniques. Treatment techniques of epithelial proliferation remain inadequate, with many affected eyes still being lost to intractable glaucoma. Fibrous ingrowth is generally less destructive to the eye than epithelial proliferation but is associated with substantial morbidity including glaucoma and vitreous traction.

EPITHELIAL PROLIFERATION

The original description of epithelialization of the anterior segment is often credited to Collins and Cross in 1892.[1] Epithelialization was grouped by Perera in 1937 into three categories: pearl tumors, posttraumatic cysts of the iris, and epithelial downgrowth.[2]

Pearl tumors occur most often after penetrating trauma in which epithelial elements associated with a cilium are implanted into the eye.[3] The epithelial wall of the pearl cyst may be keratinized, contributing to its pearly luster and opacity. Pearl tumors may remain rather dormant for extended periods of time but may expand to fill the anterior chamber and cause a secondary angle-closure glaucoma.

Posttraumatic cysts of the iris or *epithelial inclusion cysts* are thought to occur when surface epithelium is implanted into the eye as a result of surgical or accidental trauma.[4-7] They may develop months or even years after the original trauma. It is believed that the iris provides nutritional support for the epithelial cells. The cyst wall may have various degrees of pigmentation. These cysts are often translucent, and large epithelial cells and cellular debris may be visible in the cavity of the cyst with the aid of a biomicroscope. They may demonstrate progressive growth filling the pupil and anterior chamber (Fig. 131–1).

Epithelial downgrowth may occur when surface epithelium is given the opportunity to grow into the anterior chamber. It occurs most commonly after cataract extraction.[8-12] It has also been reported following penetrating keratoplasty,[13-17] ocular trauma, placement of transcorneal sutures,[18] and excision of a pterygium.[11] Epithelial downgrowth has been reported to have an incidence between 0.06 and 0.12 percent in large consecutive series of cataract operations.[8-11] In one series of 1500 consecutive aphakic penetrating keratoplasties, epithelial downgrowth occurred in four cases, or 0.27 percent.[14] Thus the incidence may be higher in aphakic eyes that later require penetrating keratoplasty. Epithelial downgrowth has been described as early as 4 days after cataract extraction and as long as 10 yr after surgery.[19] Most cases are noted within the first 12 mo after intraocular surgery.

A series of 124 patients with histologically proven epithelial downgrowth occurring between 1953 and 1983 was recently reviewed at the Massachusetts Eye and Ear Infirmary.[11] Eighteen cases resulted from accidental trauma, and 106 cases from surgical trauma. Ninety-one followed cataract extraction and 13 followed penetrating keratoplasty. A substantial decline in the incidence of epithelial downgrowth after cataract surgery was observed in the course of this series.

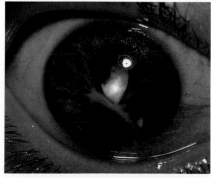

Figure 131–1. A traumatic epithelial cyst resulting from penetrating trauma fills lower half of the anterior chamber. (Courtesy of David Donaldson, M.D.)

Others have investigated the prevalence of epithelial downgrowth in a series of eyes requiring enucleation after cataract surgery.[20, 21] This prevalence has ranged between 17 and 26 percent. Epithelial downgrowth thus may be decreasing in incidence with modern microsurgical techniques, yet it still represents an important cause of eyes being lost after cataract surgery.

Pathogenesis

A large number of experimental studies have attempted to simulate the conditions responsible for the development of epithelial proliferation.[19, 22, 23] Perera was able to produce epithelial cysts by implanting a tongue flap of corneal and conjunctival epithelium into the anterior chamber.[2] Actual epithelial downgrowth has been harder to reproduce in the laboratory. Patz and colleagues did produce epithelial downgrowth in murine eyes with the aid of a carcinogen, methylcholanthrene.[23] Other successful animal models have been developed using reverse corneal autografts or organ culture models.[24–28] Despite all of these efforts in the laboratory, the greatest understanding of this entity has been gained by clinical pathologic correlation in affected patients.

A major risk factor for the development of epithelial downgrowth is delayed closure or dehiscence of the cataract incision, creating a tract for entry of surface epithelium.[29, 30] Recognized associated risk factors include a shallow anterior chamber, which places the invading epithelium in close proximity to the supportive iris. Hypotony and the associated plasmoid aqueous may provide more support to the growth of epithelium than normal aqueous. Inadvertent filtration blebs and fistulas are often present.[31] Incarcerated iris, vitreous, retained lens material, or tags of surface epithelium may prevent wound healing and thus promote downgrowth. The use of corneoscleral sutures and better wound closure has resulted in a marked decline in the incidence of downgrowth. Large silk sutures placed too deeply were thought to create a possible tract for epithelial invasion.[32, 33] Fornix-based conjunctival flaps were thought to place the proliferating cut edge of limbal epithelium in close proximity to the healing cataract incision. Many investigators thus advocated the use of limbus-based conjunctival flaps at cataract surgery.[34] Introduction of surgical instruments into the anterior chamber used for conjunctival dissection has been suggested as a possible risk factor.[35] Others have recognized that healthy corneal endothelium has a protective role against epithelial downgrowth by contact inhibition.[22, 36] It has also been suggested that the aphakic state is itself in some way a risk factor for epithelialization.[37] Reports of epithelial downgrowth involving an intact lens capsule are rare.[38] Epithelial downgrowth has been reported to include an anterior chamber intraocular lens implant.[39] Evidence also suggests that anticoagulant therapy and the delayed formation of a fibrin plug within the healing wound may be risk factors for epithelialization.[11]

Diagnosis of Epithelialization

Diagnosis of a pearl cyst or posttraumatic epithelial cyst is based on the characteristic clinical appearance in conjunction with a history of penetrating trauma. Evidence of previous trauma may be subtle, making the diagnosis more difficult. An aspirate of cyst contents may be obtained during surgical intervention. The diagnosis of an epithelial cyst can be confirmed with cytologic examination of the aspirate, looking for large epithelial cells that have been desquamated from the inner wall of the cyst.

In earlier decades, the diagnosis of epithelialization following cataract surgery was usually not made until the eye was enucleated and examined pathologically. Earlier diagnosis is now possible because clinicians have recognized the early signs of epithelialization, perhaps resulting in fewer eyes requiring enucleation.[40–42] Clinical signs include a faint gray line on the posterior surface of the cornea, which represents the advancing edge of the epithelial sheet, and chronic inflammation. Many eyes have a fistula, and careful examination of the surgical or traumatic wound with 2 percent fluorescein is important. The pupil may be updrawn, and vitreous may be incarcerated in the wound (Fig. 131–2). The normal iris architecture may be blunted from the epithelial sheet. In order to establish a definitive diagnosis of epithelialization, some have advocated obtaining a sector iridectomy biopsy specimen,[43] aspiration of the anterior chamber, or curetting of the posterior corneal surface to obtain an epithelial cell specimen.[44] A major advance in the diagnosis and treatment of epithelialization involves applying photocoagulation burns to the iris in suspected cases.[45] Areas of epithelial membrane turn white. Commonly used settings on the argon laser are 0.2 sec, 200 to 500 μm spot size, and 200 to 500 mW. Higher energy levels may be needed to penetrate hazy corneas (Fig. 131–3). This technique is also used to outline the extent of the epithelial membrane on the iris surface for preoperative planning.

Specular microscopic findings of the leading edge of the epithelial sheet have been described, providing an additional clinical means of confirming the diagnosis.[46]

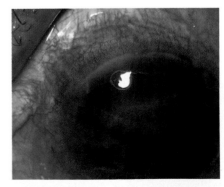

Figure 131–2. Epithelial downgrowth. Grayish retrocorneal membrane characteristic of epithelial downgrowth in an aphakic eye. (Courtesy of David Donaldson, M.D.)

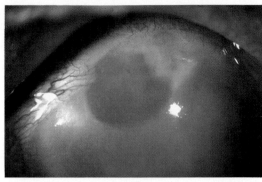

Figure 131–3. Argon laser—epithelial downgrowth. Argon laser photocoagulation of the epithelial membrane on the iris surface demonstrates characteristic whitening.

When specular microscopy is performed at the scalloped margin of the advancing epithelial membrane, an interface between intact endothelium and affected areas may be appreciated. Focusing slightly deeper in the areas of suspected epithelial membrane may reveal the outline of epithelial cells.

Histopathology

Epithelial downgrowth is recognized pathologically by the presence of nonkeratinized stratified squamous epithelium in a diffuse blanket on the iris surface.[47, 48] This epithelial membrane may extend onto the cornea, hyaloid face, posterior surface of the iris ciliary body, or even peripheral retina.[49] The epithelial membrane tends to be several cell layers in thickness on the iris and ciliary body and often thinner on the cornea (Fig. 131–4). Cells also tend to be plumper on uveal tissue compared with the cornea. Blood vessels are absent within the epithelial sheet, and the epithelial cells receive nourishment from the underlying iris or aqueous. Blood vessels may be present in the posterior corneal stroma overlying the epithelial membrane. Scanning electron microscopy of these invasive epithelial membranes demonstrates increased numbers of tonofilaments at the leading edge of the sheet of cells, suggesting actual migration of cells.[50] This epithelial sheet results in destruction of underlying endothelial cells and disorganization and destruction of trabecular meshwork.[48, 51] Goblet cells may be present, suggesting a conjunctival source for the epithelium. Electron microscopic findings of the epithelial membrane after penetrating keratoplasty are suggestive of corneal epithelium, including the absence of goblet cells.[52]

Epithelialization of the Anterior Chamber and Glaucoma

Virtually all eyes with epithelial downgrowth develop a secondary glaucoma.[37] Dysfunction of anterior chamber angle structures may be masked by an open fistula or inadvertent filtration resulting in low pressures. Fis-

tulous tracts eventually tend to close, resulting in high intraocular pressures.

Glaucoma can occur by several mechanisms. As the epithelial membrane advances over angle structures, secondary open-angle glaucoma results. This epithelial membrane results in secondary disorganization of the trabecular meshwork. Many of these eyes have preexisting peripheral synechiae from a shallow anterior chamber. Progressive anterior synechiae may develop with contraction of the epithelial membrane and chronic inflammation, causing secondary angle-closure glaucoma. Pupillary block can occur as the epithelial membrane advances across the iris to the anterior hyaloid.

Management

Pearl tumors are rarely treated because they occur infrequently and can remain unchanged for extended periods. En bloc surgical excision of the cyst and involved iris is indicated if enlargement threatens other intraocular structures.[3]

Posttraumatic epithelial cysts usually require surgical intervention for progressive enlargement. Diffuse epithelial downgrowth should be treated as early as possible to provide the best opportunity to eradicate the invading epithelium completely.

In the first half of this century, epithelialization was commonly treated with radiation therapy in the range of 2500 to 3000 rad.[40, 53–56] Encouraging results were reported by some investigators using radiation therapy for epithelial cysts. Many of these eyes were phakic, however, and this form of treatment was abandoned because of radiation effects on the crystalline lens and other structures. Poor results were reported with radiation therapy and diffuse epithelial downgrowth after cataract surgery.

Posttraumatic cysts may be amenable to en bloc excision.[6, 57, 58] However, this procedure carries the risk

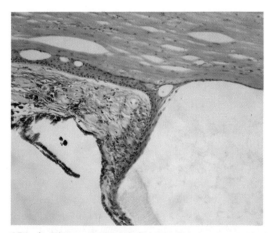

Figure 131–4. Histopathology of epithelial downgrowth demonstrating the epithelial membrane on the iris and posterior surface of the cornea with broad peripheral anterior synechiae. (Courtesy of David Donaldson, M.D.)

of releasing contents of the cyst into the eye and creating diffuse epithelialization.[59] A preferred method of dealing with posttraumatic cysts is evacuation of the cyst contents with a syringe and needle passed through the limbus.[60–62] The cyst often has a point of attachment in the anterior chamber angle. Gonioscopy is used to confirm this anatomy to guide the needle through the limbus into the cyst. The anterior chamber is filled with air as the cyst is collapsed. The air serves to protect other intraocular contents when subsequent cryotherapy is performed. Cryotherapy is applied in a double freeze-thaw technique to help obliterate epithelial cells lining the collapsed cyst wall. Alternatively, the collapsed cyst wall may be surgically excised.[63] Others have advocated reinjecting the collapsed cyst with radioactive agents[64] or caustic agents such as iodine, phenol, or trichloroacetic acid to obliterate the inner layer of epithelial cells.[65] The risk to other ocular contents if the caustic agent is released into the eye has limited the popularity of this technique. Diathermy has also been used to eradicate epithelium lining the collapsed cyst wall.[66] The surface of the collapsed cyst wall may be "painted" with photocoagulation spots using the argon laser.[67–69] This may help to obliterate epithelial cells and keep the cyst in a collapsed state. Collapsing a traumatic epithelial cyst with laser energy is not recommended because the release of cyst contents into the anterior chamber can result in a severe reaction with elevated pressure and even diffuse epithelialization.

The importance of early diagnosis and treatment of epithelial downgrowth cannot be overemphasized. Pioneering efforts in the surgical management of these difficult eyes have been made by Maumenee and coworkers,[12, 45, 70] Sullivan,[71–73] and others.[74–76] Maumenee and colleagues reported a series of 40 consecutive eyes with epithelial downgrowth undergoing surgical treatment.[12] Eleven eyes (27 percent) in this series achieved 20/50 vision or better with successfully controlled glaucoma. All eyes in this series were diagnosed when less than 25 percent of the cornea was involved. This remarkable result is probably due to the involved surgical approach to eliminate invading epithelium, coupled with an early diagnosis. Even with early diagnosis and treatment, morbidity remains high. Five eyes in this series required enucleation, and five had persistent hypotony or atrophy. Even if useful vision is not achieved with surgical intervention, the need for enucleation is reduced.[11]

The management of epithelial downgrowth as outlined below in stepwise fashion is modeled after the approach by Maumenee and coworkers:[12, 42, 45, 70, 77, 78]

1. Extent of epithelial invasion is determined with argon laser application to the iris. Fluorescein solution is used to test for a fistula. Intraoperatively, a scratch incision into Bowman's membrane may be helpful to outline the extent of corneal involvement.

2. The use of osmotic agents intraoperatively may reduce unwanted vitreous loss.

3. Sharp dissection of a fornix-based conjunctival flap is performed. A limbal incision is made posterior to the original section. If a fistula is present, the incision may be placed to bisect the fistula.

4. The fistula is resected.

5. The involved posterior corneal surface is treated with cryotherapy. A double freeze-thaw technique is used. Detachment of Descemet's membrane is avoided by allowing complete thawing of the ice ball before removing the cryoprobe. Alternative methods involve swabbing the posterior corneal surface with absolute alcohol or scraping the membrane off the posterior corneal surface.

6. Involved areas of iris and vitreous are resected. Modern vitrectomy instrumentation is used. Involved ciliary body and angle structures are resected or treated with cryotherapy after wound closure. We favor the use of cryotherapy.

7. Wound closure is watertight. If a fistula was resected, a hinged scleral flap may aid in closure (Fig. 131–5).

Postoperatively, corticosteroids are frequently administered. Cycloplegics and aqueous suppressants are used as needed for inflammation and control of intraocular pressure.

Management of glaucoma represents a major long-term challenge. Affected eyes have multiple risk factors for failing standard filtration surgery techniques. In a reported case with active epithelialization, a filtration operation with adjunctive 5-fluorouracil failed once 5-fluorouracil administration was stopped, and the epithelial membrane advanced once again.[79] Cyclodestructive procedures are commonly used when pressure is uncontrolled with medical therapy.

Corneal decompensation occurs frequently. Corneal transplantation performed simultaneously with the primary procedure to eradicate the epithelial membrane has been reported.[80] We favor delaying corneal transplantation. Some eyes may not require penetrating keratoplasty. Also, success with penetrating keratoplasty is improved once the epithelial membrane is eliminated and glaucoma is controlled.

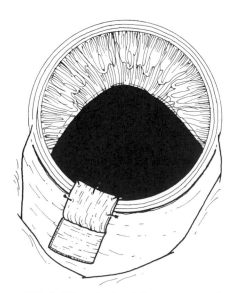

Figure 131–5. Hinged scleral flap to close a fistula.

FIBROUS PROLIFERATION

The term *fibrous ingrowth* is synonymous with stromal ingrowth or stromal overgrowth.[81] The term *retrocorneal membrane* is used by some authors for fibrous ingrowth, especially following penetrating keratoplasty.[82–85] Fibrous ingrowth and epithelial downgrowth occur under similar circumstances after anterior segment trauma or surgery when wound healing has been poor. Fibrous ingrowth has been reported after penetrating keratoplasty, cataract surgery, glaucoma filtration surgery, and penetrating trauma to the globe.[81, 86, 87]

Clinical Manifestations

Patients presenting with fibrous ingrowth typically demonstrate a translucent membrane on the posterior surface of the cornea adjacent to the limbal or corneal wound. Swan has described this grayish fibrous membrane as having the appearance of woven cloth.[81] The edges of the membrane tend to have tonguelike projections rather than the rolled edge of epithelial membranes.

Fibrous ingrowth may occur in a limited fashion or may be massive, with resulting loss of the eye. In two series of eyes requiring enucleation after cataract extraction, fibrous ingrowth was present in 33 percent[30] and 36 percent.[86] In the second series, epithelial downgrowth occurred in only 26 percent of eyes enucleated after cataract surgery, and the researcher concluded that fibrous ingrowth is a more common cause of eyes being lost after cataract surgery than epithelial downgrowth. Others have concluded that epithelial downgrowth occurs more frequently in enucleated eyes after surgical or other trauma. Weiner and colleagues found that fibrous ingrowth coexisted with epithelial downgrowth in as many as 55 percent of eyes enucleated after surgical intervention.[11] It is therefore difficult to conclude that fibrous ingrowth results in more eyes being lost than does epithelial downgrowth. It is generally accepted that fibrous ingrowth occurs more frequently than epithelial downgrowth. In eyes examined at autopsy, fibrous ingrowth was present in 84 percent that had had cataract surgery and vitreous incarceration in the wound.[88] Because of the relatively indolent nature of fibrous ingrowth compared with epithelial downgrowth, a smaller percentage of eyes with fibrous ingrowth eventually require enucleation.

Glaucoma is a frequent complication of fibrous ingrowth.[81, 88] Fibrous membranes tend to be less progressive than membranes in epithelial downgrowth, however, with less tendency for the fibrous membrane to cover angle structures and extend onto the anterior iris surface. Glaucoma occurs in fibrous ingrowth, with contraction of fibrous membranes or contraction of vitreous strands enveloped with fibrous membranes. Peripheral anterior synechiae may result from this contraction. Glaucoma can also occur from associated inflammation or hemorrhage.

Posterior segment sequelae resulting from tractional forces produced by fibrous membranes include retinal tears or detachments and cystoid macular edema.[87]

Pathogenesis

Fibrous ingrowth and epithelial downgrowth share many risk factors, yet the mechanisms favoring the development of each are not clearly understood. Epithelial downgrowth presumably requires that at some point a full-thickness wound defect and hypotony be present to allow the invasion of surface epithelium. A fistulous tract is often found in association with epithelial downgrowth but is not a characteristic finding in fibrous ingrowth.

Fibroplasia is recognized as a necessary part of the reparative phase of surgical or accidental trauma. Swan and Christensen have proposed several factors that set the stage for uncontrolled fibroplasia resulting in fibrous ingrowth.[81, 89] Prolonged inflammation is recognized as an important risk factor for fibrous ingrowth. Poor wound apposition resulting from tissue incarceration or improperly placed sutures is also a recognized risk factor. Henderson observed that normal healing of limbal wounds involves downgrowth of subepithelial or corneal stromal connective tissue to the inner margin of the wound.[90] Further ingrowth of connective tissue appears to be inhibited when the inner wound margins are bridged by endothelium by the second postoperative week. Therefore, damaged corneal endothelium is also a risk factor for stromal ingrowth even with a well-apposed wound. Henderson also suggested that posterior limbal incisions were associated with fibrous ingrowth, whereas more anterior limbal incisions with poor healing were prone to develop epithelial downgrowth.[90] Swan suggested that more posteriorly placed incisions are more often associated with hemorrhage and that hemorrhage is the important risk factor for fibrous ingrowth.[81]

The source of fibroblasts in fibrous ingrowth is believed to be either subepithelial connective tissue or corneal stromal fibroblasts. Metaplastic corneal endothelium and blood mononuclear cells are other suggested sources.[81] Studies of the healing of limbal and corneal incisions confirm the role of subepithelial connective tissue and stromal keratocytes in normal healing.[29, 30] Overgrowth of these cells under proper conditions provides an obvious mechanism for fibrous ingrowth. Substantial evidence also suggests that corneal endothelium can undergo fibrous metaplasia, resulting in certain retrocorneal membranes. This has been described in several conditions, including vitreous touch syndrome,[91] as well as after vitrectomy[92] and after penetrating keratoplasty. Such retrocorneal membranes should be considered as a separate entity from actual ingrowth of fibroblasts. One interesting case report describes a double-layered fibrous membrane representing a retrocorneal membrane from metaplastic endothelium and ingrowth of fibroblasts.[93]

Management

There is no specific treatment for fibrous ingrowth. Attention is directed at the complicating sequelae without necessarily eradicating the fibrous membrane as is necessary in epithelial downgrowth. Secondary glaucoma is managed medically or surgically as necessary. Penetrating keratoplasty may be required for visual rehabilitation. Release of vitreous traction by vitrectomy or YAG laser lysis may be indicated.

REFERENCES

1. Collins ET, Cross FR: Two cases of epithelial implantation cyst in the anterior chamber after extraction of cataract. Trans Ophthal Soc UK 12:175, 1892.
2. Perera C: Epithelium in the anterior chamber of the eye after operation and injury. Trans Am Acad Ophthal Otol 42:142, 1937.
3. Sitchevska O, Payne BF: Pearl cysts of the iris. Am J Ophthalmol 34:833, 1951.
4. Mulligan HR: Traumatic cyst of the iris. Los Angeles Society of Ophthalmology Otology. Am J Ophthalmol 88:1286, 1981.
5. Coston TO: Epithelial implantation cysts. Trans Am Ophthalmol Soc 72:181, 1974.
6. Boruchoff SA, Kenyon KR, Foulks GN, Green WR: Epithelial cyst of the iris following penetrating keratoplasty. Br J Ophthalmol 64:440, 1980.
7. Farmer SB, Kaline RE: Epithelial implantation cyst of the iris. Ophthalmology 88:1286, 1981.
8. Theobald GD, Haas JS: Epithelial invasion of the anterior chamber following cataract extraction. Trans Am Acad Ophthalmol Otol 52:470, 1948.
9. Bernardino VB, Kim JC, Smith TR: Epithelialization of the anterior chamber after cataract extraction. Arch Ophthalmol 82:742, 1969.
10. Payne BF: Epithelialization of the anterior segment after cataract extractions. Am J Ophthalmol 45:182, 1958.
11. Weiner MJ, Trentacoste J, Pon DM, et al: Epithelial downgrowth: A 30-year clinicopathological review. Br J Ophthalmol 73:6, 1989.
12. Maumenee AE, Paton D, Morse PH, et al: Review of 40 histologically proven cases of epithelial downgrowth following cataract extraction and suggested surgical management. Am J Ophthalmol 69:598, 1970.
13. Leibowitz HM, Elliott JH, Boruchoff SA: Epithelialization of the anterior chamber following penetrating keratoplasty. Arch Ophthalmol 78:613, 1967.
14. Sugar A, Meyer RF, Hood I: Epithelial downgrowth following penetrating keratoplasty in the aphake. Arch Ophthalmol 95:464, 1977.
15. Sidrys LA, Demong T: Epithelial downgrowth after penetrating keratoplasty. Can J Ophthalmol 17:29, 1982.
16. Avni I, Blumenthal M, Belkin M: Epithelial invasion of the anterior chamber following repeated keratoplasty. Metab Pediatr Systemic Ophthalmol 6:337, 1982.
17. Feder RS, Krachmer JH: The diagnosis of epithelial downgrowth after keratoplasty. Am J Ophthalmol 99:697, 1985.
18. Abbott RI, Spencer WH: Epithelialization of the anterior chamber after transcorneal (McCannell) suture. Arch Ophthalmol 96:482, 1978.
19. Regan EF: Epithelial invasion of the anterior chamber. Trans Am Ophthalmol Soc 55:741, 1957.
20. Schulze RR, Duke JR: Causes of enucleation following cataract extraction. Arch Ophthalmol 73:74, 1965.
21. Blodi FC: Causes and frequency of enucleation after cataract extraction. Presented at the 112th Annual Meeting of the AMA, Atlantic City, NJ, June 16–20, 1963.
22. Terry TL, Chisholm JF Jr, Schonberg AL: Studies on surface-epithelium invasion of the anterior segment of the eye. 22:1083, 1939.
23. Patz A, Wulff L, Rogers S: Experimental production of epithelial invasion of the anterior chamber. Am J Ophthalmol 47:815, 1959.
24. Smith DR, Blasier MS, Shea M: An experimental model of epithelialization of the anterior chamber. Can J Ophthalmol 2:158, 1967.
25. Burris TE, Nordquist RE, Rowsey JJ: Model of epithelial downgrowth. I: Clinical correlations and light microscopy. Cornea 2:227, 1983.
26. Burris TE, Nordquist RE, Rowsey JJ: Model of epithelial downgrowth. II: Scanning and transmission electron microscopy of corneal epithelialization. Cornea 3:141, 1984.
27. Burris TE, Nordquist RE, Rowsey JJ: Model of epithelial downgrowth. III: Scanning and transmission electron microscopy of iris epithelialization. Cornea 4:249, 1985–86.
28. Davanger M, Olsen EG: Experimental epithelial ingrowth: Epithelial/endothelial interaction through a corneal perforation, studied in organ culture. Acta Ophthalmol 63:443, 1985.
29. Dunnington JH: Healing of incisions for cataract extraction. Am J Ophthalmol 34:36, 1951.
30. Dunnington JH: Wound rupture with tissue incarceration. In: Transactions of the New Orleans Academy of Ophthalmology, Symposium on Diseases and Surgery of the Lens. St. Louis, CV Mosby, 1957.
31. Swan KC, Campbell L: Unintentional filtration following cataract surgery. Arch Ophthalmol 71:77, 1964.
32. Lyle DJ: Society proceedings. Am J Ophthalmol 34:899, 1951.
33. Allen JC, Duehr PA: Sutures and epithelial downgrowth. Am J Ophthalmol 66:293, 1968.
34. Christensen L: Epithelialization of the anterior chamber. In: Transactions of the New Orleans Academy of Ophthalmology, Symposium on Cataracts. St. Louis, CV Mosby, 1965.
35. Ferry AP: The possible role of epithelium-bearing surgical instruments in pathogenesis of epithelialization of the anterior chamber. Ann Ophthalmol 3:1089, 1971.
36. Cameron JD, Flaxman BA, Yanoff M: In vitro studies of corneal wound healing: Epithelial-endothelial interactions. Invest Ophthalmol 12:575, 1974.
37. Epstein DL: Epithelialization of the anterior chamber. In Epstein DL (ed): Chandler & Grant's Glaucoma, 3rd ed. Philadelphia, Lea & Febiger, 1986, pp 348–351.
38. Bruner WE, Green WR, Stark WJ: A case of epithelial ingrowth primarily involving the lens capsule. Ophthalmic Surg 17:483, 1986.
39. Samples JR, Van Buskirk EM: Epithelial ingrowth on an intraocular lens. Ophthalmic Surg 15:869, 1984.
40. Vail D: Epithelial downgrowth into the anterior chamber following cataract extraction arrested by radium treatment. Trans Am Ophthalmol Soc 56:606, 1958.
41. Calhoun FP Jr: The clinical recognition and treatment of epithelialization of the anterior chamber following cataract extraction. Trans Am Ophthalmol Soc 47:498, 1949.
42. Maumenee AE, Shannon CR: Epithelial invasion of the anterior chamber. Am J Ophthalmol 41:929, 1956.
43. Dixon WS, Speakman JS: Epithelial downgrowth following cataract surgery. Arch Ophthalmol 84:303, 1970.
44. Calhoun FP: An aid to the clinical diagnosis of epithelial downgrowth into the anterior chamber following cataract extraction. Am J Ophthalmol 61:1055, 1966.
45. Maumenee AE: Treatment of epithelial downgrowth and intraocular fistula following cataract extraction. Trans Am Ophthalmol Soc 62:153, 1964.
46. Smith RE, Parrett C: Specular microscopy of epithelial downgrowth. Arch Ophthalmol 96:1222, 1978.
47. Spencer WH, Font RL, Green WR, et al: Ophthalmic Pathology: An Atlas and Textbook, 3rd ed. Philadelphia, WB Saunders, 1985, pp 511–514.
48. Zavala EY, Binder PS: The pathologic findings of epithelial ingrowth. Arch Ophthalmol 98:2007, 1980.
49. Vannas S: Epithelial downgrowth into the anterior chamber and deep into the eye. Arch Ophthalmol 35:190, 1957.
50. Iwamoto T, Srinivasan BD, DeVoe AG: Electron microscopy of epithelial downgrowth. Ann Ophthalmol 9:1095, 1977.
51. Jensen P, Minckler DS, Chandler JW: Epithelial ingrowth. Arch Ophthalmol 95:837, 1977.
52. Yamaguchi T, Polack FM, Valenti J: Electron microscopy study of epithelial downgrowth after penetrating keratoplasty. Br J Ophthalmol 65:374, 1981.
53. Pincus MH: Epithelial invasion of anterior chamber following cataract extraction: Effect of radiation therapy. Arch Ophthalmol 43:509, 1950.
54. Smith JW, DeVoe AG: New York Academy of Medicine, Section of Ophthalmology, and The New York Roentgen Society. Arch Ophthalmol 48:527, 1952.

55. Dollfus M, Vail D: Roentgen therapy of epithelial invasion cyst of iris and anterior chamber. Arch Ophthalmol 77:86, 1967.

56. Gallardo E, Weidenheim CW: Epithelial membrane in anterior chamber after cataract surgery. Am J Ophthalmol 39:868, 1955.

57. Sugar HS: Deep lamellar resection of intra and extraocular epithelial implantation cyst. Am J Ophthalmol 76:451, 1973.

58. Sugar HS: Further experience with posterior lamellar resection of the cornea for epithelial implantation cyst. Am J Ophthalmol 46:291, 1967.

59. Harbin TS Jr, Maumenee AE: Epithelial downgrowth after surgery for epithelial cyst. Am J Ophthalmol 78:1, 1974.

60. Hogan MJ, Goodner EK: Surgical treatment of epithelial cysts of the anterior chamber. Arch Ophthalmol 64:286, 1960.

61. Ferry AP, Naghadi MR: Cryosurgical removal of epithelial cyst of iris and anterior chamber. Arch Ophthalmol 77:86, 1967.

62. Bruner WE, Michels RG, Stark WJ, Maumenee AE: Management of epithelial cysts of the anterior chamber. Ophthalmic Surg 12:279, 1981.

63. Bennet T, D'Amico RA: Epithelial inclusion cyst of iris after keratoplasty. Am J Ophthalmol 77:87, 1974.

64. Shaffer RN: Alpha irradiation: Effect of astatine of the anterior segment and on an epithelial cyst. Trans Am Ophthalmol Soc 50:607, 1952.

65. Alger EM: Large implantation cyst of the iris treated by aspiration and injection of iodine. Arch Ophthalmol 7:984, 1932.

66. Vail D: Treatment of cysts of the iris with diathermy coagulation. Trans Am Ophthalmol Soc 51:371, 1953.

67. Cleasby GW: Photocoagulation of iris-ciliary body epithelial cysts. Trans Am Acad Ophthalmol Otol 75:638, 1971.

68. Scholz RT, Kelley JS: Argon laser photocoagulation treatment of iris cysts following penetrating keratoplasty. Arch Ophthalmol 100:926, 1982.

69. Okun E, Mandell A: Photocoagulation as a treatment of epithelial implantation cysts following cataract surgery. Trans Am Ophthalmol Soc 72:170, 1974.

70. Stark WJ, Michels RG, Maumenee AE, et al: Surgical management of epithelial ingrowth. Am J Ophthalmol 85:772, 1978.

71. Sullivan GL: Epithelialization of the anterior chamber following cataract extraction: A new approach to treatment. Trans Am Ophthalmol Soc 56:606, 1958.

72. Sullivan GL: Radical anterior segment surgery for epithelial invasion of the anterior chamber: Report of three cases. Trans Am Acad Ophthalmol Otol 83:216, 1977.

73. Sullivan GL: Epithelial proliferation and anterior chamber cysts after cataract surgery. In Theodore FH (ed): Complications After Cataract Surgery. Boston, Little, Brown & Co, 1965, p 232.

74. Long JC, Tyner GS: Three cases of epithelial invasion of the anterior chamber treated surgically. Arch Ophthalmol 58:396, 1957.

75. Brown SI: Treatment of advanced epithelial downgrowth. Trans Am Acad Ophthalmol Otol 77:618, 1973.

76. Friedman AH: Radical anterior segment surgery for epithelial invasion of the anterior chamber: Report of three cases. Trans Am Acad Ophthalmol Otol 83:216, 1977.

77. Stark WJ: Management of epithelial downgrowth and cysts. Dev Ophthalmol 5:64, 1981.

78. Smith P, Stark WJ, Maumenee AE, Green WR: Epithelial fibrous, and endothelial proliferation. In Ritch R, Shields MB, Krupin J (eds): The Glaucomas, Vol. 73. St. Louis, CV Mosby, 1989, p 1299.

79. Loane ME, Weinreb RN: Glaucoma secondary to epithelial downgrowth and 5-fluorouracil. Ophthalmic Surg 21:704, 1990.

80. Brown SI: Results of excision of advanced epithelial downgrowth. Ophthalmology 86:321, 1979.

81. Swan KC: Fibroblastic ingrowth following cataract extraction. Arch Ophthalmol 89:445, 1973.

82. Brown SI, Kitano S: Pathogenesis of the retrocorneal membrane. Arch Ophthalmol 75:518, 1966.

83. Sherrard ES, Rycroft PV: Retrocorneal membranes. I: Their origin and structure. Br J Ophthalmol 51:379, 1967.

84. Sherrard ES, Rycroft PV: Retrocorneal membranes. II: Factors influencing their growth. Br J Ophthalmol 51:387, 1967.

85. Michels RG, Kenyon KR, Maumenee AE: Retrocorneal fibrous membranes. Invest Ophthalmol 11:822, 1972.

86. Allen JC: Epithelial and stromal ingrowths. Am J Ophthalmol 65:179, 1968.

87. McDonnell PJ, Zenaida CC, Green WR: Vitreous incarceration complicating cataract surgery: A light and electron microscopic study. Ophthalmology 93:247, 1986.

88. Friedman AH, Henkind P: Corneal stromal overgrowth after cataract extraction. Br J Ophthalmol 54:528, 1970.

89. Christensen L: Pathogenesis of surgical complications—The role of fibroplasia. In: Transactions of the New Orleans Academy of Ophthalmology, Symposium on Cataracts. St. Louis, CV Mosby, 1965.

90. Henderson T: A histological study of the normal healing of wounds after cataract extraction. Ophthalmol Rev 26:127, 1907.

91. Snip RC, Kenyon KR, Green WR: Retrocorneal fibrous membrane in the vitreous touch syndrome. Am J Ophthalmol 79:233, 1975.

92. Kenyon KR, Stark WJ, Stone DL: Corneal endothelial degeneration and fibrous proliferation after pars plana vitrectomy. Am J Ophthalmol 81:486, 1976.

93. Bloomfield SE, Jakobiec FA, Iwamoto T: Fibrous ingrowth with retrocorneal membrane. Ophthalmology 88:459, 1981.

Chapter 132

■

Neovascular Glaucoma

MARTIN WAND

Over the past century, our knowledge about neovascular glaucoma (NVG), paralleling the accrual of knowledge in all of medicine, has followed an exponential growth curve. The first documentable allusion to this disorder was in 1875 when Pagenstecher[223] referred to an eye with intraocular bleeding and elevated intraocular pressure (IOP) as having hemorrhagic glaucoma. In the absence of any knowledge concerning the anatomy or pathophysiology of NVG, a confusing array of terms appeared in the literature to identify vastly different disorders with superficial similarities. Historically, the terms hemorrhagic glaucoma, thrombotic glaucoma, congestive glaucoma, rubeotic glaucoma, and diabetic hemorrhagic glaucoma all referred to NVG as we now understand it.

It was not until 1906 that Coats[61] put our knowledge of NVG on a sound anatomic basis, when he described the histologic findings of new vessels on the irides of eyes with central retinal vein occlusion (CRVO). In 1928, Salus[247] described similar new vessels on the irides of eyes of diabetic patients. In 1937, after the introduction of clinical gonioscopy, Kurz[278] correlated his clinical observation of fine new vessels in the angle with the histologic finding of connective tissue along these vessels. He felt that the contraction of this connective tissue along these new vessels was the cause of synechial angle closure. In 1963 Weiss, Shaffer, and Nehrenberg[298] proposed the term neovascular glaucoma because the glaucoma is caused by the new vessels rather than the inconsistently present intraocular bleeding. This term has since found universal acceptance. Walton and Grant,[286] in 1968, proposed the more accurate and appropriate term neovascularization of the iris (NVI) rather than rubeosis iridis. Although this has not yet found wide acceptance, it is the correct terminology and NVI is used here instead of rubeosis iridis.

Over the last 2 decades, there has been an explosion of knowledge concerning the treatment as well as the pathophysiology of this disorder. Starting with the introduction of modern panretinal photocoagulation (PRP) by Aiello and associates[4] in 1967, many cases of NVG are now treatable, and even more important, preventable. We are now on the threshold of elucidating the basic mechanisms of angiogenesis. The key to earlier and even better treatment, total prevention, lies in the molecular and genetic basis of angiogenesis, which is being investigated by scientists around the world.

CLINICAL MANIFESTATION

In the prototypical picture of NVG, the eye is painful and photophobic. Visual acuity is often at the counting fingers to hand motion level, and the IOP may be 60 mmHg or higher. There is moderate-to-marked conjunctival congestion, frequently associated with a steamy cornea. The new vessels on the iris and the ectropion uveae are often visible even through a cloudy cornea. Variable degrees of synechial angle-closure are present. It would be difficult to miss the diagnosis in such an eye (Fig. 132–1). However, the success in treating NVG is in detecting it at its earliest stages so that appropriate preventive measures can be taken. The first visible signs of incipient NVG are tiny tufts of new vessels at the pupillary margin. These vessels enlarge and become clinically visible knuckles of fine vessels, appearing similar to a glomerulus (Fig. 132–2). Unless one maintains a high index of suspicion and looks carefully under high magnification at the slit lamp, it is very easy to overlook these vessels and miss the potential opportunity to prevent the development of NVG. In darkly pigmented irides, it is especially difficult to detect early pupillary NVI. If a contact gonioscopy lens is used at the initial examination, even light pressure on the lens is sufficient to collapse these neovascular tufts and render them clinically invisible.[292] It had been previously thought that angle neovascularization could not occur without NVI developing first in the pupillary margin.[288] However, dark irides may conceal early pupillary NVI on slit-lamp examination, but new vessels may be visible on gonios-

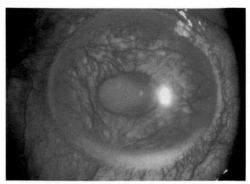

Figure 132–1. Advanced fulminant neovascular glaucoma with marked conjunctival congestion, corneal haze from elevated intraocular pressure, neovascularization of the iris, and ectropion uvea.

copy. Thus, it is imperative to perform gonioscopy in all eyes that have the potential of developing NVG.

When there are other passageways for aqueous to enter the anterior chamber, bypassing the pupil, such as the presence of a peripheral iridectomy, it is important to examine the iris surrounding these openings. Since aqueous would preferentially pass through these openings, NVI could well appear there before appearing at the pupillary margin. It seems that the greatest aqueous-tissue contact occurs where NVI first begins. There has been a report of an elderly man with diabetes mellitus who had a previous surgical peripheral iridectomy, and NVI was present at the edges of the surgical iridectomy before any NVI could be seen at the pupil.[292] As NVI progresses, new vessels extend from the pupillary tufts in an irregular, meandering manner. New vessels, at least clinically, appear on the surface of the iris. In elderly people with atrophic irides and in people with light irides, normal iris vessels are sometimes visible, but, if one looks carefully, these vessels are within the stroma of the iris and have a more radial orientation. Occasionally, with inflammation and secondary engorgement, it may be difficult if not impossible to tell if iris vessels are abnormal. When new vessels reach the iris

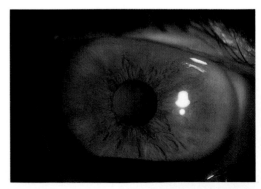

Figure 132–2. The earliest manifestations of neovascularization of the iris (NVI) at the pupillary margin, although visible on high magnification with the slit lamp, are not visible in printed photographs. This eye has slightly more advanced NVI at the pupillary margin.

collarette, the collarette vessel, which is often normally present but not visible, may become engorged and part of the rubeotic vasculature. At this stage, and more commonly at more advanced stages, it is possible to see effacement of the normal iris surface architecture, resulting in a relatively smooth iris. When these new vessels reach the angle, they cross the ciliary body band and scleral spur onto the trabecular meshwork (Fig. 132–3). Chandler and Grant[55] have long taught that if a blood vessel crosses over the scleral spur onto the trabecular meshwork, the vessel is abnormal; all normal vessels remain behind the scleral spur.[55] This axiom has withstood the test of time. Occasionally, new vessels seem to arise from the major arterial circle of the iris and cross onto the trabecular meshwork.

At the angle, the larger vessels, after crossing the scleral spur, arborize with very fine capillaries over several clock hours of the trabecular meshwork, which is analogous to a tree trunk with branches overhead. Again, a high index of suspicion and careful examination are necessary to see these early fine angle vessels. The higher magnification and higher light intensity offered by the slit lamp with the Goldmann goniolens facilitates the examination. Until new vessels in the angle cover a significant portion of the trabecular meshwork, the IOP may be completely normal. A fibrovascular membrane, which is invisible on gonioscopy, accompanies these new angle vessels and may block enough of the trabecular meshwork to cause a secondary form of open angle glaucoma (OAG) at this time. This fibrovascular membrane along these new angle vessels has a tendency to contract and pull the vessels taut, bridging the angle initially, and then tenting the iris toward the trabecular meshwork (Fig. 132–4). As these peripheral anterior synechiae coalesce, synechial angle-closure occurs. The radial traction along the surface of the iris pulls the posterior pigment layer of the iris around the pupillary margin onto the anterior iris surface, commonly, though inaccurately, known as ectropion uveae. As a corollary, when one sees ectropion uveae in NVG, one can presume that there is synechial angle-closure in the same meridian. Sometimes, there is so much traction that the iris almost disappears from view, mimicking aniridia.

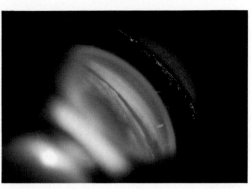

Figure 132–4. Goniophotograph showing new vessels covering all of the visible trabecular meshwork with early synechial angle-closure 1:30.

As the scattered areas of synechial closure coalesce, there is total angle-closure. The picture of a very smooth, zippered-up, line of iridocorneal adhesion is pathognomonic (Fig. 132–5). After this end stage of NVG is reached, there can be a remarkable decrease in the number of new vessels visible in the angle and on the iris (Fig. 132–6). When a prominent pigmented Schwalbe's line is present, a totally closed angle in NVG can be mistaken by even an experienced gonioscopist as a normal "open" angle.

Attempts have been made to classify and quantitate NVI.[179, 277, 297] Such a grading system could be valuable in clinical staging, following progression, when comparing patients, and when evaluating the efficacy of therapy. Unfortunately, such a classification has not been widely accepted.

Having presented this orderly picture of progressive neovascularization, it goes without saying that great variability in the clinical picture and the rate of progression constitute the rule rather than the exception. Usually, the vision is extremely poor because of the edematous cornea and the primary disorder underlying the NVG. The visual acuity can sometimes be remarkably good, 20/40 or even better, if the corneal endothelium is healthy and the primary disorder does not significantly

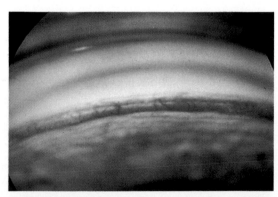

Figure 132–3. Goniophotograph showing new angle vessels crossing over the ciliary body band and scleral spur and arborizing over the trabecular meshwork. (From Wand M, Hutchinson BT: The surgical management of neovascular glaucoma. Perspect Ophthalmology 4:147, 1980. Copyright ANKHO International.)

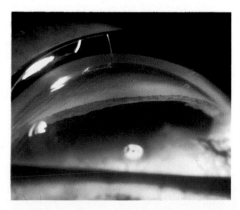

Figure 132–5. Late-stage neovascular glaucoma with total synechial angle-closure and the typical picture of a smooth line of iridocorneal adhesion. The irregular dark line is the edge of the ectropion uvea. (From Wand M, Hutchinson BT: The surgical management of neovascular glaucoma. Perspect Ophthalmology 4:147, 1980. Copyright ANKHO International.)

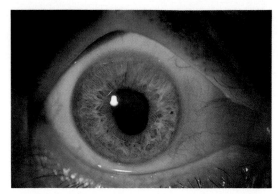

Figure 132–6. End-stage neovascular glaucoma with no light perception and total synechial angle-closure. There is no visible neovascularization of the iris, and other than the ectropion uvea, the eye looks normal.

involve the macula. The IOP is usually high, but in some causes of NVG, such as carotid artery obstructive disease (CAOD), the IOP may be normal or even subnormal. If the patient is young and the endothelium is healthy, the cornea may remain clear with an IOP as high as 60 mmHg. The time sequence is also quite variable.

NVI may progress to total synechial angle-closure within days, or it may remain stationary with no angle involvement for years. This quiescent stage may also suddenly become active after years of inactivity. Although the clinical picture of NVG from different primary causes is not distinguishable, and each case of NVG shows its individual pattern of progression, NVI from CRVO, as a group, seems to be more fulminant in appearance and rapid in course than that from other causes. This clinical impression has been confirmed anatomically by liquid rubber injection into the vasculature of eye bank eyes with NVG; it was found that the new iris vessels that developed after CRVO were larger, coarser, and more irregular than the new iris vessels that developed from diabetic retinopathy[154] (Fig. 132–7). Some correlation seems to exist between how "angry" these new vessels look and how quickly the neovascularization progresses. Most important, there may be complete arrest or even total regression of the NVI at any stage.[107, 189] Parenthetically, any synechial angle-closure is, of course, permanent. This unpredictable course of NVG makes the evaluation of various treatment modalities difficult. As a result, only studies with large numbers of patients with proper controls can provide reliable results.

DIFFERENTIAL DIAGNOSIS

As already stressed, the key aim in the treatment of NVG is early diagnosis, so that the currently optimal effective treatment regimen can be instituted. In the differential diagnosis, there are two stages to consider: the early stage, in which only NVI is present, and the late stage, in which there is elevated IOP, a cloudy cornea, and vascular congestion. In both stages, a com-

plete patient history and careful examination of both eyes usually provide the answer. For true NVG, the history is critical. Diabetes mellitus in the patient or family; history of previous loss of vision, suggesting old CRVO or retinal detachment; or history of hypertension or arteriosclerosis, suggesting possible CAOD, are all significant. Even a misleadingly benign-appearing posterior segment should not deter one from considering one of these major causes of NVI.

There are several entities to consider in the differential diagnosis of prominent iris vessels. NVI may be present in Fuchs' heterochromic cyclitis. The eye is usually white and quiet. The iris vessels tend to be extremely fine, thin-walled, and fragile. Spontaneous hyphemas may occur but do so more often with manipulation of the eye, such as during a gonioscopic examination or after paracentesis. These vessels may cross over the scleral spur onto the trabecular meshwork, but they only rarely cause synechial angle-closure or NVG. Secondary glaucoma may occur but is probably on the basis of the trabeculitis.[226] Histologic studies show localized thickening of the iris vessel walls caused by hyalinization and proliferation of the endothelium, resulting in decreased lumen size and vascular profusion.[106] Fluorescein studies have shown leakage from the iris vessels, narrowed radial iris vessels, and ischemic iris sectors, confirming localized areas of iris hypoxia as a cause of the NVI.[244]

NVI may also be present in pseudoexfoliation syndrome. Electron microscopic studies have shown endothelial thickening with decreased lumen size and fenestration of vessel walls,[239] accounting for the fluorescein leakage seen in the irides of some eyes.[284] True NVG has not been reported. In all likelihood, the NVI occasionally seen after retinal detachment or strabismus surgery is a result of trauma to the anterior ciliary vessels, which also results in localized anterior segment hypoxia.[244]

Finally, inflammatory conditions can cause prominent iris vessels, which are sometimes impossible to differentiate clinically from progressive NVI. This is especially true in diabetes mellitus after cataract extraction, when a profound iritis and secondary vascular engorgement can simulate fulminant NVG. In view of the important

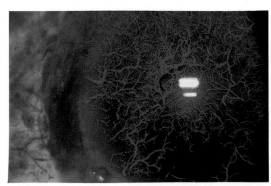

Figure 132–7. Liquid rubber injection mold of new vessels in an autopsy eye with neovascular glaucoma. (Courtesy of Vicente L. Jocson, M.D.)

role that certain cellular components of inflammation plays in the angiogenesis process, it is not surprising that inflammation could cause engorgement and dilatation of iris vessels, especially in eyes that already have some compromised retinal circulation. In any case, with topical steroid therapy, pseudo-NVI resolves, but true NVI persists.

In the late stages with elevated IOP and a cloudy cornea, there is another list of differential diagnoses. Although the underlying cause of true NVG is usually of long-term duration, such as PDR or CRVO, the presenting signs and symptoms are often precipitous. It is not unusual for a patient to present for the first time with an inflamed eye and IOP 60 mmHg or higher. Acute angle-closure must be considered high on the differential list. Gonioscopy may be impossible, even with the use of systemic hyperosmotics and topical glycerin. However, it is almost always possible to see the engorged iris vessels through the hazy cornea. More important, gonioscopy of the fellow eye provides the clue, because narrow angles and angle-closure glaucoma tend to be a bilateral disorder. Many surgical or laser iridectomies have been performed inadvertently on eyes with unrecognized NVG. Conversely, Figure 132–8 shows an elderly woman with all the findings of NVG in one eye and a normal fellow eye with a deep anterior chamber angle. She was found to have intumescent cataract and secondary angle-closure glaucoma with inflammation. After a neodymium-yttrium-aluminum-garnet (Nd.YAG) laser iridectomy and resolution of the angle-closure, the "NVI" completely disappeared (Fig. 132–9). An opaque media may prevent visualization of the posterior segment, and the diagnosis may be difficult. Hidden intraocular tumors,[286, 306] chronic retinal detachment, and other degenerative conditions[288] must be considered. Any cause of intraocular bleeding, especially with a hyphema, may be confused with NVG. Ghost cell glaucoma, presenting after trauma or surgical procedures, should be considered.[49] This diagnosis is usually made easier because there is a khaki-colored hypopyon in the anterior chamber which covers the

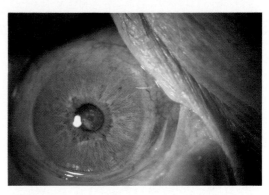

Figure 132–9. Same eye after a neodymium-yttrium-aluminum garnet (Nd.YAG) laser iridectomy that resolved the angle-closure glaucoma.

trabecular meshwork on gonioscopy. The difficulty arises when a superimposed hyphema prevents this observation. The history and paracentesis with phase-contrast microscopy of the aspirate confirm this diagnosis.

FLUORESCEIN STUDIES

There is good evidence that functional derangement of the vascular endothelium, as evidenced by leakage of fluorescein, occurs before any structural changes and well before clinically visible neovascularization. Therefore, various fluorescein studies play an important clinical and research role in NVG.

Iris fluorescein angiography shows leakage from damaged iris vessels (Fig. 132–10) long before new vessels can be detected on slit-lamp examination (Fig. 132–11). It has been shown that normal eyes can have pupillary tufts with fluorescein leakage and that the incidence seemingly increases with age.[13] In addition, patients with pseudoexfoliation,[284] myotonic dystrophy,[62] or abnormal insulin secretion[196] can also show abnormal pupillary tufts with fluorescein leakage. However, in these benign forms of vascular incompetence, the fluorescein leakage

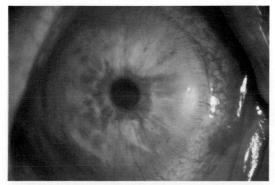

Figure 132–8. An 86-year-old woman with hand motion vision, intraocular pressure 76 mmHg, a congested eye with edematous cornea, and engorged vessels on the iris that appear to be neovascularization of the iris. The fellow eye had a normal depth anterior chamber. She had an intumescent cataract with secondary angle-closure glaucoma mimicking neovascular glaucoma.

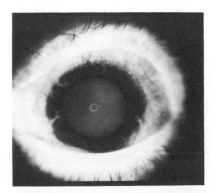

Figure 132–10. Iris fluorescein angiogram showing leakage from new iris vessels that were missed initially on careful slit-lamp examination. Normal irides, especially in elderly people, may show leakage in the pupillary region, but these leaking vessels are more peripheral and are abnormal.

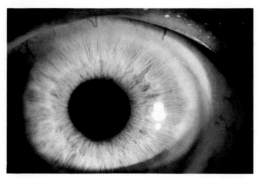

Figure 132–11. Same eye as in Figure 132–10. Very early NVI that was initially missed on careful slit-lamp examination.

occurs only at the pupillary margins; the leakage is minimal; and the leakage fades rapidly after the injection.[248] In contrast, in pathologic states, fluorescein leakage occurs throughout the iris and persists and increases with time.[153]

Iris fluorescein angiography may be performed at the same time as the fundus angiography.[248] The newer fundus cameras have an anterior segment lens that can be flipped into position for anterior segment pictures. After taking the early transit fundus photographs, the iris photographs are taken. In most eyes with NVI, a high index of suspicion with diligent observation makes iris fluorescein angiography unnecessary. However, NVI can be detected on fluorescein iris angiography in 37 per cent of eyes before the subsequent development of clinically visible new vessels.[248] In eyes prior to vitrectomy for complications of diabetic retinopathy, 94 percent showed no clinical findings of NVI but had fluorescein leakage from iris vessels.[80] If capillary dropout is noted on fundus angiography in eyes with diabetic retinopathy or CRVO, and NVI is not clinically detectable, iris angiography should be performed at the same time.

High-power fluorescein gonioscopy has demonstrated leakage of new angle vessels before they are readily visible.[165] Leakage of fluorescein from the pupillary margin usually occurs before there is leakage in the angle, confirming clinical observations that new vessel formation at the pupillary margin generally occurs before angle involvement.[292] Clinically, however, the value of fluorescein iris angioscopy must still be proved.

Of greater potential clinical value is posterior vitreous fluorophotometry. There seems to be a correlation between alteration of the blood-retinal barrier (as detected by vitreous fluorophotometry) and the severity of the retinopathy, duration of diabetes mellitus, and metabolic control of the diabetes.[66, 104, 148] At this date, however, the therapeutic implications of this test remain to be seen.

PATHOLOGY

The anterior segment histopathology of NVG, regardless of the cause, is the same.[104, 288] The only minor deviations are in CRVO, where the new vessels may be more engorged, and in diabetes mellitus, where there are characteristic iris pigment epithelium cystoid changes from accumulation of glycogen.[104] The neovascularization process begins as endothelial budding from capillaries of the minor arterial circle at the pupil. Clinically, this neovascularization appears to progress sequentially from the pupil to the periphery. However, histologically, once the process starts at the pupillary margin, new endothelial buds may appear from vessels anywhere in the iris, including the major arterial circle in the iris root.[104] These endothelial buds progress to become glomerulus-like vascular tufts. These capillary tufts are not unique to NVG. As mentioned, elderly people without known diseases[13] and people with myotonic dystrophy may have pupillary tufts as well.[62] These tufts leak fluorescein, confirming that they are indeed new vessels.[196] These new vessels are essentially very thin-walled endothelial cells without a muscular layer or much adventitia or supportive tissue. There are gaps between and fenestrations in these endothelial cells,[274a, 284] allowing leakage of fluorescein, and presumably, other substances as well.[174] In vivo, these new vessels appear to be on the surface of the iris. Histologically, new vessels have a tendency to be thin walled and to be located toward the surface of the iris, but they can be anywhere within the stroma of the iris (Fig. 132–12).[104]

The existence of a fibrovascular membrane has been known for a long time. This membrane consists of proliferating myofibroblasts, which are fibroblasts with smooth muscle differentiation.[155] These cells are clinically transparent and are only hinted at by the aforementioned flattening of the usual iris surface architecture. Scanning electron microscopy shows the uniform presence of this membrane wherever there are new vessels. Anatomically, the new vessels are not on the surface of the iris but are actually beneath this layer of myofibroblasts (see Fig. 132–12). The pervasiveness of this membrane explains why there can be increased IOP despite the gonioscopic appearance of a normal open angle or only slight angle neovascularization disproportionate to the degree of pressure elevation. The contractile smooth muscle components explain the effacement of the iris surface, the development of ectropion uveae, the formation of peripheral anterior synechiae,

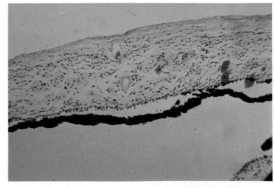

Figure 132–12. Hematoxylin and eosin section (100 ×) of the iris with neovascularization of the iris. Note the new vessel on the iris surface but beneath the fibrovascular membrane.

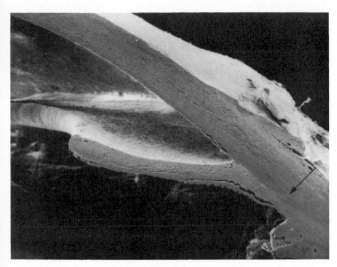

Figure 132–13. Scanning electron micrograph (20 ×) showing the fibrovascular membrane that has produced a very smooth iris surface. The contraction of this membrane has completely closed the angle (*arrow* shows the compressed trabecular meshwork) and has started to pull the posterior pigment layer over the pupillary edge and onto the anterior iris surface (ectropion uvea). (From John T, Sassani JW, Eagle RC Jr: The myofibroblastic component of rubeosis iridis. Ophthalmology 90:721, 1983. Copyright American Academy of Ophthalmology.)

vessels, hiding them from observation.[105] A fibrotic, nonresponsive iris and a fixed dilated pupil are often seen in late NVG. As mentioned, before total synechial angle-closure, the membrane can obstruct the trabecular meshwork and produce a secondary open-angle glaucoma (Fig. 132–15). Further contraction results in synechial angle-closure with iridocorneal touch. When the neovascularization process is stopped, such as with PRP, the new vessels regress, but synechial angle-closure remains.

In some cases of synechial angle-closure of long duration, endothelium and Descemet's membrane may extend from the cornea across the synechiae onto the iris surface.[105] Scanning electronmicroscopic studies have confirmed that this endothelium is contiguous to and originates from the corneal endothelium.[215] Such endothelialization of the iris is also seen in the iridocorneal endothelial syndrome[50] and after trauma[105] and may represent a pathogenic mechanism that is common to violation of the barrier between the cornea and the iris, such as with synechial angle-closure. This closed angle with few or no visible new vessels and covered with endothelium can easily be mistaken for a normal open angle, and the term pseudoangle is most appropriate.

and ultimately, synechial angle-closure[155] (Fig. 132–13). As this membrane continues to contract on the surface of the iris, the posterior pigment layer of the iris is pulled around the pupillary margin onto the anterior surface, causing ectropion uveae and pupillary distortion. The sphincter muscle can also be pulled anteriorly, resulting in ectropion of the sphincter (Fig. 132–14). Contraction may be so extensive that the iris is displaced forward or totally retracted from view. In such cases, the ciliary processes may be visible on gonioscopy. This contraction can also compress and embed the new

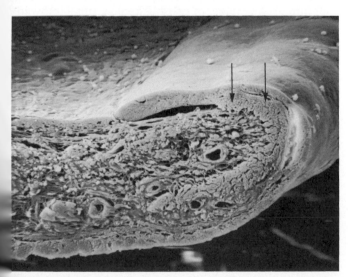

Figure 132–14. Scanning electron micrograph (160 ×) showing the marked ectropion uvea and ectropion of the sphincter muscle (*arrows*). (Courtesy of Ralph C. Eagle Jr, M.D.)

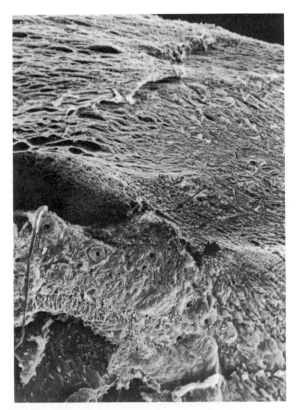

Figure 132–15. Scanning electron micrograph (110 ×). Early synechial angle closure in neovascular glaucoma. The fibrovascular membrane is partially obstructing the anterior chamber angle that is still open *(large single arrow).* Part of the trabecular meshwork is already obstructed *(double arrows);* Schlemm's canal is superior to the trabecular meshwork. (From Wand M: Neovascular glaucoma. *In* Ritch R, Shields MB, Krupin T [eds]: The Glaucomas. St Louis, CV Mosby, 1989. Copyright The C. V. Mosby Company.)

PATHOGENESIS

Since the last review of the literature on angiogenesis only 3 yr ago,[291] there has been a staggering amount of new information. Fundamental to our understanding angiogenesis is understanding how normal new blood vessels form. New vessel formation is one of the fundamental biologic processes necessary for embryogenesis and placenta formation, normal growth and development, wound healing, as well as tumor growth and a variety of other pathologies. New vessel formation, whether in normal development, tumor growth, or NVI, appears to occur in the same sequence.[310] First, endothelial cells from venules or capillaries release enzymes that disrupt the adjacent basement membrane. Adjacent endothelial cells from existing vessels migrate toward the source of the angiogenic stimulus, while more distal cells undergo proliferation. The endothelial cells then elongate, and lumen formation occurs. Finally, new basement membrane forms, and pericytes surround the new capillaries to form mature new vessels.

In 1948, Michaelson[203] postulated the existence of a vasoformative factor, "X-factor," which controlled normal development of new vessels during embryogenesis. Ashton and associates[11] in 1954 suggested that the retinal ischemia in retrolental fibroplasia might result in excess amounts of this factor, which in turn would lead to retinal neovascularization. In 1956, Wise[301] proposed that retinal capillary or venous obstruction resulted in hypoxia of the retinal cells; if the hypoxic cells did not die, they would produce a vasoformative factor. Ashton[10] agreed that the prerequisite for neovascularization was hypoxic metabolism, and he further speculated that the vasoformative factor from this hypoxic metabolism could diffuse anteriorly to stimulate NVI. Earlier, Ashton[11] had demonstrated that the vasoobliteration seen in retrolental fibroplasia was comparable with the capillary closure or nonperfusion seen in diabetic retinopathy. Clinically, it has been confirmed that widespread capillary occlusion and chronic tissue hypoxia are almost always present when there is neovascularization.[32, 225] Experimental radiation retinopathy in monkeys has shown large areas of retinal capillary non-perfusion in eyes which developed NVG.[145]

In 1963, Folkman hypothesized that solid tumors produce a substance which could stimulate new vessel formation.[94] Subsequently, several investigators independently identified and isolated a soluble substance from solid neoplasms capable of stimulating neovascularization and popularized the term "tumor angiogenesis factor" (TAF).[95, 98, 118] It has been demonstrated that a TAF can cause NVI and retinal neovascularization at a distance from intraocular tumors implanted in the eye.[89, 108] Although a specific TAF has never been isolated, angiogenic activity has now been found in retinal tissue extracts from almost all mammalian species.[57, 84, 112, 119, 234] In addition, aqueous and vitreous from human eyes with proliferative neovascularization have been shown to have vasoproliferative activity in tissue culture studies.[111, 119]

Angiogenesis Factors

To date, several major families of angiogenesis factor (AF) have been identified. The best studied group are the acidic and basic fibroblast growth factors (FGF), characterized by their affinity to heparin.[96, 259] Their amino acid sequences have been identified; their genes have been cloned and sequenced; and their receptors have been identified.[259] FGFs have been isolated from many different human tissues. They cause endothelial cells to release basement membrane–degrading enzymes, and they stimulate endothelial cell migration and mitosis.[167]

Another major group are the angiogenins, a 14,400-dalton single chain protein. Its amino acid sequence,[281] three-dimensional structure,[123] and amino acid residue that is critical for angiogenic activity[124] have been identified. It has a 68 percent overall homology to human pancreatic RNase[281] and has been isolated from human tumor and human and bovine plasma. Finally, a gene for angiogenin has been cloned from and a specific inhibitor for angiogenin has been purified and isolated from human placenta.[281] Angiogenin has no known direct effect on in vitro endothelial cells, suggesting that it may act through a third cell type or factor.[167]

Besides these two major AFs, many other polypeptide AFs have been isolated and studied.[96, 167] In addition, a large number of nonpolypeptide substances have angiogenic activity. Various biogenic amines, including histamine, acetylcholine, and serotonin, can stimulate neovascularization.[309] Certain lipids, specifically, prostaglandins of the E series, are potent stimulators of neovascularization and may even be a common mediating agent for different AFs.[19, 100, 311] Prostaglandin levels are elevated in tumors,[19] wounds, inflammatory exudates, activated macrophages,[311] activated leukocytes,[20] and immunocompetent lymphocytes.[260] Interestingly, immunologic ocular inflammation produced by serum albumin[255] and commerical insulin[254] produce a clinical picture similar to that of PDR. Antiinflammatory drugs that inhibit the effects of prostaglandins, indomethycin[69] and methylprednisolone,[199] and irradiation, which induces leukopenia,[114] all reduce experimental neovascularization. However, it is still not clear if prostaglandins act directly on endothelial cells or if they act indirectly through macrophages.[310] Suffice it to say that there have been a myriad of AFs isolated, but some semblance of order is beginning to emerge.

Antiangiogenesis Factors

Because the control of angiogenesis is so critical, much effort has gone into identifying antiangiogenesis factors (anti-AFs). Starting with research into normally avascular tissues, vitreous,[33, 276] cartilage,[208] lens,[300] and aorta-derived[81] macromolecules have been isolated. These macromolecules are capable of inhibiting angiogenesis in vivo and capillary endothelial cell proliferation and migration in vitro. Heparin has been found to be essential to the activity of a number of anti-AFs.[310] When combined with certain steroids, such as hydrocortisone or dexamethasone, a potent anti-AF is produced.[65, 97] RPE has been shown to produce an anti-AF that inhibits endothelial cell migration.[63] In addition, after PRP, RPE produces an inhibitor of the protease urokinase that is important in basement membrane degradation.[113] Orlidge and D'Amore[221] have shown that pericytes inhibit angiogenesis; this observation suggests that with maturation of new vessels, there is autoregulation that prevents the additional growth of vessels. Furthermore, loss of pericytes in the course of diabetic retinopathy may therefore permit subsequent vessel growth.[67a] Not all the known AFs or anti-AFs have been mentioned here, and certainly many more will be isolated and characterized in the future.

The multiplicity of AFs and anti-AFs suggests that vessel formation is an enormously complex process, with alternate pathways and multiple checks and balances at each step.[310] A number of inhibitors may control new vessel formation in the normal state. However, when the need arises (e.g., with injury, inflammation, or tumor stimulation), angiogenesis can quickly be activated. The AFs isolated from tumors and other angiogenic diseases do not differ from normal tissue isolates, and the new vessels in disease and physiologic growth are morphologically similar.[231] It appears that the only difference between pathologic and normal angiogenesis is that the mechanism for halting angiogenesis is either not active or ineffective in diseased states.

It has been postulated that an "X-factor" may exist, which is a normal constituent of the eye but, under abnormal circumstances, could cause angiogenesis.[203] This "X-factor," like TAF, has eluded identification to date, but current knowledge allows a tenable theory why PRP may be effective in arresting and reversing NVI. It has been shown the RPE releases a substance that inhibits angiogenesis.[110] PRP produces chorioretinal scars. The RPE in the scars may release anti-AFs.[109] It is also possible that PRP destroys the source of AFs (e.g., acidic and basic FGF), and that both pathways account for the beneficial effects of PRP. The exact way in which PRP works has yet to be revealed.

CAUSES OF NEOVASCULAR GLAUCOMA

Over the past 20 yr, there have been comprehensive reviews on NVG.[291] Each review has tried to list the disorders known to cause or at least be associated with NVG, with the highest count in the 40s.[90] There have since been more reports of entities that purportedly cause NVG. However, it has become abundantly clear that wherever NVI progresses to NVG, there is almost always widespread posterior segment hyoxia or localized anterior segment hypoxia.

Rather than compiling lists of entities that can cause NVI, it now seems more rewarding to review the major groups of disorders that can lead to NVG. In one review

of patients with NVG admitted in the 1960s to a Danish hospital, 43 percent had glaucoma attributed to diabetic retinopathy, 37 percent had glaucoma attributed to CRVO, and the rest had miscellaneous causes.[188] Surprisingly, despite the widespread use of PRP, the picture has not changed greatly. In 1984, of 208 consecutive cases of NVG diagnosed over 4 yr, 36 percent were caused by CRVO, 32 percent by diabetic retinopathy, and 13 percent by CAOD.[39] At the present time, probably one third of the cases of NVG are attributable to CRVO, one third to diabetic retinopathy, and one third to diverse causes, with CAOD being prominent.

Central Retinal Vein Occlusion

It has been known since at least the time of von Graefe[129] that CRVO can be associated with NVG. Numerous studies have reported widely varying incidences of this complication, ranging from 15 to 65 percent, with an average of about 30 percent.[117] Investigators have found that CRVO can be divided into two distinct entities, based on the presence or absence of retinal ischemia.[125] The group without retinal ischemia is termed nonischemic retinopathy (Figs. 132–16 and 132–17), and the group with retinal ischemia is termed ischemic retinopathy (Figs. 132–18 and 132–19). This differentiation has been confirmed using fundus fluorescein angiography.[180, 181]

The natural history of untreated CRVO is that essentially none of the nonischemic eyes progress on to NVG,[129, 191, 275] whereas 18[182] to 60 percent[191] of eyes in the ischemic group do so. The greater the degree of capillary nonperfusion (hence, retinal hypoxia), the greater will be the chances of developing neovascularization.[129, 171] Recent studies with experimental branch retinal vein occlusion in miniature pigs have shown that the resultant vasoproliferative microangiopathy was associated with decreased preretinal oxygen levels, confirming that the ischemic areas were indeed hypoxic.[230] An overall incidence of NVG of 40 percent for the ischemic type of CRVO is supported by the largest least-biased study.[129] NVG can appear at any time from 2 wk to 2 yr after the initial occlusion,[193] but

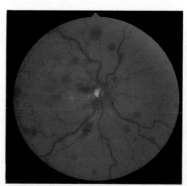

Figure 132–16. Nonischemic central retinal vein occlusion.

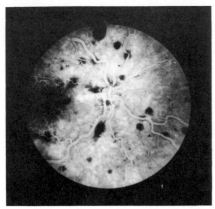

Figure 132–17. Fundus fluorescein angiogram of eye in Figure 132–16. There is good retinal perfusion; the dark spots are the intraretinal hemorrhages blocking out the fluorescence.

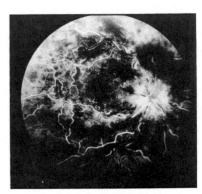

Figure 132–19. Fundus fluorescein angiogram of eye in Figure 132–18. There are extensive areas of capillary nonperfusion as well as areas of blocked fluorescence from the intraretinal hemorrhages.

in more than 80 percent of the cases, NVI and NVG appear within the first 6 mo after the CRVO.[129]

The clinical appearance of the retina can be deceiving in determining the perfusion status. A fluorescein angiogram is imperative in the diagnosis and, ultimately, the treatment of CRVO. Clinically, it is sometimes not possible to determine how much capillary nonperfusion occurs, because retinal hemorrhages block out flourescence in 30 percent of the initial fluorescein angiograms.[129] When retinal hemorrhages prevent adequate visualization of the ischemic retina and it is erroneously interpreted as being normal, patients may be falsely reassured, only to develop NVG later (Figs. 132–20 and 132–21). When it is not possible to determine the extent of the ischemia on initial fluorescein, the patient must be followed carefully and frequently, and repeat fluorescein studies must be performed, if necessary, while the retinal hemorrhages clear. The nonischemic CRVO can convert to the ischemic type.[129] Around 10 percent convert within a median time of 8 mo,[233] but much longer intervals are possible.

It has been shown that electroretinography (ERG) could be an accurate predictor of which eyes would develop NVI after CRVO.[15, 246] Instead of measuring morphologic changes, as with fluorescein angiography, ERG measures the "functional consequences" of retinal ischemia as reflected in decreased retinal sensitivity.[34]

Different parameters of the ERG have been studied[156, 160]; however, by using multiple discriminant analysis combining four ERG parameters, a false-positive prediction rate of only 14 percent has been reported.[35] There are as yet no studies to indicate the beneficial effects of initiating PRP on the basis of ERG before any NVI develops. ERG may allow early treatment for a potentially devastating problem. Quantitative measurement of a relative afferent pupillary defect is also a measure of decreased retinal sensitivity from ischemia and, as such, seems to correlate well with ERG changes in being able to differentiate ischemic from nonischemic CRVO.[127]

Twenty percent of human eyes have a two-trunked central retinal vein,[126] and either of the two trunks may occlude. When that happens, it appears to behave just like CRVO.[8, 129] In general, there must be ischemia in over at least half of the retina to cause NVI.[129] For that reason, NVG is extremely rare with branch retinal vein occlusion (BRVO)[194] and macular retinal vein occlusion.[129] However, cases of NVG have been reported after BRVO.[190]

There appears to be an association between CRVO and preexisting OAG. This relationship has been confirmed in many studies, and the incidence ranges from 6 to 66 percent.[186] In the largest series published, in-

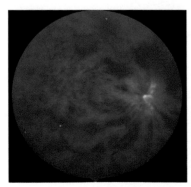

Figure 132–18. Ischemic central retinal vein occlusion.

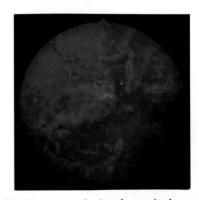

Figure 132–20. Central retinal vein occlusion with extensive intraretinal hemorrhages.

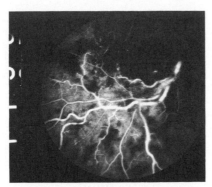

Figure 132–21. Fundus fluorescein angiogram of the eye shown in Figure 132–20. With the extensive intraretinal hemorrhages, it was not possible to determine the extent of retinal ischemia. In such cases, when the retinal hemorrhages clear, the fluorescein angiogram should be repeated.

volving 360 patients with CRVO, there was a 23 percent incidence of primary OAG or ocular hypertension.[129] The association between CRVO and primary OAG seems to be age related, with up to 75 percent of patients older than 65 yr of age with CRVO having concomitant OAG.[283] There may be an explanation for this apparent difference between older and younger patients. In a study of 12 young (average age 29 yr) patients with CRVO, although none had daytime IOP above 21 mmHg, 11 of 12 had diurnal fluctuation greater than 21 mmHg, with some IOPs up to 30 mmHg.[280] In addition, eight patients had a maximum diurnal swing in the IOP greater than 8 mmHg. This study supports the belief that elevated IOPs may play an important role in the cause of CRVO in both young and elderly patients and points out that some cases of OAG, especially in young patients, may be missed if the applanation tension is not taken at different times in the day. However, there is no consensus with regard to whether or not the presence of OAG influences the ultimate development of NVG.[129, 191]

Diabetes Mellitus

Diabetes mellitus is one of the leading causes of blindness in the United States today.[26] In the adult group (approximately 20 to 60 yr of age), it is *the* leading cause of new blindness and is one of the major causes of NVG. Most blindness is due to PDR, with only 5 percent of the blindness being due to NVG.[101] In a thorough epidemiologic study on a Danish island, the prevelance of NVG was 2.1 percent of all diabetics and 21.3 percent of all diabetics with PDR.[214] In the only study to date on the incidence of PDR meeting the current treatment criteria, the estimated annual incidence in the United States is 34,800,[152] resulting in an estimated annual incidence of approximately 7500 cases of NVG from diabetes mellitus in the United States. Despite the 1976 Diabetic Retinopathy Study, which showed the beneficial effects of PRP in preventing severe visual loss, there has not been a significant decrease in the incidence of NVG from diabetes

mellitus;[39, 188] in part, this may be due to the increasing incidence of diabetes.[22]

The association between NVI and diabetes mellitus was first made by Salus in 1928.[247] In 1939, Fehrmann[85] correlated NVI with the presence of retinal neovascularization. Subsequent studies on unselected diabetic populations found that the incidence of NVI ranged from 1[9] to 17 percent.[188] In eyes with PDR, the incidence of NVI goes up to 65 percent.[217] In a histologic study of unselected eyes removed from patients with diabetes mellitus, 95 percent of the eyes were found to have NVI, and of these, 90 percent had retinal neovascularization.[305] It is now well accepted that NVI is associated with retinal hypoxia and PDR.[136] It was shown that the conjunctival oxygen tension in diabetics with PDR is significantly lower than in diabetics with nonproliferative diabetic retinopathy (NPDR), which is significantly lower than in diabetics with no retinopathy.[196]

Clinically, there can be significant retinal hypoxia with very little visible sign of PDR. Fundus fluorescein angiography is often necessary to show capillary nonperfusion. Even then, the posterior pole may appear remarkably benign, and it is imperative to examine the peripheral retina on angioscopy and to take peripheral photographs on the angiograms (Figs. 132–22 and 132–23).

There are two major groups of diabetes mellitus. Type I or insulin-dependent diabetes, previously known as juvenile onset diabetes, comprises approximately 15 percent and type II or noninsulin-dependent diabetes, previously known as maturity or adult-onset diabetes, comprises approximately 80 percent of the total. The remaining 5 percent consists of other types of diabetes, such as secondary diabetes mellitus. Regardless of the type of diabetes, it seems that the major factor in the onset of diabetic retinopathy is the duration of diabetes. In type I diabetes, 10 percent have retinopathy after 10 yr, 50 percent after 15 yr, and 90 percent after 25 years.[45] In type II diabetes, retinopathy seems to occur sooner than in type I diabetes.[211] After 10 yr, up to 50 percent have retinopathy.[45]

Despite the difference in the onset of retinopathy between type I and type II diabetes, studies have shown that these long-term complications are due to the metabolic derangement (hyperglycemia) rather than from

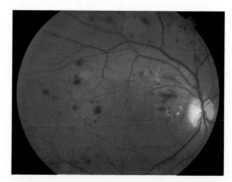

Figure 132–22. A 51-year-old woman with a 10-yr history of type II diabetes mellitus. The fundus shows nonproliferative diabetic retinopathy.

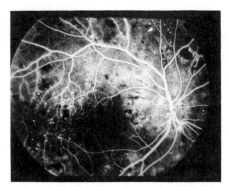

Figure 132–23. Fundus fluorescein angiogram of the eye shown in Figure 132–22, displaying extensive capillary dropout and retinal ischemia that was not apparent on fundoscopy.

genetic differences between these two types of diabetes.[27, 266] It is beyond the scope of this chapter to review the literature on this subject, but it is important to state that diabetologists and ophthalmologists agree that tight metabolic control of diabetes mellitus is important in preventing or delaying the microvascular complications of diabetes[264] and ultimately, therefore, in preventing NVG. The National Institute of Health-sponsored Diabetes Control and Complications Trial (DCCT) is designed to answer this important question.[278]

There is also now convincing evidence that concomitant hypertension in diabetic patients results in greater frequency and greater severity of diabetic retinopathy.[173, 274] Therefore, controlling hypertension is potentially important in the prevention of ocular complications of diabetes mellitus.

After NVG develops in one eye of a diabetic patient, the natural history without treatment is that the fellow eye almost inevitably develops it as well.[216] Bilateral NVI or NVG in an adult is almost always caused by diabetic retinopathy.[105] The time interval between the onset of diabetes mellitus and the development of retinopathy is known, but the time sequence between development of retinopathy and the appearance of NVI is not known. The time interval between the onset of NVI and NVG in untreated cases varies from 1 mo to more than 3 yr.[189] Furthermore, it is unpredictable as to which untreated eyes with NVI will ultimately progress to NVG. There are well-documented cases of spontaneous regression of diabetic retinopathy.[107] In eyes with early changes of microaneurysms and hemorrhages, 45 percent were found to return to retinopathy-free status at least once during regular annual ophthalmic examinations.[210] In up to 26 percent of eyes, NVI may spontaneously disappear in 5 yr.[189] This unpredictable course of NVI and NVG due to diabetic retinopathy makes the evaluation of any prophylactic treatment for NVI and NVG difficult at best.

Postcataract Extraction in Patients with Diabetes Mellitus

Capillary drop-out and retinal hypoxia make the eye with diabetic retinopathy especially vulnerable to further insult. Surgical procedures such as cataract extraction and vitrectomy add considerable risk to the development of NVG in such eyes. NVG has not been reported as a complication in large series of intracapsular cataract extraction (ICCE) in unselected populations.[150] However, diabetic patients who had undergone ICCE in one eye, with the fellow eye serving as the unoperated control, had a significant increase in postoperative NVI-NVG (7.8 percent versus 0 percent).[5] In patients with preoperative PDR, the risks of developing postoperative NVI-NVG was even greater (40 percent versus 0 percent). The preoperative presence of PDR also carries significantly greater risk of developing NVG after vitrectomy.[201, 218] Extracapsular cataract extraction (ECCE) in diabetics does not seem to be associated with an increased incidence of postoperative NVG,[228] but primary capsulotomy at the time of ECCE does seem to predispose them toward the postoperative development of NVG.[228] Thus, it appears that both active PDR as a source of some AF and removal of the diffusion barrier, through ICCE or ECCE with capsulotomy, are necessary predisposing factors toward the development of NVG. There is some question whether the posterior capsule or the anterior hyaloid membrane is the critical diffusion barrier,[290] because if only the lens capsule was the effective barrier, then one would have to assume that the zonules are an effective functional if not anatomic barrier as well. If the hyaloid membrane was the effective barrier, the assumption about the zonules would not be necessary. Regardless, the importance of the posterior capsule-anterior hyaloid barrier was shown in a report of three cases of NVG developing after Nd.YAG laser capsulotomy in diabetic patients.[296] The fundus was not visualized before the capsulotomy in their patients, but when NVG was noted, two had PDR and one had NPDR. Other concomitant causes of retinal ischemia in that case were not noted. In another report, in eight patients with NPDR who developed PDR after ECCE, only two patients developed NVG, and both had a broken posterior capsule that required a vitrectomy.[151] Bovine lens capsule has been shown to produce an inhibitor to endothelial cell proliferation, and it is thought that an intact lens capsule may provide a source of anti-AF besides being a static barrier to aqueous flow.[109, 300] Clearly, the role of the posterior capsule versus the hyaloid has not yet been settled.

The posterior capsule–anterior hyaloid barrier is only relative[151] and can be overwhelmed if there is a great amount of AF; for example, it is common to see NVG in phakic patients with extensive posterior segment ischemia. If this barrier is removed or disrupted, such as with ICCE or ECCE with capsulotomy, enough AF may then diffuse forward to stimulate NVI. Inflammation from cataract surgery or laser capsulotomy may contribute as well. Whenever possible, adequate PRP should be performed in any diabetic patient with early PDR before cataract extraction.[7] When cataract surgery is performed in a diabetic patient or in a patient who has had CRVO, the procedure should be a planned ECCE, with or without a posterior chamber intraocular lens implant. We have not seen NVG develop in diabetic patients who have had adequate PRP prior to cataract surgery. Diabetics and patients who have had CRVO should be followed carefully after cataract surgery so that NVI can be detected early and appropriate treatment can be started.

Postvitrectomy for Complications of Diabetic Retinopathy

Modern pars plana vitrectomy heralded a new era in the treatment of complications of diabetic retinopathy.[187] Initially, concurrent lens surgery was often performed whether or not a cataract was present. It soon became clear that concurrent lensectomy significantly increased the risks of developing postoperative NVI and NVG. Large series of vitrectomies in diabetic patients showed a two-fold[25] to three-fold[238] increased risk of developing NVI if lensectomy was performed; however, not all studies found this association.[1, 58]

Long before the advent of vitrectomy, it had been known that chronic retinal detachment is a significant cause of NVG.[104] Several studies have mentioned the importance of retinal detachment as a cause of postvitrectomy NVI and NVG.[2, 51, 249] However, the often-cited large studies did not consider the role of postoperative retinal detachment as a cause of postvitrectomy NVG.[238] In one study, the records of 255 consecutive vitrectomies were reviewed; 81 of the vitrectomies were performed for complications of diabetic retinopathy and 175 were performed for nondiabetes–related problems that served as controls in the study.[294] Sixty-five different preoperative, intraoperative, and postoperative parameters were statistically analyzed, and only postoperative retinal detachment had a significant correlation with the development of NVI and NVG postvitrectomy. In the diabetic group, 83 percent of the eyes with retinal detachment developed NVI-NVG versus 2 percent of the eyes with an attached retina. For comparison, it was noted that 2 percent of eyes with severe PDR in the Diabetic Retinopathy Vitrectomy Study progressed on to NVG even without vitrectomy.[71] In the control group, 19 percent of the eyes with retinal detachment developed NVI and NVG, versus none of the eyes with attached retinas.[294] Aphakia alone did not correlate significantly with the development of NVI and NVG. However, aphakia combined with retinal detachment was associated with an even greater risk of developing NVI and NVG (92 percent) in the diabetic group.[294] In a series of 15 diabetic patients undergoing combined cataract extraction, posterior chamber intraocular lens implant, and pars plana vitrectomy, the only case of postoperative NVI was in an eye with chronic inoperable retinal detachment.[172]

It is clear that both diabetic retinopathy and retinal detachment are important causes of NVI and NVG, and when both conditions coexist, there is an even greater stimulus for neovascularization. As has been pointed out earlier, the lens-posterior capsule-anterior hyaloid is a relative, but important, diffusion barrier for the anterior passage of the AF.[290, 296] When the stimulus for neovascularization has not been eliminated, such as with reattachment of the retina and adequate PRP, the presence or absence of a barrier against the AF has clinical significance. However, if there is no source of this AF, then the presence or absence of this lens-hyaloid barrier is academic. An attached retina does not mean that the stimulus for neovascularization is not present. Cases have been reported in which NVI was present after vitrectomy, despite an attached retina.[172, 294] With postvitrectomy PRP, there was regression of the NVI.[172, 294] The conclusion is that after vitrectomy for complications of PDR, an attached retina with adequate PRP is of paramount importance in preventing NVG; lensectomy per se is of secondary importance.

Carotid Artery Occlusive Disease (CAOD)

There have been numerous reports on NVG resulting from occlusion of the common carotid, internal carotid, and ophthalmic artery.[3, 64, 265, 303] Despite these reports, it had been believed that CAOD is not a common cause of NVG, because enough collateral circulation usually develops to prevent severe retinal ischemia.[117] We now know that CAOD is the third most common cause of NVG, accounting for at least 13 percent of the cases.[39] This figure may be low because COAD may be an unrecognized component of CRVO and diabetic retinopathy. Demonstrable common or internal carotid artery atherosclerosis is present in up to 37 percent of patients with CRVO.[41] The incidence is 50 percent for the ischemic type of CRVO and 17 percent for the nonischemic type.[41] In one series, 6 of 12 patients who presented with CRVO had CAOD requiring endarterectomy.[183] Forty percent of patients diagnosed with CAOD presented with CRVO in the same study.

NVG actually represents only one manifestation of CAOD. The spectrum ranges from transient ischemic attack,[137] to hypoperfusion retinopathy[130] (previously called venous stasis retinopathy[161]) to ocular ischemic syndrome.[169] It has been proposed that the term chronic ocular ischemia should be used for this confusing array of terms.[267] It has been estimated that evidence of chronic ocular ischemia will be found in 4[166] to 18 percent[162] of patients with CAOD. These patients will usually be seen by an ophthalmologist first, and it is imperative to consider this condition in a patient with NVG.

There are several unique aspects of NVG from CAOD. Decreased perfusion of the ciliary body from CAOD significantly decreases aqueous production.[14, 142, 273] Thus, despite extensive synechial angle-closure, the IOP may be normal or even low (Fig. 132–23).[64, 142, 273] One study found that only one third of the eyes with NVG from CAOD had an elevated IOP.[40] In every case of NVG with low IOP disproportionate to the extent of angle-closure, CAOD must be considered in the absence of retinal detachment.[64] After endarerectomy or carotid bypass surgery, aqueous production often returns to the normal preischemic level. IOP can

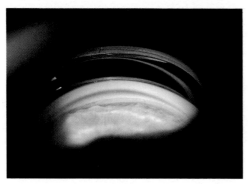

Figure 132–24. A 67-year-old woman, on a routine eye examination, was noted to have a visual acuity of 20/40 and an intraocular pressure of 18 mmHg. Extensive neovascularization of the iris with almost total synechial angle-closure was also noted. Photograph shows the inferior angle that has extensive peripheral anterior synechiae and angle neovascularization; the rest of the angle not shown was closed. She was found to have 80 to 99 percent closure of both internal carotid arteries. After successful carotid endarterectomies on both sides, her intraocular pressure increased to 36 mmHg despite antiglaucoma medications.

increase dramatically, despite the seemingly paradoxic regression of the NVI (Fig. 132–24).[64, 242, 307]

CAOD should also be considered when there is markedly asymmetric diabetic retinopathy, when there is no effect on NVI after adequate PRP, and whenever there is no apparent cause for the NVG. It is beyond the scope of this chapter to review the diagnostic and therapeutic measures for CAOD. Both carotid bypass surgery and endarterectomy have associated, albeit low, morbidity and mortality,[37, 270, 271] and bypass procedures do not increase ocular perfusion as much as endarterectomy.[163] For symptomatic patients, these procedures would seem justifiable because resolution of ocular ischemic findings, including NVG, are well documented.[135, 163, 166, 213] For asymptomatic patients with NVG, carotid surgery is not recommended.

Other vascular disorders such as aortic arch syndrome (Takayasu's syndrome),[30] carotid-cavernous sinus fistula,[268, 298] temporal arteritis,[28, 302] Wyburn-Mason syndrome,[77] congenital atrial vitreous communication of the retina,[68] and postembolization treatment of dural shunts[90] have in common decreased blood flow to the ophthalmic and central retinal artery with secondary retinal-ocular ischemia. In general, occlusive vascular diseases involving the eye are probably underdiagnosed as a primary or aggravating cause of NVG.

Central Retinal Artery Occlusion (CRAO)

The association between NVG and CRAO was first noted in 1874.[185] The incidence has been variously cited as between 1 and 17 percent.[72, 75, 128] If some of these studies are analyzed in greater detail, a more consistent figure emerges. In the largest (171 patients) reported series,[157a] branch retinal artery occlusion (BRAO) and CRAO are included together in the analysis; if only CRAO is considered, the incidence of NVG in that study is 6.8 percent. In another series,[128] 10 of 64 eyes (16 percent) with CRAO developed NVG, but 9 of them had CAOD; 1 of 64 (2 percent) with only CRAO developed NVG. A number of factors suggest that the incidence might be lower than the reported 17 percent.[72] Some of the cases reported may not have been NVG, because the NVI was determined clinically and gonioscopy was not done. Also, some of the reported cases could have had ophthalmic artery obstruction and other cases may have had CAOD.[250] In a prospective study,[75] 5 of 33 (15.2 percent) consecutive patients with CRAO developed NVG. However, two of seven patients who had any ocular neovascularization (five patients with NVG, one patient with NVI only, and one patient with optic disc neovascularization) also had concurrent ipsilateral CAOD. If these two patients with CAOD had NVG, the incidence of NVG after CRAO alone would have been 9 percent. Thus the true incidence of CRAO is probably higher than the previously accepted 2 percent and is lower than the extremely high 17 percent. Without a definitive study, we would estimate that the incidence of NVG due to CRAO alone is between 5 and 10 percent.

With CRAO, there is destruction of the inner retinal layer and capillary endothelium.[235] This explains why there is generally no retinal neovascularization in CRAO. Cases in which there is neovascularization of the disc after CRAO are rare,[31, 73, 144] and the new vessels may come from the choroidal circulation.[144] A more important consideration is that with no viable retinal tissue, the eye should not be capable of inducing a neovascular response elsewhere.[131] If this is so, it is unclear why there is NVI-NVG at all with CRAO. It has been proposed that there is first CAOD, which causes anterior segment ischemia which leads to NVI and secondary NVG.[128] At the same time, the decreased perfusion of the central retinal artery makes it susceptible to occlusion, especially if there is increased IOP from the already existent NVI. In support of this theory, several studies of eyes with CRAO and NVG have found CAOD in 45 percent,[256] 90 percent and 100 percent[40] of these eyes. Thus, rather than CRAO causing NVG, it is believed that more likely NVG from CAOD contributes toward the CRAO.

This is clearly not the only explanation of NVG from CRAO. There are documented cases of NVG that did not have concomitant CAOD.[38, 72, 75] Although some feel that the NVG from CRAO is a different entity from CRVO,[138, 302] the histology is exactly the same. Ultimately, it is believed that retinal ischemia or anterior segment ischemia from CAOD are the causes. The beneficial effect of PRP in NVG from CRAO also support this concept.[74, 282]

INTRAOCULAR TUMOR

Malignant Melanoma

The association between NVG and untreated malignant melanoma was first noted in 1944.[82] The incidence in subsequent studies has ranged from 0.5 to 15 percent.[52, 195, 304] The occurrence of NVI correlates with increased tumor size, tumor necrosis, or extent of overlying retinal detachment.[44, 52, 164] With newer treatment modalities for uveal melanomas, specifically helium ion irradiation[164] and photocoagulation with hematoporphyrin,[184] the incidence of NVI-NVG does not seem to be any lower. Since various forms of irradiation are also known to cause NVI-NVG,[116, 157, 222] it is not possible to determine if the NVI-NVG in these reports were due to the tumor, the irradiation, or the secondary tumor necrosis. In any case, it is clear that the larger the tumor with the greater retinal involvement, the greater will be the chances of developing NVI and NVG. Associated retinal detachment or tumor necrosis, either spontaneous or radiation induced, are certainly contributory factors. All of these factors have in common production of some degree of retinal hypoxia. However, one case report suggests that the production of some AF from an intraocular tumor can also play a significant role in the development of NVG. Shields and Prioa[258] reported a case of uniocular NVG in an eye with a primary epithelioid melanoma of the iris. When the tumor was totally excised, the NVI completely disappeared.

The incidence of NVG with malignant melanoma is not high, and malignant melanoma as a cause of NVG is relatively low on the list of differential diagnosis. Nevertheless, in an eye with NVG in which the posterior segment is not visible due to opaque media, malignant melanoma must be considered, especially in the absence of diabetic retinopathy in the contralateral eye or a past history of CRVO in the ipsilateral eye.

Retinoblastoma

The association between retinoblastoma and glaucoma was first noted in 1965.[141] The incidence of NVI in eyes enucleated for retinoblastoma has been reported to be from 30 to 72 percent.[105, 286, 306] There is a significant association between the presence of NVI and tumor involvement of the choroid[286] and of the posterior pole.[306] In fact, the posterior pole involvement was so consistent that it was possible to predict the presence or absence of NVI by histologic examination of the posterior pole only.[306] It was also found that the duration of retinoblastoma was associated with the development of NVI.[286] In children who present with opaque media and NVI or NVG, one must consider occult retinoblastoma high on the list. Ultrasound, computed tomography (CT) scans, and other appropriate studies must be performed.

Other Tumors

NVI has also been described in eyes with metastatic tumors[88] and reticulum cell sarcoma,[269] and in these cases, the direct effect of tumor-secreted AF may be the cause of the new vessels.[258]

POSTRETINAL DETACHMENT SURGERY

Chronic retinal detachment is a well-known cause of NVG.[105] In one study, retinal detachment was found to be the second most common cause (23 percent) of NVI in a series of 105 enucleated eyes with NVG.[251] In children younger than 5 yr of age, retinal detachment was also found to be the second most common cause (32 percent) of NVI.[286] As previously mentioned, persistent retinal detachment is the major cause of postvitrectomy NVI and NVG.[294] Several conditions thought to cause NVG may, in fact, act through the common pathway of secondary retinal detachment. For example, NVG associated with Coats' disease is often associated with retinal detachment.[61, 251, 286] Other reported causes such as X-linked juvenile retinoschisis[143] and post laser coreoplasty in Marfan's syndrome[53] also had retinal detachment as a common denominator. Retinal detachment must be considered if an obvious cause of NVG cannot be found, because the retina must be reattached, if possible, as the first step in the treatment of NVG.

MISCELLANOUS CAUSES

It no longer seems instructive to compile a long list of conditions found to be associated with NVI. Now that we have a better understanding of the pathophysiology of this condition, we know that there are several common pathways, such as chronic retinal detachment and extensive capillary nonperfusion with resultant retinal hypoxia. In addition to CRVO, sickle cell retinopathy,[29, 103] Stickler's syndrome,[308] the newly reported autosomal dominant neovascular inflammatory vitreoretinopathy,[21] and other as yet unreported retinal diseases produce NVG by the retinal hypoxia pathway. Decreased ocular perfusion, such as with CAOD, is yet another common pathway. For instance, reported cases of optic disc glioma causing NVG probably are due to the enlarging tumor compressing ciliary and retinal vessels with resultant retinal hypoxia.[43] More localized anterior segment perfusion compromise has been shown to be the cause of NVI in Fuchs' heterochromic iridocyclitis[226, 244] and pseudoexfoliation syndrome.[239] There has not been any documented case of NVG from these two entities, perhaps because the vascular occlusion and secondary hypoxia are so limited. The association between scleritis and NVG is also probably due to secondary vascular occlusion.[299] Finally, direct stimulation of iris vessels by intraocular tumor secreted AF is yet another pathway.[258] As more ocular conditions associated with NVG are found, a careful search should be made for chronic diffuse retinal or anterior segment hypoxia, which must be resolved before the secondary glaucoma can be treated properly.

MANAGEMENT

As recently as 1974, no methods were known to prevent or treat NVG.[182, 220] Since 1974, many review articles have appeared on the management of NVG,[23, 46, 243, 295] but preventive treatment has received little attention.[46, 289]

Prophylactic Treatment

Over 4500 yr ago, Huang Ti said "the superior physician helps before the early budding of the disease . . . the inferior physician begins to help when the disease has already developed." Nowhere else in ophthalmology is this more valid than with NVG.

With CRVO, all patients should have a fluorescein angiogram. If it is of the ischemic type, PRP should be performed as soon as possible. If there are retinal hemorrhages preventing photocoagulation, the patient should be followed carefully and treated as soon as the hemorrhages are clear. Nonischemic CRVO should also be followed carefully, because they can become ischemic. Without PRP, approximately 40 percent of the ischemic type of CRVO proceed on to NVG.[129] In several early studies involving small numbers of patients with xenon photocoagulation, none of the patients with CRVO treated with PRP developed NVG.[170, 198] The untreated control patients developed NVG at the expected incidence. Similar results were noted in a small study using the argon and xenon coagulator.[140] The largest, and most convincing, study to date is a series of 100 eyes with ischemic type CRVO.[192] All eyes received early argon PRP, and none developed NVG. In general, the visual outcome is unchanged whether or not PRP is performed, since the visual acuity has been determined by the primary vascular accident.[170] However, the majority of the treated patients show some improvement in the visual acuity.[241] OAG should also be well controlled, especially in the higher risk elderly patients. Since there is frequently a low IOP in eyes after a CRVO, all eyes with CRVO should be considered suspect and should be followed accordingly.

For NVG to develop in diabetes mellitus, there must be retinal hypoxia associated with PDR.[136] It has been well documented that the major factor in the onset of PDR is the duration of the diabetes mellitus.[45, 211] Although definitive evidence is still lacking, there is evidence to suggest that near-normal glycemia is associated with later development and lesser severity of diabetic retinopathy.[227, 274] Thus, the achievement of euglycemia is an important preventative measure. Once diabetic retinopathy is present, many studies have shown the beneficial effects of PRP on causing regression of NVI.[149] It has been shown that PRP in diabetic patients prevents the later development of NVI, angle neovascularization, and NVG.[292] Perhaps the most important prophylactic treatment for NVG in diabetics is regular ophthalmic examinations. The National Diabetes Advisory Board recommends that all newly diagnosed patients with type II diabetes and all patients with type I diabetes lasting for longer than 5 yr should have an annual examination done by an ophthalmologist.[212]

Several new medications offer hope for the successful prevention of diabetic retinopathy. When these medi-

cations become available, there will be a true prophylactic treatment for NVI-NVG from diabetic retinopathy.

Prophylactic therapy in CAOD is not aimed at preventing NVI since this is generally not possible, but rather at considering this diagnosis as a cause of NVG. CAOD should always be considered if there is asymmetric severity of diabetic retinopathy between two eyes, in any case of NVG in which the IOP is normal or subnormal, in which adequate PRP has not caused regression of the NVI, or when there is no other apparent cause. If unsuspected CAOD is detected, and appropriate therapy is instituted, potential stroke or death could be averted.

Since NVG has been reported to occur anywhere from 1 wk to 5 mo after CRAO,[75, 128] patients with CRAO should be followed carefully for at least 6 mo and PRP should be instituted when NVI is first noted.

Frequently, the causes of NVG may be multifactorial, including diabetes mellitus, hypertension, CAOD, and CRVO or some combination thereof. Control of hypertension, blood sugar, and cholesterol levels as well as a strong clinical suspicion for occult CAOD are the best prophylaxis for the patient against NVG.

Therapeutic: Early Stage

In the therapy of NVG, the critical aspect is early detection of NVI. Thus, every patient with diabetes, regardless of duration, as well as every patient who has had a CRVO or a CRAO should have a careful slit-lamp examination of the iris, especially the pupillary margin. Once NVI is discovered, and there is little or no angle involvement, the mainstay in early therapy is PRP.

How PRP produces its beneficial effects remains unclear. For the different theories on how photocoagulation might work, see *Principles and Practice of Ophthalmology: Basic Sciences*, Chapter 117. Since retinal ischemia is critical to the development of NVI, PRP must somehow eliminate the source or antagonize the effects of the AFs. The effectiveness of various lasers is more dependent on the amount of retina treated than on the type of laser employed.[132] This is in agreement with studies that have shown that other forms of retinal destruction such as xenon arc photocoagulation,[70] retinal diathermy,[9] and retinal cryotherapy[36, 197] also have beneficial effects on preventing and causing regression of NVI.

In practice, the most common cause of "failed" PRP is inadequate photocoagulation. It is estimated that during standard PRP, only 13 percent of the total retinal area is treated.[215a] According to the guidelines of the Diabetic Retinopathy Study, a total of 1200 to 1600 500-μ burns should be applied randomly over the peripheral retina.[70] However, more than this number of photocoagulation burns may be necessary to effect regression of neovascularization.[263a] The most recent DRS report shows that eyes that had more PRP had less risk of visual loss than did eyes with less PRP.[158] Twelve hundred spots represents less than one-quarter of the total confluent 500-μ spots that can be placed on the average extramacular retinal area of a human eye.[16] Many retinal specialists believe that a minimum of 1500 to 2000 spots using the Rodenstock wide-angle fundus contact lens is necessary to constitute adequate PRP. The Rodenstock lens produces an 670-μ size retinal lesion,[236] thus a correspondingly greater number of lesions need to be produced if the Goldmann lens (500-μ retinal spot) is employed (Fig. 132–25). If there is some opacity in the media, or if there are retinal hemorrhages present, the krypton laser is frequently more effective than argon laser treatment.

When adequate PRP is performed early in the course of NVI, there is ample documentation that there is regression of the NVI in CRVO[47] and PDR.[149, 159] PRP has also been shown to cause regression of NVI and appears to reduce the incidence of NVG after CRAO.[74] However, the results of PRP in CRAO are not nearly as impressive as in CRVO or PDR.[75] In eyes with radiation-induced ocular ischemia, PRP decreased the risk of developing NVG 6.4 times compared with similar eyes not receiving PRP.[12] Even with CAOD, in which the hypoxia may not be limited to the retina alone, PRP can still produce a diminution of NVI until more definitive therapy can be instituted.[54, 79] Thus, PRP is the most important early treatment for NVI and NVG. Obviously, if the cause is a detached retina or an ocular tumor, the therapy must be directed at the primary causes.

ENDOPHOTOCOAGULATION

There are situations in which it is not possible to perform preoperative PRP in an eye with NVI, and intraocular surgery (e.g., cataract extraction or vitrectomy) must be performed. Increased postoperative risks of developing NVG in such a situation have already been noted, and postoperative vitreous hemorrhages could prevent any postoperative photocoagulation. Argon endophotocoagulation is an effective method to perform intraoperative PRP.[92] Recently, a method for performing endophotocoagulation with indirect ophthalmoscopy has been described; this technique allows better visualization of the fundus.[121] Endophotocoagulation can be just as effective as standard photocoagulation, and this procedure is now used extensively, especially during vitrectomy.[42, 56, 155a, 200] In high-risk eyes, endophotocoagulation is valuable in providing a "head-start" on retinal photocoagulation. In many cases, further photocoagulation needs to be performed via the slit lamp at a later time.[289]

PANRETINAL CRYOTHERAPY

In cases in which the cornea, lens, or vitreous is too hazy to allow adequate PRP, there is a role for panretinal cryotherapy (PRC).[36, 197, 209, 220] A 360-degree peritomy is performed with isolation of the four rectus muscles.[36, 197] A 2.5 mm retinal cryoprobe is used, with the first row of application just anterior to the equator, three spots between each rectus muscle. Two additional rows of cryoapplications are placed posteriorly so that the third row is just outside the major vascular arcades. A total of 32 to 54 applications are commonly employed.[36, 197] This is done under direct visualization, and the tip is in contact with the sclera until $-70°C$ is achieved, approximately 5 to 10 sec, depending on the probe. If 40 cryo spots are applied, it has been estimated that 39 percent of the available retina would be treated[285] which would be significantly more area than with the average PRP.[16]

In the largest series to date, 27 eyes with NVG (nine of which had previous PRP) were treated, and 55 percent had stabilization or improvement of vision, 55 percent had reduction of IOP, and 70 percent had stabilization or regression of NVI after 12 mo.[36] As might be expected, cryopexy over an area of retinal detachment has no effect since the retina is not affected by the freezing. This is a major operation that produces significantly more inflammation and blood-retinal barrier breakdown than PRP, as shown by vitreous fluorophotometry.[147] Potential complications include traction and exudative retinal detachment and vitreous hemorrhage.[36, 285] However, PRC seems to have an added, although as yet unexplained, benefit of facilitating the clearance of existing vitreous blood.[209, 220, 253, 285] Increased influx of macrophages after PRC may be an explanation.[299a]

GONIOPHOTOCOAGULATION

Direct laser treatment of NVI before development of NVG has been investigated by several researchers with mixed results.[67, 262] A 73 percent overall success rate as defined by elimination of angle vessels in the treated area, prevention of further angle-closure in the treated area, and maintenance of IOP below 25 mmHg was reported by Simmons and associates.[262] However, 38 percent of their eyes also had concurrent PRP or PRC, and there was no breakdown of the success rate with and without this adjuvant therapy. The natural history of untreated diabetic retinopathy is rather unpredictable, and spontaneous arrest and even regression of NVI of up to one third of the eyes is well known.[107, 189] One study evaluated preoperative goniophotocoagulation on

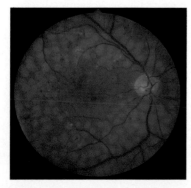

Figure 132–25. Example of adequate panretinal photocoagulation. Note the almost confluent areas of photocoagulation spots. A total of 1500 to 2000 spots should be applied if using the Rodenstock lens (800-μ spot size); if the Goldmann lens (500-μ spot size) is used, proportionately more spots should be applied.

the success of filtration surgery but found no beneficial effect.[6]

When goniophotocoagulation was first introduced in 1977, the role and efficacy of PRP in the treatment of NVG was still being evaluated. It was believed that there might be cases in which goniophotocoagulation might provide "a period of grace to delay imminent synechial angle-closure until the definitive effect of the PRP can manifest itself".[289] However, since then, in a limited number of patients in whom it was not possible to perform PRP, goniophotocoagulation alone has not proved to be beneficial in preventing synechial angle-closure and, at times, have caused increased inflammation and seemingly more rapid progression of angle neovascularization. At this stage, until a prospective randomized study is performed, the role of goniophotocoagulation in the treatment of NVG remains unclear.

MEDICAL THERAPY

Before synechial angle-closure has occurred, it is possible to have a secondary OAG from the fibrovascular membrane accompanying the angle vessels blocking the trabecular meshwork. Concomitant OAG may be present as well, especially in a patient with CRVO or diabetic retinopathy. Under these circumstances, all of the standard antiglaucoma medications (including miotics or adrenergic agents) will be effective to some degree in lowering the IOP, but one should not be lulled into a false sense of security with medical control. Unless PRP is performed, the angle can relentlessly close. Although there is no scientific evidence, clinically, the two medications that are of the greatest use during this period are topical atropine 1 percent twice per day to decrease ocular congestion[288] and topical steroids four times per day to decrease ocular inflammation.[288]

Therapeutic: Late Stage

PANRETINAL PHOTOCOAGULATION

When synechial angle-closure has already occurred, this is considered the late stage. If at all possible, PRP or PRC should still be performed to eliminate the stimulus for new vessel formation. Synechial angle-closure cannot be reversed with PRP, but further closure can be prevented. Regression of NVI can occur within days of completed PRP. Without elimination of the stimulus for new vessel formation, filtration surgery is more likely to fail. Once PRP has been completed, it is important to allow adequate time to elapse to permit regression of the NVI. At least 1 wk, and preferably 3 to 4 wk, should elapse between completed PRP and filtration surgery. Generally, eyes with NVG in the absence of concomitant OAG do not have as compromised optic nerve heads as in advanced chronic OAG and can tolerate pressures below 50 mmHg for this time span.[293] If possible, adequate disc perfusion should be confirmed by observing for the absence of central retinal artery pulsation.[293]

MEDICAL THERAPY

With extensive synechial angle-closure, any of the medication acting on aqueous outflow (e.g., pilocarpine, phospholine iodide, or adrenergic agents) are useless, and, in fact, contraindicated because they increase hyperemia and inflammation. Medications that decrease aqueous production, such as topical β-blockers and carbonic anhydrase inhibitors, are beneficial but do not lower the IOP to a normal range in the face of a closed angle. Topical apraclonidine, an α-adrenergic agonist, may be used on a short-term basis (days to weeks), but the effectiveness of long-term use has not yet been reported. Osmotic agents can be used intermittently to clear the cornea enough for treatment or diagnosis. The most important medications remain topical atropine and topical steroids to decrease congestion and inflammation and prepare the eye for definitive surgery.

CONVENTIONAL SURGERY

If there are engorged iris vessels at the time of surgery, intraoperative and postoperative hemorrhages are likely to occur. In addition, the presence of active neovascularization leads to late bleb failure through conjunctival scarring at the filtration site. Previously, the main thrust of surgery was to control intraoperative bleeding through different types of cautery or lasers[291] or even to completely bypass the whole anterior segment with a pars plana filtration technique.[263] To prevent postoperative scarring of the filtration bleb, β-irradiation[48] and subconjunctival injection of 5-fluorouracil (5-FU)[240, 279] have been tried. There have been many other interesting and even novel surgical techniques, but the number of cases involved are small and the follow-up has been too short to provide any meaningful information. These reports have been reviewed[117, 288] and are of historical interest only. It is well accepted now that whatever the surgical procedure, preoperative PRP or PRC should be performed whenever possible.[6, 91, 175, 207]

FILTRATION TECHNIQUE

After adequate PRP, topical atropine, and steroids, and enough time for the eye to quiet down, the patient is ready for surgery. If the IOP is very high, osmotic agents may be used preoperatively (if the general medical status permits) to avoid sudden surgical decompression of a hard eye. Retrobulbar anesthesia with epinephrine plus orbital massage is preferred to soften the eye further and to reduce vascular congestion. For the different surgical techniques, see Chapter 143.

A full-thickness procedure (e.g., a trephine or posterior lip sclerectomy) or a guarded procedure (e.g., a trabeculectomy) may be performed, depending on the surgeon's choice. The results appear to be the same regardless of which procedure is used.[6] When the peripheral iridectomy is performed, if some new vessels remain on the iris, preiridectomy cautery to the iris is possible when the iris is lifted by the forceps. Not infrequently, even with this precaution, some bleeding occurs with the iris surgery. Irrigation of the anterior chamber with balanced saline solution via the previously made paracentesis incision usually keeps the anterior chamber clear until the bleeding stops spontaneously. Occasionally, topical epinephrine may be necessary, but postiridectomy cautery to the iris or ciliary body should be avoided. Topical steroids and antibiotics are applied, and a single eye patch and protective shield are placed over the eye. Postoperative medications include topical atropine two to three times per day, topical steroids four to six times per day, and topical antibiotics four times per day. Using standard filtration techniques with preoperative PRP, surgical success (IOP less than 25 mmHg on one medication or less[6]) has been reported as 67 percent,[6] 77 percent,[87] and 100 percent.[59] With 5-FU, surgical success has been reported as 68 percent.[240] In this study, the role of preoperative PRP was not stated, but the authors had the "impression that appropriate PRP increased the chance of successful filter in eyes with NVG."[240]

Postoperatively, the filtration bleb tends to be more limited in size, appears less succulent, and often has a characteristic ring of conjunctival and episcleral vessels that delineate the base of the bleb (Fig. 132–26).[293] Since PRP would not be expected to ablate all of the ischemic retina, it is logical that some AFs would still be present. The base of the filtration bleb is probably the new main interface between the aqueous-borne AFs and the potential vascular bed. The IOP in successful filtration with NVG tends to be somewhat higher than with OAG, but since the optic nerve is usually not as compromised in NVG, a slightly higher postoperative IOP is often tolerable.

Valve Implant Surgery

Filtration surgery in NVG should be reserved for eyes that have useful vision, bearing in mind that almost any vision is worth preserving in eyes with PDR. Because one of the major problems with filtration surgery in NVG is failure of the filtration bleb through episcleral scarring, some physical means to maintain an opening between the anterior chamber and the subconjunctival space has formed the basis for various seton surgical techniques. Countless different materials have been tried, including many kinds of sutures, metals, and plastics in various sheet, tube, or wire forms. None of them worked very well, and their history has been

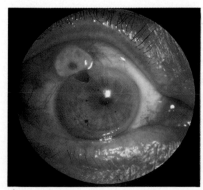

Figure 132–26. Even with adequate panretinal photocoagulation, some angiogenesis factor(s) may still present in the eye. With successful filtration surgery, there is often a ring of injected episcleral vessels around the base of the filtration bleb.

reviewed.[288] With the development of newer nonallergenic plastics, and the knowledge on how previous stents and valves have failed, a new group of implants have been developed for use with NVG and other refractory glaucomas. When conventional surgery fails or is not possible because of excessive conjunctival scarring, some type of valve implant surgery may be indicated. The different types of setons currently available and the actual surgical techniques are described in Chapter 146.

The number of patients involved in some of the studies involving eyes with NVG are too small to adequately evaluate. In 59 eyes using a simple silicone tube, there was a reported 63 percent success in controlling IOP (< 25 mmHg).[138a] With the Molteno implant, there was an 83 percent success in controlling the IOP (< 20 mmHg) in 24 eyes with NVG.[207] In another series using the single plate Molteno technique, there was 47 percent success rate in 15 eyes of patients with NVG.[205] Eleven of these eyes had preoperative PRP, but the success rate was not broken down by this adjuvant therapy. Of significance is that 9 of the 15 eyes (60 percent) had some type of severe complication, including choroidal hemorrhage (two eyes), phthisis or hypotony (two eyes), and traction retinal detachment (one eye).[205] The largest reported series of valve implant surgery utilizes the Krupin-Denver valve.[175] To date, 79 eyes with NVG have been operated on with 67 percent success in controlling IOP (< 24 mmHg), with a mean follow-up of 23 mo. This success rate was exactly the same as that reported in another study utilizing the Krupin-Denver valve in nine eyes with NVG.[99] With the new Krupin valve and scleral exoplant, there is a reported success (< 20 mmHg) in 30 of 39 eyes (77 percent); all eyes had preoperative PRP (37 eyes) or PRC (two eyes).[177]

The problems with all these stent and valve procedures remain the same: early postoperative hypotony, blockage of the internal fistula, and blockage of the external filtration site. Postoperative hypotony, flat anterior chamber, and all its attendant complications are problems common to all filtration procedures. Modifications of the Molteno technique using two stages[207] or suture intubation of the silicone tube[78] and the Krupin valve are methods of avoiding early postoperative hypotony, but unfortunately, are not uniformly successful. Obstruction of the internal fistula is unique to the usage of a drainage device and is especially frequent in NVG, in which intraocular blood and fibrovascular membranes can block the opening of the tube.[177, 205] When the blockage is at the tube opening, a combination of the argon and Nd.YAG lasers can be used to pull and cut the iris or membrane away from the opening. One report noted an intense foreign body-giant cell reaction around the Supramed portion of the Krupin-Denver valve and raises the question of tolerance to these intraocular devices.[93] The problem of conjunctival scarring is also common to all filtration procedures. In human[272] and animal[120] studies, fibrosis of the outflow system was the main course of filtration failure.

ANTIFIBROTIC AGENTS

There is greater promise at the moment in the employment of 5-FU, which is an antimetabolite and which, through its antifibroblastic activities, seems to decrease the incidence of bleb failures.[134] Subconjunctival injections of 5-FU seem to be less toxic than topical administration.[133] Employing subconjunctival 5-FU, there is a reported 2-yr success rate of 62 percent in 29 eyes with NVG. The real key in the ultimate success of filtration surgery in NVG is the prevention of filtration bleb scarring. Whether preoperative elimination of the angiogenesis (and fibroblastic) factors through PRP, the postoperative use of antifibroblastic agents, or the use of various mechanical devices is the answer to successful filtration remains to be seen. Only prospective studies comparing these different methods will give us the answer. Until we know, the primary thrust of surgical intervention in NVG must begin with adequate PRP or PRC.

END-STAGE NEOVASCULAR GLAUCOMA

When there is total synechial angle-closure and there is no useful vision remaining, there is no indication for surgical intervention, and control of pain becomes the primary therapeutic aim.

Medical Treatment

Most often, the combination of topical atropine 1 percent twice a day, and topical steroids four times a day, provides enough symptomatic relief, despite IOPs as high as 60 mmHg, that no other treatment is necessary. When there is corneal microcystic edema, the combination of these drops with a bandage soft contact lens is frequently effective.

Ciliodestructive Procedures

CYCLOCRYOTHERAPY

When medical therapy does not provide symptomatic relief in end-stage NVG, one of the ciliodestructive procedures should be considered. Cyclocryotherapy (CCT) produces its hypotensive effect by destruction of the secretory ciliary epithelium.[232] The first patients with NVG treated with CCT was in 1972.[115] All three eyes had transient (months) lowering of the IOP, aggravation of the NVI, and relief of ocular pain. The relief of pain is one of the major benefits of CCT and may occur despite persistent corneal edema and high intraocular pressures.[29, 117] In the first large series of CCT on eyes with NVG, there was a 63 percent success in 38 eyes in controlling the IOP, but almost 40 percent had posttreatment hypotony.[86] This high complication rate was confirmed in another large series in which 34 percent achieved IOP 25 mmHg or less, but 34 percent developed phthisis and 57 percent lost all light perception.[176] These studies employed either 360 degrees of CCT or nonstandardized techniques. When a standardized treatment protocol was introduced in 1973,[18] sensible comparison of data between studies became possible. With this standardized protocol, only 180 percent of the ciliary

body is treated at one time, employing six spots of freezing, 2.5 mm posterior to the limbus. The 3.5-mm probe is allowed to reach −60 to −80°C and is left in place for 1 min each. Employing this technique, 45 percent of 43 eyes with NVG had good IOP control, but 33 percent lost all light perception and another 25 percent had a significant decrease in vision.[17] Thus, the complication is lower with this technique but is still unacceptably high. In addition, there has been a report of sympathetic ophthalmia following CCT.[245] At this time, we believe that CCT should be reserved for the final effort in the treatment of NVG. If saving functional vision is not a factor, and relief of pain is the main consideration, CCT is a useful technique.

CYCLODIATHERMY

Cyclodiathermy has been tried in several small series and in one large series of 100 eyes.[287] The success rate (< 25 mmHg) matched the phthisis rate: 5 percent, an unacceptable benefit:complication ratio. More recently, diathermy under direct visualization of the ciliary body through scleral flap dissection has been tried.[237] Unfortunately, the benefit:complication ratio is not any better. At this stage, cyclodiathermy appears to be more destructive than CCT without offering any real advantages.

DIRECT LASER CYCLOPHOTOCOAGULATION

There are a number of advantages to a ciliodestructive procedure performed under direct visualization. There is better control and titration of the ciliary processes destroyed, retreatment can be directed at the functional ciliary processes, and the trabecular meshwork is not damaged. This procedure can be done transpupil[206] or with endoscopy.[257] By the former approach, the cornea must be clear, the pupil must be markedly dilated from ectropion uveae, or a large sector iridectomy is already present so that the ciliary processes are visible with a goniolens. Even then, only the anterior aspect of the ciliary processes are accessible to treatment, and this is often not enough to control the IOP. The argon laser settings are 100 μ, 0.1 sec, and approximately 500 to 1000 mW to produce confluent whitening of all visible ciliary processes. There has been transient success in lowering the IOP, but the numbers are too small to report. The endoscopic approach has the disadvantages of requiring an aphakic eye, and a vitrectomy has to be performed with all the potential complications of an invasive procedure. The reported cases are very few in number[24, 224] but seem encouraging to date. At the present time, the role of direct cyclophotocoagulation is secondary and could be tried if other procedures fail.

ND-YAG LASER TRANSCLERAL CYCLOPHOTOCOAGULATION (TSCP)

Two types of thermal mode Nd-YAG lasers are available for TSCP: noncontact[83, 122] and contact.[7, 252] With the noncontact system, a slit lamp is used to deliver their energy. In a report of 100 cases, 27 of whom had NVG, the success in controlling the IOP was only 15 percent for the eyes with NVG.[122] More important, they found less elevation of the IOP in the immediate post-treatment period and less inflammation and pain than after CCT. A case of sympathetic ophthalmia has been reported after noncontact Nd.YAG TSCP. This particular case had had two failed trabeculectomies, but the temporal sequence was consistent with the laser treatment as the inciting event.[76]

With the contact system, there is a report of 140 eyes treated, 45 of whom had NVG.[252] An IOP less than 19 mmHg was achieved in 40 percent of the eyes with NVG. It was also noted that 50 percent of the serious complications were in eyes with NVG, including one eye with phthisis and one with traction retinal detachment.

OTHER CYCLODESTRUCTIVE PROCEDURES

High intensity ultrasound[261] and intraocular carbon dioxide photocoagulation[204] have been used to destroy the ciliary processes as well. The success and complications for ultrasound have been similar to CCT.[261] There has not been a prospective randomized controlled study comparing the different ciliodestructive procedures. It is our belief that all of these should be reserved for the last attempt in saving an eye. However, in the limited experience with contact Nd.YAG TSCP, the eye is remarkably quiet and comfortable after the treatment compared with CCT. Until shown otherwise, this seems to be the ciliodestructive treatment of choice for NVG at the present time.

Pituitary Ablation

For historical interests only, pituitary ablation as a treatment for diabetic retinopathy should also be mentioned. In 1953, there was a report of regression of diabetic retinopathy in a woman who developed postpartum pituitary necrosis.[229] However, this patient had only background diabetic retinopathy, which is known to frequently undergo spontaneous regression.[107, 189] Based on this one case report, numerous studies have been published,[291] but all had been faulted with being uncontrolled or having too few patients to achieve statistical significance.[101] Pituitary ablation is a destructive procedure with high morbidity and mortality and without clear-cut evidence that it is beneficial: it should be relegated to the realms of medical history.

Alcohol Injection

We have not found any case in which pain could not be controlled with a combination of topical atropine and steroid or, infrequently, a cyclodestructive procedure. However, others have used retrobulbar alcohol injection with long-lasting relief of pain.[202] The major complications are temporary blepharoptosis or external ophthalmoplegia.[219] Rarely, enucleation may have to be performed for intractable pain.

REFERENCES

1. Aaberg TM: Pars plana vitrectomy for diabetic traction retinal detachment. Am Acad Ophthalmol 88:639, 1981.
2. Aaberg TM, Van Horn DL: Late complications of pars plana vitreous surgery. Ophthalmology 85:126, 1978.
3. Abedin S, Simmons RJ: Neovascular glaucoma in systemic occlusive vascular disease. Ann Ophthalmol 14:284, 1982.
4. Aiello LM, Beetham WP, Balodimos MC, et al: Ruby laser photocoagulation and treatment of diabetic proliferating retinopathy. In Goldberg MF, Fine SL (eds): Symposium On The Treatment Of Diabetic Retinopathy, Pub. No. 1890. Washington, DC, U.S. Public Health Service, 1969, pp 437–463.
5. Aiello LM, Wand M, Liang G: Neovascular glaucoma and vitreous hemorrhage following cataract surgery in patients with diabetes mellitus. Ophthalmology 90:814, 1983.
6. Allen RC, Bellows AR, Hutchinson BT, et al: Filtration surgery in the treatment of neovascular glaucoma. Ophthalmology 89:1181, 1982.
7. Allingham RR, de Kater AW, Bellows AR, et al: Probe placement and power levels in contact transscleral neodymium YAG cyclophotocoagulation. Arch Ophthalmol 108:738, 1990.
8. Appiah AP, Trempe CL: Differences in contributory factors among hemicentral, central, and branch retinal vein occlusions. Ophthalmology 96:365, 1989.
9. Armaly MF, Baloglou PJ: Diabetes and the eye. I: Changes in the anterior segment. Arch Ophthalmol 77:485, 1967.
10. Ashton N: Retinal vascularization in health and disease. Am J Ophthalmol 44:7, 1957.
11. Ashton N, Ward B, Serpell G: Effect of oxygen on developing retinal vessels with particular reference to the problem of retolental fibroplasia. Br J Ophthalmol 38:397, 1954.
12. Augsburger JJ, Magargal LE, Roth SE, et al: Panretinal photocoagulation for radiation-induced ocular ischemia. Ophthalmic Surg 18:589, 1987.
13. Bagessen LH: Fluorescein angiography of the iris in diabetics and nondiabetics. Acta Ophthalmol 47:449, 1969.
14. Barany E: Influence of local arterial blood pressure on aqueous humor and intraocular pressure. Acta Ophthalmol 24:337, 1946.
15. Barber C, Galloway NR, Reacher M, et al: The role of the electroretinogram in the management of central retinal vein occlusion. Doc Ophthalmol Proc Ser 40:149, 1984.
16. Barr CC: Estimation of the maximum number of argon laser burns possible in panretinal photocoagulation. Am J Ophthalmol 97:697, 1984.
17. Bellows AR: Cyclocryotherapy for glaucoma. Int Ophthalmol Clin 21:99, 1981.
18. Bellows AR, Grant WM: Cyclocryotherapy in advanced inadequately controlled glaucoma. Am J Ophthalmol 75:679, 1973.
19. Ben Ezra D: Neovasculogenic ability of prostaglandins, growth factors, and synthetic chemoattractants. Am J Ophthalmol 86:455, 1978.
20. Ben Ezra D: Neovasculogenesis: Triggering factors and possible mechanisms. Surv Ophthalmol 24:167, 1979.
21. Bennett SR, Folk JC, Kimura AE, et al: Autosomal dominant neovascular inflammatory vitreoretinopathy. Ophthalmology 97:1125, 1990.
22. Benson WE, Brown GC, Tasman W: Diabetic retinopathy: Demography. In Benson WE, Brown GC, Tasman W (eds): Diabetes and its Ocular Complications. Philadelphia, WB Saunders, 1988, pp 1–5.
23. Blach RK, Hitchings RA, Laatikainen L: Thrombitic glaucoma: Prophylaxis and management. Trans Ophthalmol Soc UK 97:275, 1977.
24. Blacharski PA, Charles S: Endocyclophotocoagulation. Ophthalmic Laser Surg 2:13, 1987.
25. Blankenship G, Cortez R, Machemer R: The lens and pars plana vitrectomy for diabetic retinopathy complications. Arch Ophthalmol 97:1263, 1979.
26. Blankenship GW, Skyler JS: Diabetic retinopathy: A general survey. Diabetes Care 1:127, 1978.
27. Bloodworth JMB Jr, Engerman RL: Diabetic microangiopathy in the experimentally-diabetic dog and its prevention by careful control with insulin. Diabetes 22:290, 1973.
28. Boberg-Ans J, Vesti Nielsen N: Neovascular glaucoma as the primary ocular complication in temporal arteritis. Glaucoma 8:138, 1986.
29. Boniuk M: Cryotherapy in neovascular glaucoma. Trans Am Acad Ophthalmol Otolaryngol 78:337, 1974.

30. Bouzas MA: Les manifestations oculaires de la maladie de Takayasu avant et après l'opération. Bull Soc Ophthalmol Fr 69:560, 1969.

31. Bovino JA, Marcus DF, Nelsen PT: Optic disk neovascularization and rubeosis iridis after surgical resection of the optic nerve. Am J Ophthalmol 106:231, 1988.

32. Branch Vein Occlusion Study Group: Argon laser scatter photocoagulation for prevention of neovascularization and vitreous hemorrhage in branch vein occlusion. Arch Ophthalmol 104:34, 1986.

33. Brem S, Preis I, Langer R, et al: Inhibition of neovascularization by an extract derived from vitreous. Am J Ophthalmol 84:323, 1977.

34. Bresnick GH: Following up patients with central retinal vein occlusion. Arch Ophthalmol 106:324, 1988.

35. Breton ME, Quinn GE, Keene SS, et al: Electroretinogram parameters at presentation as predictors of rubeosis in central retinal vein occlusion patients. Ophthalmology 96:1343, 1989.

36. Brodell LP, Olk RJ, Arribas NP, et al: Neovascular glaucoma: A retrospective analysis of treatment with peripheral panretinal cryotherapy. Ophthalmic Surg 18:200, 1987.

37. Brott TG, Labutta RJ, Kempczinski RF: Changing patterns in the practice of carotid endarterectomy in a large metropolitan area. JAMA 255:2609, 1986.

38. Brown GC: Isolated central retinal artery obstruction in association with ocular neovascularization. Am J Ophthalmol 96:110, 1983.

39. Brown GC, Magargal LE, Schachat A, et al: Neovascular glaucoma: Etiologic considerations. Ophthalmology 91:315, 1984.

40. Brown GC, Magargal LE, Simeone FA, et al: Arterial obstruction and ocular neovascularization. Ophthalmology 89:139, 1982.

41. Brown GC, Shah HG, Magargal LE, et al: Central retinal vein obstruction and carotid artery disease. Ophthalmology 91:1627, 1984.

42. Brucker AJ, Hoffman ME, Neuyas HJ, et al: New instrumentation for fluid-air exchange. Retina 3:135, 1983.

43. Buchanan TAS, Hoyt WF: Optic nerve glioma and neovascular glaucoma: Report of a case. Br J Ophthalmol 66:96, 1982.

44. Bujara K: Necrotic malignant melanomas of the choroid and ciliary body: A clinicopathological and statistical study. Graefes Arch Clin Exp Ophthalmol 291:40, 1982.

45. Caird RI, Pirie A, Ramsell TG: Diabetes And The Eye. Oxford, England, Blackwell Scientific Publications, 1968, p 76.

46. Cairns JE: Rationale for therapy in neovascular glaucoma. Trans Ophthalmol Soc UK 101:184, 1981.

47. Callahan MA, Hilton GF: Photocoagulation and rubeosis iridis. Am J Ophthalmol 78:873, 1974.

48. Cameron ME: Thrombotic glaucoma successfully treated. Trans Ophthalmol Soc UK 93:537, 1973.

49. Campbell DG, Simmons RJ, Grant WM: Ghost cells as a cause of glaucoma. Am J Ophthalmol 81:441, 1976.

50. Campbell DG, Shields MB, Smith TR: The corneal endothelium and the spectrum of essential iris atrophy. Am J Ophthalmol 86:317, 1978.

51. Canny CLB, O'Hanley GP, Wells GA: Pars plana vitrectomy for the complications of diabetic retinopathy: A report on 131 cases. Can J Ophthalmol 20:11, 1985.

52. Cappin JM: Malignant melanoma and rubeosis iridis. Br J Ophthalmol 57:815, 1973.

53. Carroll RP, Landers MB: Pinwheel rubeosis iridis following argon laser coreoplasty. Ann Ophthalmol 7:357, 1975.

54. Carter JE: Panretinal photocoagulation for progressive ocular neovascularization secondary to occlusion of the common carotid artery. Ann Ophthalmol 16:572, 1984.

55. Chandler PA, Grant WM: Lectures On Glaucoma. Philadelphia, Lea & Febiger, 1965, p 268.

56. Charles S, Wang C: A motorized gas injector for vitreous surgery. Arch Ophthalmol 99:1398, 1981.

57. Chen CH, Chen SC: Angiogenic activity of vitreous and retinal extract. Invest Ophthalmol Vis Sci 19:596, 1980.

58. Chu KM, Chen TT, Lee PY: Clinical results of pars plana vitrectomy in posterior-segment disorders. Ann Ophthalmol 17:686, 1985.

59. Clearkin LG: Recent experience in the management of neovascular glaucoma by pan-retinal photocoagulation and trabeculectomy. Eye 1:397, 1987.

60. Coats G: Further cases of thrombosis of the central vein. Roy Lond Ophthalmic Hosp Rep 16:516, 1906.

61. Coats G: Forms of retinal disease with massive exudation. Roy Lond Ophthalmic Hosp Rep 17:440, 1908.

62. Cobb B, Shilling JS, Chisholm IH: Vascular tufts at the pupillary margin in myotinic dystrophy. Am J Ophthalmol 69:573, 1970.

63. Connor T, Roberts A, Sporn M, et al: RPE cells synthesize and release transforming growth factor-beta, a modulator of endothelial cell growth and wound healing. Invest Ophthalmol Vis Sci 29:307, 1988.

64. Coppeto J, Wand M: Neovascular glaucoma and carotid vascular occlusion. Am J Ophthalmol 99:567, 1985.

65. Crum R, Szabo S, Folkman J: A new class of steroids inhibits angiogenesis in the presence of heparin or a heparin fragment. Science 230:1375, 1985.

66. Cunha-Vaz JG: Blood-retinal barriers in health and disease. Trans Ophthalmol Soc UK 100:337, 1980.

67. DalFiume E, Saccol G, Verzella F: Rubeosis iridea trattamento mediante fotocoagulatore laser ad argon. Arch Rass Ital Ottal 3:19, 1973.

67a. D'Amore PA: Capillary growth: A two-cell system. Cancer Biol 3:49, 1992.

68. DeJong PTVMP: Neovascular glaucoma and the occurrence of twin vessels in congenital arteriovenous communications of the retina. Doc Ophthalmol 68:205, 1988.

69. Deutsch TA, Hughes WF: Suppressive effects of indomethacin on thermally induced neovascularization of rabbit corneas. Am J Ophthalmol 87:436, 1979.

70. Diabetic Retinopathy Study Research Group: Preliminary report on effects of photocoagulation therapy. Am J Ophthalmol 81:383, 1976.

71. Diabetic Retinopathy Vitrectomy Study Group: Two-year course of visual acuity in severe proliferative diabetic retinopathy with conventional management. Ophthalmology 92:492, 1985.

72. Duker JS, Brown GC: Iris neovascularization associated with obstruction of the central retinal artery. Ophthalmology 95:1244, 1988.

73. Duker JS, Brown GC: Neovascularization of the optic disc associated with obstruction of the central retinal artery. Ophthalmology 96:87, 1989.

74. Duker JS, Brown GC: The efficacy of panretinal photocoagulation for neovascularization of the iris after central retinal artery obstruction. Ophthalmology 96:92, 1989.

75. Duker JS, Sivalingam A, Brown GC: A prospective study of acute central retinal artery obstruction: The incidence of secondary ocular neovascularization. Arch Ophthalmol 109:339, 1991.

76. Edward DP, Brown SVL, Higginbotham E, et al: Sympathetic ophthalmia following neodymium: YAG cyclotherapy. Ophthalmic Surg 20:544, 1989.

77. Effron L, Zakov ZN, Tomsak RL: Neovascular glaucoma as a complication of the Wyburn-Mason syndrome. J Clin Neuro Ophthalmol 5:95, 1985.

78. Egbert PR, Lieberman MF: Internal suture occlusion of the molteno glaucoma implant for the prevention of post-operative hypotony. Ophthalmol Surg 20:53, 1989.

79. Eggleston TF, Bohling CA, Eggleston HC, et al: Photocoagulation for ocular ischemia associated with carotid artery occlusion. Ann Ophthalmol 12:84, 1980.

80. Ehrenberg M, McCuen BW, Schindler RH, et al: Rubeosis iridis: Preoperative iris fluorescein angiography and periocular steroids. Ophthalmology 91:321, 1984.

81. Eisenstein R, Goren SB, Shumacher B, et al: The inhibition of corneal vascularization with aortic extracts in rabbits. Am J Ophthalmol 88:1005, 1979.

82. Ellett EC: Metastatic carcinoma of choroid. III: Rubeosis iridis with melanoma of the choroid and secondary glaucoma. Am J Ophthalmol 27:726, 1944.

83. Fankhauser F, Vander Zypen E, Kwasniewska S, et al: Transcleral cyclophotocoagulation using a neodymium YAG laser. Ophthalmic Surg 17:94, 1986.

84. Federman JL, Brown GC, Feldberg NT, et al: Experimental ocular angiogenesis. Am J Ophthalmol 89:231, 1980.

85. Fehrmann H: Uber rubeosis iridis diabetica und ihre allegemeinmedizinische Bedeutung; mit anatomischem Befund. Graefes Arch Clin Exp Ophthalmol 140:354, 1939.

86. Feibel RM, Bigger JF: Rubeosis iridis and neovascular glaucoma. Am J Ophthalmol 74:862, 1972.

87. Fernandez-Vigo J, Castro J, Cordido M: Treatment of diabetic neovascular glaucoma by panretinal ablation and trabeculectomy. Acta Ophthalmol 66:612, 1988.

88. Ferry AP, Font RL: Carcinoma metastatic to the eye and orbit. Arch Ophthalmol 93:472, 1975.

89. Finkelstein D, Brem S, Patz A, et al: Experimental retinal neovascularization induced by intravitreal tumors. Am J Ophthalmol 83:660, 1987.

90. Fiore PM, Latina MA, Shingleton BJ, et al: The dural shunt syndrome. I: Management of glaucoma. Ophthalmology 97:57, 1990.

91. Flanagan DW, Blach RK: Place of panretinal photocoagulation and trabeculectomy in the management of neovascular glaucoma. Br J Ophthalmol 67:526, 1983.

92. Fleischman JA, Swartz M, Dixon JA: Argon laser endophotocoagulation: An intraoperative trans-pars plana technique. Arch Ophthalmol 99:1610, 1981.

93. Folberg R, Hargett NA, Weaver JE, et al: Filtering valve implant for neovascular glaucoma in proliferative diabetic retinopathy. Ophthalmology 89:286, 1982.

94. Folkman J: The vascularization of tumors. Sci Am 234:59, 1976.

95. Folkman J, Haudenschild C: Angiogenesis by capillary endothelial cell in culture. Trans Ophthalmol Soc UK 100:346, 1980.

96. Folkman J, Klagsbrun M: Angiogenic factors. Science 23:442, 1987.

97. Folkman J, Langer R, Linhardt RJ, et al: Angiogenesis inhibition and tumor regression caused by heparin or a heparin fragment in the presence of cortisone. Science 221:719, 1983.

98. Folkman J, Merler E, Abernathy C, et al: Isolation of a tumor factor responsible for angiogenesis. J Exp Med 133:275, 1971.

99. Forestier F, Salvanet-Bouccara A: An evaluation of the Krupin-Denver valve implant in glaucoma. Glaucoma 8:92, 1986.

100. Form DM, Auerbach R: PGE_2 and angiogenesis. Proc Soc Exp Biol Med 172:214, 1983.

101. Frank RN: Diabetic retinopathy. In Ryan ST, Smith RE (eds): Selected Topics on the Eye in Systemic Disease. New York, Grune & Stratton, 1974, pp 65–118.

102. Fromer CH, Klintworth GK: An evaluation of the role of leukocytes in the pathogenesis of experimentally induced corneal vascularization. Am J Pathol 82:157, 1976.

103. Galinos S, Rabb MF, Goldberg MF, et al: Hemoglobin SC disease and iris atrophy. Am J Ophthalmol 75:421, 1973.

104. Gartner S, Henkind P: Neovascularization of the iris (rubeosis iridis). Surv Ophthalmol 22:291, 1978.

105. Gartner S, Taffet S, Friedman AH: The association of rubeosis iridis with endothelialisation of the anterior chamber: Report of a clinical case with histopathological review of 16 additional cases. Br J Ophthalmol 61:267, 1977.

106. Georgiades G: Les lesions de l'iris hétérochromique en général. Bull Mem Soc Fr d'Ophthalmologie 77:465, 1964.

107. Gerritzen FM: The course of diabetic retinopathy: A longitudinal study. Diabetes 22:122, 1973.

108. Gimbrone MA, Leapman SB, Cotran RS, et al: Tumor angiogenesis: Iris neovascularization at a distance from experimental intraocular tumors. J Natl Cancer Inst 50:219, 1973.

109. Glaser BM: Extracellular modulating factors and the control of intraocular neovascularization. Arch Ophthalmol 106:603, 1988.

110. Glaser BM, Campochiaro PA, Davis JO, et al: Retinal pigment epithelial cells release an inhibitor of neovascularization. Arch Ophthalmol 103:1870, 1985.

111. Glaser BM, D'Amore PA, Michels RG: The effect of human intraocular fluid on vascular endothelial cell migration. Ophthalmology 88:986, 1981.

112. Glaser BM, D'Amore PA, Michels RG, et al: The demonstration of angiogenic activity from ocular tissues. Ophthalmology 87:440, 1980.

113. Glaser BM, Hayashi H, Krause WG: A protease inhibitor accumulates within the vitreous following pan retinal photocoagulation (PRP) in primates: Possible mechanism for the effect of PRP on retinal neovascularization. Invest Ophthalmol Vis Sci 29:180, 1988.

114. Glatt HJ, Vu MT, Burger PC, et al: Effect of irradiation on vascularization of corneas grafted onto chorioallantoic membranes. Invest Ophthalmol Vis Sci 26:1533, 1985.

115. Goldstein AL, Ide CH: Cyclocryotherapy for secondary glaucoma due to rubeosis iridis. Mo Med 69:736, 1972.

116. Gragoudas ES, Seddon J, Goitein M, et al: Current results of proton beam irradiation of uveal melanomas. Ophthalmology 92:284, 1985.

117. Grant WM: Management of neovascular glaucoma. In Leopold IH (ed): Symposium on Ocular Therapy, vol. 7. St. Louis, CV Mosby, 1974, pp 36–61.

118. Greenblatt M, Shubik P: Tumor angiogenesis: Transfilter diffusion studies in the hamster by the transparent chamber technique. J Natl Cancer Inst 41:111, 1968.

119. Gu QX, Fry GL, Lata GF, et al: Ocular neovascularization. Arch Ophthalmol 103:111, 1985.

120. Haas JS, Peyman GA, Lim J: Experimental evaluation of a posterior drainage system. Ophthalmic Surg 14:494, 1983.

121. Hampton GR: Argon endophotocoagulation with indirect ophthalmolscopy. Arch Ophthalmol 105:132, 1987.

122. Hampton C, Shields MB, Miller KN, et al: Evaluation of a protocol for transscleral neodymium: YAG cyclophotocoagulation in one hundred patients. Ophthalmology 97:910, 1990.

123. Harper JW, Vallee BL: Conformational characterization of human angiogenin by limited proteolysis. J Protein Chem 7:355, 1988.

124. Harper JW, Vallee BL: A covalent angiogenin/ribonuclease hybrid with a fourth disulfide bond generated by regional mutagenesis. Biochemistry 28:1875, 1989.

125. Hayreh SS: Classification of central retinal vein occlusion. Ophthalmology 90:458, 1983.

126. Hayreh SS, Hayreh MS: Hemi-central retinal vein occlusion. Arch Ophthalmol 98:1600, 1980.

127. Hayreh SS, Klugman MR, Podhajsky P, et al: Electroretinography in central retinal vein occlusion: Correlation of electroretinographic changes with pupillary abnormalities. Graefes Arch Clin Exp Ophthalmol 227:549, 1989.

128. Hayreh SS, Podhajsky P: Ocular neovascularization with retinal vascular occlusion. II: Occurrence in central and branch retinal artery occlusion. Arch Ophthalmol 100:1585, 1982.

129. Hayreh SS, Rojas P, Kodhajsky P, et al: Ocular neovascularization with retinal vascular occlusion. III: Incidence of ocular neovascularization with retinal vein occlusion. Ophthalmology 90:488, 1983.

130. Hedges TR: Ophthalmoscopic findings in internal carotid artery occlusion. Johns Hopkins Med J 111:89, 1962.

131. Henkind P, Wise GN: Retinal neovascularization, collaterals, and vascular shunts. Br J Ophthalmol 58:413, 1974.

132. Hercules B, Bayed I, Lucas S, et al: Peripheral retinal ablation in the treatment of proliferative diabetic retinopathy: A three-year interim report of a randomized, controlled study using the argon laser. Br J Ophthalmol 61:555, 1977.

133. Heuer DK, Gressel MG, Parrish RK II, et al: Topical fluorouracil. II: Postoperative administration in an animal model of glaucoma filtering surgery. Arch Ophthalmol 104:132, 1986.

134. Heuer DK, Parrish RK II, Gressel MG, et al: 5-Fluorouracil and glaucoma filtering surgery. III: Intermediate follow-up of a pilot study. Ophthalmology 93:1537, 1986.

135. Higgins RA: Neovascular glaucoma associated with ocular hypoperfusion secondary to carotid artery disease. Australian J Ophthalmol 12:155, 1984.

136. Hohl RD, Barnett DM: Diabetic hemorrhagic glaucoma. Diabetes 19:994, 1970.

137. Hollenhorst RW: Ocular manifestations of insufficiency or thrombosis of the internal carotid artery. Trans Am Ophthalmol Soc 56:472, 1958.

138. Holm A, Sachs J, Wilson A: Glaucoma secondary to occlusion of central retinal artery. Am J Ophthalmol 48:530, 1959.

138a. Honrubia FM, Gomez ML, Hernandez A, Grijalbo MP: Long term results of silicone tube filtering surgery for eyes with neovascular glaucoma. Am J Ophthalmology 97:501, 1984.

139. Hoskins HD: Neovascular glaucoma: Current concepts. Trans Am Acad Ophthalmol Otolaryngol 78:330, 1974.

140. Hovener G: Photocoagulation for central retinal vein occlusion. Klin Monatsbl Augenheilkd 173:392, 1978.

141. Howard GM, Ellsworth RM: Differential diagnosis of retinoblastoma. Am J Ophthalmol 60:618, 1965.

142. Huckman MS, Haas J: Reversed flow through the ophthalmic artery as a cause of rubeosis iridis. Am J Ophthalmol 74:1094, 1972.

143. Hung Y, Hilton GF: Neovascular glaucoma in a patient with X-linked juvenile retinoschisis. Ann Ophthalmol 12:1054, 1980.

144. Hutchins RK, Gittinger JW, Weiter JJ: Optic disk and iris neovascularization after surgical interruption of the retinal circulation. [Letter] Am J Ophthalmol 101:616, 1986.

145. Irvine AR, Wood IS: Radiation retinopathy as an experimental model for ischemic proliferative retinopathy and rubeosis iridis. Am J Ophthalmol 103:790, 1987.

146. Isenberg SJ, McRee WE, Jedrzynski MS: Conjunctival hypoxia in diabetes mellitus. Invest Ophthalmol Vis Sci 27:1512, 1986.

147. Jaccoma EH, Conway BP, Campochiaro PA: Cryotherapy causes extensive breakdown of the blood-retinal barrier. Arch Ophthalmol 103:1728, 1985.

148. Jackson WE, Chase P, Garg SK, et al: Vitreous fluorophotometry in insulin-dependent diabetes mellitus: Correlation with microalbuminuria and diastolic blood pressure. Arch Ophthalmol 108:1733, 1990.

149. Jacobson DR, Murphy RP, Rosenthal AR: The treatment of angle neovascularization with panretinal photocoagulation. Ophthalmology 86:1270, 1979.

150. Jaffe NS: Cataract Surgery And Its Complications. St. Louis, CV Mosby, 1972.

151. Jaffe GJ, Burton TC: Progression of nonproliferative diabetic retinopathy following cataract extraction. Arch Ophthalmol 106:745, 1988.

152. Javitt JC, O'Connor SS, Sommer AR: Incidence of proliferative diabetic retinopathy in the United States population. Invest Ophthalmol Vis Sci 29(Suppl):259, 1988.

153. Jensen VA, Lundbock K: Fluorescein angiography of the iris in recent and long-term diabetes: Preliminary communication. Acta Ophthalmol 46:584, 1968.

154. Jocson VL: Microvascular injection studies in rubeosis iridis and neovascular glaucoma. Am J Ophthalmol 83:508, 1977.

155. John T, Sassani JW, Eagle RC: The myofibroblastic component of rubeosis iridis. Ophthalmology 90:721, 1983.

155a. Johnson RN, Irvine AR, Wood IS: Endolaser, cryopexy, and retinal reattachment in the air-filled eye: A clinicopathologic correlation. Ophthalmology 105:231, 1987.

156. Johnson MA, Marcus S, Elman MJ, et al: Neovascularization in central retinal vein occlusion: Electroretinographic findings. Arch Ophthalmol 106:348, 1988.

157. Jones RF: Glaucoma following radiotherapy. Br J Ophthalmology 42:636, 1958.

157a. Katjalainen K: Occlusion of the central retinal artery and retinal branch arterioles: A clinical, tomographic, and fluorescein angiographic study of 175 patients. Acta Ophthalmol Suppl 109:9, 1971.

158. Kaufman SC, Ferris FL III, Seigel DG, et al: Factors associated with visual outcome after photocoagulation for diabetic retinopathy. Diabetic Retinopathy Study Report No. 13. Invest Ophthalmol Vis Sci 30:23, 1989.

159. Kaufman SC, Ferris FL III, Swartz M. Diabetic Retinopathy Study Research Group: Intraocular pressure following panretinal photocoagulation for diabetic retinopathy. Arch Ophthalmol 105:807, 1987.

160. Kaye SB, Harding SP: Early electroretinography in unilateral central retinal vein occlusion as a predictor of rubeosis iridis. Arch Ophthalmol 106:353, 1988.

161. Kearns TP, Hollenhorst RW: Venous-stasis retinopathy of occlusive disease of the carotid artery. Proc Mayo Clin 38:304, 1963.

162. Kearns TP, Siekert RG, Sundt TM: The ocular aspects of bypass surgery of the carotid artery. Mayo Clin Proc 54:3, 1979.

163. Kearns TP, Young BR, Piepgras DG: Resolution of venous stasis retinopathy after carotid artery bypass surgery. Mayo Clin Proc 55:342, 1980.

164. Kim MK, Char DH, Castro JL, et al: Neovascular glaucoma after helium ion irradiation for uveal melanoma. Ophthalmology 93:189, 1986.

165. Kimura R: Fluorescein goniophotography. Glaucoma 2:359, 1980.

166. Kiser WD, Gonder J, Magargal LE, et al: Recovery of vision following treatment of the ocular ischemic syndrome. Ann Ophthalmol 15:305, 1983.

167. Klagsbrun M, D'Amore PA: Regulators of angiogenesis. Annu Rev Physiol 53:217, 1991.

168. Knowles HC Jr: The problem of the relation of the control of diabetes to the development of vascular disease. Trans Am Clin Climatol Assoc 76:142, 1964.

169. Knox DL: Ischemic ocular inflammation. Am J Ophthalmol 60:995, 1965.

170. Kohner EM, Laatikainen L, Oughton J: The management of central retinal vein occlusion. Ophthalmology 90:484, 1983.

171. Kohner EM, Shilling JS, Hamilton AM: The role of avascular retina in new vessel formation. Metab Ophthalmol 1:15, 1976.

172. Kokame GT, Flynn HW, Blankenship GW: Posterior chamber intraocular lens implantation during diabetic pars plana vitrectomy. Ophthalmology 96:603, 1989.

173. Kornerup T: Blood pressure and diabetic retinopathy. Acta Ophthalmol 35:163, 1957.

174. Kottow MW: Anterior Segment Fluorescein Angiography. Baltimore, Williams & Wilkins, 1978, pp 129–151.

175. Krupin T, Kaufman P, Mandell AI, et al: Long-term results of valve implants in filtering surgery for eyes with neovascular glaucoma. Am J Ophthalmol 95:775, 1983.

176. Krupin T, Mitchell KB, Becker B: Cyclocryotherapy in neovascular glaucoma. Am J Ophthalmol 86:24, 1978.

177. Krupin T, Ritch R, Camras CB, et al: A long Krupin-Denver valve implant attached to a 180° scleral explant for glaucoma surgery. Ophthalmology 95:1174, 1988.

178. Kurz O: Zur Rubeosis iridis diabetica. Arch Augenheilkd 110:284, 1937.

179. Laatikainen L: Development and classification of rubeosis iridis in diabetic eye disease. Br J Ophthalmol 63:156, 1979.

180. Laatikainen L, Blach RK: Behavior of the iris vasculature in central retinal vein occlusion: A fluorescein angiographic study of the vascular response of the retina and the iris. Br J Ophthalmol 61:272, 1977.

181. Laatikainen L, Kohner EM: Fluorescein angiography and its prognostic significance in central retinal vein occlusion. Br J Ophthalmol 64:411, 1976.

182. Laatikainen L, Kohner EM, Khoury D, et al: Panretinal photocoagulation in central retinal vein occlusion: A randomized controlled clinical study. Br J Ophthalmol 61:741, 1977.

183. Lazzaro EC: Retinal-vein occlusions: Carotid artery evaluation indicated. Ann Ophthalmol 18:116, 1986.

184. Lewis RA, Tse DT, Phelps CD, et al: Neovascular glaucoma after photoradiation therapy for uveal melanoma. Arch Ophthalmol 102:839, 1984.

185. Loring EG: Remarks on embolism. Am J Med Sci 67:313, 1874.

186. Luntz M, Schenker HI: Retinal vascular accidents in glaucoma and ocular hypertension. Surv Ophthalmol 25:163, 1980.

187. Machemer R, Beuttner H, Norton EWD, et al: Vitrectomy: A pars plana approach. Trans Am Acad Ophthalmol Otolaryngol 75:813, 1971.

188. Madsen PH: Haemorrhagic glaucoma: Comparative study in diabetic and non-diabetic patients. Br J Ophthalmol 55:444, 1971.

189. Madsen PH: Rubeosis of the iris and haemorrhagic glaucoma in patients with proliferative diabetic retinopathy. Br J Ophthalmol 55:369, 1971.

190. Magargal LE, Brown GC, Augsburger JJ, et al: Neovascular glaucoma following branch retinal vein obstruction. Glaucoma 3:333, 1981.

191. Magargal LE, Brown GC, Augsburger JJ, et al: Neovascular glaucoma following central retinal vein obstruction. Ophthalmology 88:1095, 1981.

192. Magargal LE, Brown GC, Augsburger JJ, et al: Efficacy of panretinal photocoagulation in preventing neovascular glaucoma following ischemic central retinal vein obstruction. Am Acad Ophthalmol 89:780, 1982.

193. Magargal LE, Donoso LA, Sanborn GE: Retinal ischemia and risk of neovascularization following central retinal vein obstruction. Ophthalmology 89:1241, 1982.

194. Magargal LE, Sanborn GE, Kimmel AS, et al: Temporal branch retinal vein obstruction: A review. Ophthalmic Surg 17:240, 1986.

195. Makley TA, Teed RW: Unsuspected intraocular malignant melanoma. Arch Ophthalmol 60:475, 1950.

196. Mason GI: Iris neovascular tufts: Relationship to rubeosis, insulin, and hypotony. Arch Ophthalmol 97:2346, 1979.

197. May DR, Bergstrom TJ, Parmet AJ, et al: Treatment of neovascular glaucoma with transscleral panretinal cryotherapy. Ophthalmology 87:1106, 1980.

198. May DR, Klein ML, Peyman GA, et al: Xenon arc panretinal photocoagulation for central retinal vein occlusion: A randomised prospective study. Br J Ophthalmol 63:725, 1979.

199. McAuslan BR, Gole GA: Cellular and molecular mechanisms in angiogenesis. Trans Ophthalmol Soc UK 100:354, 1980.

200. Michels RG: Vitrectomy techniques in retinal re-attachment surgery. Ophthalmology 86:556, 1979.

201. Michels RG: Vitrectomy for complications of diabetic retinopathy. Arch Ophthalmol 96:237, 1978.

202. Michaels RG, Maumenee AE: Retrobulbar alcohol injection in seeing eyes. Trans Am Acad Ophthalmol Otol 77:164, 1973.

203. Michaelson IC: The mode of development of the vascular system of the retina with some observations of its significance in certain retinal diseases. Trans Ophthalmol Soc UK 68:137, 1948.

204. Miller JB, Smith MR, Boyer DS: Intraocular carbon dioxide laser photocautery. Ophthalmology 87:1112, 1980.

205. Minckler DS, Heuer DK, Hasty B, et al: Clinical experience with the single-plate Molteno implant in complicated glaucomas. Ophthalmology 95:1181, 1988.

206. Mochizuki M: Transpupillary cyclophotocoagulation in hemorrhagic glaucoma: A case report. Jpn J Ophthalmol 19:191, 1975.

207. Molteno ACB, Haddad PJ: The visual outcome in cases of neovascular glaucoma. Aust N Z J Ophthalmol 13:329, 1985.

208. Moses MA, Sudhalter J, Langer R: Identification of an inhibitor of neovascularization from cartilage. Science 248:1408, 1990.

209. Mosier MA, Del Piero E, Gheewala SM: Anterior retinal cryotherapy in diabetic vitreous hemorrhage. Am J Ophthalmol 100:440, 1985.

210. Murphy RP, Maguire M, Vitale S, et al: Retrogression of early diabetic retinopathy. Invest Ophthalmol Vis Sci 29(Suppl):259, 1988.

211. Nathan DM, Singer DE, Godine JE, et al: Retinopathy in older type II diabetics: Association with glucose control. Diabetes 35:797, 1986.

212. National Diabetes Advisory Board: The prevention and treatment of five complications of diabetes: A guide for primary care physicians. Metabolism 33:15, 1984.

213. Neupert JR, Brubaker RF, Kearns TP, et al: Rapid resolution of venous stasis retinopathy after carotid endarterectomy. Am J Ophthalmol 81:600, 1976.

214. Nielsen NV: The prevalence of glaucoma and ocular hypertension in type I and II diabetes mellitus: An epidemiological study of diabetes mellitus on the island of Falster, Denmark. Acta Ophthalmol 61:662, 1983.

215. Nomura T: Pathology of anterior chamber angle in diabetic neovascular glaucoma: Extension of corneal endothelium onto iris surface. Jpn J Ophthalmol 27:193, 1983.

215a. Ogden TE, Rickhof FT, Benkwith SM: Correlation of histologic and electroretinographic changes in peripheral retinal ablation in the rhesus monkey. Am J Ophthalmol 81:1272, 1976.

216. Ohrt V: Glaucoma due to rubeosis iridis diabetica. Ophthalmologica 142:356, 1961.

217. Ohrt V: The frequency of rubeosis iridis in diabetic patients. Acta Ophthalmol 49:301, 1971.

218. Oldendoerp J, Spitznas M: Factors influencing the results of vitreous surgery in diabetic retinopathy. I: Iris rubeosis and/or active neovascularization at the fundus. Graefes Arch Clin Exp Ophthalmol 227:1, 1989.

219. Olurin O, Osuntokun O: Complications of retrobulbar alcohol injections. Ann Ophthalmol 10:474, 1978.

220. Oosterhuis JA, Bijlmer-Gorter H: Cryotreatment in proliferative diabetic retinopathy. Ophthalmologica 181:81, 1980.

221. Orlidge A, D'Amore PA: Inhibition of capillary endothelial cell growth by pericytes and smooth muscle cells. J Cell Biol 105:1455, 1987.

222. Packer S, Rotman M, Salanitro P: Iodine-125 irradiation of choroidal melanoma: Clinical experience. Ophthalmology 91:1700, 1984.

223. Pagenstecher M: Beitrage zur Lehre vom hamorrhagischen Glaucom. Graefes Arch Ophthalmol 17:98, 1871.

224. Patel A, Thompson JT, Michels RG, et al: Endolaser treatment of the ciliary body for uncontrolled glaucoma. Ophthalmology 93:825, 1986.

225. Patz A, Yassur Y, Fine SL, et al: Branch retinal venous occlusion. Trans Am Acad Ophthalmol Otolaryngol 83:373, 1977.

226. Perry HD, Yanoff M, Scheie HG: Rubeosis in Fuchs heterochromic iridocyclitis. Arch Ophthalmol 93:337, 1975.

227. Pirart J: Diabetes mellitus and its degenerative complications: A prospective study of 4400 patients observed between 1947 and 1973. Diabetes Care 1:168, 252, 1978.

228. Poliner LS, Christianson DJ, Escoffery RF, et al: Neovascular glaucoma after intracapsular and extracapsular cataract extraction in diabetic patients. Am J Ophthalmol 100:637, 1985.

229. Poulsen JE: The Houssay phenomenon in man: Recovery from retinopathy in a case of diabetes with Simmonds' disease. Diabetes 2:7, 1953.

230. Pournaras CJ, Tsacopoulos M, Strommer K, et al: Experimental retinal branch vein occlusion in miniature pigs induces local tissue hypoxia and vasoproliferative microangiopathy. Ophthalmology 97:1321, 1990.

231. Presta M, Rifkin DB: New aspects of blood vessel growth: Tumor and tissue-derived angiogenesis factors. Haemostasis 18:6, 1988.

232. Quigley HA: Histologic and physiologic studies of cyclocryotherapy in primate and human eyes. Am J Ophthalmol 82:722, 1976.

233. Quinlan PM, Elman MJ, Bhatt AK, et al: The national course of central retinal vein occlusion. Am J Ophthalmol 110:118, 1990.

234. Raymond L, Jacobson B: Isolation and identification of stimulatory and inhibitory cell growth factors in bovine vitreous. Exp Eye Res 34:267, 1982.

235. Reinecke RD, Kuwabara T, Cogan DG, et al: Retinal vascular patterns. V: Experimental ischemia of the cat eye. Arch Ophthalmol 67:470, 1962.

236. Reddy VM, Zamora VM, Olk RJ: A comparison of the size of the burn produced by Rodenstock and Goldmann contact lenses. Am J Ophthalmol 112:212, 1991.

237. Riaskoff S, Pameyer JH: Results of the treatment of neovascular glaucoma by diathermy of the dissected ciliary body. Doc Ophthalmol 48:277, 1979.

238. Rice TA, Michels RG, McQuire MG, et al: The effect of lensectomy on the incidence of iris neovascularization and neovascular glaucoma after vitrectomy for diabetic retinopathy. Am J Ophthalmol 85:1, 1983.

239. Ringvold A, Davanger M: Iris neovascularisation in eyes with pseudoexfoliation syndrome. Br J Ophthalmol 65:138, 1981.

240. Rockwood EJ, Parrish RK, Heuer DK, et al: Glaucoma filtering surgery with 5-fluorouracil. Ophthalmology 94:1071, 1987.

241. Romem M, Isakow I: Photocoagulation in retinal vein occlusion. Ann Ophthalmol 13:1057, 1981.

242. Rosenberg PR, Walsh JB, Zimmerman RD: Neovascular glaucoma and carotid bruits. J Clin Neuro Ophthalmol 4:459, 1984.

243. Ryan SJ: An approach to the management of neovascularization of the iris and secondary glaucoma. Tr Am Ophthalmol Soc 78:107, 1980.

244. Saari M, Vuorre I, Nieminen H: Fuchs's heterochromic cyclitis: A simultaneous bilateral fluorescein angiographic study of the iris. Br J Ophthalmol 62:715, 1978.

245. Sabates R: Choroiditis compatible with the histopathologic diagnosis of sympathetic ophthalmia following cyclocryotherapy of neovascular glaucoma. Ophthalmic Surg 19:176, 1988.

246. Sabates R, Hirose T, McMeel JW: Electroretinography in the prognosis and classification of central retinal vein occlusion. Arch Ophthalmol 101:232, 1983.

247. Salus R: Rubeosis iridis diabetica, eine bisher unbekannte diabetische Irisveranderung. Med Klin 24:256, 1928.

248. Sanborn GE, Symes DJ, Magargal LE: Fundus-iris fluorescein angiography: Evaluation of its use in the diagnosis of rubeosis iridis. Ann Ophthalmol 18:52, 1986.

249. Scader JJ, Blumenkranz MS, Blankenship G: Regression of diabetic rubeosis iridis following successful surgical reattachment of the retina by vitrectomy. Retina 2:193, 1982.

250. Schachat AP: Discussion of iris neovascularization associated with obstruction of the central retinal artery. Ophthalmology 95:1249, 1988.

251. Schulze RR: Rubeosis iridis. Am J Ophthalmol 63:487, 1967.

252. Schuman JS, Puliafito CA, Allingham RR, et al: Contact transscleral continuous wave neodymium: YAG laser cyclophotocoagulation. Ophthalmology 97:571, 1990.

253. Segato T, Piermarocchi S, Midena E, et al: Retinal cryotherapy in the management of proliferative diabetic retinopathy. Am J Ophthalmol 98:240, 1984.

254. Shabo AL, Maxwell DS: Insulin-induced immunogenic retinopathy resembling retinitis proliferans of diabetes. Trans Am Acad Ophthalmol Otolaryngol 81:497, 1976.

255. Shabo AL, Maxwell DS: Experimental immunogenic proliferative retinopathy in monkeys. Am J Ophthalmol 83:471, 1977.

256. Shah HG, Brown GC, Goldberg RE: Digital subtraction carotid angiography and retinal arterial obstruction. Ophthalmology 92:68, 1985.

257. Shields MB: Cyclodestructive surgery for glaucoma: Past, present, and future. Trans Am Ophthalmol Soc 23:285, 1985.

258. Shields MB, Proia AD: Neovascular glaucoma associated with an iris melanoma: A clinicopathologic report. Arch Ophthalmol 105:672, 1987.

259. Shing Y, Folkman J, Sullivan R, et al: Heparin affinity: Purification of a tumor-derived capillary endothelial cell growth factor. Science 223:1296, 1984.

260. Sidkey YA, Auerbach R: Lymphocyte-induced angiogenesis: A quantitative and sensitive assay of the graft-vs-host reaction. J Exp Med 141:1084, 1975.

261. Silverman RH, Vogelsang B, Rondeau MJ, et al: Therapeutic ultrasound for the treatment of glaucoma. Am J Ophthalmol 111:327, 1991.

262. Simmons RJ, Depperman SR, Dueker DK: The role of goniophotocoagulation in neovascularization of the anterior chamber angle. Ophthalmology 87:79, 1980.

263. Sinclair SH, Aaberg TM, Meredith TA: A pars plana filtering procedure combined with lensectomy and vitrectomy for neovascular glaucoma. Am J Ophthalmol 93:185, 1982.

263a. Singerman L, Weaver D: The risk of proliferative diabetic retinopathy in juvenile onset diabetes. Retina 1:181, 1981.

264. Skyler JS: Complications of diabetes mellitus: Relationship to metabolic dysfunction. Diabetes Care 2:499, 1979.

265. Smith JL: Unilateral glaucoma in carotid occlusive disease. JAMA 182:683, 1962.

266. Steffes MW, Sutherland DER, Goetz FC, et al: Studies of kidney and muscle biopsy specimens from identical twins discordant for type I diabetes mellitus. N Engl J Med 312:1282, 1985.

267. Sturrock GD, Mueller HR: Chronic ocular ischaemia. Br J Ophthalmol 68:716, 1984.

268. Sugar HS: Neovascular glaucoma after carotid-cavernous fistula formation. Ann Ophthalmol 11:1667, 1979.

269. Sullivan ST, Dallow RL: Intraocular reticulum cell sarcoma. Ann Ophthalmol 9:401, 1977.

270. Sundt TM, Whisnant JP, Fode NC, et al: Results, complications, and follow-up of 415 bypass operations for occlusive disease of the carotid system. Mayo Clin Proc 60:230, 1985.

271. Sundt TM, Whisnant JP, Houser OW, et al: Prospective study of the effectiveness and durability of carotid endarterectomy. Mayo Clin Proc 65:625, 1990.

272. Sutton GE, Popp JC, Records RE: Krupin-Denver valve and neovascular glaucoma. Trans Ophthalmol Soc UK 102:119, 1982.

273. Swan KC, Raff J: Changes in the eye and orbit following carotid ligation. Trans Am Ophthalmol Soc 49:435, 1951.

274. Szabo AJ, Stewart AG, Joron GE: Factors associated with increased prevalence of diabetic retinopathy. Can Med Assoc J 97:286, 1967.

274a. Tamara T: Electron microscopic study on the small blood vessels in rubeosis diabetica. Jpn J Ophthalmol 13:65, 1969.

275. Tasman W, Magargal LE, Augsberger JJ: Effects of argon laser photocoagulation or rubeosis iridis and angle neovascularization. Ophthalmology 87:400, 1980.

276. Taylor CM, Weiss JB, McLaughlin B, et al: Increased procollagenase activating angiogenic factor in the vitreous humour of oxygen treated kittens. Br J Ophthalmol 72:2, 1988.

277. Teich SA, Walsh JB: A grading system for neovascularization: Prognostic implications for treatment. Ophthalmology 88:1102, 1981.

278. The DCCT Research Group: The Diabetes Control and Complications Trial (DCCT): Results of feasibility study. Diabetes Care 10:1, 1987.

279. The Fluorouracil Filtering Surgery Study Group: Fluorouracil filtering surgery study one-year follow-up. Am J Ophthalmol 108:625, 1989.

280. Chew EY, Trope GE, Mitchell BJ: Diurnal intraocular pressure in young patients with central retinal vein occlusion. Ophthalmology 94:1545, 1987.

281. Vallee BL, Riordan JF: Chemical and biochemical properties of human angiogenin. Adv Exp Med Biol 234:41, 1988.

282. Vander JF, Brown GC, Benson WE: Iris neovascularization after central retinal artery obstruction despite previous panretinal photocoagulation for diabetic retinopathy. Am J Ophthalmol 109:464, 1990.

283. Vannas S: Discussion of Bertelsen TI: The relationship between thrombosis in the retinal vein and primary glaucoma. Acta Ophthalmol 39:603, 1961.

284. Vannas A: Fluorescein angiography of the vessels of the iris in pseudo-exfoliation of the lens capsule, capsular glaucoma, and some other forms of glaucoma. Acta Ophthalmol 105(Suppl):9, 1969.

285. Vernon SA, Cheng H: Panretinal cryotherapy in neovascular disease. Br J Ophthalmol 72:401, 1988.

286. Walton DS, Grant WM: Retinoblastoma and iris neovascularization. Am J Ophthalmol 65:598, 1968.

287. Walton DS, Grant WM: Penetrating cyclodiathermy for filtration. Arch Ophthalmol 83:47, 1970.

288. Wand M: Neovascular glaucoma. In Ritch R, Shields MB (eds): The Secondary Glaucomas. St. Louis, CV Mosby, 1982, pp 162–193.

289. Wand M: Treatment of neovascular glaucoma. In Jakobiec FA, Sigelman J (eds): Advanced Techniques in Ocular Surgery. Philadelphia, WB Saunders, 1984, pp 169–182.

290. Wand M: Hyaloid membrane vs. posterior capsule as a protective barrier. Arch Ophthalmol 103:1112, 1985.

291. Wand M: Neovascular glaucoma. In Ritch R, Shields MB, Kurpin T (eds): The Glaucomas. St. Louis, CV Mosby, 1989, p 1063.

292. Wand M, Dueker DK, Aiello LM, et al: Effects of panretinal photocoagulation on rubeosis iridis, angle neovascularization, and neovascular glaucoma. Am J Ophthalmol 86:332, 1978.

293. Wand M, Hutchinson BT: The surgical management of neovascular glaucoma. Perspect Ophthalmol 4:147, 1980.

294. Wand M, Madigan JC, Gaudio AR, et al: Neovascular glaucoma following pars plana vitrectomy for complications of diabetic retinopathy. Ophthalmic Surg 21:113, 1990.

295. Weber PA: Neovascular glaucoma, current management. Surv Ophthalmol 25:149, 1981.

296. Weinreb RN, Wasserstrom JP, Parker W: Neovascular glaucoma following neodymium:YAG laser posterior capsulotomy. Arch Ophthalmol 104:730, 1986.

297. Weiss DI, Gold D: Neofibrovascularization of iris and anterior chamber angle: A clinical classification. Ann Ophthalmol 10:488, 1978.

298. Weiss DI, Shaffer RN, Nehrenberg TR: Neovascular glaucoma complicating carotid-cavernous fistula. Arch Ophthalmol 69:304, 1963.

299. Wilhelmus KR, Grierson I, Watson PG: Histopathologic and clinical associations of scleritis and glaucoma. Am J Ophthalmol 91:697, 1981.

299a. Williams DF, Burke JW, Williams EA: Clearance of experimental vitreous hemorrhage after panretinal cryotherapy related to macrophage influx. Arch Ophthalmol 108:585, 1986.

300. Williams GA, Eisenstein R, Schumacher B, et al: Inhibitor of vascular endothelial cell growth in the lens. Am J Ophthalmol 92:366, 1984.

301. Wise GN: Retinal neovascularization. Trans Am Ophthalmol Soc 54:729, 1956.

302. Wolter JR: Secondary glaucoma in cranial arteritis. Am J Ophthalmol 59:625, 1965.

303. Yablonski ME, Jacobson J, Goldfarb M: Glaucoma and bilateral carotid artery occlusion. Glaucoma 7:19, 1985.

304. Yanoff M: Mechanisms of glaucoma in eyes with uveal melanoma. Int Ophthalmol Clin 12:51, 1972.

305. Yanoff M, Fine BS: Ocular Pathology: A Text And Atlas. New York, Harper & Row, 1975, p 339.

306. Yoshizumi MO, Thomas JV, Smith TR: Glaucoma-inducing mechanisms in eyes with retinoblastoma. Arch Ophthalmol 96:105, 1978.

307. Young LHY, Appen RE: Ischemic oculopathy: A manifestation of carotid artery disease. Arch Neurol 18:358, 1981.

308. Young NJA, Hitchings RA, Sehmi K, et al: Stickler's syndrome and neovascular glaucoma. Br J Ophthalmol 63:826, 1979.

309. Zauberman H, Michaelson IC, Bergmann F, et al: Stimulation of neovascularization of the cornea by biogenic amines. Exp Eye Res 8:77, 1969.

310. Zetter BR: Angiogenesis: State of the art. Chest 93:159S, 1988.

311. Ziche M, Jones J, Gullino P: Role of prostaglandin E1 and copper in angiogenesis. J Natl Cancer Inst 69:475, 1982.

Chapter 133

∎

Glaucoma Following Cataract Surgery

JOSEPH H. KRUG, JR.

There does not appear to be a specific trend for intraocular pressure (IOP) after uncomplicated cataract extraction. However, early transient and chronic elevations of IOP do occur and can threaten vision. The glaucomas considered in this chapter are related by their development after cataract extraction. They differ in time course, etiology, and natural history. For this reason, the terms *pseudophakic glaucoma* and *aphakic glaucoma* are abandoned in favor of the general category of glaucomas in pseudophakia. The glaucomas are broadly described as predominantly open angle or closed angle in mechanism. However, it is possible for open-angle and closed-angle components to occur simultaneously. Specific glaucomas in which a closed angle evolves from a predominantly open angle are discussed. The rapidity of postsurgical onset and natural history are emphasized as important differential diagnostic clues to specific etiologies, and how the presence or absence of preexisting glaucoma can alter the likelihood of postoperative IOP elevations is reviewed. It is hoped that appreciation of the varied forms of glaucoma will lead to their early recognition and appropriate therapeutic intervention.

EARLY, TRANSIENT POSTOPERATIVE ELEVATIONS IN INTRAOCULAR PRESSURE

It is not uncommon to recognize an acute and transient elevation of IOP after uncomplicated cataract extraction. The IOP rise typically reaches its maximum at 3 to 8 hr postoperatively and returns to preoperative levels after 24 to 48 hr.[16, 27, 45, 82, 95] Increased IOP can be accompanied by nausea or vomiting and moderate to severe eye and brow pain that can be masked by long-acting retrobulbar anesthetics. It is not unusual for the IOP to have normalized by the first postoperative examination, leaving only the history of discomfort and perhaps corneal folds as evidence of the event. However, Hayreh has suggested that postoperative nonarteritic ischemic optic neuropathy may be related to exaggerated IOP elevations, with subsequent embarrassment of optic nerve head blood flow.[49] These IOP elevations are statistically more common and generally higher in patients with compromised trabecular meshwork function, as in primary open-angle glaucoma.[47, 76, 104, 125] In these patients, consideration is given to the alternative surgical approaches discussed in Chapter 148. The

pathogenesis of early and transient elevation of IOP is multifactorial and is discussed later.

Mechanical Deformation of the Anterior Chamber Angle Tissues

Before the advent of improved fine suture material and microsurgical techniques for tight wound closure, the most common postoperative pressure problem encountered by cataract surgeons was hypotony associated with wound leaks. In a discussion of this topic, Galin and colleagues pointed out that although McLean was performing cataract surgery using only preplaced 6–0 silk sutures (the predominant technique of the time), elevated IOP was rare on the first postoperative day.[41] However, after the introduction of fine suture closure and beveled incisions, postoperative IOP elevations became more common.[40, 94, 122]

Rich reported significant IOP elevation in the absence of α-chymotrypsin in 100 percent of patients studied.[95] The maximum pressure effect occurred at a mean time of 6 to 8 hr postoperatively. A deliberate attempt at tight wound closure was made at the time of surgery, raising a question about whether the pressure increase was the result of mechanical compression of the outflow system or merely preventing the effect of a postoperative wound leak in maintaining IOP control. Kirsch and coworkers explored this subject and described a gonioscopically visible ridge at the internal edge of a cataract incision resembling an inverted snowbank.[66] Intraoperative gonioscopy revealed that the ridge was present even before sutures were placed, suggesting that the tightness or placement of the sutures was not critical. Proposed mechanisms for the ridge included malposition of the internal lip of the corneal incision, inward cupping of Descemet's membrane, or corneal endothelial physiomechanical changes secondary to the incision, corneal edema, or a combination of these. For 2 wk, the ridge obscures visualization of the angle structures. Whether the corneal ridge simply obscures the view of the angle or creates clinically significant trabecular dysfunction is still a matter of debate. It is, however, associated with peripheral anterior synechia, hyphema, and vitreous adhesions.

Campbell and Grant examined the effect of corneoscleral sutures in the absence of corneal section on outflow facility in enucleated human eyes.[19] They found a decrease of approximately 50 percent in outflow facil-

1511

ity. This was associated with histologic sections demonstrating distortion and compression of underlying trabecular meshwork and collapse of Schlemm's canal. Outflow facility returned to baseline when the sutures were removed. Melamed used cationized ferritin perfusion as a tracer to define regional changes in aqueous flow through the trabecular meshwork.[77, 78] He found collapse of trabecular beams and loss of trabecular spaces in sutured regions. These changes were associated with reduced staining with cationized ferritin in the areas adjacent to Schlemm's canal. In contrast, unsutured areas of the trabecular meshwork showed diffuse staining outlining the entire outflow system.

Rich hoped to avoid trabecular involvement and decrease the incidence of IOP elevations by anteriorizing the wounds to clear cornea but continued to note postoperative IOP elevations.[94]

In contrast, Rothkoff and colleagues were able to demonstrate a decrease in the incidence of IOP elevations when corneal wounds were used instead of limbal wounds.[99]

Corticosteroid-Induced Glaucoma

Corticosteroids are typically prescribed after cataract extraction, so the principles of corticosteroid-induced glaucomas (see Chap. 129) must always be considered in these patients.

When a significant inflammatory response is noted postoperatively, high levels of corticosteroids are prescribed. Clinicians must recognize the effect that uveitis can have on both aqueous production and outflow facility. Corticosteroids influence each independently and therefore can have a profound effect on IOP independent of their ability to produce corticosteroid-induced glaucoma.

When corticosteroid-induced glaucoma does develop, the duration of drug use can be as short as 3 days but more commonly is 2 to 3 wk in cases of topical administration.[127] In general, the propensity for IOP elevation is correlated with antiinflammatory potency, frequency of application, and drug concentration.[90] Patients with primary open-angle glaucoma are especially sensitive to the IOP effects of corticosteroids, compared with patients with pseudoexfoliation glaucoma, who tend to respond like normal persons. Most patients who develop IOP elevations return to baseline IOP over days to weeks with the cessation of the corticosteroid medication. In rare patients, the effect persists and requires standard medical therapy for open-angle glaucoma. Because discontinuation of steroids is often required to normalize IOP, an obvious inherent risk is associated with posteriorly placed depot injections.

Alpha-Chymotrypsin

Alpha-chymotrypsin is a 23,000-dalton endopeptidase obtained from bovine pancreas; it hydrolyzes ester and peptide bonds. Alpha-chymotrypsin was introduced to the practice of ophthalmology when Baraquer reported that intracapsular cataract extraction was facilitated by enzymatic zonulysis.[7] That α-chymotrypsin is commonly associated with a rise in IOP after cataract extraction is well described.[41, 63, 65, 69] Kirsch first reported α-chymotrypsin–induced elevations of IOP in a controlled study of 343 nonglaucomatous patients.[63] In the first postoperative week, 72.5 percent of those patients in whom α-chymotrypsin was used versus 23.6 percent of the controls developed IOP elevations. Treatment to lower IOP was withheld during the postoperative period, and the natural history of the IOP elevation observed. The longest duration noted was 19 days. A small subgroup of patients with known glaucoma was similarly treated, with 80 percent of the α-chymotrypsin patients and 57.1 percent of the controls developing increased IOP. Packer and colleagues, in their study of nonglaucomatous patients, showed 69 percent of patients developing IOP greater than 25 mmHg and 29 percent of patients greater than 40 mmHg at 24 hr.[86] IOP as high as 56 mmHg at 24 hr and 75 mmHg at 36 hr postoperatively were noted. Patients with preexisting glaucoma may be at increased risk for elevations in IOP,[69] although this has not been universally noted.[43, 108]

Kirsh performed tonography before and after instillation of pilocarpine in patients with enzymatic glaucoma and confirmed the abnormally low facility of outflow associated with the hypertensive period,[64] and Jocson demonstrated an absence of long-term consequences of α-chymotrypsin on outflow facility.[58]

Both volume and concentration of the enzyme have been implicated in the production of enzymatic glaucoma.[8, 41, 65] Therefore, using minimum volumes of 1:10,000 versus 1:5000 solution may be associated with a decreased incidence of enzymatic glaucoma. Irrigation of the anterior chamber may decrease the load of zonular fragments to be cleared through the trabecular meshwork.

Viscoelastic Agents

Sodium hyaluronate is a large polysaccharide molecule of varying molecular weight that is a physiologic component of human vitreous as well as other connective tissues. In the 1970s, Balazs and coworkers evaluated its usefulness as a substitute for human vitreous and demonstrated its lack of antigenicity or inflammatory potential.[5] Miller and Stegmann reported on its use in anterior segment surgery.[80] Viscoelastic agents are now commonly used to maintain the anterior chamber, protect the corneal endothelium, and improve access to the capsular bag. The viscoelastic substances that are useful in ophthalmologic surgery share certain rheologic properties including viscosity, molecular volume, chain length, molecular rigidity, and shear, which may also be responsible for their tendency to induce or exaggerate IOP elevations after cataract extraction.[70] In a prospective study evaluating IOP rise at 6, 24, 48, and 72 hr, Naeser and colleagues found both an increased percentage of patients and an exaggeration of the IOP elevation and time course in sodium hyaluronate–treated eyes compared with controls in normal, nonglaucomatous patients.[82] Fifty-seven percent versus 44 percent of patients experienced an IOP increase greater than 5 mmHg at 6 hr despite meticulous aspiration of all sodium hyaluronate. Forty-three percent versus 19 percent of patients have experienced IOP greater than 26 mmHg, and 7 percent versus 0 percent of patients suffered IOP greater than 40 mmHg. It is important to note that no patient in either group had IOP elevation at 1 to 3 days. This may explain the conflicting results when IOP was not found to be elevated at the first postoperative (1 day) visit.[53] IOP greater than 60 mmHg has been reported and may last for 48 to 72 hr.[6] The mechanism by which sodium hyaluronate increases postoperative IOP is thought to be related to mechanical obstruction of the trabecular meshwork. When sodium hyaluronate was instilled into the anterior chamber of enucleated human eyes, a 65 percent reduction of outflow facility was noted.[11] Vigorous irrigation of the anterior chamber did not reverse this effect; however, irrigation with hyaluronidase restored normal outflow facility. When 9–0 nylon suture was used to simulate a cataract wound, outflow facility further deteriorated, leading investigators to speculate an exaggeration of the effect with a deformation of the cataract wound.[19] A number of investigators have noted dampening of the IOP effect when an anterior chamber washout is attempted.[42, 84] The effect is unpredictable, however, and great care should therefore be exercised in patients with compromised optic nerve function.[10]

Early, transient elevations of IOP after cataract extraction are frequent and multifactorial. Wound deformation may act in concert with α-chymotrypsin or viscoelastic agents to cause profound short-term IOP elevation. The role of increased surgical trauma in patients with glaucoma is unclear. In addition, fibrin and other serum proteins, red blood cells, prostaglandins, and inflammatory cells may contribute. In most cases, the peak hypertensive period is past when a patient is first examined postoperatively. When IOP remains dangerously elevated, β-blockers and carbonic anhydrase inhibitors offer the best short-term control. Hyperosmotic agents may also have a role. Miotics should be avoided if possible because of their effect on the blood-aqueous barrier. The efficacy of apraclonidine in this clinical setting has now been established.[131]

Intracameral acetylcholine[51, 100] and carbachol[52, 71] have been reported to be effective prophylaxis against postoperative IOP rise. It is noteworthy that neither has been associated with an increase in postoperative inflammation. Pilocarpine gel has been shown to be efficacious in this situation.[100] Beta-blockers[12, 46, 85, 87, 89, 94, 100, 120, 130] and carbonic anhydrase inhibitors have demonstrated variable efficacy.[86]

Prophylaxis appears prudent, especially in patients with compromised optic nerve function and known trabecular meshwork dysfunction (e.g., primary open-angle glaucoma), if there are no contraindications. McGuigan and colleagues found a 7-mmHg or greater rise in IOP in 62 percent of glaucomatous eyes versus only 10 percent of control eyes at 24 hr, with an average increase

in IOP of 10.2 mmHg at 24 hr.[76] The average short-term IOP was 33 mmHg. Ruiz and associates noted, while evaluating methods of prophylaxis against elevated IOP, that 55 percent of their patients receiving placebo demonstrated IOP of greater than 25 mmHg at 24 hr.[100]

Complete removal of sodium hyaluronate, minimal iris manipulation, and complete cortical cleanup are advisable. Examination at 6 to 8 hr increases the likelihood that episodes of elevated IOP will be observed.

Hyphema

Most hyphemas occur in the first few days after cataract surgery. These early postoperative hyphemas are generally well handled by the trabecular meshwork and do not constitute a pressure risk.[46] Fortunately, when elevations of IOP do occur in this setting, they tend to be transient. Patients may notice blurred vision,[13] but unless there is a significant rise in IOP, they will be otherwise asymptomatic and pain free. The source of bleeding in the immediate postoperative period appears to be either the iris or iris root or the corneoscleral incision. Bleeding tends to be more common with more posteriorly located corneoscleral wounds. As in hyphemas not associated with surgery, the mechanism of IOP elevation is mechanical obstruction of the trabecular meshwork with red blood cells, fibrin, and other blood proteins.

Patients with an underlying trabecular dysfunction (e.g., primary open-angle glaucoma) potentially experience higher and more prolonged IOP elevation postoperatively owing to hyphema. Additional medical therapy is occasionally necessary. It is generally possible to control the secondary glaucoma medically, but anterior chamber irrigation is occasionally necessary. Beta-blockers and carbonic anhydrase inhibitors are preferred, but hyperosmotic agents can be used to temporize. Apraclonidine may also be useful in this clinical setting. Pilocarpine tends to aggravate the inflammatory component of this process. Although control of dangerous levels of IOP is paramount, efforts should be made to allow the greatest possible aqueous flow to encourage passage of red blood cells through the trabecular meshwork. Corticosteroids should be used judiciously because they may produce trabecular meshwork dysfunction.

Late-onset hyphemas most commonly occur as a result of fine arborizing neovascularization of the inner aspect of the cataract incision.[57, 109, 118, 126] These blood vessels are fragile and can bleed spontaneously or as a result of minor trauma such as eye rubbing. In one study, the average time between surgery and presentation was 4 yr.[57] Patients most often complained of painless blurring of vision, especially on awakening. This symptom usually resolved over several hours. Pain and photophobia were also described in the constellation of symptoms associated with Swan's syndrome.[118] Care must be exercised during the examination because active bleeding can be provoked with dynamic gonioscopy. When the bleeding stops and the blood clears, the offending blood vessels can be gonioscopically visualized and ablated using argon laser goniophotocoagulation[92] or limbal cryopexy.[118]

In addition to this mechanism, posterior chamber intraocular lens haptics may erode into the ciliary sulcus,[74] causing late-onset hyphema. More commonly, anterior chamber intraocular lenses may produce hyphemas[68] in association with uveitis and IOP elevation ("UGH" syndrome).[34, 59, 132]

Ghost Cell Glaucoma

Although fresh red blood cells may induce an immediate and generally transient elevation of IOP, late-onset secondary glaucoma may present as a consequence of retained intraocular blood. Ghost cell glaucoma was first described by Campbell and colleagues in 1976.[20] Obstruction of the trabecular meshwork by degenerative spherical erythrocytes (erythroclasts) occurs as a consequence of the loss of pliability enjoyed by biconcave fresh erythrocytes. Erythroclasts are resistant to passage through the trabecular meshwork. Generally, the degeneration of red blood cells occurs in the vitreous cavity and therefore requires disruption of the anterior hyaloid face. While in the vitreous, red blood cells lose hemoglobin and convert to spherical transparent cell remnants whose plasma membranes are stippled with denatured hemoglobin clumps known as *Heinz bodies*. These characteristics, visible in phase-contrast microscopy of anterior chamber aspirates, can be useful if the diagnosis is in doubt.[117] The transformation tends to occur over weeks to months. The anterior hyaloid face serves as a barrier to passage from the vitreous cavity to the anterior chamber. In the setting of cataract extraction, any event that places blood in the vitreous cavity can be responsible for the subsequent emergence of ghost cell glaucoma.[116] Examples include postoperative hyphema associated with extracapsular cataract extraction, complicated by vitreous loss. The vitreous loss is associated with a violation of the anterior hyaloid face. The immediate postoperative period can be complicated by fresh red blood cells causing IOP elevation, but this is not necessary. Typically, one to three wk later, IOP elevation can occur secondary to ghost cell–induced obstruction of the trabecular meshwork.

The anterior chamber contains floating tan cells, which can be easily mistaken for white blood cells. If a pseudohypopyon is present, ghost cell glaucoma may be confused with an inflammatory process. Diagnostic clues include the absence of keratoprecipitates and a limited response to steroids. The candy-stripe sign refers to the passive layering out of the tan erythroclasts and fresh red blood cells.

Medical treatment may provide sufficient therapy for self-limited disease, but surgical intervention is most often necessary. Anterior chamber washout alone can temporize, but IOP again increases after 1 to 3 days unless vitrectomy is included to eradicate the reservoir of ghost cells in the vitreous cavity.[17, 116]

INFLAMMATION

Glaucoma associated with noninfectious intraocular inflammation can occur postoperatively as a result of the surgical procedure itself (see Lens Particle, Retained Cortex) or secondary to the implanted intraocular lens. It also occurs as an exacerbation of an underlying uveitic process. In this section, we concentrate on intraocular lens–induced inflammation. It is noteworthy that breakdown of the blood-aqueous barrier due to surgical manipulation is frequently encountered postoperatively but is rarely associated with a long-term inflammatory response or IOP elevation.

Historically important causes of noninfectious intraocular-related toxicity are residual polishing compounds.[79] The resulting postoperative sterile hypopyon typically presents only a few days after surgery and therefore can be confused with bacterial endophthalmitis. Ethylene oxide[111] and γ-radiation sterilization were also associated with pronounced postoperative inflammatory responses.

The physical properties of early intraocular lenses were often associated with mechanical irritation of ocular tissue and resultant breakdown of the blood-aqueous barrier, leading to chronic postoperative inflammation. The most notable examples were the warpage of the foot plates of some injection-molded lenses[33, 34] and imperfect finishing of poorly lathe-cut lenses, resulting in serrated or sharp edges.[4, 60] Proper sizing of these early lenses was critical, and even then rigid lenses often eroded deeply into the ciliary body.[75, 81] Highly flexible or undersized anterior chamber lenses were associated with the mobile lens syndrome and recurrent angle and iris trauma.[91] Peripheral anterior synechiae and "cocooning" at points of contact with the lens haptic can also be encountered.[4, 91, 136] Iris-supported lenses were notorious for iris chafing and erosion caused by excessive uveal contact.[67] Ellington is credited with bringing our attention to a syndrome whose constellation of signs was long present.[34] The "UGH" syndrome is characterized by *u*veitis, *g*laucoma, and *h*yphema.

Management of these related processes requires steroids to quiet the inflammatory process, mydriatics, and on rare occasions miotics to arrest iris movement. Antiglaucoma medications used are predominantly β-blockers and carbonic anhydrase inhibitors (miotics should generally be avoided because of their effect on the blood-aqueous barrier). If bleeding sites are visible, argon laser photocoagulation can be attempted. In cases with persistent inflammation, elevated IOP, toxicity of lens material, corneal decompensation, or evidence of physical bioincompatibility, then lens removal or exchange is necessary.

LENS PARTICLE, RETAINED CORTEX

After planned or unplanned extracapsular cataract extraction, retained cortical material may induce an inflammatory reaction and glaucoma. Liberated cortical material has been shown to effectively block trabecular outflow pathways in enucleated human eyes.[37] The additive role of high-molecular-weight soluble lens proteins, macrophages, and other cellular responses to the lens material is not clear.[98]

Clinically, cortical material may be visible in the anterior chamber and typically appears as fluffy white material. In addition, an often associated inflammatory response can be significant. If the amount of retained cortical material or the inflammatory response is disproportionate to the degree of IOP elevation, diagnostic paracentesis can be performed with microscopic examination for lens material and macrophages. A hiatus of days to weeks before the onset of IOP elevation is typical. The level and severity of glaucoma seem to be correlated with the load of cortical material. Significant amounts of cortex can be sequestered out of sight in the capsular bag.[35] The infrequency of lens particle glaucoma implies an inherent capacity of the normal trabecular meshwork to handle this material.

Medications that suppress aqueous production (β-blockers, carbonic anhydrase inhibitors, apraclonidine) are most useful in managing this disorder. Miotics should be avoided. Corticosteroids are useful to treat the inflammatory response and prevent synechial formation but should be tapered carefully. The use of excessive steroids can actually delay the clearance of lens material. If medical therapy is insufficient, then surgical aspiration of lens material is required.

"Phacoanaphylactic" uveitis with glaucoma has been described but is extremely rare. The onset is usually between 1 and 14 days after surgery. Treatment involves IOP stabilization, steroids to quiet the eye, and surgical intervention for complete removal of the offending lens material.

PIGMENTARY GLAUCOMA

Coincident with the increased frequency of posterior chamber intraocular lens implantation was the recognition of a new postoperative glaucoma associated with pigment dispersion. Unlike pigmentary glaucoma, described by Sugar in 1940,[112] this process is not limited to myopic eyes, is not bilateral, and occurs in eyes after intraocular lens implantation. Posterior chamber intraocular lenses are most typically implicated, but iris-supported lens-induced pigmentary glaucoma has been described.[6, 21]

Onset can be immediate and associated with markedly increased IOP or can be delayed by several months.[134] The mechanism of disease appears to be mechanical rubbing of the iris pigment epithelium by the implant with pigment release and trabecular dysfunction. When tonographic outflow facility has been measured, decreased outflow facility has been noted. However, clinical and experimental studies do not support the role of pigment dispersion alone in the pathogenesis of the trabecular dysfunction encountered in both idiopathic and intraocular lens-related pigmentary glaucoma.[36]

Iris transillumination defects classically tend to occur in areas of the haptic and adjacent to the optic edge and not in a radial midperipheral location.[102] In one study, four of six cases were associated with anteriorly angulated intraocular lenses.[102] Intraocular lens-related pigmentary glaucoma is often associated with lens decentration[134] or traumatic insertion. On gonioscopy, the angle of the involved eye tends to be dramatically laden with pigment, especially inferiorly, compared with the contralateral eye. Pigment dusting of the lens, iris, and corneal endothelium occurs. In blue irides, the iris can assume a gray discoloration.[54] Most cases are controlled medically, and the condition may improve over time. This complication should be avoided with "in the bag" placement of intraocular lenses.

VITREOUS-INDUCED GLAUCOMA

Loose vitreous filling the anterior chamber is a rare cause of secondary glaucoma after cataract extraction. As first described by Grant in 1963, this open-angle mechanism is not to be confused with vitreous-induced pupillary block.[44] Grant reported four cases and experimentally supported the contention that the disease was related to a mechanical obstruction of the trabecular meshwork by vitreous. Perfusion experiments using enucleated human eyes demonstrated decreased facility of outflow associated with vitreous completely filling the anterior chamber. Samples and Van Buskirk reported three additional cases characterized by a poor response to medical intervention.[103] Only one of these three cases occurred after cataract extraction, however. All three responded to vitrectomy, supporting the role of the vitreous in the development of elevated IOP. Vitreous-induced glaucoma generally develops over weeks to months or longer. In these cases, vitreous typically occupies the entire anterior chamber. On gonioscopy, vitreous is in contact with trabecular meshwork structures. It is at times difficult to appreciate the vitreous when there are few visible anatomic landmarks. However, close inspection may reveal pigment and cells suspended in its matrix.

Simmons reported spontaneous resolution of vitreous-induced glaucoma over months.[107] Grant[44] pointed out that mydriasis or miosis combined with hyperosmotic agents can be used to eliminate vitreotrabecular contact. Caution must be exercised in the diagnosis of vitreous-induced glaucoma because it remains a diagnosis of exclusion. Vitreous-induced glaucoma is anatomically unlikely without posterior capsular disruption either during the procedure or after YAG laser capsulotomy.

PREEXISTING AND UNSUSPECTED CHRONIC ANGLE CLOSURE

The existence of a significant degree of peripheral anterior synechiae can be associated with normal IOP, especially on a single determination. Outflow facility calculations have shown that approximately half of a normal trabecular meshwork can support normal or nearly normal IOP. However, the added insult of viscoelastic agents or wound deformation can result in profound IOP elevations. In addition, the aqueous misdirection syndrome is more likely to occur in these patients. Specific clinical entities are reviewed next.

Pupillary Block

Relative pupillary block occurring in phakic patients is due to the anatomic relationship between the iris and the crystalline lens, which offers increased resistance to the passage of aqueous from the posterior to the anterior chamber. In aphakic and pseudophakic patients, a functional anatomic pupillary block can exist, but one frequently encounters synechial formation between the iris and other ocular structures, typically the hyaloid, lens remnants including the posterior capsule, and the implanted intraocular lens.[50, 113, 114] Furthermore, the integrity of the eye, having been violated postoperatively, may no longer be a closed system, the implications of which are both mechanistic and therapeutic and shall be explored.

Aphakic pupillary block was first described by Bowman in 1863.[14] Aphakic pupillary block typically presents as iris bombe with angle closure. The anterior chamber is shallowed peripherally to a greater extent than centrally. Irregular shallowing of the anterior chamber may be seen in cases in which broad iridovitreal adhesions result in loculation of aqueous pools posterior to the iris, resulting in segmental pupillary block. The least reliable clinical feature of aphakic pupillary block is IOP.[3] Fifty percent of patients with aphakic pupillary block in one series had an IOP of less than 21 mmHg. "Normal" pressures most commonly resulted from wound leak, choroidal detachments associated with increased uveoscleral outflow, and inhibition of aqueous production. A number of conditions predisposed to the development of aphakic pupillary block. Historically, wound leak is very important.[29] Ninety-two percent of Cotliers series had wound leak, pupillary block, and choroidal detachments.[29] Wound leak results in shallowing of the anterior chamber, which is prominent both centrally and peripherally. It is often associated with hypotony and choroidal detachments. The cycle is then exaggerated by ciliary body rotation and displacement of vitreous, which can further promote pupillary block. A wound leak is confirmed in the presence of a positive Seidel's test.

Inflammation also predisposes to aqueous hyposecretion, pupillary membranes, and iridovitreal adhesions. Aphakia is often marked by broad adhesions of the vitreous to the iris,[113] thus the popularity of the term *iridovitreal block*. In round-pupil intracapsular cataract extractions, the development of functional and synechial pupillary block is increased.[22, 23, 114] Prolapse of an intact hyaloid face through the round pupil results in pupillary block.[61] The vitreous itself can block a patent iridec-

tomy.[105] It appears likely that for a vitreous-related episode of pupillary block, an intact hyaloid face is necessary because aqueous is capable of percolating through a broken hyaloid face.[26] However, inflammatory membranes or lens remnants may cause pupillary block in the presence of a violated hyaloid face. Placement of peripheral iridectomy is important but should not be too centrally located.[119] Lack of a basal iridectomy leaves an iris root remnant, which can be susceptible to hyaloid adhesions and blockage of the coloboma.

The time course of presentation is variable. Pupillary block may present in the immediate postoperative period[32, 50, 88] but has been described weeks to years after surgery.[61] Unfortunately, many cases are asymptomatic and are recognized at the time of routine examination.[106, 123]

Glaucoma may also result from air injected at the time of surgery.[135] Barkan observed air-induced pupillary block with iris bombe in a postoperative patient in 1938[9] and confirmed this mechanism in an animal model. Jaffe and Light proposed that air acts as a noncompressible space-occupying mass, especially in the presence of preoperative osmotic hypotonia, and is forced into apposition with the iris in either the anterior or posterior chamber, resulting in pupillary block.[56]

Pseudophakic Pupillary Block

Ridley is credited with developing modern intraocular lens rehabilitation of patients with cataract. It is apropos that he, too, is responsible for the first report of pseudophakic pupillary block. In pseudophakic pupillary block, the principles are the same but the anatomic position of the intraocular lens and the surgical condition of the eye may vary. In lenses that occupy the pupil, as in iris fixation lenses[62, 129] and rigid uniplanar anterior chamber lenses,[81, 123] the incidence of pupillary block is so high that peripheral iridectomy is considered requisite. Despite a patent peripheral iridectomy, pupillary block is still possible. The peripheral iridectomy can be occluded by vitreous,[21] inflammatory membranes, or lens remnants. Intraocular lens rotation can be responsible for peripheral iridectomy obstruction and pupillary block even with meticulous sizing of the implant.[81] The peripheral iridectomy may be involved in an iris tuck or prolapse.[81] Loculation of posterior aqueous pools with segmental pupillary block can be evident in quadrants not protected by patent peripheral iridectomy. Imperforate peripheral iridectomies are, of course, nonfunctional.

With the popularity of posterior chamber intraocular lenses, peripheral iridectomy has become less common. This is the result of confidence that pseudophakic pupillary block will not occur and concern about increasing trauma and bleeding. Pupillary block in this setting is still possible, however.[28] Inflammatory membranes and hyphema may be responsible for pupillary seclusion. Zonular dehiscence with an intact posterior capsule may be associated with vitreous prolapse and pupillary block.[133] Vitreous can prolapse through an intentional

(YAG laser capsulotomy) or inadvertent posterior capsular rent. In one study, diabetes mellitus was present in 6 of 12 patients[101] in whom pupillary block was associated with uncomplicated extracapsular cataract extraction with a posterior chamber intraocular lens and may be another risk factor for pseudophakic pupillary block glaucoma.[128] Many have advocated placement of a peripheral iridectomy even in uncomplicated extracapsular cataract extractions, although it should be noted that obstruction of a peripheral iridectomy is still possible by previously described mechanisms.

Angle closure can occur through mechanisms other than pupillary block. Late-onset progressive peripheral anterior synechiae have been reported with posterior chamber intraocular lenses.[39, 124] The mechanism is related to posterior "pushing" with closure of the overlying angle by the haptics of a posterior chamber intraocular lens. The incidence of peripheral anterior synechiae is higher (65 to 80 percent) with 10-degree anterior vaulted haptics[39] and when these lenses are sulcus supported.[83] In most cases, peripheral anterior synechiae are noted early and are nonprogressive. Anterior chamber intraocular lenses are also responsible for loss of functional trabecular meshwork through fibrosis and cocooning of the lens haptics.[91] Chronic uveitis may be associated with peripheral anterior synechiae or pupillary seclusion and pupillary block.

Pupillary block may be broken by mydriasis, but ultimately, peripheral iridotomy is necessary. Initially, β-blockers, carbonic anhydrase inhibitors, and hyperosmotic agents are useful in controlling IOP. The use of apraclonidine in this situation is also attractive but needs further investigation to confirm its effectiveness. Pilocarpine should only be used with caution. Steroids are effective in controlling inflammation. Efforts should be made to treat underlying conditions including severe inflammation and wound leak. If the condition is not treated appropriately, permanent difficulties with IOP control can emerge as a serious sequel to unrecognized pupillary block.[31]

Aqueous Misdirection Syndrome

Although more commonly encountered after filtration or combined cataract and glaucoma surgery, aqueous misdirection syndrome can be a sequel to standard extracapsular cataract extraction.[28, 48, 72, 105] It typically appears early in the postoperative course, but its presentation can be delayed by weeks to years.[30, 115] It may occur spontaneously or in association with the addition of a miotic agent[24, 96] or the cessation of cycloplegia. The principles and treatment of this syndrome are reviewed in Chapter 145. It is very important to emphasize that low or normal IOP is possible with clinical aqueous misdirection syndrome in the presence of an inadvertent filtering bleb, a wound leak, or choroidal detachments.

Standard medical treatment does not appear to be as successful in pseudophakic patients but should be attempted. Nd.YAG laser disruption of the posterior capsule or hyaloid face or both is an option in these patients and should be exercised before surgical vitrectomy.[15, 25, 38, 72, 97, 106, 121]

NEOVASCULAR GLAUCOMA

Neovascular glaucoma is rarely considered among the complications of cataract extraction. One retrospective study noted that neovascular glaucoma developed in diabetic patients after cataract extraction in 13 of 146 eyes after intracapsular cataract extraction (8.9 percent), 2 of 17 eyes after extracapsular cataract extraction with primary posterior capsulotomy (11.8 percent), and 0 of 53 eyes after extracapsular cataract extraction without primary capsulotomy.[93] These data seem to suggest the role of violating the integrity of the posterior capsule in promoting iris neovascularization. Reports have also described progression from nonproliferative to proliferative diabetic retinopathy after cataract extraction.[1, 55] For a more detailed discussion of neovascular glaucoma, see Chapter 132.

EPITHELIAL DOWNGROWTH

Epithelial and fibrous downgrowth as causes of late postoperative glaucoma are fortunately rare. Their decline in frequency is primarily related to improved wound closure, after it was appreciated that wound leaks[73, 110] and tissue incarceration[2] were associated with epithelial downgrowth.

In its earliest stage, epithelial downgrowth can be difficult to diagnose unless specifically considered. It is often associated with a persistent "uveitis" that does not respond to corticosteroid therapy. As the process continues, a characteristically scalloped migrating line of epithelium appears on the corneal endothelium. The iris is also involved in the migration of epithelial cells. The anterior chamber angle initially is anatomically open but physiologically obstructed. Over time, however, it begins to form peripheral anterior synechiae. The diagnosis of epithelial downgrowth is based on the clinical appearance but can be supported by both the argon laser, which when directed at areas of involved iris blanches the overlying epithelium,[73, 110] and anterior chamber paracentesis, which reveals circulating epithelial cells.[18]

Treatment is complicated and often unsatisfactory and is considered in detail in Chapter 184.

REFERENCES

1. Aiello LM, Wand M, Liang G: Neovascular glaucoma and vitreous hemorrhage following cataract surgery in patients with diabetes mellitus. Ophthalmology 90:7, 1983.
2. Allen JC: Epithelial and stromal ingrowths. Am J Ophthalmol 65:179 1968.
3. Anderson DR, Forster RK, Lewis ML: Laser iridotomy for aphakic pupillary block. Arch Ophthalmol 93:343, 1975.
4. Apple DJ, Brems RN, Park RB, et al: Anterior chamber lenses. Part I: Complications and pathology and a review of designs. J Cataract Refract Surg 13:157, 1987.

5. Balazs EA, Freeman MI, Kloti R: Hyaluronic acid and the replacement of vitreous and aqueous humor. Med Probl Ophthalmol 10:3, 1972.

6. Ballin N, Weiss DM: Pigment dispersion and intraocular pressure elevation in pseudophakia. Ann Ophthalmol 14:627, 1982.

7. Baraquer J: Totale Linsenex traktion Nach Suflosung Der Zonula durch Alpha-chymotrypsin Enzymatiche Zonulyse. Klin Monatsbl Augenheild 133:609, 1958.

8. Baraquer J, Rutlan J: Enzymatic zonulolysis and postoperative ocular hypertension. Am J Ophthalmol 63:159, 1967.

9. Barkan O: Glaucoma Caused by air blockade. Am J Ophthalmol 34:567, 1951.

10. Barron BA, Busin M, Page C, et al: Comparison of the effects of Viscoat and Healon on postoperative intraocular pressure. Am J Ophthalmol 100:377, 1985.

11. Berson FG, Patterson MM, Epstein DL: Obstruction of Aqueous Outflow by Sodium hyaluronate in enucleated human eyes. Am J Ophthalmol 95:668, 1983.

12. Biedner BZ, Rosenblatt I, David R, Sachs V: The effect of timolol on early increased intraocular pressure after cataract extraction. Glaucoma 4:53, 1982.

13. Binkhorst CD: Five hundred planned extracapsular extractions with irido-capsular and iris clip lens implantation in senile cataract. Ophthalmic Surg 8:37, 1977.

14. Bowman W: On extraction of cataract by a traction instrument with iridectomy with remarks on capsular obstructions and their treatment. Ophthalmic Hospital Reports 4:332, 1863.

15. Brown RH, Lynch MG, Tearse JE, Nunn RD: Neodymium-YAG Vitreous Surgery for phakic and pseudophakic malignant glaucoma. Arch Ophthalmol 104:1464, 1986.

16. Brown SVL, Tye JG, McPherson SD Jr: Intraocular pressure after intracapsular cataract extraction. Ophthalmic Surg 15:389, 1984.

17. Brucker AJ, Michels RG, Green WR: Pars plana vitrectomy in the management of blood-induced glaucoma with vitreous hemorrhage. Ann Ophthalmol 10:1427, 1978.

18. Calhoun FP Jr: An aid to the clinical diagnosis of epithelial downgrowth into the anterior chamber following cataract extraction. Am J Ophthalmol 61:1055, 1966.

19. Campbell DG, Grant WM: Trabecular deformation and reduction of outflow facility due to cataract and penetrating keratoplasty sutures [Abstract]. Invest Ophthalmol Vis Sci 18(Suppl):126, 1977.

20. Campbell DG, Simmons RJ, Grant WM: Ghost cells as a cause of glaucoma. Am J Ophthalmol 81:441, 1976.

21. Cashwell LF, Reed JW: Glaucoma management in pseudophakia. South Med J 79:10, 1986.

22. Chandler PA: Glaucoma from pupillary block in aphakia. Arch Ophthalmol 67:14, 1962.

23. Chandler PA: Glaucoma in aphakia. Trans Am Acad Ophthalmol Otolaryngol 67:483, 1963.

24. Chandler PA, Grant WM: Mydriatic-cycloplegic treatment in malignant glaucoma. Arch Ophthalmol 68:353, 1962.

25. Chandler PA, Grant WM: Malignant glaucoma medical and surgical treatment. Am J Ophthalmol 66:495, 1968.

26. Chandler PA, Johnson CC: A neglected cause of secondary glaucoma in eyes in which the lens is absent or subluxated. Arch Ophthalmol 37:740, 1947.

27. Cherfan GM, Rich WJ, Wright G: Raised intraocular pressure and other problems with sodium hyaluronate and cataract surgery. Trans Ophthalmol Soc UK 103:277, 1983.

28. Cohen JS, Osher RJ, Weber P, Faulkner JD: Complications of extracapsular cataract surgery. Ophthalmology 91:826, 1984.

29. Cotlier E: Aphakic flat anterior chamber. II: Effect of spontaneous reformation and medical therapy. Arch Ophthalmol 87:124, 1972.

30. Cotlier E, Herman S: Aphakic flat anterior chamber. Arch Ophthalmol 86:506, 1971.

31. Cotlier E: Aphakic flat anterior chamber. III: Effect of inflation of the anterior chamber and drainage of choroidal detachment. Arch Ophthalmol 88:15, 1972.

32. Cotlier E: Aphakic flat anterior chamber. IV: Treatment of pupillary block by iridectomy. Arch Ophthalmol 88:22, 1972.

33. Drews RC: Inflammatory response, endophthalmitis, corneal dystrophy, glaucoma, retinal detachment, dislocation, refractive error, lens removal, and enucleation. Symposium on Surgical Procedures 85:164, 1978.

34. Ellingson T: Complications with the Choyce Mark VIII anterior chamber lens implant (uveitis—glaucoma—hyphema). Am Intraocular Implant Soc J 3:199, 1977.

35. Epstein DL: Diagnosis and management of lens-induced glaucoma. Ophthalmology 89:3, 1982.

36. Epstein DL, Freddo TF, Anderson J, et al: Experimental obstruction to aqueous outflow by pigment particles in living monkeys. Invest Ophthalmol Vis Sci 27:387, 1986.

37. Epstein DL, Jedziniak JA, Grant WM: Obstruction of aqueous outflow by lens particles and by heavy-molecular-weight soluble lens proteins. Invest Ophthalmol Vis Sci 17:3, 272.

38. Epstein DL, Steinert RF, Puliafito CA: Neodymium-YAG laser therapy to the anterior hyaloid in aphakic malignant (ciliovitreal block) glaucoma. Am J Ophthalmol 98:137, 1984.

39. Evans RB: Peripheral anterior synechia overlying the haptics of posterior chamber lenses. Ophthalmology 97:415, 1990.

40. Francois J, Verbraeken H: Complications in 1,000 consecutive intracapsular cataract extractions. Ophthalmologica 180:121, 1980.

41. Galin MA, Barasch KR, Harris LS: Enzymatic zonulolysis and intraocular pressure. Am J Ophthalmol 61:690, 1966.

42. Glasser DB, Matsuda M, Edelhauser HF: A comparison of the efficacy and toxicity of and intraocular pressure response to viscous solutions in the anterior chamber. Arch Ophthalmol 104:1819, 1986.

43. Gombos GM, Oliver M: Cataract extraction with enzymatic zonulolysis in glaucomatous eyes. Am J Ophthalmol 64:68, 1968.

44. Grant WM: Open-angle glaucoma associated with vitreous filling the anterior chamber. Trans Am Ophthalmol Soc 61:197, 1963.

45. Gross JG, Meyer DR, Robin AL, et al: Increased intraocular pressure in the immediate postoperative period after extracapsular cataract extraction. Am J Ophthalmol 105:466, 1988.

46. Haimann MH, Phelps CD: Prophylactic timolol for the prevention of high intraocular pressure after cataract extraction. Ophthalmology 88:233, 1981.

47. Handa J, Henry JC, Krupin T, Keates E: Extracapsular cataract extraction with posterior chamber lens implantation in patients with glaucoma. Arch Ophthalmol 105:765, 1987.

48. Hanish SJ, Lamberg RL, Gordon JM: Malignant glaucoma following cataract extraction and intraocular lens implant. Ophthalmic Surg 13:713, 1982.

49. Hayreh SS: Anterior ischemic optic neuropathy. IV: Occurrence after cataract extraction. Arch Ophthalmol 98:1410, 1980.

50. Hitchings RA: Acute aphakia pupillary block glaucoma: An alternative surgical approach. Br J Ophthalmol 63:31, 1979.

51. Hollands RH, Drance SM, Schulzer M: The effect of acetylcholine on early postoperative intraocular pressure. Am J Ophthalmol 103:749, 1987.

52. Hollands RH, Drance SM, Schulzer M: The effect of intracameral carbachol on intraocular pressure after cataract extraction. Am J Ophthalmol 104:225, 1987.

53. Holmberg AS, Philipson BT: Sodium hyaluronate in cataract surgery. I: Report on the use of Healon in two different types of intracapsular cataract surgery. Ophthalmology 91:45, 1984.

54. Huber C: The gray iris syndrome. Arch Ophthalmol 102:397, 1984.

55. Jaffe GJ, Burton TC: Progression of non-proliferative diabetic retinopathy following cataract extraction. Arch Ophthalmol 106:745, 1988.

56. Jaffe NS, Light DS: The danger of air pupillary block glaucoma in cataract surgery with osmotic hypotonia. Arch Ophthalmol 76:633, 1966.

57. Jarstad JS, Hardwig, PW: Intraocular hemorrhage from wound neovascularization years after anterior segment surgery (Swan syndrome). Can J Ophthalmol 22:271, 1987.

58. Jocson VL: Tonography and gonioscopy before and after cataract extraction with alpha chymotrypsin. Am J Ophthalmol 60:318, 1965.

59. Johnson SH, Kratz RP, Olson PF: Iris transillumination defect and microhyphema syndrome. Am Intraocular Implant Soc J 10:425, 1984.

60. Keates RH, Ehrlich DR: "Lenses of chance" complications of anterior chamber implants. Ophthalmology 85:408, 1978.

61. Kessing Sv V, Rasmussen KE: Aphakic glaucoma. Acta Ophthalmol 55:717, 1977.
62. Kielar RA, Stambaugh JL: Pupillary block glaucoma following intraocular lens implantation. Ophthalmic Surg 13:647, 1982.
63. Kirsch RE: Glaucoma following cataract extraction associated with use of alpha-chymotrypsin. Arch Ophthalmol 72:612, 1964.
64. Kirsch RE: Further Studies on glaucoma following cataract extraction associated with the use of alpha-chymotrypsin. Trans Am Acad Ophthalmol Otolaryngol 69:1011, 1965.
65. Kirsch RE: Dose relationship of alpha chymotrypsin in production of glaucoma after cataract extraction. Arch Ophthalmol 75:774, 1966.
66. Kirsch RE, Levine O, Singer JA: Ridge at internal edge of cataract incision. Arch Ophthalmol 94:2098, 1976.
67. Kraff MC, Lieberman HL: Experience with the large circular loop medallion lens and a critical comparison with the suture medallion lens: A report of 300 Cases. Ophthalmic Surg 8:89, 1989.
68. Kratz RP, Mazzaocco TR, Davidson B, Colvard DM: A comparative analysis of anterior chamber, iris-supported, capsule-fixated, and posterior chamber intraocular lenses following cataract extraction by phacoemulsification. Ophthalmology 88:56, 1981.
69. Lantz JM, Quigley JH: Effects of alpha chymotrypsin. Can J Ophthalmol 8:339, 1973.
70. Liesegang TJ: Viscoelastic substances in ophthalmology. Surv Ophthalmol 34:268, 1990.
71. Linn DK, Zimmerman TJ, Nardin GF, et al: Effect of intracameral carbachol on intraocular pressure after cataract extraction. Am J Ophthalmol 107:133, 1989.
72. Lynch MG, Brown RH, Michels RG, et al: Surgical vitrectomy for pseudophakic malignant glaucoma. Am J Ophthalmol 102:149, 1986.
73. Maumenee AE: Treatment of epithelial downgrowth and intraocular fistula following cataract extraction. Trans Am Ophthalmol Soc 62:153, 1964.
74. McDonnell PJ, Champion R, Green WR: Location and composition of haptics of posterior chamber intraocular lenses. Ophthalmology 94:136, 1987.
75. McDonnel PJ, Green WR, Maumenee AE, Iliff WJ: Pathology of intraocular lenses in 33 eye examined postmortems. Ophthalmology 90:386, 1983.
76. McGuigan LJB, Gottsch J, Stark WJ, et al: Extracapsular cataract extraction and posterior chamber lens implantation in eyes with preexisting glaucoma. Arch Ophthalmol 104:1301, 1986.
77. Melamed S: Use of cationized ferritin to trace aqueous humor outflow. Exp Eye Res 43:273, 1986.
78. Melamed S: Alteration of trabecular aqueous flow after cataract extraction. Ophthalmic Surg 18:878, 1987.
79. Meltzer DW: Sterile hypopyon following intraocular lens surgery. Arch Ophthalmol 98:100, 1980.
80. Miller D, Stegmann R: Use of sodium hyaluronate in human intraocular lens implantation. Ann Ophthalmol 13:811, 1981.
81. Moses L: Complications of rigid anterior chamber implants. Ophthalmology 91:820, 1984.
82. Naeser K, Thim K, Hansen TE, et al: Intraocular pressure in the first days after implantation of posterior chamber lenses with the use of sodium hyaluronate (Healon). Acta Ophthalmol 64:331, 1986.
83. Naylor G, Morrell AJ, Sutton GA, Pearce JL: Intercapsular versus extracapsular cataract extraction. Ophthalmic Surg 20:766, 1989.
84. Olivius E, Thorburn W: Intraocular pressure after surgery with Healon. Am Intraocul Implant Soc J 11:480, 1985.
85. Ostbaum JA, Galin MA: The effects of timolol on cataract extraction and intraocular pressure. Am J Ophthalmol 88:1017, 1979.
86. Packer AJ, Fraioli AJ, Epstein DL: The effect of timolol and acetazolamide on transient intraocular pressure elevation following cataract extraction with alpha-chymotrypsin. Ophthalmology 88:3, 1981.
87. Passo MS, Ernest JT, Goldstick TK: Hyaluronate increases intraocular pressure when used in cataract extraction. Br J Ophthalmol 69:572, 1985.
88. Patti JC, Cinotti AA: Iris photocoagulation therapy of aphakic pupillary block. Arch Ophthalmol 93:347, 1975.
89. Percival SPB: Complications from use of sodium hyaluronate (Healonid) in anterior segment surgery. Br J Ophthalmol 66:714, 1982.
90. Podos SM, Krupin T, Assef C, Becker B: Topically administered corticosteroid preparations: Comparison of intraocular pressure effects. Arch Ophthalmol 86:251, 1971.
91. Poleski SA, Willis WE: Angle-supported intraocular lenses: A goniophotographic study. Ophthalmology 91:838, 1984.
92. Petrelli EA, Wiznia RA: Argon laser photocoagulation of inner wound vascularization after cataract extraction. Am J Ophthalmol 84:58, 1977.
93. Poliner LS, Christianson DJ, Escoffery RF, et al: Neovascular glaucoma after intracapsular and extracapsular cataract extraction in diabetic patients. Am J Ophthalmol 100:637, 1985.
94. Rich WJ: Further studies on early post-operative ocular hypertension following cataract extraction. Trans Ophthalmol Soc UK 89:639, 1969.
95. Rich WJ, Radtke ND, Cohan BE: Early ocular hypertension after cataract extraction. Br J Ophthalmol 58:725, 1975.
96. Rieser JC, Schwartz B: Miotic induced malignant glaucoma. Arch Ophthalmol 87:706, 1972.
97. Risco JM, Tomey KF, Perkins TW: Laser capsulotomy through intraocular lens positioning holes in anterior aqueous misdirection. Arch Ophthalmol 107:1569, 1989.
98. Rosenbaum JT, Samples JR, Seymour B, et al: Chemotactic activity of lens proteins and the pathogenesis of phacolytic glaucoma. Arch Ophthalmol 105:1582, 1987.
99. Rothkoff L, Biedner B, Blumenthal M: The effect of corneal section on early increased intraocular pressure after cataract extraction. Am J Ophthalmol 85:337, 1978.
100. Ruiz RS, Wilson CA, Musgrove KH, Prager TC: Management of increased intraocular pressure after cataract extraction. Am J Ophthalmol 103:487, 1987.
101. Samples JR, Bellows AR, Rosenquist RC, et al: Pupillary block with posterior chamber intraocular lenses. Arch Ophthalmol 105:335, 1987.
102. Samples JR, Van Buskirk EM: Pigmentary glaucoma associated with posterior chamber intraocular lenses. Am J Ophthalmol 100:385, 1985.
103. Samples JR, Van Buskirk ME: Open-angle glaucoma associated with vitreous humor filling the anterior chamber. Am J Ophthalmol 102:759, 1986.
104. Savage JA, Thomas JV, Belcher CD: Extracapsular cataract extraction and posterior chamber intraocular lens implantation in glaucomatous eyes. Ophthalmology 92:1506, 1985.
105. Shaffer RN: The role of vitreous detachment in aphakia and malignant glaucoma. Trans Am Acad Ophthalmol Otolaryngol 58:217, 1954.
106. Shrader CE, Belcher CD, Thomas JV, et al: Pupillary and iridovitreal block in pseudophakic eyes. Ophthalmology 91:831, 1984.
107. Simmons RJ: The vitreous in glaucoma. Trans Ophthalmol Soc UK 95:422, 1975.
108. Skalka HW: Alpha-chymotrypsin glaucoma. Ann Ophthalmol 8:151, 1976.
109. Speakman JS: Recurrent hyphema after surgery. Can J Ophthalmol 10:299, 1975.
110. Stark WJ, Micheles RG, Maumenee AE, Cupples H: Surgical management of epithelium ingrowth. Am J Ophthalmol 85:772, 1978.
111. Stark WJ, Rosenblum P, Maumenee AE, Cowan CL: Postoperative inflammatory reactions to intraocular lenses sterilized with ethylene oxide. Ophthalmology 87:385, 1980.
112. Sugar SH: Concerning the chamber angle in gonioscopy. Am J Ophthalmol 23:853, 1940.
113. Sugar SH: Pupillary block in aphakic eyes. Am J Ophthalmol 46:831, 1958.
114. Sugar SH: Pupillary block and pupil-block glaucoma following cataract extraction. Am J Ophthalmol 61:435, 1966.
115. Sugar SH: Bilateral aphakic malignant glaucoma. Arch Ophthalmol 87:347, 1972.
116. Summers CG, Lindstrom RL: Ghost cell glaucoma following lens implantation. Am Intraocular Implant Soc J 9:429, 1983.

117. Summers CG, Lindstrom RL, Cameron JD: Phase contrast microscopy: Diagnosis of ghost cell glaucoma following cataract extraction. Surv Ophthalmol 28:342, 1984.
118. Swan KC: Hyphema due to wound vascularization after cataract extraction. Arch Ophthalmol 89:87, 1973.
119. Swan KC: Relationship of basal iridectomy to shallow chamber following cataract extraction. Arch Ophthalmol 69:85, 1963.
120. Timida T, Tuberville AW, Wood TO: Timolol and postoperative intraocular pressure. Am Intraocular Implant Soc J 10:180, 1984.
121. Tomey KR, Senft SH, Antonios SR, et al: Aqueous misdirection and flat chamber after posterior chamber implants with and without trabeculectomy. Arch Ophthalmol 105:770, 1987.
122. Tuberville A, Tomoda T, Nissenkorn I, Wood TO: Postsurgical intraocular pressure elevation. Am Intraocular Implant Soc J 9:309, 1983.
123. Van Buskirk EM: Pupillary block after intraocular lens implantation. Am J Ophthalmol 95:55, 1983.
124. Van Buskirk EM: Late onset, progressive, peripheral anterior synechiae with posterior chamber intraocular lenses. Ophthalmic Surg 18:115, 1987.
125. Vu MT, Shields MB: The early postoperative pressure course in glaucoma patients following cataract surgery. Ophthalmic Surg 19:467, 1988.
126. Watzke RC: Intraocular hemorrhage from wound vascularization following cataract surgery. Trans Am Ophthalmol Soc 72:242, 1974.
127. Weinreb PN, Pulansky JR, Kramer SG, Baxter JD: Acute effects of dexamethasone on intraocular pressure in glaucoma. Invest Ophthalmol Vis Sci 26:170, 1985.
128. Weinreb RN, Wasserstrom JP, Forman JS, Ritch R: Pseudophakic pupillary block with angle-closure glaucoma in diabetic patients. Am J Ophthalmol 102:325, 1986.
129. Werner D, Kaback M: Pseudophakic pupillary-block glaucoma. Ophthalmology 61:329, 1977.
130. West DR, Lischwe TD, Thompson VM, Ide CH: Comparative efficacy of the β-blockers for the prevention of increased intraocular pressure after cataract extraction. Am J Ophthalmol 106:168, 1988.
131. Wiles SB, MacKenzie D, Ide CH: Control intraocular pressure with apraclonidine hydrochloride after cataract extraction. Am J Ophthalmol 111:184, 1991.
132. Wiley RG, Neville RG, Martin WG: Late postoperative hemorrhage following intracapsular cataract extraction with the 10 LAB 912 anterior chamber lens. Am Intraocular Implant Soc J 9:466, 1983.
133. Willis DA, Stewart RH, Kimbrough RL: Pupillary block associated with posterior chamber lenses. Ophthalmic Surg 16:108, 1985.
134. Woodhams T, Lester JC: Pigmentary dispersion glaucoma secondary to posterior chamber intraocular lenses. Ann Ophthalmol 16:852, 1984.
135. Wyman GJ: Glaucoma induced by air injections into the anterior chamber. Am J Ophthalmol 37:424, 1954.
136. Yeo JH, Jakobiec FA, Pukorny K: The ultrastructure of anterior intraocular lens "cocoon membrane." Ophthalmology 90:410, 1983.

Chapter 134

■

Malignant Glaucoma

MARSHALL N. CYRLIN

The term *malignant glaucoma* was first used by von Graefe[1] to describe a rare and severe form of glaucoma that followed ocular surgery. This complication was associated with elevated intraocular pressure and shallowing or flattening of the anterior chamber. The word *malignant* was used to characterize the uniformly poor visual prognosis. The current definition has been expanded to include *classic malignant glaucoma* as well as glaucomas occurring in other clinical situations. Classic malignant glaucoma is usually associated with the secondary glaucoma that follows incisional surgery for primary angle-closure glaucoma in phakic patients. Persistence of malignant glaucoma after cataract extraction in the classic form and the occurrence of malignant glaucoma after cataract surgery have been termed *aphakic malignant glaucoma*. The diagnosis *nonphakic malignant glaucoma* has been suggested for both aphakic and pseudophakic types.[2] The term *malignant-like glaucoma* has been proposed for cases with a known cause, other than aqueous trapped within the vitreous, for marked forward position of the lens/vitreous.[2]

Malignant glaucoma in its various clinical presentations exhibits

1. Shallowing or flattening of the peripheral and central anterior chamber

2. Increased intraocular pressure
3. Lack of lowering of the intraocular pressure in response to miotic treatment
4. Lowering of intraocular pressure or cure with mydriatic-cycloplegic treatment in many cases
5. Response to specific vitreous surgery
6. Absence of pupillary block

The term *malignant glaucoma* is undesirable to some clinicians because to patients it may suggest a neoplastic process and it is not related to the underlying mechanisms of the disease. For these reasons, various other terms based on presumed pathophysiologic mechanisms, such as *aqueous misdirection syndrome, ciliary block glaucoma,*[3, 4] and *direct lens block glaucoma*[5] have been proposed. Nonetheless, the term *malignant glaucoma* remains useful because it is readily understood by most clinicians to define the classic syndrome.

CLINICAL MANIFESTATIONS

The spectrum of disorders known as malignant glaucoma is divided into classic malignant glaucoma and other entities that share some or all of its clinical findings.

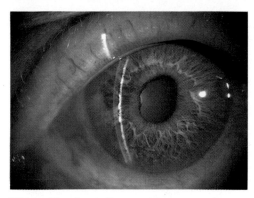

Figure 134–1. Classic malignant glaucoma with central and peripheral flat chamber after surgical peripheral iridectomy.

Classic Malignant Glaucoma

Classic malignant glaucoma following intraocular surgery has been noted to occur in 0.6 to 4 percent of eyes with a diagnosis of acute angle-closure glaucoma.[6–8] It typically develops after surgical peripheral iridectomy or filtering (full-thickness sclerectomy or trabeculectomy) surgery in phakic patients (Figs. 134–1 and 134–2). Shallowing of the chamber and elevated intraocular pressure may occur during the surgery, immediately afterward, following the cessation of cycloplegics,[9] after the initiation of miotics,[9, 10] or a considerable time later.[11–14] If one eye develops malignant glaucoma after surgery, the contralateral eye will probably do likewise. The chance of developing malignant glaucoma after surgery for angle-closure glaucoma is the highest when some of the angle remains closed at the time of the operation, regardless of whether or not the intraocular pressure has been reduced before surgery.[9]

The onset of malignant glaucoma is attended by anterior displacement of the iris-lens diaphragm, resulting in shallowing of the central as well as peripheral anterior chamber. The intraocular pressure may elevate to 40 to 60 mmHg or greater. Miotics are ineffective and may further increase the pressure. Conventional filtering surgery in patients who have had previous peripheral iridectomy does not reverse the process.

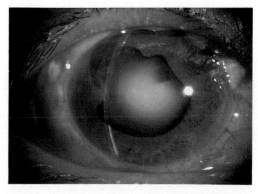

Figure 134–2. Classic malignant glaucoma with central and peripheral flat chamber after sector iridectomy and subsequent trabeculectomy.

Nonphakic Malignant Glaucoma

Malignant glaucoma in aphakia has been used to describe malignant glaucoma in patients with persistence of preexisting malignant glaucoma after cataract extraction as well as in patients with malignant glaucoma occurring de novo after routine cataract extraction. Cataract extraction as a treatment for classic malignant glaucoma was initially used by Rheindorf (1877).[15] Chandler (1950)[16] was the first to note that in those cases in which lens extraction was curative, vitreous loss occurred during the procedure. If vitreous was not lost, the patient had persistence of the classic malignant glaucoma. Shaffer (1954)[17] emphasized the importance of the vitreous in phakic and aphakic eyes with malignant glaucoma. He found that deep vitreous incision could be curative and proposed that posteriorly directed aqueous accumulated behind a vitreous detachment, leading to anterior displacement of the lens-iris diaphragm and angle closure.

Reports of nonphakic malignant glaucoma have increased during the past few decades. It has been noted after cataract surgery in eyes without preexisting glaucoma[7] and in eyes with anterior chamber intraocular lens implants at the time of cataract extraction.[18] In the latter circumstance, an initiating factor may be posterior displacement of the iris against the vitreous face by the intraocular lens. Malignant glaucoma has been described in eyes with posterior chamber implants and in patients who have had combined posterior chamber intraocular lens and filtration surgery.[19–24] Pseudophakic malignant glaucoma needs to be considered in postoperative patients with central shallowing of the anterior chamber and in patients with a shallow chamber and pressures in the teens or greater after a combined trabeculectomy and implant procedure.[25]

Other Malignant Glaucomas

Numerous clinical entities share some or all of the findings of classic phakic and nonphakic malignant glaucoma. Malignant glaucoma, malignant-like glaucoma,[2] and terms defining them by their presumed pathophysiologic mechanisms have been described by various authors. An extensive review of case reports in the literature has been presented by Luntz and Rosenblatt.[26]

Malignant glaucoma has been reported to occur under the following circumstances:

    I. Spontaneously[27, 28]
    II. After miotics
        A. With prior surgery
            1. Iridectomy[29]
            2. Filtration[10]
        B. Without prior surgery[30]
    III. After laser in glaucoma patients
        A. Following laser iridectomy
            1. Narrow angle[2]
            2. Acute angle closure[31]
            3. Chronic angle closure[32]
        B. Following laser suture lysis after trabeculectomy[33]

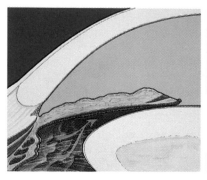 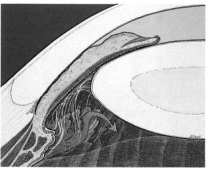

A   B

Figure 134–3. A, Normal pathway of aqueous flow from posterior chamber toward anterior chamber (arrows). B, Posterior aqueous diversion toward vitreous (arrows) in an eye with malignant glaucoma. The zonules are lax, the lens shifted forward, and the central and peripheral chamber shallowed. (Courtesy of Dr. B. T. Hutchinson.)

IV. Following trauma[5]
V. Associated with retinal disease
   A. Retinopathy of prematurity[34, 35]
   B. After retinal detachment surgery[36]
   C. After central vein occlusion[37]
VI. Associated with inflammation[5]
VII. Associated with infection
   A. Fungal keratomycosis[38]
   B. *Nocardia asteroides*[39]

PATHOGENESIS

The constellation of clinical findings in malignant glaucoma and its various presentations are believed to be the end result of aqueous misdirection or posterior aqueous diversion (Fig. 134–3). As mentioned earlier, Shaffer recognized early the effects of aqueous accumulation in the vitreous and its possible role in the pathogenesis of classic malignant glaucoma.[17] By strict definition, malignant glaucoma is not caused by pupillary block and is not cured by laser or surgical iridectomy. Mechanisms that involve various contributions of the lens or zonules, ciliary processes, anterior hyaloid face, or vitreous body have been proposed.

The term *ciliary block* has been used as an alternative to malignant glaucoma to emphasize the presumed role of the ciliary processes in blocking the forward flow of aqueous in many cases.[3, 4] It has been noted that swollen, anteriorly displaced ciliary processes may be pressed up against the lens or against abnormally forward vitreous in phakic patients, or ciliary processes may be touching or adherent to vitreous in aphakic patients (Fig. 134–4).[8] Anterior displacement of the lens has also been attributed to ciliary muscle contraction[5] or laxity of the zonules.[28, 40] Swelling, spasm, or displacement of the ciliary processes could then be further aggravated by miotics or inflammation. Direct lens block, as proposed by Levene,[5] would result from anterior displacement of the lens with flattening of both the peripheral and central anterior chamber and represents a more severe form of angle closure than the pupillary block type. To emphasize ciliary or direct lens block as the primary mechanism in malignant glaucoma underestimates the role of the vitreous, which is probably of greater importance.

Fatt has shown in animal eyes, in vitro, that as pressure is increased on the vitreous gel the vitreous becomes dehydrated and fluid conductivity is decreased.[41] In experimental perfusion studies in enucleated normal human eyes, Epstein and others have demonstrated a decrease in the permeability of the anterior hyaloid and vitreous gel to the anterior movement of fluid only at increased pressures.[42, 43] It was proposed that this resistance to the forward flow could be further increased by a reduction of anterior hyaloid surface area caused by apposition to the peripheral lens or ciliary body. Malignant glaucoma would result from a persistent expansion of the vitreous volume rather than from isolated pockets of trapped aqueous. Quigley has hypothesized a vicious cycle of elevated pressure, vitreous compaction and dehydration, further reduction in fluid conductivity, and shallowing of the chamber.[44] The final common pathway of the various contributing factors in malignant glaucoma is a self-perpetuating expansion of the vitreous (Fig. 134–5).

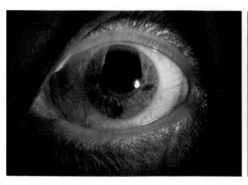 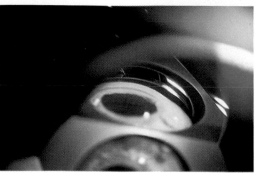

A   B

Figure 134–4. A, Aphakic malignant glaucoma, not relieved by multiple laser iridectomies, in an eye with an intact vitreous face bulging forward, totally flat anterior chamber, and intraocular pressure of 50 mmHg. B, Gonioscopic view of flattened ciliary processes adherent to vitreous. (Courtesy of Dr. P. A. Weber.)

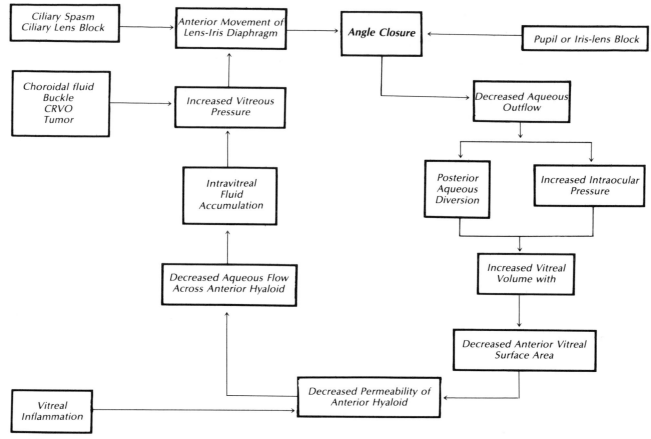

Figure 134–5. Possible mechanisms in malignant glaucoma emphasizing the role of the vitreous in maintaining the disease process. (CRVO, central retinal vein occlusion.) (From Luntz MH, Rosenblatt M: Malignant glaucoma. Surv Ophthalmol 32:73, 1987.)

DIFFERENTIAL DIAGNOSIS

Malignant glaucoma is distinguished by a postoperative flat anterior chamber in an eye with normal or elevated intraocular pressure. The diagnoses it is most commonly confused with are pupillary block, choroidal effusion, and suprachoroidal hemorrhage (Table 134–1).

Pupillary Block

Pupillary block glaucoma is often the most difficult situation to differentiate from malignant glaucoma. In pupillary block glaucoma, the pressure is usually elevated and the anterior chamber is shallow to flat. The anterior chamber in pupillary block glaucoma tends to remain deeper centrally than peripherally in comparison

Table 134–1. DIFFERENTIAL DIAGNOSIS OF MALIGNANT GLAUCOMA

	Malignant Glaucoma	Choroidal Separation	Pupillary Block	Suprachoroidal Hemorrhage
Anterior chamber	Flat or shallow	Flat or shallow	Flat or shallow	Flat or shallow
Intraocular pressure	Normal or elevated	Subnormal	Normal or elevated	Normal or elevated
Fundus appearance	No choroidal elevation	Large, smooth, light-brown choroidal elevations	Normal	Dark-brown or dark-red choroidal elevations
Suprachoroidal fluid	Absent	Straw-colored fluid present	Absent	Light-red or dark-red blood present
Relief by drainage of suprachoroidal fluid	No	Yes	No	Yes
Relief by iridectomy	No	No	Yes	No
Patent iridectomy	Yes	Yes	No	Yes
Onset	At surgery or first 5 days postoperatively, but sometimes weeks to months postoperatively	First 5 days postoperatively, occasionally later	Early or late postoperatively	At surgery or first 5 days postoperatively, rarely later

From Simmons RJ, Thomas JV, Yaqub MK: Malignant glaucoma. *In* Ritch R, Shields MB, Krupin T (eds): The Glaucomas. St. Louis, CV Mosby, 1989.

with malignant glaucoma, in which axial shallowing occurs as well. This is not a pathognomonic finding, however, and marked axial shallowing may be noted in some patients on strong miotics. First to be evaluated is the presence and patency of an iris coloboma. This can usually be determined by careful slit-lamp examination. Previously made iridectomies should be full thickness and not occluded by ciliary processes, inflammatory debris, the anterior hyaloid face, vitreous, retained lens material, or intraocular lenses. In selected cases, in relatively quiet eyes, injection of 10 ml of 5 percent aqueous solution of fluorescein into the antecubital vein can be used as a simple clinical test to establish the presence or absence of a communication between the posterior and anterior chamber.[45] Normally, in approximately 30 seconds the fluorescein is seen seeping through the pupil during slit-lamp examination. In malignant glaucoma, fluorescein-tinged aqueous is seen to pool in the posterior segment, posterior to the lens in phakic individuals, or posterior to the vitreous face, pseudophakos, or inflammatory membrane in nonphakic patients.[46] If a patent communication between the posterior and anterior chambers cannot be determined with certainty, another iridectomy should be created, preferably with the argon or neodymium:yttrium-aluminum-garnet (Nd.YAG) laser. In cases of pupillary block glaucoma, the anterior chamber will deepen after laser treatment.

Choroidal Effusion

Choroidal effusion is associated with a shallow or flat anterior chamber following filtering surgery. The intraocular pressure is usually low. On ophthalmoscopy, light-brown peripheral choroidal elevations that contain a straw-colored fluid are generally visible. If visibility is poor or they cannot be discerned, ultrasonography may be needed. With rare exception, fluid is not present in the suprachoroidal space in patients with malignant glaucoma.[6] Posterior sclerotomies with drainage of the choroidal fluid and anterior chamber reformation through paracentesis are curative in cases of effusion.

Suprachoroidal Hemorrhage

Suprachoroidal hemorrhage presents with a shallow or flat chamber at the time of surgery or usually within 1 week. The intraocular pressure is normal or elevated. Sudden onset of ocular pain and increased inflammation are characteristic. Findings on examination are similar to choroidal effusion except for a darker brown or dark-red appearance of the choroidal elevations. When posterior sclerotomies and drainage are performed, bright- or dark-red blood is obtained.

Overfiltration and Wound Leak

Overfiltration and wound leak are also associated with shallow or flat postoperative anterior chambers and are usually not confused with malignant glaucoma. In both cases, the pressure is low. Overfiltration is associated with a well-formed filtration bleb. A wound leak is identified by a positive Seidel's sign and a small bleb. Choroidal effusions may or may not be present.

MANAGEMENT

Medical and surgical management of malignant glaucoma has greatly improved with advances in our understanding of the pathophysiologic mechanisms of this disease in its various presentations. As noted previously, cataract extraction alone as an early treatment for phakic malignant glaucoma did not prove successful.[15] The role of the vitreous was better appreciated when cataract extraction with vitreous loss or disruption proved curative.[16, 17] Early attempts at treatment with miotics proved equally unsuccessful.[8] As has been discussed, these drugs may actually worsen or precipitate malignant glaucoma. Chandler and Grant (1962) advocated the effective use of cycloplegic-mydriatic drugs.[40] Weiss and colleagues (1963)[47] suggested treatment with intravenous hyperosmotic agents. Oral and topical aqueous suppressants have been added to our pharmacologic armamentarium.

Medical Treatment

Current medical treatment consists of atropine (1 to 4 percent) drops q.i.d., phenylephrine (2.5 to 10 percent) drops q.i.d., a topical β-blocker (timolol, bunolol, betaxolol, metipranolol, or carteolol) b.i.d., and an oral carbonic anhydrase inhibitor (acetazolamide, 250 mg q.i.d. or 500 mg sequel b.i.d., or methazolamide, 50 mg b.i.d.). In phakic patients, the atropine paralyzes the sphincter muscle of the ciliary body. The phenylephrine stimulates the α-adrenergic receptors of the longitudinal muscle of the ciliary muscle. This combination tightens the zonules and helps to pull the anteriorly displaced lens posteriorly. The result would presumably reduce "direct lens block" or "ciliary block" and increase the surface area of the anterior hyaloid. The β-blockers and carbonic anhydrase inhibitors lower intraocular pressure by decreasing the volume of posterior aqueous diversion and further compaction of the vitreous. An oral osmotic agent (50 percent glycerol or isosorbide) or intravenous 20 percent mannitol in a dosage of 1 to 2 g/kg can be administered, with caution, every 12 to 24 hours. The osmotic agents serve to further reduce vitreous volume, deepen the anterior chamber, and possibly increase vitreous permeability. Topical steroids may also be helpful in reducing inflammation.[48] Oral steroids have been recommended for some cases of nonclassic (pseudomalignant) glaucoma.[49]

Medical therapy has been reported to be curative in 50 percent of patients within 5 days.[6, 7] Following resolution, administration of at least one drop of atropine daily may be required indefinitely to prevent relapse.[9]

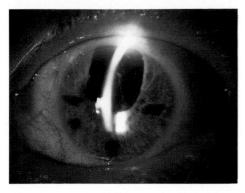

Figure 134–6. Relief of aphakic malignant glaucoma (see Fig. 134–4) with Nd.YAG laser to the superior vitreous face. Chamber deepened after laser. (Courtesy of Dr. P. A. Weber.)

Laser and Cyclocryotherapy

Argon laser treatment of the ciliary processes, with or without adjunctive medical therapy, has been advocated for phakic and aphakic malignant glaucoma.[50, 51] The Nd.YAG laser has been used to treat the anterior hyaloid or posterior lens capsules in cases of aphakic or pseudophakic malignant glaucoma.[22, 52] Cyclocryotherapy has also been reported as a treatment for malignant glaucoma.[53] The rationale for the previously mentioned procedures is to relieve ciliary block or the disruption of the anterior hyaloid face by thermal or mechanical means (Fig. 134–6).

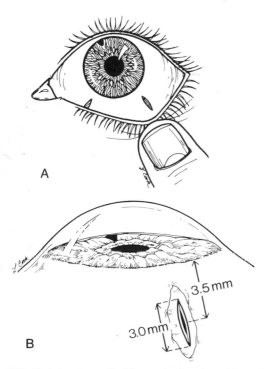

Figure 134–7. Sclerotomy incisions. A, Relationship to limbus. B, Size of sclerotomy incision and its distance from limbus. (From Simmons RJ, Thomas JV, Yaqub MK: Malignant glaucoma. In Ritch R, Shields MB, Krupin T [eds]: The Glaucomas. St. Louis, CV Mosby, 1989.)

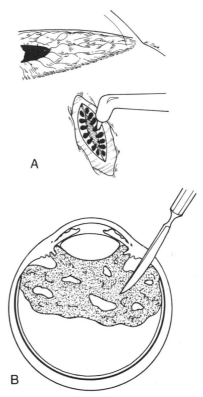

Figure 134–8. Sclerotomy technique. A, Diathermy is placed at inner edges of scleral wound to cauterize inner scleral layers, as well as vessels in adjacent wound. Diathermy should not be applied directly to choroid, because it may cause and stimulate bleeding. B, Wheeler's knife is used to pierce uvea and enter vitreous cavity. Knife should be kept away from lens by aiming it toward optic nerve head. (From Simmons RJ, Thomas JV, Yaqub MK: Malignant glaucoma. In Ritch R, Shields MB, Krupin T [eds]: The Glaucomas. St. Louis, CV Mosby, 1989.)

Surgical Therapy

When medical or laser therapy is not successful in relieving malignant glaucoma, vitreous surgery is indicated. Simmons has advocated a "surgical confirmation procedure" in which other diagnostic possibilities such as pupillary block or choroidal effusion are ruled out in the operating room before proceeding with vitreous surgery.[8] Radial incisions are made through the sclera to the suprachoroidal space, about 3 mm in length with their centers carefully measured 3.5 mm from the limbus in both inferior quadrants (Fig. 134–7). If the straw-colored fluid of choroidal effusion or blood is found, the fluid is drained and the procedure terminated. If no fluid is found, a posterior sclerotomy is made at one of the sites (Fig. 134–8). Simmons emphasizes that the success of Chandler's manual deep vitreous surgery method is dependent on exacting attention given to all of the details (Fig. 134–9).[7, 8] Luntz and colleagues, to the contrary, have described cases in which suprachoroidal effusion and vitreous loculation of aqueous have occurred simultaneously, necessitating drainage of both the suprachoroidal space and vitreous cavities.[54] Automated mechanical vitrectomy through a posterior sclerotomy in a phakic eye or through a limbal approach in

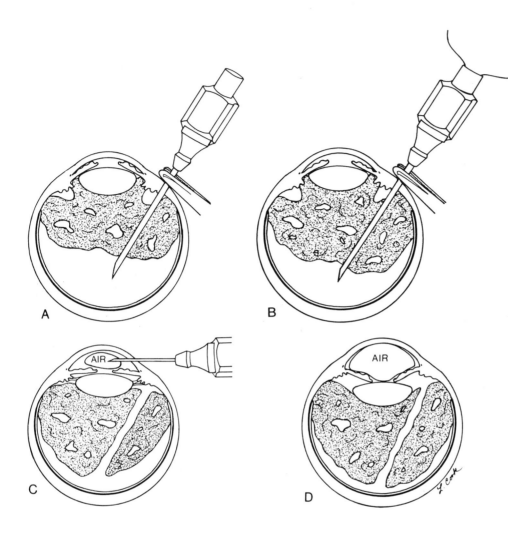

Figure 134–9. Sclerotomy technique. *A,* An 18-gauge needle is inserted 12 mm from the needle point. A hemostat guard to control depth of needle is shown. *B,* A syringe is attached to an 18-gauge needle, and 1.0 to 1.5 ml of vitreous is aspirated. *C,* Air bubble is placed in anterior chamber to deepen it. *D,* Size of air bubble should be large enough to deepen chamber to a depth greater than usually encountered in a normal myopic eye. (From Simmons RJ, Thomas JV, Yaqub MK: Malignant glaucoma. *In* Ritch R, Shields MB, Krupin T [eds]: The Glaucomas. St. Louis, CV Mosby, 1989.)

Figure 134–10. *A,* Posterior sclerotomy with disruption of the anterior hyaloid face and automated mechanical vitrectomy for malignant glaucoma. *B,* Deepening of anterior chamber with viscoelastic agent *(arrow)* through a paracentesis after vitrectomy. (Courtesy of Dr. B. T. Hutchinson.)

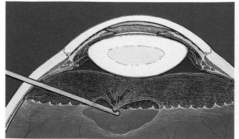

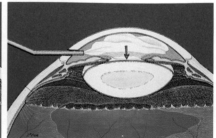

a nonphakic eye has been reported as an alternative to the manual method.[55-59] The rationale for vitreous surgery is disruption of the anterior hyaloid face, reduction of vitreous volume, and deepening of the anterior chamber (Fig. 134–10).

Management of the Contralateral Eye

After an episode of malignant glaucoma in one eye, the risk of malignant glaucoma in the contralateral eye is significant if surgery is needed following an acute angle-closure attack.[60] It may be advisable to create a laser iridectomy in the fellow eye, without pretreatment with miotics, before surgical intervention on the involved eye.[8]

REFERENCES

1. von Graefe A: Beitrage zur pathologie und therapie des glaucoma. Arch Ophthalmol 15:108, 1869.
2. Levene R: Malignant glaucoma: Proposed definition and classification. In Shields MB, Pollack I, Kolker A (eds): Perspectives in Glaucoma. Transactions of the First Scientific Meeting of the American Glaucoma Society. Thorofare, NJ, Slack, 1988, pp 243–350.
3. Weiss DI, Shaffer RN: Ciliary block (malignant) glaucoma. Trans Am Acad Ophthalmol Otol 76:450, 1972.
4. Shaffer RN, Hoskins HD Jr: Ciliary block (malignant) glaucoma. Ophthalmology 85:215, 1978.
5. Levene R: A new concept of malignant glaucoma. Arch Ophthalmol 87:497, 1972.
6. Chandler PA, Simmons RJ, Grant WM: Malignant glaucoma: Medical and surgical treatment. Am J Ophthalmol 66:495, 1968.
7. Simmons RJ: Malignant glaucoma. Br J Ophthalmol 56:263, 1972.
8. Simmons RJ, Thomas JV, Yaqub MK: Malignant glaucoma. In Ritch R, Shields MB, Krupin T (eds): The Glaucomas. St. Louis, CV Mosby, 1989, pp 1251–1263.
9. Simmons RJ: Malignant glaucoma. In Epstein DL (ed): Chandler and Grant's Glaucoma. Philadelphia, Lea & Febiger, 1986, pp 264–278.
10. Merritt JC: Malignant glaucoma induced by miotics postoperatively in open-angle glaucoma. Arch Ophthalmol 95:1988, 1977.
11. Hoshiwara I: Case report of simultaneous malignant glaucoma occurring 3 years after glaucoma surgery. Arch Ophthalmol 72:601, 1964.
12. Gorin G: Angle-closure glaucoma induced by miotics. Am J Ophthalmol 62:1063, 1966.
13. Jafar MS, Tomey KF: Malignant glaucoma manifesting bilaterally 15 months after peripheral iridectomy. Glaucoma 4:177, 1982.
14. Ellis PP: Malignant glaucoma occurring 16 years after successful filtering surgery. Ann Ophthalmol 16:177, 1984.
15. Rheindorf O: Uber glaukom. Klin Monatsbl Augenheilkd 25:148, 1887.
16. Chandler PA: Malignant glaucoma. Trans Am Ophthalmol Soc 48:128, 1950.
17. Shaffer RN: The role of vitreous detachment in aphakic and malignant glaucoma. Trans Am Acad Ophthalmol Otol 58:217, 1954.
18. Hanish SJ, Lamberg RL, Gordon JM: Malignant glaucoma following cataract extraction and intraocular lens implant. Ophthalmic Surg 13:713, 1982.
19. Tomey KF, Senft SH, Antonios SR, et al: Aqueous misdirection and flat chamber after posterior chamber implants with and without trabeculectomy. Arch Ophthalmol 105:770, 1987.
20. Duy TP, Wollensak J: Ciliary block (malignant) glaucoma following posterior chamber lens implantation. Ophthalmic Surg 18:741, 1987.
21. Dickens CJ, Shaffer RN: The medical treatment of ciliary block

22. Risco JM, Tomey KF, Perkins TW: Laser capsulotomy through intraocular lens positioning holes in anterior aqueous misdirection. Arch Ophthalmol 107:1569, 1989.
23. Reed JE, Thomas JV, Lytle RA, et al: Malignant glaucoma induced by an intraocular lens. Ophthalmic Surg 21:177, 1990.
24. Boreham C: Combined extracapsular cataract extraction and posterior chamber intraocular lens implantation and trabeculectomy. Aust N Z J Ophthalmol 15:201, 1987.
25. Epstein DL: Pseudophakic malignant glaucoma—Is it really pseudo-malignant? Am J Ophthalmol 103:231, 1987.
26. Luntz MH, Rosenblatt M: Malignant glaucoma. Surv Ophthalmol 32:73, 1987.
27. Schwartz AL, Anderson DR: "Malignant glaucoma" in an eye with no antecedent operation or miotics. Arch Ophthalmol 93:379, 1975.
28. Lowe RF: Malignant glaucoma related to primary angle closure glaucoma. Aust N Z J Ophthalmol 7:11, 1979.
29. Pecora JL: Malignant glaucoma worsened by miotics in a postoperative angle-closure glaucoma patient. Ann Ophthalmol 11:1412, 1979.
30. Rieser JC, Schwartz B: Miotic-induced malignant glaucoma. Arch Ophthalmol 87:706, 1972.
31. Brooks AM, Harper CA, Gillies WE: Occurrence of malignant glaucoma after laser iridotomy. Br J Ophthalmol 73:617, 1989.
32. Robinson A, Prialnic M, Deutsch D, et al: The onset of malignant glaucoma after prophylactic laser iridotomy. Am J Ophthalmol 110:95, 1990.
33. DiSclafani M, Liebmann JM, Ritch R: Malignant glaucoma following argon laser release of scleral flap sutures after trabeculectomy. Am J Ophthalmol 108:597, 1989.
34. Pollard AF: Secondary angle closure glaucoma in cicatricial retrolental fibroplasia. Am J Ophthalmol 89:651, 1980.
35. Kushner BJ: Ciliary block in retinopathy of prematurity. Arch Ophthalmol 100:1078, 1982.
36. Weiss IS, Deiter PD: Malignant glaucoma syndrome following retinal detachment surgery. Ann Ophthalmol 6:1099, 1974.
37. Weber PA, Cohen JS, Baker D: Central retinal vein occlusion and malignant glaucoma. Arch Ophthalmol 105:635, 1987.
38. Jones BR: Principles in the management of oculomycosis. Trans Am Acad Ophthalmol Otol 79:15, 1975.
39. Lass JH, Thoft RA, Bellows AR, et al: Exogeneous nocardia asteroides endophthalmitis associated with malignant glaucoma. Ann Ophthalmol 13:317, 1981.
40. Chandler PA, Grant WM: Mydriatic-cycloplegic treatment in malignant glaucoma. Arch Ophthalmol 68:353, 1962.
41. Fatt I: Hydraulic flow conductivity of the vitreous gel. Invest Ophthalmol Vis Sci 16:555, 1977.
42. Epstein DL, Hashimoto JM, Anderson PJ, Grant WM: Experimental perfusions through the anterior and vitreous chambers with possible relationships to malignant glaucoma. Am J Ophthalmol 88:1078, 1979.
43. Epstein DL: Malignant glaucoma. In Jacobiec FA, Sigelman J (eds): Advanced Techniques in Ocular Surgery. Philadelphia, WB Saunders, 1984, pp 158–168.
44. Quigley HA: Malignant glaucoma and fluid flow rate. [Editorial] Am J Ophthalmol 89:879, 1980.
45. Ray RR, Binkhorst RD: The diagnosis of pupillary block glaucoma by intravenous injection of fluorescein. Am J Ophthalmol 61:481, 1966.
46. Spaeth GL: Flat anterior chamber. In Sherwood MB, Spaeth GL (eds): Complications of Glaucoma Therapy. Thorofare, NJ, Slack, 1990, pp 229–236.
47. Weiss DI, Shaffer RN, Harrington DO: Treatment of malignant glaucoma with intravenous mannitol infusion: Medical reformation of the anterior chamber by means of an osmotic agent: A preliminary report. Arch Ophthalmol 69:154, 1963.
48. Phelps CD: Angle closure glaucoma secondary to ciliary body swelling. Arch Ophthalmol 92:287, 1974.
49. Beckman H, Blau RP: Oral steroid therapy for ciliary (pseudo-malignant) glaucoma. Glaucoma 3:169, 1981.
50. Herschler J: Laser shrinkage of the ciliary processes: A treatment for malignant (ciliary block) glaucoma. Ophthalmology 87:1155, 1980.

glaucoma after extracapsular cataract extraction. Am J Ophthalmol 103:237, 1987.

51. Weber PA, Henry MA, Kapetansky FM, et al: Argon laser treatment of the ciliary processes in aphakic glaucoma with flat anterior chamber. Am J Ophthalmol 97:82, 1984.
52. Epstein DL, Steinert RF, Puliafito CA: Neodymium-YAG laser therapy to the anterior hyaloid in aphakic malignant (ciliovitreal block) glaucoma. Am J Ophthalmol 98:137, 1984.
53. Benedikt O: A new operative method for the treatment of malignant glaucoma. Klin Monatsbl Augenheilkd 170:665, 1977.
54. Luntz MH, Harrison R, Schenker H: Management of secondary glaucoma. In Glaucoma Surgery. Baltimore, Williams & Wilkins, 1984, pp 107–116.
55. Boke W, Teichmann KD, Junge W: Experiences with ciliary block ("malignant") glaucoma. Klin Monatsbl Augenheilkd 177:407, 1980.
56. Koerner FH: Anterior pars plana vitrectomy in ciliary and iris block glaucoma. Graefes Arch Clin Exp Ophthalmol 214:119, 1980.
57. Weiss H, Shin DH, Kollarits CR: Vitrectomy for malignant (ciliary block) glaucomas. Int Ophthalmol Clin 21:113, 1981.
58. Momeda S, Hayashi H, Oshima K: Anterior pars plana vitrectomy for phakic malignant glaucoma. Jpn J Ophthalmol 27:73, 1983.
59. Lynch MG, Brown RH, Michels RG, et al: Surgical vitrectomy for pseudophakic malignant glaucoma. Am J Ophthalmol 102:148, 1986.
60. Shields MD: Glaucomas following ocular surgery. In Textbook of Glaucoma. Baltimore, Williams & Wilkins, 1992, pp 400–406.

Chapter 135

▼

Nanophthalmos: Guidelines for Diagnosis and Therapy

OMAH S. SINGH and SANDRA J. SOFINSKI

Nanophthalmos is a rare form of pure microphthalmos that results from arrested development of the globe after closure of the embryonic fissure.[1] Microphthalmos represents a spectrum of phenotypes with variable penetrance, manifesting as primary anophthalmos with lack of a clinically detectable eyeball; microphthalmos with cyst, caused by failure of the embryonic fissure to close at the 7- to 14-mm stage; complicated microphthalmos, associated with ocular and systemic anomalies; and pure microphthalmos, also referred to as nanophthalmos, which is not generally associated with ocular or systemic anomalies.[1–9]

Nanophthalmos is usually bilateral and may be inherited in sporadic, autosomal dominant, or autosomal recessive fashions.[1–9] Nanophthalmos is derived from the Greek word "nano," meaning dwarf, and represents an eye reduced in volume but otherwise grossly normal in form and function.[1–8]

CHARACTERISTICS

Clinical characteristics of the eye in nanophthalmos usually include a narrow palpebral fissure with a deeply set eyeball in a small orbit (Fig. 135–1). Marked hypermetropia is characteristic, but lesser ranges of hypermetropia, emmetropia, and rarely myopia have been reported.[1–8] Typically, the young nanophthalmic patient is extremely hyperopic and has good visual acuity corrected by glasses resembling aphakic spectacles. The globe demonstrates reduced total axial length (14 to

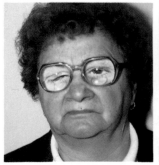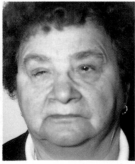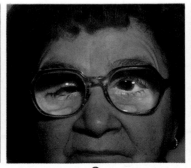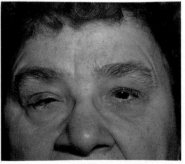

A   B   C   D

Figure 135–1. A–D, A 64-year-old white woman experienced external characteristics of nanophthalmos including deeply set eyes in small bony orbits, narrow palpebral fissures, and hyperopic refractive correction resembling aphakic spectacles.

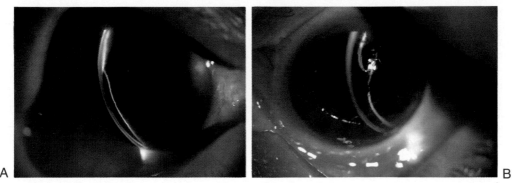

Figure 135–2. *A* and *B*, The parallelopiped of light demonstrates asymmetric stages of anterior chamber shallowing by slit-lamp examination.

20.50 mm),* small equatorial and transverse diameters, with reduced ocular volume to two thirds that of the normal eye.[1, 10] The corneal diameter may be normal or reduced (10 to 11.5 mm), and the crystalline lens has a normal volume. In the young nanophthalmic patient the anterior chamber is open in the presence of prominent iris convexity. Progressive anterior chamber shallowing and narrowing of the angle occurs with the onset of angle-closure during the fourth to sixth decades (Fig. 135–2).[11] The posterior segment may appear normal, but varying degrees of macular hypoplasia associated with nystagmus and strabismus may occur. The choroid may show maldevelopment, and the sclera is abnormally thickened with reduced permeability to protein, thus

predisposing nanophthalmic patients to choroidal effusion and nonrhegmatogenous retinal detachments.[1, 5, 12–14] Goldmann applanation tensions may reveal a wide ocular pulse (8 to 12 mmHg) consistent with thickened sclera and impaired drainage of vortex veins. The fundus may exhibit bone spicule changes of the retinal pigment epithelium, resembling a retinitis pigmentosa pattern (Fig. 135–3).[1, 15]

Nanophthalmos is not characteristically associated with systemic abnormalities. However, one case reports the association of nanophthalmos and cryptorchidism.[16] This is hypothesized to result from abnormal forebrain development leading to failure of the fetal hypothalamic gonadotrophin axis.

CLINICAL SIGNIFICANCE

Nanophthalmos may present clinically with reduced penetrance, making milder forms of this disorder diffi-

---

* The axial length criteria cited by Duke-Elder have been expanded to identify eyes with similar anatomic characteristics which are clinically associated with a suboptimal response to routine medical or surgical intervention like those of the original nanophthalmos subset.

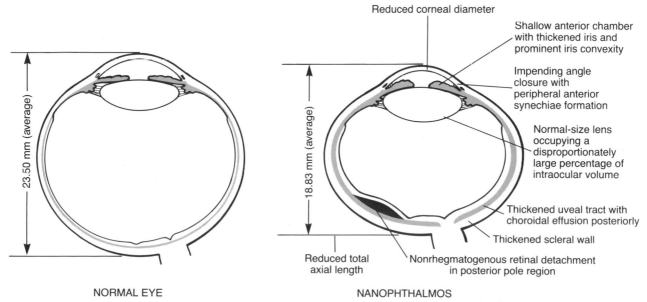

NORMAL EYE   NANOPHTHALMOS

Figure 135–3. The eye in nanophthalmos has these ocular features: (1) reduced corneal diameter; (2) shallow anterior chamber with thickened iris and prominent iris convexity; (3) impending angle closure with peripheral anterior synechiae formation; (4) a crystalline lens of normal size occupying a disproportionately large percentage of intraocular volume; (5) a thickened uveal tract with choroidal effusion occurring posteriorly; (6) a thickened scleral wall; (7) nonrhegmatogenous retinal detachment affecting the posterior pole region; and (8) reduced total axial length of 18.83 mm (compared with the normal axial length of 23.50 mm, average).

cult to recognize unless the examiner maintains a high index of suspicion. While open-angle glaucoma and pseudoexfoliation have been associated with nanophthalmos, these eyes often present with angle-closure glaucoma in the fourth to sixth decades of life. However, these eyes often develop posterior segment complications during or immediately after conventional anterior segment surgical intervention for glaucoma or cataract, with blinding consequences.[17-19] Both choroidal effusion and retinal detachment may occur preoperatively, intraoperatively, or postoperatively and lead to decreased visual acuity that does not respond to conventional therapy.[5, 20, 21] In 1982, a series of 15 nanophthalmic eyes requiring glaucoma surgery were examined. Nine eyes of 15 (60 percent) failed to achieve tension control; 13

Table 135–1. 1990 NANOPHTHALMOS DATA*

I. Sex
   N = 40 patients
   16 patients (male)
   24 patients (female)

II. Age†
   N = 40 patients
   Average = 55.2 years; median = 58 years; range = 25 to 77 years

III. Corneal Diameter (mm)
   N = 47 eyes of 24 patients
   Average = +10.56; median = +10.50; range = +9.5 to 12.00

IV. Anterior Chamber Depth (mm)‡
   N = 48 eyes of 25 patients
   Average = 1.91; median = 2.25; range = 0.50 to 4.60

V. Refractive Error (Diopters)
   N = 74 eyes of 37 patients
   Average = +10.00; median = +10.00; range = −3.50 to +24.00

VI. Axial Length (mm)
   N = 78 eyes of 40 patients
   Average +18.83; median = +19.50; range = +15.00 to 20.50

VII. Crystalline Lens Anterior-Posterior Diameter (mm)
   N = 42 eyes of 23 patients
   Average = 4.68; median = 4.25; range = 3.0 to 5.9

VIII. Crystalline Lens; Eye Volume Ratio
   N = 46 eyes of 23 patients
   Average = 24.68%; median = 23.60%; range = 16.60 to 37.60%

IX. Combined Thicknesses of Scleral and Choroidal Layers (mm)
   N = 22 eyes of 12 patients
   Average = 2.80; median = 2.25; range = 1.37 to 4.00

*Patients comprising our nanophthalmos subset originated through a variety of referral networks over approximately 30 yr of practice and include but are not limited to:
   1. Patients referred for the evaluation or treatment of angle-closure and open-angle glaucoma.
   2. Patients referred as blood relatives of an index case affected by nanophthalmos.
   3. Patients with posterior segment findings consistent with the diagnosis of nanophthalmos (e.g., choroidal effusion or nonrhegmatogenous retinal detachment) referred from a retinal practice.
†Patient age refers to the age at time of initial presentation, which may or may not correlate with the age at the time of diagnosis of nanophthalmos.
‡Twenty additional eyes showed clinically shallow chamber depths measuring less than two corneal thicknesses.

Table 135–2. COMPARATIVE OCULAR ANATOMY

Parameter	Normal Adult Human Eye[10]	1990 Nanophthalmos Eyes
Horizontal corneal diameter (mm)	11.7 mm	N = 47 eyes of 24 patients Average = 10.56; median = 10.50; range = 9.50 to 12.00
Anterior chamber Depth	3.5 mm	N = 48 eyes of 25 patients Average = 1.91; median = 2.25; range = 0.5 to 4.60
Axial length (mm)	23.6 mm	N = 78 eyes of 40 patients Average = 18.83; median = +19.50; range = 15.00 to 20.50
Crystalline lens with anterior-posterior diameter (mm)	4.11 to 4.77 mm[61]	N = 42 eyes of 23 patients Average = 4.68; median = 4.25; range = 3.0 to 5.9
Crystalline lens; eye volume ratio[11]	3.1 to 4.4%[11]	N = 46 eyes of 23 patients Average = 24.68%; median = 23.60%; range = 16.60 to 37.60%
Combined thicknesses of scleral and choroidal layers (mm)	1.01 mm	N = 22 eyes of 12 patients Average = 2.80; median = 2.25; range = 1.37 to 4.00

of 15 eyes (86.6 percent) suffered visual loss following surgery; and 6 of 13 eyes (46 percent) had visual loss to counting fingers at 6' or less.[17] In the same report, of 6 eyes undergoing cataract surgery, only 50 percent showed visual improvement postoperatively.[17]

In the authors' 1990 series, 14 eyes of 12 patients with nanophthalmos underwent cataract surgery. Of these, 11 of 14 (79 percent) showed visual improvement postoperatively; 2 of 14 (14 percent) showed decreased visual acuity; and 1/14 (7 percent) showed no change in visual acuity, which was thought to be due to preexisting retinal dysfunction or age-related macular degeneration. In these eyes preoperative prophylactic vortex vein decompression was performed on 2 of 14 (14 percent); anterior sclerotomy was performed on 2 of 14 (14 percent); and 2 of 14 (14 percent) required intraoperative management for malignant glaucoma. Five eyes of five patients with nanophthalmos underwent filtration surgery. Of these, 4 of 5 (80 percent) achieved glaucoma control; 1 of 5 (20 percent) required additional procedures for control of glaucoma; and 1 of 5 (20 percent) suffered visual loss following surgery, and this loss was attributed to progressive cataract formation. Proper preoperative diagnosis and therapy of nanophthalmos can help to avert disastrous consequences and improve the outcome to medical and surgical management (Tables 135–1 and 135–2).

EXAMINATION TECHNIQUES IN THE NANOPHTHALMIC PATIENT

The diagnosis of nanophthalmos is based on clinical criteria and detailed measurement of ocular parameters. The patient usually presents for evaluation of narrow-angle glaucoma, either suspect or acute, or with choroidal effusion with or without retinal detachment causing visual impairment. There may be a history of familial blindness from angle-closure glaucoma or a history of disastrous consequences of the fellow eye resulting from intraocular surgery.[17] Refractive error is determined by standard refraction techniques. The external horizontal corneal diameter is measured by ruler or calipers. The presence of nystagmus or strabismus is documented by Hirschberg measurement.[22] Anterior chamber depth is measured axially and peripherally in the method described by Van Herrick and associates.[23] Measurements may be supplemented by Haag-Streit pachymetry, B-scan ultrasound, and magnetic resonance imaging when available. Intraocular pressure readings are obtained by Goldmann applanation tonometry, and the width of the ocular pulse is noted. When possible, tonography is performed to document the facility of outflow. Careful notations are made regarding the degree of iris convexity and the anterior chamber angle configuration by gonioscopy using Koeppe or Goldmann lenses in all cases. The standard 16- to 18-mm Koeppe lens may be too large for some eyes with microcornea, reduced anterior segment dimensions, and narrow palpebral fissures. In these cases, the 12-mm pediatric Koeppe lens may facilitate the examination. Tilting the Koeppe lens toward the quadrant under examination assists in evaluating areas of the angle that lie peripherally to areas of prominent iris convexity (Fig. 135–4). Eyes affected by nanophthalmos may exhibit variable degrees of angle-closure that may progress over time. When possible, anterior segment and goniophotos are obtained, and these provide documentation of angle structures and assist in future comparisons. A Zeiss or Posner 4-mirror lens may be utilized for compression gonioscopy to distinguish appositional areas from synechial areas of closure.

Waterbath B-scan ultrasound (and magnetic resonance imaging, when available) achieves accurate measurements of the axial length of the globe; dimensions of the crystalline lens; the condition of the posterior segment including choroidal and scleral thickness measurement; and the presence and extent of choroidal effusion or retinal detachment.[74] The measurements are used to calculate lens:eye volume ratios in the manner described by Kimbrough and associates.[11] Lens volume is calculated by a formula of 4/3 AB,[2] in which A represents one half of the thickness of the crystalline lens and B represents the radius of the lens. The formula $4/3R^3$ is used to calculate eye volume in which R represents the radius of the globe. The lens:eye volume ratio is greater (10 to 32 percent) in nanophthalmic eyes compared with emmetropic eyes (3 to 4 percent).[10]

If the angle is nonoccludable, mydriasis may assist in evaluation of the posterior segment. The optic discs are characteristically small and pink as seen in hyperopia, unless there is associated glaucomatous damage. Baseline stereo disc photos and automated visual fields are obtained at this time for the purposes of future comparison. In cases in which there is advanced glaucomatous damage, nonautomated visual fields may assist in assessing glaucomatous progression. An evaluation of the posterior segments may reveal bone-spicule changes that resemble a retinitis pigmentosa–like pattern. Direct or indirect ophthalmoscopy may reveal low-lying peripheral choroidal detachment with or without associated nonrhegmatogenous retinal detachment. In some cases the choroidal detachment may involve the posterior pole, producing a macular fold and thus reducing visual acuity.[25] In eyes that cannot be dilated or in which media opacification limits the view, B-scan ultrasound (and magnetic resonance imaging) can assist in accurately determining the thickness of the sclera and choroid layers and the presence of posterior segment abnormalities associated with nanophthalmos.

MECHANISM OF ANGLE-CLOSURE IN NANOPHTHALMOS

Anatomic characteristics of nanophthalmic eyes that predispose to angle-closure include high degrees of hypermetropia, small corneal diameter, shallow anterior chamber, prominent iris convexity, reduced axial length, and a normal or large crystalline lens that causes anterior segment crowding by occupying a disproportionately large volume of the globe.[3, 11, 17] In normal eyes, choroidal effusion may be frequently seen as a postoperative phenomena, but in nanophthalmic eyes choroidal effusion is frequently seen preoperatively and may explain presenting symptoms of decreased visual acuity, angle-closure, and even abnormal retinal pigmentation.[5] Several investigators have suggested the following mechanism by which preoperative choroidal effusion contributes to angle-closure.[5, 11, 17] Annular choroidal detachment may be associated with detachment, elevation, and forward rotation of the ciliary body, which results in relaxed tension of the zonule on the crystalline lens.[11] When the lens moves forward, increased iridolenticular apposition and relative pupillary block occurs (Fig. 135–5).[11] The development of choroidal effusion in nanophthalmic patients between the ages of 40 and 70 yr correlates well with the frequent occurrence of angle-closure glaucoma.[5]

Whereas nanophthalmos is characteristically associ-

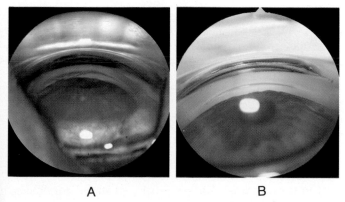

Figure 135–4. A and B, Koeppe gonioscopy demonstrates prominent iris convexity and asymmetric stages of angle closure in both eyes.

A   B

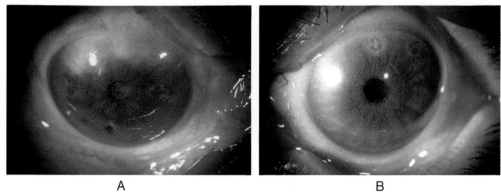

A   B

Figure 135–5. *A* and *B,* The anterior segment examination demonstrates superior corneal opacification corresponding to areas of iridocorneal apposition during acute angle-closure glaucoma in the right eye. Patent iridotomies present inferiorly in the right eye and superiorly in the left eye were created by argon and subsequent neodymium-yttrium-aluminum-garnet (Nd.YAG) lasers.

ated with angle-closure glaucoma, open-angle glaucoma may occur as well. There is a report of bilateral pseudoexfoliation syndrome occurring in a sibling with nanophthalmos from a consanguineous family and a report of two patients with nanophthalmos associated with open-angle glaucoma.[18, 19]

The association of retinal detachment with high degrees of hyperopia was first recorded in 1951 by Witmer.[26] Brockhurst first reported the association of uveal effusion and nonrhegmatogenous retinal detachment with nanophthalmos.[5, 6] In a series of five patients, there was a poor visual outcome with conventional surgical treatment. Oral steroid therapy has been noted to produce resolution of choroidal effusion and nonrhegmatogenous retinal detachment in some cases.[5, 6] Subretinal fluid analysis in one case of massive uveal effusion with secondary retinal detachment demonstrated a protein content of more than three-fold greater than plasma, an absence of cells, low potassium concentration, and one type of acid phosphatase enzyme. This suggested derivation from plasma and not from inflammation.[27] The absence of hyaluronic acid in the subretinal fluid strongly suggests a nonrhegmatogenous etiology.[5, 6]

The pathophysiology of choroidal effusion involves an increased transudation of fluid and protein molecules from the intravascular choriocapillaris to the suprachoroidal space. The volume of effusion increases when water molecules enter the extravascular space to balance the osmotic gradient. Nonrhegmatogenous retinal detachments with "shifting fluid" phenomena may occur. Causes of choroidal effusion include hypotony, inflammation, trauma, and increased orbital or elevated episcleral venous pressure.[5, 28, 32] Since the eye has no lymphatic drainage system, vortex veins are instrumental in draining the suprachoroidal space. Shaffer has hypothesized that the abnormally thickened sclera found in nanophthalmic eyes impedes outflow through the vortex veins, thus resulting in choroidal effusion with subsequent retinal detachment.[29] Impedance of venous outflow by thickened sclera is supported by a wide ocular pulse pressure that is frequently noted in the nanophthalmic eye.[29]

Choroidal detachment may occur insidiously in asymptomatic nanophthalmic eyes during the third to

fifth decades of life.[5] These eyes usually have increased intraocular pressures that offset the increased venous pressure in the choroidal space. When the globe is suddenly decompressed during glaucoma or cataract surgery, the choroidal effusion and retinal detachment may be precipitated or exacerbated intraoperatively, thus requiring emergent decompression of the suprachoroidal space in a congested globe.[30] Brockhurst introduced the vortex vein decompression technique, which should be performed 4 to 6 wk before planned intraocular surgery.[30] This procedure permits controlled drainage of the suprachoroidal space, which allows spontaneous retinal reattachment to occur and reduces the risk of a disastrous visual outcome at the time of planned intraocular surgery. These eyes should be followed carefully by ultrasound B-scan evaluation, and if choroidal effusion persists, anterior sclerotomies are recommended at the time of planned glaucoma or cataract surgery.[32]

Gass described the idiopathic uveal effusion syndrome in nine patients.[33] He hypothesized that aging and hormonal changes in collagen and ground substance of patients with abnormal congenitally thickened sclera may inhibit transscleral protein transport[33, 34] and postulated that the barrier effect of the sclera was more important than the vortex vein obstruction effect.[34] He achieved successful resolution of uveal and retinal detachments by performing 5 × 7 mm, two-third thickness sclerectomies in four quadrants, avoiding the vortex veins and without decompressing the vortex veins. Central 1-mm sclerotomies, without choroidal puncture, were placed to decompress the suprachoroidal space, but no drainage of subretinal fluid was attempted. This technique has been applied successfully in some cases of nanophthalmic uveal effusion.[34, 35] Laboratory investigations have revealed abnormalities in nanophthalmic sclera that may explain the reduced protein transport and the subsequent development of uveal effusion. Light and transmission electron microscopy have demonstrated a disordered arrangement of collagen lamellae.[12] Histologic analysis has shown increased levels of proteoglycan surrounding collagen fibrils, which may influence their abnormal arrangement.[12]

Histochemical studies on sclera obtained from a patient with nanophthalmos have shown increased fibronectin staining, with higher fibronectin levels confirmed by tissue culture compared with normal sclera.[13, 14] High levels of fibronectin found in nanophthalmos have been hypothesized to play a role in the abnormal development of its sclera.[14]

CLASSIFICATION OF THE NANOPHTHALMIC PATIENT BASED ON GONIOSCOPIC FINDINGS AND INTRAOCULAR PRESSURE

At the time of the initial evaluation, nanophthalmic eyes are placed into one of three categories, based on the appearance of the angle on gonioscopy and intraocular pressure as follows[17]:

1. The angle is completely open gonioscopically with marked iris convexity characteristic of nanophthalmos and tension of less than or equal to 20 mmHg.
2. The angle appears partially closed with tension of less than or equal to 20 mmHg.
3. The angle is partially or totally closed with tension of greater than 20 mmHg.

Observation at frequent intervals every 3 to 4 mo is recommended for the nanophthalmic eye without glaucoma or posterior segment abnormalities in category 1. The frequency of evaluation is determined by the patient's age, the degree of iris convexity, the narrowness of the angle, and any evidence of appositional closure. In categories 2 and 3, where there is evidence of impending or early closure, the frequency of observation is increased, and treatment is initiated when there is evidence of a progression of angle-closure.

Medical Therapy

STEROIDS

Uncontrolled intraocular pressure is treated using all currently available glaucoma medications. In cases in which choroidal effusion contributes to angle-closure, oral steroids in doses of 1 to 2 g/kg of body weight per day on a tapering regimen have been utilized with some success.[5] Nanophthalmic eyes frequently present with attacks of acute angle-closure glaucoma, and of these, approximately two thirds are bilateral in occurrence.[17] Chronic open-angle glaucoma may also occur in these eyes.[17–19]

MIOTICS

Pilocarpine is the mainstay of initial therapy and is utilized in most eyes before laser or surgical intervention. For the treatment of suspected angle-closure glaucoma, in addition to other pressure reducing agents, a test dose of topical 1 percent pilocarpine solution is applied. Repeat evaluation by slit lamp and gonioscopy is performed 45 to 90 min thereafter. A favorable clinical response is evidenced by anterior chamber deepening and a wider angle configuration. If shallowing of the anterior chamber or exacerbation of angle-closure occurs, pilocarpine is not readministered. For the treatment of pressure elevation in open-angle glaucoma, pilocarpine therapy is usually initiated with 1 percent topical solution on a q.i.d. basis, but a higher concentration (e.g., 4 percent) and more frequent administration (e.g., every 2 hr while awake) are titrated according to the clinical response. If pilocarpine is utilized for pressure control, the patient's pressure and angle configuration should be checked several days following initiation to confirm a favorable response. Approximately half of the eyes require continued miotic therapy following successful laser application in the form of iridotomy or goniophotocoagulation.

The response of nanophthalmic eyes to pilocarpine is unpredictable. In some, there is a widening of the angle with concomitant decrease in intraocular pressure. In others, miotics appear to shallow the anterior chamber, narrow the angle, and increase the relative pupillary block.[36] In a few eyes, the anterior chamber widened following discontinuation of miotic therapy.

MYDRIATIC AND CYCLOPLEGIC THERAPY

Unlike other eyes with narrow-angle glaucoma, nanophthalmic eyes may exhibit a paradoxic effect to mydriatic (Phenylephrine 2.5 percent) and cycloplegic (Scopolamine 0.25 percent, atropine 1 percent, and cyclopentolate 1 percent) therapy, with deepening of the anterior chamber and reduction of intraocular pressure. Cycloplegics may relax the ciliary muscles and tighten the zonules, thus moving the lens-iris diaphragm posteriorly. This tends to deepen the anterior chamber; decrease relative pupillary block; and restore the normal pathway for aqueous flow anteriorly, consistent with therapy used to treat malignant glaucoma (aqueous diversion syndrome).

SYMPATHOMIMETICS AND BETA-BLOCKERS

Beta blockade in the form of timolol (Timoptic) may lower intraocular pressure by reduction of aqueous production but usually has no significant effect on angle configuration. Epinephrine and its derivatives may have no effect on intraocular pressure control or angle configuration, but in some cases the anterior chamber may deepen and the angle may widen with concomitant reduction of intraocular pressure.

CARBONIC ANHYDRASE INHIBITORS

Carbonic anhydrase inhibitors (Diamox and Neptazane) reduce aqueous production. They are utilized, in conjunction with other medications, in the medical treatment of glaucoma and prior to laser or surgical intervention. Some nanophthalmic eyes have demonstrated deepening of the anterior chamber with widening of the angle following treatment with Diamox.

HYPEROSMOTICS

Hyperosmotics, including oral glycerol (Osmoglyn), isosorbide (Ismotic), and intravenous Mannitol can be useful on a short-term basis to improve pressure control (e.g., during an acute attack of angle-closure).

LASER THERAPY

Two forms of laser therapy recommended for the treatment of angle-closure are iridotomy (iridectomy) and gonioplasty.

Nanophthalmic eyes in acute angle-closure respond poorly to conventional surgical iridectomy. The development of choroidal effusion, retinal detachment, malignant glaucoma, and decreased visual acuity have all been reported.[17] Laser iridotomy combined with appropriate medical therapy is the procedure of choice to break pupillary block and deepen the anterior chamber in the treatment of angle-closure glaucoma. The laser is used to create a hole, which reestablishes communication between the posterior and anterior chambers to relieve relative pupillary block. The iridotomy is checked for patency by slit-lamp evaluation, including retroillumination (Fig. 135–6). Nanophthalmic irides are clinically thicker than are their normal counterparts, and several treatment sessions may be required to achieve a patent opening. Brown irides may require higher power settings when compared with the lighter blue irides, and previously patent iridotomies can undergo subsequent spontaneous closure. Usually, an iridotomy that remains patent at 6 wk following therapy will not close.

Both Nd.YAG and argon lasers can be used to produce iridotomies, and in most cases we prefer the former. Care must be taken to create an iridotomy peripherally and to avoid damage to the lens of a phakic eye.

The technique of laser iridotomy is modified for eyes in acute angle-closure, because the iris is often closely apposed to the cornea. In this situation argon laser is preferred for the initial iridotomy to benefit from anterior chamber deepening that occurs due to the gonioplasty effect, while avoiding potential endothelial damage that can result from pulsed laser energy in close proximity to corneal tissue. In eyes with iridocorneal touch or very shallow anterior chambers, the iridotomy is placed more centrally than usual. Once pupillary block is relieved and the anterior chamber is deepened, it is often possible to perform a second iridotomy at a more peripheral location.

LASER GONIOPLASTY (IRIDOPLASTY)

Laser gonioplasty (iridoplasty) utilizes low power argon laser therapy to contract the peripheral iris stroma, thus flattening the iris with subsequent widening of the angle.[37–48] Standard laser settings of 200-μ spot size, 200-mW power, and 0.2-sec duration are used. The Goldmann 3 mirror lens is utilized to stabilize the eye and permit visualization of the angle during laser application. The energy level is titrated to the iris response at the initial settings. Usually, 1 to 2 quadrants are treated at any one time, because treatment of larger areas may result in ballooning of the iris in opposite clock hours with exacerbation of angle-closure. Gonioplasty is a relatively atraumatic procedure and can be repeated as often as needed.

Postoperative Care

Following laser iridotomy, patients are maintained on miotics and preoperative glaucoma medications. Laser gonioplasty is associated with minimal inflammation, and topical steroid therapy is tapered and discontinued over a period of 1 wk, unless there is evidence of persistent inflammation. The intraocular pressure is rechecked within 24 to 48 hr postoperatively to detect any pressure spike, and iridotomies are examined for patency. If the iridotomy shows evidence of early closure, laser therapy is repeated and the postoperative steroid regimen is continued. Rarely, laser iridotomy is unsuccessful in breaking the pupillary block associated with acute angle-closure glaucoma, and surgical iridectomy is required. Topical steroids and continuance of glaucoma medications help to reduce intraocular inflammation

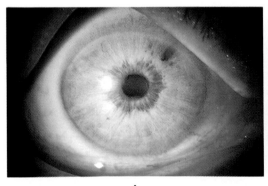
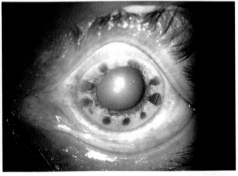

A   B

Figure 135–6. *A* and *B,* Anterior segment examination displays asymmetric shallowing of the anterior chambers associated with angle closure in both eyes. A patent laser iridotomy is present superonasally in the right eye, and prominent gonioplasty markings were placed in the midperipheral iris in the left eye to widen the angle.

while controlling intraocular pressure, thus enhancing the safety of subsequent ocular surgery. In general, glaucoma medications are continued after all laser procedures. Compared with laser iridotomy, laser gonioplasty is not associated with significant complications, and the patients' pressures can be checked at longer intervals following this treatment.

SURGICAL STRATEGIES IN NANOPHTHALMOS

A. Prophylactic posterior segment surgery
   1. Posterior scleral resection ± posterior sclerotomy
   2. Vortex vein decompression
   3. Indications for posterior segment intervention
B. Prophylactic anterior segment surgery
   1. Anterior sclerotomies
   2. Indications for anterior sclerotomies
   3. The surgical technique of anterior sclerotomy
C. Glaucoma filtration surgery
   1. Surgical peripheral iridectomy
   2. Adjunctive surgical procedures
      a. Intraoperative gonioscopy
      b. Anterior chamber deepening by the method of Paul A. Chandler, M.D.
   3. "Tight" trabeculectomy with adjunctive 5-FU therapy
   4. Additional options for glaucoma control
      a. Cyclocryotherapy
      b. Setons
      c. Nd.YAG cyclodestruction
D. Cataract surgery
   1. Indications
   2. Methods of cataract extraction
      a. Intracapsular technique
      b. Extracapsular technique ± IOL
      c. Phacoemulsification technique ± IOL
E. Combined cataract and glaucoma surgery
   1. ECCE/IOL/trabeculectomy
   2. Phacofiltration/IOL
   3. Cataract extraction ± IOL/cyclodialysis
F. Postoperative care
G. Surgical complications in nanophthalmos

When anterior segment surgery is deemed necessary or beneficial for the patient affected by nanophthalmos, posterior segment consultation is obtained. If choroidal effusion is suspected or identified preoperatively, a decision is made regarding the need for systemic steroid therapy, with or without posterior segment surgery to decompress the suprachoroidal space, in an attempt to prevent or minimize vision threatening posterior segment complications.[5] Prophylactic posterior segment surgery in the form of scleral resection, with or without vortex vein decompression, is optimally performed by the retinal surgeon 4 to 6 wk prior to the planned anterior segment procedure. These elective posterior segment prophylactic procedures, and anterior sclerotomies performed at the time of the planned anterior segment surgery, are indicated in the following five situations in the presence of thickened choroid with or without uveal effusion:

1. Choroidal effusion associated with nonrhegmatogenous retinal detachment that causes loss of central visual acuity or constriction of the visual field (e.g., macular fold).
2. Impending angle-closure glaucoma with annular choroidal detachment.
3. Prior to elective cataract surgery with or without an intraocular lens.[49]
4. Prior to elective glaucoma filtration surgery.
5. Prior to elective cataract and filtration surgery with or without an intraocular lens.

For detailed information regarding the surgical techniques of scleral resection and vortex vein decompression,[30, 31] the reader is referred to Chapter 143.

At the time of the planned anterior segment surgery, anterior sclerotomies may be indicated to decompress the suprachoroidal space and drain preexisting or developing choroidal effusion(s), thus reducing the chance of vision threatening posterior segment complications (Fig. 135–7). Our initial approach involved resection of two full thickness scleral triangles located in the inferonasal and inferotemporal quadrants, but our recent modifications have shown successful results with the base of the scleral triangles remaining attached to adjoining sclera. We have incorporated the technique of

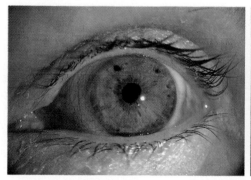
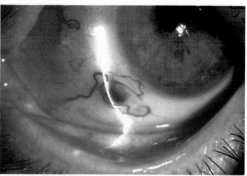

A   B

Figure 135–7. A and B, The anterior segment in the right eye shows patent peripheral iridotomies superiorly, whereas the left eye shows an anterior sclerotomy inferonasally formed prior to proceeding with cataract extraction.

anterior sclerotomy in our nanophthalmos protocol since 1978.[17] This technique has been supported by others.[19]

Anterior sclerotomies are indicated in the following three situations:

1. If the eye undergoing a planned anterior segment intraocular surgical procedure shows signs of anterior chamber shallowing related to positive vitreous pressure, our recommendations are to close the eye and perform anterior sclerotomies with the intention of resuming the planned procedure after the pressure differential resolves.

2. In the presence of thickened sclera and choroid, with or without uveal effusion, scleral resection with or without vortex vein decompression is indicated 4 to 6 wk prior, and anterior sclerotomies performed directly preceding the planned anterior segment surgery.

3. In acute or chronic angle-closure glaucoma unresponsive to laser iridotomy in nanophthalmic eyes, anterior sclerotomy may be indicated to drain the suprachoroidal space prior to proceeding with surgical peripheral iridectomy.

We have found that not all nanophthalmic eyes develop posterior segment complications. In the absence of preexisting glaucoma, with normal angle configuration and normal posterior segment findings, intraoperative and postoperative complications are uncommon, and prophylactic anterior sclerotomies do not appear to be indicated prior to proceeding with planned cataract surgery.

OPERATIVE TECHNIQUE OF ANTERIOR SCLEROTOMY

The operative technique of anterior sclerotomy begins with superior rotation of the eye and generous exposure of the inferior quadrants. A radial conjunctival incision is created to expose the underlying sclera. The globe is fixated with Bishop-Harmon forceps, and using a No. 15 Bard-Parker blade, a full-thickness equilateral triangular scleral flap is created, with its apex directed anteriorly and centered 5 mm posterior to the surgical limbus overlying the pars plana region. The sides measure 3 mm in length and are hinged at the base (Fig. 135–8). The apex of the triangle is grasped with forceps and the flap is dissected posteriorly with the No. 15 Bard-Parker blade to expose the underlying choroid (Fig. 135–9). Meticulous hemostasis is maintained with the aid of monopolar diathermy (Fig. 135–10), and care is taken to avoid inadvertent incisions into the choroid that may result in bleeding. When dissection is completed, a cyclodialysis spatula is advanced in a course tangential to the peripheral suprachoroidal space (nasally and temporally) to drain potential pockets of sequestered fluid (Fig. 135–11). Cautery is applied to the edges of the cut sclera to permit slight wound gape for continued choroidal drainage during the postoperative period. The scleral flap is reposited. In the presence of large amounts of choroidal effusion, in which the risk of posterior segment complications is high, two anterior

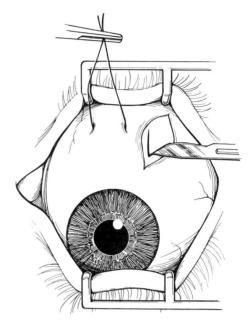

Figure 135–8. The globe is rotated superiorly and fixated with a Bishop-Harmon forcep while a radial conjunctival incision is created in the inferior temporal (or nasal) quadrant to expose the underlying sclera. A full-thickness equilateral triangular scleral flap is created with its apex directed anteriorly and centered 5 mm posterior to the surgical limbus overlying the pars plana region.

sclerotomies are created and the scleral flaps are resected (Table 135–3).

Attention is then turned to the anterior segment, and the proposed surgery is performed. Following completion of the glaucoma or cataract surgery, the sclerotomies are reexamined. In the absence of bleeding or

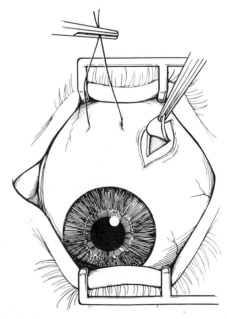

Figure 135–9. The apex of the triangle is grasped with a Pierse-Hoskin forcep and the flap is dissected posteriorly with a Bard-Parker No. 15 blade to expose the underlying choroid.

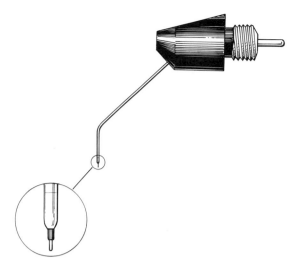

Figure 135–10. Meticulous hemostasis is achieved with the aid of monopolar diathermy (MIRA, Inc.).

Table 135–3. INSTRUMENTS AND SUPPLIES UTILIZED FOR ANTERIOR SCLEROTOMY

1. Sharp-point knife
2. Blunt, ⅝-inch, 25-gauge needle
3. Control syringe of 5-ml volume filled with balanced salt solution
4. Pierse-Hoskin tissue forceps
5. Sharp Westcott scissors
6. Calipers
7. Bipolar pencil cautery (Mentor)
8. Monopolar underwater diathermy (MIRA, Inc.)
9. Elschnig fixation forceps
10. No. 15 Bard-Parker blade
11. 10-0 nylon suture
12. 8-0 Vicryl suture
13. Needle holder(s)
14. Simmons-Kimbrough cyclodialysis spatula (0.5 mm)

exudation of fluid, the overlying conjunctiva is closed with 10-0 nylon sutures in interrupted fashion (Fig. 135–12). Complications related to the anterior sclerotomy procedure performed in this fashion are uncommon in the authors' experience. Several reports have documented its effectiveness in reducing the incidence of operative and postoperative complications in nanophthalmic eyes.[17, 19, 49, 50]

In cases involving angle-closure that do not respond to laser intervention, the technique of surgical peripheral iridectomy is performed in the manner described by Chandler and Grant.[51] In nanophthalmic eyes that require glaucoma surgery, operative gonioscopy and anterior chamber deepening are useful adjuncts in selective cases for determining whether a peripheral iridectomy

or filtration surgery would be most likely to succeed in the eye being treated (Figs. 135–13 and 135–14). Based on the findings of Chandler and Simmons, if there are 4 clock hours or less of synechial closure, with satisfactory pressure control on maximally tolerated medical therapy, peripheral iridectomy is the procedure of choice. If 6 clock hours or more are closed, with inadequately controlled pressures on maximally tolerated medical therapy, then filtration surgery should be performed.[51, 52]

When glaucoma filtration surgery is performed in eyes affected by nanophthalmos, there is a significant risk of posterior segment complications, even after prophylactic posterior scleral resection and anterior sclerotomies have been created. We currently advocate the creation of a "tight trabeculectomy," with a gradual reduction of intraocular pressure during the postoperative period by the technique of laser suture lysis (Fig. 135–15).[53] This helps to avoid sudden decompression of the globe and reduces the risk of choroidal effusion and retinal detachment associated with visual loss. Postoperative adjunctive therapy with 5-fluorouracil can inhibit the fibro-

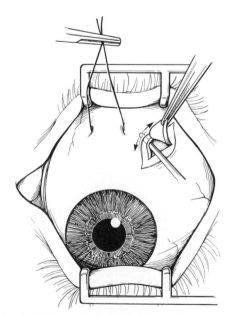

Figure 135–11. The cyclodialysis spatula is advanced along a course tangential to the sclera (nasally and temporally) to drain sequestered pockets of fluid in the suprachoroidal spaces.

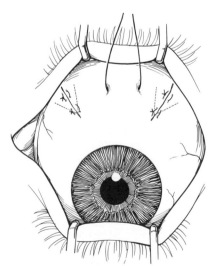

Figure 135–12. The conjunctival incisions are closed with 10–0 nylon sutures in interrupted fashion.

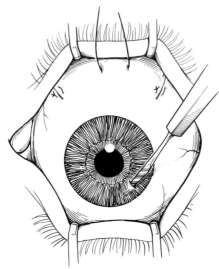

Figure 135–13. A beveled paracentesis is created in the peripheral cornea with the aid of a sharp-pointed knife.

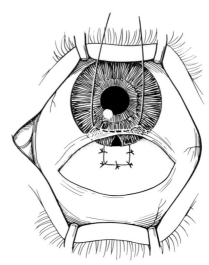

Figure 135–15. Placement of interrupted 10–0 nylon sutures through the scleral flap creates a "tight trabeculectomy" which allows gradual reduction of intraocular pressure through sequential laser suture lysis during the postoperative period.

vascular response often associated with bleb failure, thus enhancing the ultimate success of the filtration procedure.[54-56] Graded digital pressure maneuvers during the postoperative period can assist in achieving target tension control.[57] Additional details regarding the strategy and techniques of glaucoma filtration surgery are provided in Chapter 143.

Options for glaucoma control in eyes with poor visual potential or following several unsuccessful attempts to establish adequate filtration include cyclocryotherapy, setons, and Nd.YAG cyclophotocoagulation to the ciliary body region.

Indications for cataract surgery in eyes affected by nanophthalmos are essentially the same as those in normal eyes, but the risk of poor visual outcome is significantly greater.[17, 19, 58] Nanophthalmic eyes developing angle-closure in the fourth to sixth decades may

be susceptible to earlier cataract formation, and present for surgical visual rehabilitation earlier compared with age-matched normals. Although newer diagnostic techniques have allowed earlier confirmation of nanophthalmos (Fig. 135–16), and new operative techniques (anterior sclerotomy and vortex vein decompression) have lessened the incidence of anterior and posterior segment complications, significant risk still exists. Hyperosmotics may be used to reduce the intraocular pressure and decompress the vitreous cavity preoperatively. In the absence of glaucoma, or in the presence of glaucoma controlled on maximally tolerated medical therapy, with open or partially open angles and normal posterior segment findings, extracapsular cataract extraction with posterior chamber lens implantation is our recommended procedure. In the presence of thickened choroid or sclera with or without uveal effusion, we recommend elective vortex vein decompression at 4 to 6 wk prior to

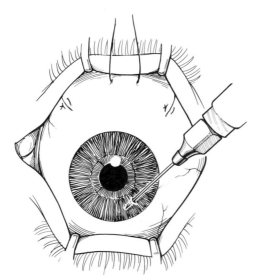

Figure 135–14. Anterior chamber deepening is accomplished by introducing balanced salt solution contained in a 5-ml syringe through the beveled paracentesis.

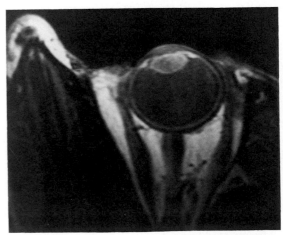

Figure 135–16. T$_1$-weighted image of a nanophthalmic eye. (Courtesy of Dr. Hong-Ming Cheng, Howe Laboratory of Ophthalmology, Harvard Medical School, Boston, MA.)

cataract extraction. At surgery, anterior sclerotomies may be utilized if indicated. Compared with intracapsular cryophake cataract extraction, extracapsular cataract extraction or phacoemulsification with posterior chamber lens implantation is associated with fewer complications. Phacoemulsification with posterior chamber lens implantation utilizes smaller incisions and reduces the risk of intraoperative and postoperative expulsive choroidal hemorrhages. However, the crowded anterior segment anatomy in nanophthalmos makes this technique more difficult. In select cases that demonstrate unremitting positive vitreous pressure or crowded anterior segment anatomy intraoperatively, despite prophylactic sclerotomies, one may elect to omit implantation of an intraocular lens. Postoperative refractive correction can be achieved by means of contact lenses, aphakic spectacles, and even secondary intraocular lens implantation at a future date. The reduced axial lengths characteristic of the eye in nanophthalmos correlate with highly hyperopic, aphakic refractive corrections (e.g., +23.00 to +24.00 diopters), unless the disparity is somewhat reduced by increased corneal curvatures.

In the presence of visually significant cataract with glaucoma uncontrolled on maximally tolerated medical therapy, and in the absence of choroidal thickening or effusion, a combined extracapsular cataract extraction, posterior chamber lens implantation, and "tight" trabeculectomy are indicated.[53, 59] The technique of "phacofiltration" involves cataract extraction by phacoemulsification combined with the creation of a trabeculectomy and implantation of an intraocular lens through a small incision.[59] We have found that this is an effective method of achieving glaucoma control and visual restoration, while preserving conjunctiva for future filtration surgery, as needed. If there is marked choroidal thickening or choroidal effusion, in conjunction with anterior chamber shallowing, elective, four-quadrant vortex vein decompression with or without scleral resection is recommended 4 to 6 wk prior to anterior segment surgery. At the time of anterior segment surgery, if there is still a very shallow anterior chamber or thickened choroid, anterior sclerotomies should be performed followed by cataract extraction, using phacoemulsification or extracapsular method, combined with posterior chamber lens implantation and "tight trabeculectomy." Eyes with visually significant cataract formation and uncontrolled glaucoma, which lack sufficient conjunctiva for filtration surgery, can achieve visual restoration and glaucoma control through combined cataract extraction with intraocular lens implantation and cyclodialysis.[50] The cyclodialysis procedure usually involves 2 to 3 clock hours of angle in a quadrant opposite the cataract wound.

Postoperative Care

When anterior segment surgery is completed, subtenon's injections of antibiotics, such as gentamycin and cefazolin, are delivered unless contraindicated by a history of adverse reaction. Subtenon's injections of depesteroids (Celestone Soluspan) at the surgeon's discretion, are placed 180 degrees opposite the limbal wound. Postoperative care following a cataract or a combined cataract and glaucoma surgery involves generous application of topical steroids to reduce inflammation and ocular congestion. Topical antibiotic therapy is tapered over a 1-wk period following uncomplicated cataract surgery but is continued indefinitely on a qd–bid basis as prophylaxis to infection in the presence of a functioning glaucoma filter. Adjunctive therapies such as 5-fluorouracil, laser suture lysis, and digital massage may be utilized to enhance filtration success.[53–57] Glaucoma medications may be introduced, as needed, to achieve adequate pressure control. For a thorough discussion of postoperative care following glaucoma filtration surgery, the authors refer to Chapter 143.

Complications

Vigilant observation is indicated during the postoperative period following anterior segment surgery in eyes affected by nanophthalmos. These eyes may develop crowding of the anterior segment anatomy or angle-closure that may require peripheral iridotomy, if this is not present at the time of surgery. A patent peripheral iridotomy prevents angle-closure on the basis of a pupillary block. In some situations, retained peripheral cortical material following cataract extraction may effectively occlude small, peripheral laser iridotomies, but larger surgical peripheral iridectomies remain patent and facilitate stabilization of fluid dynamics. Pseudophakic malignant glaucoma has been reported in four eyes with reduced axial lengths, which were implanted with posterior chamber intraocular lens optics measuring 7 mm in diameter.[60] To avoid this rare complication, we recommend the use of posterior chamber lenses with optics measuring 6 mm or less in diameter. Complications of surgery in nanophthalmos include corneal decompensation, flat anterior chamber, pupillary block, choroidal effusion, cystoid macular edema, hypotony maculopathy, retinal detachment, failed filtration, malignant glaucoma, endophthalmitis, and blindness. For a thorough discussion regarding further management the reader is referred to Chapter 145.

CONCLUSIONS

Nanophthalmos is a rare and commonly unrecognized disorder that is associated with disastrous complications following routine surgery for glaucoma and cataract. Early detection requires a high index of suspicion by the examiner. Prophylactic scleral resection with optional posterior sclerotomy, vortex vein decompression, and anterior sclerotomies are newer techniques that are used to make surgery safer in these eyes. Correct diagnosis with implementation of therapeutic guidelines has improved the outcome of medical and surgical management of nanophthalmos.

REFERENCES

1. Duke-Elder S: Anomalies in the size of the eye. *In* Duke-Elder S: System of Ophthalmology, vol 3, pt 2. St. Louis, CV Mosby, 1964, p 488.
2. O'Grady RB: Nanophthalmos. Am J Ophthalmol 71:1251, 1971.
3. Calhoun FP Jr: The management of glaucoma in nanophthalmos. Trans Am Ophthalmol Soc 73:97, 1975.
4. Zamorani G: Microftalmo E Glaucoma. Boll Oculist 39:746, 1960.
5. Brockhurst RJ: Nanophthalmos with uveal effusion: A new clinical entity. Trans Am Ophthalmol Soc 72:371, 1974.
6. Cross HE, Yoder F: Familial nanophthalmos. Am J Ophthalmol 81:300, 1976.
7. Duggan JW, Hassard DTR: Familial microphthalmos classification and definition of terms. Trans Can Ophth Soc 24:210, 1961.
8. Weiss H, Kousseff BG, Ross MA, et al: Simple microphthalmos. Arch Ophthalmol 107:1624, 1989.
9. Warburg M: Genetics of microphthalmos. Int Ophthalmol 4:45, 1981.
10. Wilmer HA, Scammon RE: Growth of the components of the human eyeball. Arch Ophthalmol 43:599, 1950.
11. Kimbrough RL, Trempe CL, Brockhurst RJ, et al: Angle closure glaucoma in nanophthalmos. Am J Ophthalmol 88:572, 1979.
12. Trelstad RL, Silberman NN, Brockhurst RJ: Nanophthalmic sclera. Arch Ophthalmol 100:1935, 1982.
13. Yue BY, Duvall, J Goldberg MF, et al: Nanophthalmic sclera: Morphologic and tissue culture studies. Ophthalmology 93:534, 1986.
14. Yue BY, Kurosawa A, Duvall J, et al: Nanophthalmic sclera fibronectin studies. Ophthalmology 95:56, 1988.
15. Ghose S, Sachdev M, Kumar H: Bilateral nanophthalmos, pigmentary retinal dystrophy and angle closure glaucoma. Br J Ophthalmol 69:624, 1982.
16. Barad RF, Nelson LB, Cowchock FS, et al: Nanophthalmos associated with cryptorchidism. Ann Ophthalmol 17:284, 1985.
17. Singh OS, Simmons RJ, Brockhurst RJ, et al: Nanophthalmos: A perspective on identification and therapy. Ophthalmology 89:1006, 1982.
18. Diehl DL, et al: Nanophthalmos in sisters, one with exfoliation syndrome. Can J Ophthalmol 24:327, 1989.
19. Jin JC, Anderson D: Laser and unsutured sclerostomy in nanophthalmos. Am J Ophthalmol 109:575, 1990.
20. Gass DJ, et al: Idiopathic serous detachment of the choroid, ciliary body, and retina (uveal effusion syndrome). Ophthalmology 89:1018, 1982.
21. Ryan EA, Zqaan J, Chylack LT: Nanophthalmos with uveal effusion: Clinical and embryologic considerations. Ophthalmology 89:1013, 1982.
22. Von Noorden GK: Von Noorden, Maumenee's Atlas of Strabismus, 3rd ed. St. Louis, CV Mosby, 1977.
23. Van Herrick W, Shaffer RN, Schwartz A: Estimation of width of angle of anterior chamber. Am J Ophthalmol 68:626, 1969.
24. Jalkh AE, Avila MP, Trempe CL, et al: Diffuse choroidal thickening detected by ultrasonography in various ocular disorders. Retina 3:277, 1983.
25. Spitznas M, et al: Hereditary posterior nanophthalmos with papillomacular fold and high hyperopia. Arch Ophthalmol 101:413, 1982.
26. Witmer VR: Hohe Hypermetropie und Ablatio. Ophthalmologica 121:178, 1951.
27. Brockhurst RJ, Lam K: Uveal effusion II: Report of a case with analysis of subretinal fluid. Arch Ophthalmol 90:399, 1973.
28. Ruiz RS, Salmonsen PC: Expulsive choroidal effusion: A complication of intraocular surgery. Arch Ophthalmol 94:69, 1976.
29. Shaffer RN: Discussion. *In* Calhoun FP Jr: The management of glaucoma in nanophthalmos. Trans Am Ophthalmol Soc 73:119–122, 1975.
30. Brockhurst RJ: Vortex vein decompression for nanophthalmic uveal effusion. Arch Ophthalmol 89:1987, 1980.
31. Brockhurst RJ: Vortex vein decompression. *In* Thomas JV(ed): Contemporary Glaucoma Surgery, 1st ed. St. Louis, CV Mosby, 1990.
32. Singh OS: 'Nanophthalmos Identification and Therapy.' Presentation at Massachusetts Eye and Ear Infirmary, May, 1990.
33. Gass DJ, Jallow S: Idiopathic serous detachment of the choroid, ciliary body, and retina (uveal effusion syndrome). Ophthalmology 89:1018, 1982.
34. Gass DJ: Uveal effusion syndrome: A new hypothesis concerning pathogenesis and technique of surgical treatment. Trans Am Ophthalmol 81:246, 1982.
35. Allen K, Meyers S, Zegarra H: Nanophthalmic uveal effusion. Retina 8:145, 1988.
36. Wilkie J, Drance SM, Schulzer M: The effects of miotics on anterior chamber depth. Am J Ophthalmol 68:78, 1969.
37. Simmons RJ, Kimbrough RL, Belcher CD: Gonioplasty for selected cases of angle-closure glaucoma. Doc Ophthal Proc 22:200, 1980.
38. Sellem EA, Belcher CD, Thomas JV, et al: Quelques techniques particulières de photocoagulation à L'argon du segment antérieur. J Fr Ophthalmol 8:497, 1986.
39. Simmons RJ: Nanophthalmos, diagnosis and treatment. *In* Epstein DL(ed): Chandler and Grant's Glaucoma. Philadelphia, Lea & Febiger, 1979.
40. Simmons RJ, Kimbrough RL, Belcher CD: Laser gonioplasty for special problems in angle closure glaucoma. *In* Symposium on Glaucoma. Trans New Orleans Acad Ophthalmol St. Louis, CV Mosby 13:220, 1981.
41. Belcher CD, Simmons RJ, Thomas JV: Other uses of laser in the anterior segment of the eye. *In* Zimmerman TJ(ed): International Ophthalmology Clinics, vol 24, Boston, Little, Brown, 1984, p 121.
42. Simmons RJ, Simmons RB: Gonioplasty. *In* Photocoagulation in Glaucoma and Anterior Segment Disease. Baltimore, Williams & Wilkins, 1984, p 122.
43. Simmons RJ, Singh OS: Gonioplasty (iridoretraction). *In* Wilensky JT (ed): Laser Therapy in Glaucoma. East Norwalk, CT, Appleton-Century-Crofts, 1985, p 47.
44. Simmons RJ, Savage JA, Belcher CD, et al: Usual and unusual uses of laser in glaucoma. *In* Symposium on the Laser in Ophthalmology and Glaucoma Update. Trans New Orleans Acad Ophthalmol St. Louis, CV Mosby, 1985, p 154.
45. Simmons RJ: Nanophthalmos diagnosis and treatment. (gonioplasty). *In* Epstein DL(ed): Chandler and Grant's Glaucoma, 3rd ed. Philadelphia, Lea & Febiger, 1986, p 251.
46. Simmons RJ, Brown SV, Sharpe ED, et al: The role of lasers in glaucoma management: General introduction. *In* McAllister JA, Williams RP(eds): Glaucoma, vol.2. London, Butterworths, 1986, p 169.
47. Smith PD, Simmons RJ: Argon laser therapy of the primary and secondary angle-closure glaucomas. *In* McAllister JA, Williams RP (eds). Glaucoma, vol 2. London, Butterworths, 1986, p 180.
48. Spurny RC, Simmons RJ: Unusual uses of the argon laser in glaucoma. *In* McAllister JA, Williams RP(eds): Glaucoma, vol 2. London, Butterworths, 1986, p 194.
49. Singh OS, Simmons RJ: Glaucoma surgical techniques in nanophthalmos. *In* Thomas JV(ed): Contemporary Glaucoma Surgery, 1st ed. St. Louis, CV Mosby, 1990.
50. Brockhurst RJ: Cataract surgery in nanophthalmic eyes. Arch Ophthalmol 108:965, 1990.
51. Chandler PA, Grant WM: Surgical Procedures and Treatment of Complications in Surgery: Lectures on Glaucoma. Philadelphia, Lea & Febiger, 1965, pp 381–406.
52. Chandler PA, Simmons RJ: Anterior chamber deepening for gonioscopy at time of surgery. Arch Ophthalmol 74:177, 1965.
53. Savage JA, Condon GP, Lyttle RA, et al: Laser suture lysis after trabeculectomy. Ophthalmology 95:1631, 1988.
54. Heuer DK, Parrish RK, Gressel MG, et al: 5-Fluorouracil and glaucoma filtering surgery II: A pilot study. Ophthalmology 91:384, 1984.
55. Heuer DK, Parrish RK, Gressel MG, et al: 5-Fluorouracil and glaucoma filtering surgery III: Intermediate follow-up of a pilot study. Ophthalmology 93:1537, 1986.
56. Rockwood EJ, Parrish RK, Heuer DK, et al: Galucoma filtering surgery with 5-fluorouracil. Ophthalmology 94:1971, 1987.
57. Cashwell LF, Simmons RJ: Adjunctive techniques to glaucoma filtering surgery. Perspect Ophthalmology 4(2):115, 1980.
58. Susanna R: Implantation of an intraocular lens in a case of nanophthalmos. CLAO 13:117, 1987.
59. Simmons RJ, et al: Personal communication, 1990.
60. Reed JE, Thomas JV, Lytle RA, et al: Malignant glaucoma induced by an intraocular lens. Ophthal Surg 21:177, 1990.
61. Duke-Elder S: The anatomy of the visual system. *In* System of Ophthalmology, vol. 2. St. Louis, CV Mosby, 1961, p 312.

Chapter 136

∎

Penetrating Keratoplasty and Glaucoma

PAUL P. LEE, R. RAND ALLINGHAM, and PETER J. McDONNELL

Penetrating keratoplasty has become a commonly performed procedure, with nearly 36,000 transplants in 1987.[1] The 1-yr graft survival rate is 80 to 90 percent under certain conditions. It is one of the most successful of all transplants.[2] As a result, penetrating keratoplasty has been increasingly used at earlier stages in a wider range of ocular disorders for visual rehabilitation. Since the early 1980s, the leading indications for keratoplasty have been pseudophakic and aphakic bullous keratopathy (18 and 11 percent, respectively) and corneal regrafts (15 percent).[3, 4] Other indications for penetrating keratoplasty are listed in Table 136–1. As more grafts are performed, however, the number of patients with problems associated with keratoplasty will continue to rise.

Complications associated with keratoplasty include glaucoma, graft melt, endophthalmitis, increased susceptibility to trauma, choroidal hemorrhage, macular edema, graft failure, retinal detachment, and worsening of other ocular disorders.[5, 6] One of the most vexing problems is increased intraocular pressure (IOP). The leading cause of enucleation (46 percent) after corneal transplantation is secondary glaucoma.[5] Clinical glaucoma after keratoplasty ranges from nearly nonexistent for grafts for keratoconus[7] to 52 percent for pseudophakic or aphakic bullous keratopathy.[8] As the number of both total grafts and grafts for aphakic and pseudophakic keratoplasty increases, the management of postkeratoplasty glaucoma will become more important.

GLAUCOMA ASSESSMENT IN PATIENTS UNDERGOING KERATOPLASTY

It was only in the 1960s, with the development of instruments that allowed routine monitoring of IOP immediately after keratoplasty, that the problem of keratoplasty-associated glaucoma became widely recognized.[9–11] Postoperative glaucoma, astigmatism, and irregular corneal surfaces secondary to corneal edema, scarring, and epithelial irregularities before and after keratoplasty make reliable Goldmann's applanation tonometry unreliable.[10] When the graft is clear, usually well after the operation, both Goldmann's tonometry and Schiotz tonometry[12] may be useful.

The MacKay-Marg tonometer and pneumotonometer permit reliable assessment of IOP pre- and postoperatively. The definition of postkeratoplasty or keratoplasty-associated glaucoma currently focuses on the level of IOP,[9] frequently without reference to other parameters used to assess patients with glaucoma. In large part, this has been because of the difficulty in assessing the visual field and neuroretinal structures in eyes with corneal disease sufficient to require keratoplasty. Further, postoperative astigmatism and refractive changes often preclude reliable postoperative assessment and comparison of the visual field, and analysis of the optic nerve and nerve fiber layer may not be possible until after surgery.

Although no study has explicitly investigated the feasibility of performing visual field testing and neuroretinal examinations in these patients, a few studies suggest that it may be possible in some patients.[13, 14] In one study, of 17 patients with eyes undergoing Molteno's implantation, 8 (47 percent) had reliable automated visual fields pre- and postoperatively and 14 (82 percent) had a view sufficient to monitor the optic nerve head.[13] In another study, ten eyes undergoing laser trabeculoplasty with clear grafts 2 years after keratoplasty were reliably monitored with visual field testing.[14] Therefore, future efforts to study glaucoma associated with pene-

Table 136–1. INDICATIONS FOR PENETRATING KERATOPLASTY AND ASSOCIATED CHRONIC GLAUCOMA RATES (IOP)

Indication[3, 4]	Rate	Mean Follow-up Period	References
Pseudophakic bullous keratopathy	18–53%	1–3 yr	7, 8, 17, 19, 74
Corneal regraft	45–50%	0.5–2.5 yr	19, 21, 75
Aphakic bullous keratopathy	20–70%	0.5–3 yr	7, 8, 16–19, 21, 23
Trauma	9–55%	0.5–2.5 yr	21, 23
Fuchs's dystrophy	0–37%	1 yr (min)	7, 19
Ulcerative disease	50% (n = 2)	1 yr (min)	23
Keratoconus	0–12%	1 yr (min)	7, 19, 23
Scarring	No data	No data	No data
Viral keratitis	20–75%	1–2.5 yr	19, 23, 21

trating keratoplasty may include evaluation of standard parameters in addition to IOP. Similarly, past studies cited in this chapter need to be evaluated with this limitation in mind.

Gonioscopy is another important component of the evaluation of patients with glaucoma to assess the status and structure of the filtration angle. Corneal pathology frequently precludes preoperative assessment, even after topical glycerin is used to reduce corneal edema. Postoperatively, the size of the graft and corneal astigmatism may pose difficulties in attempting gonioscopy. However, evaluation of the angle is critical in helping determine the mechanism of glaucoma after keratoplasty. Most published studies in this area do not specify whether gonioscopy was performed routinely in the postoperative setting.

FACTORS IN KERATOPLASTY-ASSOCIATED GLAUCOMA

After 20 yr, much has been learned about the behavior of the IOP after keratoplasty, including some of the risk factors for increased IOP and some possible mechanisms for postkeratoplasty glaucoma. Unfortunately, a multivariate analysis required to separate possible confounding factors has not been carried out. Thus, both our understanding of postkeratoplasty glaucoma and the rationale for treatment are incomplete and subject to continuing change.

An excellent illustration of this evolution in thought comes from the initial description of the pressure response to keratoplasty. Among the first important points made was the bimodal nature (early and late) of IOP increases after keratoplasty and the predictive role of early pressure rises within the first week in the development of late glaucoma occurring months to years later.[15, 16] In one study of early IOP elevation in 71 consecutive keratoplasties, 53 (75 percent) had IOP higher than 21 mmHg during the first postoperative week.[15] In another study, 37 of 81 eyes (46 percent) undergoing keratoplasty combined with cataract extraction or for aphakic bullous keratopathy had IOP greater than 35 mmHg during the first week.[16] In this study, those eyes with an early elevation of pressure were more likely (76 percent) than those without such a spike (61 percent) to develop persistently elevated pressures at 6 mo.[16]

Overshadowed in the flurry of excitement about these initial descriptions of IOP elevations after keratoplasty was the fact that these differences, and thus the predictive ability of early pressure rises, were not statistically significant. A later study by another group showed that only 36 percent (33 of 91) of eyes that developed late glaucoma at a mean follow-up of 3 yr had early IOP spikes in the first week, although 75 percent of eyes with early spikes would subsequently develop late pressure problems.[17] Later studies suggested that changes in operative techniques and postoperative care could diminish the incidence of both early and late IOP spikes.[9, 17] It is evident that even the description of

postkeratoplasty glaucoma is dependent on additional factors, such as the preoperative condition of the eye, the operative technique used, and the postoperative care.

Unaddressed in this context is the role of race in keratoplasty-associated glaucoma. Blacks are more likely than whites to develop glaucoma, at an earlier age and often of a more severe nature. How this observation relates to glaucoma after penetrating keratoplasty has not been explored.

Spectrum of Disease

An approach that may be helpful in organizing our understanding of postkeratoplasty glaucoma is to consider what is known about these glaucomas. The following statements are generally recognized as true:

1. Postkeratoplasty glaucoma occurs much more frequently in patients with preexisting glaucoma.[17, 18]
2. Aphakic and pseudophakic eyes are at increased risk for developing postkeratoplasty glaucoma, as are, to a lesser extent, eyes undergoing corneal regrafts.[17–19]
3. Steroids have a role in both preventing and inducing postkeratoplasty glaucoma in a significant portion of patients.[8, 17, 19, 21–23]
4. Synechial angle closure occurs in many, if not most, eyes with keratoplasty-associated glaucoma.[13, 23]
5. The part played by conformative changes within the anterior chamber changes induced by penetrating keratoplasty is uncertain.[24–32]

When evaluated in light of the relative risks from a purely glaucoma perspective, the relative incidence of late-onset glaucoma after penetrating keratoplasty for different conditions (see Table 136–1) becomes more understandable. Certain conditions, such as keratoconus, generally occur in young phakic patients without prior surgery. In these eyes, initial transplants have a low incidence of late glaucoma. In contrast, penetrating keratoplasty in a patient with aphakic bullous keratopathy after intracapsular cataract extraction, with vitreous in the anterior chamber, represents major surgery on an eye that has had previous surgery; such surgery may itself predispose to the development of glaucoma.

Mechanisms that have been implicated in the development of keratoplasty-associated glaucoma can thus be understood by reference to principles present for other forms of glaucoma. Keratoplasty-associated glaucoma may represent a spectrum of glaucomas caused by specific etiologies. As such, this offers hope for prevention and improved treatment for glaucoma in eyes following penetrating keratoplasty.

Proposed Mechanisms

Although the list of possible mechanisms is lengthy (Table 136–2), certain mechanisms are more common than others.

The three major preoperative factors affecting th

Table 136–2. MECHANISMS OF INCREASED IOP AFTER KERATOPLASTY

Open-Angle Glaucoma
Early onset
  Preexisting open-angle glaucoma
  Enzyme induced
  Viscoelastic induced
  Hyphema
  Outflow reduction due to trabecular collapse
Intermediate onset
  Vitreous in anterior chamber
  Hyphema
  Inflammation
  Steroid induced
  Ghost cell
  Rejection
Late onset
  Primary open angle glaucoma
  Ghost cell
  Epithelial ingrowth
  Steroid induced
  Rejection

Angle-Closure Glaucoma
Early onset
  Preexisting peripheral anterior synechiae
  Pupillary block
  Malignant glaucoma
Late onset
  Pupillary block
  Malignant glaucoma
  Progressive synechial closure

risk of developing keratoplasty-associated glaucoma are the presence or absence of preoperative glaucoma, the phakic status of the eye, and the size of the graft compared with the host (Table 136–3). The two major postoperative risk factors are the use of steroids and progressive synechial angle closure (Table 136–4).

PREOPERATIVE FACTORS

Although the three factors noted in Table 136–3 have been observed in several studies in the past 20 yr, no

Table 136–3. FACTORS ASSOCIATED WITH ELEVATED IOP

	Aphakic (%)	Pseudophakic (%)	Phakic (%)
Phakic status			
Early rise[10]	89	Unknown	18
Late rise[17–19]	35–53	16–39	4–20
Preoperative glaucoma			
Early rise[16, 18, 21]			
With	48–82		
Without	17–41		
Late rise[8, 16, 18, 21, 23, 74]			
With	76–100	38–40	
Without	10–56	25–50	
Graft size (all without preoperative glaucoma)			
Early rise[22, 28, 30]			
Same size	29–56		6–25
Oversize	8–45		0–4
Late rise[22, 28]			
Same size	31–47		24
Oversize	10–42		16

Table 136–4. POSTOPERATIVE FACTORS IN ELEVATED IOP

	%	Patient Population
Steroid Response		
Krontz and Wood[20]	60	Acute nonangle glaucoma after combined surgery
Goldberg et al[21]	23	Mixed
Thoft et al[23]	17	Aphakic bullous keratopathy/pseudophakic bullous keratopathy
Foulks[17]	7	Mixed
Kirkness and Moshegov[19]	5	Mixed
Peripheral Anterior Synechiae Formation		
Thoft et al[23]	100	Aphakic bullous keratopathy/pseudophakic bullous keratopathy (not clear whether done in all)
Lass and Paven-Langston[51]	100	Mixed
McDonnell et al[13]	76	Mixed
Waring[37]	46	Mixed
Foulks[17]	14	Mixed
Cohen et al[36]	40	Unknown

study has conducted a multivariate analysis to separate interactions that may exist. For example, aphakic eyes may be more likely to have preoperative glaucoma than phakic eyes. Although this factor can be controlled to some degree by looking at the incidence of preoperative glaucoma among a subset of patients (e.g., with aphakia or pseudophakia, as in Table 136–3), this method lacks the ability to generalize to other patient groups. Similarly, nearly all of the work in oversize grafting has been in eyes without preexisting glaucoma (see Table 136–3). Although this approach allows for the most uncluttered analysis, it omits critical data in the group shown to be at highest risk—aphakic patients with preoperative glaucoma—without any firm assurance that the data are readily transferable between groups. We would thus anticipate that a future study would have sufficient data and numbers to allow us to address these questions in a statistically more significant manner. However, relatively few surgeons have sufficient numbers of patients to permit such an analysis.

Phakic Status

At least four studies provide sufficient data to allow us to determine the part played by the eye's phakic status in keratoplasties performed by the same surgeon.[10, 17–19] However, none of these studies provide sufficient information to allow us to subcategorize by either the presence of preoperative glaucoma or the use of oversize grafting. Thus, recognizing the possible confounding role played by the other two factors, it is clear that both in the immediate postoperative period and at follow-up to 3 yr, aphakic eyes have the highest rate of elevated IOP. Pseudophakic eyes appear to have an intermediate position, and naturally phakic eyes have the lowest rate. As such, we should expect, and so inform our patients, that the risk of elevated IOP among all aphakic patients is at least 40 percent. Indeed, with longer follow-up, this risk may be even higher.

The mechanisms underlying this well-known predisposition are not known. A partial explanation is the higher rate of preoperative glaucoma among aphakic eyes compared with phakic eyes, given the importance of preoperative glaucoma (discussed later). However, when data are stratified to control for the presence of preoperative glaucoma, Foulks[17] found that aphakia was still an independent variable for the risk of postoperative IOP elevation. Olson,[24] Olson and Kaufman,[25] and Zimmerman and colleagues[26] suggest that the size of the graft may be an important factor because of anterior segment structural changes induced by keratoplasty. Zimmerman was able to show that the depth of suture placement had no effect on outflow facility in phakic human eye bank eyes undergoing penetrating keratoplasty. However, unlike through-and-through sutures, nonpenetrating sutures produced a 37 percent decrease in outflow facility in aphakic eye bank eyes.[26] It was hypothesized that the lens provides the trabecular meshwork with some form of support that is lost when the lens is removed. This loss of trabecular support in conjunction with distortive forces induced by the keratoplasty may increase aqueous outflow resistance. A clinical trial to test this hypothesis was discontinued because of persistent suture tract leaks among eyes with through-and-through sutures.[27] A subsequent study showed that the same effect as through-and-through sutures could safely be achieved by using a 0.5-mm oversize graft.[28]

How these factors interact is unknown at this time. Nevertheless, it does appear that phakic status is a favorable prognostic factor in reducing the development of keratoplasty-associated IOP elevations.

Preoperative Glaucoma

The role of preoperative glaucoma in predisposing to elevated IOP after keratoplasty has been examined in detail only among aphakic and pseudophakic eyes (see Table 136–3). Although one study states that preoperative glaucoma is significantly associated with postoperative IOP elevation among phakic eyes as well as aphakic,[17] insufficient data are published to allow us to determine the amount of difference. Part of the reason why most studies have concentrated on aphakic and pseudophakic eyes may be the high percentage of keratoplasties performed on aphakic and pseudophakic eyes as well as the relatively low incidence of glaucoma among diseases in phakic eyes with a need for keratoplasty. Similarly, phakic eyes, by definition, have had at least one fewer operation and may have had no prior operations. Nevertheless, it is clear that aphakic eyes with clinically controlled glaucoma preoperatively have at least a 75 percent risk of losing IOP control postoperatively (see Table 136–3). It is interesting that the rate of IOP derangement in pseudophakic eyes does not appear to be influenced by the preoperative status of the eye (see Table 136–3).

The explanations for this phenomenon are even more hypothetical than for phakic eyes. Again, it can be argued that aphakic eyes undergoing penetrating keratoplasty are even more disordered than pseudophakic eyes and that keratoplasty thus represents a greater insult to the eye. It could be that pseudophakic eyes provide more posterior support to the trabecular meshwork than aphakic eyes, so that the postulated trabecular meshwork distortion is less significant in pseudophakic eyes.

Operating on eyes without adequate pressure control preoperatively is ill advised. One can expect an even greater frequency and severity of IOP problems in these eyes. The use of combined glaucoma and keratoplasty procedures is being investigated. However, data are insufficient to properly evaluate the efficacy of these interventions in eyes with uncontrolled pressures at the time of operation (see Surgical Approaches, later).

Use of Oversize Grafts

Studies on the role of oversize grafts have been confined almost exclusively to eyes without preoperative glaucoma (see Table 136–3) and mainly in the immediate postoperative period. Because many of these studies investigated small numbers of eyes, the failure of some studies to find a statistically significant difference may not mean that the concept supporting oversize grafting is invalid. Similarly, the failure of the studies investigating the chronic elevation of IOP to find a statistically significant difference[29b] should be evaluated with this in mind, because both suggest a trend toward a protective effect of oversize grafting. Nevertheless, it is clear that the concept of oversize grafting has not been definitively proven.

Since its original suggestion by Franchesetti in 1949[31] and its theoretical testing by Olson,[24] Olson and Kaufman,[25] and Zimmerman,[26] the use of oversize grafting has now become standard practice. As Olson[32, 33] has pointed out, the actual size of the button removed can vary depending on which surface (endothelial or epithelial) is trephined or cut and what the pressure of the eye is (when removed from the host or from a whole-eye donor) at that moment. Therefore, the degree that grafts are oversized (or not) may vary. As such, any conclusion that can be drawn must be tentative.

POSTOPERATIVE FACTORS

The two major postoperative influences cited in altering the course after keratoplasty are the presence of synechial closure of the angle and the dual role played by steroids (see Table 136–4). These represent two mechanisms by which the preoperative factors noted earlier may cause elevated IOP after keratoplasty.

Peripheral Anterior Synechiae

Progressive angle closure carries a poor prognosis for pressure control and graft survival.[17, 19, 34] Table 136–4 shows some of the reported rates of peripheral anterior synechiae formation as a percentage of eyes that have

IOP elevation. Other studies have shown that the presence of peripheral anterior synechiae may indicate a need to undergo later surgery; in one series, five of eight eyes with peripheral anterior synechiae subsequently needed surgical intervention for glaucoma at a follow-up of 3 mo to 27 yr.[35]

The importance of progressive synechial closure has led many surgeons to recommend lysis of synechiae at the time of grafting. Further, intraoperative iridoplasty and synechialysis, perhaps as part of an anterior chamber reconstruction, have been reported to be successful in reducing the incidence of continued progressive synechial closure after keratoplasty.[36, 37] Thus, the need to be aware of synechial formation and to try to prevent it is well recognized.

Progressive angle-closure offers an attractive mechanism to explain keratoplasty-associated glaucoma, particularly among those without preoperative glaucoma. Some studies demonstrated that it is present in all eyes with elevated IOP after keratoplasty.[23] None of the reports supporting the role of oversize grafts, aphakia, or the preoperative presence of glaucoma involved routine gonioscopy of angle structures. One major study that did conduct routine gonioscopy found that only 14 percent of eyes with elevated IOP could have their disorder explained by progressive synechial closure.[17]

Steroids

Before the elucidation of the role of immune and inflammatory factors in graft rejection and inflammatory glaucomas, the use of steroids in the postoperative period was not emphasized. The use of potent steroids at frequent intervals was reported to reduce the perceived rate of acute or early IOP elevation.[23] However, with the recognition of the need for steroids to reduce inflammation and decrease allograft rejection came the awareness that a certain proportion of IOP elevations represented steroid responsiveness among patients (see Table 136–4).

The reported rate of steroid-responsive glaucoma ranges from 5 to 60 percent (see Table 136–4). Other studies have recognized the importance of this factor by noting its "occasional" occurrence or that the first therapeutic step should be to reduce the dose of steroids.[22] Insufficient information exists to draw any conclusions about the interrelationships between the role of steroids and the preoperative factors noted earlier.

Unanswered Questions

Many questions remain about whether additional mechanisms are at work in keratoplasty-associated glaucoma. In the most comprehensive study, 91 of 502 eyes (1 percent) developed chronic postoperative glaucoma.[17] However, only 32 eyes developed postoperative glaucoma but did not have preoperative glaucoma. The proportion of cases in which progressive angle closure, acute angle closure, steroid-induced glaucoma, or allograft rejection was involved is unstated. However, because these known causes added up to 28 cases, at one extreme only 4 of 502 (1 percent) eyes could have developed open-angle glaucoma over a number of years. Although this may be unlikely, it does suggest that previously described mechanisms for other forms of glaucoma may indeed be able to explain a large proportion of eyes with new-onset keratoplasty-associated glaucoma.

This question, like many of the other reservations about available information in this chapter, seeks an answer in a large study with multivariate analysis. We could then seek to answer questions about exactly what the relative risk factors are for elevated IOP and glaucoma after keratoplasty and how we can best modify them.

TREATMENT MODALITIES

Glaucoma associated with penetrating keratoplasty is often difficult to control,[38, 39] largely because of the underlying nature of the ocular conditions necessitating the transplant and the postoperative complications associated with keratoplasty. For example, aphakic glaucoma, even in the absence of a corneal graft and the presence of an open angle, is often difficult to control. Similarly, angle closure postoperatively reduces the number and effectiveness of treatment approaches. Thus, a critical consideration is the prevention of those mechanisms that may contribute to the development of postoperative glaucoma.

Despite our best efforts at prevention, patients with grafts will develop glaucoma. The available options today are much broader and potentially more effective than those of just 15 yr ago. They include medical treatment, laser trabeculoplasty, laser iris manipulation, filtering surgery, implant surgery, laser ablation of the ciliary structures, cryoablation, and focused ultrasound ablation.

A related issue is the effect of penetrating keratoplasty on eyes with preexisting glaucoma and functioning filtering operations. As noted earlier, keratoplasty in eyes with preoperative glaucoma results in reduced glaucoma control in a significant number of patients. Here too, however, little is known about an important effect of keratoplasty—namely, the effect of keratoplasty on filtering blebs.

The control of glaucoma, however, is only one consideration. The effect of glaucoma treatment on rejection episodes, graft clarity, and graft survival is as important to patients, because the grafts are usually performed in an attempt to increase visual function. Some believe that glaucoma is a risk factor for graft failure,[40] but whether the effect is due to the glaucoma, the treatment given, or both is unknown. The available data on the effects of various surgical approaches come from studies with a small number of cases (maximum of 28).[13, 14, 17, 41–48] More importantly, no investigations have addressed the effect of topical and systemic glaucoma medications on graft rejection, graft clarity, and graft survival, even though timolol and pilocarpine are potentially toxic to the epithelium.[49, 50]

Medical Therapy

Unlike virgin eyes with chronic open-angle glaucoma, eyes with penetrating keratoplasty-associated glaucoma have had at least one major operation, with significant alterations in anterior structures. Treatment is directed at the underlying cause, if the cause can be discerned. If it cannot, during the acute phase, medical therapy is the initial treatment of choice.

BETA-BLOCKERS

The reduction of aqueous production by β-blockers is helpful in patients who can tolerate their use.[51, 52] Even in aphakic eyes with partial synechial angle-closure, timolol was found to reduce IOP to less than 22 mmHg in 70 percent (9 of 13) of eyes, from a mean baseline of 39.7 mmHg.[51] Further data on the effectiveness of β-blocker therapy in keratoplasty-associated glaucoma have not been published, but widespread experience suggests that it is effective.

EPINEPHRINE

The use of adrenergic agents is limited by several considerations. First, because many eyes are aphakic, the risk of inducing cystoid macular edema is significant.[53] Second, the additive effect to topical β-blockers is minimal, particularly with nonselective agents such as timolol or levobunolol.[54, 55] Third, the presence of synechial closure would limit one proposed mechanism of action, that of increasing conventional outflow. Fourth, it is possible that induced alterations in the ocular-blood barrier, particularly in the presence of inflammation, may have some effect on graft survival or clarity. Thus, the use of epinephrine compounds should be limited to specific patients and clinical situations, such as phakic patients who have open angles and who are not concurrently using nonselective β-blockers.

PARASYMPATHOMIMETICS

Both direct- and indirect-acting agents are useful in the treatment of keratoplasty-associated glaucoma.[9, 56] However, because they act by increasing conventional outflow through the trabecular meshwork, their effectiveness is markedly reduced in the presence of significant synechial angle closure.

α-AGONISTS

Apraclonidine, an α_2-agonist, has been approved by the Food and Drug Administration for use in the perioperative period for laser trabeculoplasty and posterior capsulotomy.[57, 58] Experience suggests that it can be a useful adjunct, particularly in an acute setting, for keratoplasty-associated glaucoma. Apraclonidine appears to be additive to β-blockers; thus, it may become a useful addition to our medical therapy approach, particularly in the early postoperative period.

CARBONIC ANHYDRASE INHIBITORS

Before the development of topical β-blockers, carbonic anhydrase inhibitors were considered the most effective form of medical treatment for keratoplasty-associated glaucoma. They remain effective in the large majority of patients, albeit at the risk of well-known systemic side effects.

STEROIDS

Steroids are needed to reduce postoperative inflammation and to prevent and treat graft rejection. Experience has shown that steroids can be helpful in reducing IOP postoperatively.[23] However, they can also cause steroid-induced glaucoma. Thus, patients with increased IOP postoperatively must be assessed for the possible need to either decrease or increase steroids after ruling out other causes of elevated IOP. If the cause of elevated IOP is in question, as for example in the presence of mild inflammation 2 weeks postoperatively, one possible approach is to give potent steroids frequently for 48 hours. If the IOP is elevated because of inflammation, IOP reduction should be observed; however, if it is not, then steroids could be tapered to the minimum amount and strength possible to ensure graft survival.

Laser Therapy

The use of argon and ythrium-aluminum-garnet (YAG) lasers is dictated by the clinical condition. In those patients who develop pupillary block, malignant glaucoma, progressive synechial angle-closure, or increased IOP with no prior laser trabeculoplasty, laser treatment can be beneficial. The use of neodymium.YAG (Nd.YAG) lasers for cycloablation is discussed later.

PUPILLARY BLOCK AND MALIGNANT GLAUCOMA

A patent peripheral iridectomy is often created at the time of penetrating keratoplasty. In aphakic eyes or those with intraocular lenses, it is mandatory. In those situations in which a complete iridectomy was not performed or a patent iridectomy has subsequently been closed by inflammation or scarring, a laser iridotomy can be performed to prevent acute and chronic angle-closure glaucoma. Indeed, 6 percent of cases of elevated IOP in one series were due to acute angle closure.[17]

Malignant (ciliary block, aqueous diversion) glaucoma can be treated with the YAG laser in aphakic and pseudophakic eyes.[59] The aim is to disrupt the anterior vitreous hyaloid face.[59] In the keratoplasty setting, differentiation from pupillary block can be particularly difficult, because postoperative inflammation and the effects of intraoperative iris manipulation can result in loculated aqueous pockets posteriorly. The presence of a patent iridectomy is mandatory to rule out a pupillary block mechanism before initiating treatment for malignant glaucoma.

LASER IRIDOPLASTY/GONIOPLASTY

The finding of progressive synechial angle closure after penetrating keratoplasty is an ominous sign because it represents potentially worsening glaucoma over time. Although a few eyes with progressive synechiae may not develop IOP elevation, those that do are extremely difficult to manage.[17] Although there have been no reports of laser gonioplasty after keratoplasty, its successful use in other settings with chronic or secondary angle-closure, with or without trabeculectomy,[60, 61] suggests that this may be a potentially useful approach, particularly given the initial results of intraoperative synechialysis (discussed later).

LASER TRABECULOPLASTY

In selected eyes, laser trabeculoplasty after penetrating keratoplasty may be helpful. Van Meter and colleagues performed laser trabeculoplasty in ten eyes an average of 25 mo after penetrating keratoplasty; the IOP was reduced more than 5 mmHg in eight eyes (mean of 9.1 mmHg), with a mean follow-up of 23 mo.[14] Both eyes without peripheral anterior synechiae and six of eight eyes with them were successfully treated. Eyes without prekeratoplasty glaucoma had a mean pressure reduction of 46 percent. Four eyes with preoperative glaucoma had a mean decrease of 15 percent; however, whether these eyes had prior laser trabeculoplasty was unstated.[14]

In another study, Gross and colleagues performed laser trabeculoplasty in 20 aphakic and pseudophakic eyes after grafting.[62] At 9 months, only 45 percent had an IOP less than 22 mmHg and only 10 percent met both vision and pressure criteria for success.[62] Thus, laser trabeculoplasty is less successful in aphakic and pseudophakic eyes and in eyes with large amounts of peripheral anterior synechiae, which limit the amount of treatable angle. In other eyes, particularly those without prekeratoplasty glaucoma, laser trabeculoplasty should be considered.

Surgical Approaches

The need for surgical intervention in eyes with keratoplasty-associated glaucoma has been estimated at 12 to 57 percent.[17, 21, 62, 63] Among phakic eyes receiving grafts for inactive interstitial keratitis, the lowest rate of 12 percent at an average follow-up of 3.7 yr was observed.[35] Among a mixed population of patients, Foulks reported a rate of 24 percent at 3 yr.[17] Not surprisingly, among a mixed population of eyes undergoing repeat grafting, Goldberg and colleagues reported a higher rate of 35 percent at a follow-up of only 7 to 30 mo.[21] Finally, among seven eyes that had congenital glaucoma (having had previous glaucoma operations) and that received grafts when the patients were adults, four required additional glaucoma surgery after the keratoplasty and the other three required medical therapy.[63]

Because penetrating keratoplasty is often performed on seriously compromised eyes and is itself a major alteration of ocular structures, surgery is often difficult and less successful. In many eyes, the conjunctiva is scarred. In many cases, the eyes are aphakic or pseudophakic. As a result, many eyes are poor candidates for filtration surgery, and implant surgery or cilioablative procedures may be required.

FILTRATION SURGERY

The use of trabeculectomy has been investigated in a limited number of studies.[17, 42, 62, 64] As can be seen in Table 136–5, the reported success rate ranges from 27 to 80 percent. The success of trabeculectomy is influenced by the same factors that alter its success in the nonkeratoplasty setting. Gilvarry and colleagues reported, for example, that the success rate was four times greater in eyes that had only one graft performed as opposed to those with two or more.[42] Similarly, aphakic eyes tend to fare much worse than phakic eyes. In addition, eyes with angles closed by peripheral anterior synechiae fare worse than eyes without.[42] Thus, the less anterior segment architecture has been disturbed, the more successful intervention becomes.

The timing of the operation should be based on a patient's clinical condition. Although some have advocated early trabeculectomy in these patients on the basis of early IOP rises,[64] the effectiveness does not appear to be increased by doing so. As an alternative, Insler and associates reported that 43 percent (three of seven) of eyes had an IOP less than 21 mmHg when combined keratoplasty and trabeculectomy were performed, at a mean follow-up of 16 mo.[65]

Performing filtration surgery appears to pose a risk to the graft. Among eyes in which the surgery succeeds, the rate of graft failure at 3 yr ranges from 11 to 20 percent.[17, 42] How many failures could be expected in any case is uncertain; this phenomenon could potentially represent the natural history of grafts in these eyes.

Table 136–5. TRABECULECTOMY

Investigators	Success (%)	Criteria	Mean Follow-up	Patient Population
Foulks[17]	80	IOP	3 yr	Mixed
Gilvarry et al[42]	51	IOP	3 yr	Mixed
Gross et al[62]	27	IOP and VA	9 mo	Aphakic/pseudophakic
Kushwaha and Pual[64]	53	IOP	1 yr	Mixed (immediate operation within 2 weeks of penetrating keratoplasty)

IOP, intraocular pressure; VA, visual acuity.

However, in eyes that failed filtration surgery, the rate of graft failure at 3 years has been reported to be as high as 59 percent.[42] Whether such failures are due to the need for further intervention, the results of the operation itself, or a combination of factors is not clear. Nevertheless, this observation does suggest the gravity of unsuccessful filtration surgery in eyes having undergone keratoplasty.

CYCLODIALYSIS

The success rate of cyclodialysis ranges from 22 to 35 percent.[62, 64] Among aphakic and pseudophakic eyes, 35 percent achieved a pressure of 21 mmHg or less at 9 mo,[62] whereas 22 percent of a mixed population were successful at an unknown length of follow-up in another study.[64] When combined with visual criteria, however, the rate of success fell to 15 percent after 9 mo.[62]

SYNECHIALYSIS

With the recent repopularization of surgical lysis of peripheral anterior synechiae,[66, 67] the application of this technique may prove useful in the treatment of progressive angle-closure after keratoplasty. Performing iridoplasty and synechialysis at the time of keratoplasty reduces the number of patients in whom progressive closure occurs after surgery.[36] As mentioned earlier, many others have noted the importance of performing intraoperative synechialyis when possible and preventing postoperative anterior or peripheral anterior synechiae.

Performing synechialyis may increase the risk of inducing graft failure. In one case in which graft failure was mentioned, synechialysis preceded graft failure.[41]

PROSTHETIC DEVICES

Because of the refractory nature of many forms of secondary glaucoma, several prosthetic devices designed to be implanted in the eye have been developed to overcome the eye's healing responses to filtration and other surgery. These have become more widely used for keratoplasty-associated glaucoma, in an attempt to salvage useful vision in eyes before performing ciliodestructive procedures.[13]

Molteno's Implant

Molteno's plate implantation appears to be a promising technique (Figs. 136–1 and 136–2). In 17 eyes, 16 aphakic or pseudoaphakic and 13 having had prior glaucoma operations, 12 eyes achieved an IOP of less than 21 mmHg after one implant; 2 of 3 eyes (of the unsuccessful 5 eyes) undergoing a second implant also achieved IOP control, with a mean follow-up of 13 mo and ranging to 28 mo. This finding offers hope for patients with keratoplasty-associated glaucoma.[13]

The disadvantage of this procedure, however, is the occurrence of graft rejection in a high percentage (7 of 17) of eyes, progressing to failure in 5 (29 percent) eyes. Thus, although 12 of 17 eyes had the same or better

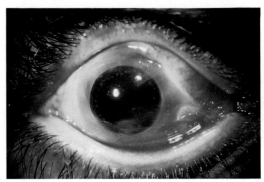

Figure 136–1. Low-power photo of a Molteno's tube in an eye with penetrating keratoplasty.

vision after placement of a Molteno's plate, 5 suffered a decrease in vision.[12] Of the 12 eyes with successful pressure control, three had a decrease in vision due to graft failure.

Schocket's Tube

Schocket's tube implantation has also been used to try to preserve visual function while controlling IOP.[45, 46, 62] Its potential usefulness was suggested in the original report of Schocket's tube, in which four of five eyes, including two aphakic eyes and one with keratoplasty, were successfully controlled despite the presence of 360 degrees of synechial angle-closure.[68] Subsequent groups have noted a success rate of 50 to 100 percent in keratoplasty-associated glaucoma.[45, 46, 62, 68]

In an initial report, Kirkness noted that 91 percent (10 of 11) of aphakic eyes had IOP control at a follow-up ranging from 3 to 24 mo, despite the fact that an average of 5.1 procedures were performed before receiving the implant.[45] An expanded report showed that among 20 aphakic eyes monitored for an average of 26 mo (range of 6 to 60), all having undergone prior glaucoma surgery, 16 eyes achieved successful control.[46] The 4-year survival probability was estimated at 68 percent.[46] Six eyes had a single-stage procedure, and 14 had a two-stage procedure; results were better with the two-stage procedure.[46] Interestingly, of the 14 two-stage procedures, three involved a combined tube implant and

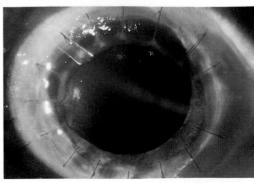

Figure 136–2. Higher-power view of eye with a Molteno's tube in position.

keratoplasty, suggesting that combined surgery may be useful in the future in selected eyes.[46]

In another series of six aphakic or pseudophakic eyes, Schocket's tube implantation not only resulted in an IOP of less than 21 mmHg but visual stability in 83 percent (five eyes) during a 9-month follow-up period.[62] Although two of these eyes required a revision, this intervention was the most successful of any type among all the possible approaches performed. Nine of nine eyes in another series, at a mean follow-up of 10.7 mo, had successful IOP control after a modified Schocket's tube implant, with a mean IOP of 15 mmHg.[69]

The rate of graft failure during the follow-up periods noted earlier ranged up to 20 percent.[45, 46] Again, whether this represents what would have occurred without tube placement or is a result of the surgery or the tube placement is unknown. However, concern has been raised about the role of implant devices in altering the blood-ocular barrier in inducing or increasing the rate of graft rejections and graft failure.[19, 45, 46]

CILIODESTRUCTIVE PROCEDURES

Long ago, end-stage glaucoma in eyes undergoing keratoplasty was often treated by enucleation or functional denervation with retrobulbar alcohol. Less than 25 yr ago, the development of cyclocryotherapy created another option. Since that time, modern technology has created additional instruments and methods to lower eye pressure through destructive means. Putting aside concerns of the mechanisms of cryotherapy and its newer counterparts (see Chapter 147), these are often successful in lowering the IOP to acceptable ranges.

Cryotherapy

The success rate for IOP control ranges from 38 to 100 percent at follow-ups ranging to 3 yr (Table 136–6).[13, 17, 19, 22, 43, 44, 62, 64] Again, the rate of success is lower in aphakic and pseudophakic eyes.[62] Although highly successful from an IOP viewpoint, cryotherapy carries significant morbidity. In one series, 14 percent of eyes receiving cryotherapy lost more than two Snellen's lines of visual acuity within 9 months.[62]

Vitreous hemorrhage, retinal detachment, choroidal detachment, cystoid macular edema, uveitis, phthisis, and graft failure are among the reported side effects.[13,] [43, 44] The rate of phthisis is from 0 to 14 percent at follow-up ranging to a mean of 19.4 mo.[43, 44, 62, 70] As importantly, the rate of graft failure is quite high, from 7 to 80 percent in series with a follow-up of at least 10 mo.[13, 17, 43, 44] In part, failure may be due to injuring the corneal endothelium. In many cases, these eyes are already severely compromised and graft failure might not be unexpected; for example, 8 of 36 (22 percent) eyes in one study had corneal clouding even before cryotherapy.[44] Three other studies report rates of graft failure of 41 to 80 percent at follow-up ranging from 10 mo to 3 years.[13, 17, 43] Thus, cryotherapy carries significant risk to the graft as well as the eye.

Laser Cycloablation

Refinement of transscleral cyclophotocoagulation has raised hope of offering a more controlled and less morbid approach for IOP control. Success rates from 50 to 100 percent have been reported at median follow-up from 6 to 18 mo.[47, 48, 62] Not surprisingly, aphakic and pseudophakic eyes appear to fare somewhat worse,[62] although one study suggests that short-term IOP control (minimum of 3 mo, median of 6 mo follow-up) was achieved in six of six aphakic and three of three pseudophakic eyes.[48]

Although laser cycloablation has been reported to be less morbid than cryotherapy in some series,[71] the rate of graft clouding and failure has been reported to range from 22 percent at a follow-up median of 6 mo to 42 percent at a follow-up median of 18 mo.[47, 48] Further, visual loss of greater than two lines of Snellen's acuity has also been reported among eyes that are successfully treated.[62] Thus, what role laser cyclophotocoagulation will have in the management of keratoplasty-associated glaucoma has yet to be determined.

High-Intensity, Focused Ultrasound

A few centers in the United States and Europe have explored the use of ultrasound as a means of destroying the ciliary body and processes to reduce IOP. Its use in keratoplasty-associated glaucoma has not been reported, though a success rate of 60 percent at 1 yr by IOP criteria was reported for 34 eyes with nonuveitic, nonneovascular secondary angle closure.[72] Concern exists, however, about the impact of ultrasound waves on the graft and its subsequent functioning.[73]

Table 136–6. CRYOTHERAPY

Investigators	Success (%)	Criteria	Mean Follow-up	Patient Population
Binder et al[44]	100	IOP	19.4 mo	Mixed
Foulks[17]	88	IOP	3 yr	Mixed
Tragakis et al[78]	69	IOP	20 mo	Mixed
West et al[43]	86	IOP	10 mo	Mixed
Gross et al[62]	41	IOP and VA	9 mo	Aphakic/pseudophakic
	77	IOP only		
Kirkness and Moshegov[19]	62	IOP	N/A	Mixed
Kushwaha and Pual[64]	61	IOP	1 yr	Early/mixed

IOP, intraocular pressure; VA, visual acuity.

CONCLUSION

In eyes with preexisting glaucoma, either medically uncontrolled or only controllable with multiple medications, we recommend surgical management to lower IOP in advance (preferably) or at the time of keratoplasty. Such an approach may blunt the early IOP rise and possibly avoid the need for later glaucoma surgery jeopardizing a clear graft. The decision about which procedure to perform in conjunction with, before, or after keratoplasty requires careful consideration of a patient's status and the options available to the surgeon.

Glaucoma associated with penetrating keratoplasty is a common and growing problem. Although much has been learned in the past 20 yr, much more still needs to be discovered. With our level of knowledge, we can draw certain tentative conclusions.

First, the incidence of keratoplasty-associated glaucoma varies widely depending on the cause of the corneal disease. Second, eyes with preexisting glaucoma have high rate of loss of IOP control after keratoplasty. Third, although the underlying mechanisms are unclear, several discrete interventions can be undertaken intra- and postoperatively to try to control IOP. Fourth, current methods of treatment leave much to be desired. In particular, eyes requiring surgery face not only the risk of unsuccessful surgery but also the risk of graft decompensation, even when pressure control is achieved.

REFERENCES

1. Eye Bank Association of America: Eye Banking Activity: 1987. Washington DC, Eye Bank Association of America, 1988.
2. Council on Scientific Affairs: Report of the organ transplant council: Corneal transplantation. JAMA 259:719, 1988.
3. Robin JB, Gindi JJ, Koh K, et al: An update of the indications for penetrating keratoplasty. Arch Ophthalmol 104:87, 1986.
4. Mohamadi P, McDonnell JM, Irvine JA, et al: Changing indications for penetrating keratoplasty, 1984–88. [Letter] Am J Ophthalmol 107:551, 1989.
5. Lang GK, Green WR: Clinicopathologic studies of keratoplasty eyes obtained surgically. Cornea 4:229, 1985.
6. Stark WJ, Bruner WE, Maumenee AE: Surgery of the cornea. In Rice TA, Michels RG, Stark WJ (eds): Ophthalmic Surgery. St. Louis, CV Mosby, 1984, pp 129–36.
7. Polack FM: Glaucoma in keratoplasty. Cornea 7:67, 1988.
8. Schanzlin DJ, Robin JB, Gomez DS, et al: Results of penetrating keratoplasty for aphakic and pseudophakic bullous keratopathy. Am J Ophthalmol 98:302, 1984.
9. Olson RJ: Glaucoma associated with penetrating keratoplasty. In Ritch R, Shields MB, Krupin T. (eds): The Glaucomas. St. Louis, CV Mosby, 1989, pp 1337–1347.
10. Irvine AR, Kaufman HE: Intraocular pressure following penetrating keratoplasty. Am J Ophthalmol 68:835, 1969.
11. Wind CA, Kaufman HE: Validity of MacKay-Marg tonometry following penetrating keratoplasty in man. Am J Ophthalmol 72:117, 1971.
12. Buxton JN, Riechers RJ, Aaron SD: Corneal grafts and their effect upon the applanation Schiotz disparity. Arch Ophthalmol 86:28, 1971.
13. McDonnell PJ, Robin JB, Schanzlin DJ, et al: Molteno implant for control of glaucoma in eyes after penetrating keratoplasty. Ophthalmology 95:364, 1988.
14. Van Meter WS, Allen RC, Waring GO, Stulting RD: Laser trabeculoplasty for glaucoma in aphakic and pseudophakic eyes after penetrating keratoplasty. Arch Ophthalmol 106:185, 1988.
15. Olson RJ, Kaufman HE: Intraocular pressure and corneal thickness after penetrating keratoplasty. Am J Ophthalmol 86:97, 1978.
16. Olson RJ, Kaufman HE: Prognostic factors of intraocular pressure after aphakic keratoplasty. Am J Ophthalmol 86:510, 1978.
17. Foulks GN: Glaucoma associated with penetrating keratoplasty. Ophthalmology 94:871, 1987.
18. Karesh JW, Nirankari VS: Factors associated with glaucoma after penetrating keratoplasty. Am J Ophthalmol 96:160, 1983.
19. Kirkness CM, Moshegov C: Post-keratoplasty glaucoma. Eye 2 (Suppl):919, 1988.
20. Krontz DP, Wood TO: Corneal decompensation following acute angle-closure glaucoma. Ophthalmic Surg 19:334, 1988.
21. Goldberg DB, Schanzlin DJ, Brown SI: Incidence of increased intraocular pressure after keratoplasty. Am J Ophthalmol 92:372, 1981.
22. Heidemann DG, Sugar A, Meyer RF, Musch DC: Oversized donor grafts in penetrating keratoplasty. Arch Ophthalmol 103:1807, 1985.
23. Thoft RA, Gordon JM, Dohlman CH: Glaucoma following keratoplasty. Trans Am Acad Opthalmol Otol 78:OP-352, 1974.
24. Olson RJ: Aphakic keratoplasty. Arch Ophthalmol 96:2274, 1978.
25. Olson RJ, Kaufman HE: A mathematical description of causative factors and prevention of elevated intraocular pressure after keratoplasty. Invest Ophthalmol Vis Sci 16:1085, 1977.
26. Zimmerman TJ, Krupin T, Brodzki W, Waltman SR: The effect of suture depth on outflow facility in penetrating keratoplasty. Arch Ophthalmol 96:505, 1978.
27. Zimmerman TJ, Waltman SR, Sachs U, Kaufman HE: Intraocular pressure after aphakic penetrating keratoplasty: Through-and-through suturing. Ophthalmic Surg 10:49, 1979.
28. Bourne WM, Davison JA, O'Fallon WM: The effects of oversize donor buttons on postoperative intraocular pressure and corneal curvature in aphakic penetrating keratoplasty. Ophthalmology 89:242, 1982.
29. Zimmerman T, Olson R, Waltman S, Kaufman H: Transplant size and elevated intraocular pressure. Arch Ophthalmol 96:2231, 1978.
30. Perl T, Charlton KH, Binder PS: Disparate diameter grafting. Ophthalmology 88:774, 1981.
31. Foulks GN, Perry HD, Dohlman CH: Oversize corneal donor grafts in penetrating keratoplasty. Ophthalmology 86:490, 1979.
32. Olson RJ: Discussion. Ophthalmology 88:780, 1981.
33. Olson RJ: Variation in corneal graft size related to trephine technique. Arch Ophthalmol 97:1323, 1979.
34. Polack FM: Keratoplasty in aphakic eyes with corneal edema. Ophthalmic Surg 11:701, 1980.
35. Rabb MF, Fine M: Penetrating keratoplasty in interstitial keratitis. Am J Ophthalmol 67:907, 1969.
36. Cohen EJ, Kenyon KR, Dohlman CH: Iridoplasty for prevention of post-keratoplasty angle closure and glaucoma. Ophthalmic Surg 13:994, 1982.
37. Waring GO: Management of pseudophakic corneal edema with reconstruction of the anterior ocular segment. Arch Ophthalmol 105:709, 1987.
38. Wood TO, West C, Kaufman HE: Control of intraocular pressure in penetrating keratoplasty. Am J Ophthalmol 74:724, 1972.
39. Olson RJ, Zimmerman TJ, Kaufman HE: Elevated intraocular pressure after aphakic keratoplasty: Iatrogenic disease and prevention. Ann Ophthalmol 1978, p 931.
40. Paton D: The prognosis of penetrating keratoplasty. Ophthalmic Surg 7:36, 1976.
41. Lemp MA, Pfister RR, Dohlman CH: The effect of intraocular surgery on clear corneal grafts. Am J Ophthalmol 70:719, 1970.
42. Gilvarry AME, Kirkness CM, Steele AD, et al: The management of post-keratoplasty glaucoma by trabeculectomy. Eye 3:713, 1989.
43. West CE, Wood TO, Kaufman HE: Cyclocryotherapy for glaucoma pre- or postpenetrating keratoplasty. Am J Ophthalmol 76:485, 1973.
44. Binder PS, Abel R, Kaufman HE: Cyclocryotherapy for glaucoma after penetrating keratoplasty. Am J Ophthalmol 79:489, 1975.
45. Kirkness CM: Penetrating keratoplasty, glaucoma and silicone drainage tubing. Dev Ophthalmol 14:161, 1987.
46. Kirkness CM, Ling Y, Rice NSC: The use of silicone drainage tubing to control post-keratoplasty glaucoma. Eye 2:583, 1988.

47. Cohen EJ, Schwartz LW, Luskind RD, et al: Neodymium:YAG laser transcleral cyclophotocoagulation for glaucoma after penetrating keratoplasty. Ophthalmic Surg 20:713, 1989.
48. Levy NS, Bonney RC: Transscleral YAG cyclophotocoagulation of the ciliary body for persistently high intraocular pressure following penetrating keratoplasty. Cornea 8:178, 1989.
49. Wilson RP, Spaeth GL, Poryzees EM: The place of timolol in the practice of ophthalmology. Ophthalmology 87:451, 1980.
50. Johnson DH, Kenyon KR, Epstein DL, Van Buskirk EM: Corneal changes during pilocarpine gel therapy. Am J Ophthalmol 101:13, 1986.
51. Lass JH, Paven-Langston D: Timolol therapy in secondary angle-closure glaucoma post penetrating keratoplasty. Ophthalmology 86:51, 1979.
52. Olson RJ, Kaufman HE, Zimmerman TJ: Effects of timolol and daranide on elevated intraocular pressure after aphakic keratoplasty. Ann Ophthalmol 1979, p 1833.
53. Thomas JV, Gragoudas ES, Blair NP, Lapus JV: Correlation of epinephrine use and macular edema in aphakic glaucomatous eyes. Arch Ophthalmol 96:625, 1978.
54. Thomas JV, Epstein DL: Timolol and epinephrine in primary open angle glaucoma. Arch Ophthalmol 99:91, 1981.
55. Parrow KA, Hong YJ, Shin DH, et al: Is it worthwhile to add dipivefrin HC1 0.1% to topical β_1-, β_2-blocker therapy? Ophthalmology 98:1338, 1989.
56. Shields MB: Textbook of Glaucoma, 2nd ed. Baltimore, Williams & Wilkins, 1987, pp 374–382.
57. Pollack IP, Brown RH, Crandall AS, et al: Prevention of the rise in intraocular pressure following neodymium-YAG posterior capsulotomy using topical 1% apraclonidine. Arch Ophthalmol 106:754, 1988.
58. Brown RH, Stewart RH, Lynch MG, et al: ALO 2145 reduces the intraocular pressure elevation after anterior segment laser surgery. Ophthalmology 95:378, 1988.
59. Epstein DL, Steinert RF, Puliafito CA: Neodymium-YAG laser therapy to the anterior hyaloid in aphakic malignant (ciliovitreal block) glaucoma. Am J Ophthalmol 98:137, 1984.
60. Kandarakis A, Zimmerman T: Non-pupillary block angle-closure glaucoma and their treatment by laser. Ann Ophthalmol 16:914, 1984.
61. Fu YA, Liaw ZC: Argon laser gonioplasty with trabeculoplasty for chronic angle-closure glaucoma. Ann Ophthalmol 19:419, 1987.
62. Gross RL, Feldman RM, Spaeth GL, et al: Surgical therapy of chronic glaucoma in aphakia and pseudoaphakia. Ophthalmology 95:1195, 1988.
63. Huang SCM, Soong HK, Brenz RM, et al: Problems associated with penetrating keratoplasty for corneal edema in congenital glaucoma. Ophthalmic Surg 20:399, 1989.
64. Kushwaha DC, Pual AK: Incidence and management of glaucoma in post operative cases of penetrating keratoplasty. Indian J Ophthalmol 29:167, 1981.
65. Insler MS, Cooper HD, Kastl PR, Caldwell DR: Penetrating keratoplasty with trabeculectomy. Am J Ophthalmol 100:593, 1985.
66. Campbell DG, Vela MA: Modern goniosynechialysis for the treatment of synechial angle-closure glaucoma. Ophthalmology 91:1052, 1984.
67. Shingleton BJ, Chan MA, Bellows AR, Thomas JV: Surgical goniosynechialysis for angle-closure glaucoma, Ophthalmology 97:551, 1990.
68. Schocket SS, Nirankari VS, Lakhanpal V, et al: Anterior chamber tube shunt to an encircling band in the treatment of neovascular glaucoma and other refractory glaucomas. Ophthalmology 92:553, 1985.
69. Omi CA, de Almeida GV, Cohen R, et al: Modified Schocket implant for refractory glaucoma. Ophthalmology 98:211, 1991.
70. Wilson SE, Kaufman HE: Graft failure after penetrating keratoplasty. Surg Ophthalmol 34:325, 1990.
71. Schuman JS, Puliafito CA, Allingham RR, et al: Contact transscleral continuous wave neodymium-YAG laser cyclophotocoagulation. Ophthalmology 97:571, 1990.
72. Burgess SEP, Silverman RH, Coleman DJ, et al: Treatment of glaucoma with high-intensity focused ultrasound. Ophthalmology 93:831, 1986.
73. McDonnell PJ, Quigley HA, Green WR: Effect of therapeutic ultrasound on intraocular lenses. Ophthalmic Surg 17:655, 1986.
74. Waring GO, Welch SN, Cavagh MD, et al: Results of penetrating keratoplasty in 123 eyes with pseudophakic or aphakic corneal edema. Ophthalmology 90:25, 1983.
75. Robinson CH: Indications, complications and programs for repeat penetrating keratoplasty. Ophthalmic Surg 10:27, 1979.
76. Feldman ST, Frucht-Perry J, Brown SI: Corneal transplantation in microphthalmic eyes. Am J Ophthalmol 104:164, 1987.
77. Crawford GJ, Stulting RD, Cavanagh HD, Waring GO: Penetrating keratoplasty in the management of iridocorneal endothelial syndrome. Cornea 8:34, 1929.
78. Tragakis MP, Brown SI: The significance of new anterior synechiae after corneal transplantation. Am J Ophthalmol 74:523, 1972.

Chapter 137

■

Glaucoma Associated with Disorders of the Retina, Vitreous, and Choroid

SANDRA J. SOFINSKI and JOSEPH F. BURKE JR.

GENERAL PRINCIPLES

The relationship of glaucoma to disorders of the posterior segment is complex and multifaceted. Glaucoma represents a significant challenge to the successful diagnosis, treatment, and management of several posterior segment disorders. The spectrum of glaucoma-related conditions associated with disorders of the retina, vitreous, and choroid are best understood in terms of mechanism and treatment. Mechanisms of glaucoma include open-angle glaucoma (primary and secondary); closed-angle glaucoma (in the presence or absence of pupillary block); and glaucoma caused by increased episcleral venous pressure. These relationships are further classified into three major categories: glaucoma associated with posterior segment disorders on the basis of a common underlying etiology; glaucoma caused by posterior segment disorders; and glaucoma resulting from the treatment of posterior segment disorders. Posterior segment disorders arising from the treatment of glaucoma are discussed in Chapter 145. Whenever possible, the reader is referred to the appropriate sections in this compendium in which topics are explored in greater detail.

Examination of the Patient

The association of glaucoma and posterior segment disorders creates unique challenges in the diagnosis and management of both disorders. The presence of one can confound the diagnosis or impair the treatment of the other. Examiners must be constantly aware of the possibility that the two coexist in one patient when searching for the cause of visual impairment or glaucoma. A thorough, baseline ophthalmic examination including biomicroscopy, gonioscopy, dilated fundoscopic evaluation, and peripheral retinal examination should be conducted on all new patients as well as those presenting with a change in symptoms or new onset visual loss. Baseline central and peripheral visual fields as well as stereo disc photographs should be obtained for the purposes of future comparison. Refractive errors, tilted discs, optic nerve head drusen, and chorioretinal degeneration associated with axial myopia are some posterior segment conditions that can mimic visual field defects found in glaucoma.[1] Unexpected visual field changes that do not correlate with optic nerve head pathology or that cannot be explained on the basis of patient or examiner error should be investigated with dilated fundoscopic evaluation, because subclinical retinal detachment can present in this fashion. Unexpected, asymmetric decreases or elevations of pressure associated with uveitis, which do not respond to medical therapy may be signs of retinal detachment that require fundoscopic evaluation.[2]

Clues to the diagnosis of glaucoma or retinal detachment can often be obtained from an examination of the fellow eye, because both can manifest as bilateral diseases. Glaucoma may be difficult to detect in the presence of retinal detachment because of hypotony, inflammation, or media opacification. Preexisting glaucoma will not interfere with anatomic repair of retinal detachment but may limit visual potential postoperatively.[3] Preoperative diagnosis of preexisting glaucomatous damage is important in at least two ways: (1) identification of eyes that are predisposed to, but least able to, tolerate elevations of pressure during the operative and postoperative periods; and (2) counseling of patients regarding limited visual potential expectations postoperatively. A detailed examination of the optic nerve in the presence of miotic pupils or nystagmus can be performed by direct ophthalmoscopy through a Koeppe lens.[4] Frequently, cataract coexists with glaucoma, and media opacification becomes a significant impediment to posterior segment evaluation. In this situation, B-scan ultrasound becomes a valuable adjunct in the determination of retinal tears or detachment.[5]

Miotic therapy for glaucoma may interfere with adequate pupillary dilation needed for posterior segment evaluation. To facilitate peripheral retinal evaluation, miotic therapy may be withheld for 24 to 48 hr in the case of direct-acting miotics and slightly longer in the case of indirect-acting miotics to enable greater response to mydriatic agents.

Symptoms of flashes or floaters need to be investigated for the presence of retinal tear or detachment in all patients, and especially if miotic therapy has recently been started or increased in a patient with glaucoma. Subjective symptoms of flashes may be explained on the basis of posterior vitreous detachment, and floaters may represent entoptic phenomenon enhanced by miotic-induced pupillary miosis in patients who are taking pilocarpine or echothiophate iodide.

Role of Miotic Therapy of Glaucoma in Relation to Retinal Detachment

There are several reports in the literature of retinal detachment developing shortly after the initiation or incremental increase of miotic therapy.[6–10] While some support the perception of miotic therapy with retinal detachment, no large, prospective study with matched controls has ever been undertaken to prove or disprove a cause-and-effect relationship.[11] Patient care can be optimized while affording maximum protection to the examiner by adhering to the following recommendations:

1. Patients who manifest symptoms suggestive of posterior segment pathology (flashes of light or floaters) should have dilated posterior segment and peripheral retinal evaluation prior to the initiation of miotic therapy.

2. Patients who manifest posterior segment pathology or conditions that may predispose to retinal tear or detachment (i.e., aphakic or pseudophakic eyes with any retinal break, and phakic eyes with horseshoe breaks or dialyses) should be informed of the option of prophylactic therapy before the institution of miotic therapy.

3. All patients should be informed of the need for and possible risks associated with miotic therapy prior to the initiation of therapy. Patients should be informed regarding symptoms and signs of retinal detachment and the need for prompt evaluation.

GLAUCOMA ASSOCIATED WITH DISORDERS OF THE POSTERIOR SEGMENT ON THE BASIS OF A COMMON UNDERLYING CAUSE OR FOR REASONS UNKNOWN

Primary Open-Angle Glaucoma Associated with Rhegmatogenous Retinal Detachment

Intraocular pressure following retinal detachment may be reduced, unchanged, or elevated compared with the fellow eye. A study involving 604 patients with uncomplicated unilateral retinal detachment identified relative hypotony of 1.3 mmHg in 40 percent of the eyes compared with the normal fellow eye.[12] A series of investigators have found pressure asymmetry occurring in patients with unilateral retinal detachment compared with the fellow eye as follows: lower pressure, 64.2 percent; equal pressure, 26 percent; higher pressure, 9.8 percent.[12]

The prevalence of primary open-angle glaucoma (POAG) in the general population has been reported to range from 0.84 to 1.1 percent.[13-15] Several investigators have noted a higher prevalence of primary open-angle glaucoma occurring in patients with nontraumatic, rhegmatogenous retinal detachments when compared with the general population.[16, 17] In 1955, Becker reported bilateral tonographic and clinical data regarding 530 patients with retinal detachment and found that POAG was present in 5.8 percent.[16] In 1977, Phelps and Burton evaluated 817 patients undergoing primary retinal detachment repair and found that POAG was present in 4 percent.[17] Langham and Regan found reduced intraocular pressures, decreased outflow facilities, and decreased rates of aqueous humor formation in eyes with retinal detachment and their counterparts, compared with a control population.[18] Evidence to support the genetic association of POAG and retinal detachment on a multiple allelic basis is derived from a study involving 30 patients with nontraumatic retinal detachment.[19] Two factors predisposing to POAG—large cup:disc ratio[20] and topical steroid responsiveness[21]—were found to be significantly correlated with nontraumatic, rhegmatogenous retinal detachment, compared with their respective prevalences in the nonglaucomatous population.

Glaucoma Associated with Nanophthalmos

(The reader is referred to Chapter 135 for a more detailed discussion.)

Nanophthalmos is an inheritable ocular disorder in which the dimensions of the globe, except for the crystalline lens, are reduced in scale to approximately two thirds that of normal. The eye is otherwise normal in form and function.[22-24] Usually, high degrees of hyperopia are discovered through cycloplegic refraction; however, myopia and emmetropia may rarely be encountered.[22, 25] By expanded definition, the axial length as measured through quantitative biometry is less than or equal to 20.5 mm.[194]

Mechanisms of glaucoma associated with nanophthalmos are open-angle glaucoma[25]; primary angle-closure glaucoma on the basis of pupillary block[26]; secondary angle-closure resulting from ciliochoroidal thickening and effusion[23, 27]; increased episcleral venous pressure associated with impaired drainage of vortex veins through abnormally thickened sclera[23]; and malignant glaucoma following intraocular surgery.[23, 25]

Ocular features that predispose to the development of glaucoma include a crystalline lens of normal volume occupying a disproportionately large percentage of ocular volume (24 percent compared with normal 4 percent),[26, 28] thus creating anterior segment crowding. Progressive anterior chamber shallowing and narrowing of the angle occurs with the onset of angle-closure during the fourth to sixth decades, hence the need for frequent gonioscopic evaluation and documentation.[26] Shaffer suggested that abnormally thickened sclera in nanophthalmos could cause choroidal effusion by reduced permeability to protein and impairing outflow through vortex veins.[29] Since then, laboratory investigations have demonstrated abnormally arranged and thickened scleral fibers to support this theory.[30-32]

Brockhurst was the first person to identify choroidal effusion and nonrhegmatogenous retinal detachment occurring spontaneously in asymptomatic nanophthalmos patients.[27] Reduced visual outcome resulting from sudden, unexpected, choroidal effusion and nonrhegmatogenous retinal detachment occurring during routine glaucoma or cataract surgery in 15 patients with nanophthalmos was reported by Singh and associates in 1982.[25] Eighty-seven percent had visual loss; 46 percent were reduced to counting fingers vision or less; and 60 percent failed to achieve glaucoma control. The complications responsible for visual loss and filtration failure were related to choroidal effusion, retinal detachment, malignant glaucoma, and flat anterior chamber.[25] Techniques to promote controlled drainage of the suprachoroidal space, retinal reattachment, and reduced risk of visual loss during intraocular surgery have been developed. Brockhurst introduced vortex vein decompression,[33, 34] and later Gass proposed scleral resection.[35] Posterior segment consultation is recommended before planned anterior segment surgery in patients affected by nanophthalmos. If choroidal thickening or effusion is detected, it is recommended that elective scleral resection (with or without vortex vein decompression) be performed 4 to 6 wk prior to planned anterior segment surgery.[33-35] Oral steroid therapy is an alternative treatment option that has met with some success.[25, 33] The technique of anterior sclerotomy has been advocated by Singh and associates and Simmons[24-36] before or during intraocular surgical procedures as enhanced prophylaxis against ciliochoroidal effusion in the following circumstances:

1. Despite previous scleral resection, the eye demonstrates persistent choroidal thickening (as detected by ultrasound evaluation).

2. The eye has a history of angle-closure glaucoma that does not respond to laser iridotomy.

3. The eye demonstrates anterior chamber shallowing due to positive vitreous pressure during the intraocular procedure.

Open-angle glaucoma responds well to conventional therapy, including topical β-blockers, miotics, and carbonic anhydrase inhibitors. Acute or chronic angle-closure glaucoma on the basis of pupillary block is best treated with medical therapy to achieve pressure control followed by laser iridotomy to relieve the pupillary block.[25] Caution is advised because pupillary block occurring in nanophthalmic eyes may be improved or exacerbated by miotic therapy.[37] When cases of pupillary block do not respond to pilocarpine therapy, a concomitant choroidal effusion is invoked as a possible mechanism that contributes to angle-closure. In this event, nanophthalmic eyes may respond to cycloplegic agents by deepening the anterior chamber and by widening of the angle, which is similar to the response seen in malignant glaucoma.[25] Laser gonioplasty is advocated to widen the angle and achieve pressure reduction while helping to prevent the permanent formation of peripheral anterior synechiae and resultant angle-closure.[24, 38]

Glaucoma Associated with the Iris Retraction Syndrome

In 1984 Campbell reported nine patients with traumatic rhegmatogenous retinal detachment, hypotony, seclusion of the pupil, and retraction of the peripheral iris.[39] Other associated findings were ciliochoroidal detachment, inflammation, progressive cataract formation, and proliferative vitreoretinopathy.[39] Two types of clinical manifestations were identified: (1) angle-closure secondary to iris bombé with elevation of intraocular pressure (which could revert to), (2) iris retraction with deep anterior chamber and relative hypotony under the influence of pharmacologic aqueous suppressants. Initially, vitreous traction was theorized to explain the iris retraction.[40] However, Campbell suggested a hydrodynamic theory of hypotony caused by decreased aqueous production and a functioning fluid removal mechanism associated with a rhegmatogenous retinal detachment. Several investigators have noted the association of hypotony with retinal detachment[18, 41, 42] and have proposed the existence of a subretinal fluid pump.[42, 43] In the iris retraction syndrome, the subretinal fluid removal mechanism apparently equals or exceeds aqueous production after the addition of an aqueous suppressant. This, in association with secondary inflammation, ciliochoroidal detachment, and outpouring of protein and cells into the aqueous, contributes to seclusion of the pupil and iris retraction. The goal of therapy is retinal reattachment, but in Campbell's series, only two underwent successful reattachment and six of nine were considered to be inoperable due to proliferative vitreoretinopathy. Preoperatively, posterior synechiae may be broken pharmacologically, and glaucoma may be controlled by topical β-blockers, carbonic anhydrase inhibitors, and hyperosmotics, when necessary. Although some patients developed permanent peripheral anterior synechiae, three patients had open-angle glaucoma.

Glaucoma Associated with Retinopathy of Prematurity, Familial Exudative Vitreoretinopathy, and Coat's Disease (see Chaps. 62 and 268)

Retinopathy of prematurity (ROP) has increased in incidence as a potentially blinding disease because of the increased survival of very small, premature infants of low birth weight and gestational age in modern neonatal intensive care units.[44] In 1981, it was predicted that 30 percent of infants with birth weight less than or equal to 1000 g would develop the severe stages of ROP and that 8 percent would become blind.[45] The most frequent complication of ROP is secondary glaucoma, which develops in 25 to 33 percent of cases throughout the lifetime of the patient.[46]

Several mechanisms are responsible for glaucoma, which occurs in ROP. Angle-closure glaucoma can occur in untreated ROP stage V, secondary to the anterior displacement of the lens-iris diaphragm caused by contraction of retrolental membranes during 3 to 6 mo of age but may occur in adulthood as well.[47, 48] Secondary angle-closure glaucoma has been reported on the basis of ciliary block[49] and neovascular glaucoma.[47, 49] Inflammation occurring in eyes affected by ROP can result in posterior synechiae formation, which may contribute to angle-closure on the basis of pupillary block with resultant peripheral anterior synechiae formation.[50] Methods of treatment including iridectomy,[50] lensectomy,[51] topical corticosteroids,[50] and cycloplegics[49] have not been totally successful in achieving glaucoma control. Ciliary body detachment with decreased aqueous production secondary to centripetal traction from retrolental membranes may contribute to decreased intraocular pressure.[51] Measurements of preoperative intraocular pressure in stage V ROP have not been useful predictors of glaucoma control following surgical reattachment of the retina.[51]

In an effort to identify anterior segment abnormalities that could explain other mechanisms of glaucoma, Hartnett and associates[51] prospectively examined 27 eyes of 17 premature infants with stage IV and stage V ROP. Among the findings were angle-closure greater than 180 degrees in approximately 12 percent; prominent Schwalbe's line in 15 percent; prominent iris convexity in 58 percent; hypopigmentation of the iris root in 73 percent; a translucent or Barkan's-type membrane in 69 percent; posterior synechiae in 62 percent; visible iris or angle vessels in 46 percent; and pigment clumping in the angle recess in 46 percent.[51]

In addition to ROP, familial exudative vitreoretinopathy,[52] and Coat's disease[53] are examples of other disorders that can be associated with posterior segment ischemia and can result in angle-closure on the basis of neovascular glaucoma in children and adolescents. For a more detailed discussion of these disorders and others involving posterior segment ischemia and neovascular glaucoma, the reader is referred to Chapter 132.

Glaucoma Associated with Persistent Hyperplastic Primary Vitreous

Persistent hyperplastic primary vitreous (PHPV) is a congenital ocular disorder that affects infants of normal birth weight and gestational age and is mostly unilateral (90 percent) in occurrence.[54] Embryologically, a persistent tunica vasculosa lentis (the hyaloid artery, vasa hyaloidea propria, and anterior ciliary vessels) fails to undergo spontaneous regression. Anterior and posterior forms have been described with corresponding predispositions to glaucoma.[55]

The anterior form of PHPV may manifest clinically with leukocoria, microphthalmos, shallow anterior chamber, elongated ciliary processes, and engorged iris vessels. Initially, the lens is clear but cataract formation may develop. Remnants of the tunica vasculosa lentis may grow into the lens through a rent in the posterior capsule and lead to sudden hydrostatic expansion of an intumescent lens with precipitation of secondary angle-closure glaucoma. Concurrent vitreous hemorrhage may contribute to glaucoma by inflammatory or ghost cell mechanisms.[55] The contralateral eye is at risk for open-angle glaucoma.[56]

Ocular findings in the posterior form of PHPV include microcornea, embryonic filtration angle abnormalities, vitreous membranes, stalks, retinal folds, and tractional retinal detachment. The involved eye is at risk for open-angle glaucoma.[55]

Early surgical intervention is recommended for preservation of eyes affected by PHPV with characteristics of progressive cataract formation and shallowing of the anterior chamber.[57] Surgical objectives accomplished by closed-system vitrectomy techniques are clearing of the visual axis and relief of ciliary body traction by removal of retrolenticular fibrovascular membranes and lenticular material. Relative contraindications to surgical intervention in eyes affected by PHPV are severe microphthalmos; longstanding intractable glaucoma; hemorrhage; or minimal involvement by PHPV with no evidence of progressive change.[57]

Pigmentary Dispersion Syndrome Glaucoma and Its Association to Retinal Detachment

The association of pigmentary dispersion syndrome (PDS) with glaucoma is well known.[58] It has been suggested that there is an increased prevalence of pigmentary dispersion-related glaucoma with rhegmatogenous retinal detachment, although this has never been proved. Bracket and Chermet were the first persons to suggest an association of pigmentary dispersion-related glaucoma and retinal detachment in their presentation of 19 patients affected by both disorders but offered no statistical analysis.[59] Scheie and Cameron found no significant correlation of retinal detachment with glaucoma in a retrospective study of 407 patients affected by the pigmentary dispersion syndrome in that the incidence of retinal detachment was approximately equal in the glaucomatous (6 percent) and nonglaucomatous (6.6 percent) subsets.[60]

Eyes with rhegmatogenous retinal detachment have been found to have pigmentation of the angle structures in several studies, but no association with preexisting glaucoma has been proved statistically. Sebestyen prospectively examined 160 eyes with preoperative rhegmatogenous retinal detachment but no prior history of glaucoma and found that 22.5 percent had marked pigmentation of the trabeculum or peripheral anterior synechiae, or both, associated with postoperative pressure elevations.[61] Syrdalen conducted a prospective gonioscopic evaluation of 267 patients diagnosed with rhegmatogenous retinal detachment and found no significant difference in the degree of pigmentation when compared with the fellow eyes if complicated detachments were excluded from consideration.[61] Rodriguez-Gonzales found the pigmentary dispersion syndrome, with or without glaucoma, in 10 percent of 1532 eyes affected by retinal detachment.[62]

Glaucoma Associated with Retinitis Pigmentosa

The association of glaucoma with retinitis pigmentosa is not well defined. Several investigators have reported an incidence ranging from 2 to 12 percent, but these lack documentation regarding the type of glaucoma and the pattern of inheritance of retinitis pigmentosa.[63, 64] Phelps reported treating three patients with dominantly inherited retinitis pigmentosa and glaucoma that was described as primary angle-closure in two cases and congenital glaucoma in the third case inherited from the parent who was not affected by retinitis pigmentosa.[65] Visual field loss associated with retinitis pigmentosa may be similar to that found in POAG but can usually be differentiated on the basis of detailed clinical correlation of optic nerve head excavation, notching, and pallor. In cases that cannot be easily distinguished clinically, electrophysiologic testing may be useful.

Glaucoma Associated with Stickler's Syndrome

Stickler's syndrome is an autosomal dominant connective tissue disorder that was reported in 1965 and includes ocular, orofacial, and generalized skeletal findings.[66] Major ocular features include myopia, open-angle glaucoma, cataract, vitreoretinal degeneration, perivascular pigmentary retinopathy, and retinal detachment that is resistant to repair.[67] Orofacial findings include midfacial flattening and the Pierre-Robin malformation complex (micrognathia, cleft palate, and glossoptosis). Skeletal abnormalities include joint enlargement, hyperextensibility, arthritis, and mild spondyloepiphyseal dysplasia.[67]

Wagner's disease is an autosomal dominant ocular disorder that was identified in 1938 and is characterized by features of moderate to high myopia, cataract, strabismus, and vitreoretinal degeneration.[68] Patients who are affected by Stickler's disorder or Wagner's disorder have a similar-appearing vitreoretinal degeneration that can manifest clinically as an "optically empty vitreous cavity" on biomicroscopy; however, patients who are affected by Wagner's disease do not have associated systemic abnormalities or a predisposition to retinal detachment.[69]

Patients who are affected by Stickler's syndrome benefit from periodic, thorough ophthalmologic examinations with peripheral retinal evaluation. This allows for early detection and treatment of glaucoma, retinal breaks, or detachment as possible prophylaxis to blindness. Phelps recommends that miotic therapy should be avoided in these individuals to reduce the risk of retinal detachment.[70] The open-angle glaucoma noted in several patients affected by Stickler's syndrome is associated with mild-to-moderate elevations in pressure that have responded to medical therapy.[70] Evaluation of optic nerve head excavation, progression, and corresponding visual field changes can be difficult to interpret in the presence of lenticular opacification and myopic chorioretinal degeneration, which can cause visual field defects resembling those found in glaucoma.[70]

Glaucoma Associated with Diabetes Mellitus

Several investigators have noted an increased prevalence ranging from 6 to 11 percent of POAG in patients with diabetes compared with the control population.[71–75] Ingersheimer first suggested that ocular hypotony in diabetes might contribute to the development of diabetic retinopathy.[76] Becker found a significant correlation between elevated intraocular pressure (greater than or equal to 20 mmHg) and lack of proliferative retinopathy in a clinical comparison of diabetic patients older than 40 yr of age, thus supporting a protective effect of elevated intraocular pressure against the development of proliferative diabetic retinopathy.[72] Others have suggested that the relationship of POAG and diabetic retinopathy involves many variables and that no simple relationship can be implied.[77]

Glaucoma Associated with Central Retinal Vein Occlusion

Mechanisms of glaucoma described in cases of central retinal vein occlusion (CRVO) include POAG,[78] secondary angle-closure,[79, 80] and primary angle-closure on the basis of pupillary block,[80] but only POAG has been documented to be associated with CRVO.[78–81] In 1960, a study involving 186 patients diagnosed with retinal vein occlusion reported an association of POAG in 42 percent of patients with CRVO and 10 percent of patients with branch retinal vein occlusion.[78] In 1972, Hyams and Newman described two cases of angle-closure glaucoma following CRVO in which the unaffected fellow eyes had normal pressures and nonoccludable angles.[81] Topical pilocarpine therapy was instituted, which deepened both angles slightly and achieved a mild reduction in pressure. One case resolved while the other progressed to neovascular glaucoma. In 1973, Grant reported seven cases of temporary shallowing of the anterior chamber with reversible angle closure glaucoma occurring after occlusion of the central retinal vein.[79] In 1977, Bloome reported two cases of unilateral transient angle-closure following CRVO. Several investigators have noted the reversal of secondary angle-closure and concomitant reduction in pressure following short-term treatment with cycloplegics and carbonic anhydrase inhibitors.[79, 80]

Ocular examination may reveal unilateral anterior chamber shallowing and angle narrowing compared with the fellow eye. If sufficient narrowing occurs to block the outflow pathway, pressure elevation may be noted. The onset of anatomical narrowing usually follows the CRVO event by a range of 3 days, but others have reported onset as late as 2 yr.[82] If the fellow angle appears occludable, one must rule out angle-closure on the basis of a pupillary block. A posterior segment evaluation may reveal retinal hemorrhages in the nerve fiber layer and cotton wool spots. There commonly occurs dilatation and tortuosity of the retinal veins in the regions where they share a common adventitial sheath with their corresponding retinal arteriole. The degree of retinal ischemia as evaluated by fluorescein angiography can help to determine whether the pattern is more consistent with ischemic (hemorrhagic) or non-ischemic (venous-stasis) retinopathy.[83] If the ischemic pattern is identified, panretinal photocoagulation is the preferred treatment, as 45 percent of these, left untreated, progress to neovascular glaucoma.[83] A careful follow-up evaluation of the patient with applanation pressures, biomicroscopy, and fundus evaluation is indicated at least monthly for the first 3 mo to identify new vessel formation and pressure elevation at the earliest stages that are amenable to treatment.

Mechanisms proposed to explain the anterior chamber shallowing following CRVO are transudation of fluid from the retinal vessels, which increases the volume of the vitreous cavity, and choroidal edema with resultant effusion and ciliary body detachment.[79, 80] Both of these mechanisms involve forward displacement of the lens-iris diaphragm and secondary angle closure. Hyams and Neumann[81] invoked angle-closure on the basis of pupillary block, but several cases reported by Grant failed to respond to peripheral iridectomy.[79]

The angle-closure usually widens gradually over a period of several weeks. Treatment with topical cycloplegics help to resolve the condition by relaxing the ciliary muscle, tightening the zonule, and moving the lens-iris diaphragm posteriorly. Pressure reduction may be achieved by topical β-blockers, carbonic anhydrase inhibitors, and hyperosmotics, as needed. Topical steroid preparations may help to resolve the inflammatory component of the choroidal effusion and thus assist in resolving the angle-closure on this basis.[84]

Glaucoma Associated with Ocular Trauma (see Chap. 125)

Ocular trauma and its sequelae may cause glaucoma in a variety of ways: trauma to angle structures, including angle recession[85]; transient obstruction of the trabecular meshwork by white blood cells (cell) and serum (flare) that result from disruption of the blood-aqueous barrier[86]; inflammation associated with prostaglandin release[87]; glaucoma-related complications of hyphema[88]; and retinal detachment.[89, 90]

Blunt ocular trauma may cause a tear between the circular and longitudinal muscles of the ciliary body, which may be associated with iridodialysis, cyclodialysis, and increased depth of the anterior chamber (Fig. 137–1).[85] In a prospective study involving 267 patients who developed retinal detachment following ocular trauma, there was a significantly higher association in males compared with females.[89] Anterior chamber angle abnormalities were present in 55.6 percent of males and 60 percent of females with traumatic retinal detachment, but there was no major difference in the degree of angle pigmentation noted when compared with the fellow eyes.[89] Chronic monocular "open-angle" glaucoma may develop insidiously months or years later, despite a history of seemingly uneventful recovery during the immediate period following ocular trauma.[85] It is recommended that patients with a history of ocular trauma undergo a thorough ocular evaluation, including gonioscopy and dilated fundoscopic evaluation with scleral depression, when possible, to detect evidence of angle trauma or retinal detachment. Patients must be warned regarding the possibility that future glaucoma may develop and of the need for a periodic examination.

Glaucoma Associated with Tumors of the Posterior Segment (Melanoma, Retinoblastoma, and Choroidal Hemangioma) (see Chaps. 259, 260, 268, and 270)

Glaucoma can be an important indicator of posterior segment neoplasia. Fraser and Font found that 3 percent of eyes with vitreous hemorrhage harbored a choroidal melanoma.[91] Yanoff found that 20 percent of eyes diagnosed with choroidal malignant melanoma presented clinically with glaucoma.[92] In 37 percent of these eyes with glaucoma, media opacification prevented detection of the tumors prior to enucleation. It is recommended that an ultrasound evaluation be used in eyes with dense media to aid in the detection of choroidal melanoma or retinal detachment before invasive action is taken.[92]

Several mechanisms of glaucoma associated with choroidal melanoma have been identified.[92] In one group, the mechanism of glaucoma was related to obstruction of the outflow pathway by (1) direct invasion of the angle structures in association with melanomas involving the ciliary body and iris structures; (2) obstruction of the trabecular meshwork by melanoma cells and macrophages that have ingested melanin pigment released from necrotic melanoma cells (melanomalytic glaucoma).[92] In the second group, the mechanism of glaucoma was related to inflammation, posterior synechiae formation, and chronic angle-closure on the basis of pupillary block with resultant peripheral anterior synechiae formation. In this second group, large choroidal melanomas associated with total retinal detachment caused anterior displacement of the iris-lens diaphragm.

Neovascular glaucoma is considered to be the most common mechanism by which secondary angle-closure with formation of peripheral anterior synechiae occurs in association with choroidal melanoma and retinal detachment.[92]

In a retrospective study of 149 eyes with retinoblastoma, glaucoma was detected clinically in 23 percent and histopathologically in 50 percent.[93] The most com-

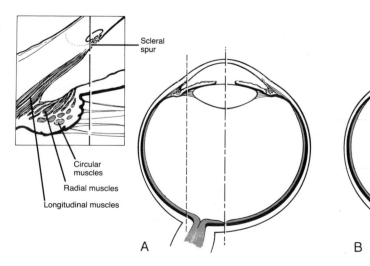

Figure 137–1. Mechanisms of glaucoma associated with disorders of the retina, vitreous, and choroid. *A,* Angle recession caused by a tear between the radial and longitudinal muscles of the ciliary body. Note the deep anterior chamber and iris retrodisplacement. A line parallel to the visual axis drawn through the scleral spur transects anteriorly to the first ciliary process. *B,* Ocular anatomy depicting the normal relationship of the ciliary body to the angle structures. A line parallel to the visual axis drawn through the scleral spur transects the first ciliary process.

Scleral spur

Circular muscles

Radial muscles

Longitudinal muscles

mon mechanism of glaucoma associated with retinoblastoma is rubeosis iridis, leading to angle-closure and neovascular glaucoma.[93, 94] Other mechanisms of glaucoma are secondary angle-closure with pupillary block related to massive exudative retinal detachment and secondary open-angle glaucoma caused by obstruction of the anterior chamber angle by necrotic, neoplastic, or inflammatory cells.[93] Once neovascular glaucoma develops in eyes affected by retinoblastoma, medical management usually fails and enucleation is required.[94]

Two mechanisms of glaucoma have been proposed to explain glaucoma occurring in patients with choroidal hemangiomas associated with Sturge-Weber syndrome. Early onset glaucoma is thought to be related to a developmental abnormality of the anterior chamber angle similar to primary congenital glaucoma,[95] whereas glaucoma that occurs later in life is explained by elevated episcleral venous pressure caused by small arteriovenous fistulas occurring in episcleral vessels.[96]

Glaucoma Associated with Ocular Metastatic Disease (Metastases Originating from Primary Carcinoma of the Lung, Breast, Kidney, Rectum; Leukemia, and Reticulum Cell Sarcoma)

By virtue of the abundant blood supply through approximately 20 short posterior ciliary arteries, the posterior segment of the eye is involved more frequently as a site of metastatic disease than the anterior segment.[97] Metastases to the anterior segment tend to occur along the horizontal meridiens of the iris or ciliary body, consistent with the blood supply through two long posterior ciliary arteries that are located at the 3 and 9 o'clock position.[97] Glaucoma is reported more frequently as a symptom of ocular metastatic disease affecting the anterior segment (56 percent) compared with the posterior segment (1 percent).[97, 98]

Some secondary open-angle mechanisms of glaucoma that occur in anterior segment metastatic disease are obstruction of the anterior chamber angle by a sheet of tumor cells that infiltrate the trabecular meshwork and emissary vessels. Secondary angle-closure may occur from tumor-related obstruction of the angle, peripheral anterior synechiae formation, and the development of neovascular glaucoma.[97]

Mechanisms of glaucoma occurring in posterior segment metastatic disease are secondary angle-closure resulting from increased posterior segment volume and ciliochoroidal effusion; retinal and choroidal detachment; and neovascular glaucoma.[98]

In order of decreasing frequency, the sites of primary carcinoma responsible for ocular metastatic disease are the lung, breast, kidney, and rectum.[97] Posterior segment metastases usually appear clinically as small, multifocal, grayish elevations.[97] Glaucoma arising from ocular metastatic disease is treated with pressure-reducing agents (topical β-blockers, oral carbonic anhydrase inhibitors, and systemic hyperosmotic agents, as needed). Secondary angle-closure glaucoma on the basis of suspected ciliochoroidal effusion is treated with topical cycloplegics, corticosteroids, and aqueous suppressants, as needed.

Ocular involvement in leukemia most frequently affects the choroid and retina with retinal and vitreous hemorrhages, but anterior segment involvement with iris infiltration, hyphema, and glaucoma may rarely occur as the initial manifestation.[99] Following diagnostic anterior chamber paracentesis, irradiation usually promotes resolution of the ocular findings, and pressure reduction is achieved by aqueous suppressants and topical corticosteroids.

Intraocular reticulum cell sarcoma (histiocytic lymphoma) is considered to be a B-cell lymphoma that is a rare cause of uveitis and is usually recalcitrant to conventional corticosteroid therapy.[100] It characteristically manifests in patients older than 40 yr of age with symptoms of uveitis affecting the posterior segment (vitritis) to a greater degree than the anterior segment (iridocyclitis), with choroidal or retinal infiltrates. It may be unilateral or bilateral in occurrence. Secondary glaucoma and corneal edema may preclude adequate fundus examination.[100] Pars plana vitrectomy is diagnostic and therapeutic in terms of obtaining a cytologic diagnosis and in clearing the visual axis. A search for central nervous system involvement is indicated through computed axial tomography (CT) or magnetic resonance imaging (MRI), especially in the setting of neurologic symptoms. Treatment entails irradiation to the eye, brain, and spinal chord. The application of intrathecal chemotherapeutic agents is optional. It is uncertain whether reticulum cell sarcoma represents a primary or metastatic tumor of the eye, central nervous system, or other site.[101, 102]

Glaucoma Associated with Hemorrhagic Complications of Age-Related Macular Degeneration (ARMD)

Rarely, spontaneous massive hemorrhagic retinal or choroidal detachment may be caused by a disciform macular degenerative lesion. Secondary angle-closure glaucoma may result from anterior displacement of the lens-iris diaphragm with anterior rotation of the ciliary body.[103-105] This condition was first identified by Parsons in 1906, and 17 cases have been reported to date.[104] Risk factors include systemic hypertension, a primary (e.g., neoplastic disorder) or secondary clotting disorder (e.g., anticoagulant induced).[104, 107]

Patients usually present emergently with ocular pain of abrupt onset, accompanied by occasional nausea and vomiting, and no prior history of surgical intervention. Vision is usually reduced to light perception or hand motion, but there may commonly be no light perception. Applanation pressure is usually elevated and, when in the 60 to 70 range, may be accompanied by corneal edema and marked shallowing of the anterior chamber. Angle-closure is seen by gonioscopic examination.[104]

Gonioscopic examination of the fellow eye usually reveals an anterior chamber of normal depth with a nonoccludable angle. Posterior segment evaluation may not be possible because of massive vitreous hemorrhage which has broken through Bruch's membrane with concomitant choroidal and retinal separation. An evaluation of the fellow eye may show drusen, hemorrhages, and retinal pigment epithelial changes.[104]

An examiner should be reluctant to explain total hemorrhagic retinal or choroidal detachment with vitreous hemorrhage on the basis of ARMD, because these conditions are a rare occurrence.[104] Although suprachoroidal hemorrhage can occur during or after surgical intervention, in the absence of recent surgery one must rule out melanoma of the ciliary body or choroid.

Posterior segment consultation and ultrasound evaluation, in particular, may help to differentiate ARMD from choroidal melanoma.[108] "Kissing choroidal" configuration, absent vascularity, sound attenuation, and decreasing size on serial examination are more representative of ARMD compared with the regular structure and low internal reflectivity of uveal melanoma.[108] If the possibility of uveal melanoma cannot be ruled out, enucleation may be considered, particularly in the absence of useful vision. If melanoma has been ruled out, treatment of the secondary glaucoma is mainly for the relief of pain and preservation of the globe as the visual prognosis is not favorable. In one study, only two of 17 eyes retained vision in the range of light perception to hand motion, whereas 10 of 17 underwent enucleation for relief of pain.[104]

The disrupted retinal architecture that occurs in ARMD with vitreous hemorrhage may limit peripheral as well as central visual potential.[104] Initial medical therapy for pressure reduction includes topical β-blockers, carbonic anhydrase inhibitors, and hyperosmotics as tolerated. Topical steroids may help to reduce the inflammatory component. In the event of a blind and painful eye, medical therapy commonly fails and retrobulbar alcohol injections are required for relief of pain. Transscleral neodymium yttrium aluminum garnet (Nd.YAG) cyclodestruction or cyclocryotherapy may be employed, at the discretion of the clinician and in accordance with the patient's wishes.

If the fellow eye is affected by ARMD in the form of a disciform lesion and the patient is taking oral anticoagulant therapy, an internal medicine consultation should be obtained. The possibility of discontinuing anticoagulants to reduce the risk of a similar hemorrhagic episode in the fellow eye may be considered.[104]

Glaucoma Associated with AIDS

Ocular manifestations of AIDS include opportunistic infections and neoplastic proliferation resulting from a major disorder of cellular immunity.[109, 110] Common ocular involvement in AIDS includes conjunctival Kaposi's sarcoma, cotton wool spots, retinal periphlebitis, and cytomegalovirus retinitis.[109] Retinitis associated with cytomegalovirus and herpes viruses may result in acute retinal necrosis, uveitis, rhegmatogenous, and nonrhegmatogenous retinal detachment and is a significant cause of visual loss. Other immunocompromised involvement can include herpes zoster ophthalmicus, cryptococcal choroiditis, choroidal *Mycobacterium avium intracellulare, Histoplasma capsulatum* chorioretinitis, toxoplasmosis, syphilis, and *Pneumocystis carinii* retinitis.[110]

AIDS-related chorioretinal perivasculitis, ischemia, and necrosis contribute to ciliochoroidal effusion and detachment, which permits anterior rotation of the ciliary body around the scleral spur thus resulting in secondary angle-closure glaucoma.[111–113]

Two patients with secondary angle-closure on the basis of AIDS-related ciliochoroidal effusions have been described.[113] One patient presented with bilateral secondary angle-closure as the initial manifestation of AIDS.[113] Surgical peripheral iridectomies failed to relieve the angle-closure in the absence of a pupillary block mechanism. The authors have recommended that a careful history and clinical examination will help to identify secondary angle-closure. This is optimally treated with topical cycloplegics to relax the ciliary muscle, tighten the zonule, and move the lens-iris diaphragm posteriorly, thus opening the angle and deepening the chamber.[113] Uncontrolled pressure elevations should be managed with topical β-blockers, carbonic anhydrase inhibitors, and hyperosmotics, if needed. Attention to AIDS-related posterior segment involvement with ganciclovir[114] should be instituted for CMV-retinitis and choroidal effusion, if present. Topical steroids should be used with caution to resolve the inflammatory component of the ciliochoroidal effusion, and only when covered by appropriate antiviral therapy.

Glaucoma Associated with Amyloidosis (see Chap. 241)

Primary familial amyloidosis (PFA) is a generalized systemic disorder that may have neurologic, cardiac, and renal involvement and is inherited in an autosomal dominant fashion.[115] Ocular manifestations of PFA include bilateral secondary open-angle glaucoma, progressive vitreous opacities, and lattice corneal dystrophy type II.[115, 116]

The glaucoma typically develops during the third through fifth decades of life and is thought to be caused by trabecular meshwork obstruction by amyloid fibrils as identified in electron microscopy of trabeculectomy specimens. Anterior segment features of glaucoma associated with PFA that may also occur in pigmentary and exfoliative glaucomas include pigment dusting of the corneal endothelial surface and trabecular meshwork with iris transillumination defects. Progressive vitreous opacification associated with PFA may reduce visual acuity and obscure the assessment of glaucomatous progression through visual field testing or direct evaluation of the optic nerves. The glaucoma associated with PFA usually responds to conventional medical and surgical management, although trabeculectomy sites may become obstructed by amyloid fibrils.[115]

Glaucoma Associated with Uveitis

Uveitis may precede or follow retinal detachment. It may cause ciliary body shutdown with reduced aqueous humor formation and hypotony, or it can interfere with outflow pathways thus leading to pressure elevation. Chronic uveitis that is left untreated or that does not respond to corticosteroid therapy may precipitate formation of posterior synechiae and iris bombé leading to pupillary block and peripheral anterior synechiae. The resultant angle-closure glaucoma may require medical therapy, iridotomy formation, and possible filtration surgery to achieve control. In cases of recurrent or recalcitrant uveitis, a high index of suspicion should be maintained, and a thorough search should be conducted to rule out an infectious etiology that may respond to antibiotic therapy.

Gonioscopic evaluation of patients affected by uveitic glaucoma in association with ocular or systemic inflammatory disease may reveal iridocyclitis, peripheral anterior synechiae formation, and precipitates on the trabecular meshwork. These should be distinguished from the syndrome of inflammatory precipitates on the trabecular meshwork (IPTM), as described by Chandler and Grant.[117, 118] IPTM is an open-angle glaucoma with precipitates on the trabecular meshwork and irregular peripheral anterior synechiae. It occurs in the setting of minimal or absent inflammation and does not have other signs of ocular or systemic involvement. Glaucoma associated with IPTM may respond well to intensive corticosteroid therapy, alone, or in combination with conventional pressure-reducing medications.[118] However, the goal of therapy for uveitic glaucoma secondary to an underlying disorder is treatment of the primary disease process. Intraocular pressure is controlled through conventional glaucoma medications, and reduction of inflammation is achieved through the judicious use of topical corticosteroids.

Caution is advised when treating uveitis with corticosteroids because of the possibility of precipitating corticosteroid-induced glaucoma in susceptible individuals, which is difficult to distinguish from inflammatory glaucoma.[119] Uveitis has been identified as an important mechanism contributing to glaucoma in Schwartz's syndrome,[120] iris retraction syndrome,[39] ROP,[52] and others that feature long-standing retinal detachment with possible formation of posterior and anterior synechiae.

A retrospective study of 532 cases of sarcoidosis in the southeastern United States found ocular manifestations present in 38 percent.[121] Ocular involvement was second only to pulmonary involvement as a presenting symptom. Chronic granulomatous uveitis was the most common abnormality and was found in 53 percent; secondary uveitic glaucoma occurred in 11 percent.[121] Anterior segment involvement occurred in 85 percent, whereas posterior segment involvement was found in 25 percent, usually manifesting as chorioretinitis or periphlebitis. Central nervous system involvement by sarcoidosis occurred more frequently in patients with posterior segment findings.[121]

Glaucoma may occur in the setting of congenital or acquired ocular syphilis through a variety of mechanisms.[122, 123] Both anterior and posterior segments may be affected, and glaucoma may occur on the basis of inflammation (uveitis) in both early and late interstitial keratitis associated with congenital syphilis. Other mechanisms cited in the development of glaucoma related to interstitial keratitis are open-angle glaucoma resulting from increased pigmentation and "hyalinization" of the trabecular meshwork; secondary irregular angle-closure related to peripheral anterior synechiae (PAS) formation; and intraepithelial cysts of the iris and ciliary body that result in narrowing of the angle.[122, 123] The open-angle glaucoma related to a dysfunctional trabecular meshwork usually fails to respond to medical therapy and may require filtration surgery. Secondary angle-closure related to PAS formation and uveal cysts may respond to peripheral iridotomy with pressure reduction through glaucoma medications. Cases of chronic or extensive angle-closure may also require filtration surgery.[122, 123]

Other disorders affecting the posterior segment that have been associated with secondary glaucoma on a uveitic basis include, but are not limited to, toxoplasmosis,[124] Vogt-Koyanagi-Harada syndrome,[125] sympathetic ophthalmia,[126] Behçet's disease,[127] toxocariasis,[128] cytomegalic inclusion disease retinitis,[129] mumps,[130] coccidiodomycosis,[131] onchocerciasis,[132] leprosy,[133] tuberculosis,[133, 134] and the AIDS-related opportunistic infections.[109–114]

Glaucoma Associated with Orbital and Extraorbital Vascular Factors that Result in Elevated Episcleral Venous Pressure

Interference with physiologic pathways of aqueous recycling through venous return may be caused by abnormalities in the orbit (dural shunt syndrome)[135] or along the great vessels of the heart (superior vena caval syndrome)[136] that may result in elevated venous pressure and secondary glaucoma. In these settings, the mechanisms of secondary glaucoma may manifest as choroidal effusion with anterior rotation of the ciliary body and secondary angle-closure without pupillary block; CRVO; and ischemic damage to the trabecular meshwork. Prolonged ischemia may result in neovascularization and neovascular glaucoma.[137] A full discussion of glaucoma associated with orbital and extraorbital vascular disease is beyond the scope of this chapter, and the reader is referred to Chapter 130.

GLAUCOMA CAUSED BY DISORDERS OF THE RETINA, VITREOUS, AND CHOROID

Glaucoma Associated with Neovascularization

A full discussion of the numerous causes of posterior segment ischemia, which may lead to ocular neovascularization, is beyond the scope of this chapter, and the reader is referred to Chapter 132.

Rubeosis iridis and neovascular glaucoma are commonly the result of posterior segment ischemia with blinding consequences unless detected early and treated aggressively with retinal ablative therapy.[138]

Glaucoma is a frequent complication following posterior segment surgery. Various investigators report the incidence of neovascular glaucoma during the postoperative period following pars plana vitrectomy procedures, ranging between 11 and 28 percent,[139–141] and the incidence of secondary open-angle glaucoma (e.g., hemolytic, ghost cell), ranging between 15 and 26 percent.[139, 140] Several investigators have noted an increased incidence of postoperative rubeosis iridis and neovascular glaucoma following intraocular procedures in diabetic patients who are aphakic or who lack an intact posterior capsule ranging from 32 to 40 percent.[141, 142]

Glaucoma Associated with Schwartz's Syndrome

Open-angle glaucoma secondary to rhegmatogenous retinal detachment was described by Schwartz in 1973.[120] He presented 11 patients with unilateral open-angle glaucoma and retinal detachment in whom the history and postoperative course indicated that the untreated retinal detachment preceded and actually caused the secondary open-angle glaucoma. A younger age group, compared with that of the usual group of patients affected by retinal detachment, was noted with half of the cases preceded by a history of direct ocular trauma.

In the affected eyes, intraocular pressure ranged from 29 to 55 mmHg, with the fellow eye remaining in the range of normal intraocular pressure. In most cases, attention was directed at treatment of concomitant iridocyclitis and glaucoma, which were unresponsive to medical management (including corticosteroids). Despite the duration of the detachment, all pressure elevations resolved within days to weeks following the successful repair of the detachment.

Several theories have been postulated to explain the glaucoma associated with Schwartz's syndrome on the basis of reduced aqueous outflow facility.[120, 143, 144] Schwartz hypothesized that iridocyclitis could cause a reduction in outflow facility, which could contribute to an elevated intraocular pressure in the presence of normal or reduced aqueous production.[120] Davidorf proposed that retinal breaks could release retinal pigment epithelial cells that could then migrate anteriorly with the aqueous humor to obstruct the trabecular meshwork.[143] More recently, Matsuo isolated photoreceptor outer segments and inflammatory cells in aqueous humor aspirates of seven patients who met the criteria for Schwartz's syndrome.[144] He has hypothesized that photoreceptor outer segments pass through the retinal break and gain access to aqueous outflow pathways, thus producing outflow obstruction.

Glaucoma Associated with Complications of Intraocular Hemorrhage (Hemolytic, Ghost Cell, Hemosiderotic, and Sickle Cell Hemoglobinopathy)

Mechanisms of glaucoma associated with intraocular hemorrhage unrelated to posterior segment ischemia usually include the secondary open-angle glaucomas: hemolytic,[145] ghost cell,[146] and hemosiderotic glaucoma.[147] All three can cause persistent elevations of pressure that may require medical or surgical therapy. Hemolytic glaucoma is caused by an obstruction of the trabecular meshwork by fragments of hemolyzed red blood cells and hemoglobin-laden macrophages and typically presents from 5 to 7 days or later after intraocular hemorrhage. Ghost cell glaucoma is caused by an obstruction of the trabecular meshwork by tan-colored degenerating red blood cells that may have been sequestered in the vitreous cavity and communicate with the aqueous outflow pathways through a rent or disruption in the vitreous face. It typically presents from 11 to 14 days after ocular trauma or surgery accompanied by intraocular hemorrhage. Hemosiderotic glaucoma accompanies recurrent or long-standing intraocular hemorrhage, during which iron breakdown products from degenerating red blood cells accumulate within trabecular meshwork and other endothelial cells to cause degenerative changes accompanied by elevations of pressure. Both hemolytic and ghost cell glaucoma may respond to medical management in the form of topical β-blockers, carbonic anhydrase inhibitors, or hyperosmotics, as indicated, but anterior chamber washout or vitrectomy may be required. Hemosiderotic glaucoma may respond to surgical evacuation of blood in the early stages, but once panocular degenerative changes occur, enucleation is usually required because of uncontrolled glaucoma.

Patients with hyphema in the setting of known or suspected sickle cell hemoglobinopathy or sickle cell trait are at greater risk for uncontrolled glaucoma and corneal blood staining.[148] Intracameral red blood cells (even in microscopic amounts) become sickled under conditions of relative hypoxia and acidemia compared with the blood stream. These sickled cells obstruct the trabecular meshwork and cause elevation of intraocular pressure. Persistent elevations of intraocular pressure contribute to posterior and anterior segment ischemia, which precipitates a self-perpetuating cycle of more sickling and greater ischemia. Elevations of intraocular pressure are treated with conventional pressure-lowering medications with the following exceptions: carbonic anhydrase inhibitors (Diamox) are omitted to avoid metabolic acidosis, which may produce further sickling; systemic hyperosmotic agents are administered only once in any 24-hr period to avoid systemic hyperviscosity with increased sickling of small vessels supplying the optic nerve.[148]

Although medical therapy usually achieves adequate pressure control, patients experiencing persistent pressure elevations of more than 24 mmHg for longer than 24 hr are at significant risk for visual loss secondary to optic nerve ischemia. Surgical intervention in the form of anterior chamber washout and/or filtration surgery may be indicated.[149]

GLAUCOMA RESULTING FROM THE TREATMENT OF DISORDERS OF THE RETINA, VITREOUS, AND CHOROID

Glaucoma Resulting from Angle-Closure Secondary to the Repair of Retinal Detachment by Scleral Buckle

Narrowing of the anterior chamber and corresponding angle, ranging in incidence from 14.4 to 50 percent, has been described following scleral buckle placement for the repair of retinal detachment.[150–152] A lower estimate of the incidence of actual angle-closure, ranging from 2.1 to 14.4 percent, has been reported.[17, 152–155] The mechanism of angle-closure is postulated to occur from anterior rotation of the ciliary body at the scleral spur as a result of ciliochoroidal effusion and detachment.[156, 157] Fluid accumulation in the suprachoroidal space may result from surgical manipulation, inflammation, relative ischemia, and impedance of vortex venous outflow.[152, 158–160] Pupillary block is not usually a mechanism and can be excluded by history and clinical examination (Fig. 137–2).

During the immediate postoperative period following retinal detachment surgery, eyes are usually tender and exhibit varying degrees of conjunctival chemosis and injection. Corneal edema may or may not be present depending on many variables, including the intraocular pressure, endothelial cell integrity, age of the patient, and surgical trauma. Goldmann or Perkins applanation pressures are the most reliable methods of determining intraocular pressure, and emphasis should be placed on identifying dangerous elevations of pressure rather than on absolute accuracy in the presence of corneal irregularities.[161, 162] Anterior chamber reaction may re-

veal mild cell and flare. Pupillary block is usually bilateral in predisposition, and this can usually be ruled out through biomicroscopic and gonioscopic evaluation of the chamber and angle with comparison to the fellow eye. If pupillary block remains a possibility, laser iridotomy may be both diagnostic and therapeutic.[162]

Posterior segment evaluation by indirect or direct ophthalmoscopy, or ultrasound, may not reveal clinically detectable ciliochoroidal detachment, but this does not rule out its causative etiology, because effusion is rarely detected clinically.[161, 162]

Frequent pressure checks daily or more frequently, if indicated, are recommended during the immediate postoperative period to detect dangerously high elevations in pressure (>30 mmHg) that could compromise the integrity of the optic nerve. Many cases show spontaneous resolution during 1 to 3 days postoperatively,[163, 164] but uncontrolled pressure elevations are best managed medically with a combination of topical β-blockers, carbonic anhydrase inhibitors, cycloplegics, and hyperosmotics, as indicated. Topical and oral steroids may help to reduce the inflammatory component but should be used with caution because of the possibility of side effects including untoward psychotropic reactions, physiologic disturbances, and steroid-induced glaucoma in susceptible individuals.[22, 119] Cycloplegics help to relax the ciliary muscle, tighten the zonules, and move the lens-iris diaphragm posteriorly, thus relieving angle-closure. Miotics have not been effective and may actually exacerbate the angle-closure by increasing congestion and anterior rotation of angle structures.

The decision to perform surgical drainage of ciliochoroidal effusion depends on many factors but is supported by several previously failed attempts at medical resolution with persistence of angle-closure for more than 4 days.[164] The general goal of surgical intervention is to prevent permanent damage to angle structures by the formation of peripheral anterior synechiae. In contrast, varying degrees of angle narrowing in the absence of peripheral anterior synechiae formation can be well tolerated and managed medically, if necessary, for several weeks until resolution occurs.[164] In some cases of secondary angle-narrowing or closure, which are unresponsive to medical therapy, laser gonioplasty (developed by Simmons[38]) can be utilized to open the angle.

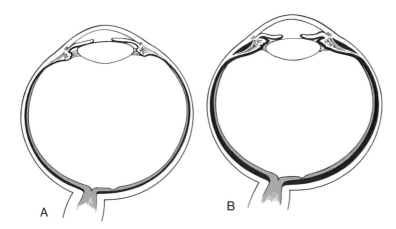

Figure 137–2. The concept of secondary angle-closure on the basis of ciliochoroidal effusion and detachment compared with primary angle-closure on the basis of pupillary block. *A,* Primary angle-closure related to pupillary block. Note the prominent iris bowing with shallowing of the anterior chamber and angle-closure on the basis of pupillary block. Treatment is with medical reduction of intraocular pressure (as indicated) and laser peripheral iridotomy. *B,* Secondary angle-closure related to ciliochoroidal effusion and detachment. Note the swelling and anterior rotation of the ciliary processes about the scleral spur (with occasional diffuse choroidal thickening and detachment to create secondary angle-closure without pupillary block. Treatment is with medical reduction of intraocular pressure (as indicated), in addition to topical cycloplegic and corticosteroid therapy.

prevent formation of peripheral anterior synechiae, and achieve pressure reduction, providing that permanent damage has not already occurred to the angle structures. Other indications for drainage of choroidal effusion or reformation of the anterior chamber include flat anterior chamber with lenticular-corneal endothelial touch and the presence of "kissing choroidal configuration" with macular detachment.

Glaucoma Resulting from Angle-Closure Secondary to Panretinal Photocoagulation

Panretinal photocoagulation (PRP) is a well-recognized treatment for reducing the stimulus, which leads to vision-threatening neovascularization formation in disease states associated with posterior segment ischemia.[165] Experimental studies using xenon and ruby laser photocoagulation in rabbit eyes have demonstrated acute intraocular pressure elevations from 400 to 900 mmHg for 0.3 msec in the former and 10 to 40 mmHg for 0.3 msec in the latter.[166, 167] A retrospective study of 30 patients who underwent argon or xenon panretinal photocoagulation for the treatment of diabetic retinopathy reported that 33 percent developed angle-closure and 66 percent developed narrowing of the angle, which resolved in 3 to 4 days.[168] Although the incidence of complications following argon panretinal photocoagulation arc thought to bc rcduccd with treatment sessions separated by 2 wk or more compared with the sessions completed over a 1- to 3-day period, the following complications[169-172] were still reported: choroidal detachment, 81 percent; anterior chamber shallowing, 38 percent; exudative retinal detachment, 12 percent; and increased intraocular pressure, 7 percent.

During panretinal photocoagulation, light energy is converted to thermal energy, which creates an inflammatory process that results in the disruption of the blood retinal barrier at the level of the retinal vessels and the retinal pigment epithelium.[166, 167] This promotes ciliochoroidal effusion and detachment, which allows anterior rotation of the ciliary body, relaxation of the zonule, forward displacement of the lens-iris diaphragm, and angle narrowing or closure. Pupillary block must be ruled out by a history and clinical examination but is not usually a mechanism.[170]

Patients usually report little or no ocular discomfort or visual disturbance. A clinical examination may show a clear cornea, but corneal edema may accompany elevations of intraocular pressure. Applanation pressure may be normal or elevated in the range of 20 to 50 mmHg. Biomicroscopy may show a shallow or closed angle with anterior, annular ciliochoroidal detachment.[170]

In the absence of pupillary block, the treatment is primarily medical, with topical cycloplegic therapy to relax the ciliary muscle, tighten the zonule, and move the lens-iris diaphragm posteriorly, thus opening the angle.[170] Acute elevations of pressure that pose a risk to visual function (e.g., >30 mmHg) may be treated with topical β-blockers, carbonic anhydrase inhibitors, and

hyperosmotic therapy, as indicated. Topical steroid application may enhance resolution of the effusion by reducing the inflammatory component. Most cases resolve spontaneously over a period of 4 to 14 days.[170, 171]

Glaucoma Resulting from Secondary Angle-Closure Associated with Intravitreal Gas Tamponade

The use of intravitreal gas for retinal tamponade was first introduced in 1911 by Ohm[173] and later utilized in 1938 by Rosengren[174] for retinal tamponade in conjunction with surface or penetrating diathermy and drainage of subretinal fluid. In 1973, Norton[175] introduced intravitreal application of sulfur hexafluoride (SF6) gas for retinal tamponade in cases requiring long-acting intravitreal gas tamponade. In 1973, Vygantas and Peyman[176, 177] introduced octofluorocyclopropane (C3F8) for intravitreal tamponade. Both SF6 and C3F8 are inert, lipid-soluble gases that expand and increase their volume within the vitreous cavity. Their volume expansion occurs as a result of nitrogen diffusion from body tissues and blood into the gas pocket until equilibrium is achieved.[173, 176-178] Intraocular air is not useful as a long-acting retinal tamponade, because it does not expand and it is absorbed from the vitreous cavity over a 4-day period.[175] SF6 (M.W. 146) expands to twice its original volume over the first 24 to 36 hr and lasts for 14 days.[179] C3F8 (M.W. 200) expands to four times its original volume over the first 18 to 36 hr and lasts 4 to 6 wk.[180] During pneumatic retinoplexy procedures, it is not uncommon to experience elevations in intraocular pressure to 80 mmHg for several minutes' duration during the introduction of intravitreal gas, which is relieved by factors such as outflow of aqueous and stretching of scleral fibers.[181] Some complications of expandable intravitreal gas tamponade include central retinal artery occlusion, acute open-angle glaucoma, and acute pupillary block glaucoma.[184] The results of intravitreal sulfur hexafluoride gas in conjunction with 101 vitrectomies performed on 87 eyes reported ocular hypertension in 45 eyes, with a significantly higher incidence in eyes receiving 100 percent SF6 compared with lesser gas concentrations.[184] Twenty-six of 101 eyes developed transient fibrinous exudation (with a greater incidence noted in diabetic patients), which contributed to pupillary block and angle-closure. Eleven of 101 eyes developed presumed central retinal artery occlusion, which manifested as elevated intraocular pressure in 10 eyes and a total loss of vision in another eye on the first postoperative day.[184]

To avoid or minimize complications resulting from elevation of intraocular pressure, it is recommended that no more than 50 percent of the volume of the vitreous cavity be replaced with "pure SF6" gas, or alternatively, utilizing a mixture of 15 percent SF6: 85 percent air that is considered to be an equilibrium concentration that minimizes gas expansion while providing the benefits of long duration of action (Burke).

Certain underlying conditions predispose to postoperative elevations of pressure because of reduced outflow facility or increased susceptibility to ischemia in the presence of a compromised vascular supply. Expandable gases should be used with caution in patients with diabetes or glaucoma because of their increased susceptibility to damage from pressure elevation.[183]

Schiotz pressure measurements are inaccurate because of altered scleral rigidity following retinal surgery[182] and high displacement errors that occur in eyes harboring a compressible gas.[183] The most accurate method of pressure measurement is with Goldmann, Perkins, or MaCay-Marg low-displacement tonometry units.[178] Frequent pressure monitoring is recommended during the early postoperative period following intravitreal gas injection, particularly during the rate of maximal gas expansion. It may be necessary to reduce abrupt elevations in pressure with a vitreous tap through the pars plana to avoid serious visual complications. Institution of medical therapy in the form of topical β-blockers, carbonic anhydrase inhibitors, and even hyperosmotics may be needed on a temporary basis to achieve pressure control.

Table 137–1. MECHANISMS OF GLAUCOMA ASSOCIATED WITH DISORDERS OF THE RETINA, VITREOUS, AND CHOROID

Primary Open-Angle Glaucoma
1. Nanophthalmos
2. Rhegmatogenous retinal detachment
3. Diabetes mellitus

Primary Angle-Closure (Related to Pupillary Block)
1. Nanophthalmos
2. AIDS
3. Central retinal vein occlusion
4. Fibrin pupillary block associated with intravitreal gas
5. Retinopathy of prematurity
6. Fibrin pupillary block following pars plana vitrectomy (especially in patients affected by diabetes mellitus)
7. Intravitreal silicone oil

Secondary Angle-Closure (Related to Ciliochoroidal Swelling or Effusion)
1. Nanophthalmos
2. AIDS
3. Panretinal photocoagulation
4. Scleral buckle procedures
5. Central retinal vein occlusion
6. Retinopathy of prematurity
7. Primary ocular tumors
8. Metastatic ocular tumors

Secondary Open-Angle Glaucoma (Related to Obstruction of the Trabecular Meshwork)
1. Melanomalytic (choroidal melanoma)
2. Photoreceptor-induced (Schwartz's syndrome)
3. Intraocular silicone-related
4. Hemolytic
5. Ghost cell
6. Hemosiderotic
7. Pigmentary dispersion glaucoma
8. Amyloidosis
9. Serum (cell and flare)
10. Primary ocular tumors
11. Metastatic ocular tumors
12. Corticosteroid-induced
13. Sickle cell hemoglobinopathy related
14. Leukemia
15. Syphilis

Neovascular Glaucoma (All Processes Associated with Posterior Segment Ischemia Including but not Limited to the Following)
1. Diabetes mellitus
2. Branch retinal vein occlusion
3. Central retinal vein occlusion
4. Central retinal artery occlusion
5. Branch retinal artery occlusion
5. Retinopathy of prematurity
6. Familial exudative vitreoretinopathy
7. Coat's disease

8. Sickle cell hemoglobinopathy
9. Eales' disease
10. Primary ocular tumors
11. Metastatic ocular tumors
12. Carotid ischemia
13. Dural shunt syndrome
14. Superior vena caval syndrome
15. Giant cell arteritis*
16. Systemic lupus erythematosus*
17. Vogt-Koyanagi-Harada's disease
18. Sympathetic ophthalmia
19. Sarcoidosis*
20. Norrie's disease*
21. Takayasu's disease*
22. Incontinentia pigmenti*
23. Leber's miliary aneurysms*
24. Retinal embolization (i.e., talc)*
25. Long-standing retinal detachment*

Increased Episcleral Venous Pressure
1. Nanophthalmos
2. Choroidal hemangioma associated with Sturge-Weber disease
3. Dural shunt syndrome
4. Superior vena caval syndrome

Trauma Related
1. Angle recession
2. Hemolytic
3. Ghost cell
4. Hemosiderotic
5. Serum (cell and flare)
6. Prostaglandin-induced

Inflammation (Uveitic) Related
1. Iris retraction syndrome
2. Schwartz's syndrome
3. Retinopathy of prematurity
4. Sarcoidosis
5. Syphilis
6. Toxoplasmosis
7. Vogt-Koyanagi-Harada syndrome
8. Behçet's disease
9. Sympathetic uveitis
10. Toxocariasis
11. Mumps
12. Onchocerciasis
13. Coccidiodomycosis
14. Leprosy
15. Tuberculosis
16. Reticulum cell sarcoma (histiocytic lymphoma)
17. AIDS-related retinopathy and associated opportunistic infections

*Data from Jampol LM: Proliferative retinopathies. Surv Ophthalmol 25:1, 1980.

We advocate pressure checks on at least a daily basis, thereafter, during the period of volume expansion, unless indicated more frequently by unexpected pressure rises or inadequate responses to therapeutic intervention. Caution is advised concerning air travel for patients harboring intravitreal gases. A prospective study of simulated air travel with monkeys containing intravitreal gas volumes as small as 0.25 ml following vitrectomy and air/fluid exchange showed an average intraocular pressure elevation of 42 mmHg associated with complications of central retinal artery occlusion and visual loss.[182] Some recommend that air travel should be postponed until all intraocular gas has resorbed or take precautions to ensure that cabin pressure is maintained at 2000 ft (706 mmHg).[182] Others recommend that patients who harbor greater than or equal to 1 ml of expansile gas should avoid air travel completely.[178]

Glaucoma Associated with Intravitreal Silicone Application
(see Chap. 101)

Silicone oil insufflation for the treatment of complex retinal detachment was introduced by Cibis in 1962.[185] Since then, indications and techniques have evolved to include intravitreal silicone as an adjunct to vitrectomy, membrane peeling, endophotocoagulation, and scleral buckling for the treatment of retinal detachment and advanced vitreoretinopathy.[186-188] Intravitreal silicone has been implicated in both short- and long-term elevations of intraocular pressure, primarily on the basis of secondary open-angle glaucoma. A retrospective analysis of 48 patients treated with pars plana vitrectomy and intravitreal silicone injection for repair of vitreoretinopathy showed that 56 percent of patients had an intraocular pressure elevation of at least 10 mmHg between 6 hr and 60 days during the postoperative period.[189] Of these, pressure elevation resolved either spontaneously or with the aid of temporary medical therapy in 56 percent of patients. Twenty-two percent required removal of silicone oil, and 22 percent required extended medical management.

Angle-closure with pupillary block related to intravitreal silicone oil has been reported.[190] Performance of an inferior peripheral iridotomy by laser or surgical means may be necessary to reestablish communication between the anterior and posterior chambers.

Anatomic success rates in reattaching the retina have been reported between 64 and 66 percent, and complications associated with silicone oil placement over a 1- to 3-yr period of follow-up include cataract, 60 percent; glaucoma, 17 percent; and keratopathy, 12.3 percent.[187] Histopathologic findings in eyes enucleated following intravitreal silicone placement over a period of 5 to 12 yr have shown blockage of the trabecular meshwork by macrophages that had phagocytized silicone. Silicone was also present in the vitreous, preretinal membranes, optic disc, iris, and choroid.[191, 192] The most common cause of enucleation following silicone placement was for intractable secondary glaucoma (Table 137–1).[193]

REFERENCES

1. Epstein DL (ed): Chandler and Grant's Glaucoma, 3rd ed. Philadelphia, Lea & Febiger, 1986, p 86.
2. Epstein DL (ed): Chandler and Grant's Glaucoma, 3rd ed. Philadelphia, Lea & Febiger, 1986, p 374.
3. Burton TC, Lambert RW Jr: A predictive model for visual recovery following retinal detachment surgery. Ophthalmology 85:619, 1978.
4. Epstein DL (ed): Chandler and Grant's Glaucoma, 3rd ed. Philadelphia, Lea & Febiger, 1986, p 88.
5. Gitter KA, Meyer D, Sarin LK: Ultrasound to evaluate eyes with opaque media. Am J Ophthalmol 64:100, 1967.
6. Lemke HH, Pischel DK: Retinal detachments after the use of phospholine iodide. Trans Pac Coast Oto-ophthalmol Soc 47:157, 1966.
7. Ackerman AL: Retinal detachments and miotic therapy. In Pruett RL, Regan CDJ (eds): Retinal Congress. New York, Appleton-Century-Crofts, 1972, p 533.
8. Kraushar MF, Podell DL: "Miotic-induced" retinal detachment. In Pruett RL, Regan CDJ (eds): Retinal Congress. New York, Appleton-Century-Crofts, 1972, p 541.
9. Pape LG, Forbes M: Retinal detachment and miotic therapy. Am J Ophthalmol 85:558, 1978.
10. Beasley H, Fraunfelder FT: Retinal detachments and topical ocular miotics. Ophthalmology 86:95, 1979.
11. Kraushar MF, Steinberg JA: Miotics and retinal detachment: Upgrading the community standard. Surv Ophthalmol 35(4):311, 1991.
12. Burton TC, Arafat NT, Phelps CD: Intraocular pressure in retinal detachment. Int Ophthalmol 1:147, 1979.
13. Bankes JL, Perkins ES, Tsolakis S, Wright JE: Bedford glaucoma survey. Br Med J 1:791, 1968.
14. Hollows FC, Graham PA: Intraocular pressure, glaucoma, and glaucoma suspects in a defined population. Br J Ophthalmol 50:570, 1966.
15. Leske MC, Rosenthal J: Epidemiologic aspects of open angle glaucoma. Am J Epidemiol 109:250, 1979.
16. Becker B: Discussion of Smith JL: Retinal detachment and glaucoma. Trans Am Acad Ophthalmol-otolaryngol 67:731, 1963.
17. Phelps CD, Burton TC: Glaucoma and retinal detachment. Arch Ophthalmol 95:418, 1977.
18. Langham ME, Regan CDJ: Circulatory changes associated with the onset of primary retinal detachment. Arch Ophthalmol 81:820, 1969.
19. Shammas HF, Halassa AH, Faris BM: Variations in intraocular pressure, cup:disc ratio, and steroid responsiveness in the retinal detachment population. Arch Ophthalmol 94:1108, 1976.
20. Armaly MF: Cup/disc ratio in early open angle glaucoma. Doc Ophthalmol 26:526, 1969.
21. Armaly MF: Inheritance of dexamethasone hypertension and glaucoma. Arch Ophthalmol 77:747, 1967.
22. Duke-Elder S: Anomalies in the size of the eye. In System of Ophthalmology, vol. 3, pt 2. St. Louis, CV Mosby, 1964, p 488.
23. Calhoun FP Jr: The management of glaucoma in nanophthalmos. Trans Am Ophthalmol Soc 73:97, 1975.
24. Simmons RJ: Nanophthalmos, diagnosis and treatment. In Epstein DL (ed): Chandler and Grant's Glaucoma, 3rd ed. Philadelphia, Lea & Febiger, 1986.
25. Singh OS, Simmons RJ, Brockhurst RJ, et al: Nanophthalmos: A perspective on identification and therapy. Ophthalmology 89:1006, 1982.
26. Kimbrough RL, Trempe CL, Brockhurst RJ, et al: Angle closure glaucoma in nanophthalmos. Am J Ophthalmol 88:572, 1979.
27. Brockhurst RJ: Nanophthalmos with uveal effusion: A new clinical entity. Trans Am Ophthalmol Soc 72:371, 1974.
28. Wilmer HA, Scammon RE: Growth of the components of the human eyeball. Arch Ophthalmol 43:599, 1950.
29. Shaffer R: Discussion of Calhoun FP Jr: The management of glaucoma in nanophthalmos. Trans Am Ophthalmol Soc 73:97, 1975.
30. Trelstad RL, Silberman NN, Brockhurst RJ: Nanophthalmic sclera. Arch Ophthalmol 100:1935, 1982.

31. Yue BY, Duvall J, Goldberg MF, et al: Nanophthalmic sclera: Morphologic and tissue culture studies. Ophthalmology 93:534, 1986.

32. Yue BY, Kurosawa A, Duvall J, et al: Nanophthalmic sclera fibronectin studies. Ophthalmology 95:56, 1988.

33. Brockhurst RJ: Vortex vein decompression for nanophthalmic uveal effusion. Arch Ophthalmol 89:1987, 1980.

34. Brockhurst RJ: Vortex vein decompression. In Thomas JV (ed): Contemporary Glaucoma Surgery, 1st ed. St. Louis, CV Mosby, 1990.

35. Gass DJ: Uveal effusion syndrome: A new hypothesis concerning pathogenesis and technique of surgical treatment. Trans Am Ophthalmol 81:246, 1982.

36. Singh OS: Nanophthalmos. In Thomas JV (ed): Contemporary Glaucoma Surgery, 1st ed. St. Louis, CV Mosby, 1991.

37. Wilkie J, Drance SM, Schulzer M: The effects of miotics on anterior chamber depth. Am J Ophthalmol 68:78, 1969.

38. Simmons RJ, Kimbrough RL, Belcher CD: Gonioplasty for selected cases of angle closure glaucoma. Doc Ophthalmol 22:200, 1980.

39. Campbell DG: Iris retraction associated with rhegmatogenous retinal detachment syndrome and hypotony. Arch Ophthalmol 102:1457, 1984.

40. Donaldson DD: Atlas of External Diseases of the Eye, vol. 4. St. Louis, CV Mosby, 1973, p 58.

41. Duke-Elder WS: System of Ophthalmology, vol. X. St. Louis, CV Mosby, 1967, p 808.

42. Dobbie JC: A study of the intraocular fluid dynamics in retinal detachment. Arch Ophthalmol 69:159, 1963.

43. Frambach DA, Marmor MF: The rate and route of fluid absorption from the subretinal space of the rabbit. Invest Ophthalmol Vis Sci 22:292, 1982.

44. Shokat M, Reisner SH, Krikler R, et al: Retinopathy of prematurity: Incidence and risk factors. Pediatrics 72:159, 1983.

45. Phelps DL: Vision loss due to retinopathy of prematurity. Lancet 1:606, 1981.

46. Blodi FC: Symposium: Retrolental fibroplasia (retinopathy of prematurity). Trans Am Acad Ophthalmol-otolaryngol 59:35, 1955.

47. Walton DS: Retrolental fibroplasia with glaucoma. In Epstein DL (ed): Chandler and Grant's Glaucoma, 3rd ed. Philadelphia, Lea & Febiger, 1986, p 518.

48. Cohen J, Alfano JE, Boshes LD, Palmgren C: Clinical evaluation of school-age children with retrolental fibroplasia. Am J Ophthalmol 57:41, 1964.

49. Kushner BJ: Ciliary block glaucoma in retinopathy of prematurity. Arch Ophthalmol 100:1078, 1982.

50. Kushner BJ, Sondheimer S: Medical treatment of glaucoma associated with cicatricial retinopathy of prematurity. Am J Ophthalmol 94:313, 1982.

51. Hartnett ME, Gilbert MM, Richardson TM, et al: Anterior segment evaluation of infants with retinopathy of prematurity. Ophthalmology 97:122, 1989.

52. Criswick VG, Schepens CL: Familial exudative vitreoretinopathy. Am J Ophthalmol 68:578, 1961.

53. Ridley ME, Shields JA, Brown GC, et al: Coat's disease: Evaluation of management. Ophthalmology 89:1381, 1982.

54. Reese AB: Persistent hyperplastic primary vitreous (PHPV). Am J Ophthalmol 40:317, 1955.

55. Pruett RC, Schepens CL: Posterior hyperplastic primary vitreous. Am J Ophthalmol 69:535, 1970.

56. Awan KJ, Humayun M: Changes in the contralateral eye in uncomplicated persistent hyperplastic primary vitreous in adults. Am J Ophthalmol 99:122, 1985.

57. Stark WJ, Lindsey PS, Fagadau WR, Michels RG: Persistent hyperplastic primary vitreous surgical treatment. Ophthalmology 90:452, 1983.

58. Sugar HS: Pigmentary glaucoma: A 25-year review. Am J Ophthalmol 62:499, 1966.

59. Bracket A, Chermet M: Association glaucome pigmentaire et decollement de retine. Ann Ocul 207:451, 1974.

60. Scheie HG, Cameron JD: Personal communication. In Ritch R, Shields MB (eds): The Secondary Glaucomas. St. Louis, CV Mosby, 1982, p 158.

61. Sebestyen JG, Schepens CL, Rosenthal ML: Retinal detachment and glaucoma. I: Tonometric and gonioscopic study of 160 cases. Arch Ophthalmol 67:736, 1962.

62. Rodriguez-Gonzalez A: Personal communication. In Ritch R, Shields MB (eds): The Secondary Glaucomas. St. Louis, CV Mosby, 1982, p 158.

63. Gartner S, Schlossman A: Retinitis pigmentosa associated with glaucoma. Am J Ophthalmol 32:1337, 1949.

64. Kogbe OI, Follmann P: Investigations into aqueous humor dynamics in primary pigmentary degeneration of the retina. Ophthalmologica 171:165, 1975.

65. Phelps CD: Glaucoma associated with disorders of the retina. In Ritch R, Shields MB (eds): The Secondary Glaucomas. St. Louis, CV Mosby, 1982, p 158.

66. Stickler GB, et al: Hereditary progressive arthro-ophthalmopathy. Mayo Clin Proc 40:433, 1966.

67. Blair NP, Albert DM, Liberfarb RM, Hirose T: Hereditary progressive arthro-ophthalmopathy of Stickler. Am J Ophthalmol 88:876, 1979.

68. Wagner H: Ein bisher un bekanntes Erblei den des Anges (hereditary vitreoretinal degeneration) beobachet in Kanton Zurich. Klin Monatsbl Augenheilkd 100:840, 1938.

69. Maumenee IH: Vitreoretinal degeneration as a sign of generalized connective tissue diseases. Am J Ophthalmol 88:432, 1979.

70. Phelps CD: Glaucoma associated with retinal disorders. In Ritch R, Shields MB (eds): The Secondary Glaucomas. St. Louis, CV Mosby, 1982, p 159.

71. Armstrong JR, Daily RK, Dobson HL, Girard LJ: The incidence of glaucoma in diabetes mellitus: A comparison with the incidence of glaucoma in the general population. Am J Ophthalmol 50:55, 1960.

72. Becker B: Diabetes mellitus and primary open-angle glaucoma. The XXVII Edward Jackson Memorial Lecture. Am J Ophthalmol 71:1, 1971.

73. Lieb WA, Stark N, Jelinek MB, Malzi R: Diabetes mellitus and glaucoma. Acta Ophthalmol Suppl 94, 1967.

74. Leske MC, Podgor MJ: Intraocular pressure, cardiovascular risk variables, and visual field defects. Am J Epidemiol 118:280, 1983.

75. Klein BEK, Klein R, Moss SE: Intraocular pressure in diabetic persons. Ophthalmology 91:1356, 1984.

76. Ingersheimer J: Intraocular pressure and its relation to retinal extravasation. Arch Ophthalmol 32:50, 1944.

77. Armaly MF, Baloglou PJ: Diabetes mellitus and the eye. II: Intraocular pressure and aqueous outflow facility. Arch Ophthalmol 77:493, 1967.

78. Vannas S, Tarkkanen A: Retinal vein occlusion and glaucoma. Br J Ophthalmol 44:583, 1960.

79. Grant WM: Shallowing of the anterior chamber following occlusion of the central retinal vein. Am J Ophthalmol 75:384, 1973.

80. Bloome MA: Transient angle closure glaucoma in central retinal vein occlusion. Ann Ophthalmol 9:44, 1977.

81. Hyams SW, Neumann E: Transient angle-closure glaucoma after retinal vein occlusion. Br J Ophthalmol 56:353, 1972.

82. Phelps CD: Glaucoma associated with disorders of the retina. In Ritch R, Shields MB (eds): The Secondary Glaucomas. St. Louis, CV Mosby, 1982, p 152.

83. Magargal LE, Donoso LA, Sanborn GE: Retinal ischemia and risk of neovascularization following central retinal vein obstruction. Ophthalmology 89:1241, 1982.

84. Epstein DL: Chandler and Grant's Glaucoma, 3rd ed. Philadelphia, Lea & Febiger, 1986, p 289.

85. Wolff SM, Zimmerman LE: Chronic secondary glaucoma: Associated with retrodisplacement of the iris root and deepening of the anterior chamber secondary to contusion. Am J Ophthalmol 54:547, 1962.

86. Epstein DL, Hashimoto JM, Grant WM: Serum obstruction of aqueous outflow in enucleated eyes. Am J Ophthalmol 86:101, 1978.

87. Podos SM, Becker B, Kass MA: Prostaglandin synthesis, inhibition, and intraocular pressure. Invest Ophthalmol 12:430, 1973.

88. Phelps CD, Watzke RC: Hemolytic glaucoma. Am J Ophthalmol 80:690, 1975.

89. Syrdalen P: Trauma and retinal detachment: The anterior chamber angle with special reference to width, pigmentation, and traumatic ruptures. Acta Ophthalmol 48:1006, 1970.

90. Cox MS, Schepens CL, Freeman HM: Retinal detachment due to ocular contusion. Arch Ophthalmol 76:678, 1966.
91. Fraser DJ Jr, Font RL: Ocular inflammation and hemorrhage as initial manifestations of uveal malignant melanoma: Incidence and prognosis. Arch Ophthalmol 97:1311, 1979.
92. Yanoff M: Glaucoma mechanisms in ocular malignant melanomas. Am J Ophthalmol 70:898, 1970.
93. Yoshizumi MO, Thomas JV, Smith TR: Glaucoma-inducing mechanisms in eyes with retinoblastoma. Arch Ophthalmol 96:105, 1978.
94. Walton DS, Grant WM: Retinoblastoma and iris neovascularization. Am J Ophthalmol 65:598, 1968.
95. Weiss DI: Dual origin of glaucoma in encephalotrigeminal haemangiomatosis. Trans Ophthalmolol Soc UK 93:477, 1973.
96. Phelps CD: The pathogenesis of glaucoma in Sturge-Weber syndrome. Ophthalmology 85:276, 1978.
97. Ferry AP, Font RL: Carcinoma metastatic to the eye and orbit. II: A clinicopathologic study of 26 patients with carcinoma metastatic to the anterior segment of the eye. Arch Ophthalmol 93:472, 1975.
98. Shields CL, Shields JA, Shields MB, Augsburger JJ: Prevalence and mechanisms of secondary intraocular pressure elevation in eyes with intraocular tumors. Ophthalmology 94:839, 1987.
99. Zakka KA, Yee RD, Shorr N, et al: Leukemic iris infiltration. Am J Ophthalmol 89:204, 1980.
100. Michels RG, Knox DL, Erozan YS, Green WR: Intraocular reticulum cell sarcoma: Diagnosis by pars plana vitrectomy. Arch Ophthalmol 93:1331, 1975.
101. Kennerdell JS, Johnson BL, Wisotzkey HM: Vitreous cellular reaction. Arch Ophthalmol 93:1341, 1975.
102. Char DH, Margolis L, Newman AB: Ocular reticulum cell sarcoma. Am J Ophthalmol 91:480, 1981.
103. Parsons JH: The Pathology of the Eye. III: General Pathology, Part 1. London, Hodder & Stoughton, 1904, p 1087.
104. Pesin SR, Katz LJ, Augsburger JJ, et al: Acute angle-closure glaucoma from spontaneous massive hemorrhagic retinal or choroidal detachment: An updated diagnostic and therapeutic approach. Ophthalmology 97:76, 1990.
105. Wood WJ, Smith TR: Senile disciform macular degeneration complicated by massive hemorrhagic retinal detachment and angle closure glaucoma. Retina 3:296, 1983.
106. Brown GC, Tasman WS, Shields JA: Massive subretinal hemorrhage and anticoagulant therapy. Can J Ophthalmol 17:227, 1982.
107. El Baba F, Jarrett WH II, Harbin TS Jr, et al: Massive hemorrhage complicating age-related macular degeneration: Clinicopathologic correlation and role of anticoagulants. Ophthalmology 93:1581, 1986.
108. Shammas HJ: Atlas of Ophthalmic Ultrasonography and Biometry. St. Louis, CV Mosby, 1984, p 82.
109. Holland GN, Pepose JS, Pettit TH, et al: Acquired immune deficiency syndrome: Ocular manifestations. Ophthalmology 90:859, 1983.
110. Palestine AG, Rodrigues MM, Macher AM, et al: Ophthalmic involvement in acquired immunodeficiency syndrome. Ophthalmology 91:1092, 1984.
111. Brubaker RF, Pederson JE: Ciliochoroidal detachment. Surv Ophthalmol 27:281, 1983.
112. Phelps CD: Angle-closure glaucoma secondary to ciliary body swelling. Arch Ophthalmol 92:287, 1974.
113. Ullman S, Wilson RP, Schwartz L: Bilateral angle-closure glaucoma in association with the acquired immune deficiency syndrome. Am J Ophthalmol 101:419, 1986.
114. Holland GN, Sidikaro Y, Kreiger AE, et al: Treatment of cytomegalovirus retinopathy with ganciclovir. Ophthalmology 94:815, 1987.
115. Epstein DL (ed): Amyloidosis and open-angle glaucoma. In Chandler and Grant's Glaucoma, 3rd ed. St. Louis, CV Mosby, 1986, p 198.
116. Tsukahara ST, Matsuo T: Secondary glaucoma accompanied with primary familial amyloidosis. Ophthalmologica 175:250, 1977.
117. Chandler PA, Grant WM: Inflammatory precipitates of the trabecular meshwork. In Chandler PA, Grant WM (eds): Lectures on Glaucoma. Philadelphia, Lea & Febiger, 1965, p 257.
118. Roth M, Simmons RJ: Glaucoma associated with precipitates of the trabecular meshwork. Ophthalmology 86:1613, 1979.
119. Epstein DL (ed): Chandler and Grant's Glaucoma, 3rd ed. Philadelphia, Lea & Febiger, 1986, pp 403–404.
120. Schwartz A: Chronic open-angle glaucoma secondary to rhegmatogenous retinal detachment. Am J Ophthalmol 75:205, 1973.
121. Obernauf CD, Shaw HE, Syndor CF, Klintworth GK: Sarcoidosis and its ophthalmic manifestations. Am J Ophthalmol 86:648, 1978.
122. Duke-Elder S (ed): System of Ophthalmology, vol. 9. St. Louis, CV Mosby, 1966, p 292.
123. Lichter PR, Shaffer RN: Interstitial keratitis and glaucoma. Am J Ophthalmol 68:241, 1969.
124. O'Connor GR: Manifestations and management of ocular toxoplasmosis. Bull N Y Acad Med 50(2):192, 1974.
125. Ohno S, Char DH, Kimura SJ, O'Connor GR: Vogt-Koyanagi-Harada syndrome. Am J Ophthalmol 83:735, 1977.
126. Makley TA, Azar A: Sympathetic ophthalmia. Arch Ophthalmol 96:257, 1978.
127. Colvard DM, Robertson DM, O'Duffy JD: The ocular manifestations of Behçet's disease. Arch Ophthalmol 95:1813, 1977.
128. Shields JA: Ocular toxocariasis: A review. Surv Ophthalmol 28:361, 1984.
129. Merritt JC, Callender CO: Adult cytomegalic inclusion retinitis. Ann Ophthalmol 10:1059, 1978.
130. Riffenburgh RS: Iritis and glaucoma associated with mumps. Arch Ophthalmol 51:702, 1954.
131. Pettit TH, Learn RN, Foos RY: Intraocular coccidiodomycosis. Arch Ophthalmol 77:655, 1967.
132. Ben-Sira I, Yassur Y: Ocular onchocerciasis in Malawi. Br J Ophthalmol 56:617, 1972.
133. Malla OK, Brandt F, Auten JGF: Ocular findings in leprosy patients in an institution in Nepal (Khokana). Br J Ophthalmol 65:226, 1981.
134. Fountain JA, Werner RB: Tuberculosis retinal vasculitis. Retina 4:48, 1984.
135. Grove AS Jr: The dural shunt syndrome: Pathophysiology and clinical course. Ophthalmology 91:31, 1984.
136. Alfano JE, Alfano PA: Glaucoma and superior vena caval syndrome. Am J Ophthalmol 42:685, 1956.
137. Weiss DI, Shaffer RN, Nehrenberg TR: Neovascular glaucoma complicating carotid-cavernous fistula. Arch Ophthalmol 69:60, 1963.
138. Dueker DK: Neovascular glaucoma. In Epstein DL (ed): Chandler and Grant's Glaucoma, 3rd ed. Philadelphia, Lea & Febiger, 1986, p 378.
139. Aaberg TM, Van Horn D: Late complications of pars plana vitreous surgery. Ophthalmology 85:126, 1978.
140. Ghartley KN, Tolentino FI, Freeman HM, et al: Closed vitreous surgery. XVII: Results and complications of pars plana vitrectomy. Arch Ophthalmol 98:1248, 1980.
141. Aiello LM, Wand M, Liang G: Neovascular glaucoma and vitreous hemorrhage following cataract surgery in patients with diabetes mellitus. Ophthalmology 90:814, 1983.
142. Schachat AP, Oyakawa RT, Michels RG, Rice TA: Complications of vitreous surgery for diabetic retinopathy. II: Postoperative complications. Ophthalmology 90:522, 1983.
143. Davidorf FH: Retinal pigment epithelial glaucoma. Ophthalmol Dig 38:11, 1976.
144. Matsuo N, Takabatake M, Ueno H, et al: Photoreceptor outer segments in the aqueous humor in rhegmatogenous retinal detachment. Am J Ophthalmol 101:673, 1986.
145. Phelps CD, Watzke RC: Hemolytic glaucoma. Am J Ophthalmol 80:690, 1975.
146. Campbell DG: Ghost-cell glaucoma following trauma. Ophthalmology 88:115, 1981.
147. Vannas S: Hemosiderosis in eyes with secondary glaucoma after delayed intraocular hemorrhages. Acta Ophthalmol 38:254, 1960.
148. Goldberg MF: The diagnosis and treatment of sickled erythrocytes in human hyphemas. Trans Am Ophthalmol Soc 76:481, 1978.
149. Deutsch TA, Weinreb RN, Goldberg MF: Indications for surgical management of hyphemas in patients with sickle cell trait. Arch Ophthalmol 102:566–569, 1984.

150. Fiore JV Jr, Newton JC: Anterior segment changes following the scleral buckle procedure. Arch Ophthalmol 84:284, 1970.

151. Hartley RE, Marsh RJ: Anterior chamber depth changes after retinal detachment. Br J Ophthalmol 57:546, 1973.

152. Boniuk M, Zimmerman LE: Pathologic anatomy of complications. In Schepens CL, Regan CD (eds): Controversial Aspects of the Management of Retinal Detachment. Boston, Little, Brown, 1965, p 286.

153. Smith TR: Acute glaucoma developing after scleral buckle procedures. Am J Ophthalmol 64:1907, 1967.

154. Krieger AE, Hodgkinson J, Frederick AR, et al: The results of retinal detachment surgery: Analysis of 286 operations with a broad scleral buckle. Arch Ophthalmol 86:385, 1971.

155. Holland PM, Smith TR: Broad scleral buckle in the management of retinal detachments with giant tears. Am J Ophthalmol 83:518, 1977.

156. Perez RN, Phelps CD, Burton TC: Angle closure glaucoma following scleral buckle operations. Trans Am Acad Ophthalmol Otolaryngol 81:247, 1976.

157. Chandler P, Grant WM: Lectures on Glaucoma. Philadelphia, Lea & Febiger, 1965, p 204.

158. Hayreh SS, Baines JAB: Occlusion of the vortex veins: An experimental study. Br J Ophthalmol 57:217, 1973.

159. Diddie KR, Ernest JT: Uveal blood flow after 360 degree constriction in the rabbit. Arch Ophthalmol 98:729, 1980.

160. Phelps CD: Angle-closure glaucoma secondary to ciliary body swelling. Arch Ophthalmol 92:287, 1974.

161. Pemberton JW: Schiotz-applanation disparity following retinal detachment surgery. Arch Ophthalmol 81:535, 1969.

162. Epstein DL (ed): Chandler and Grant's Glaucoma, 3rd ed. St. Louis, CV Mosby, 1986, p 403.

163. Davis MD: Complications and pathology. In Schepens CL, Regan CDJ (eds): Controversial Aspects of the Management of Retinal Detachment. Boston, Little, Brown, 1965, p 237.

164. Simmons RJ: Angle closure glaucoma after scleral buckling operations for separated retina. In Epstein DL (ed): Chandler and Grant's Glaucoma, 3rd ed. Philadelphia, Lea & Febiger, 1986, p 279.

165. The Diabetic Retinopathy Study Research Group: Photocoagulation treatment of proliferative diabetic retinopathy: The second report of diabetic retinopathy study findings. Ophthalmology 85:82, 1978.

166. Fraunfelder FT, Viernstein LJ: Intraocular pressure variation during xenon and ruby laser photocoagulation. Am J Ophthalmol 71:1261, 1971.

167. McNair J, Fraunfelder FT, Wilson RS, et al: Acute pressure changes and possible secondary tissue changes due to laser or xenon photocoagulation. Am J Ophthalmol 77:13, 1974.

168. Mensher JH: Anterior chamber depth alteration after retinal photocoagulation. Arch Ophthalmol 95:113, 1977.

169. Huamonte FU, Peyman GA, Goldberg MF, et al: Immediate fundus complications after retinal scatter photocoagulation. I: Clinical picture and pathogenesis. Ophthalmic Surg 7:88, 1976.

170. Blondeau P, Pavan PR, Phelps CD: Acute pressure elevation following panretinal photocoagulation. Arch Ophthalmol 99:1239, 1981.

171. Liang JC, Huamonte FU: Reduction of immediate complications after panretinal photocoagulation. Retina 4:166, 1984.

172. Doft BH, Blankenship GW: Single versus multiple treatment sessions of argon laser panretinal photocoagulation for proliferative diabetic retinopathy. Ophthalmology 89:772, 1982.

173. Killey FP, Edelhauser HF, Aaberg TM: Intraocular sulfurhexafluoride and octofluorocyclobutane effects on intraocular pressure and vitreous volume. Arch Ophthalmol 96:511, 1978.

174. Rosengren B: The results of treatment of detachment of the retina with diathermy and injection of air into the vitreous. Acta Ophthalmol 16:573, 1938.

175. Norton EWD: Intraocular gas in the management of selected retinal detachments. Trans Am Acad Ophthalmol Otolaryngol 77:85, 1973.

176. Vygantas CM, Peyman GA, Daily MJ, et al: Octofluorocyclobutane and other gases for vitreous replacement. Arch Ophthalmol 90:235, 1973.

177. Peyman GA, Vygantas CM, Bennett TO, et al: Octofluorobutane in vitreous and aqueous humor replacement. Arch Ophthalmol 93:1191, 1976.

178. Aronowitz LD, Brubaker RF: Effects of intraocular gas on intraocular pressure. Arch Ophthalmol 94:1191, 1976.

179. Fineberg E, Machemer R, Sullivan P, et al: Sulfur hexafluoride in owl monkey vitreous cavity. Am J Ophthalmol 79:67, 1975.

180. Lincoff A, Haft D, Liggett P, et al: Intravitreal expansion of perfluorocarbon bubbles. Arch Ophthalmol 98:1646, 1980.

181. Hilton GF, Grizzard S: Pneumatic retinopexy: A two-step outpatient operation without conjunctival incision. Ophthalmology 93:626, 1986.

182. Dieckert JP, O'Connor PS, Schacklett DE, et al: Air travel and intraocular gas. Ophthalmology 93:642, 1986.

183. Sabates WI, Abrams GW, Swanson DE, Norton EWD: The use of intraocular gases: The results of sulfur hexafluoride gas in retinal detachment surgery. Ophthalmology 88:447, 1981.

184. Abrams GW, Swanson DE, Sabates WI, et al: The results of sulfur hexafluoride gas in vitreous surgery. Am J Ophthalmol 94:165, 1982.

185. Cibis PA, Becker B, Okun E, Canaan S: The use of liquid silicone in retinal detachment surgery. Arch Ophthalmol 68:590, 1962.

186. Watzke RC: Silicone retinopiesis for retinal detachment: A long-term clinical evaluation. Arch Ophthalmol 77:185, 1967.

187. Chan C, Okun E: The question of ocular tolerance to intravitreal liquid silicone: A long-term analysis. Ophthalmology 93:651, 1986.

188. McCuen BW II, Landers MB, Machemer R: The use of silicone oil following failed vitrectomy for retinal detachment with advanced proliferative vitreoretinopathy. Ophthalmology 92:1029, 1985.

189. de Corral LR, Cohen SB, Peyman GA: Effect of intravitreal silicone oil on intraocular pressure. Ophthalmic Surg 18:446, 1987.

190. Ando F: Intraocular hypertension resulting from pupillary block by silicone oil. [Correspondence] Am J Ophthalmol 99:87, 1985.

191. Ni C, Wen-Ji W, Albert D, Schepens CL: Histopathologic findings in a human eye after 12 years. Arch Ophthalmol 101:1399, 1983.

192. Rentsch FJ: Electromicroscopical aspects of acid compartments of the ground substance of collagen in different cases of intravitreal tissue proliferation. Dev Ophthalmol 2:385, 1981.

193. Alexandris E, Daniel H: Results of silicone oil injection into the vitreous. Dev Ophthalmol 2:24, 1981.

194. Singh OS, Sofinski SJ: Personal communication, 1991.

Chapter 138

■

Medical Management of Glaucoma

ROBERT C. ALLEN

For ophthalmologists using medical treatment to lower intraocular pressure (IOP) in patients who have glaucoma or are at high risk for developing glaucoma, the current era might be described as both the best of times and the worst of times. It is encouraging that we now have numerous drugs at our disposal, including those with long histories of excellent safety and efficacy as well as newer agents that potentially allow better tailoring of individual treatment regimens for each patient. Complementing the enlarged armamentarium are other advances such as the continually improving ability to monitor visual function quantitatively in most patients with automated static visual fields, a much greater knowledge about barriers to compliance with medical treatment, and the more convenient dosing schedule and tolerable profile of side effects of current topical ophthalmic medications. It is an even more propitious time to advocate medical therapy because clinical research trials now show a probable protective effect of topical medication and allow our clinical decisions to be more scientifically based. Reconciled with these advances, however, are the qualifications that lead some clinicians to believe that this is a very difficult period in which to initiate and sustain medical therapy. The reasons for this position include the continued awareness of very high rates of glaucoma in eyes with statistically normal IOP, patients' and physicians' continued interest in the earlier use of interventional treatment such as laser procedures or trabeculectomy, and lingering controversy about the ability of medical therapy to prevent visual field damage with long-term follow-up. Added to these considerations are the societal concerns and increasing knowledge about systemic side effects of even our best topical antiglaucoma drugs and the combined pressure of government, third-party payers, and the public to lower health care costs at a time when medicines are becoming increasingly more expensive.

In order to cope effectively with these seemingly paradoxical issues, ophthalmologists must remain familiar with a wide body of increasingly complex literature on new drugs and must be receptive to changing indications for the use of medical treatment in the future based on the results of long-term clinical trials. This chapter presents an overview of current medical management of glaucoma, reviews pertinent studies, and provides some insight into new developments as well as the potential for modification of currently available therapy.

BASIS FOR MEDICAL TREATMENT

The primary goal in the treatment of glaucoma is to prevent loss of visual function caused by damage to the optic nerve. Whether or not the damage is always pressure-induced remains debatable, but elevated IOP is just one of several significant risk factors that have a causal relationship to the production of glaucomatous field loss.[1-4] Our therapeutic approaches, however, are currently limited to reducing IOP. This approach of lowering a potentially harmful pressure might apply to patients with both documented optic nerve damage and visual field loss as well as patients with elevated IOP or other well-described risk factors so that treatment is indicated to prevent the onset of damage.[5] Therefore, for the purposes of our discussion on medical therapeutics, glaucoma is addressed along with the diagnosis of glaucoma suspect and ocular hypertension.[6]

This approach certainly implies a bias that high IOP can potentially harm visual function but also begs the question of whether reducing IOP by either a certain physiologic percentage or to an absolute level within the statistically normal range will lower or remove the potential for damage. Although the answer is at first intuitive, currently available data continue to be inconclusive.

Retrospective studies of medical therapy for established glaucoma have been relatively consistent in showing that lowering IOP has a beneficial effect on preventing the progression of field loss,[8-11] although at least one study offers an opposing viewpoint.[12]

Another important question about the efficacy of medical therapy and attempted lowering of IOP concerns the treatment of glaucoma suspects or so-called ocular hypertensives. Like the previously cited studies on treatment of established glaucoma, some data have shown a beneficial effect of medical treatment in preventing visual field loss in suspected glaucoma,[13-15] but the majority of the studies show an equivocal effect of long-term medical treatment in preventing field loss.[16-21] Prospective studies of this important question are helpful in formulating guidelines for treating such cases. In a study by Epstein and colleagues,[22] patients were prospectively randomized to treatment with timolol or no treatment and were monitored for as long as 7 yr. The investigators found a statistically valid and protective result of medical treatment in this group of glaucoma suspects; 17 nontreated patients failed (based on their study criteria of field loss, IOP greater than 30, or progressive cupping), and only 9 patients failed in the group receiving treatment. Although the study has been criticized for allowing treatment to be considered a failure based solely on pressure criteria (IOP greater than 30), the trend of the findings is quite clear despite any statistical weaknesses. If more liberal inclusion criteria were used, such as considering the patients who discontinued treatment because of side effects or pregnancy as "nontreated patients," 11 of 13 patients having visual field loss progression were not taking timolol, and only 2 of 13 were being treated. These findings were further substantiated in a study by Kass and colleagues[23] in which 62 pairs of eyes were randomized so that one eye was treated with timolol and one eye was treated with placebo. Eighteen placebo-treated eyes became worse versus eight in the treatment group, which is not only statistically significant but very surprising because the contralateral β-blocker effect blunted the treatment effect difference between eyes. On an average, there was a 2.3 mmHg difference between eyes, which, although small in magnitude, in this well-controlled prospective study appeared to prevent or at least delay damage in most of the eyes studied.

Two qualifications about these studies should be considered before applying the results to the treatment of patients in a clinical practice. First, a Canadian study with a design similar to the Epstein investigation found a nearly equal number of failures in the treatment and non-treatment groups.[24] Although this study was the only one to use automated perimetry throughout the research, different perimeters were used in the baseline and follow-up examinations. Additionally, the baseline pressures in this group differed from those in the Epstein study, with untreated patients in the Canadian study showing baseline pressure of 26.1 mmHg versus 23.9 mmHg in the Epstein study. Therefore, because both groups were treated with the same drug and had similar percentage reductions in pressure, the absolute level of pressure was lower by almost 2 mmHg in the Boston group. Coincidentally, baseline pressures in these two different populations are very similar to the hypothetical stratification reported by Kass and coworkers using survival curve analysis and revealing different predicted times to failure (Fig. 138–1). The 2 mmHg difference in baseline pressure was also nearly comparable with the difference between eyes in the Kass study, providing one possible explanation for lack of a treatment effect in the patients with the higher IOP. Second, one must always consider the fact that in epidemiologic terms, all of these studies are relatively small surveys, and because of the complexities and differences in designs, it is possible that when dealing with a treatment effect that may be manifested by only a 2 mmHg difference in pressure, one or all of the studies may have shown a particular result merely by chance.

It is important to remember that in these studies, many patients had very high IOP, large cups, asymmetric cupping, and a positive family history (as high as 44 percent). Therefore, if we can insert some pragmatic perspective, it would seem that in patients at risk of

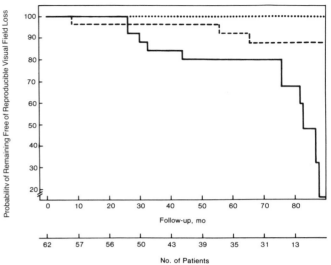

Figure 138–1. Probability of remaining free of reproducible visual field loss. The development of reproducible glaucomatous visual field lost over time at different levels of intraocular pressure irrespective of treatment. Dotted line indicates intraocular pressure to be 16 to 20.4 mmHg during the study; broken line, intraocular pressure 20.5 to 23.4 mmHg; and solid line, intraocular pressure 23.5 to 36.4 mmHg. Intraocular pressure groups were determined by dividing the eyes into three equal groups. Kaplan-Meier method. (From Kass MA, Gordon MO, Hoff MR, et al: Topical timolol administration reduces the incidence of glaucomatous damage in ocular hypertensive individuals: A randomized double-masked long-term clinical trial. Arch Ophthalmol 107:1592, 1989. Copyright 1989, American Medical Association.)

having visual field loss due to the presence of significant non–pressure-related risk factors, lowering the IOP from levels in the high 20s using tolerable medication is appropriate.

Prevention of visual field loss, although justified, may be considered by some to be trivial in terms of the net effect on functional visual acuity or daily living patterns. However, histopathologic data reveal that axonal loss as great as 35 percent may precede the appearance of kinetic visual field defects[25] and a 20 percent loss of large retinal ganglion cells may be present with static visual field loss of 5 decibels (dB).[26] This reminds us that visual field testing is a poor barometer for detecting early ocular damage and underscores the need for improved psychophysical tests for both diagnosis and follow-up.

Interventional Treatment Before Medical Treatment

Surgical therapy with trabeculectomy has been shown to be effective in many studies,[27–31] but its risk:benefit ratio has traditionally been believed to be inferior to that of medicine and probably laser trabeculoplasty. Although the appropriate sequence for laser procedures and surgery after the failure of medical therapy is currently under investigation by the National Institutes of Health in a multicenter protocol entitled the Advanced Glaucoma Intervention Study, the question of whether surgery should be performed before medical treatment has already been addressed in previous clinical trials. Two prospective studies[32, 33] and one retrospective study[34] have shown that lowering IOP with trabeculectomy gives superior results to medical therapy in terms of both magnitude of reduction and prevention of progressive visual field loss. However, both long-term follow-up[34] and even relatively short follow-up[33] have shown that the progression of lens opacities is much more common in the surgery group than in the medical group. This observation implies that this form of surgical treatment not only needs further study but also may only be applicable to a certain target group of patients willing to accept the expectation of mild decreases in visual acuity following trabeculectomy. Until more prospective studies and longer follow-up are available, it seems that the risk:benefit ratio for medical therapy will remain more favorable. In the past, analysis of this ratio has not been mitigated by the effect of so-called "quality of life" as a potential benefit from reducing or avoiding medications, but it is hoped that future studies will address this issue.

One of the studies cited earlier[33] showed very little difference in efficacy between argon laser trabeculoplasty and medical treatment. Preliminary results of a National Institutes of Health–sponsored trial, the Glaucoma Laser Trial, suggest possible differences between medical and laser treatment.[35] Using this protocol, in which eyes in eligible patients were randomized to either stepped medical management or full 360-degree argon laser trabeculoplasty, trabeculotomy was successfully avoided in 89 percent of the eyes treated with laser plus adjunctive stepped medications. This compares with successful avoidance of 66 percent of the eyes initially treated with medicines in stepped fashion surgery as well as the next step (which would be laser). Unfortunately, the laser-treated eyes had more therapeutic alternatives available (argon laser trabeculoplasty plus multiple medications) than did the medication-treated eyes, which had only the same number of medical steps, so this type of analysis seems to be problematic. If treatment with a single medication only (epinephrine product, miotic, or β-blocker) is considered, 51 percent of the eyes treated with medications did not require additional steps, whereas laser was successful in preventing the need for adjunctive therapy in only 44 percent of the patients. The main problem with the entire study is that patients have been monitored for only 2 yr, which, based on well-documented data showing that progression may take several decades, represents a very small segment of total therapeusis during a patient's lifetime. More worrisome is the fact that visual field changes were twice as frequent in the eyes receiving laser first than in the medically treated eyes, but because only 18 eyes exhibited field loss in this short follow-up period, the different prevalence did not reach statistical significance. Many ophthalmologists have disagreed on whether to use argon laser trabeculoplasty as an initial treatment, but it would seem important to inform patients about the permanent morphologic as well as biochemical changes that are probably occurring in eyes

after laser therapy as well as the fact that the data from the Glaucoma Laser Trial were gathered during a relatively brief follow-up. There is no question that IOP can be effectively lowered by early laser treatment, as shown in several other studies,[36–38] but the potential improvement in the quality of life due to avoidance of medications for a year or two must be weighed against the potential for unrecognized and possibly deleterious long-term effects from the laser treatment.

REASONS FOR FAILURE OF MEDICAL TREATMENT

Patients who undergo medical treatment for glaucoma either in investigational settings[22–24] or in clinical practice may still have progression of their disease. It seems logical that (1) the IOP reduction is intermittent owing to poor compliance, (2) the effect of the diminished IOP is jeopardized by untoward effects of the drugs, or (3) the magnitude of IOP reduction is not adequate. Most commonly, the third explanation (inadequate IOP reduction) is sought, but previously unrecognized problems with compliance are becoming more widely appreciated.

Compliance Issues

Research into compliance using electronic eye drop medication monitors has shown that defaulting rates in patients were much higher than physicians would have predicted. Pilocarpine had the most dismal compliance; one third of the patients took fewer than 75 percent of the prescribed doses, and 25 percent totally skipped 1 day/mo.[39] Although compliance is improved with timolol drops, it is still discouraging; 27 percent of patients administered fewer than 75 percent of the prescribed applications.[40] Even experienced examiners are seldom able to correctly identify patients who by design or deep denial cannot admit to their defaulting.[41] The use of medical therapy remains very dependent on good compliance by patients as well as the continual development of medications with fewer side effects and more tolerable dosing regimens. The IOP-lowering efficacy of once-daily levobunolol and timolol administration may be a significant advantage in promoting better compliance, but as previous data have suggested, improving poor compliance will remain a greater challenge than detection.

Accelerated Visual Field Loss Caused by Medical Treatment

As alluded to earlier, an unproven but still theoretically possible explanation for the failure of medical treatment to forestall visual field changes in patients with glaucoma is an untoward effect of the drug. Most eye drops used for the treatment of glaucoma are truly systemic drugs and can be detected in the serum. Although drugs approved subsequent to pilocarpine have been convincingly shown to be effective in lowering IOP, none of these have been judged by the Food and Drug Administration to be effective in preventing visual field loss. Although two of the prospective trials cited earlier[22, 23] are a step toward that goal, it would appear premature to dismiss the possibility that some of the agents could produce a systemic or locally deleterious effect on the neurovascular elements of the eye and that this effect is not adequately compensated for by the reduction in IOP.

For example, several laboratory investigations have found ophthalmic timolol to have no significant effect on retinal circulation.[42–43] However, clinical studies using automated perimetry have suggested that timolol has an adverse effect on the visual field,[44–46] in contrast to short term treatment with another β-blocker, betaxolol.[45, 46]

The final and most commonly invoked reason for the failure of medical therapy is inadequate reduction of IOP. In order to overcome this potential pitfall, it is helpful to establish a treatment strategy, with pressure-related goals and techniques to pursue and evaluate their success safely.

STRATEGY FOR MEDICAL TREATMENT

Target Range of IOP

A useful concept in treatment is the formulation of a target range of IOP as a goal of therapy whether a patient is a glaucoma suspect or has established glaucoma. As other risk factors for glaucoma in addition to IOP are increasingly recognized, IOP reduction in eyes that have not obviously sustained damage will probably receive less emphasis.[5] This trend will need to be complemented by more aggressive attempts to reduce IOP in eyes with established neuronal damage, because we are consistently finding that eyes with severe damage require very low IOP to maintain visual stability.

A target range for IOP in eyes with no detectable damage may be no reduction whatsoever. In other words, the eye is tolerating the current "high" pressure and no treatment is indicated unless the IOP escalates, at which time a trial medication period might be appropriate. It is also possible that these eyes at high risk may benefit if IOP is lowered as depicted in "survival curves" from the Kass study discussed earlier (see Fig. 138–1).

With severe damage, the target IOP range may be a statistically normal IOP or perhaps subnormal IOP (e.g., 13 to 15 mmHg). Published studies appear to verify that once a high percentage of axons are damaged, progression can occur more rapidly unless the IOP is brought down to these subnormal levels.[47] Therefore, even if therapy beyond the use of medications is required, ophthalmologists must remain forthright in both recognizing and achieving an appropriate target IOP.

With mild damage, a 15 to 20 percent reduction may produce a more physiologically normal pressure that

will prevent further optic nerve damage even if the IOP is not lowered into a statistically normal range. For example, an eye that has suffered optic nerve damage with a consistent pressure in the high 20s may adequately stabilize with a reduction to 24 mmHg, although this might at first not appear to be an acceptable therapeutic goal. For long-term goals, it is interesting to note that the retrospective study by Grant and Burke[47] showed almost a linear pressure-related treatment response in patients with normal kinetic fields and abnormal cups, with 20-yr success (nonlosers, equated with lack of blindness) highly correlating with IOP below 21 (Fig. 138–2). It is also important to realize that to achieve the target IOP range, the quality of life and risk:benefit ratio should be considered as well.

With moderate damage exhibiting consistently reproducible field defects in both hemifields, a larger percentage of IOP reduction in the range of 20 percent or more is usually required, with an absolute reduction to the high teens or low 20s. More than a single therapeutic agent certainly may be needed, but all of us are unfortunately aware of patients exhibiting progressive damage when we thought the pressure was reasonably controlled in a range of 22 to 23 mmHg. In a study reviewing stability of visual fields after trabeculectomy, one investigator stated that "despite seemingly adequate control of pressure at an average of 22 mmHg, progression of field loss occurred in nearly one third of the patients."[48] The amount of damage is probably not just related to the absolute pressure level but also to the duration of that pressure. This is a standard physical concept, and the therapeutic correlate is that mild damage that ap-

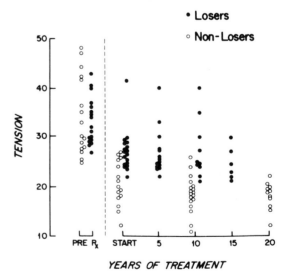

Figure 138–2. Mildly damaged eyes (stage 1) with open angles, tensions of 24 mmHg or more before treatment, and discs with abnormal cupping suggestive of glaucoma but with normal visual fields are presented as two groups that are matched approximately for pretreatment tensions but that differ fundamentally in that subsequently under treatment one group had losses of visual field but the other group did not. Under treatment, the eyes without visual field losses in the course of 10 to 20 yr generally had greater reduction of tension than did the losers. (From Grant WM, Burke JF Jr: Why do some people go blind from glaucoma? Ophthalmology 89:991, 1982.)

pears to occur quickly may denote a more susceptible optic nerve and the need for greater pressure reduction than moderate damage that has occurred over a very extended period of time.

Other factors that may represent not only risk factors for treatment of suspected glaucoma but also factors that can be reasonably used to adjust the target IOP range are age, low facility of outflow, race, and systemic vascular disease.[6, 22] Additionally, the recognition of seasonal pressure changes is important because target IOP ranges may be more difficult to achieve in the winter, when IOP tends to be slightly higher.

Trial Medication Period

Assuming that a diagnosis of glaucoma has been made or that a diagnosis of glaucoma suspect in association with enough risk factors to justify treatment is made, it is very important to initiate a trial medication period or so-called therapeutic trial. Most patients will forever remember how this therapy is introduced, and physicians should approach it in an open-ended manner. It is best to avoid comments such as "you need this medication" or "take this prescription." Most patients find it much easier to accept a suggestion such as "this medication may be a helpful treatment to reduce the pressure in your eye." Approached more as suggestion than a mandate, this trial period allows patients to deal more effectively with their grief over essentially losing the "normal" status of their eyes, feeling all the typical grief stages including anger, denial, depression, and resolution. In addition to suggesting a trial medication period, physicians should openly discuss the goals and duration of the trial as well as potential side effects, both ocular and systemic. The technique of applying the drops can easily be taught by a nurse or ancillary professional, and it is often helpful to use a diagram such as Figure 138–3. A medication card stating the times of application and the cap color is useful. In addition to maintaining effective communication with the patient, it is also wise to inform the patient's primary physician about the intended treatment, as both a courtesy and a safeguard to avoid inappropriate choices due to systemic disease or other therapy.

The trial medication period is usually best initiated with unilateral application of the medication as long as the baseline pressures are reasonably symmetric. Thus a follow-up pressure check in the treated eye may be evaluated in relation to the nontreated or control eye even if there is some contralateral pressure reduction such as would be expected with β-blocker treatment.

When assessing results of the trial medication period, a physician should also continue inquiry and offer encouragement (Table 138–1). IOP needs to be assessed in relation to the control eye as well as drug tolerance and lack of side effects. Pertinent questions should be asked, such as whether a patient is having any problem with breathing, ankle swelling, impotence, arrhythmia, or extreme lethargy after application of a β-blocker. It is also of continued importance to inquire about the

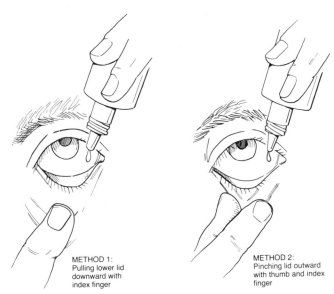

Figure 138–3. Two techniques of instilling eyedrops. (Modified from AAO patient education brochure.)

affordability of the medication and to make an overall prediction of a patient's likelihood of compliance and acceptance of this medication. Only if a physician is able to accurately assess these interpersonal and socioeconomic factors in addition to the drug's efficacy in reducing IOP will a patient likely have a long-term chance of success with medical treatment.

Evaluation of Established Treatment

Once a therapy is found to be effective, follow-up visits are best performed at different times of day so that a relative appreciation of diurnal changes can be documented. Continued surveillance of both the side effects of the ophthalmic medication and the changes in a patient's systemic medications is necessary. If IOP appears to increase, withholding the drug for several weeks should be considered to make certain that the change in IOP does not reflect loss of efficacy. If this is done, pilocarpine and acetazolamide need only be dis-

Table 138–1. ASSESSING A TRIAL MEDICATION PERIOD

Efficacy
  Intraocular pressure reduction during initial 2–3 wk
  Follow-up with diurnal variability

Safety
  Ocular side effects
  Systemic side effects
  Acquiescence of primary care physician

Compliance
  Technique of applying drops
  Use of medication schedule
  Rate of defaulting
  Affordability

continued for a few days, but β-blockers should probably be discontinued for 3 to 4 wk with an interim IOP check to make sure the IOP is not rising quickly. If the drug hiatus, or so-called drug holiday, shows that the disease or IOP is actually escalating and that the drug is not losing its effectiveness, one important principle of therapy is to switch medications instead of adding medications. The ongoing strategy is to keep the regimen as simple as possible. Although multiple medications are not always avoidable, they certainly add to the complexity and decrease compliance with the regimen. If adjunctive therapy is used, it is also important to instruct patients to wait 3 to 5 min between applying drops in the same eye.

After adjustment of medication, appropriate follow-up visits can be planned, but they are ordinarily scheduled every 3 mo for the first year or two. If a patient shows adequate stability with a plateau of IOP control, then the return visit schedule might be altered based on the amount of damage, the time estimated for the damage to occur, and the target IOP range as discussed earlier (the former and latter should be highly correlated). Once stability is reached, patients with very mild damage might be monitored once every 6 mo. Four visits a year are not unreasonable for patients with a target IOP in the high teens or low 20s and a corresponding amount of mild to moderate damage. For patients with severe damage, follow-up visits six to eight times a year might be justified. In general, visual field testing is recommended approximately every third visit to add an important assessment of visual function to careful observation of the optic nerve head for progressive cupping or disc hemorrhage.

APPROVED DRUGS FOR TREATMENT OF PRIMARY OPEN-ANGLE GLAUCOMA

Beta-Blockers

Since the introduction of timolol in 1978, topical treatment with this drug as well as four other topical β-blockers has steadily increased. First-line treatment in the initial medical management of most cases of glaucoma now consists of one of the five approved agents in this class. Although all five of these drugs are categorized as β-blockers, they have individual differences in pharmacology, efficacy, safety, tolerability, and cost (Fig. 138–4 and Table 138–2). One broad classification separates these drugs into nonselective agents that have both β_1- and β_2-receptor inhibition and relatively selective agents that have predominantly β_1-blocking ability. Although this division might seem arbitrary because it is based on the in vitro pharmacology of the drugs, there do appear to be practical clinical correlates to such a classification.

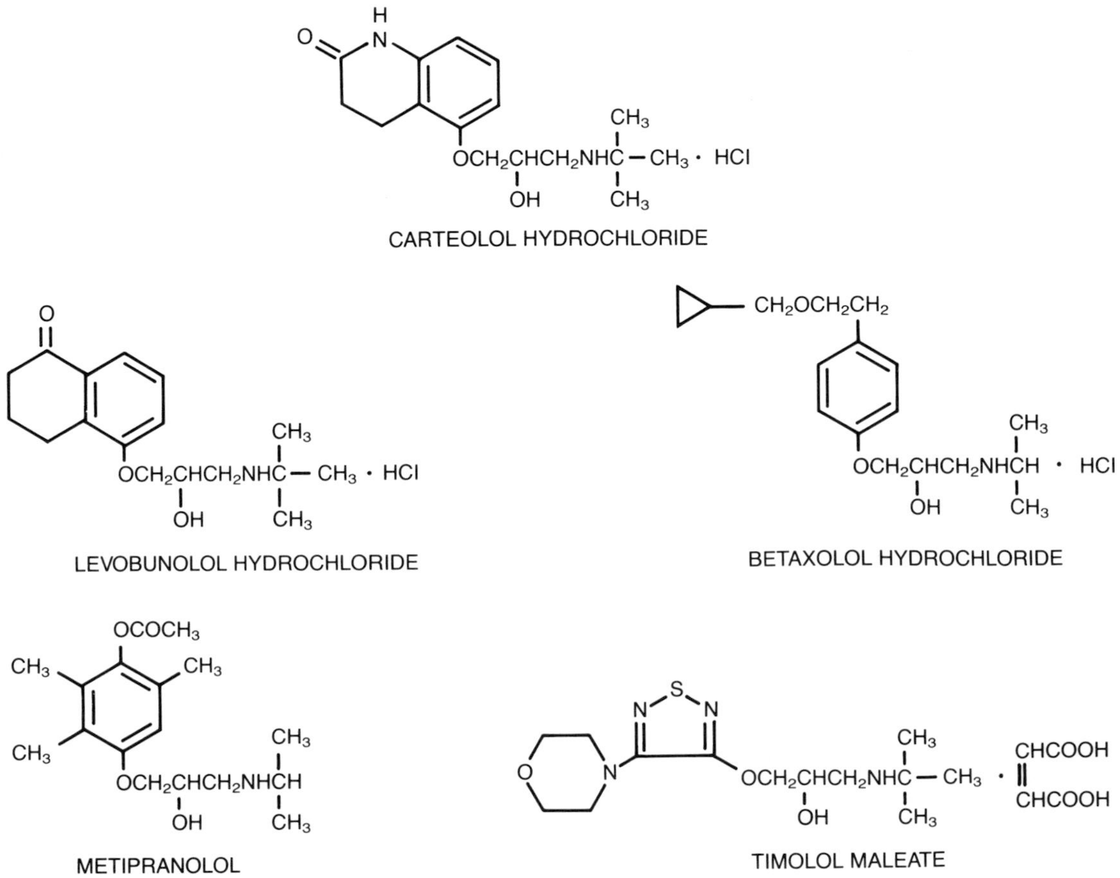

Figure 138–4. Chemical structure of β-blockers.

Table 138–2. PHARMACOLOGIC PROPERTIES OF β-BLOCKERS

	Betaxolol	Levobunolol	Carteolol	Metipranolol	Timolol
Partial agonist activity	–	–	+	–	–
Cardioselectivity	+	–	–	–	–
Membrane stabilization activity	–	–	–	–	+
Relative β-blocking potency (propranolol = 1)	1.0	14.6	10.0	1.8	4.7

Modified from Chrisp P, Sorkin EM: Ocular Carteolol. Drugs and Aging 2:58, 1992.

NONSELECTIVE AGENTS

Timolol

Timolol is an extremely potent β-adrenergic-blocking agent that can cause a rapid decline in IOP within 1 hr after topical application, and many cases can maintain a 30 to 35 percent reduction during the next 24-hr period, with a peak decrement at 3 to 4 hr.[49, 50] The mechanism of action seems to be inhibition of aqueous humor secretion,[51] and several studies have shown the lack of an effect on outflow.[52, 53] Inhibition of aqueous flow has not been found in sleeping volunteers, suggesting a therapeutically important circadian rhythm for aqueous production.[54] The initial reduction in pressure may not be sustained in all patients, and several studies have suggested that during the first year of treatment, many patients lose maximum lowering of IOP.[55] In a controlled crossover study, patients treated with timolol showed a smaller degree of IOP reduction after 3 mo. Epinephrine, on the other hand, seemed to enhance IOP-lowering effect with time.[56] Previous efforts to compare timolol with other topical agents such as epinephrine or pilocarpine have been marred by a greater drop-out rate for patients taking 4 percent pilocarpine or 1 percent epinephrine products than for patients on the β-blocker, but available data support the fact that 0.5 percent timolol is at the very least equally effective as these other classes of drugs.[57, 58]

Rapid acceptance of timolol as well as the other β-blockers has been mainly due to the convenient once- or twice-daily dosing schedule and lack of significant ocular side effects. The duration of action of the drug seems to be at least 24 hr, and it is becoming increasingly apparent that many patients can now be effectively treated with once-daily application of either the 0.5 percent solution or in many cases an even systemically safer regimen of 0.25 percent given every morning.[59, 60]

Local side effects described with timolol include irritation, allergic reaction, decreased vision, punctate keratopathy, and rare reports of uveitis, reversible myopia, pain, and cystoid macula edema. It is also important to keep in mind that because of timolol's systemic absorption, a well-described ocular hypotensive response occurs in the contralateral eye.[61] This effect may influence the results of a trial medication period using timolol in one eye and can also be a factor when timolol is used to treat open-angle glaucoma in one eye after filtration surgery in the contralateral eye. In this case, even a small decrease in the secretion of aqueous humor resulting from this contralateral effect might be deleterious. Also, the corneal anesthetic effect[62] and the ability to inhibit corneal epithelial cell migration[63] may cause ocular complications in certain patients with glaucoma and after keratoplasty.

The main drawbacks of the use of timolol seem to be the cost and associated systemic side effects. Systemic β-blockers such as propranolol are known to cause side effects related to the central nervous system. Because timolol is poorly lipid soluble and is therefore less likely to cross the blood-brain barrier and because topical application produces very low serum levels, toxicity is not expected. Many symptoms have been reported, however, including disorientation, memory impairment, anxiety, depression, fatigue, emotional lability, and hallucinations.[64–66] The target population for the use of this drug is predominantly elderly persons, and it is possible that the problems are underreported because systemic or cerebrovascular disease is cited as causing the symptoms.

Topical administration of timolol consistently reduces the heart rate and shares with systemic β-blockers the ability to worsen congestive heart failure.[66] Reports of syncope, bradyarrhythmias, heart block, fibrillation, and infarction have provoked caution about the use of timolol in patients at risk for these conditions. Other miscellaneous side effects include impotence, rashes, diarrhea, male pattern baldness, and reduction of plasma high-density lipoproteins.[67–69]

The most serious and alarming complication after topical administration of timolol as well as most of the nonselective β-blockers is exacerbation or worsening of pulmonary disease. Bronchospasm, bronchorrhea, apnea in neonates, and acute exacerbation of asthma all have been well documented after the use of timolol, and these complications can be significant and life-threatening problems.[70–76] Pulmonary function test results have worsened after administration of a single drop of topical timolol in patients with asthma, chronic obstructive pulmonary disease, and chronic bronchitis, and the use of this drug in these patients is contraindicated.[77]

If ophthalmologists judiciously exclude patients likely to have systemic medical conditions susceptible to worsening by β-blockade, timolol will continue to be an effective, convenient, and safe medication. In Caucasian patients, 0.5 percent timolol is seldom more effective in lowering IOP than 0.25 percent, and side effects from systemic blood levels can be reduced with this concentration. Punctal occlusion or lid closure has been recommended to help reduce systemic absorption and the incidence of systemic complications.[78, 79]

Levobunolol

Levobunolol is a nonselective topical β-blocker that has been used extensively since its approval by the Food and Drug Administration 7 yr ago. Available in both 0.5 percent and 0.25 percent solutions, it has been extensively tested in well-designed clinical trials, and data on long-term IOP control for up to 48 mo have been widely reported.[80–84]

Single-drop as well as 3-mo placebo-controlled studies have shown statistically significant decreases in IOP using concentrations of 0.3 to 2 percent levobunolol. Although the 0.5 percent concentration seems to be at the top of the dose-response curve for an acute effect, 1.0 and 2.0 percent levobunolol gave a sustained effect that was statistically significant for 12 hr. Levobunolol is metabolized in both rabbits and humans to dihydrolevobunolol, which has a half-life of 7 hr.[85, 86] This compound, which also has β-blocking activity, may prolong the duration of topically applied levobunolol compared with some of the other agents in this class. However, in multiple clinical trials comparing once-daily levobunolol treatment with once-daily timolol treatment, no statistical differences in success rate could be found with either the 0.5 or 0.25 percent concentrations.[59, 87] These important studies have brought attention to the fact that once-daily dosing for both timolol and levobunolol is a potentially important part of our therapeutic armamentarium and may offer a significant advantage in terms of both compliance and cost.

In clinical trials, levobunolol was well tolerated by patients, with no significant difference in the incidence of adverse effects when compared with ophthalmic timolol. Ocular side effects were similar to those previously recorded with timolol but also included blepharoconjunctivitis, transient decreased vision, and iritis. The most common reported symptoms are ocular burning and stinging.

In nearly all studies reported to date, a mean decrease in heart rate of five to ten beats per minute was noted with topical administration of levobunolol. This effect was statistically significant when compared with therapy with placebo.[81, 88] One study investigating the effects with several concentrations of levobunolol in patients with glaucoma documented decreased heart rate in 15 patients taking 0.25 percent levobunolol.[89] None of the changes in heart rate was believed to be clinically significant but do underscore the fact that levobunolol, like timolol, enters the systemic circulation and provides low-grade systemic β-blockade that may be deleterious in certain patients who are at risk because of cardiac or pulmonary problems. Accumulated data show that le-

Table 138–3. SOME CLINICAL TRIALS INVOLVING THE USE OF TWICE-DAILY METIPRANOLOL IN PATIENTS WITH GLAUCOMA OR OCULAR HYPERTENSION

Study	Patient Group	Study Design	Study Duration (Weeks)	Dosage (%) (No. of Patients)	Decrease in IOP (%)	Patients with Satisfactory IOP (%)	Patients Withdrawn Due to Inadequate IOP Control (%)	Withdrawal Due to Side Effects (%)
Uncontrolled studies								
Dausch et al[91]	COAG, OH IOP > 25 mmHg	o†	24	Met 0.3 or 0.6 [41]‡	28.8	80.5	19.5	0
Denffer[92]	OAG, NAG IOP > 22 mmHg	o	24§	Met 0.3 or 0.6 [47]‡	30.0	93.6	0	6.4
Kruse[95]	OAG, NAG IOP > 24 mmHg	o	24–48§	Met 0.3 [23] Met 0.6 [26]	33.0 34.0			0
Müller and Knobel[98]	COAG, OH IOP > 22 mmHg	o	4–16§	Met 0.1‖ [114]	25.0	87.4		
Comparisons with twice-daily Tim								
Bleckmann et al[98a]	COAG IOP > 22 mmHg	db, co†, ¶	6	Met 0.3 [20] Tim 0.25 [18]	22.0 24.0	95.0 95.0		
Ecoffet and Demailly[93]	COAG IOP ≥ 22 mmHg	r, db, p†	17	Met 0.3 or 0.6 [20]‡ Tim 0.25 or 0.5 [20]‡	20.7 17.4	75.0 65.0	25.0 35.0	0 0
Kruse[94]	COAG, NAG IOP > 24 mmHg	db, p†, ¶	4§	Met 0.25 [18] Tim 0.25 [19]	20.9 25.5		0 0	
Mertz[96]	COAG IOP > 22 mmHg	r, db, co**	6§	Met 0.25 [27] Tim 0.25 [27]	23.4 26.3			0 0
Mills and Wright[97]	OAG IOP > 22 mmHg	r, db, co**	8	Met 0.3 [10] Tim 0.25 [10]	14.8 11.5	80.0 80.0		0 0
Schmitz-Valchenberg et al[99]	COAG IOP > 21 mmHg	r, db, co†	8	Met 0.1 [20] Tim 0.25 [20]	24.0 25.0	90.0 90.0		0 0
Comparison with twice-daily Lev								
Krieglstein et al[99a]	COAG, OH IOP > 22 mmHg	r, db, p†	12	Met 0.6 [25] Lev 0.5 [21]	28.5 28.8	96.0 95.2	4 0	0 4.8

Modified from Battershill PE, Sorkin EM: Ocular metipranolol. Drugs 36:601, 1988.
*Treatment was considered satisfactory if an IOP of ≤21 mmHg was achieved.
†IOP measured after 3- to 14-day washout periods.
‡Results not analyzed separately.
§Multicenter studies.
‖Frequency of administration not stated.
¶Patients not stated to be randomized to drug treatment in this study.
**No-washout period before treatment crossover.
IOP, intraocular pressure; COAG, chronic open-angle glaucoma; OH, ocular hypertension; OAG, open-angle glaucoma; NAG, narrow-angle glaucoma; o, open; db, double-blind; co, crossover; r, randomized; p, parallel; Met, metipranolol; Tim, timolol; Lev, levobunolol.

vobunolol is an extremely potent ocular hypertensive agent and is safe in patients without cardiac or pulmonary complications.

Metipranolol

Metipranolol is a nonselective β-blocker introduced in Europe nearly 10 yr ago. It is marketed in concentrations of 0.1, 0.3, and 0.6 percent, and most studies have shown efficacy of all three concentrations when compared with 0.5 percent timolol[90-98] and levobunolol 0.5 percent (Table 138–3).[99] In one comparison with 0.5 percent timolol, the magnitude of pressure reduction seemed slightly less with metipranolol, although no statistical difference was reported.

Ocular complications reported consisted mainly of stinging on instillation in 12 to 56 percent of patients. Close attention was given to the detection of any systemic side effects, and with the exception of slightly decreased pulse, which was less than that seen with other non-selective β-blockers, no other cardiac or pulmonary problems occurred. In one study comparing metipranolol with two other β-blockers, a slightly increased reduction in forced expiratory volume was noted

with metipranolol in preselected pulmonary patients.[100] This drug will probably remain a reasonable treatment choice for some patients, and it is hoped that additional clinical experience will clarify specific advantages of this drug.

Carteolol

Carteolol is a newer agent approved in the United States after extensive use in Europe and Japan. This drug is a potent nonselective β-blocker with partial β-agonist activity, also called intrinsic sympathomimetic activity.[101] The molecule is ten times more active than the prototype agent, propranolol. In addition, it has an active metabolite, 8-hydroxy-carteolol, which has a half-life two to three times that of the parent molecule. This may allow increased bioavailability and duration of action.[102]

The efficacy of carteolol has been shown in placebo-controlled studies[103] and direct comparisons with timolol,[104-108] in which there was no significant difference in efficacy with either concentration of carteolol (Table 138–4). An exception was one study[109] that did show a slight difference between 0.25 percent timolol and car-

Table 138–4. SOME RANDOMIZED STUDIES COMPARING CARTEOLOL WITH PLACEBO OR TIMOLOL IN PATIENTS WITH GLAUCOMA OR OCULAR HYPERTENSION

Study	Patient Group	Treatment [Duration (Weeks)]	Study Design	Mean Baseline IOP (mmHg)	Mean IOP Change (mmHg) [%]	Efficacy
Comparison with placebo						
Duff and Graham[103]	12 GR	C 2% b.i.d. Pl b.i.d. [2]	db, r, co, wo	21	↓ 2.2–2.8 [11–14][a]	C>Pl
Comparisons with timolol						
Horie et al[104]	10 OH, OAG / 10 OH, OAG	C 2% b.i.d. T 0.5% b.i.d.	db, r, co	23.25 / 23.7	↓ 3.1–3.5 [13.3–14.8]*** / ↓ 3.2 [13.7]**	C=T
Maclure et al[105]	18 OAG / 17 OAG	C 2% T 0.5% [52]	sb, r, p	30 / 30	↓ 10 [33][c] / ↓ 10 [33][c]	C=T
Mills et al[106]	19 OAG / 17 OAG	C 1% T 0.25% [26]	sb, r, p, wo	25.1 / 24.2	↓ 4.6 [18]*** / ↓ 4.3 [17.7]***	C=T
Scoville et al[109]	50 OH[b] / 47 OH[b]	C 1% b.i.d. T 0.25% b.i.d. [4]	db, r, p, wo	22.75[c] / 23.75[c]	↓ 2.8 [12][c] / ↓ 4 [17][c]	C=T
Stewart et al[107]	33 OH, OAG / 39 OH, OAG / 33 OH, OAG	C 1% b.i.d. C 2% b.i.d. T 0.5% b.i.d. [12]	db, r, p, wo	25.3 / 25.3 / 24.8	↓ 6.3 [24]*** / ↓ 5.8 [23]*** / ↓ 6.5]28]***	C=T
Tsuchisaka et al[108]	20 OH, OAG / 23 OH, OAG / 19 OH, OAG	C 1% b.i.d. C 2% b.i.d. T 0.5% b.i.d. [26]	r, p, wo	20.7 / 21 / 21	↓ 1.4 [7]**c, d / ↓ 2.5 [12]**c, d / ↓ 2 [9.5]*c, d	C=T

Modified from Chrisp P, Sorkin EM: Ocular carteolol. Drugs and Aging 2:58, 1992.
a, Reduction compared with placebo.
b, All patients previously treated with timolol.
c, Results presented graphically; extrapolations only.
d, Compared with IOP after 4 wk of treatment with timolol 0.5% b.i.d.
GR, glaucoma risk (raised IOP, family history, or optic disc cupping); OH, ocular hypertension; OAG, open-angle glaucoma; b.i.d., twice daily; db, double-blind; r, randomized; co, crossover; p, parallel group; wo, washout period before treatment; sb, single-blind; ↓, decrease; ↑, increase; > indicates significantly greater efficacy (P ≤ .01); = indicates equivalent efficacy; * indicates P <.05 versus baseline; ** indicates P <.01 versus baseline; *** indicates P < .001 versus baseline.

teolol 1 percent, but this did not appear to be statistically significant, and the researchers concluded that the efficacy was comparable. A three-way comparison study evaluated the effect of carteolol, metipranolol, and timolol on pulmonary function, and slightly decreased forced expiratory volume was noted with the metipranolol and timolol when compared with carteolol.[100] Although one would theoretically expect some slight margin of safety with carteolol because of its β-agonist activity, the data documented slightly reduced forced expiratory volume with carteolol and underscores the need for caution when using any β-blocker in patients with current or past pulmonary pathology.

Another interesting theoretical effect of the partial agonist activity is potential improvement in retinal blood flow. Although early clinical studies[110] implied that enhanced retinal perfusion from carteolol may have produced improvements in visual fields, conflicting results using various laboratory techniques[111, 112] have made a blood flow effect difficult to confirm.

Overall, carteolol appears to be a very useful and safe agent. Further use may help establish whether its long duration of action and unique pharmacologic qualities make it a suitable choice for certain patient groups or for once-daily dosing.

SELECTIVE BETA-BLOCKERS

In some patients, the use of selective β-blockers has theoretical as well as clinical advantages. These agents have more affinity for the cardiac (β_1) than the pulmonary (β_2) receptors. It has been proposed that cardioselective or relatively selective β_1-blockers have found a niche in the treatment of systemic hypertension[113] and likewise are used with increasing frequency as topical agents in the treatment of glaucoma. It is now well documented that some systemic β_1-blockers, although only relatively selective, have less bronchospastic potential in patients with bronchitis, asthma, and chronic obstructive pulmonary diseases. They may also have the ability to leave ocular and systemic β_2-receptors unblocked and more responsive to endogenous and exogenous epinephrine.

Several selective β_1-blockers, including metoprolol,[114] practolol,[115] and atenolol,[116] have been found to lower IOP after topical administration; however, they have been unacceptable for chronic clinical use because of either rapid tolerance or, in the case of practolol, serious potential morbidity. Betaxolol, another relatively selective β_1-blocker, has been extensively tested and found to have potent long-term efficacy in placebo-controlled studies[117–119] as well as in masked comparisons with timolol[120–122] and levobunolol.[123] As with the other β-blockers, fluorophotometric studies have shown the mechanism of action of betaxolol to be reduction in the secretion of aqueous humor.[124]

In comparison studies with timolol, average IOP reductions with betaxolol were similar and did not display any statistically significant difference.[120, 121] However, using a quartile analysis necessitated by the number of patients requiring adjunctive therapy, one study found a high statistical significance in the 1 to 2 mmHg of difference in the pressure-lowering effects of the two drugs, with betaxolol exhibiting slightly less magnitude of effect.[122] Another study reported a significant number of patients with elevated IOP after a switch from betaxolol to timolol.[125]

Compared with levobunolol, betaxolol produced slightly (2 to 3 mmHg) less reduction in IOP.[123] This study design used morning IOP comparisons (before application of the morning dose of medication) that may have favored the levobunolol because of its apparent longer duration of action after the previous evening dose.

In addition to the many long-term studies using 0.5 percent betaxolol, a newer formulation using 0.25 percent racemic drug in a suspension (Betoptic S) has been investigated and found to be comparable in safety and efficacy to the parent molecule.[126]

Several additional studies have shown that acetazolamide,[127] pilocarpine,[120] and epinephrine[128, 129] have a useful additive effect. The additive effect when epinephrine was administered at the same time as betaxolol was somewhat surprising, because epinephrine and dipivefrin provided only a small additional effect when added to timolol in several studies investigating this combination during different time courses ranging from 3 hr to 3 mo.[130–132]

The effect of adding epinephrine to betaxolol was quite significant and accompanied by an increased facility of outflow.[128] Betaxolol has been shown in vitro to produce approximately ten times greater β_1-blockade than β_2.[133] The increased facility, also found in primates,[134] is most likely due to epinephrine's stimulation of β_2-receptors (not significantly blocked by betaxolol), which have been shown by several laboratory techniques to be present in human trabecular meshwork.[135, 136]

Stinging on instillation was the main side effect noticed with chronic use of betaxolol, and other ocular side effects were comparable to or less than those noted with the nonselective agents.

The main feature that distinguishes betaxolol and betaxolol suspension from most topical β-blockers in the nonselective category is their apparent lack of systemic side effects, a finding that has now been documented in 7 yr of approved use. Studies of nonglaucomatous[137, 138] as well as glaucomatous patients[139–141] with chronic obstructive pulmonary disease, asthma, and chronic bronchitis have shown no changes in pulmonary function with betaxolol. These same studies as well as previous reports have consistently shown timolol and other nonselective topical β-blockers to cause a decrease in pulmonary function that was most sensitively detected by measurements of the forced expiratory volume at 1 min. As with systemic treatment, even a relatively selective β_1-blocker has a potential for adverse effects in patients with severe pulmonary disease, because the β-blockers are not totally devoid of some β_2-blocking activity, and a few reports describe nonfatal pulmonary complications with betaxolol.[142, 143] However, because of the extremely worrisome incidence of pulmonary complications noted with ophthalmic timolol and anticipated with other nonselective topical β-blockers, an agent that may be less prone to affect pulmonary function would be advantageous in the many cases of geriatric-skewed glaucoma.

Although a β₁-blocker would be suspected to have some cardiac effect, further evidence that ophthalmic betaxolol is unable to offer systemic blockade comes from controlled studies showing no significant changes in pulse.[122] Timolol and other nonselective agents have been shown to decrease the pulse rate and inhibit exercise tachycardia.[144] One percent betaxolol had no effect on exercise tachycardia when administered in masked comparison.[145] Many explanations have been proposed to explain this lack of systemic effect by ophthalmic betaxolol. The drug may not be well absorbed into the circulation, may be highly protein bound, may be quickly or effectively metabolized, or may be kinetically limited by lower receptor affinity in nonocular tissue. It should be emphasized that betaxolol is used as a racemic mixture and that only the L-isomer is active. Thus, if 2 ng of both 0.5 percent ophthalmic betaxolol solution and 0.5 percent ophthalmic timolol solution entered the serum, all of the timolol would be active as the L-isomer, but the effective dose of betaxolol would only be 1 ng. The newer formulation, Betoptic S, presents an even safer alternative because the concentration of the active L-isomer is only 0.125 percent solution.

A final feature attributed to betaxolol is the absence of an effect on ocular blood flow,[146] which may be different than the effect of other β-blockers used for treating glaucoma. Based on current evidence, betaxolol seems to be an effective agent for the treatment of glaucoma and has extremely low potential for ocular and systemic side effects.

Epinephrine Products

In the late 1950s, the introduction of the epinephrine hydrochloride with an acceptable shelf-life was a welcome addition for the medical management of glaucoma. Before that time, only miotics and oral agents were available. Epinephrine is a naturally occurring sympathomimetic agonist with activity at both α- and β-receptors. Dipivefrin is a pro-drug formed from the esterification of epinephrine with two pivalic acid side chains that greatly enhance its solubility and allow it to penetrate the cornea 17 times more effectively than the parent compound. Intracameral esterases cleave the pivalic acid chains so that epinephrine is released in the aqueous. Therapeutic concentrations of intracameral epinephrine can thus be achieved with application of only one tenth of the pro-drug concentration.[147]

The efficacy of 0.1 percent dipivefrin is between that of 1 percent and 2 percent epinephrine hydrochloride, as shown in comparative trials.[148–150] The theoretical problems with the use of concomitant echothiophate and dipivefrin have not been apparent in human trials. The mechanism of action of epinephrine has been debated for many years. With recent advances in fluorophotometric techniques, earlier reports of improved outflow facility after the topical administration of epinephrine have been confirmed. This increase in outflow facility does seem to increase with chronic use and is slightly offset by what is now believed to be a net increase in secretion of aqueous.[151] Although not germane to primary open-angle glaucoma, this finding is of some practical significance in the treatment of patients with extremely poor or absent outflow, as may occur in neovascular glaucoma or secondary angle-closure glaucoma. In this setting, epinephrine can theoretically increase IOP by stimulating secretion without a compensatory improvement in outflow.

As previously mentioned, the effect of epinephrine is not always immediate, and many patients show a maximum response only after several months.[151–153] Both the epinephrine parent compound and dipivefrin can cause a 22 to 28 percent decrease in IOP. A marked difference, however, is noted in the incidence of side effects with dipivefrin and epinephrine.[147] Compared with patients on dipivefrin, the percentage of patients on epinephrine who reported local allergy, local irritation, pigmentation, madarosis, and loss of vision due to cystoid macular edema in aphakia is much higher. The commercially available preparation of dipivefrin contains sodium metabisulfite, an antioxidant preservative that may cause some hypersensitivity in asthmatic persons. This is unfortunate, because this class of drugs may be the most appropriate for initial therapy in patients who have glaucoma and reactive airway disease; although β-blockers should ideally be avoided, the potential systemic side effects of epinephrine such as bronchodilation would be desirable. Dipivefrin also causes a distinctive follicular conjunctivitis that resembles the large follicles (giant papillary conjunctivitis [GPC]) seen in some contact lens wearers.[154, 155] Systemic side effects that may result from systemic absorption of either epinephrine or dipivefrin include pallor, perspiration, syncope, and elevation of pulse and blood pressure. In one study, systemic levels of epinephrine after topical treatment with dipivefrin were found to be lower than those after administration of topical epinephrine,[156] suggesting an improved risk:benefit ratio with this derivative.

Miotics

SHORT-ACTING: PILOCARPINE DROPS

The initial use of physostigmine for glaucoma by Laqueur in 1876 represented the start of IOP-lowering therapy, and the introduction of topical pilocarpine 1 yr later provided a benchmark for safe and effective treatment during the next 100 yr. As a parasympathomimetic, pilocarpine mimics acetylcholine by its direct stimulation of the iris sphincter and ciliary muscle, both of which are cholinergically innervated. Because both have anatomic connections with the scleral spur, their stimulation and concomitant contraction would logically reduce resistance to aqueous humor outflow, as shown in primates.[157, 158]

Pilocarpine penetrates ocular tissues well. Although miosis occurs in 15 to 30 min, maximal reduction of IOP occurs in 2 to 4 hr, with a total duration of 4 to 8 hr.

We conventionally begin treatment with a low-dose solution such as 0.5 or 1 percent pilocarpine and titrate upward to achieve the maximal response. Better short-term response is noted in only a very few patients if the solution exceeds 4 percent pilocarpine. If a 6 or 8 percent solution is used, however, the duration of action may be longer, but with a corresponding higher incidence of side effects. Pilocarpine drops are prescribed every 4 to 8 hr, and most cases are well controlled on a four-times-daily schedule.

The ideal patients treated with pilocarpine are those who are older than 40 yr and who do not have significant cataracts, because decreased vision is usually worsened by miosis. In addition to miosis and spasm accommodation with associated myopia, other problems include headache, brow ache, conjunctival hyperemia, lacrimation, local allergy, twitching of the eyelids, and occasional increase in inflammation, posterior synechiae, retinal detachment, and exacerbation of pupillary block in predisposed eyes. Myopia is particularly distressful in young patients, and attempts to change optical correction are usually thwarted by the cyclic changes in accommodative magnitude.

One should not overlook the potential problem of systemic side effects resulting from administration of short-acting miotics, especially in visually handicapped patients, who can occasionally overdose themselves. Observed effects include salivation, diaphoresis, nausea, vomiting, abdominal cramping, incontinence, diarrhea, hypotension, hypertension, bradycardia, bronchospasm, and muscle weakness. Although the IOP-lowering effect of a miotic is often favorably added to the effects of a topical β-blocker, the additive systemic effect on the cardiopulmonary system can be potentially dangerous.

Four-times-daily uniocular administration of 0.5 percent pilocarpine in patients with light irides or 1 percent pilocarpine in patients with dark irides is reasonable initiation to trial medication. Punctal occlusion helps avoid systemic problems,[159] and dilation of the eye twice a year may help prevent formation of synechiae and loss of dilator muscle tone.

Carbachol, another short-acting miotic with a slightly longer duration of action, may additionally enhance cholinergic stimulation by indirectly inhibiting cholinesterase. Carbachol may be used to replace pilocarpine and very often has an enhanced effect when used in dosages of 0.75 to 3 percent solution given three times daily. As expected, symptoms of headache, hyperemia, and accommodative spasm may escalate in proportion to the degree of improvement in controlling IOP.

ALTERNATIVE DELIVERY SYSTEMS

Ocuserts

The difficulties that can occur with four to six daily applications of any topical drug in both eyes are obvious and have led to many cases of poor compliance. Although pilocarpine has been used in different vehicles as well as with soft contact lenses, the Ocusert delivery system was the first successful attempt at sustained, nonpulsed delivery of medication for the treatment of glaucoma. The Ocusert system is composed of a small wafer with two outer polymeric membrane layers surrounding a central reservoir of pilocarpine. The rate of drug delivery is controlled by the outer membranes and seems to produce stable miosis and lower IOP. Typical side effects of pilocarpine may occur with Ocuserts but are usually much less in magnitude because no large bolus of drug is administered. Any "burst" effect that may occur is caused not only by mechanical manipulation of the delivery system in the cul-de-sac but also by the application of other drugs, which, probably because of their preservatives such as benzalkonium chloride, can enhance penetration of the slowly released pilocarpine. Other side effects mirror those occurring with pilocarpine drops, with the addition of a "migrating" Ocusert or an occasional lost Ocusert.

Ocuserts are available in two strengths: 20 µg/hr and 40 µg/hr. Most patients do best when they are inserted in the evening, so that initial symptoms due to bolus release of the drug are minimized. The drug effect generally persists for 1 wk, but many Ocuserts have a shorter duration of action. Ocuserts should definitely be checked periodically after the fifth or sixth day of treatment to ensure that drug release and IOP control are adequate.

Pilocarpine Gel

Studies of compliance using dropper bottles with built-in recording devices have confirmed what ophthalmologists have suspected for a long time—patients very seldom comply with four doses of pilocarpine per day. In fact, one fourth of the doses of pilocarpine prescribed were missed in a study of a general glaucoma population.[39] A relatively new preparation that may help combat poor compliance is pilocarpine gel, a high-viscosity acrylamide gel with pilocarpine suspended in it. Its ability to reduce IOP is comparable to that noted with the administration of 4 percent pilocarpine drops four times daily. One recommended dose is one-half inch of gel, which contains a total of 2 mg of pilocarpine (only 25 percent of the amount of the drug contained in four drops of 4 percent pilocarpine in a traditional regimen) and is given before bedtime in the lower cul-de-sac. This quantity of gel may be poorly tolerated, and it may be clinically useful to start with one-eighth inch of gel.

Patients are instructed to administer the gel before bedtime so that some of the side effects are avoided during sleeping hours. Most patients enjoy stable control of IOP until their next nightly dose. The effectiveness of the drug has been documented by all published studies, and the average decline in IOP is comparable to that in patients who were previously treated with pilocarpine drops. This applies to morning IOP measurements as well as to the important afternoon measurement, when the gel's effect may have "escaped" slightly.[160–162]

It is important to recognize that the IOP of some patients will not be controlled for an entire 24-hr period. An analysis was made of individual patients' responses to pilocarpine gel, including during afternoon visits. Thirty-eight percent of patients had morning and afternoon IOP measurements that were more than 2 mmHg higher than baseline diurnal readings while taking pilocarpine drops. In a comparison of diurnal pressure, 33 percent of patients using pilocarpine eye drops had values that were more than 2 mmHg higher in the afternoon than values noted in the morning; moreover, 43 percent of patients using pilocarpine gel had similar increases in the afternoon.[148] This finding is of practical importance because many of the rises noted in the afternoon are not detected at office visits during regular hours. Some patients with severe glaucoma may have an unacceptable response to even a minimal increase in the afternoon. The gel efficacy can be enhanced by administering an extra drop of pilocarpine in patients whose response consistently lessens after 18 to 24 hr; this regimen would still be easier to comply with than prior schedules of drops given four times daily.

The gel seems to cause only minor side effects and symptoms. About 50 percent of patients in a long-term trial noted minor irritation, but only 11 percent of patients asked for treatment to be discontinued because of this irritation. Sixty-nine percent of the patients had mild blurring of vision, principally in the morning; blurring diminished throughout the day, and only 9 percent of those patients with blurring asked that treatment be discontinued because of it. Many patients complained that their eyelids stuck together in the morning, but this did not seem to be a serious problem. Overall, the gel seems to be well tolerated.

Corneal signs were noted in 20 to 40 percent of the patients in the study just mentioned. Signs included the early development of punctate keratitis, which appeared to resolve with the continued use of the gel, and the late occurrence of subtle, diffuse focal subepithelial corneal opacities. The corneal deposits appeared after 4 to 12 mo of use of the gel and were still noted after its discontinuation but were not correlated with any changes in vision.[163] A report describing similar focal subepithelial opacities after the use of pilocarpine drops has drawn attention to this new finding, which in the past may have been missed in patients on miotic therapy.[164]

Patients who have used pilocarpine gel found once-a-day administration quite convenient and strongly preferred it for this reason. Although some adverse symptoms were generated by use of the gel, miosis and decreased vision were experienced less than with the prior use of pilocarpine eye drops. With wider use of the gel, we have now also noticed that many patients need detailed and repeated instruction about proper instillation.

STRONG MIOTICS

With the introduction of Ocuserts and pilocarpine gel, it seems inappropriate to distinguish indirect-acting parasympathomimetics from other treatments by using the term *long-acting miotics*. Because the extended duration of action is no longer unique to the anticholinesterases, we prefer the term *indirect-acting* or *strong* miotic.

Strong miotics are actually divided into two subcategories: the carbamates, which include physostigmine, neostigmine, and demecarium; and the organophosphorus compounds, which are echothiophate iodide and diisopropylphosphorofluoridate (DFP).[165] These two subcategories were formerly distinguished from each other by the irreversibility of their effect, but it is now known that the carbamates are truly irreversible inhibitors, as are the organophosphorus compounds. The older distinction still has practical significance, however, because phosphorylation of the organophosphorus compounds to acetylcholinesterase is more resistant to hydrolysis than carbamoylation, thus giving them a longer duration of action.

Strong miotics are used principally because their magnitude of IOP reduction exceeds that of pilocarpine. The other advantage is the extended duration of action of all these compounds, which can be as long as 7 to 21 days with echothiophate. Although this long duration of action has been well known since strong miotics were introduced for the treatment of glaucoma in 1946, a twice-daily regimen has ordinarily been recommended. We have found that once-daily application yields IOP reductions that are indistinguishable from those obtained with twice-daily application and believe that the reduction in the frequency and amount of drug applied will reduce toxicity such as cataract formation, which is noted in chronic treatment with twice-daily echothiophate.

Other side effects of the strong miotics are essentially identical to those of shorter-acting cholinergic agents but are often more intense. Retinal detachments are rare with any of the cholinergic agents, but in theory the likelihood of detachment is higher after the use of a strong miotic.[166]

This group of topical antiglaucoma drugs also provides a valuable lesson in the appreciation of potential ocular toxicity resulting from the administration of any new drug. In 1968, Axelsson and Holmberg[167] conducted a classic study linking anterior subcapsular cataracts to therapy with echothiophate. The study took place 22 yr after the original introduction of this class of drugs and 12 yr after the introduction of echothiophate. The mechanism causing the cataracts remains unknown, but cataracts seem to be the main reason why many ophthalmologists have abandoned the use of this drug in phakic patients. The length of time it took to detect this dramatic side effect encourages clinicians to be more observant when prescribing any new agents that are being introduced. The possibility of cataracts is likely related to dose, and if these drugs are used in phakic patients, it would seem reasonable not only to use a once-daily regimen but also to use the lowest possible dose, such as 0.06 percent, if an acceptable therapeutic response is obtained.

When used in low doses with once-daily application, echothiophate and other strong miotics may still be useful and safer than filtration surgery. In patients with aphakic open-angle glaucoma, strong miotics provide an effective and convenient means of therapy at any time when pilocarpine seems to give inadequate control.

The use of strong miotics in phakic patients may best be reserved for cases in which IOP has not responded to maximum alternative medical and laser therapy. Most ophthalmologists agree that except in eyes jeopardized

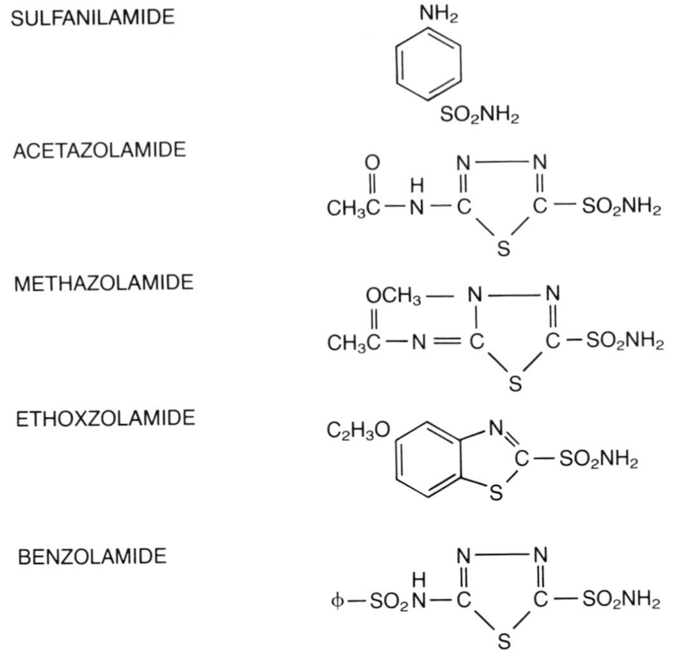

SULFANILAMIDE

ACETAZOLAMIDE

METHAZOLAMIDE

ETHOXZOLAMIDE

BENZOLAMIDE

Figure 138–5. Chemical structure of carbonic anhydrase inhibitors.

by a pressure spike after treatment with laser in the setting of advanced disease, laser trabeculoplasty is probably safer and better tolerated by phakic patients than is strong miotic therapy. It is important to remember that strong miotics should be discontinued for several weeks before intraocular surgery to prevent the possibility of severe fibrinous postoperative iritis and to minimize the inhibition of systemic pseudocholinesterases that reverse anesthetic drugs such as succinylcholine.

Carbonic Anhydrase Inhibitors

Introduced for the treatment of glaucoma in 1954,[168] acetazolamide has continued to occupy a unique, albeit tentative, place in our medical armamentarium. Although carbonic anhydrase inhibitors other than acetazolamide are now available (Fig. 138–5 and Table 138–5), this class of agents has limited efficacy in the treatment of open-angle glaucoma because of poor compliance due to systemic side effects. Particularly since the introduction of topical β-blockers, ophthalmologists more commonly realize and recognize that treatment with topical agents causes systemic side effects, but patients often fail to associate side effects with eye drops. In comparison, when patients receive metazolamide or acetazolamide, they not only make an association between their side effects and administration of the drug but may complain bitterly about the effects the drug causes. Also, the use of trabeculoplasty has at least temporarily contributed to the decline in the use of carbonic anhydrase inhibitors, but it is hoped that the use of low doses of methazolamide will continue to gain acceptance.

All carbonic anhydrase inhibitors belong to the sulfonamide family. In therapeutic doses, they are able to reduce the production of aqueous by a maximum of 50 percent, with a corresponding decrease in IOP. Universal agreement has not been reached about the mechanism of pressure reduction, but current evidence seems to favor a reduction in the accumulation of bicarbonate in the posterior chamber, with a decrease in sodium and associated fluid movement linked to the bicarbonate ion.[169] With maximum doses of these drugs, an additional decrease in IOP is caused by metabolic acidosis. Animal research indicates that the pressure-lowering effect related to shifts in bicarbonate ion is independent of changes related to the acidosis.[170]

Although a 50-mg p.o. dose of the carbonic anhydrase inhibitor methazolamide produces a slightly smaller reduction in IOP than does a 250-mg oral dose of acetazolamide, the pharmacology of the former compound has several advantages.[171–174] The slight difference in the drugs' IOP-lowering effects at these doses is probably due to the metabolic acidosis caused by acetazolamide, which can be deleterious in many clinical situations. Methazolamide has a more favorable partition coefficient, which allows enhanced systemic absorption and easier access into ocular tissues. In addition, methazolamide is only 55 percent bound to plasma protein, whereas acetazolamide is 95 percent bound. In practical terms, this means that a far smaller quantity of oral methazolamide is needed to produce therapeutic levels in target tissue (presumably the ciliary processes) as

Table 138–5. PHARMACOLOGIC PROPERTIES OF CARBONIC ANHYDRASE INHIBITORS

Name	$K_i^a \times 10^9$ (M)	pK_{a1}	Partition Coefficient to Buffer pH 7.4 Ether	CHCl₃	Solubility in H_2O (mM)	Human %† Bound to Plasma	Human $t\frac{1}{2}$‡ Plasma (hr)	km h⁻¹ × 10⁵ RBC§	km h⁻¹ × 10⁵ Aqueous Humor
Sulfanilamide	1000	10	0.15	0.02	9	10	6	136	—
Acetazolamide	6	7.4	0.14	10^{-3}	3	95	4	27	2
Methazolamide	8	7.2	0.62	0.06	5	55	15	195	8
Ethoxzolamide	1	8.1	140	25	0.04	96	6	4500	330
Benzolamide	1	3.2	0.001	10^{-4}	0.14	96	2	23	1

From Maren TH: *In* Case RM, Lingard JM, Young J (eds): Secretion: Mechanisms and Control. Manchester, U.K., Manchester University Press, 1984.
*Against pure carbonic anhydrase C, in hydration.
†At concentrations of 4–40 μM.
‡After oral dose in human.
§From free concentration in plasma to red blood cells (human).

compared with acetazolamide. Because of this difference in dose, the renal effects of carbonic anhydrase inhibition can be avoided with administration of methazolamide at doses of less than 2 mg/kg/day.

Another advantage is methazolamide's serum half-life of 15 hr, compared with the 4-hr half-life of acetazolamide. It is therefore unnecessary to give methazolamide more often than every 12 hr; this twice-a-day dosage schedule is much more convenient than that required for acetazolamide tablets. Methazolamide also undergoes predominantly hepatic rather than renal metabolism, so that dosages do not have to be adjusted in the large number of patients with renal disease.

Many well-known ocular and systemic side effects occur with administration of all the carbonic anhydrase inhibitors. These include numbness, paresthesias, malaise, anorexia, nausea, flatulence, diarrhea, depression, decreased libido, poor tolerance of carbonated beverages, myopia, hirsutism, increased serum urate, and rarely thrombocytopenia and idiosyncratic aplastic anemia. Some investigators believe that the malaise-anorexia-depression syndrome may be related to concomitant acidosis and have found some success in reducing the incidence of these complaints with the coadministration of sodium bicarbonate.[175] Patient groups in whom metabolic acidosis related to carbonic anhydrase inhibitor therapy may be a serious risk include (1) diabetic patients susceptible to ketoacidosis, (2) patients who have hepatic insufficiency and cannot tolerate the obligatory increase in serum ammonia, and (3) patients with chronic obstructive pulmonary disease, in whom increased retention of carbon dioxide can cause potentially fatal narcosis.[176–178]

An early, mild hypokalemia usually follows the institution of most carbonic anhydrase inhibitors but does not progress unless patients are taking diuretics concomitantly. The exception is the drug dichlorphenamide, which has a unique chloruretic effect that may cause chronic and potentially dangerous loss of potassium. A deformity of the forelimb has been seen in the offspring of animals given acetazolamide, and the drug should definitely be avoided by women of child-bearing age.[179]

Urolithiasis is believed to be much more common in patients taking carbonic anhydrase inhibitors, most likely because of the depressed excretion of renal citrate and the higher urine levels of calcium available to form urate stones. In a case study with controls, the incidence of renal stones was 15 times higher after treatment with acetazolamide than before its administration.[180] The incidence was 11 times higher than in the age-matched control group. The incidence of stones in this study did not seem to increase after 15 mo, suggesting that susceptible persons ordinarily experience this side effect during the first or second year of treatment, if at all. Although methazolamide has been linked to the formation of kidney stones in several patients on high doses (greater than 200 mg/day),[181] the lack of a significant renal effect with low-dose therapy seems to suggest a potentially lower risk of urolithiasis with regimens such as 50 mg b.i.d.

Carbonic anhydrase inhibitors should still be considered a relatively safe and effective form of therapy in open-angle glaucoma. A starting dose of 25 to 50 mg of methazolamide is very easily tolerated by many patients and may be a reasonable trial before laser trabeculoplasty. If a patient has some minor intolerance of this regimen, it can often be temporarily continued during therapy with the laser, in order to blunt the occasional acute IOP elevation in patients who have received laser trabeculoplasty. If the results of escalated therapy and trabeculoplasty are unacceptable and filtration surgery is to be avoided, topical medication can be increased further, possibly introducing a strong miotic drop and giving a higher dose of carbonic anhydrase inhibitors titrated to a maximally tolerated level to avoid filtration surgery.

The use of a maximum dose such as 250 mg of acetazolamide q.i.d. or 150 mg of methazolamide b.i.d. produces systemic acidosis, which is beneficial in lowering IOP but is more likely to be associated with greater systemic toxicity. Sustained-release capsules of 500 mg of acetazolamide may improve compliance when used twice daily and have been reported to give better IOP reduction, but the advantage over therapy with the less expensive 250-mg tablets has not been explained pharmacologically. Many patients younger than 40 yr tolerate carbonic anhydrase inhibitor therapy very well, and its use in this age group may provide suitable control until safer surgery or more tolerable medical treatment becomes available.[182] It is advisable to administer both methazolamide and acetazolamide after meals to decrease gastrointestinal side effects. Because blood dyscrasias have been reported after the use of both agents,[183] there has been considerable debate about whether surveillance of blood counts is justified. Despite the poor outcome in patients who develop idiosyncratic aplastic anemia,[184, 185] some patients also develop isolated neutropenia, thrombocytopenia, and pancytopenia but have an uneventful recovery if the condition is discovered and the drug withdrawn in time.[186] Because such reactions are rare, with an incidence of around 1:14,000, it would not seem justified to continue obtaining blood counts during the entire course of therapy. It is reasonable and relatively inexpensive to obtain a pretreatment complete blood count and one to two follow-up studies during the first 6 mo of treatment, when most of the serious hematologic events were noted to occur. Although some ophthalmologists believe that oral therapy with carbonic anhydrase inhibitors should be abandoned in favor of an "earlier" trabeculectomy, most surgeons would admit that the risk:benefit ratio of a trial medication period using low-dose methazolamide is superior to that of intraocular surgery.

INVESTIGATIONAL AGENTS

New drugs on the horizon for glaucoma treatment may fall into existing classes such as β-blockers or combinations of approved drugs such as a β-blocker with a miotic. However, several exciting new classes of drugs are currently being investigated with the hope that their safety and efficacy will be documented and they will be available for use in treating primary open-angle glaucoma in the very near future.

One such drug is apraclonidine hydrochloride, which is currently being used at the 1 percent concentration as an approved adjunct to laser surgery in the prevention of pressure spikes.[187] The drug is an α-agonist and seems to be a very potent agent for reducing IOP. Its only consistent side effects are systemic symptoms of dry mouth and sour taste. As one would expect from the sympathetic stimulation, some blanching of the conjunctival vessels occurs, as well as obligatory lid retraction. With respect to long-term treatment, clinical trials of efficacy have been equivocal, but a certain group of patients seem to respond for a relatively long period, and for them this drug could be a valuable adjunct to presurgical therapy.[188, 189]

Another new class of drug is the prostaglandin derivatives, with the likely candidate for approval being an analog of prostaglandin $F_{2\alpha}$. This agent effectively lowered IOP in both placebo-controlled trials and comparisons with timolol.[190] Although mild conjunctival hyperemia was noted, duration of action was sustained for 24 hr. The mechanism of action of this agent seems to be increased uveal scleral outflow, which suggests the possibility of perhaps better additivity with available agents.[191]

An effort has been made during the past 30 yr to develop a topical carbonic anhydrase inhibitor. Finally, with the ongoing synthesis of "designer drugs" for this purpose during the past 10 yr, two molecules, sezolamide (MK-417) and dorzolamide (MK-507), have been found to have excellent efficacy and adequate corneal penetration to allow at least an 8-hr duration of action.[192, 193] Both these agents have been extensively tested in animals and humans, and dorzolamide has been found to be effective in several concentrations up to 2 percent. This topical carbonic anhydrase inhibitor was effective in reducing IOP on a three-times-daily administration schedule, yielding IOP decreases from 18 to 22 percent. If these results are confirmed, this agent will probably be valuable for both the initial and adjunctive treatment of glaucoma.

SUMMARY

Many topical systemic drugs have been tried in the treatment of glaucoma, but as more nonmedical therapies such as laser trabeculoplasty and early trabeculectomy have become available, both physicians and patients have begun to be more attentive to the incidence and magnitude of drug side effects as well as the overall risk:benefit ratio. Appropriate strategies to treat selected patients with justifiable degrees of damage or risk factors for damage will be expanded by the newly available β-blockers and, it is hoped, in the future by new classes of drugs such as the prostaglandin derivatives and topical carbonic anhydrase inhibitors. As these new drugs are being developed, even the present low level of adverse reactions might be reduced, and if physicians continue to be prudent in avoiding overtreatment, medical therapy should still continue to be the most appropriate modality for the initial treatment of open-angle glaucoma.

REFERENCES

1. Pohjanpelto PEJ, Plava J: Ocular hypertension and glaucomatous optic nerve damage. Acta Ophthalmol 52:194, 1974.
2. Schwartz B, Talusan AG: Spontaneous trends in ocular pressure in untreated ocular hypertension. Arch Ophthalmol 98:105, 1980.
3. Bengtsson B: The prevalence of glaucoma. Br J Ophthalmol 65:46, 1981.
4. Anderson DR: Glaucoma: The damage caused by pressure. Am J Ophthalmol 108:485, 1989.
5. Kass MA, Hart WM Jr, Gordon M, Miller JP: Risk factors favoring the development of glaucomatous visual field loss in ocular hypertension. Surv Ophthalmol 25:155, 1980.
6. Shaffer R: "Glaucoma suspect" or "ocular hypertension"? Arch Ophthalmol 95:588, 1977.
7. Quigley HA, Maumenee AE: Long-term follow-up of treated open-angle glaucoma. Am J Ophthalmol 87:519, 1979.
8. Vogel R, Crick RP, Newson RB, et al: Association between intraocular pressure and loss of visual field in chronic simple glaucoma. Br J Ophthalmol 74:3, 1990.
9. Kolker AE: Visual prognosis in advanced glaucoma: A comparison of medical and surgical therapy for retention of vision in 101 eyes with advanced glaucoma. Trans Am Ophthalmol Soc 75:539, 1977.
10. Odberg T: Visual field prognosis in advanced glaucoma. Acta Ophthalmol 182(Suppl 65):27, 1987.
11. Kitayawa Y: Prophylactic therapy of ocular hypertension, a prospective study. Trans Ophthalmol Soc N Z 33:30, 1981.
12. Schulzer M, Mikelberg FS, Drance SM: Some observation on the relation between intraocular pressure reduction and the progression of glaucomatous visual loss. Br J Ophthalmol 71:486, 1987.
13. Becker B, Morton WR: Topical epinephrine in glaucoma suspects. Am J Ophthalmol 62:272, 1966.
14. Shin DH, Kolker AE, Kass MA, et al: Longterm epinephrine therapy of ocular hypertension. Arch Ophthalmol 94:2059, 1976.
15. Kitazawa Y: Prophylactic therapy of ocular hypertension: A prospective study. Trans Ophthalmol Soc NZ 33:30, 1981.
16. Graham PA: The definition of pre-glaucoma: A prospective study. Eye 88:153, 1969.
17. Norskov K: Routine tomometry in ophthalmic practice. II: Five-year follow-up. Acta Ophthalmol 48:873, 1970.
18. Levene RZ: Uniocular miotic therapy. Ophthalmology 79:376, 1975.
19. David R, Livingston DG, Luntz MH: Ocular hypertension: A long-term follow-up of treated and untreated patients. Br J Ophthalmol 61:668, 1977.
20. Chauhan BC, Drance SM, Douglas GR: The effect of long-term intraocular pressure reduction on the differential light sensitivity in glaucoma suspects. Invest Ophthalmol Vis Sci 29:1478, 1988.
21. Chisholm IA, Stead S, Tan L, Melenchuk JW: Prognostic indicators in ocular hypertension. Can J Ophthalmol 15:4, 1980.
22. Epstein DL, Krug JH Jr, Hertzmark E, et al: A long-term clinical trial of timolol therapy versus no treatment in the management of glaucoma suspects. Ophthalmology 96:1460, 1989.
23. Kass MA, Gordon MO, Hoff MR, et al: Topical timolol administration reduces the incidence of glaucomatous damage in ocular hypertensive individuals: A randomized, double-masked, long-term clinical trial. Arch Ophthalmol 107:1590, 1989.
24. Schulzer M, Drance SM, Douglas GR: A comparison of treated and untreated glaucoma suspects. Ophthalmology 98:301, 1991.
25. Quigley HA, Addicks EM, Green WR: Optic nerve damage in human glaucoma. III: Quantitative correlation of nerve fiber loss and visual field defect in glaucoma, ischemic neuropathy, papilledema, and toxic neuropathy. Arch Ophthalmol 100:135, 1982.
26. Quigley HA, Dunkelberger GR, Green WR: Retinal ganglion cell atrophy correlated with automated perimetry in human eyes with glaucoma. Am J Ophthalmol 107:135, 1982.
27. Roth SM, Spaeth GL, Poryzees EM, et al: The effects of postoperative corticosteroids on trabeculectomy: Long-term follow-up. ARVO Abstracts. Invest Ophthalmol Vis Sci 29(Suppl):367, 1988.
28. Greve EL, Dake CL: Four-year followup of a glaucoma operation: Prospective study of the double flap Scheie. Int Ophthalmol 1:139, 1979.

29. Werner EB, Drance SM, Schulzer M: Trabeculectomy and the progression of glaucomatous visual field loss. Arch Ophthalmol 95:1374, 1977.
30. Kidd MN, O'Connor M: Progression of field loss after trabeculectomy: A five-year follow-up. Br J Ophthalmol 69:827, 1985.
31. Rollins DF, Drance SM: Five year follow-up of trabeculectomy in the management of chronic open-angle glaucoma. In Symposium on Glaucoma: Transactions of the New Orleans Academy of Ophthalmology. St. Louis, CV Mosby, 1981, pp 295–300.
32. Migdal C, Hitchings R: Control of chronic simple glaucoma with primary medical, surgical and laser treatment. Trans Ophthalmol Soc UK 105:653, 1986.
33. Jay JL, Murray SB: Early trabeculectomy versus conventional management in primary open angle glaucoma. Br J Ophthalmol 72:881, 1988.
34. Smith RJH: The enigma of primary open angle glaucoma. Trans Ophthalmol Soc UK 105:618, 1986.
35. The Glaucoma Laser Trial Research Group: The Glaucoma Laser Trial (GLT). 2: Results of argon laser trabeculoplasty versus topical medicines. Ophthalmology 97:1403, 1990.
36. Thomas JV, El-Mofty A, Hamdy EE, et al: Argon laser trabeculoplasty as initial therapy for glaucoma. Arch Ophthalmol 102:702, 1984.
37. Rosenthal AR, Chaudhuri PR, Chiapella AP: Laser trabeculoplasty primary therapy in open-angle glaucoma: A preliminary report. Arch Ophthalmol 102:699, 1984.
38. Tuulonen A: Laser trabeculoplasty as primary therapy in chronic open-angle glaucoma. Acta Ophthalmol 62:150, 1984.
39. Kass MA, Meltzer DW, Gordon M, et al: Compliance with topical pilocarpine treatment. Am J Ophthalmol 101:515, 1986.
40. Kass MA, Gordon M, Morley RE Jr, et al: Compliance with topical timolol treatment. Am J Ophthalmol 103:188, 1987.
41. Kass MA, Gordon M, Meltzer DW: Can ophthalmologists identify patients defaulting from pilocarpine therapy? Am J Ophthalmol 101:524, 1986.
42. Pillunat LE, Stodmeister R, Wilmanns I, Metzner D: Effect of timolol on optic nerve need regulation. Ophthalmologica 193:146, 1986.
43. Grunwald JE, Furubayashi C: Effect of topical timolol maleate on the ophthalmic artery blood pressure. Invest Ophthalmol Vis Sci 30:1095, 1989.
44. Drance SM, Flammer J: Some effects of antiglaucoma drugs on visual function. In Drance SM, Neufeld AH (eds): Glaucoma Applied Pharmacology in Medical Treatment. New York, Grune & Stratton, 1984, pp 569–576.
45. Messmer C, Flammer J, Stumpfig D: Influence of betaxolol and timolol on the visual fields of patients with glaucoma. Am J Ophthalmol 112:678, 1991.
46. Collignon-Brach J: Long-term effect of ophthalmic β-adrenoceptor antagonists on intraocular pressure and retinal sensitivity in primary open-angle glaucoma. Curr Eye Res 11:1, 1992.
47. Grant WM, Burke JF Jr: Why do some people go blind from glaucoma? Ophthalmology 89:991, 1982.
48. Hart WM, Yablonski M, Kass MA, Becker B: Quantitative visual field and optic disc correlates early in glaucoma. Arch Ophthalmol 96:2209, 1978.
49. Zimmerman TJ, Kaufman HE: Timolol. A beta-adrenergic blocking agent for the treatment of glaucoma. Arch Ophthalmol 95:601, 1977.
50. Allen RC: Medical treatment of open angle glaucoma. In Weinstein G (ed): Open Angle Glaucoma. Boston, Little, Brown & Co, 1985, pp 31–48.
51. Coakes RL, Brubaker RF: The mechanism of timolol in lowering intraocular pressure in the normal eye. Arch Ophthalmol 96:2045, 1978.
52. Zimmerman TJ, Harbin R, Pett M, Kaufman HE: Timolol and facility of outflow. Invest Ophthalmol Vis Sci 16:623, 1977.
53. Sonntag JR, Brindley GO, Shields MB: Effect of timolol therapy on outflow facility. Invest Ophthalmol Vis Sci 17:293, 1978.
54. Topper JE, Brubaker RF: Effects of timolol, epinephrine, and acetazolamide on aqueous flow during sleep. Invest Ophthalmol Vis Sci 26:1315, 1985.
55. Boger WP III: Shortterm "escape" and longterm "drift": The dissipation effects of the beta adrenergic blocking agents. Surv Ophthalmol 28:235, 1983.
56. Korey MS, Hodapp E, Kass MA, et al: Timolol and epinephrine:
Long-term evaluation of concurrent administration. Arch Ophthalmol 100:742, 1982.
57. Boger WP III, Steinert RF, Puliafito CA, Pavan-Langston D: Clinical trial comparing timolol ophthalmic solution to pilocarpine in open-angle glaucoma. Am J Ophthalmol 86:8, 1978.
58. Moss AP, Ritch R, Hargett NA, et al: A comparison of the effects of timolol and epinephrine on intraocular pressure. Am J Ophthalmol 86:489, 1978.
59. Yalon M, Urinowsky E, Rothkoff L, et al: Frequency of timolol administration. Am J Ophthalmol 92:526, 1981.
60. Wandel T, Fishman D, Novack GD, et al: Ocular hypotensive efficacy of 0.25% levobunolol instilled once daily. Ophthalmology 95:252, 1988.
61. Radius RL, Diamond GR, Pollack IP, Langham ME: Timolol: A new drug for management of chronic simple glaucoma. Arch Ophthalmol 96:1003, 1978.
62. Van Buskirk EM: Adverse reactions from timolol administration. Ophthalmology 87:447, 1980.
63. Liu GS, Basu PK, Trope GE: Ultrastructural changes of the rabbit corneal epithelium and endothelium after timoptic treatment. Graefes Arch Clin Exp Ophthalmol 225:325, 1987.
64. McMahon CD, Shaffer RN, Hoskins HD Jr, Hetherington J Jr: Adverse effects experienced by patients taking timolol. Am J Ophthalmol 88:736, 1979.
65. Wilson RP, Spaeth GL, Poryzees E: The place of timolol in the practice of ophthalmology. Ophthalmology 87:451, 1980.
66. Van Buskirk EM: Adverse reactions from timolol administration. Ophthalmology 87:447, 1980.
67. Fraunfelder FT: Interim report: National registry of possible drug-induced ocular side effects. Ophthalmology 87:87, 1980.
68. Fraunfelder FT, Meyer SM, Menacker SJ: Alopecia possibly secondary to topical ophthalmic β-blocker. JAMA 263:1493, 1990.
69. Coleman AL, Diehl DLC, Jampel HD, et al: Topical timolol decreased plasma high-density lipoprotein cholesterol level. Arch Ophthalmol 108:1260, 1990.
70. Lawrsen SO, Bjerrum P: Timolol eyedrop-induced severe bronchospasm. Acta Med Scand 211:505, 1982.
71. Noyes JH, Chervinsky P: Case report: Exacerbation of asthma by timolol. Ann Allergy 45:301, 1980.
72. Guzman CA: Exacerbation of bronchorrhea induced by topical timolol [Letter]. Am Rev Respir Dis 121:899, 1980.
73. Nelson WL, Fraunfelder FT, Sills JM, et al: Adverse respiratory and cardiovascular events attributed to timolol ophthalmic solution, 1978–1985. Am J Ophthalmol 102:606, 1986.
74. Jones FL Jr, Ekberg NL: Exacerbation of asthma by timolol. N Engl J Med 301:270, 1979.
75. Burnstine RA, Felton JL, Ginther WH: Cardiorespiratory reaction to timolol maleate in pediatric patient: A case report. Ann Ophthalmol 14:905, 1982.
76. Olson RJ, Bromberg BB, Zimmerman TJ: Apneic spells associated with timolol therapy in a neonate. Am J Ophthalmol 88:120, 1979.
77. Schoene RB, Martin TR, Charan NB, French CL: Timolol-induced bronchospasm in asthmatic bronchitis. JAMA 245:1460, 1981.
78. Zimmerman TJ, Kooner KS, Kandarakis AS, Ziegler LP: Improving the therapeutic index of topically applied ocular drugs. Arch Ophthalmol 102:551, 1984.
79. Huang TC, Lee DA: Punctal occlusion and topical medications for glaucoma. Am J Ophthalmol 107:151, 1989.
80. Duzman E, Ober M, Scharrer A, Leopold IH: A clinical evaluation of the effects of topically applied levobunolol and timolol on increased intraocular pressure. Am J Ophthalmol 94:318, 1982.
81. Cinotti A, Cinotti D, Grant W, et al: Levobunolol vs timolol for open-angle glaucoma and ocular hypertension. Am J Ophthalmol 99:11, 1985.
82. Berson FG, Cohen HB, Foerster RJ, et al: Levobunolol compared with timolol for the long-term control of elevated intraocular pressure. Arch Ophthalmol 103:379, 1985.
83. Berson FG, Cinotti A, Cohen H, et al: Levobunolol: A beta-adrenoceptor antagonist effective in the long-term treatment of glaucoma. Ophthalmology 92:1271, 1985.
84. The Levobunolol Study Group: Levobunolol: A four-year study of efficacy and safety in glaucoma treatment. Ophthalmology 96:642, 1989.

85. DiCarlo FJ, Leinweber F-J, Szpiech JM, et al: Metabolism of L-bunolol. Clin Pharmacol Ther 22:858, 1977.
86. Woodward DF, Novack GD, Williams LS, et al: The ocular beta-blocking activity of dihydrolevobunolol. J Ocul Pharmacol 3:11, 1987.
87. Wandel T, Charap AD, Lewis RA, et al: Glaucoma treatment with once-daily levobunolol. Am J Ophthalmol 101:298, 1986.
88. Bensinger RE, Keates EU, Gofman JD, et al: Levobunolol: A three-month efficacy study in the treatment of glaucoma and ocular hypertension. Arch Ophthalmol 103:375, 1985.
89. Boozman FW III, Carriker R, Foerster R, et al: Long-term evaluation of 0.25% levobunolol and timolol for therapy for elevated intraocular pressure. Arch Ophthalmol 106:614, 1988.
90. Battershill PE, Sorkin EM: Ocular metipranolol. Drugs 36:601, 1988.
91. Dausch D, Brewitt H, Edelhoff R: Metipranolol eye drops: Clinical suitability in the treatment of chronic open angle glaucoma. In Merte HJ (ed): Metipranolol. New York, Springer-Verlag Wien, 1983, pp 132–147.
92. Denffer H: Efficacy and tolerance of metripranolol: Results of a multicenter long-term study. In Merte HJ (ed): Metipranolol. New York, Springer-Verlag Wien, 1983, pp 121–125.
93. Ecoffet M, Demailly P: Resultats d'une étude à moyen terme à double insu comparant le metipranolol au timolol dans le traitement du glaucome primitif à angle ouvert. J Fr Ophthalmol 10:451, 1987.
94. Kruse W: Metipranolol: A new beta-receptor blocking agent. Klin Monatsbl Augenheil 182:582, 1983.
94a. Kruse W: Results of a long-term study with metripranolol. In Merte HJ (ed): Metopranolol. New York, Springer-Verlag Wien, 1983, pp 126–131.
95. Kruse W: Metipranolol in glaucoma therapy. Der Augenarzt 3:168, 1983.
96. Mertz M: Results of a 6 weeks' multicenter double-blind trial, metripranolol versus timolol. In Merte HJ (ed): Metipranolol. New York, Springer-Verlag Wien, 1983, pp 93–105.
97. Mills KB, Wright G: A blind randomized cross-over trial comparing metipranolol 0.3% with timolol 0.25% in open-angle glaucoma: A pilot study. Br J Ophthalmol 70:39, 1986.
98. Muller O, Knobel HR: Efficacy and tolerance of metipranolol: Results of a Swiss long-term multicenter study. Klin Monatsbl Augenheilkd 188:62, 1986.
98a. Bleckmann H, Pham Duy T, Grajewski O: Therapeutic efficacy of metipranolol eye drops 0.3% versus timolol eye drops 0.25%: a double-blind cross-over study. In Merte HJ (ed): Metipranolol. New York, Springer-Verlag Wien, 1983, pp. 106–120.
99. Schmitz-Valchenberg P, Jonas J, Brambring DF: Reductions in pressure with metipranolol 0.1%. Z Prakt Augenheilk 5:171, 1984.
99a. Krieglstein GK, Novack GD, Voepel E, et al: Levobunolol and metipranolol: comparative ocular hypotensive efficacy, safety and comfort. Br J Ophthalmol 71:250–253, 1987.
100. LeJeunne CL, Hughues FC, Dufier JL, et al: Bronchial and cardiovascular effects of ocular topical β-antagonists in asthmatic subjects: Comparison of timolol, carteolol, and metipranolol. J Clin Pharmacol 29:97, 1989.
101. Chrisp P, Sorkin EM: Ocular carteolol. Drugs and Aging 2:58, 1992.
102. Wellstein A, Palm D, Wiemeer G, et al: Simple and reliable radioreceptor assay for beta-adrenoceptor antagonists and active metabolites in native human plasma. Eur J Clin Pharmacol 27:545, 1984.
103. Duff GR, Graham PA: A double-crossover trial comparing the effects of topical carteolol and placebo on intraocular pressure. Br J Ophthalmol 72:890, 1988.
104. Horie T, Takahashi O, Shirato S, Kitazawa Y: Comparison of ocular hypotensive effects of topical timolol and carteolol. Jpn J Clin Pharmacol 36:1065, 1982.
105. Maclure GM, Gregory JE, Munro AJ: Comparison of carteolol and timolol—a double blind study. Poster. Third Congress of the European Glaucoma Society, Amsterdam, May 1988.
106. Mills KB, Raines M, Joyce P: A single-blind, stratified, randomized non-crossover trial comparing carteolol 1% with timolol 0.25% in the long term management of glaucoma. Br J Clin Pract 41(Suppl 51):10, 1987.
107. Stewart WC, Shields MB, Allen RC, et al: A 3-month compar-
ison of 1% and 2% carteolol and 0.5% timolol in open-angle glaucoma. Graefes Arch Clin Exp Ophthalmol 229:258–261, 1991.
108. Tsuchisaka H, Kin K, Matsumoto S, et al: Multi-institutional evaluation of timolol and carteolol for glaucomas. Ganka Rinsho Iho 85:1136–1140, 1991.
109. Scoville B, Mueller B, White BG, Krieglstein GK: A double-masked comparison of carteolol and timolol in ocular hypertension. Am J Ophthalmol 105:150–154, 1988.
110. Flammer J, Etienne R: The effect of beta-blockers on differential light sensitivity: Preliminary results. Japanese-French Symposium on Glaucoma. May 29–30, 1985.
111. Mihara M, Matsuo N, Koyama T, Tsuji T: Studies on the retinal mean circulation time in eyes treated with carteolol (Mikelan) by means of fluorescein video-angiography and image analysis. Ther Res 10:161–167, 1989.
112. Grunwald JE, Delehanty J: Effect of topical carteolol on the normal human retinal circulation. Invest Ophthalmol Vis Sci 33:1853–1856, 1992.
113. Hoffman BB, Lefkowitz RJ: Adrenergic receptor antagonists. In Goodman AG, Rall TW, Nies AS, Taylor P (eds): Goodman & Gilman's The Pharmacological Basis of Therapeutics, 8th ed. New York, Pergamon Press, 1990, p 240.
114. Nielsen NV, Eriksen JS: Timolol and metoprolol in glaucoma: A comparison of the ocular hypotensive effect, local and systemic tolerance. Acta Ophthalmol 59:336, 1981.
115. Vale J, Phillips CI: Practolol (Eraldin) eye drops as an ocular hypotensive agent. Br J Ophthalmol 57:210, 1973.
116. Phillips CI, Gore SM, MacDonald MJ, et al: Atenolol eye drops in glaucoma: a double-masked, controlled study. Br J Ophthalmol 61:349, 1977.
117. Radius RL: Use of betaxolol in the reduction of elevated intraocular pressure. Arch Ophthalmol 101:898, 1983.
118. Caldwell DR, Salisbury CR, Guzek JP: Effects of topical betaxolol in ocular hypertensive patients. Arch Ophthalmol 102:539, 1984.
119. Feghali JG, Kaufman PL: Decreased intraocular pressure in the hypertensive human eye with betaxolol; a β-adrenergic antagonist. Am J Ophthalmol 100:777, 1985.
120. Berry DP, Van Buskirk EM, Shields MB: Betaxolol and timolol: A comparison of efficacy and side effects. Arch Ophthalmol 102:42, 1984.
121. Stewart RH, Kimbrough RL, Ward RL: Betaxolol vs timolol: A six-month double-blind comparison. Arch Ophthalmol 104:46, 1986.
122. Allen RC, Hertzmark E, Walker AM, Epstein DL: A double-masked comparison of betaxolol vs timolol in the treatment of open-angle glaucoma. Am J Ophthalmol 101:535, 1986.
123. Long DA, Johns GE, Mullen RS, et al: Levabunolol and betaxolol: A double-masked controlled comparison of efficacy and safety in patients with elevated intraocular pressure. Ophthalmology 95:735, 1988.
124. Reiss GR, Brubaker RF: The mechanism of betaxolol, a new ocular hypotensive agent. Ophthalmology 90:1369, 1983.
125. Vogel R, Tipping R, Kulaga SF Jr, et al: Changing therapy from timolol to betaxol: Effects on intraocular pressure in selected patients with glaucoma. Arch Ophthalmol 107:1303, 1989.
126. Weinreb RN, Caldwell DR, Goode SM, et al: A double-masked three-month comparison between 0.25% betaxolol suspension and 0.5% betaxolol ophthalmic solution. Am J Ophthalmol 110:189, 1990.
127. Smith JP, Weeks RH, Newland EF, Ward RL: Betaxolol and acetazolamide: Combined ocular hypotensive effect. Arch Ophthalmol 102:1794, 1984.
128. Allen RC, Epstein DL: Additive effect of betaxolol and epinephrine in primary open angle glaucoma. Arch Ophthalmol 104:1178, 1986.
129. Weinreb RN, Ritch R, Kushner FH: Effect of adding betaxolol to dipivefrin therapy. Am J Ophthalmol 101:196, 1986.
130. Thomas JV, Epstein DL: Timolol and epinephrine in primary open-angle glaucoma: Transient additive effect. Arch Ophthalmol 99:91, 1981.
131. Keates EC, Stone RA: Safety and effectiveness of concomitant administration of dipivefrin and timolol maleate. Am J Ophthalmol 91:243, 1981.
132. Cyrlin MS, Thomas JV, Epstein DL: Additive effect of epineph-

rine to timolol therapy in primary open-angle glaucoma. Arch Ophthalmol 100:414, 1982.

133. Wax MB, Molinoff PB: Distribution and properties of β-adrenergic receptors in human iris-ciliary body. Invest Ophthalmol Vis Sci 28:420, 1987.

134. Robinson JC, Kaufman PL: Effects and interactions of epinephrine, norepinephrine, timolol, and betaxolol on outflow facility in the cynomolgus monkey. Am J Ophthalmol 109:189, 1990.

135. Wax MB, Molinoff PB, Alvarado J, Polansky J: Characterization of β-adrenergic receptors in cultured human trabecular cells and in human trabecular meshwork. Invest Ophthalmol Vis Sci 30:51, 1989.

136. Jampel HD, Lynch MG, Brown RH, et al: β-Adrenergic receptors in human trabecular meshwork: Identification and autoradiographic localization. Invest Ophthalmol Vis Sci 28:772, 1987.

137. Schoene RB, Abuan T, Ward RL, Beasley CH: Effects of topical betaxolol, timolol, and placebo on pulmonary function in asthmatic bronchitis. Am J Ophthalmol 97:86, 1984.

138. Dunn TL, Gerber MJ, Shen AS et al: Timolol-induced bronchospasm: Utility of betaxolol as an alternative ocular hypotensive agent in patients with asthma. Clin Res 33:20A, 1985.

139. Van Buskirk EM, Weinreb RN, Berry DP, et al: Betaxolol in patients with glaucoma and asthma. Am J Ophthalmol 101:531, 1986.

140. Bleckmann H, Dorow P: Treatment of patients with glaucoma and obstructive airway diseases with betaxolol and placebo eye drops. Klin Monatsbl Augenheilkd 191:199, 1987.

141. Weinreb RN, Van Buskirk EM, Cherniack R, Drake MM: Long-term betaxolol therapy in glaucoma patients with pulmonary disease. Am J Ophthalmol 106:162, 1988.

142. Harris LS, Greenstein SH, Bloom AF: Respiratory difficulties with betaxolol. Am J Ophthalmol 102:274, 1986.

143. Roholt PC: Betaxolol and restrictive airway disease. Arch Ophthalmol 105:1172, 1987.

144. Doyle WJ, Weber PA, Meeks RH: Effect of topical timolol maleate on exercise performance. Arch Ophthalmol 102:1517, 1984.

145. Atkins JM, Pugh BR Jr, Timewell RM: Cardiovascular effects of topical beta-blockers during exercise. Am J Ophthalmol 99:173, 1985.

146. Pillunat L, Stodtmeister R: Effect of different antiglaucomatous drugs on ocular perfusion pressures. J Ocul Pharmacol 4:231, 1988.

147. Mandell AI, Stentz F, Kitabchi AE: Dipivalyl epinephrine: A new pro-drug in the treatment of glaucoma. Ophthalmology 85:268, 1978.

148. Krieglstein GK, Leydhecker W: The dose-response relationships of dipivalyl epinephrine in open-angle glaucoma. Graefes Arch Clin Exp Ophthalmol 205:141, 1978.

149. Kass MA, Mandell AL, Goldberg L, et al: Dipivefrin and epinephrine treatment of elevated intraocular pressure: A comparative study. Arch Ophthalmol 97:1865, 1979.

150. Kohn AN, Moss AP, Hargett NA, et al: Clinical comparison of dipivalyl epinephrine and epinephrine in the treatment of glaucoma. Am J Ophthalmol 87:196, 1979.

151. Townsend DJ, Brubaker RF: Immediate effect of epinephrine on aqueous formation in the normal human eye as measured by fluorophotometry. Invest Ophthalmol Vis Sci 19:256, 1980.

152. Garner LL, Johnstone WW, Ballintine EJ, Carroll ME: Effect of 2% levo-rotary epinephrine on the intraocular pressure of the glaucomatous eye. Arch Ophthalmol 62:230, 1959.

153. Krill AE, Newell FW, Novak M: Early and long-term effects of levo-epinephrine on ocular tension and outflow. Am J Ophthalmol 59:833, 1965.

154. Liesegang TJ: Bulbar conjunctival follicles associated with dipivefrin therapy. Ophthalmology 92:228, 1985.

155. Coleiro JA, Sigurdsson H, Lockyer JA: Follicular conjunctivitis on dipivefrin therapy for glaucoma. Eye 2:440, 1988.

156. Kerr CR, Hass I, Drance SM, et al: Cardiovascular effects of epinephrine and dipivalyl epinephrine applied topically to the eye in patients with glaucoma. Br J Ophthalmol 66:109, 1982.

157. Kaufman PL, Barany EH: Loss of acute pilocarpine effect on outflow facility following surgical disinsertion and retrodisplacement of the ciliary muscle from the scleral spur in the cynomolgus monkey. Invest Ophthalmol 15:793, 1976.

158. Kaufman PL, Barany EH: Residual pilocarpine effects on outflow facility after ciliary muscle disinsertion in the cynomolgus monkey. Invest Ophthalmol 15:558, 1976.

159. Zimmerman TJ, Kooner KS, Kandarakis AS, Ziegler LP: Improving the therapeutic index of topically applied ocular drugs. Arch Ophthalmol 102:551, 1984.

160. Goldberg I, Ashburgn FS Jr, Kass MA, Becker B: Efficacy and patient acceptance of pilocarpine gel. Am J Ophthalmol 88:843, 1979.

161. March WF, Stewart RM, Mandell AL, Bruce LA: Duration of effect of pilocarpine gel. Arch Ophthalmol 100:1270, 1982.

162. Johnson DH, Epstein DL, Allen RC, et al: A one-year multicenter clinical trial of pilocarpine gel. Am J Ophthalmol 97:723, 1984.

163. Johnson DH, Keyon KR, Epstein DL, Van Buskirk EM: Corneal changes during pilocarpine gel therapy. Am J Ophthalmol 101:13, 1986.

164. Crandall AS, Levy NS, Hoskins HD Jr, et al: Characterization of subtle corneal deposits. J Toxicol Cutan Ocul Toxicol 3:263, 1984.

165. Lutjen-Drecoll E, Kaufman PL: Biomechanics of echothiophate-induced anatomic changes in monkey aqueous outflow system. Graefes Arch Clin Exp Ophthalmol 224:564, 1986.

166. Beasley H, Fraunfelder FT: Retinal detachments and topical ocular miotics. Ophthalmology 86:95, 1979.

167. Axelsson U, Holmberg A: The frequency of cataract after miotic therapy. Acta Ophthalmol 44:421, 1966.

168. Becker B: Decrease in intraocular pressure in man by a carbonic anhydrase inhibitor, Diamox. Am J Ophthalmol 37:13, 1954.

169. Maren TH: The rates of movement of Na^+, Cl^- and HCO_3^- from plasma to posterior chamber: Effect of acetazolamide and relation to the treatment of glaucoma. Invest Ophthalmol 15:356, 1976.

170. Friedman Z, Krupin T, Becker B: Ocular and systemic effects of acetazolamide in nephrectomized rabbits. Invest Ophthalmol Vis Sci 23:209, 1982.

171. Maren TH, Haywood JR, Chapman SK, Zimmerman TJ: The pharmacology of methazolamide in relation to the treatment of glaucoma. Invest Ophthal Vis Sci 16:730, 1977.

172. Stone RA, Zimmerman TJ, Shin DH, et al: Low-dose methazolamide and intraocular pressure. Am J Ophthalmol 83:674, 1977.

173. Dahlen K, Epstein DL, Grant WM, et al: A repeated dose-response study of methazolamide in glaucoma. Arch Ophthalmol 96:2214, 1978.

174. Merkle W: Effect of methazolamide on the intraocular pressure of patients with open-angle glaucoma. Klin Monatsbl Augenheilkd 176:181, 1980.

175. Arrigg CA, Epstein DL, Giovanoni R, Grant WM: The influence of supplemental sodium acetate on carbonic anhydrase inhibitor-induced side effects. Arch Ophthalmol 99:1969, 1981.

176. Heller I, Halevy J, Cohen S, Theodor E: Significant metabolic acidosis induced by acetazolamide: Not a rare complication. Arch Intern Med 145:1815, 1985.

177. Margo CE: Acetazolamide and advanced liver disease. Am J Ophthalmol 101:611, 1986.

178. Block ER, Rostand RA: Carbonic anhydrase inhibition in glaucoma: Hazard or benefit for the chronic lunger. Surv Ophthalmol 23:169, 1978.

179. Maren TH, Ellison AC: The teratological effect of certain thiadiazoles related to acetazolamide, with a note on sulfanilamide and thiazide diuretics. Johns Hopkins Med J 130:95, 1972.

180. Kass MA, Kolker AE, Gordon M, et al: Acetazolamide and urolithiasis. Ophthalmology 88:261, 1981.

181. Shields MB, Simmons RJ: Urinary calculus during methazolamide therapy. Am J Ophthalmol 81:622, 1976.

182. Shrader CE, Thomas JV, Simmons RJ: Relationship of patient age and tolerance to carbonic anhydrase inhibitors. Am J Ophthalmol 96:730, 1983.

183. Werblin TP, Pollack IP, Liss RA: Blood dyscrasias in patients using methazolamide (Neptazane) for glaucoma. Ophthalmology 87:350, 1980.

184. Wisch N, Fischbein FI, Siegel R, et al: Aplastic anemia resulting from the use of carbonic anhydrase inhibitors. Am J Ophthalmol 75:130, 1973.

185. Zimran A, Beutler E: Can the risk of acetazolamide-induced aplastic anemia be decreased by periodic monitoring of blood cell counts? Am J Ophthalmol 104:654, 1987.
186. Fraundfelder FT, Meyer SM, Bagby GC Jr, Dreis MW: Hematologic reactions to carbonic anhydrase inhibitors. Am J Ophthalmol 100:79, 1985.
187. Abrams DA, Robin AL, Pollack IP, et al: The safety and efficacy of topical 1% ALO 2145 (p-aminoclonidine hydrochloride) in normal volunteers. Arch Ophthalmol 105:1205, 1987.
188. Jampel HD, Robin AL, Quigley HA, Pollack IP: Apraclonidine: A one-week dose-response study. Arch Ophthal 106:1069, 1988.
189. Morrison JC, Robin AL: Adjunctive glaucoma therapy: A comparison of apraclonidine to dipivefrin when added to timolol maleate. Ophthalmology 96:3, 1989.

190. Camras CB, Siebold EC, Lustgarten JS, et al: Maintained reduction of intraocular pressure by prostaglandin F$_2$-1-isopropyl ester applied in multiple doses in ocular hypertensive and glaucoma patients. Ophthalmology 96:1329, 1989.
191. Jorgen Villumsen J, Alm A: The effect of adding prostaglandin F$_2$-Isopropylester to timolol in patients with open angle glaucoma. Arch Ophthalmol 108:1102, 1990.
192. Lippa EA, Schuman JS, Higginbotham EJ, et al: MK-507 versus Sezolamide: Comparative efficacy of two topically active carbonic anhydrase inhibitors. Ophthalmology 98:308, 1991.
193. Lippa EA, Carlson LE, Ehinger B, et al: Dose response and duration of action of dorzolamide, a topical carbonic anhydrase inhibitor. Arch Ophthalmol 110:495, 1992.

Chapter 139

■

Laser Therapy of Open-Angle Glaucoma

CLAUDIA U. RICHTER

HISTORY

Laser surgery on the trabecular meshwork to lower intraocular pressure and control open-angle glaucoma has been investigated since the early 1970s. Initial investigations concentrated on treating limited extents of the trabecular meshwork with intense penetrating burns to develop a communicating channel between the anterior chamber and Schlemm's canal. Krasnow[1, 2] and Robin and Pollack[3] attempted to create holes in the trabecular meshwork with the Q-switched ruby laser to decrease outflow resistance. This technique did decrease outflow resistance and lower intraocular pressure, but for only a limited time.

Worthen and Wickham,[4, 5] Ticho,[6] and others[7-10] used the argon laser to alter the trabecular meshwork. Although intraocular pressure was frequently reduced, the results were variable and the procedure was not widely accepted. Interest in laser treatment to the trabecular meshwork abated somewhat when it was demonstrated that scarring of the trabecular meshwork, obliteration of Schlemm's canal, and secondary glaucoma could be produced in monkey eyes by treatment of the meshwork with 200 high-intensity argon laser burns.[11] However, Wise and Witter found that the intraocular pressure could be reduced reliably and predictably by evenly spaced burns around the circumference of the trabecular meshwork.[12] No attempt was made with this procedure to penetrate through the trabecular meshwork to Schlemm's canal. Since this report first appeared, argon laser trabeculoplasty has provided long-term intraocular pressure control in a high percentage of patients with open-angle glaucoma with few complications.

Investigative attention has focused on the effects of the neodymium-yttrium-aluminum-garnet (Nd.YAG) laser and the diode laser on the trabecular meshwork and their roles in the management of open-angle glaucoma.

Whereas some investigators attempted to increase outflow facility by laser treatment of the trabecular meshwork, others focused on decreasing aqueous production by laser treatment of the ciliary processes. The results of these investigations and the development of laser cycloablation are discussed in Chapter 147.

Newer laser technologies have raised the possibility of creating filtration fistulas using laser energy. The types of lasers and procedures being investigated are discussed in Chapter 140.

ARGON LASER TRABECULOPLASTY

Indications

Argon laser trabeculoplasty is usually the appropriate treatment to lower intraocular pressure in eyes with open-angle glaucoma that are uncontrolled by maximally tolerated medical therapy (Table 139–1). Argon laser

Table 139–1. INDICATIONS FOR ARGON LASER TRABECULOPLASTY

Uncontrolled intraocular pressure in open-angle glaucoma by maximal tolerated medical therapy prior to filtration surgery
Uncontrolled intraocular pressure in open-angle glaucoma following failed filtration surgery and uncontrolled by antiglaucomatous medical therapy
Initial glaucoma therapy (Glaucoma Laser Trial)
Noncompliance

trabeculoplasty is virtually always indicated for intraocular pressure control in open-angle glaucoma prior to filtration surgery.

Maximal medical therapy is usually defined as treatment with a β-adrenergic antagonist, epinephrine, a cholinergic agent (pilocarpine, carbachol, or a cholinesterase inhibitor), and a carbonic anhydrase inhibitor unless a systemic contraindication exists. Although these medications successfully lower intraocular pressure, they may also cause visual or systemic side effects significant enough to prevent patient compliance or interfere with daily activities. For instance, cholinergic therapy may induce myopia, causing visual blurring, and preclude its use. Carbonic anhydrase inhibitors may cause systemic side effects, such as lethargy, weight loss, depression, kidney stones, and even life-threatening blood dyscrasias. Recognizing the potential adverse effects of all antiglaucoma medications, maximal medical therapy in the treatment of glaucoma prior to argon laser trabeculoplasty is usually modified to include treatment only with medications that lower intraocular pressure and do not have adverse side effects for the patient (maximally tolerated medical therapy). Additionally, positive experience with argon laser trabeculoplasty for more than 10 yr has resulted in a tendency to treat patients with argon laser trabeculoplasty (ALT), or to at least discuss the possibility, prior to trying carbonic anhydrase inhibitors due to the concern about their systemic side effects.

Noncompliance with antiglaucoma medications can be an indication for argon laser trabeculoplasty. These patients may have optic nerve damage and visual field loss due to uncontrolled intraocular pressure secondary to their noncompliance. Argon laser trabeculoplasty may provide adequate intraocular pressure control and prevent this visual loss.

The success of argon laser trabeculoplasty in controlling intraocular pressure in open-angle glaucoma has inspired several studies of laser trabeculoplasty as a primary therapy in glaucoma treatment.[13–16] Intraocular pressure control with argon laser trabeculoplasty as primary therapy in open-angle glaucoma would eliminate drug-related side effects and could avoid difficulties with compliance. The Glaucoma Laser Trial[17] is a multicenter, randomized clinical trial assessing the efficacy and safety of argon laser trabeculoplasty as an alternative to treatment with topical medications for uncontrolled intraocular pressure in patients with newly diagnosed, previously untreated primary open-angle glaucoma. After 2 yr of follow-up, eyes treated with argon laser trabeculoplasty first and medications added as necessary had lower mean intraocular pressures compared with eyes treated with medications first. Additionally, eyes treated initially with argon laser trabeculoplasty required fewer medications for intraocular pressure control than eyes treated initially with medications. There were no differences in visual acuity or visual field between the two groups. Although the results of this study are encouraging, longer-term observations are necessary to determine if argon laser trabeculoplasty as the initial therapy of open-angle glaucoma preserves vision better than initial therapy with medications.

The contraindications to argon laser trabeculoplasty are few. The two absolute contraindications are total angle-closure and hazy media precluding visualization of the angle structures. Argon laser trabeculoplasty may be difficult or impossible in an uncooperative patient, but this situation is very uncommon and retrobulbar anesthesia may allow safe treatment. Secondary open-angle glaucomas that are infrequently improved by laser trabeculoplasty, such as the inflammatory glaucomas, may be contraindications. A serious complication from argon laser trabeculoplasty in one eye, such as a markedly elevated intraocular pressure elevation, may constitute a contraindication to treatment in the fellow eye. Finally, laser trabeculoplasty should be used cautiously in eyes that need urgent intraocular pressure control to preserve vision. Because the results of trabeculoplasty are not immediate, these eyes may be better treated with glaucoma filtration surgery than with argon laser trabeculoplasty.

Technique

Argon laser trabeculoplasty is an outpatient procedure that is usually well tolerated by the patient. Preoperative preparations include obtaining informed consent, prophylactic treatment for postlaser intraocular pressure elevations, topical anesthesia, and positioning the patient to maximize the patient's comfort (Table 139–2). The literature on informed consent should be clearly written for the patient to understand and should give the reasons for the procedure, the potential benefits, and the possible complications.

An acute increase in intraocular pressure after argon laser trabeculoplasty is the procedure's most serious potential complication and can result in permanent visual loss. Consequently, meticulous attention to intraocular pressure control before and after the procedure is critical to prevent further glaucoma damage. All glaucoma medications should be continued prior to laser trabeculoplasty and, 1 hr prior to the procedure, *para*-aminoclonidine should be administered. *Para*-aminoclonidine has been shown to significantly reduce the magnitude and incidence of intraocular pressure elevations following argon laser trabeculoplasty.[18, 19] If *para*-aminoclonidine is contraindicated, the patient can be given a carbonic anhydrase inhibitor or an osmotic agent such as oral glycerin or isosorbide.

Topical anesthesia with 0.5 percent proparacaine hydrochloride is usually adequate anesthesia. In very rare circumstances, poor patient cooperation or nystagmus may require retrobulbar anesthesia.

Table 139–2. PREOPERATIVE PREPARATION

Informed consent
Continue antiglaucoma medications
Para-aminoclonidine (Iopidine) 1 hr preoperatively
Proparacaine
Position the patient comfortably
Contact lens placement

Table 139–3. TECHNIQUE OF ARGON LASER TRABECULOPLASTY

Laser power	700–1200 mW
Duration	0.1 sec
Spot size	50 μ
Placement of burns	Anterior trabecular meshwork
Tissue reaction	Blanching, minimal bubble formation
Number of burns	50 over 180 degrees of trabecular meshwork circumference

The laser energy is delivered to the trabecular meshwork through a mirrored contact lens that has been filled with methylcellulose and placed on the cornea. Typically, the dome-shaped mirror angled at 59 degrees on the Goldmann three-mirror lens is used. The Ritch trabeculoplasty lens[20] is also available.

The initial laser settings are 0.1-sec duration, 50-μ spot size, and 800-mW power (Table 139–3). The desired reaction to the laser treatment is a blanching of the trabecular meshwork with or without minimal bubble formation (Fig. 139–1). The power setting is adjusted between 700 and 1200 mW to achieve this response. If only blanching is obtained with a laser burn, the reaction is adequate and no higher energy is necessary. Large bubble formation and pigment scattering indicate that the power is too high and should be lowered. Occasionally, the trabecular meshwork is very pale, and even 1200 mW power causes no discernible tissue reaction. In this situation, the trabeculoplasty session should be completed with the 1200-mW power. During a treatment session the power may need to be adjusted because the trabecular meshwork pigmentation can vary over its circumference. The power necessary to elicit the desired reaction is typically inversely proportional to the amount of pigmentation in the trabecular meshwork.

The laser burns are placed at the anterior half of the trabecular meshwork, straddling the junction of the pigmented and nonpigmented trabecular meshwork

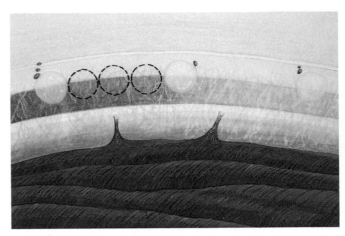

Figure 139–2. The laser burns are placed at the anterior half of the trabecular meshwork, straddling the junction of the pigmented and the nonpigmented meshwork. The appropriate spacing between laser burns and the effect of trabecular meshwork pigmentation on tissue reaction are also demonstrated.

(Fig. 139–2). Placement of burns in the anterior region of the trabecular meshwork minimizes both the postlaser intraocular rise and the postlaser formation of peripheral anterior synechiae.

Adequate visualization of the angle structures and precise focusing of the laser during the procedure are important. If the angle is narrow and visualization is difficult, a laser iridectomy will deepen the angle and facilitate the trabeculoplasty. Fine-focusing of the laser beam on the trabecular meshwork can be performed by movement of the hand holding the goniolens in conjunction with the slit-lamp control lever. A properly focused beam is important for adequate energy delivery and appears perfectly round.

Approximately 40 to 50 laser burns are placed over 180 degrees of the trabecular meshwork or 80 to 100 burns over 360 degrees. While Wise and Witter[12] initially administered 100 to 120 laser burns over the circumference of the trabecular meshwork, postlaser intraocular pressure increases were found to be a complication.[21–24] Further studies determined that the application of 50 burns over 180 or 360 degrees of the trabecular meshwork minimized the magnitude of the postlaser intraocular pressure increase and still provided long-term intraocular pressure reduction.[21, 24–27]

After argon laser trabeculoplasty (Table 139–4), *para*-aminoclonidine, which had been given 1 hr preoperatively, is administered again at the conclusion of the procedure. The intraocular pressure is then monitored for 1 to 3 hr. Any intraocular pressure elevations are treated as necessary to protect the optic nerve and visual

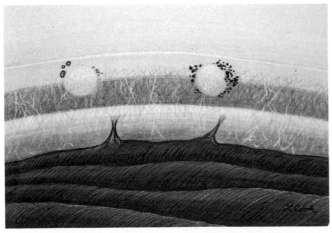

Figure 139–1. The desired tissue reaction is blanching of the trabecular meshwork, with or without minimal bubble formation, demonstrated on the left. The laser burn on the right demonstrates excessive pigment scattering, and the power should be reduced.

Table 139–4. POSTOPERATIVE MANAGEMENT

Para-aminoclonidine (Iopidine)
Continue antiglaucoma medications
Topical corticosteroids four times daily for 3 to 5 days
Measure intraocular pressure 1 hr, 24 hr, 1 wk, 4 to 6 wk, more frequently as necessary

field. The patient's preoperative glaucoma medications are continued, and topical steroids, such as 1 percent prednisolone or fluoromethalone, are prescribed about four times daily for 3 to 5 days. The patient is evaluated on the first postoperative day, at 1 wk, again at 4 to 6 wk, or sooner if the severity of the glaucoma requires it.

Complications

Complications of argon laser trabeculoplasty are fortunately relatively uncommon and usually transient. The most serious postlaser complication is elevated intraocular pressure that may cause optic nerve damage or visual field loss. Other complications include decreased vision, pain, corneal burns, hemorrhage, peripheral anterior synechiae, iritis, and a possible adverse effect on filtration surgery (Table 139–5).

Elevated Intraocular Pressure. Some level of intraocular pressure elevation occurs commonly following laser trabeculoplasty. Frequently the intraocular pressure increase is transient and less than 5 mmHg, although a small percentage of eyes can have increases greater than 20 mmHg that may be associated with loss of visual field.[24, 26] In the Glaucoma Laser Trial, 34 percent of eyes had an intraocular pressure increase of more than 5 mmHg, and 12 percent had an increase of more than 10 mmHg.[28] Most of these increases were detectable 1 hr after treatment, but a small percentage of eyes had intraocular pressure increases greater than 5 mmHg at 4 hr despite no such elevation at 1 hr.

The magnitude and frequency of elevated intraocular pressure seems to be related to the amount of treatment administered, the amount of pigmentation in the trabecular meshwork, the laser power, and placement of the laser burns. Weinreb and associates[24, 29] demonstrated that the incidence as well as the magnitude of the postoperative rise in pressure was significantly greater in eyes that had received 100 laser burns over 360 degrees compared with 50 laser burns over 180 degrees. The Glaucoma Laser Trial found that moderate or heavy pigmentation of the trabecular meshwork was the strongest risk factor for pressure increases after argon laser trabeculoplasty. Elevations of more than 10 mmHg were observed in 19 percent of eyes with moderate or heavy pigmentation in comparison with 5 percent in eyes with no pigmentation and 8 percent in eyes with mild pigmentation. Whereas the Glaucoma Laser Trial

Table 139–5. POSTOPERATIVE COMPLICATIONS OF ARGON LASER TRABECULOPLASTY

Elevated intraocular pressure
Decreased visual acuity or visual field
Pain
Corneal burns
Hemorrhage
Peripheral anterior synechiae
Iritis
Adverse effect on filtration surgery

found no correlation between intraocular pressure increases and laser power, Rouhiainen found that intraocular pressure increases greater than 10 mmHg were associated with laser power settings of 900 mW compared with power settings of 500 to 700 mW.[30] The intraocular pressure decrease 1 wk after treatment was not statistically different in the three groups. The incidence of postlaser increases in intraocular pressure is also lower when burns are placed along the anterior portion of the trabecular meshwork than when they are placed posteriorly.[25, 31]

Histopathologic examination of eyes with persistent, medically unresponsive elevation of intraocular pressure following argon laser trabeculoplasty has revealed an inflammatory response essentially confined to the trabecular meshwork.[32] The intraocular pressure increase may have resulted from inflammatory cells and debris obstructing the trabecular meshwork and reducing aqueous outflow facility. One clinical study observed that eyes with postlaser intraocular pressure increases had greater anterior chamber inflammation than eyes that had decreases in postlaser intraocular pressure.[24]

Many attempts have been made to prevent the immediate rise in postoperative intraocular pressure. Treatment with topical steroids or topical nonsteroidal antiinflammatory agents does not affect the postlaser intraocular pressure elevation.[33–37]

Para-aminoclonidine (Iopidine) administered 1 hr before and immediately after argon laser trabeculoplasty significantly reduces the frequency and magnitude of intraocular pressure increases.[18, 19] In one study, 10 percent of patients given *para*-aminoclonidine and 24 percent of patients given a placebo had an intraocular pressure spike greater than 5 mmHg after argon laser trabeculoplasty. If *para*-aminoclonidine is contraindicated, 4 percent pilocarpine,[38] a carbonic anhydrase inhibitor, or an osmotic agent may be administered to reduce the risk of an intraocular pressure increase. However, one study compared the efficacy of *para*-aminoclonidine, pilocarpine 4 percent, timolol maleate 0.5 percent, dipivefrin 0.1 percent, and acetazolamide 250 mg and found that *para*-aminoclonidine was significantly more effective in reducing the frequency of intraocular increases greater than 5 mmHg than the other antiglaucoma medications.[39]

Decreased Visual Acuity. Decreased visual acuity is usually a transient problem following argon laser trabeculoplasty and is usually caused by the goniosolution and laser flash. Occasionally, hemorrhage into the anterior chamber and iritis can be significant enough to cause decreased vision until they resolve. Visual acuity or visual field may be permanently lost by significantly elevated intraocular pressure following argon laser trabeculoplasty.[24, 26]

Pain. Discomfort is usually minimal during and following argon laser trabeculoplasty. Topical anesthesia with 0.5 percent proparacaine is almost always adequate anesthesia during the procedure. Marked iritis may cause some ocular discomfort following argon laser trabeculoplasty until it is controlled.

Corneal Burns. Corneal endothelial and epithelial

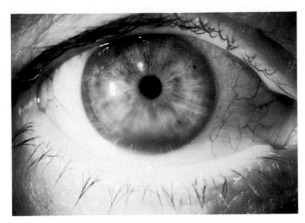

Figure 139–3. Hyphema after argon laser trabeculoplasty.

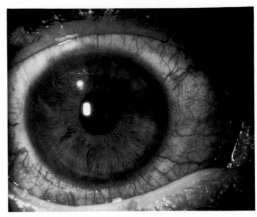

Figure 139–5. Inflammation after laser trabeculoplasty to the inferior 180 degrees of the trabecular meshwork.

burns are very uncommon with argon laser trabeculoplasty. They are more frequently seen with laser iridectomy. If they occur, they are transient and resolve within a few days. No significant change in central corneal endothelial cell density has been observed following argon laser trabeculoplasty.[40]

Hemorrhage. Hemorrhage into the anterior chamber uncommonly occurs during argon laser trabeculoplasty (Fig. 139–3). Bleeding may result from reflux of blood from Schlemm's canal or inadvertent photocoagulation of an iris root vessel or a circumferential ciliary vessel. Any bleeding is usually easily controlled by increasing pressure on the contact lens. Low-power photocoagulations (200 mW, 200 μ, 0.2 sec) can be used to control bleeding from an identifiable site.

Peripheral Anterior Synechiae. Peripheral anterior synechiae can be identified in as many as 46 percent of eyes treated with argon laser trabeculoplasty.[28] The peripheral anterior synechiae are characteristically small and peaked and may reach to the ciliary body band, scleral spur, or the trabecular meshwork (Fig. 139–4). Formation of peripheral anterior synechiae has been associated with posterior laser burns[28, 41] and higher power burns.[42] In one study, 43 percent of eyes receiving burns to the posterior trabecular meshwork developed peripheral anterior synechiae, whereas only 12 percent of eyes receiving burns to the anterior trabecular meshwork developed peripheral anterior synechiae.[41] Rouhiainen found that 40 percent of eyes treated with 800 mW of laser power developed peripheral anterior synechiae, whereas only 22 percent of eyes treated with 500 mW of laser power developed the synechiae.[42] The formation of peripheral anterior synechiae has variably been reported to have no effect on intraocular pressure reduction by argon laser trabeculoplasty[41] and to be associated with a significantly smaller intraocular pressure reduction.[42]

Iritis. Anterior iritis is very common following argon laser trabeculoplasty (Fig. 139–5),[43] and all patients are treated routinely with topical corticosteroids for 3 to 5 days. The iritis is usually mild and clears rapidly. Occasionally, the inflammation may be prolonged and may be associated with elevated intraocular pressure. A transient postlaser breakdown in the blood-aqueous barrier, as measured by fluorophotometry,[44] accompanies the inflammation. Occasionally, the only sign of inflammation may be the presence of trabecular precipitates observed gonioscopically.[45]

Effect on Filtration Surgery. One of the concerns about argon laser trabeculoplasty and the inflammation of the trabecular meshwork that it produces[32] has been that the procedure could adversely affect glaucoma-filtering surgery. Richter and associates[46] and Feldman and coworkers[47] found that the formation of encapsulated blebs following filtration surgery was associated with prior argon laser trabeculoplasty. Further studies are needed to determine if a causal relationship exists.

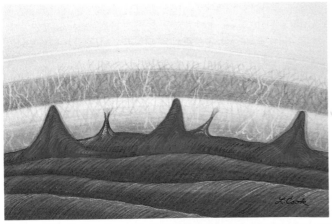

Figure 139–4. Small, peaked peripheral anterior synechiae can complicate argon laser trabeculoplasty.

Efficacy

Short-Term Efficacy. Intraocular pressure reduction does not usually occur immediately after laser trabeculoplasty but evolves over several days and weeks. The intraocular pressure reduction that may be present at 24 hr is frequently accompanied by iritis, and the contribution of this inflammation to the initial hypotensive effect is unknown. By 4 to 6 wk, however, the iritis is usually resolved, and any intraocular pressure reduction caused by the procedure is apparent.[33, 35, 37]

The efficacy of laser trabeculoplasty in controlling intraocular pressure for less than 1 yr has variously been reported to range from 65 to 97 percent. The success of laser trabeculoplasty may vary with treatment technique, prelaser intraocular pressure, aphakic or phakic status, age, race, and type of glaucoma.

Technique variations in laser trabeculoplasty that may affect the outcome of laser trabeculoplasty include the laser wavelength, laser power, location of treatment, and the number of laser burns applied. Laser trabeculoplasty is usually performed with the argon blue (488 nm) or argon green (514.5 nm) as the source of laser energy. However, the monochromatic green (514.5 nm),[48] the krypton red (647.1 nm) or yellow (568.2 nm) lasers,[49] the Nd.YAG laser (used without puncturing the trabecular meshwork),[50] and the diode laser (805 nm)[51] result in equivalent intraocular pressure reductions. Laser power[52] and placement of laser burns[53] do not appear to affect the hypotensive effect of argon laser trabeculoplasty.

Wise and Witter initially performed argon laser trabeculoplasty with 120 burns to the circumference of the trabecular meshwork.[12] However, as previously mentioned, postlaser intraocular pressure spikes were a complication, and it was found that applying 50 burns to the trabecular meshwork over 180 or 360 degrees of the angle reduced the immediate postlaser intraocular pressure increases but still provided significant longer-term intraocular pressure reduction and glaucoma control.[21, 24–27] Wilensky and Weinreb found that only 25 burns to one quadrant of the trabecular meshwork could result in a significant decrease in intraocular pressure in some eyes but that the results were more variable than with 50 burns over one half of the trabecular meshwork.[54]

If half-circumference treatment has been performed and additional pressure reduction is necessary, treatment of the untreated trabecular meshwork with argon laser trabeculoplasty may be beneficial. Horns and associates,[21] Klein,[55] and Thomas[26, 27] found similar success rates between eyes treated with 100 spots over 360 degrees in one session and eyes treated with 50 spots over 180 degrees in each of two sessions.

The absolute amount of intraocular pressure reduction by laser trabeculoplasty is frequently directly related to the prelaser intraocular pressure. Eyes with higher initial intraocular pressures often have a greater absolute decrease in intraocular pressure as a result of the procedure. However, eyes with very high prelaser intraocular pressures may require very large decreases in pressure for adequate glaucoma control, and the large decreases as a result of laser trabeculoplasty may still not be adequate to provide this control. Thomas demonstrated an intraocular pressure reduction of 40 to 50 percent,[21] and Schwartz demonstrated a 39 percent decrease[56] in eyes with intraocular pressures exceeding 30 mmHg. Eyes with pretreatment intraocular pressures below 20

mmHg had a mean decline of only 3 to 4 percent. When pretreatment intraocular pressures were between 20 and 29 mmHg, the mean decrease was between 6 and 10 mmHg and the initial success rate was 70 to 90 percent.

Aphakic eyes respond less well to argon laser trabeculoplasty than phakic eyes. Thomas demonstrated a mean decrease of 2 mmHg in aphakic eyes with open-angle glaucoma and a mean decrease of 7 mmHg in phakic eyes with open-angle glaucoma following argon laser trabeculoplasty.[27] Controlled data are not available comparing the effect of argon laser trabeculoplasty in pseudophakic eyes with phakic eyes.

The age of the patient affects the results of laser trabeculoplasty. Patients over 40 yr of age respond much more favorably than do younger patients with success rates reported near 90 percent.[27, 57, 58] Race does not appear to affect the short-term efficacy of laser trabeculoplasty[59] but may affect the long-term efficacy[60] with black patients who have a lower long-term success rate than do white patients.

The type of glaucoma also significantly influences the efficacy of laser trabeculoplasty. Primary open-angle glaucoma, glaucoma with the exfoliation syndrome,[21, 61–64] and pigmentary glaucoma[65] frequently have good intraocular pressure reductions and glaucoma control from argon laser trabeculoplasty. However, both the glaucoma associated with exfoliation syndrome and with the pigmentary dispersion syndrome may have sudden late failure of glaucoma control months following laser trabeculoplasty. Patients who have had prior glaucoma filtering surgery but have failing filtering blebs may have good intraocular pressure reductions with argon laser trabeculoplasty and control of their glaucoma.[66]

Glaucoma associated with intraocular inflammation usually does not respond well to argon laser trabeculoplasty,[21, 61, 62] although Thomas[27] reported success in three of four treated eyes. Argon laser trabeculoplasty may exacerbate the uveitis and should be used cautiously.

Patients with angle-recession glaucoma[27, 67] and glaucoma associated with the Sturge-Weber syndrome[61, 67] may have variable results with argon laser trabeculoplasty. Eyes with congenital[62, 67] or juvenile[21, 57, 68] glaucoma, iridocorneal endothelial syndrome,[27, 67] and trabeculodysgenesis[27, 67] have not had good results with laser trabeculoplasty.

Long-Term Efficacy of Argon Laser Trabeculoplasty. The excellent short-term results of laser trabeculoplasty do abate somewhat with longer follow-up, but the procedure still provides intraocular pressure control for many patients for several years. Wise reported glaucoma control in 73 percent of patients 4 yr after treatment.[69] Schwartz and associates,[60] Grinich and associates,[70] and Shingleton and coworkers[71] reported a decline in successful glaucoma control to 46 percent at 5 yr, 59 percent at 3 yr, and 52 percent at 4 yr, respectively. Schwartz also found that the success rate for black patients after 3 yr was 32 percent but was 65 percent for white patients. Ticho found a 55-percent success rate at 6 yr that then remained stable through 10 yr of follow-up.[72] The results of these studies demonstrate that the efficacy of argon laser trabeculoplasty in controlling glaucoma decreases with duration of follow-up, but also that argon laser trabeculoplasty continues to provide glaucoma control after 4 yr for approximately half the patients.

Efficacy of Retreatment. Retreatment with argon laser trabeculoplasty means additional laser therapy to the trabecular meshwork after the entire circumference of trabecular meshwork has been treated, whether in one or two sessions. If only one half of the trabecular meshwork has been treated and the glaucoma again becomes uncontrolled, additional therapy to the untreated meshwork is indicated and is frequently effective in lowering intraocular pressure[21, 26, 27, 55] but is not referred to as retreatment. The results of studies of the efficacy of argon laser trabeculoplasty retreatment when the entire trabecular meshwork circumference has been previously treated are variable.

In studies of eyes that had initially successful glaucoma control by argon laser trabeculoplasty but had a return of elevated intraocular pressure, Messner reported 36 percent of eyes had a 15 percent reduction in intraocular pressure at 6 wk, but only 21 percent had such a reduction at 6 mo.[73] Brown reported a 38-percent success rate in glaucoma control with argon laser trabeculoplasty retreatment, but that 12 percent of the treated eyes had intraocular pressure increases 10 mmHg or greater necessitating urgent surgical intervention.[74] Richter reported that 32 percent of eyes retreated were successfully controlled.[75] In eyes with initially unsuccessful laser trabeculoplasty, Starita found that 35 percent of patients had an intraocular pressure reduction of at least 3 mmHg.[76] However, Weber reported a 70-percent success rate at 1 yr with retreatment,[77] and Jorizzo found that 73 percent of eyes had a significant intraocular pressure reduction after repeat laser trabeculoplasty.[78]

These studies demonstrate that argon laser trabeculoplasty retreatment can lower intraocular pressure and provide glaucoma control for some patients, but the results are more variable and less predictable than with initial treatment. Consequently, retreatment should be performed cautiously. Patients who need urgent intraocular pressure control to prevent visual loss may need glaucoma surgery rather than argon laser trabeculoplasty retreatment.

Histology

The morphologic changes in the trabecular meshwork immediately following argon laser trabeculoplasty have been studied in nonglaucomatous cynomolgus monkeys and in human specimens obtained at trabeculectomy. In monkey eyes, Melamed and associates[79] found coagulative necrosis of treated trabecular meshwork 1 hr after treatment with disruption of trabecular beams and fragmented cells and fibrocellular tissue debris in the juxtacanalicular meshwork (Figs. 139–6 and 139–7). Many endothelial cells were rounded up, and some were actively phagocytic. Four weeks after treatment, the treated spots were detected as regions of flattened and collapsed beams covered by a cellular sheet extending

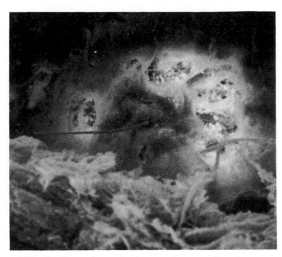

Figure 139–6. Scanning electron micrograph of argon laser trabeculoplasty lesion immediately after treatment in a cynomolgus monkey. Coagulative damage with adjacent tears of the corneal endothelium is demonstrated. (Courtesy of S. Melamed, M.D.)

from the corneal endothelium (Fig. 139–8).[80] The inner wall of Schlemm's canal beneath these regions was flat, and no vacuoles were present. Adjacent nonlasered spots had wide-open intertrabecular spaces with herniations of juxtacanalicular trabecular meshwork and of inner wall endothelium into and across the lumen of Schlemm's canal. The herniations contained chronic inflammatory cells and large vacuoles.

Specimens of human trabecular meshwork after argon laser trabeculoplasty obtained at trabeculectomy demonstrates changes similar to those seen in monkey eyes.[81]

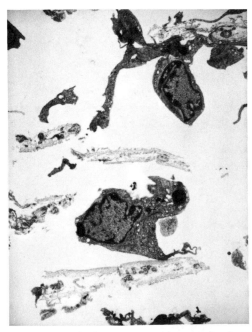

Figure 139–7. Transmission electron micrograph of argon laser trabeculoplasty lesion immediately after treatment in a cynomolgus monkey. Coagulative damage to the trabecular meshwork is demonstrated. (Courtesy of S. Melamed, M.D.)

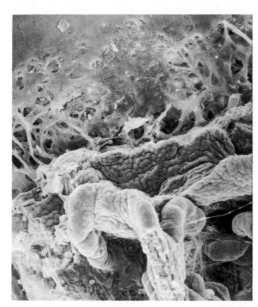

Figure 139–8. Scanning electron micrograph of argon laser trabeculoplasty lesion 4 weeks after treatment in a cynomolgus monkey. Flattening of the trabecular meshwork with extension of the corneal endothelium over the scarred lasered region is demonstrated. (Courtesy of S. Melamed, M.D.)

Early changes consisted of disruption of the trabecular beams and accumulation of cellular and fibrinous debris. The corneal endothelial cells adjacent to the laser burn showed extension of cytoplasmic processes, cytoplasmic edema, and nuclear irregularity. One week after treatment, shrinkage of treated uveal and corneoscleral trabecular meshwork occurred in a 50- to 60-μ area, with nontreated areas appearing normal. After 6 mo to 1 yr, tissues demonstrated confluent areas of fibrosis and abnormally migrating corneal endothelial cells lining the uveal meshwork and occluding the trabecular spaces.

Pathophysiology

The intraocular pressure reduction after argon laser trabeculoplasty is caused by an increase in aqueous outflow facility.[43, 82] The mechanism for this increased outflow resistance has variously been explained by a shrinkage of the inner trabecular ring and by a biologic response of the trabecular cells.

Wise initially proposed that argon laser trabeculoplasty caused shrinkage of the inner trabecular ring, resulting in separation of the trabecular sheets and opening of the aqueous channels in the trabecular meshwork.[12, 69] According to this hypothesis, multiple burns would displace the entire inner portion of the meshwork toward the anterior chamber. Schlemm's canal would be prevented from collapsing. However, in studies of 23 pairs of enucleated eyes examined equidistant between argon laser trabeculoplasty burns, no effect could be demonstrated on the cross-sectional area of Schlemm's canal or the development of its collapse.[83]

Van Buskirk has suggested that the increased facility of outflow and reduced intraocular pressure following argon laser trabeculoplasty is due to a biologic response by the trabecular endothelial cells. Trabecular meshwork preserved in organ culture and treated with laser trabeculoplasty had an alteration in the turnover or synthesis of glycosaminoglycans.[84] In addition, trabecular cell division and migration were studied using organ culture trabecular meshwork exposed to tritiated thymidine following 180-degree argon laser trabeculoplasty. Nonburned areas of the trabecular meshwork showed a marked incorporation of thymidine into trabecular-cell DNA 2 days after laser trabeculoplasty.[84, 85] The cell division indicated by this thymidine incorporation occurred predominantly in the anterior, nonfiltering region of the trabecular meshwork where it inserts into the cornea beneath Schwalbe's line. Two weeks after trabeculoplasty, the labeled cells became concentrated in the burn sites. Based on these observations, the authors suggested that the laser burns are repopulated by dividing trabecular cells and that these cells have migrated into the burn sites from a distant site, primarily the region of Schwalbe's line. The effect of an alteration in glycosaminoglycans or cell migration from the region of Schwalbe's line on intraocular pressure remains unclear.

ND.YAG LASER TRABECULOPUNCTURE

The Nd.YAG laser has been used to create an opening through the trabecular meshwork into Schlemm's canal in an effort to lower intraocular pressure. Epstein and associates found that the intraocular pressure reduction observed in adult patients was transient.[86] However, two eyes with juvenile open-angle glaucoma had dramatic intraocular pressure reductions. Robin and Pollack performed Nd.YAG laser trabeculopuncture on 22 eyes.[87] They reported significant intraocular pressure reductions at 3 mo and glaucoma control in 46 percent of eyes at 1 yr. Postoperative complications included intraocular pressure elevation, bleeding from the angle, and posterior displacement of the iris root. Further studies are needed to determine if this procedure will be a valuable adjunct in the management of open-angle glaucoma.

REFERENCES

1. Krasnov MM: Q-switched laser goniopuncture. Arch Ophthalmol 92:37, 1974.
2. Krasnov MM: Laseropuncture of anterior chamber angle in glaucoma. Am J Ophthalmol 75:674, 1973.
3. Robin AL, Pollack IP: The Q-switched ruby laser in glaucoma. Ophthalmology 91:366, 1984.
4. Wickham MG, Worthen DM: Argon laser trabeculotomy: Long-term follow-up. Ophthalmology 86:495, 1979.
5. Worthen DM, Wickham MG: Argon laser trabeculotomy. Trans Am Acad Ophthalmol Otolaryngol 78:371, 1974.
6. Ticho U, Zauberman H: Argon laser application to the angle structures in the glaucomas. Arch Ophthalmol 94:61, 1976.
7. Demailly P, Haut J, Bonnet-Boutier M: Trabeculotomie au laser à l'argon (note préliminaire). Bull Soc Ophthalmol Fr 73:259, 1973.
8. Hager H: Besondere mikrochirurgische Engriffe. II: Derste Drfahrungen mit der Argon-laser-gerat 800. Klin Monatsbl Augenheilkd 163:437, 1973.

9. Vogel MH, Schildberg P: Histologische Fruhergebnisse nach experimenteller laser Trabekulopunktur. Lkin Monatsbl Augenheilkd 163:353, 1973.

10. Zweng HC, Flocks M: Experimental photocoagulation of the anterior chamber angle: A preliminary report. Am J Ophthalmol 52:163, 1961.

11. Gaasterland D, Kupfer C: Experimental glaucoma in the rhesus monkey. Invest Ophthalmol 13:455, 1974.

12. Wise JB, Witter SL: Argon laser therapy for open angle glaucoma: A pilot study. Arch Ophthalmol 97:319, 1979.

13. Migdal C, Hitchings R: Primary therapy for chronic simple glaucoma: The role of argon laser trabeculoplasty. Trans Ophthalmol Soc UK 104:62, 1984.

14. Rosenthal AR, Chaudhuri PR, Chiapella AP: Laser trabeculoplasty primary therapy in open angle-glaucoma: A preliminary report. Arch Ophthalmol 102:699, 1984.

15. Thomas JV, El-Mofty A, Hamdy EE, et al: Argon laser trabeculoplasty as initial therapy for glaucoma. Arch Ophthalmol 102:702, 1984.

16. Zborowski L, Ritch R, Podos SM, et al: Prognostic features in laser trabeculoplasty. Acta Ophthalmol 62:142, 1984.

17. Glaucoma Laser Trial Research Group: The glaucoma laser trial (GLT). 2: Results of argon laser trabeculoplasty versus topical medicines. Ophthalmology 97:1403, 1990.

18. Robin AL, Pollack IP, House B, et al: Effect of ALO 2145 on intraocular pressure following argon laser trabeculoplasty. Arch Ophthalmol 105:646, 1987.

19. Brown RH, Stewart RH, Lynch MG, et al: ALO 2145 reduces the intraocular pressure elevation after anterior segment laser surgery. Ophthalmology 95:378, 1988.

20. Ritch R: A new lens for argon laser trabeculoplasty. Ophthalmic Surg 16:331, 1985.

21. Horns DJ, Bellows AR, Hutchinson BT, et al: Argon laser trabeculoplasty for open angle glaucoma: A retrospective study of 380 eyes. Trans Ophthalmol Soc UK 103:288, 1983.

22. Hoskins HD, Hetherington J, Minckler DS: Complications of laser trabeculoplasty in primary open-angle glaucoma. Ophthalmology 90:796, 1983.

23. Krupin T, Kolker AE, Kass MA, et al: Intraocular pressure the day of argon laser trabeculoplasty in primary open-angle glaucoma. Ophthalmology 91:361, 1984.

24. Weinreb RN, Ruderman J, Juster R, et al: Immediate intraocular pressure response to argon laser trabeculoplasty. Am J Ophthalmol 95:279, 1983.

25. Lustgarten J, Podos SM, Ritch R, et al: Laser trabeculoplasty: A prospective study of treatment parameters. Arch Ophthalmol 102:517, 1984.

26. Thomas JV, Simmons RJ, Belcher CD: Complications of argon laser trabeculoplasty. Glaucoma 4:50, 1982.

27. Thomas JV, Simmons RJ, Belcher CD: Argon laser trabeculoplasty in the pre-surgical glaucoma patient. Ophthalmology 89:187, 1982.

28. Glaucoma Laser Trial Research Group: The Glaucoma Laser Trial. I: Acute effects of argon laser trabeculoplasty on intraocular pressure. Arch Ophthalmol 107:1135, 1989.

29. Weinreb RN, Ruderman J, Juster R, et al: Influence of the number of laser burns administered on the early results of argon laser trabeculoplasty. Am J Ophthalmol 95:287, 1983.

30. Rouhiainen HJ, Terasvirta ME, Tuovinen EJ: Laser power and postoperative intraocular pressure increase in argon laser trabeculoplasty. Arch Ophthalmol 105:1352, 1987.

31. Schwartz LW, Spaeth GL, Traverso C, et al: Variation of techniques on the results of argon laser trabeculoplasty. Ophthalmology 90:781, 1983.

32. Greenidge KC, Rodrigues MM, Spaeth GL, et al: Acute intraocular pressure elevation after argon laser trabeculoplasty and iridectomy: A clinicopathologic study. Ophthalmic Surg 15:105, 1984.

33. Ruderman JM, Zweig KO, Wilensky JT, et al: Effects of corticosteroid pretreatment on argon laser trabeculoplasty. Am J Ophthalmol 96:84, 1983.

34. Hotchkiss ML, Robin AL, Pollack IP, et al: Non-steroidal anti-inflammatory agents after argon laser trabeculoplasty: A trial with flurbiprofen and indomethacin. Ophthalmology 91:969, 1984.

35. Pappas HR, Berry DP, Partamian L, et al: Topical indomethacin therapy before argon laser trabeculoplasty. Am J Ophthalmol 99:571, 1985.

36. Weinreb RN, Drake MV: Treatment parameters of laser trabeculoplasty. Trans Pacific Coast Oto-Ophthalmol Soc 64:75, 1983.

37. Weinreb RN, Robin AL, Baerveldt G, et al: Flurbiprofen pretreatment in argon laser trabeculoplasty for primary open angle glaucoma. Arch Ophthalmol 102:1629, 1984.

38. Ofner S, Samples JR, Van Buskirk EM: Pilocarpine and the increase in intraocular pressure after trabeculoplasty. Am J Ophthalmol 97:647, 1984.

39. Robin AL: Argon laser trabeculoplasty medical therapy to prevent the intraocular pressure rise associated with argon laser trabeculoplasty. Ophthalmology 22:31, 1991.

40. Traverso C, Cohen EJ, Groden LR, et al: Central corneal endothelial cell density after argon laser trabeculoplasty. Arch Ophthalmol 102:1322, 1984.

41. Traverso CE, Greenidge KC, Spaeth GL: Formation of peripheral anterior synechiae following argon laser trabeculoplasty: A prospective study to determine relationship to position of laser burns. Arch Ophthalmol 102:861, 1984.

42. Rouhiainen HJ, Terasvirta ME, Tuovinen EJ: Peripheral anterior synechiae formation after trabeculoplasty. Arch Ophthalmol 106:189, 1988.

43. Wilensky JT, Jampol LM: Laser therapy for open angle glaucoma. Ophthalmology 88:213, 1981.

44. Feller DB, Weinreb RN: Breakdown and reestablishment of blood-aqueous barrier with laser trabeculoplasty. Arch Ophthalmol 102:537, 1984.

45. Fiore PM, Melamed S, Epstein DL: Trabecular precipitates and elevated intraocular pressure following argon laser trabeculoplasty. Ophthalmic Surg 20:697, 1989.

46. Richter CU, Shingleton BJ, Bellows AR, et al: The development of encapsulated filtering blebs. Ophthalmology 95:1163, 1988.

47. Feldman RM, Gross RL, Spaeth GL, et al: Risk factors for the development of Tenon's capsule after trabeculectomy. Ophthalmology 96:336, 1989.

48. Smith J: Argon laser trabeculoplasty: Comparison of bichromatic and monochromatic wavelengths. Ophthalmology 91:355, 1984.

49. Spurny RC, Lederer CM Jr: Krypton laser trabeculoplasty: A clinical report. Arch Ophthalmol 102:1626, 1984.

50. Del Priore LV, Robin AL, Pollack IP: Long-term follow-up of neodymium YAG laser angle surgery for open-angle glaucoma. Ophthalmology 95:277, 1988.

51. Schuman JS, Puliafito CA, Allingham RA, et al: A controlled clinical trial of diode versus argon laser trabeculoplasty. Ophthalmology 97(Suppl):143, 1990.

52. Rouhiainen H, Terasvirta M: The laser power needed for optimum results in argon laser trabeculoplasty. Acta Ophthalmol 64:254, 1986.

53. Rouhiainen HJ, Terasvirta ME, Tuovinen EJ: The effect of some treatment variables on the results of trabeculoplasty. Arch Ophthalmol 106:611, 1988.

54. Wilensky JT, Weinreb RN: Low-dose trabeculoplasty. Am J Ophthalmol 95:423, 1983.

55. Klein HZ, Shields MB, Ernest JT: Two-stage argon laser trabeculoplasty in open angle glaucoma. Am J Ophthalmol 99:392, 1985.

56. Schwartz AL, Whitter ME, Bleiman B, et al: Argon laser trabecular surgery in uncontrolled phakic open angle glaucoma. Ophthalmology 88:203, 1981.

57. Forbes M, Bansal RK: Argon laser goniophotocoagulation of the trabecular meshwork in open-angle glaucoma. Trans Am Ophthalmol Soc 79:257, 1981.

58. Safran MJ, Robin AL, Pollack IP: Argon laser trabeculoplasty in younger patients with primary open angle glaucoma. Am J Ophthalmol 97:292, 1984.

59. Krupin T, Patkin R, Kurata FK, et al: Argon laser trabeculoplasty in black and white patients with primary open-angle glaucoma. Ophthalmology 93:811, 1986.

60. Schwartz AL, Love DC, Schwartz MA: Long-term follow-up of argon laser trabeculoplasty for uncontrolled open angle glaucoma. Arch Ophthalmol 103:1482, 1985.

61. Lieberman MF, Hoskins HD, Hetherington J Jr: Laser trabeculoplasty and the glaucomas. Ophthalmology 90:790, 1983.

62. Robin AL, Pollack IP: Argon laser trabeculoplasty in secondary forms of open angle glaucoma. Arch Ophthalmol 101:382, 1983.

63. Logan P, Burke E, Joyce PD, et al: Laser trabeculoplasty in the pseudoexfoliation syndrome. Trans Ophthalmol Soc UK 103:586, 1983.

64. Pohjanpelto P: Late results of laser trabeculoplasty for increased intraocular pressure. Acta Ophthalmol 61:998, 1983.
65. Lunde MW: Argon laser trabeculoplasty in pigmentary dispersion syndrome with glaucoma. Am J Ophthalmol 96:721, 1983.
66. Fellman RL, Starita RJ, Spaeth GL, et al: Argon laser trabeculoplasty following failed trabeculectomy. Ophthalmic Surg 15:195, 1984.
67. Spaeth GL, Fellman RL, Starita RJ, et al: Argon laser trabeculoplasty in the treatment of secondary glaucoma. Trans Am Ophthalmol Soc 81:325, 1983.
68. Wilensky JT, Weinreb RN: Early and late failures of argon laser trabeculoplasty. Arch Ophthalmol 101:895, 1983.
69. Wise JB: Long-term control of adult open angle glaucoma by argon laser treatment. Ophthalmology 88:197, 1981.
70. Grinich NP, Van Buskirk EM, Samples JR: Three-year efficacy of argon laser trabeculoplasty. Ophthalmology 94:858, 1987.
71. Shingleton BJ, Richter CU, Bellows AR, et al: Long-term efficacy of argon laser trabeculoplasty. Ophthalmology 94:1513, 1987.
72. Ticho U, Nesher R: Laser trabeculoplasty in glaucoma: Ten-year evaluation. Arch Ophthalmol 107:844, 1989.
73. Messner D, Siegel LI, Kass MA, et al: Repeat argon laser trabeculoplasty. Am J Ophthalmol 103:113, 1987.
74. Brown SVL, Thomas JV, Simmons RJ: Laser trabeculoplasty retreatment. Am J Ophthalmol 99:8, 1985.
75. Richter CU, Shingleton BJ, Bellows AR, et al: Retreatment with argon laser trabeculoplasty. Ophthalmology 94:1085, 1987.
76. Starita RJ, Fellman RL, Spaeth GL, et al: The effect of repeating full-circumference argon laser trabeculoplasty. Ophthalmic Surg 15:41, 1984.
77. Weber PA, Burton GD, Epitropoulos AT: Laser trabeculoplasty retreatment. Ophthalmic Surg 10:702, 1989.
78. Jorizzo PA, Samples JR, Van Buskirk EM: The effect of repeat argon laser trabeculoplasty. Am J Ophthalmol 106:682, 1988.
79. Melamed S, Pei J, Epstein DL: Short-term effect of argon laser trabeculoplasty in monkeys. Arch Ophthalmol 103:1546, 1985.
80. Melamed S, Pei J, Epstein DL: Delayed response to argon laser trabeculoplasty in monkeys. Arch Ophthalmol 104:1078, 1986.
81. Rodrigues MM, Spaeth GL, Donahoo P: Electron microscopy of argon laser therapy in phakic open-angle glaucoma. Ophthalmology 89:198, 1982.
82. Yablonski ME, Cook DJ, Gray J: A fluorophotometric study of the effect of argon laser trabeculoplasty on aqueous humor dynamics. Am J Ophthalmol 99:579, 1985.
83. Van Buskirk EM, Pond V, Rosenquist RC, et al: Argon laser trabeculoplasty: Studies on mechanism of action. Ophthalmology 91:1005, 1984.
84. Bylsma SS, Samples JR, Acott TS, et al: Trabecular cell division after argon laser trabeculoplasty. Arch Ophthalmol 106:544, 1988.
85. Acott TS, Samples JR, Bradley JMB, et al: Trabecular repopulation by anterior trabecular meshwork cells after laser trabeculoplasty. Am J Ophthalmol 107:1, 1989.
86. Epstein DL, Melamed S, Puliafito CA, Steinert RF: Neodymium YAG laser trabeculopuncture in open-angle glaucoma. Ophthalmology 92:931, 1985.
87. Robin AL, Pollack IP: Q-switched neodymium-YAG laser angle surgery in open-angle glaucoma. Arch Ophthalmol 103:793, 1985.

Chapter 140

■

Laser Therapy of Angle-Closure Glaucoma

C. DAVIS BELCHER III and LINDA J. GREFF

LASER IRIDECTOMY

For more than 100 yr, ophthalmic surgeons have known that making a hole in the iris could be curative in many types of glaucoma. The elucidation of the pathophysiologic mechanisms of relative and absolute pupillary block in the primary and some secondary angle-closure glaucomas permits us to understand the role that a full-thickness iris coloboma plays in most angle-closure glaucomas.[1–3] In cases in which relative or absolute pupillary block is the mechanism of angle-closure, the creation of a full-thickness opening in the iris permits equalization of pressures in the anterior and posterior chambers and is curative if done before the iris becomes irreversibly attached to the trabecular meshwork and angle structures (peripheral anterior synechiae).

Although surgical iridectomy has been one of the most successful of all intraocular procedures, complications occur related to its performance. Such complications can include hemorrhage, infection, wound leak, flat anterior chamber, cataract, and assorted problems related to anesthesia and hospitalization. Laser iridectomy is a safe, effective, outpatient procedure that has essentially replaced surgical iridectomy in the ophthalmic armamentarium. All eye surgeons need an understanding of the techniques, advantages, and disadvantages of creating laser iridectomies.

The possibility of utilizing laser light to perform iridectomies was realized almost coincidentally with the development of the laser in 1960. It followed logically from the attempts of Meyer-Schwickerath and others, using broad-spectrum, incoherent light sources, such as the xenon arc lamp (or even the sun) to burn full-thickness openings in the iris.[4] Lens and corneal damage resulted from the long-duration burns required to create an iridectomy. Later investigators hoped that laser sources that produced more energy in a shorter time could overcome the problems of lens and corneal damage.[5–7] The first available laser (the pulsed ruby) had few problems but little success.[8–12] A decade of exploration of laser sources and interfacing systems preceded the appearance of commercially available argon laser instruments in the early 1970s.[13–17] Improvements in instrument reliability, power output, and focusing systems led to an investigative furor in the mid to late

Table 140–1. SUMMARY OF TECHNIQUES OF LASER IRIDECTOMY

Argon Laser Iridectomy
Short-pulse technique (for dark brown eyes)
   Time = 0.02–0.05 sec   Spot size = 50 μ*
   Power = 1000–1500   No. of applications = 50–100
   mW
Long-pulse technique (for blue, hazel, or light brown eyes)
   Time = 0.2 sec   Spot size = 50 μ
   Power = 1000 mW   No. of applications = 1–30

Nd.YAG† Laser Iridectomy (for blue to light brown eyes)
   Energy = 4–6 mJ   No. of applications = 1–4 bursts of
                                   1–4 pulses per burst

Argon + Nd.YAG (for dark brown eyes, difficult perforation or
  blood dyscrasia/anticoagulant therapy)
Argon thinning of iris
   Time = 0.02–0.05 sec   Spot size = 50 μ
   Power = 1000 mW   No. of applications = 5–25
Nd.YAG perforation
   Energy = 4–5 mJ   No. of applications = 1 burst of 2–4
                                  pulses per burst

Pretreatment Regimen
Miotics
Apraclonidine (30 min before laser)
Beta-blocker (optional)
Carbonic anhydrase inhibitor (optional)
Oral osmotic (rare)
Topical anesthetic

Posttreatment Regimen
Apraclonidine
Topical steroids qid × 3 days
Avoid miotics postlaser treatment if possible to avoid synechiae
Others prn

*Note that all laser settings listed assume concomitant contact lens use.
Power and duration should be increased accordingly if a lens is not used.
†Nd.YAG, neodymium-yttrium-aluminum-garnet.

1970s.[18–22] Despite the inertia all surgical advances must overcome, the success of these investigations made argon iridectomy a preferred alternative to surgical iridectomy.[23–29] Currently, the neodymium:yttrium-aluminum-garnet (Nd.YAG)[30–56] or combined argon and Nd.YAG iridectomy[57–62] supersede the argon laser alone, especially in certain clinical settings. Along the way it became obvious that other coherent light sources, such as the krypton laser, the Q-switched ruby laser, the organic dye laser, and the diode laser could create successful iridectomies in a safe and efficient fashion.[63–66] The lack of widespread availability of these instruments has limited their clinical utility.

Many techniques for the performance of laser iridectomy have evolved using the argon and Nd.YAG lasers that are available in the United States and Europe.[67–77]

In this chapter we present two techniques for argon laser iridectomy, a technique for Nd.YAG laser iridectomy, and a technique for combined argon and Nd.YAG laser iridectomy. Alternative approaches are available, but those described here have worked well in the authors' hands. The techniques are summarized in Table 140–1.

Indications

Argon laser iridectomy, Nd.YAG laser iridectomy, and the combined approach can be used as an alternative to surgical iridectomy in almost any situation in which iridectomy is necessary. Indications are listed in Table 140–2.

In some situations, it may be inadvisable or impossible to safely accomplish a laser iridectomy. In the setting of ongoing inflammation or rubeosis in which it is imperative to create a long-standing iridectomy, the surgical approach should probably best be chosen. This is a rare event at present.

In the presence of corneal edema or other corneal opacification, it may be impossible to obtain a clear view of the target tissue. Topical glycerin could be used to try to clear the cornea. A surgical iridectomy may have to be considered if the cornea does not clear adequately.

The patient who is unable to cooperate by maintaining firm fixation may present an undue hazard for the performance of this procedure unless a retrobulbar injection is chosen. Use of the Abraham or Wise contact lens may help.

In the presence of a shallow anterior chamber, it may be difficult to obtain a full-thickness hole without creating overlying corneal lesions that both prevent completion of the iridectomy and can potentially lead to permanent corneal changes.

Although aphakic or pseudophakic pupillary block is often cited as an excellent indication for laser iridectomy, it may be difficult to safely perform this procedure because the chamber may be shallow or flat. In cases like this, it is best to pick the deepest part of the anterior chamber and try to create an iridectomy in that location, even when it is not in the superior location or in the far periphery. Often the area immediately adjacent to the haptic of an anterior chamber lens is most satisfactory. Laser gonioplasty can also be tried in these situations (see later). Part of the difficulty in creating a successful iridectomy in this clinical situation is that the position of the hyaloid face with respect to the posterior iris surface is unknown. If an area is chosen for an iridectomy in which the hyaloid is adherent, it may be impossible for the aqueous to pass through if an iris

Table 140–2. INDICATIONS FOR LASER IRIDECTOMY

Angle-closure glaucoma
  Acute, subacute, chronic
Narrow "occludable" angle
Combined mechanism glaucoma
Imperforate surgical iridectomy
Pupillary block (iridovitreal block after cataract surgery)
Surgical iridectomy refused
Nanophthalmos
Surgical iridectomy cannot be safely performed
Fellow eye in malignant "ciliary block" glaucoma
Fellow eye after complicated surgical iridectomy
Suspected malignant "ciliary block" glaucoma

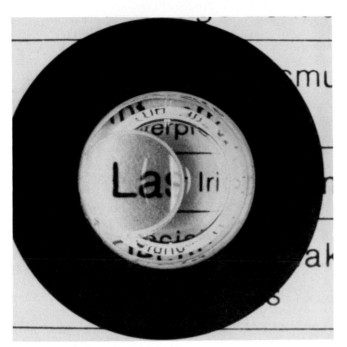

Figure 140–1. Abraham iridectomy lens.

hole alone is created. The adhesion of the anterior hyaloid to the posterior iris may prevent access of the aqueous to the iridectomy.

The Nd.YAG laser can be used in such cases to open the hyaloid.[2] It may be necessary to repeat the iridectomy several times because of recurrent vitreous occlusion in the postlaser period. Nd.YAG laser iridectomies alone or in combination may be better in eyes with "sticky" anterior segments, but no laser technique is uniformly successful in this setting. Additionally at times, aqueous seems to be sequestered in different quadrants, and more than one iridectomy may be necessary to achieve full deepening of the anterior chamber in different segments of the eye.

Technique

In the evolution of the argon iridectomy techniques, there have been a few momentous landmarks. The first was the introduction of the Abraham iridectomy lens,[70] as shown in Figure 140–1. This is a + 66.0-diopter button lens that decreases the spot size, thus increasing the power density. The second major advance was the realization of the importance of adequate miosis to give a thin and fixed target site. It was later realized that iridectomies created with high-power, long-duration burns (0.5 to 1 sec) enlarge greatly with time, and an opening that is initially small can become monstrous. When these were placed in the palpebral fissure, as many early iridectomies were, a second pupil could be created with undesirable optical effects (Fig. 140–2).

The successful creation of a laser iridectomy involves a series of steps, as listed in Table 140–3.

Miosis. All patients should be treated with pilocarpine 4 percent drops or an equivalent agent until the pupil is immobile. In most cases pilocarpine 4 percent administered every 5 min for three applications beginning 30 min to 1 hr before laser therapy accomplishes this goal. In dark brown irides, additional pilocarpine may be required. Patients already using miotics need to be examined to ensure that the pupil is, indeed, immobile and not reactive to light. This is best checked at the slit lamp. Miosis places the iris on stretch, thinning it to allow easier perforation and fixating it to prevent the iris from "flowing" toward the iridectomy site, especially with argon techniques. This unwanted iris movement can result in peaking of the pupil. Peaking can relieve pupillary block and permit the anterior chamber to deepen, giving a false sense of having created a full-thickness iridectomy.

Other Premedications. A serious potential complication of iridectomy is a posttreatment pressure spike.[78-81] Postlaser pressure spikes can occur with all photosurgical procedures done in the anterior segment of the eye, including iridectomy, trabeculoplasty, gonioplasty, and

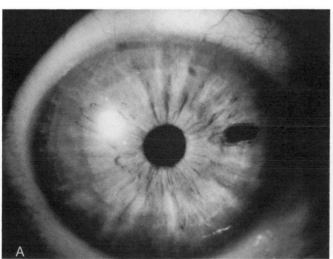

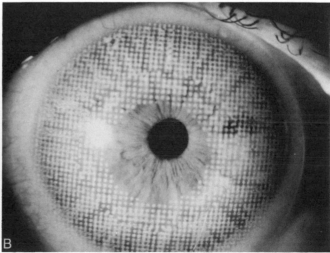

Figure 140–2. A, Large argon laser iridectomy in palpebral fissure caused unwanted optical effect. B, Elimination of unwanted optical effect ("second pupil") by application of cosmetic contact lens.

Table 140–3. SURGICAL SEQUENCE

Preoperative miotics (pilocarpine 4% q 5 min × 3)
Other premedication (apraclonidine, β-blocker, CAI*)
Anesthesia (proparacaine, cocaine, retrobulbar)
Use of contact lens (Abraham, Wise)
Choice of iridectomy site
Choice of laser and performance of iridectomy
Postoperative medications (topical, steroids)
Postoperative follow-up
    Same day—postlaser gonioscopy and dilatation
    24–48 hr—check IOP,† slit-lamp examination
    6 wk—check IOP, slit-lamp examination, gonioscopy

*CAI, carbonic anhydrase inhibitor.
†IOP, intraocular pressure.

capsulotomy. It is important to try to *prevent* pressure spikes from occurring and to treat them aggressively when they do occur.[82-85]

We routinely use apraclonidine 30 min to 1 hr before laser treatment. This is very helpful for preventing pressure spikes. Topical β-blockers and carbonic anhydrase inhibitors are also helpful. If the patient has advanced glaucoma with cupping and field loss, an oral osmotic agent (e.g., isosorbide) is additionally strongly considered.

The prelaser and postlaser techniques and medications for the Nd.YAG laser iridectomy or the combined argon and Nd.YAG iridectomy are essentially the same as for argon iridectomy only. One principal difference is that with the pure Nd.YAG approach, it is wise to be certain that patients are not taking anticoagulants, such as coumadin or aspirin, before doing the laser therapy. This laser functions primarily in a "cutting" mode and does not have the same coagulative effects on vessels as the argon laser.

Anesthesia. Topical anesthesia with proparacaine 0.5 percent or cocaine 4 percent is usually adequate. Retrobulbar anesthesia is very rarely required. With older laser techniques (e.g., Abraham's hump technique), the very long duration of the burns caused more pain and the potential for motion, and the use of retrobulbar anesthesia was somewhat more common. It is rarely used today.

Use of Contact Lens. The Abraham iridectomy lens (see Fig. 140–1) is essential in the production of iridectomies with the argon techniques.[70] It is very helpful in the Nd.YAG or combined argon and Nd.YAG approaches. Other contact lenses have been manufactured for this purpose, but the Abraham iridectomy lens is the benchmark against which they must be measured. A similar lens (the Wise lens) with a much stronger magnifying optic (+102 diopters) has also been introduced.[77] Many surgeons find this lens helpful; however, the great amount of magnification brought about gives a very limited depth of focus, and it is more difficult to use. It greatly augments the power of the laser impact, however, and is an excellent alternative lens for those skilled in its use.

The Abraham lens is a modified Goldmann type fundus lens with a flat glass plate bonded to its anterior surface. The glass plate has a +66.0-diopter plano

convex button bonded into a decentered 8-mm hole. The front surface of this lens is coated with an antireflective coating, which improves energy transmission by reducing reflecting losses and slightly increasing brightness and contrast to the transmitted image. When the laser beam is directed through the button of the Abraham lens, the beam spot size becomes approximately one half of that which would occur without the lens. By decreasing the diameter of the spot size at the iris level by a factor of two, the power and density increase by a factor of 4, thus facilitating the production of a full-thickness iris hole. The advantages of the use of this lens are: (1) the lens brings about concentration of energy at the iris level as mentioned earlier; (2) the lens acts as a heat sink, decreasing the number of epithelial corneal burns with the argon techniques; (3) the lens acts as a speculum, keeping the lids apart, allowing for easier treatment of the superior half of the iris; (4) the lens provides limited control of ocular movement; and (5) the lens provides magnification of the target site with less loss of depth of field, which occurs if magnification is increased by the use of the slit-lamp magnification controls.

It is possible to buy an Abraham iridectomy lens specifically designed for argon or Nd.YAG use, but in our experience, the one designed for the argon iridectomy can be used for both without difficulty.

Choice of Iridectomy Site. In general, iridectomies should be performed in the upper nasal quadrant, as close to the limbus as possible (Fig. 140–3). Late stretching with resultant enlargement of the iridectomy can occur. Placing the iridectomy under the lid helps to prevent a "second pupil" effect if hole enlargement occurs (see Fig. 140–2).

Initially, iridectomies were created approximately one third of the way from the limbus to the pupil, but with time, we have now realized that it is possible in many cases to go much further peripherally. Such placement usually hides the iridectomy under the peripheral corneal haze once miosis has worn off.

With argon techniques, it is important to avoid the position directly at 12 o'clock, because gas bubbles can preclude adequate visualization and make completion of the iridectomy in one sitting impossible. Usually a site at approximately a 1 o'clock position in a right eye

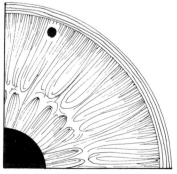

Figure 140–3. Ideal laser iridectomy location in the far periphery of one of the superior quadrants of the eye.

and an 11 o'clock position in a left eye is chosen. One iridectomy, if patent, is usually sufficient. Additionally, some believe that a target site in an iris crypt makes penetration easier.

With argon techniques, blue eyes can be challenging. A blue eye is a series of white cords with intervening gray stromal patches. It is most helpful if an area that is broad, dark, and gray is chosen as the target to allow for adequate absorption of laser energy. With blue eyes and utilizing the Nd.YAG laser only techniques, visible blood vessels should be avoided.

Adequate focusing requires a clear view. Patients with microcystic edema or mild Fuch's dystrophy can have a laser iridectomy successfully performed if clear areas of cornea are chosen. Glycerin, preceded by topical pro-paracaine 0.5 percent may be instilled directly on the eye or placed in the laser contact lens itself to aid in clearing the cornea. This should be done 5 to 15 min before using laser therapy. Antiglaucoma medications can also be tried.

With the use of the argon laser, direct the beam at all times away from the macula or optic nerve head to avoid inadvertent photocoagulation.

Performance of the Iridectomy

Argon Laser Iridectomy—Chipping Away Technique. The chipping away technique has two variants, one for the extremely dark brown eye (short-pulse) and the other for the caucasian eye (long-pulse). The short-pulse technique uses a time per laser impact one tenth that of the long-pulse technique. The shorter pulse prevents the formation of bubbles in the anterior chamber, which can impede completion of the iridectomy. Less pigment dispersion into the anterior chamber also results from the shorter application time.

The parameters for both techniques are listed in Table 140–4. With the considerations discussed earlier in mind, direct the laser beam at the chosen site with the beam centered in the button on the Abraham contact lens. The beam must also be as perpendicular to the lens as possible. Exact perpendicularity to the surface of the iris cannot be achieved, as the beam must be directed away from the posterior pole and angled either temporally or nasally. One or more burns are placed, and the reaction of the iris is judged. If an adequate reaction, indicated by good initial penetration of the depths of

Table 140–4. PARAMETERS FOR ARGON LASER IRIDECTOMY

Chipping Away Technique—Long Pulse (Light-Colored Irides)
Spot Size = 50 μ
Power = 700–1500 mW
Time = 0.2 sec
Applications = variable number (~ 1–30)

Chipping Away Technique—Short Pulse (Dark Brown Irides)
Spot Size = 50 μ
Power = 1000–1500 mW
Time = 0.02–0.05 sec
Applications = 50–100

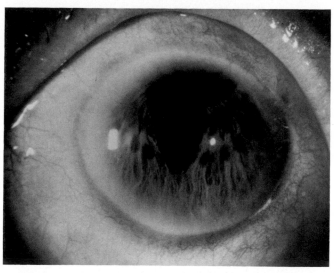

Figure 140–4. Optical iridectomy performed with neodymium-yttrium-aluminum-garnet (Nd.YAG) laser when argon laser pupilloplasty (see round burns on the iris surface) has failed.

the iris is achieved, further applications are superimposed one on top of another until full penetration is achieved. This requires many more laser applications with the short-pulse technique than with the long-pulse technique. Occasionally, it is necessary to increase the power. For unknown reasons, on rare occasions, there are seemingly "dead" areas on the surface of the iris, where it is impossible to perform an iridectomy. Fortunately, just a few laser applications at a nearby area usually successfully produce a full-thickness hole.

Additionally, there are a few extremely dark brown irides in which full-thickness perforation with the argon laser alone can be quite difficult. These are perhaps more suited for the combined technique discussed later.

During the production of argon iridectomies, bubbles may form. With patience on the part of the physician and the patient, these float up and out of the way. In general, laser iridectomy can be continued, firing the laser straight through the bubble at the target site. As full-thickness iris penetration is achieved, clouds of pigment liberated from the pigmented epithelium are washed forward as aqueous moves from the posterior chamber to the anterior chamber. Some people call this pigment streaming "smoke signals."

Nd.YAG Laser Iridectomy Technique. Since the rapid introduction of the Nd.YAG laser for posterior capsulotomies, many surgeons have used these instruments as well for laser iridectomies (Fig. 140–4). The principal reason for the rapid increase in popularity of the Nd.YAG iridectomy or the combined argon and Nd.YAG iridectomy is that iridectomies performed with this technique have a much lower incidence of closure in the postlaser period than do those performed with argon techniques only.[35, 36, 39, 48] In the absence of inflammation or rubeosis, it is rare for a well-performed Nd.YAG iridectomy or combined method iridectomy to close. In the presence of rubeosis or inflammation, it is highly likely that an iridectomy done by any laser technique will close, but one done by the combined

Table 140–5. PARAMETERS FOR ND.YAG* LASER IRIDECTOMY

Energy = 4–6 mJ
Applications = 1–4 bursts that contain 1–4 pulses per
burst

*Nd.YAG, neodymium-yttrium-aluminum-garnet.

argon and Nd.YAG technique has the least chance of closing because of its size and the mechanism of its production. Table 140–5 lists the parameters for the Nd.YAG laser iridectomy.

Nd.YAG laser techniques are dependent on the specific Nd.YAG laser unit available. Argon lasers are essentially a "commodity," and one behaves very much like another. This is not true with Nd.YAG lasers.

The authors use a Coherent 7970 Nd.YAG laser photodisruptor, which has the ability to produce up to three pulses in a row with an interval of 20 μsec between pulses. With lasers that can produce only a single shot, it may be necessary to use a greater initial energy (e.g., 10 mJ) to effectively bring about an iridectomy with Nd.YAG energy alone. The performance of an iridectomy with the Nd.YAG laser is straightforward. An upper nasal location is usually selected.

With a blue eye, the iridectomy can usually be accomplished with one burst of three shots at 5 to 6 mJ (Fig. 140–5). A second shot is rarely required.

With a light brown eye, the same parameters are usually effective, but more than one shot may be required. If subsequent shots are required and there is some question as to whether the iridectomy is patent, the authors choose to aim using single shots only at the edge of the iris defect to try to avoid any possibility of damaging the anterior lens capsule.

Most Nd.YAG lasers come with double helium-neon aiming beams. These beams are in general focused so that when the two visible helium neon spots come precisely together, optical breakdown takes place

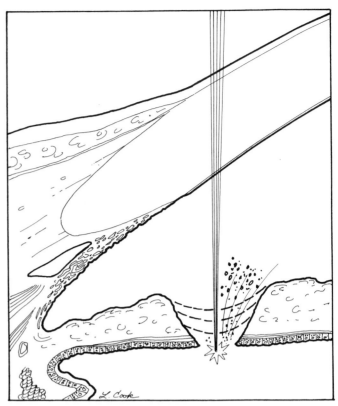

Figure 140–6. Nd.YAG iridectomy created by focusing deep into the stroma. Optical breakdown is produced, and the shock and acoustic waves cause the iridectomy to form.

slightly posteriorly. These instruments, however, are set for this to happen usually at relatively low energies somewhere between 1 and 2 mJ. As energy is increased on the Nd.YAG laser, the point of optical breakdown comes further forward and has moved markedly forward at the intermediate energy ranges of 4 to 6 mJ used for an iridectomy. For this reason, when performing an iridectomy, we bring the two helium neon spots together in precise focus in the depths of the iris stroma and then focus posteriorly, separating the dots slightly, thus bringing optical breakdown into focus approximately on the target stroma (Fig. 140–6). There is a certain imprecision built into this, and the exact point at which the iridectomy can be most efficiently achieved is determined with experience with each individual laser unit.

Argon and Nd.YAG Laser Combined Iridectomy. We prefer to use the argon and Nd.YAG combined

Table 140–6. PARAMETERS FOR COMBINED ARGON AND ND.YAG* LASER IRIDECTOMY

Argon Thinning of the Iris
Time = 0.02–0.05 sec
Power = 1000 mW
Spot Size = 50 μ
No. of Applications = 5–25

Nd.YAG Perforation of the Iris
Energy = 4–5 mJ
No. of Applications = 1 burst of 2–4 pulses per burst

*Nd.YAG, neodymium-yttrium-aluminum-garnet.

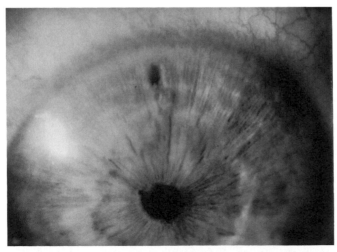

Figure 140–5. Nd.YAG laser iridectomy in a blue eye. When the pupil resumes its normal position, the iridectomy is located in the far periphery.

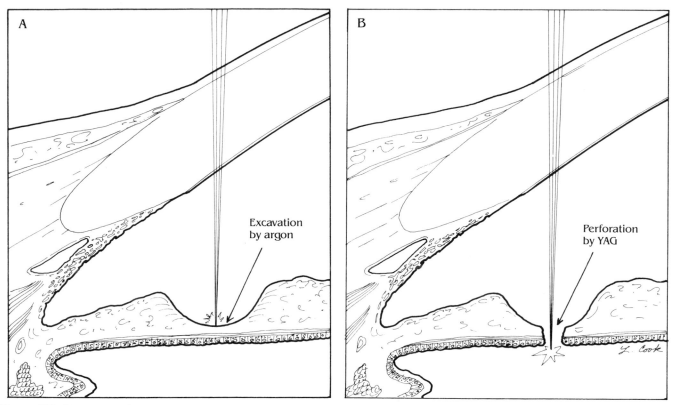

Figure 140–7. *A,* Approximately 80 percent of the surface of a thick brown iris is excavated with the use of the argon laser. *B,* The Nd.YAG laser is then used to perforate the remaining iris substance.

technique in both light and dark brown irides and to reserve the Nd.YAG only technique for blue eyes, for which it is the technique of choice.

With the combined technique, the argon laser is used with very short pulses to chip out a small opening down to two thirds to three fourths the depth of the iris stroma (Table 140–6). Then, the Nd.YAG laser completes the procedure, utilizing the same focusing caveats mentioned earlier (Fig. 140–7). This creates larger and "neater" iridectomies than the ragged ones seen in

deeply pigmented eyes created with the Nd.YAG laser alone (Fig. 140–8).[60]

The end-point of the iridectomy made with an argon laser should be visualization of the anterior lens capsule and a deepening of the anterior chamber. A false deepening, however, can occur with peaking of the pupil. The block resumes when the pupil resumes its normal configuration. Likewise, the observance of a bright red reflex, while encouraging, is not satisfactory, because there can still be a thin layer of overlying stroma

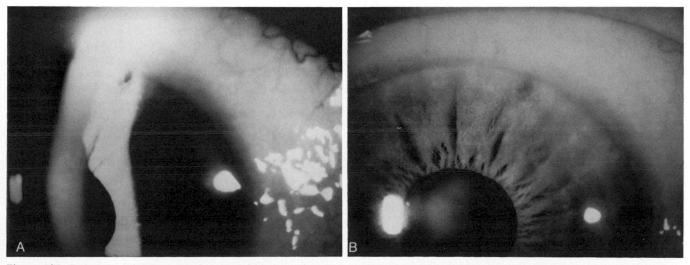

Figure 140–8. *A,* A combined-mechanism laser iridectomy in a dark brown eye. *B,* The location of the combined-mechanism iridectomy when the pupil resumes its normal size. Note its location in the far periphery under the peripheral limbal haze.

impermeable to aqueous. Visualization of the lens capsule ensures a full-thickness opening. Isolated, small stromal strands bridging the wound should be ignored. Small amounts of pigment in the base can be removed by chipping them away, but often this only rearranges them in the opening and does not result in their removal. If, after a few attempts at removing pigment from the base of the hole, success is not achieved, the procedure should be terminated and a new site should be selected.

With a Nd.YAG laser iridectomy, a direct view of the small iris opening is sufficient. It is not necessary (nor is it usually possible) to view the lens capsule through a hole made with this technique.

Although a rare situation, if penetration is not achieved in any site, the patient can be asked to return in 1 or 2 wk, and repeated attempts can be made. It is often best to complete an iridectomy with the Nd.YAG laser if there is great difficulty achieving it with the argon laser alone.

Postlaser Treatment

The postlaser follow-up begins immediately after the laser iridectomy is completed. The intraocular pressure should be determined before the patient leaves the office, because pressure spikes are frequent. These usually subside within 48 hr.

Postlaser treatment depends on the general glaucoma status of the eye. Topical prednisolone acetate 1 percent is given four times a day for 3 days. Whenever possible, it is best to avoid the use of pilocarpine in the postlaser period, because this encourages the formation of posterior synechiae. A need for long-term glaucoma medication can be assessed when the result of the iridectomy becomes known.

The question of whether to dilate in the postlaser period is controversial. The angle is examined gonioscopically before and after dilatation, thus confirming the success of the iridectomy and excluding the possibility of a plateau iris syndrome.[86] With argon laser iridectomy, we prefer to dilate all patients immediately after laser therapy is completed if the anterior capsule is visualized and the angle is open. This prevents inflammatory material from causing posterior synechiae to develop from the pupil to the lens or from the edges of the iridectomy to the lens. In addition, there is typically pigment debris at the base of the iridectomy upon its completion, and this material frequently can be made to fall out merely by dilating the pupil. With Nd.YAG iridectomy or argon and Nd.YAG iridectomy, there is less tendency for posterior synechial formation, and dilatation immediately after laser treatment is used less frequently.

If dilatation fails to remove and loosen pigment debris from the iridectomy site and if there is danger that the hole may close, the patient may be returned immediately for laser therapy, and the debris is removed. This can be done either with argon laser therapy or with the very low energy Nd.YAG laser treatment.

The most critical reason for careful intermediate-term follow-up is the possibility of closure of initially successful iridectomies. This can happen up to 40 percent of the time with the argon technique.[35, 36, 48] This is the primary reason why Nd.YAG techniques have become increasingly popular.

Closure is defined as the defect becoming smaller by 50 percent or more and, thus, is not always a measure of true total closure. Closure, when it occurs, does so almost always within the first 6 to 8 wk after argon laser therapy, except in the case of patients with inflammatory eye disease or anterior segment neovascularization. In these disease states and rarely in other patients, closure of an initially successful iridectomy can occur at any time. Very rarely does an argon laser iridectomy close, however, after 6 wk, unless one of these two entities is present. If closure does occur, the iridectomy can be reopened using the parameters for the argon laser or Nd.YAG laser as listed in Table 140–7. We find that use of the Nd.YAG single pulse mode is most satisfactory.

Complications

The postlaser intraocular pressure spike and the potential for closure of laser iridectomies are the two biggest potential problems. All other problems are relatively infrequent and usually minor. Complications can be divided as to frequency of occurrence and those that are common to argon and Nd.YAG techniques alone or in combination.[35, 54, 82, 85, 87–95] These complications are summarized in Table 140–8.

Table 140–7. SETTINGS TO REOPEN IRIDECTOMIES

Argon Laser Settings to Reopen Iridectomies
Spot Size = 50 μ
Power = 200–1000 mW
Time = 0.05–0.2 sec
Applications = variable number

Nd.YAG* Laser Settings to Reopen Iridectomies
Energy = 1–4 mJ
Applications = usually 1 shot of single burst

*Nd.YAG, neodymium-yttrium-aluminum-garnet.

Table 140–8. COMPLICATIONS OF LASER IRIDECTOMY

Complications Usually Associated with Argon Techniques Only
Increase size of iridectomy with time
Corneal burns (epithelial and endothelial)
Retinal burns

Complications Usually Associated with Nd.YAG* Techniques Only
Bleeding

Complications Common to Argon and Nd.YAG Techniques
Increased intraocular pressure
Closure of iridectomy
Posterior synechiae
Corneal epithelial defect
Iritis
Lens opacification

*Nd.YAG, neodymium-yttrium-aluminum-garnet.

LASER GONIOPLASTY

Gonioplasty is the contracture of peripheral iris stroma by argon laser application (Fig. 140–9). Contracting the midperipheral iris with laser energy is an alternative to laser iridectomies when such therapies fail or as an adjunct to medical therapy.[96] Termed laserogonioplasty by Krasnov and Hagar in 1974, this technique widens the angle in subacute and chronic angle-closure glaucoma.[97, 98] Kimbrough reported successful treatment of angle-closure in nanophthalmos using this technique of iris photocoagulation.[99] Its usefulness has been described by Simmons in the management of plateau iris syndrome, acute and chronic angle-closure, and in iris convexity prior to laser trabeculoplasty.[100, 101] Angle-closure following retinal detachment surgery is another use of this technique.[102] Fiore and associates have described its use in shallowed angles in dural shunt syn-

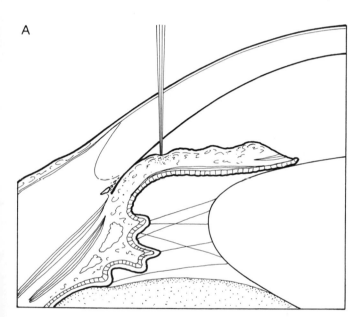

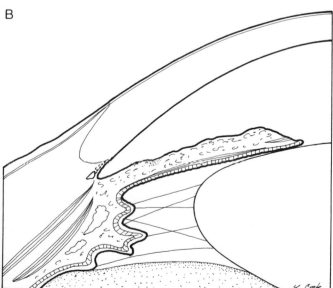

Figure 140–9. *A,* Argon laser application to the iris surface in the gonioplasty technique. *B,* Widening of the angle brought about by the contracture of the iris stroma in the gonioplasty technique.

Table 140–9. INDICATIONS FOR ARGON GONIOPLASTY

Open-angle glaucoma
  Adjunct to laser trabeculoplasty
Angle-closure glaucoma
  Laser iridectomy not immediately possible secondary to corneal bedewing or patient refusal
  Iridovitreal block
  Plateau iris syndrome
  Persistent PAS* after laser iridectomy in pupillary block glaucoma
  Anterior segment crowding
    Nanophthalmos
    Postscleral buckling
    Postpanretinal ablation
    Dural shunt syndrome
    Lens intumescence or anterior lens displacement
Miscellaneous
  Reopening closed cyclodialysis cleft
  Closure of inadvertent cyclodialysis cleft

*PAS, peripheral anterior synechiae.

drome.[103] Synonymous terms are gonioplasty, laser iris retraction, iridoplasty, and iridoretraction.

Indications

Gonioplasty can be used to prevent or treat pupillary and nonpupillary block-angle closure glaucoma. Gonioplasty can break an acute pupillary block when corneal bedewing precludes a successful laser iridectomy. Recurrent pseudophakic pupillary or iridovitreal block has been treated successfully with gonioplasty.[2]

The best use of gonioplasty is in the nonpupillary block glaucomas.[104, 105] Perhaps the most common use of gonioplasty is in plateau iris syndrome, in which a high iris insertion can block the trabecular meshwork with pupil dilatation. Peripherally placed contraction burns pull the iris from the angle. This same technique can be used in narrow nonoccludable angles to make crucial landmarks visible for successful laser trabeculoplasty.[106–109]

In nanophthalmos, crowding of the anterior segment is relieved with laser gonioplasty.[99, 110–112] Miotics are used with caution in these cases because of the increased risk of relative pupillary block. Carbonic anhydrase inhibitors, epinephrine, β-blockers, and osmotics can be tried at first. Gonioplasty is the preferred technique in the initial stages of progressive angle narrowing or localized appositional closure in these eyes. Gonioplasty can also be tried following imperforate laser iridectomy. Singh and associates reported a series of 32 nanophthalmic eyes.[113] In that series, gonioplasty was used initially when there was evidence of progressive narrowing and chronic asymptomatic partial angle-closure. It was also used successfully in cases in which laser therapy failed to produce a patent iridectomy. Glaucoma control and prevention of further angle-closure was achieved in 91.6 percent of 12 eyes treated with gonioplasty.

Other nonpupillary block glaucomas such as after scleral buckling procedures and dural shunt-induced shallowing of the anterior chamber have been managed with the use of gonioplasty (Table 140–9).

Technique

Burns by argon laser are applied directly without a lens or with an Abraham iridectomy lens or indirectly with a Goldmann four-mirror goniolens (Fig. 140–10).[101, 107, 114] Topical proparacaine 0.5 percent is the only required anesthetic. An argon laser beam is directed to the peripheral iris 1.5 mm from the iris root. In cases of iridocorneal touch, the spot is directed to the portion of the anterior chamber that is open and marched toward the periphery as the iris pulls away from the cornea. The goal of visible sustained iris contracture and flattening of the surrounding iris is achieved by using 100 to 300 mW of power for 0.2 sec as a 200- to 250-μ spot size. Release of pigment indicates the use of too much power, and a lack of contracture indicates the use of too little power. In plateau iris syndrome or in cases of 360-degree angle narrowing, the application area is 360 degrees. Sectoral burns can be used for focal areas of closure or narrowing. We prefer a single row of burns, although others advocate two concentric rows. Burns should be one to one and a half-spot size apart (10 to

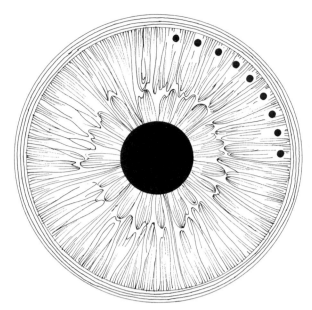

Figure 140–11. Location and spacing of argon laser applications in the gonioplasty technique.

15 spots per quadrant) (Fig. 140–11). Care is taken to avoid prominent iris vessels. Table 140–10 summarizes the technique for gonioplasty.

Gonioplasty is less permanent than laser iridectomy, and retreatment may be necessary. Carpel and associates described "subiridotomy" focal burns for more permanent results using 750 mW, 0.2-sec duration, 100-μ spot size, and an Abraham lens.[115] We believe that the latter technique may lead to through-and-through burns or to progressive iris atrophy with its inherent optical problems.

Postoperative Management

Postoperatively, prednisolone acetate 1 percent should be instilled every hour while the patient is awake for 48 hr, four times per day for 5 days, and should then be discontinued. Postlaser pressure elevation is ameliorated with pre- and post-dose apraclonidine instillation. Intraocular pressure should be monitored for 1 to 2 hr after laser treatment and again in 24 hr. We recommend gonioscopy within the first 24 hr. The patient is examined again in 1, 3, and 6 mo, at which time gonioscopy is repeated.

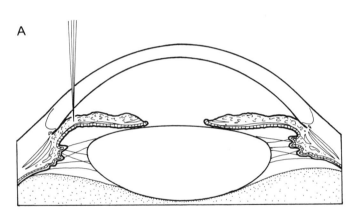

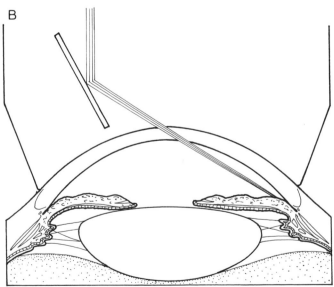

Figure 140–10. *A,* Direct applications of the argon laser in the gonioplasty technique. *B,* Indirect applications of the argon laser in the gonioplasty technique with the use of the angle mirror of the Goldmann lens.

Table 140–10. PARAMETERS FOR ARGON GONIOPLASTY

Time	Power	Size	Separation
0.2 sec	100–300 mW	200–250 μ	Single row of 1–1.5 spot sizes (10–15 spots per quadrant)
Goal:	Visible sustained iris contracture and flattening of the surrounding iris		
Avoid:	Pigment release or excessive contracture		

Table 140–11. COMPLICATIONS OF ARGON GONIOPLASTY

Transient iritis
Peripheral anterior synechiae
Pupillary distortion
Intraocular pressure spike
Iris atrophy
Full-thickness iridectomy

Complications

The complications of gonioplasty are minimal.[101, 107, 116] Mild transient iritis is not uncommon. Pupillary distortion, bleeding, and transient ciliary body shutdown have been seen. Fu and Llaw reported focal peaking, and peripheral anterior synechiae in the lasered areas have occurred in 61 percent in one series.[109] These same authors reported a permanent intraocular pressure elevation in two of 31 eyes (6 percent). A transient intraocular pressure rise within 24 hr is more common. Table 140–11 summarizes gonioplasty complications.

CONCLUSION

Laser iridectomy and gonioplasty are both effective and safe office procedures for treatment of the narrow-angle glaucomas. Laser iridectomy is the initial procedure of choice in most cases. Laser gonioplasty is valuable for breaking peripheral anterior synechiae and for relieving angle-closure glaucoma in eyes with residual PAS after a patent laser iridectomy or eyes in which pupillary block is not the causative mechanism for angle-closure. Both have proven usefulness in the treatment of angle-closure glaucoma and may delay or prevent the need for surgical intervention.

REFERENCES

1. Kolker AE, Hetherington J Jr: Becker-Shaffer's Diagnosis and Therapy of the Glaucoma, 5th ed. St. Louis, CV Mosby, 1983.
2. Shrader CE, Belcher CD III, Thomas JV, et al: Pupillary and iridovitreal block in pseudophakic eyes. Ophthalmology 91:831, 1984.
3. Epstein DL (ed): Chandler and Grant's Glaucoma, 3rd ed. Philadelphia, Lea & Febiger, 1986.
4. Meyer-Schwickerath G: Erfahrungen mit der lichtokoagulation der netzhaut und der irs. Doc Ophthalmol 10:91, 1956.
5. McDonald JE, Light A: Photocoagulation of iris and retina. Arch Ophthalmol 60:384, 1958.
6. Hogan MF, Schwartz A: Experimental photocoagulation of the iris of guinea pigs: A pilot study. Am J Ophthalmol 49:629, 1960.
7. Pollack IP, Patz A: Argon laser iridotomy: An experimental and clinical study. Ophthalmic Surg 7:22, 1976.
8. Flocks M, Zweng HC: Laser coagulation of ocular tissues. Arch Ophthalmol 72:604, 1964.
9. Snyder WB: Laser coagulation of the anterior segment. Arch Ophthalmol 77:93, 1967.
10. Hallman VL, Perkins ES, Watts GK, et al: Laser irradiation of the anterior segment of the eye. II: Monkey eyes. Exp Eye Res 8:1, 1969.
11. Perkins ES: Laser iridotomy for secondary glaucoma. Trans Ophthalmol Soc UK 91:777, 1971.
12. Perkins ES, Brown NAD: Iridotomy with a ruby laser. Br J Ophthalmol 57:487, 1973.
13. Campbell CJ, Rittler MC, Innis RE, et al: Ocular effects produced by experimental lasers. III: Neodymium laser. Am J Ophthalmol 66:614, 1968.
14. L'Esperance FA Jr: An ophthalmic argon laser photocoagulation system: Design, construction and laboratory investigations. Trans Am Ophthalmol Soc 66:827, 1968.
15. Zweng HC, Paris GL, Vassiliadis A, et al: Laser photocoagulation of the iris. Arch Ophthalmol 84:193, 1970.
16. Beckman H, Barraco R, Sugar S, et al: Laser iridectomies. Am J Ophthalmol 72:393, 1971.
17. Beckman H, Sugar HS: Laser iridectomy therapy of glaucoma. Arch Ophthalmol 90:453, 1973.
18. L'Esperance FA, James WA: Argon laser photocoagulation of iris abnormalities. Trans Am Acad Ophthalmol Otolarlygol 9:191, 1975.
19. Schwartz LW, Rodrigues MM, Spaeth GL, et al: Argon laser iridotomy in the treatment of patients with primary angle closure glaucoma or pupillary block glaucoma: A clinicopathologic study. Ophthalmology 85:294, 1978.
20. van der Zypen E, Fankhauser F, Bebie H: On the effects of different laser energy sources upon the iris of the pigmented and the albino rabbit. Int Ophthalmol 1:39, 1978.
21. van der Zypen E, Fankhauser F, Bebie H, et al: Changes in the ultrastructure of the iris after irradiation with intense light: A study of long-term effects after irradiation with argon ion, Nd:YAG and Q-switched ruby lasers. Adv Ophthalmol 39:59, 1979.
22. Yassur Y, Melamed S, Cohen S, et al: Laser iridotomy in closed angle glaucoma. Arch Ophthalmol 97:1920, 1979.
23. Podos SM, Kels BD, Moss AP, et al: Continuous wave argon laser iridectomy in angle closure glaucoma. Am J Ophthalmol 88:836, 1979.
24. Pollack IP: Use of argon laser energy to produce iridotomies. Trans Am Ophthalmol Soc 77:674, 1979.
25. Pollack IP: Use of argon laser energy to produce iridotomies. Ophthalmic Surg 11:506, 1980.
26. Mendelkorn RM, Mendelsohn AD, Olander KW, et al: Short exposure time in argon laser iridotomy. Ophthalmic Surg 12:805, 1981.
27. Quigley HA: Longterm follow up of laser iridotomy. Ophthalmology 88:218, 1981.
28. Ritch R: Argon laser treatment for medically unresponsive attacks of angle closure glaucoma. Am J Ophthalmol 94:197, 1982.
29. Forman JS, Ritch R, Dunn MW, Szymd L: Pupillary block following posterior chamber lens implantation. Ophthalmic Laser Ther 2:85, 1987.
30. Fankhauser R, Roussel P, Setffen J, et al: Clinical studies on the efficiency of high power laser radiation upon some structures of the anterior segment of the eye (neodymium:YAG Q-switched). Int Ophthalmol 3.3:129, 1981.
31. Fankhauser F, Lortscher H, van der Zypen E: Chemical studies on high and low power laser radiation upon some structures of the anterior and posterior segments of the eye. Int Ophthalmol 5:15, 1982.
32. Cambie E, De Bleecker C: Outpatient Nd:YAG laser iridectomy for angle-closure glaucoma. Bull Soc Belge Ophthalmol 210:231, 1984.
33. Klapper RM: Q-switched neodymium:YAG laser iridotomy. Ophthalmology 91:1017, 1984.
34. Latina MA, Puliafito CA, Steinert RR, Epstein DL: Experimental iridotomy with the Q-switched neodymium:YAG laser. Arch Ophthalmol 102:1211, 1984.
35. Pollack IP, Robin AL, Dragon DM, et al: Use of the neodymium:YAG laser to create iridotomies in monkeys and humans. Trans Am Ophthalmol Soc 82:307, 1984.
36. Kandarakis A, Zimmerman TJ: Non-pupillary block angle-closure glaucomas and their treatment by laser. Part I: Description. Ann Ophthalmol 16:1005, 1984.
37. Kandarakis A, Zimmerman TJ: Non-pupillary block angle-closure glaucomas and their treatment by laser. Part II: Laser gonioplasty technique. Ann Ophthalmol 16:914, 1984.
38. Dragon DM, Robin AL, Pollack IP, et al: Neodymium:YAG laser iridotomy in the cynomolgus monkey. Invest Ophthalmol Vis Sci 26:789, 1985.
39. McAllister JA, Schwartz LW, Moster M, et al: Laser peripheral

iridectomy comparing Q-switched neodymium:YAG with argon. Trans Ophthalmol Soc UK 104:67, 1985.

40. Richardson TM, Brown SV, Thomas JV, et al: Shock-wave effect on anterior segment structures following experimental neodymium:YAG laser iridectomy. Ophthalmology 92:1387, 1985.

41. Rodrigues MM, Spaeth GL, Moster M, et al: Histopathology of neodymium:YAG laser iridectomy in humans. Ophthalmology 92:1696, 1985.

42. Tomey KF: Efficacy and safety of neodymium:YAG laser iridotomy in angle closure glaucoma. Glaucoma 7:107, 1985.

43. Brazier DJ: Neodymium:YAG laser iridotomy. J R Soc Med 79:658, 1986.

44. Cinotti DJ, Reiter DJ, Maltzman BA, et al: Neodymium:YAG laser therapy for pseudophakic pupillary block. J Cataract Refract Surg 12:174, 1986.

45. Gailitis R, Peyman GA, Pulido J, et al: Prostaglandin release following Nd:YAG iridotomy in rabbits. Ophthalmic Surg 17:467, 1986.

46. Haut J, Gaven I, Moulin F, et al: Study of the first hundred phakic eyes treated by peripheral iridotomy using the Nd:YAG laser. Int Ophthalmol 9:227, 1986.

47. Moster MR, Schwartz LW, Spaeth GL, et al: Laser iridectomy: A controlled study comparing argon and neodymium:YAG. Ophthalmology 93:20, 1986.

48. Same as Ref. 47.

49. Robin AL, Arkell S, Gilbert SM, et al: Q-switched neodymium:YAG laser iridotomy: A field trial with a portable laser system. Arch Ophthalmol 104:526, 1986.

50. Robin AL, Pollack IP: Q-switched neodymium:YAG laser iridotomy in patients in whom the argon laser fails. Arch Ophthalmol 104:531, 1986.

51. Schrems W, Denninger U: Fluorophotometric studies of hydrodynamics following YAG laser iridotomy. Fortschr Ophthalmol 83:575, 1986.

52. Schrems W, Glaab-Schrems E, Hofmann G: Is YAG laser iridotomy suitable for the prevention of glaucoma attacks? Klin Monatsbl Augenheilkd 189:402, 1986.

53. Schrems W, Zeuss R, Leydhecker W: Effect of neodymium:YAG laser treatment of glaucoma on endothelial cell density of the cornea. Klin Monatsbl Augenheilkd 188:272, 1986.

54. Schwartz LW, Moster MR, Spaeth GL, et al: Neodymium:YAG laser iridectomies in glaucoma associated with closed or occludable angles. Am J Ophthalmol 102:41, 1986.

55. Albuquerque M, Belcher CD III, Tomlinson CP: Success of neodymium:YAG laser iridectomy. Ophthalmic Laser Ther 2:239, 1987.

56. Schrems W, Belcher CD, Tomlinson CP: Neodymium:YAG laser iridectomy: A report of 200 cases. Ophthalmic Laser Ther 2:33, 1987.

57. Krasnov MM: Q-switched ("cool") lasers in ophthalmology. Int Ophthalmol Clin 16:29, 1976.

58. Verworst F, Brihaye M, de Jong P, et al: Treatment of the iris with argon laser and pulsed neodymium:YAG laser: Preliminary note. Bull Soc Belge Ophthalmol 203:151, 1982.

59. Del Priore LV, Robin AL, Pollack IP: Neodymium:YAG and argon laser iridotomy. Long-term follow-up in a prospective, randomized clinical trial. Ophthalmology 95:1207, 1988.

60. Naveh-Floman N, Blumenthal M: A modified technique for serial use of argon and neodymium:YAG lasers in laser iridotomy. Am J Ophthalmol 100:485, 1985.

61. Park C, Rhee SW: The effect of combined application of argon and Nd:YAG lasers on iridectomy in rabbits. Korean J Ophthalmol 3:47, 1989.

62. Goins K, Schmeisser E, Smith T: Argon laser pretreatment in Nd:YAG iridotomy. Ophthalmic Surg 21:497, 1990.

63. Bass MS, Cleary CB, Perkins ES, et al: Single treatment laser iridotomy. Br J Ophthalmol 63:29, 1979.

64. Bonney CH, Gaasterland DE: Low-energy, Q-switched ruby laser iridotomies in Maccaca mulata. Invest Ophthalmol Vis Sci 18:278, 1979.

65. Pollack IP, Robin AL: Iridotomies in cynomolgus monkeys using a Q-switched ruby laser. Trans Am Ophthalmol Soc 78:88, 1980.

66. Wishart PK, Hitchings RA: Neodymium:YAG laser and dye laser iridotomy—A comparative study. Trans Ophthalmol Soc UK 105:521, 1986.

67. Khuri CH: Argon laser iridectomies. Am J Ophthalmol 76:490, 1973.

68. Abraham RK, Miller GL: Outpatient argon laser iridectomy for angle closure glaucoma: A two-year study. Trans Am Acad Ophthalmol Otolaryngol 79:OP-529, 1975.

69. Abraham RK: Procedure for outpatient argon laser iridectomies for angle closure glaucoma. Int Ophthalmol Clin 16:1, 1976.

70. Abraham PK, Munnerly C: Laser iridotomy. Improved methodology with a new iridotomy lens. Ophthalmology 86(Suppl):126, 1979.

71. Ritch R, Palmberg P: Argon laser iridectomy in densely pigmented irides. Am J Ophthalmol 93:800, 1982.

72. Belcher CD: Laser iridectomy. In Belcher CD, Thomas JV, Simmons RJ (eds): Photocoagulation in Glaucoma and Anterior Segment Disease. Baltimore, Williams & Wilkins, 1984.

73. Pollack IP: Current concepts in laser iridotomy. Int Ophthalmol Clin 24:153, 1984.

74. Payer H: YAG laser iris hole at 6 o'clock in the periphery in the treatment of prevention of closed angle glaucoma and plateau iris and in pupillary block (posterior iris surface-blocking mechanisms). Klin Monatsbl Augenheilk 189:404, 1986.

75. Singh OS (ed): Anterior segment laser section: Laser iridectomy (iridotomy). Ophthalmic Laser Ther 1:113, 1986.

76. Weiblinger RP: Clinical literature highlights on argon and neodymium:YAG laser iridectomy. Ophthalmic Laser Ther 1:237, 1986.

77. Wise JD, Munnerly CR, Erickson PJ: A high efficiency laser iridotomy-sphincterotomy lens. Am J Ophthalmol 101:546, 1986.

78. Schrems W, Van Dorp HP, Mager S, et al: The effect of prostaglandin inhibitors on the laser-induced disruption of the blood aqueous barrier in the rabbit. Graefes Arch Clin Exp Ophthalmol 221:61, 1983.

79. Schrems W, Van Dorp HP, Mechler W, et al: The time course of laser-induced disruption of the blood-aqueous barrier in the rabbit. Graefes Arch Clin Exp Ophthalmol 221:65, 1983.

80. Krupin T, Stone RA, Cohen BH, et al: Acute intraocular pressure response to argon laser iridotomy. Ophthalmology 92:922, 1985.

81. Taniguchi T, Rho SH, Gotoh Y, et al: Intraocular pressure rise following Q-switched neodymium:YAG laser iridotomy. Ophthalmic Laser Ther 2:99, 1987.

82. Schrems W, Eichelbronner O, Krieglstein GK: The immediate IOP response of Nd:YAG laser iridotomy and its prophylactic treatability. Acta Ophthalmol (Copenh) 62:673, 1984.

83. Fourman S: Effects of topical ALO 2145 (p-aminoclonidine hydrochloride, aplonidine hydrochloride) on the acute intraocular pressure rise after argon laser iridotomy (Letter). Arch Ophthalmol 106:307, 1988.

84. Kitazawa Y, Taniguchi T, Sugiyama K: Use of apraclonidine to reduce acute intraocular pressure rise following Q-switched Nd:YAG laser iridotomy. Ophthalmic Surg 20:49, 1989.

85. Robin AL: Medical management of acute post-operative intraocular pressure rises associated with anterior segment ophthalmic laser surgery. Int Ophthalmol 30:102, 1990.

86. Wand M, Grant WM, Simmons RJ, et al: Plateau iris syndrome. Trans Am Acad Ophthalmol Otolaryngol 83:122, 1977.

87. Cooper RL, Constable IJ: Prevention of corneal burns during high energy laser iridotomy. Am J Ophthalmol 91:534, 1981.

88. Gilbert CM, Robin AL, Pollack IP: Hyphema complicating neodymium:YAG laser iridotomy. Ophthalmology 91:1123, 1984.

89. Gaasterland DE, Rodriguez MM, Thomas G: Threshold for lens damage during Q-switched Nd:YAG laser iridectomy: A study of rhesus monkey eyes. Ophthalmology 92:1616, 1985.

90. Welch DB, Apple DJ, Mendelsohn AD, et al: Lens injury following iridotomy with a Q-switched neodymium:YAG laser. Arch Ophthalmol 104:123, 1986.

91. Seedor JA, Greenidge KC, Dunn MW: Neodymium:YAG laser iridectomy and acute cataract formation in the rabbit. Ophthalmic Surg 17:478, 1986.

92. Kublin J, Simmons RJ: Use of tinted soft contact lenses to eliminate monocular diplopia secondary to laser iridectomies. Ophthalmic Laser Ther 2:111, 1987.

93. Maltzman BA, Agin M: Argon peripheral iridotomy and cataract formation. Ann Ophthalmol 20:28, 1988.

94. Schwartz AL, Martin NF, Weber PA: Corneal decompensation after argon laser iridectomy. Arch Ophthalmol 106:1572, 1988.

95. Berger CM, Lee DA, Christensen RE: Anterior lens capsule perforation and zonular rupture after Nd:YAG laser iridotomy. Am J Ophthalmol 107:674, 1989.

96. Blumenthal M, Floman N, Treister G: Laser iris retraction for narrow-angle glaucoma. Glaucoma 4:47, 1982.

97. Krasnov MM, Saprykin PI, Klatt A: Laserogonioplasty in glaucoma. Vestn Oftalmol 2:30, 1974.

98. Hagar H: Zur Lasermikrochirurgie bei Glaukom [Lasertrabekulopunktur (LTP), tangentiale Irisbasiskoagulation (TIK), Pupillenerweiterung und Verlangerung]. Klin Monatsbl Augenheilkd 167:18, 1975.

99. Kimbrough RL, Trempe CS, Brockhurst RJ, et al: Angle-closure glaucoma in nanophthalmos. Am J Ophthalmol 88:572, 1979.

100. Simmons RJ, Kimbrough RL, Belcher CD: Gonioplasty for selected cases of angle-closure glaucoma. Docum Ophthalmol Proc Series 22:200, 1980.

101. Simmons RJ, Kimbrough RL, Belcher CD, et al: Laser gonioplasty for special problems in angle closure glaucoma. In New Orleans Academy of Ophthalmology (ed): Symposium on Glaucoma, Vol. 220, 1981.

102. Burton TC, Folk JC: Laser iris retraction for angle-closure glaucoma after retinal detachment surgery. Ophthalmology 95:742, 1988.

103. Fiore PM, Latina MA, Shingleton BJ, et al: The dural shunt syndrome. Part I: Management of glaucoma. Ophthalmology 97:56, 1990.

104. Robin AL, Pollack IP: A comparison of neodymium:YAG and argon laser iridotomies. Ophthalmology 91:1011, 1984.

105. Rockwood EJ, Meyers SM, Meisler DM, et al: Treatment of selected cases of pupillary block with YAG laser iridotomies (Letter). Ophthalmic Surg 15:968, 1984.

106. Higgins RA: Laser trabeculoplasty: Early experience with a new procedure. Aust J Ophthalmol 11:169, 1983.

107. Simmons RJ, Simmons RB: Gonioplasty. In Belcher CD, Thomas JV, Simmons RJ (eds): Photocoagulation in Glaucoma and Anterior Segment Disease. Baltimore, Williams & Wilkins, 1984.

108. Higgins RA: Two years' experience with laser trabeculoplasty. Aust N Z Ophthalmol 13:237, 1985.

109. Fu YA, Llaw ZC: Argon laser gonioplasty with trabeculoplasty for chronic angle closure glaucoma. Ann Ophthalmol 19:419, 1987.

110. Brockhurst RJ: Nanophthalmos with uveal effusion: A new clinical entity. Arch Ophthalmol 93:1289, 1975.

111. Calhoun FP Jr: The management of glaucoma in nanophthalmos. Trans Am Ophthalmol Soc 73:97, 1975.

112. Simmons RJ: Nanophthalmos, diagnosis and treatment. In Chandler PA, Grant WM (eds): Glaucoma. Philadelphia, Lea & Febiger, 1979.

113. Singh OS, Simmons RJ, Brockhurst RJ, et al: Nanophthalmos: A perspective on identification and therapy. Ophthalmology 89:9, 1982.

114. Perkins ES, Brown NAD: Laser treatment of glaucoma. In Amarlic P (ed): International Glaucoma Symposium. Albi, France, 1974. Marseilles, Diffusion Générale de Librairie, 1975.

115. Carpel EF, Brown DJ: Permanent iridoplasty. Am J Ophthalmol 96:113, 1983.

116. Reibaldi A, Uva MG, Scuderi GL: Laser and glaucoma: Our experience. Ophthalmologica 191:84, 1985.

Chapter 141

■

Laser Filtration Surgery

MARK A. LATINA and JEAN-BERNARD CHARLES

Glaucoma filtration surgery, first introduced by McKenzie[1, 2] in the 19th century, has been continually modified and refined in order to improve surgical success.[3–6] Within the past decade, the laser has been used after glaucoma filtration surgery as a modality to treat hypofunctioning filtration blebs and to reestablish the patency of occluded sclerostomies.[7–9] Previous conventional surgical approaches to revise surgical glaucoma filters, introduced by Swan,[10] can now be performed with a laser on an outpatient basis without entering the eye with instruments.

As ophthalmologists have become more sophisticated in the use of lasers in the eye and with the development of new types of lasers, the ability to perform filtration surgery entirely with a laser has generated considerable interest (Fig. 141–1). Laser filtration surgery has several potential advantages over conventional filtration surgery. First, complications resulting from filtration surgery can be reduced by using smaller incisions or even avoiding entry into the eye by using an ab-interno goniolens approach. Second, the long-term success of filtration surgery may be enhanced by minimizing ma-

nipulation of ocular tissues, especially the conjunctiva, which can lead to inflammation, scarring, and eventual failure of filtration blebs. Two approaches to laser sclerostomy procedures have evolved, ab-externo and ab-interno.

In ab-externo laser sclerostomy procedures, the fistula is created from the subconjunctival side either by directly focusing the laser onto the exposed sclera overlying the trabecular meshwork and Schlemm's canal or by placing a fiberoptic laser probe in physical proximity to the sclera at the intended sclerostomy site. The carbon dioxide, excimer, and holmium lasers have been used in human eyes to create ab-externo sclerostomies.

In the ab-interno approach, a fistula is created starting from within the anterior chamber. One approach uses a slit-lamp/goniolens delivery system. The laser energy is delivered through the goniolens to the sclera in the area of the trabecular meshwork to produce a fistula. The ability to create a scleral fistula using only a light beam to penetrate the eye would be a significant advantage over conventional filtration surgery because no surgical instruments would be required to enter the eye. Because

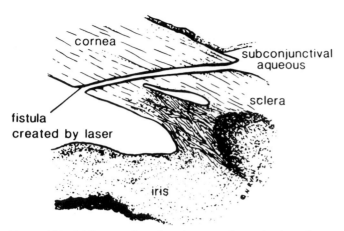

Figure 141–1. Diagram for sclerostomy performed using a laser. (Courtesy of W. March, M.D.)

only the light beam penetrates the eye with this approach, it is essential that the wavelength emitted by the laser be transmitted through the ocular media (i.e., cornea and aqueous). Various types of lasers have been used with this technique, including argon, Q-switched Nd.YAG, and flashlamp pumped dye lasers.

A second ab-interno technique uses a fiberoptic delivery system. A fiberoptic probe is inserted through a corneal or limbal incision, maneuvered across the anterior chamber, and placed against the sclera in the area of the trabecular meshwork. Laser energy is then directly applied to the sclera to create the sclerostomy. Virtually any laser that can be coupled to a fiberoptic delivery system could be used for this approach. The continuous-wave Nd.YAG, argon-ion, holmium, erbium-YAG, excimer, and flashlamp pumped dye lasers have been the principal lasers used with this technique.

AB-INTERNO LASER SCLEROSTOMY USING A GONIOLENS

Argon Laser Sclerostomy

L'Esperance was the first to report a noninvasive ab-interno laser sclerostomy procedure.[11] Energy from an argon laser was directed by a goniolens to perform an "internal laser trabeculosclerostomy" on three blind human eyes. First, using a 30-gauge needle to pass through the subconjunctival space to the sclera, L'Esperance injected India ink in the trabecular meshwork at the future filtration site in order to enhance tissue absorption of argon laser energy. The argon laser was then focused onto the dyed region at a power setting of 600 to 800 mW, an exposure time of 0.5 sec, and a spot size of 50 μm. Laser tissue ablation resulted in a marked thermal effect that caused shrinkage of the sclera, corneal striae, and significant astigmatism lasting several weeks. Other complications encountered included postoperative iritis or iridocyclitis and intraocular pressure (IOP) elevation necessitating antiglaucoma medications. These filters failed within 7 days.

Q-Switched Nd.YAG Laser Sclerostomy

Fifteen years later, in 1984, interest in laser sclerostomy surgery was revived by March and colleagues, who used a high-powered Q-switched Nd.YAG laser to perform sclerostomies on human cadaver eyes.[12] The Q-switched ophthalmic Nd.YAG laser is a short-pulsed (12 nsec) near-infrared laser emitting at a wavelength of 1064 nm. The extremely short pulse characteristic of the Q-switched Nd.YAG laser produces an explosion of the tissue at the point of focus into a collection of ions known as *plasma*. This nonthermal process, termed *optical breakdown*, occurs by nonlinear absorption and is independent of tissue pigmentation. Based on the ability of the Q-switched Nd.YAG laser to "cut" tissue without coagulation, March hypothesized that sclerostomies could be created without causing thermal damage to surrounding tissues.

Using six human cadaver eyes whose corneas had been trephined to expose the trabecular meshwork more completely, March was able to achieve perforation of the sclera with a Coherent 9900 Nd.YAG laser set at 15 to 16 mJ of energy, 12-nsec pulse, and nine-salvo burst; an additional laser system, the LASAG Microrupter YAG laser, was also used and set at 52 to 53 mJ of energy in multimode, 12-nsec pulse, and nine-salvo burst.[12] The sclerostomies were placed anterior to the trabecular meshwork. Descemet's membrane was perforated with the focus-offset dial on the LASAG laser set at 1 D; then it was set at 9 D for the remainder of the procedure. March found that at least 3312 mJ of energy was required to create a sclerostomy (Fig. 141–2). Optimal perforations were obtained at energy levels that exceeded 26,000 mJ.

Several months later, March and colleagues performed a successful sclerostomy procedure on the eye of a living human.[13] The patient had a malignant choroid

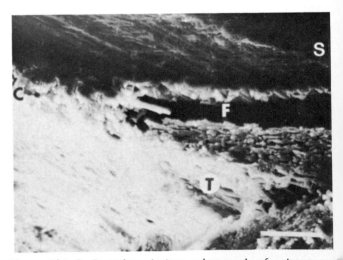

Figure 141–2. Scanning electron micrograph of a transverse section of an incision at internal ostium of sclerostomy made with a Q-switch Nd. YAG laser. (F, fistula; C, cornea; S, sclera, T, trabecular meshwork, bar = 50 μm.) (From March WF: Histologic study of Nd.YAG laser sclerostomy. Arch Ophthalmol 103:862, 1985. Copyright 1985, American Medical Association.)

melanoma that was 1.5 cm in diameter, had received prior radiation therapy, and was scheduled to have an enucleation. The sclerostomy was performed 25 hr before the enucleation using a LASAG Microruptor set at 53 mJ of energy in multimode, 12 nsec, and single pulses. In order to place the sclerostomy posterior the limbal-conjunctival insertion, March and associates developed an improved goniolens[14, 15] (Fig. 141–3) that could withstand high laser pulse energies with its mirror set at 68 degrees, in contrast to the Zeiss and Goldmann lenses, whose mirrors are set at 62 and 59 degrees, respectively. With this lens, March was able to place the sclerostomy approximately 2 mm posterior to the limbal-conjunctival interface. The conjunctiva overlying the future sclerostomy site was initially elevated with subconjunctival injection of 2 per cent lidocaine. Scleral perforation required approximately 15,800 mJ. The sclerostomy measured 0.7 mm in diameter, and careful histologic examination revealed no complications such as hemorrhage or distance effects of the Nd.YAG shock wave from this procedure in a single eye. Intraocular pressure fell immediately to 2 mmHg, and a filtering bleb was noted.

In order to assess the long-term outcome of the Nd.YAG laser filtration procedure, Gherezghiher and coworkers[16] performed a Nd.YAG laser sclerostomy procedure in four cynomolgus monkeys. One eye of each animal was treated with laser, and the other eye was used as a control. A Coherent 9900 Nd.YAG laser was set to deliver 15 to 16 mJ of energy at 12-nsec pulses and nine-burst salvo. The procedure was similar to the approach used by March, described earlier. Two primates were treated with approximately 23 and 24 J of energy; the other two received 12 and 14 J. IOP measurements and tonography were performed 1 wk later and monthly thereafter. A significant reduction of IOP in the treated eyes was associated with a significant

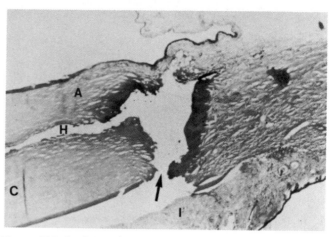

Figure 141–4. Light micrograph of rabbit corneosclera function after silver-stabilized protein injection into the sclera and Nd.YAG laser sclerostomy. The arrow denotes a fistula. The dark color of the silver injection (A) has penetrated halfway through the rabbit's sclera. (C, cornea; I, iris.) (From March WF: Silver oxide in YAG sclerostomy. Lasers Surg Med 7:354, 1987.)

increase in outflow facility. The sclerostomy remained patent for more than 180 days. Scanning electron microscopic examination of the cornea revealed no significant damage to the central cornea, iris, or lens in the treated eyes. However, mild endothelial cell loss was noted at the site of treatment at the peripheral cornea and in the area immediately posterior to the sclerostomy, in addition to a focal break in Descemet's membrane. The major concern about March's procedure was the potential for collateral damage to surrounding tissues resulting from the photoacoustic effect produced by the high pulse energies required to create a sclerostomy.

Subsequently, March and coworkers used a LASAG Microrupter II to perforate the sclera. To improve success and reduce the pulse energy required, March injected the sclera with silver oxide to enhance the laser energy absorption characteristics of the sclera.[17] Ten microliters of Argyrol 20 per cent was injected intrasclerally at the limbus with a special 30-gauge needle in 24 albino rabbit eyes at the future sclerostomy site. Four 20-msec pulses followed by one 12-msec multimode pulse of 135 mJ of energy produced perforation in every case (Fig. 141–4). With the longer 20-msec pulse, the laser-tissue interaction is primarily thermal rather than photodisruptive. Thus, the silver oxide acts like a dye that absorbs the Nd.YAG laser energy, making it possible to ablate tissue with greater efficiency. Even though high-power settings in the Nd.YAG laser sclerostomy procedure appear safe, lower power requirements would make the procedure more clinically acceptable.

Pulsed Dye Laser Sclerostomy

To maximize the efficiency and effectiveness of scleral ablation, Latina and colleagues[18] introduced the concept of dye-matched laser ablation using a flashlamp pumped

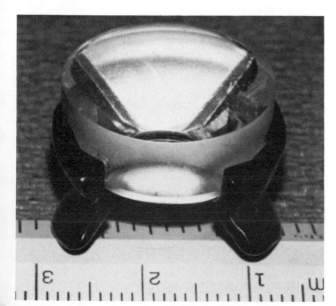

Figure 141–3. Contact glass for filtration (CGF) lens. (From March WF, Gherezghiher T, Koss MC, et al: Design of a new contact lens for YAG laser filtering procedures. Ophthalmic Surg 18:513, 1987.)

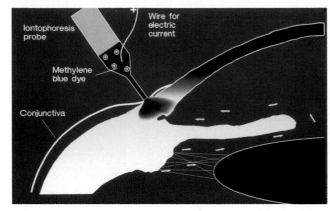

Figure 141–5. Schematic representation of iontophoresis of methylene blue dye into the sclera at the limbus. (From Arch Ophthalmol 108:1747, 1990. Copyright 1990, American Medical Association.)

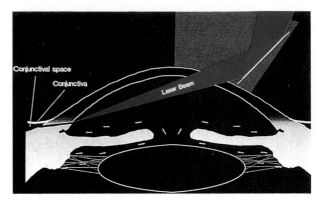

Figure 141–7. Schematic representation of a laser beam directed through a goniolens onto the dyed scleral region to create a full-thickness fistula. (From Latina MA, et al: Experimental ab-interno sclerostomies using a pulsed-dye laser and goniolens. Arch Ophthalmol 108:1747, 1990. Copyright 1990, American Medical Association.)

dye laser, also called a *pulsed dye laser*. As the name implies, these are pulsed lasers that emit visible light with pulse widths in the microsecond range. The emission wavelength can be "tuned" by changing the circulating laser dye. By selecting the appropriate wavelength and pulse width, scleral perforation can be achieved at significantly lower laser energy levels.

To enhance the optical absorption of the sclera, Latina and associates[19] used iontophoresis to deposit methylene blue dye with an absorption peak at 688 nm into the sclera noninvasively (Figs. 141–5 and 141–6). Using a flashlamp pumped dye laser emitting at 666 nm, pulse energies of 50 and 150 mJ, a pulse duration of 1.2 or 20 μsec, and a 200 μm spot size, the pulsed dye laser sclerostomy procedure was performed using a slit-lamp goniolens delivery (Fig. 141–7) in 50 rabbit eyes. An average of 12 pulses was required for perforation. Fistulas were easier to create with the shorter 1.2-μm pulse duration. Reported postoperative inflammation was minimal, and hyphema, cyclodialysis, and retinal detachment were not observed. Histologic examination revealed a 20- to 150-μm zone of thermal damage surrounding the fistula (Fig. 141–8). A human clinical trial using the method of dye-enhanced ablation with a pulsed dye laser is now in progress.

Krypton Red Laser Sclerostomy

Applying the concept of dye-enhanced ablation, March[20] used the continuous-wave krypton red laser emitting at 647 nm to perform a laser sclerostomy after dying the sclera with methylene blue by iontophoresis. The conjunctiva overlying the future sclerostomy site was raised with a subconjunctival injection of sodium hyaluronate. The laser aiming beam was focused by a goniolens anterior to the trabecular meshwork, and the focal point was buried into the sclera. The krypton laser was first used to coagulate scleral tissue up to the innermost corneal stroma. The Q-switched Nd.YAG laser was then used to perforate the poorly stained Descemet's membrane and complete the sclerostomy. For the krypton laser, an average of 10 pulses at 1000 mW of power, a spot size of 50 μm, and a pulse duration of 0.2 sec were sufficient. An average of four pulses of 25 mJ with the Nd.YAG laser was then required to complete the sclerostomy.

Of the 70 patients who underwent this procedure, 50 patients maintained permanent filtration and lowered IOP. The longest follow-up of a functioning filter was 2 yr. One patient with neovascular glaucoma had a functioning filter for 8 mo of follow-up. The filtering fistulas promptly sealed in the other 20 patients. Reported complications have been few and of minor consequence. Two patients had inadvertent conjunctival perforations that were successfully treated with a bandage contact lens. Small hemorrhages occurred in 5 per cent of the patients with open-angle glaucoma. Eyes with neovascular glaucoma invariably had significant hemorrhages, but these never prevented completion of the procedure.

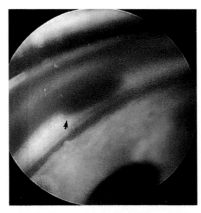

Figure 141–6. Gonioscopic view of methylene blue–dyed sclera *(arrow)*. Kawa Camera, × 2. (From Latina MA, et al: Experimental ab-interno sclerostomies using a pulsed-dye laser and goniolens. Arch Ophthalmol 108:1747, 1990. Copyright 1990, American Medical Association.)

INVASIVE AB-INTERNO LASER SCLEROSTOMY USING FIBEROPTIC DELIVERY

Fiberoptic ab-interno sclerostomy permits intraocular delivery of wavelengths of laser light that are normally absorbed by the cornea and aqueous humor. However, entry into the eye, albeit via a small incision, is required.

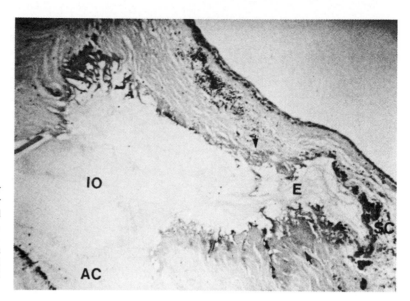

Figure 141–8. Photomicrograph of ab-interno laser sclerostomy in a rabbit using a pulsed-dye laser. Laser parameters are 1.5 μsec, 75 mJ, 100-μm spot size, and seven pulses to perforate. (IO, internal ostium; AC, anterior chamber; E, external ostium.) (From Latina MA, et al: Experimental ab-interno sclerostomies using a pulsed-dye laser and goniolens. Arch Ophthalmol 108:1748, 1990. Copyright 1990, American Medical Association.)

and a viscoelastic agent must routinely be used to maintain the anterior chamber. The ab-interno laser sclerostomy procedure using a fiberoptic laser probe has been reported by several investigators using argon-ion laser with ultraviolet optics, high-power argon, Nd.YAG, excimer, and holmium and flashlamp pumped dye lasers.

Argon-Ion Laser With Ultraviolet Optics

Gaasterland and colleagues[21] produced sclerostomies in bovine eyes using an argon laser with ultraviolet intracavitary optics capable of emitting ultraviolet light between 333- and 363-nm wavelengths. Ultraviolet radiation was used because of the higher energy and shorter absorption depth characteristics of photons at this wavelength as compared with visible light. They studied both ab-interno and ab-externo sclerostomy techniques using a 200-μm-diameter fiber. The fiber that was used had two different distal ends: a cleaved end and another end with a 500-μm ball lens. Using the 200-μm cleaved fiber, 0.6 to 1.5 J of energy with a power setting of 0.5 W and 0.1 sec duration, they successfully created the sclerostomies. Both the ab-interno and ab-externo perforations required the same amount of energy using this type of fiber. Using the 500-μm ball lens fiberoptic probe, 5.1 to 10.4 J were necessary with a laser power of 2.0 W for at least 0.1 sec duration. Both ab-interno and ab-externo perforations required equivalent amounts of energy with this fiberoptic probe as well. When the fiberoptic probe was moved into the sclerostomy, aqueous was noted to pass freely through the sclerostomy into the subconjunctival space.

High-Power Argon-Ion Laser

Blue-green argon laser radiation has also been used to create ab-interno sclerostomies. Jaffe and colleagues used a high-powered 15-W water-cooled argon laser coupled to a 300-μm quartz fiberoptic delivery system in pigmented rabbits.[22] The conjunctiva in the area of the proposed sclerostomy was elevated with sodium hyaluronate. The anterior chamber was then deepened with the same viscoelastic substance through a paracentesis site made 180 degrees from the future sclerostomy site. The fiberoptic probe was then inserted through the paracentesis site and positioned into the angle 180 degrees away, stopping approximately 0.5 mm from the trabecular meshwork. Single pulses varying from 5 to 15 W set with a pulse duration of 0.1 sec were used to create full-thickness sclerostomies. The number of pulses necessary for perforation ranged from one to four. At lower energy levels, more pulses were required. The average amount of energy required to produce a sclerostomy was calculated to be 1.7 ± 0.4 J. This average total amount of energy was similar to that reported by March and associates[12] using a noncontact laser and by Gaasterland and coworkers[21] using a contact argon laser. The high-power density of the laser caused not only ablation but also thermal cauterization. No intraoperative complications such as conjunctival perforation, lens damage, hyphema, or subconjunctival hemorrhage were reported.

Postoperatively, transient localized corneal edema, focal iris atrophy, and mild anterior segment inflammation lasting 2 to 3 days were detected. Histologically, the diameter of the fistula was approximately 400 μm. In an effort to demonstrate the zone of thermal damage, Jaffe's group used tritiated thymidine to label sites of cellular proliferation as a response to laser damage. A 125-μm-diameter zone of damage surrounding the sclerostomy site was demonstrated.

In brief, using a high-powered continuous-wave argon laser, Jaffe's group was able to create a sclerostomy by thermal ablation in the absence of an adjunctive absorbent medium. However, the presence of transient corneal edema and focal iris atrophy signaled significant thermal diffusion into surrounding tissue.

Jaffe and coworkers subsequently used the same technique to create an ab-interno sclerostomy in a patient undergoing enucleation for a blind, painful eye.[23] Despite the presence of diffuse rubeosis, 360-degree peripheral anterior synechiae, and superior conjunctival scarring, the workers created the sclerostomy without complications. Six laser applications were required using 8 W per pulse and 0.1-sec pulse duration. The eye was enucleated immediately after the laser procedure. Histologic analysis demonstrated a patent fistula 300 μm in diameter. Tissue damage was noted in the area within 150 μm of the sclerostomy. The overlying conjunctiva remained intact.

Nd.YAG Laser With Sapphire Probe

An important development in ab-interno laser filtration surgery was the advent of the Nd.YAG laser coupled with a sapphire crystal–tipped fiberoptic delivery system (Fig. 141–9). These crystals readily transmit Nd.YAG laser light and have low thermal conductivity and a high melting temperature.[24] Any change in the geometric design of these crystals alters the shape and focal point of the laser beam, providing beam configurations appropriate for cutting or coagulating tissue. When used in direct contact with the tissue, these sapphire crystal–tipped probes allow for more precise delivery of the laser energy with less tissue damage.[25] The use of the continuous-wave Nd.YAG laser with a sapphire-tipped probe has been approved by the Food and Drug Administration for performing laser sclerostomy.

The CLX 60-W (Surgical Laser Technologies) continuous-wave Nd.YAG laser has been used to perform laser sclerostomies in animal as well as human eyes.[26–28] Because it is necessary in these procedures to enter the anterior chamber with the fiberoptic probe, retrobulbar anesthesia is necessary, and the procedure should be performed under sterile conditions with an operating microscope. The conjunctiva is elevated to prevent inadvertent conjunctival perforation, using a 30-gauge needle and either balanced salt solution or a viscoelastic agent. If the inferonasal quadrant is chosen as the future sclerostomy site, a 1.5-mm incision is then made at the superotemporal limbus using a sharp blade. The viscoelastic agent is injected into the anterior chamber in the area of the future fistula. The laser probe with a tip diameter of 200 μm is introduced through the limbal incision into the anterior chamber to abut the angle 180 degrees away in the area of Schwalbe's line. It is important to avoid the trabecular meshwork, if possible, in order to minimize scleral wound healing, inflammation, and iris incarceration. Gonioscopic control with a Zeiss four-mirror goniolens is helpful but is usually not necessary for adequate sclerostomy placement.

Three to five pulses of 800 mJ (8 W × 0.1 sec) or one to two pulses of 2.4 J (12 W × 0.2 sec) have usually been required to complete corneoscleral perforation. The end-point of the procedure can be determined by observing the flow of viscoelastic substance into the subconjunctival space and by observing the tip of the laser probe with its red helium-neon aiming beam in the subconjunctival space. A 10–0 nylon suture may be required to close the limbal wound.

Postoperatively, while awake, all patients must be treated with 1 per cent prednisolone acetate, topical antibiotic, and 1 per cent atropine sulfate solutions every 2 hr.

Wilson and colleagues used the primate model to perform contact laser sclerostomies with the CLX 60-W continuous-wave Nd.YAG laser system.[27] Three to five pulses of 800 mJ (8 W × 0.1 sec) or one or two pulses of 2.4 J (12 W × 0.2 sec) were required to achieve perforation. The procedure caused minimal conjunctival trauma and allowed sclerostomies to be performed at any location in the angle.

Wilson and Javitt used the same technique described earlier with the continuous-wave contact Nd.YAG laser to create ab-interno sclerostomies in five patients with aphakia, glaucoma, and chronic inflammation.[28] Between three and five pulses of 800 mJ or one or two pulses of 2.4 J were used to create the scleral fistula. Adjunctive 5-fluorouracil was administered postoperatively during a 3-wk period as tolerated. After a follow-up period of 24 to 28 mo, three of the five patients had IOP less than 20 mmHg with adjunctive antiglaucoma medications. The sclerostomy failed owing to vitreous plugging in one patient and chronic intraocular inflammation in the fifth patient. Because this approach created a fairly large full-thickness sclerostomy, severe hypotony was routinely observed postoperatively and drainage of choroidal effusions was necessary in several cases.

Higginbotham and colleagues compared the efficacy and complications of synthetic sapphire contact Nd.YAG laser sclerostomies with those noted with standard ab-externo thermal sclerostomies in rabbits.[2] The ab-interno Nd.YAG fiberoptic contact laser filtration group was found to have a longer duration of functioning blebs when compared with the ab-externo thermosclerostomy group. Higginbotham's technique was similar to that described by Jaffe and Federman

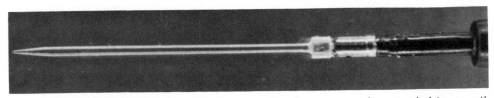

Figure 141–9. Synthetic sapphire probe used to perform ab-interno filtration surgery when coupled to a continuous-wave Nd.YAG laser. The probe is manufactured by Surgical Laser Technologies, Inc. (From Ophthalmol Clin North Am 12:629, 1989.)

except that the entry site for the fiberoptic probe was 90 degrees away from the future sclerostomy site in order to avoid passing the probe across the pupil and directly over the lens. Despite this modification, some eyes had localized damage to the corneal endothelium and stroma as well as iris and lenticular damage. These complications were more frequent with the contact ab-interno procedure. No iatrogenic bleb leaks were encountered. Histologically, a cellular reaction was noted around the sclerostomy created by the Nd.YAG contact laser, but it was less than the cellular reaction in the eyes that had undergone ab-externo thermal sclerostomy. In the patients undergoing contact laser sclerostomy, the cellular reaction was a consequence of the thermal and cauterizing effect of the continuous-wave Nd.YAG laser.

Excimer Laser Ab-Interno Sclerostomy

Excimer lasers have also been used to create ab-interno sclerostomies.[30, 33] Excimer lasers emit high-powered pulsed ultraviolet radiation at various wavelengths from 193 to 351 nm. Ablation of tissue at these short wavelengths occurs through a process referred to as *photoablation*. Photoablation results from the strong absorption of these wavelengths by protein and produces minimal thermal damage to the surrounding tissues.

Berlin and colleagues, using an excimer laser emitting at 308 nm coupled to an ultraviolet-grade silica optical fiber, succeeded in creating ab-interno contact sclerostomies in 16 rabbit eyes.[30] Penetration of the sclera was accomplished with a pulse repetition rate of 20 Hz (Fig. 141–10). The number of required pulses varied depending on the fluence. The repetition rate with a fluence of 2.5 J/cm² was 80 Hz and with a fluence of 2.1 J/cm² was 120 Hz. Once penetration was achieved, the repetition

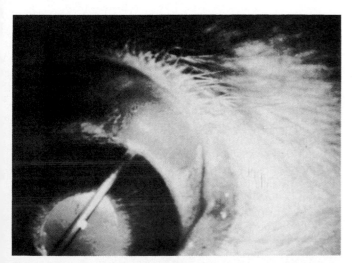

Figure 141–10. Ab-interno sclerostomy performed using an excimer laser emitting at 308 nm delivered via a 400-μm fiber crossing the anterior chamber to the corneoscleral angle of a rabbit's eye. (From Berlin MS: Excimer laser goniophotoablation. Lasers Light Ophthalmol 2:20, 1988.)

rate was lowered to 5 Hz until the subtenon space was entered. During the process of laser sclerostomy formation, gas bubbles were noted in the anterior chamber. Transient hyphema developed in six eyes, and a conjunctival buttonhole in one eye sealed spontaneously. Tissue damage was noted in the cornea, iris, or lens in all eyes. Bleb flattening occurred between 5 days to 3 mo, but the scleral fistula remained histologically open in all the eyes that were monitored for 10 months.

AB-EXTERNO LASER SCLEROSTOMY

In ab-externo laser sclerostomy procedures, the fistula is created from the subconjunctival side either by directly focusing the laser onto the exposed sclera overlying the trabecular meshwork and Schlemm's canal or by placing a fiberoptic laser probe in physical proximity to the sclera at the intended sclerostomy site. Compared with ab-interno sclerostomies using a fiberoptic delivery, entry into the eye is avoided using the ab-externo approach. The major disadvantage of ab-externo sclerostomies compared with ab-interno sclerostomies is the need for conjunctival manipulation. This may vary from the need for a routine conjunctival flap, which does not significantly improve morbidity over the standard trabeculectomy, to the use of a subconjunctival fiberoptic delivery probe, as in the case of the thulium-holmium-doped YAG (THC:YAG) laser, which reduces significant conjunctival dissection. The carbon dioxide laser, excimer laser, and holmium laser have been used to create ab-externo laser sclerostomies in the eyes of humans.

Carbon Dioxide Laser

In 1971, a rapid superpulsed carbon dioxide industrial laser system was used for the first time to perform corneal and scleral dissection in rabbits.[31] This effort led to the development of a small ophthalmic carbon dioxide laser system capable of delivering either continuous-wave or rapid superpulsed-mode carbon dioxide laser energy through a Zeiss operating microscope directly onto the eye. With an emission wavelength of 10.6 μm, the carbon dioxide laser beam is principally absorbed by water. The high water content of the sclera limits tissue penetration depth with this laser to approximately 20 μm, thus protecting underlying tissue from damage.

Ab-externo carbon dioxide laser sclerostomy procedures, using the rapid superpulsed mode, were performed on five patients with glaucoma refractory to medical therapy.[32] Dissection of a limbus-based flap of conjunctiva and Tenon's capsule was first carried out to expose the underlying sclera. A partial-thickness laser scleral incision was made adjacent to the superior corneal limbus to outline a 5 × 5-mm flap that was dissected with a conventional lamellar dissector. The resultant scleral bed was then treated with the laser to create a 1.5-mm hole into the anterior chamber anterior to the scleral spur. The laser was set at a repetition rate of 120 pulses per second, a pulse width of 150 msec, a spot size of 600 μm, 35 mJ per pulse, and an average power of 5 W. The procedure was completed with a surgical iridectomy followed by closure of the scleral and conjunctival wounds using four 10–0 Supramid sutures to tie the scleral flap and 8–0 collagen sutures to close the conjunctival incision.

On the first postoperative day, one eye had a flat chamber due to a leaking conjunctival flap; it was successfully repaired, with subsequent re-formation of the anterior chamber. No other complications were encountered. The surgical field was notably bloodless, presumably because of the coagulative properties of this laser. The coagulative property of the carbon dioxide laser could theoretically be useful in eyes with neovascular glaucoma, a condition in which intraoperative bleeding is common. At the 6-mo follow-up period, all five eyes had a diffuse, flat bleb with IOP less than 20 mmHg. Four of the eyes required no medication for IOP control, and the fifth one, which had the initial complication of conjunctival leakage and flat chamber, was successfully treated with timolol 0.25 per cent for postoperative IOP control. This procedure never gained acceptance because of the lack of availability of the pulsed carbon dioxide laser and the need for a conventional conjunctival flap. Thus, this procedure merely replaced a mechanical punch with an expensive laser to perform the actual sclerostomy.

Excimer Partial External Trabeculotomy

A nonpenetrating ab-externo trabeculotomy procedure was developed by Seiler and colleagues using an excimer laser.[33] In this group's partial external trabeculotomy (Fig. 141–11), dissection of a flap of conjunctival and Tenon's capsule was carried out as described earlier. The laser was set at 193-nm pulsed emission and focused

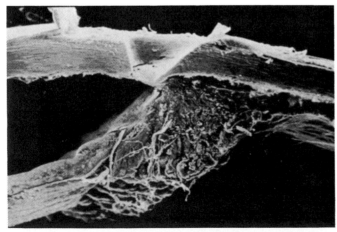

Figure 141–11. Scanning electron micrograph of an excimer laser partial external trabeculectomy demonstrating ablation of the sclera with preservation of the trabecular meshwork. (Courtesy of T. Seiler, M.D.)

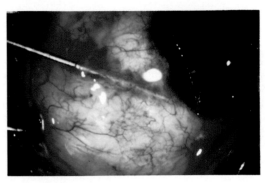

Figure 141–12. Fiberoptic probe is introduced into subconjunctival space and advanced to the limbus. Holmium laser energy is emitted perpendicular to the axis of the probe. (Courtesy of Sunrise Technology, CA.)

onto the sclera in the area overlying Schlemm's canal. Scleral ablation was performed until Schlemm's canal was penetrated. The major advantage of this laser procedure over other ab-externo approaches is that the trabecular meshwork can be preserved because of the strong absorption of 193-nm radiation by aqueous, which is encountered on entering Schlemm's canal. This self-limiting procedure effectively produces a nonpenetrating trabeculectomy without damage to the trabecular meshwork or surrounding tissues. Clinical trials to assess the long-term efficacy and complications of this procedure in humans are currently in progress in the United States and Germany.

THC:YAG Laser Sclerostomy

The THC:YAG laser is the most recent addition to the laser sclerostomy armamentarium. This pulsed laser emits at a wavelength of 2.1 μm in the near-infrared region, and its beam is highly absorbed by water. Hoskins and associates[34] created sclerostomies using a specially designed fiberoptic probe that is placed subconjunctivally (Fig. 141–12).

The specially designed fiberoptic delivery probe has the diameter of a 26-gauge needle and focuses the laser beam perpendicular to the axis of the probe. The spot size at the tip of the probe is 200 μm. The probe is advanced through the subconjunctival space to the limbus through a 25-gauge conjunctival incision made 10 to 15 mm posterior to the limbus. The conjunctiva may be elevated by subconjunctival injection of a viscoelastic substance before inserting the fiberoptic probe. The probe is then positioned so that the emitted laser beam is applied on the sclera in the limbal area and directed into the anterior chamber. The laser pulses at 5 Hz and is set at 80 to 100 mJ per pulse. Six to 50 pulses are usually required to penetrate the sclera. Penetration of the anterior chamber is usually accompanied by gas bubble formation in the aqueous humor adjacent to the sclerostomy and shallowing of the anterior chamber. The conjunctiva may be closed with 10–0 nylon suture at the site of penetration as needed. A previously made

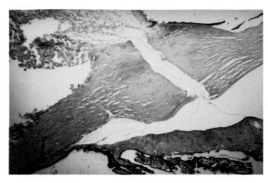

Figure 141–13. Histopathology of ab-externo THC:YAG laser sclerostomy without an iridectomy. (From Hoskins HD, et al: Subconjunctival THC:YAG laser limbal sclerostomy ab externo in the rabbit. Ophthalmic Surg 21:591, 1990.)

paracentesis is used to re-form the anterior chamber and to raise the bleb. Histopathology of a holmium sclerostomy (Fig. 141–13) reveals a zone of thermal damage of at least 300 μm, which is equivalent to the size of the fistula. Whether a large zone of thermal damage is advantageous to the healing process is unknown at this time.

The procedure can be performed on an outpatient basis in the minor surgery room using a microscope. However, as with a majority of laser filtration procedures, it should be emphasized that this intervention is tantamount to a full-thickness filtration procedure with all its attendant complications such as hypotony, hyphema, choroid effusion, flat anterior chamber, postoperative inflammation, and iatrogenic caractogenesis. For that reason, the conservative approach of admitting such patients to the hospital for close observation during the immediate postoperative period would not be objectionable. A clinical trial to assess the efficacy and complications of this new therapeutic modality is currently in progress.

CONCLUSIONS

Scientific research and interest in the area of laser sclerostomy are growing. Several novel techniques using various types of laser systems have shown significant potential for efficacious therapeutic application that could revolutionize the clinical management of glaucoma. The distinct advantages of laser sclerostomy procedures are evident. Many of these procedures can be performed on an outpatient basis or in a minor surgery room setting. The operating time is significantly less than required for conventional filtration procedures. Procedures using the pulsed dye laser with a goniolens delivery require no entry into the eye with instruments, and the holmium laser requires only minimal conjunctival manipulation. Thus, these procedures can be performed using only topical anesthesia and can be readily repeated. Furthermore, most sites around the limbus are accessible to create a sclerostomy, even in the inferonasal quadrant. Additionally, because conjunctival incisions are minimized in these procedures, some of the complications associated with the use of 5-fluorouracil may be significantly reduced.

Despite all these advantages, serious complications can occur in laser sclerostomy surgery. It is yet unclear which type of laser sclerostomy approach, ab-interno or ab-externo, and which type of laser procedure will gain wide acceptance in clinical practice. After sufficient advances in this area in the future and after laser sclerostomy surgery becomes an acceptable alternative treatment of glaucoma, earlier surgical intervention using one or more of these techniques in the management of glaucoma and prevention of visual loss is a distinct possibility.

REFERENCES

1. Katz LJ, Spaeth GC: Filtration surgery. In Ritch R, Shields M, Krupid T (eds): The Glaucomas. St. Louis, CV Mosby, 1989, p 653.
2. Morales J, Ritch R: Conventional surgical iridectomy. In Ritch R, Shields M, Krupid T (eds): The Glaucomas. St. Louis, CV Mosby, 1989, p 645.
3. Sugar HS: Experimental trabeculotomy in glaucoma. Am J Ophthalmol 51:623, 1961.
4. Cairns JE: Trabeculotomy. Trans Am Acad Ophthalmol Otolaryngol 66:673, 1968.
5. Schwartz AL, Anderson D: Surgical techniques: Trabecular surgery. Arch Ophthalmol 92:134, 1974.
6. Mills KB: Trabeculectomy: A retrospective long-term follow-up of 444 cases. Br J Ophthalmol 65:790, 1981.
7. Ticho V, Ivory M: Reopening of occluded filtering blebs with argon laser photocoagulation. Am J Ophthalmol 94:413, 1977.
8. Van Buskirk EM: Reopening filtration fistulas with the argon laser. Am J Ophthalmol 94:1, 1982.
9. Cohn HC, Aron-Rosa D, et al: Reopening blocked trabeculectomy sites with the YAG laser. Am J Ophthalmol 95:293, 1983.
10. Swan KC: Reopening of nonfunctioning filters: Simplified surgical techniques. Trans Am Acad Ophthalmol Otolaryngol 79:342, 1975.
11. L'Esperance FA Jr: Ophthalmic Lasers: Photocoagulation, Photoradiation and Surgery, 2nd ed. St. Louis, CV Mosby, 1983, pp 538–543.
12. March WF, Gherezghiher T, Koss MC, et al: Experimental YAG laser sclerostomy. Arch Ophthalmol 102:1834, 1984.
13. March WF, Gherezghiher T, Koss MC, et al: Histologic study of a neodymium:YAG laser sclerostomy. Arch Ophthalmol 103:860, 1985.
14. March WF, Gherezghiher T, Koss MC, et al: Design of a new contact lens for YAG laser filtering procedures. Ophthalmic Surg 16:328, 1985.
15. March WF, LaFuente H, Rol P: Improved goniolens for YAG sclerostomy. Ophthalmic Surg 18:513, 1987.
16. Gherezghiher T, March MF, Koss MC, et al: Neodymium-YAG laser sclerostomy in primates. Arch Ophthalmol 103:1543, 1985.
17. March WF, Shaver RP, Gherezghiher T, et al: Silver oxide in YAG sclerostomy. Lasers Surg Med 7:353, 1987.
18. Latina MA, Long F, Deutsch T, et al: Dye-enhanced ablation of sclera using a pulsed dye laser. Invest Ophthalmol Vis Sci 27(AVRO Suppl):254, 1986.
19. Latina MA, Goode S, de Kater AW, et al: Experimental sclerostomies using a pulsed-dye laser. Lasers Surg Med 8:233, 1988.
20. March WF: Long-term follow-up of patients undergoing laser sclerostomy. Ophthalmic Laser Ther 2:161, 1987.
21. Gaasterland DE, Hennings DR, Boutacoff TA, et al: Ab interno and ab externo filtering operations by laser contact surgery. Ophthalmic Surg 18:24, 1987.
22. Jaffe GJ, Williams GA, Mieler WF, et al: Ab interno sclerostomy with a high-powered argon endolaser. Am J Ophthalmol 106:391, 1988.
23. Jaffe GH, Mieler WF, Radius RL, et al: Ab interno sclerostomy

with a high-powered argon endolaser. Arch Ophthalmol 107:1183, 1989.

24. Daikuzono N, Joffe SN: Artificial sapphire probe for contact photocoagulation and tissue vaporization with the Nd:YAG laser. Med Instrum 19:173, 1985.

25. Joffe SN: Contact neodymium:YAG laser surgery in gastroenterology: A preliminary report. Laser Surg Med 6:155, 1986.

26. Federman JL, Wilson RP, Ando F, et al: Contact laser: Thermal sclerostomy ab interno. Ophthalmic Surg 18:726, 1987.

27. Wilson RP, Javitt JC, Federman JL, et al: Contact Nd:YAG laser thermal sclerostomy ab interno in primates. Ophthalmology 95(Suppl):168, 1988.

28. Wilson RP, Javitt JC: Ab interno laser sclerostomy in aphakic patients with glaucoma and chronic inflammation. Am J Ophthalmol 110:178, 1990.

29. Higginbotham EJ, Kao G, Peyman G: Internal sclerostomy with

the Nd:YAG contact laser versus thermal sclerostomy in rabbits. Ophthalmology 95:385, 1988.

30. Berlin MS, Rajacich G, Duffy M, et al: Excimer laser photoablation in glaucoma filtering surgery. Am J Ophthalmol 103:713, 1987.

31. Beckman H, Rota A, Barraco R, et al: Limbectomies, keratectomies and keratostomies performed with a rapid-pulsed carbon dioxide laser. Am J Ophthalmol 71:1277, 1971.

32. Beckman H, Fuller TA: Carbon dioxide laser scleral dissection and filtering procedure for glaucoma. Am J Ophthalmol 88:114, 1979.

33. Seiler T, Kriogerawski M, Bende F, Wollensak J: Partial external trabeculectomy. Klin Monatsbl Augenheilkd 195:216–220, 1989.

34. Hoskins HD, Iwach AG, Drake MV, et al: Subconjunctival THC:YAG laser limbal sclerostomy ab externo in the rabbit. Ophthalmic Surg 21:589, 1990.

Chapter 142

■

Peripheral Iridectomy and Chamber Deepening

M. ROY WILSON

Prior to the advent of laser therapy, conventional surgical peripheral iridectomy had long been the treatment of pupillary block glaucoma in angle-closure. Von Graefe[1] first introduced surgical sector iridectomies for the treatment of acute glaucoma in 1857. However, peripheral iridectomy did not gain widespread acceptance until the concept of relative pupillary block was explained by Curran[2] in 1920. Shortly thereafter, Barkan[3] introduced an anatomic classification of the cause of glaucoma, and surgical peripheral iridectomy became established as the treatment of choice for primary angle-closure glaucoma.

INDICATIONS

Conventional surgical peripheral iridectomy is indicated in most situations in which a laser iridectomy has repeatedly failed or is not feasible. Repeated closure of a laser iridectomy occurs most commonly when chronic uveitis is present. A laser iridectomy may not be feasible for a variety of reasons: (1) lack of laser equipment, (2) breakdown of laser equipment, (3) patient unable or unwilling to cooperate, (4) inability to adequately visualize iris because of corneal edema or opacity, or (5) presence of shallow or flat anterior chamber with broad cornea-iris contact. A surgical peripheral iridectomy is also indicated in situations in which iris tissue is necessary for pathologic analysis and as an adjunct to glaucoma filtering surgery and cataract surgery. Our discussion of surgical peripheral iridectomy in this chapter is limited to its role in the treatment of angle-closure glaucoma.

PREOPERATIVE CONSIDERATIONS

Pupillary constriction should be attempted prior to surgery with 2 percent pilocarpine instilled topically every 30 min for 3 doses. If pupillary constriction is not achieved with this regimen, overdosing with pilocarpine should be avoided and surgery should proceed. To reduce the risk of postoperative bacterial endophthalmitis, topical gentamycin should also be instilled every 30 min for 3 doses before surgery.

Local anesthesia with retrobulbar or peribulbar block combined with a lid block is desirable. General anesthesia should be reserved only for uncooperative patients.

SURGICAL TECHNIQUE

A superior rectus bridle suture of 4–0 silk is placed and fastened to the drapes. A paracentesis is made through clear cornea at 10 or 2 o'clock with a Wheeler knife or simply a sharp blade. The incision can be made either at the limbus under a conjunctival flap or through clear cornea. Prolapsing iris tissue is more difficult with the clear cornea incision. However, the conjunctiva, which might be needed later for filtration surgery, is spared, and there is less potential for bleeding than in the limbal approach. An additional consideration is that when there is extensive peripheral anterior synechiae extending far anteriorly, the limbal approach may be too far posterior to properly perform an iridectomy.

The corneal incision is made in one of the superior quadrants just anterior to the limbal corneal vessels.

This incision should be perpendicular to the surface, should be approximately 3-mm wide, and should extend through two thirds of the corneal thickness. In the limbal approach, a small fornix-based conjunctival flap is made in one of the superior quadrants, and the incision is placed approximately 1 to 1.5 mm behind the corneolimbal junction. This incision should also be approximately 3-mm wide and two thirds deep but may be beveled slightly anteriorly.

A suture of 10–0 nylon is preplaced through the groove and looped out of the wound (Fig. 142–1A). While the assistant spreads apart the lips of the groove by grasping the two parts of the suture with tying forceps, Descemet's membrane is penetrated with a sharp blade, and the anterior chamber is entered (see Fig. 142–1B). Care is taken to ensure that the internal opening is nearly as wide as the external incision (see Fig. 142–1C).

The assistant may facilitate prolapse of the iris by pulling on the preplaced suture and by exerting gentle pressure on the posterior lip of the incision. Once the iris has prolapsed, it is grasped with fine forceps and is cut using Vannas or de Wecker scissors (see Fig. 142–1D). If the iris does not prolapse, the anterior chamber must be entered with fine, nontoothed forceps, and the iris must be grasped and gently lifted out of the incision for surgical excision. The excised tissue should be inspected for the presence of the pigment epithelium.

Reposition of the iris is usually achieved by gentle massage over the peripheral cornea radially with a blunt cannula or muscle hook (see Fig. 142–1E). Irrigation with acetylcholine through the previously made paracentesis may facilitate this process. Occasionally, it may be necessary to gently push the iris tissue back into the anterior chamber with an iris spatula. Care must be taken to avoid inserting instruments into the anterior chamber through the incision site, because this may inadvertently damage the lens. After successful repositioning of the iris, the iridectomy should be visible and the pupil should be round and central (see Fig. 142–1F). If necessary, the anterior chamber can be reformed by injecting balanced salt solution through the paracentesis site.

The preplaced suture is then tightened and tied to reapproximate the wound (see Fig. 142–1G). The suture is cut close to the knot, and the knot is buried. If the limbal approach is used, the conjunctiva is brought over the wound and is closed with a 7–0 Vicryl suture. Subconjunctival antibiotics and corticosteroids are injected inferiorly as well as topical administration of these medications.

POSTOPERATIVE MANAGEMENT

The postoperative management is straightforward. Slit-lamp examination should be performed during the morning after surgery. The patency of the iridectomy and the intraocular pressure are assessed. Topical antibiotic and steroid drops are administered four times per day, and the steroid is tapered as the degree of inflam-mation warrants. A short-acting cycloplegic agent such as Mydriacyl 1 percent or Cyclogyl 1 percent may be administered twice daily if the eye is inflamed to minimize the chances of posterior synechiae formation. However, a rise in postdilatation pressure may occur if plateau iris configuration is present or if the lens is large and the iris stroma crowds the angle. Intraocular pressure should therefore be re-measured after dilatation. Gonioscopy should be performed in the early postoperative period to evaluate the effect of the procedure.

COMMON COMPLICATIONS

Intraoperative

Serious intraoperative complications are rare when correct surgical techniques are utilized. Bleeding from the iris may occur but is usually self-limiting. The presence of rubeosis iridis increases the likelihood of a more significant hemorrhage, and consideration should be given to gently cauterizing these vessels before cutting iris tissue.[4] The Simmons-Savage diathermy is well suited for this purpose. Bleeding from the ciliary body is most commonly caused by inadvertent excision because of a limbal incision that is too far posterior. If excessive bleeding is encountered, a drop of epinephrine 1:1000 may be applied. Injection of a large air bubble into the anterior chamber may also be effective in controlling the hemorrhage. Injection of sodium hyaluronate and other viscoelastic agents offer excellent hemostasis, but their widespread use must be cautioned because of the tendency for a postoperative intraocular pressure rise. Large amounts of hemorrhage or viscoelastic agents should be removed by irrigation with a balanced salt solution through the paracentesis before the operative wound is closed.

Vitreous loss may also occur because of a limbal incision that is too far posterior. If this occurs, it is best to close the wound and go to another surgical site to perform a peripheral iridectomy through a more anterior approach.

Postoperative

HYPHEMA

Hyphema may occur because of persistent bleeding from the iris or ciliary body. These hyphemas are usually mild and require no treatment.

CATARACT

Lens damage during the procedure results in rapid formation or progression of a cataract. However, even when definite evidence of direct lens trauma from surgery is lacking, eyes that have had a peripheral iridectomy appear to be at increased risk for progressive cataract formation.[5–9]

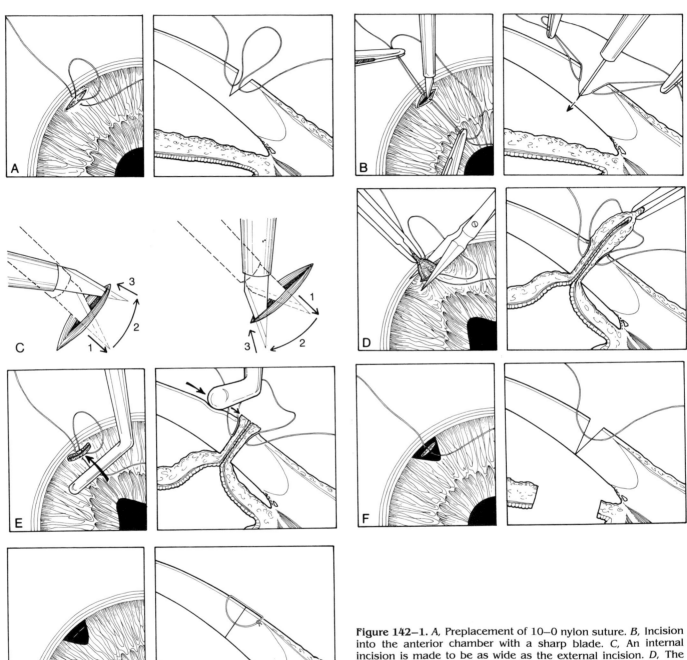

Figure 142–1. *A,* Preplacement of 10–0 nylon suture. *B,* Incision into the anterior chamber with a sharp blade. *C,* An internal incision is made to be as wide as the external incision. *D,* The prolapsed iris is grasped and cut. *E,* Massaging the peripheral cornea with a blunt instrument. *F,* A picture of the successful iridectomy. *G,* The preplaced suture is tied, and the knot is buried.

SHALLOW ANTERIOR CHAMBER

A shallow anterior chamber is often caused by a wound leak. A Seidel test with 2 percent fluorescein should be performed for confirmation. If the result is negative, malignant glaucoma or choroidal effusion should be suspected. If the result is positive, immediate attention must be paid to reform the anterior chamber and to repair the wound.

PERSISTENT INCREASED INTRAOCULAR PRESSURE

The intraocular pressure may remain elevated despite a surgical peripheral iridectomy if the iridectomy is imperforate, if synechial angle-closure is present, if the iridectomy is blocked by vitreous, if plateau iris syndrome is present, or if malignant glaucoma develops. A re-operation or adjunctive laser treatment is indicated if the iridectomy is imperforate or blocked by vitreous. Filtration surgery is indicated if synechial angle-closure is present. The management of plateau iris syndrome and malignant glaucoma are discussed in Chapters 120 and 134.

MISCELLANEOUS

Endophthalmitis as well as all the complications of intraocular surgery may occur, although these are extremely rare. Complaints of uniocular diplopia, photophobia, and glare have been reported after peripheral iridectomies.[10, 11]

SECTOR IRIDECTOMY

A sector iridectomy should be considered rather than a peripheral iridectomy when there is a need for a large optical opening. This may be the situation when the visual axis is occluded by a membrane, when the pupil is displaced, or when visual access to the retinal periphery is necessary for examination or treatment of retinal disease. The procedure is similar to performing a peripheral iridectomy, except that the initial entry incision is larger to allow the iris to be grasped close to the pupillary margin. The iris is then withdrawn until the pupillary margin is exposed. Alternatively, after the iris has prolapsed, a hand-over-hand technique may be used until the sphincter has been exteriorized. Excision of the iris is performed with a single cut (Fig. 142–2).

CHAMBER DEEPENING

Conventional surgical iridectomy may not be appropriate in all situations for which a laser iridectomy is indicated but not possible. If extensive synechial angle-closure is present, an iridectomy may not be adequate to control the intraocular pressure, and filtration surgery may be required. Before the advent of the laser, the potential complications associated with surgery necessitated a choice being made between performing a surgical

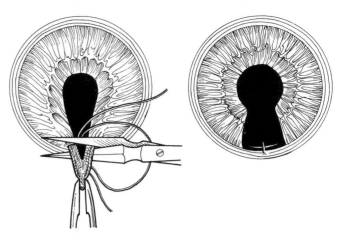

Figure 142–2. Excision of the iris for a sector iridectomy.

iridectomy and possibly requiring a second operation or performing filtration surgery with its associated increased risks when perhaps a peripheral iridectomy would have been adequate. Laser technology has retired this earlier argument of iridectomy versus filtering operation. A laser iridectomy, if feasible, can be tried in almost all cases of primary angle-closure glaucoma; filtration surgery, if necessary, can be performed subsequently. Having performed the initial laser iridectomy will not have added significantly to the overall potential complication rate and probably will not have affected the success rate of a subsequent filter. When laser iridectomy is not feasible, the prior dilemma of peripheral iridectomy versus filtration surgery resurfaces.

The original application of anterior chamber deepening and intraoperative gonioscopy was to help the surgeon to decide whether to perform an iridectomy or a filtering operation.[12–14] Appositional closure of the angle was eliminated by the chamber deepening, and the degree of permanent anterior synechiae was assessed by gonioscopy. The extent of synechial closure was the major contributing factor to the choice of operation.

Anterior chamber deepening and intraoperative gonioscopy are rarely used today for their original purpose and as originally described. The ability to artificially widen the angle and distinguish between appositional and synechial closure with the Zeiss four-mirror goniolens and indentation gonioscopy has made it possible to accurately assess the angle preoperatively in most cases.[15] However, indentation gonioscopy is not possible when the anterior chamber is excessively shallow or if the patient is not cooperative. Anterior chamber deepening and intraoperative gonioscopy may thus prove to be extremely helpful in selected circumstances in helping to determine whether to perform a surgical iridectomy or a glaucoma-filtering operation. Additionally, modifications in technique have allowed the concepts of chamber deepening and intraoperative gonioscopy to be adapted for other purposes.

Intraoperative gonioscopy during surgery for angle-closure glaucoma was first introduced by Shaffer in 1957.[12] The concept of chamber deepening before gonioscopy was introduced by Ogino in 1961.[13] Chandler and Simmons refined and popularized both techniques in 1965.[14] In Chandler's technique, after a paracentesis is made, as much aqueous as possible is evacuated from both the anterior and posterior chambers. The anterior chamber is then artificially deepened with an injection of saline solution through the paracentesis. Gonioscopy is performed using the Koeppe lens, a hand-held microscope, and a Barkan light.

The Koeppe lens provides an unsurpassed view of the angle. However, the hand-held biomicroscope and Barkan light source are not commonly available in many operating rooms. A Zeiss goniolens and operating microscope have thus been substituted by many surgeons. Another modern modification has been the use of sodium hyaluronate in place of saline to deepen the anterior chamber. Because of its viscosity, aqueous evacuation is less critical when sodium hyaluronate is used. Protection of the corneal endothelium and hemostasis are other advantages provided by sodium hyaluronate. These features have made it safer to insert instruments into the anterior chamber and have thus allowed chamber deepening with intraoperative gonioscopy to be used for therapeutic purposes as well as diagnostic purposes.

The concept of lysing synechiae (goniosynechialysis) is not new, but the generally poor success rate combined with the technically difficult and hazardous surgical techniques have caused most surgeons to abandon the procedure. Campbell and Vela have reintroduced the procedure using modern surgical techniques and instruments.[16] Chamber deepening is initially performed using sodium hyaluronate instead of saline. Using direct visualization as provided by the Barkan goniotomy lens system with a fiberoptic headlight and magnifying loupes, peripheral anterior synechiae are separated with a curved irrigating cyclodialysis spatula.

A modification of this procedure may also be used for internal revisions of filtration sites that have become occluded by fibrous membranes. In this procedure, a Ziegler knife is inserted into the anterior chamber and used to slice an opening through the obstructing membrane using direct visualization.

Anterior chamber deepening and intraoperative gonioscopy have played important roles in our surgical management of angle-closure glaucoma. Although the advent of laser technology has obviated its original use, except in situations in which a laser iridectomy is not feasible, the concepts of anterior chamber deepening and intraoperative gonioscopy are still valuable. Modern surgical advances have allowed a broadening of their indication for use, and these techniques remain as useful adjuncts in the careful evaluation and surgical treatment of glaucoma.

REFERENCES

1. Von Graefe A: Veber die Iridectomie be: Glaucom und uber den glaucomatosen Process. Graefes Arch Clin Exp Ophthalmol 3:456, 1857.
2. Curran EJ: A new operation for glaucoma involving a new principle in the etiology and treatment of chronic primary glaucoma. Arch Ophthalmol 49:131, 1920.
3. Barkan O: Glaucoma: Classification, causes, and surgical control. Am J Ophthalmol 21:1099, 1938.
4. Hersh SB, Kass MA: Iridectomy in rubeosis iridis. Ophthalmic Surg 7:19, 1976.
5. Sugar HS: Cataract formation and refractive changes after surgery for angle-closure glaucoma. Am J Ophthalmol 69:747, 1970.
6. Godel V, Regenbogen L: Cataractogenic factors in patients with primary angle-closure glaucoma after peripheral iridectomy. Am J Ophthalmol 83:180, 1977.
7. Floman N, Berson D, Landau L: Peripheral iridectomy in closed angle glaucoma—Late complications. Br J Ophthalmol 61:101, 1977.
8. Krupin T, Mitchell KB, Johnson MF, Becker B: The long-term effects of iridectomy for primary acute angle-closure glaucoma. Am J Ophthalmol 86:506, 1978.
9. Bobrow JC, Drews RC: Long-term results of peripheral iridectomies. Glaucoma 3:319, 1981.
10. Luke S: Complications of peripheral iridectomy. Can J Ophthalmol 4:346, 1969.
11. Go FJ, Kitazawa Y: Complications of peripheral iridectomy in primary angle-closure glaucoma. Jpn J Ophthalmol 25:222, 1981.
12. Shaffer RN: Operating room gonioscopy in angle closure glaucoma surgery. Trans Am Ophthalmol Soc 55:59–64, 1957.
13. Ogino N: On the angle of the anterior chamber in closed-angle glaucoma with the anterior chamber deepening method by injection of saline solution. Acta Soc Ophthalmol Jpn 65:1673–1681, 1961.
14. Chandler PA, Simmons RJ: Anterior chamber deepening for gonioscopy at time of surgery. Arch Ophthalmol 74:177–190, 1965.
15. Forbes M: Gonioscopy with corneal indentation. Arch Ophthalmol 76:488–492, 1966.
16. Campbell DG, Vela A: Modern goniosynechialysis for the treatment of synechial angle closure glaucoma. Ophthalmology 91:1052–1060, 1984.

Chapter 143

∎

Glaucoma Filtration Surgery

R. RAND ALLINGHAM, JOEL S. SCHUMAN, SANDRA J. SOFINSKI,
DAVID L. EPSTEIN, and RICHARD J. SIMMONS

INTRODUCTION AND PHILOSOPHY

Glaucoma filtration surgery is an art as well as a science. Those involved in the medical and surgical management of patients with glaucoma in the Harvard system look to the late Paul A. Chandler and W. Morton Grant as leaders who taught many of today's approaches and philosophies. Chandler and Grant emphasized the case method of study.[1] This involved critical evaluation and analysis of individual cases, from which they were able to draw profound conclusions. This method was and is helpful in analyzing all aspects of glaucoma care. It is important to remember that glaucoma filtering surgery is a multivariate technique. Caution is advised before drawing conclusions based on statistical analysis of glaucoma filtration surgery, because many differences exist in the surgical approach as well as the patient population. Surgical options include choosing a guarded trabeculectomy versus a full-thickness procedure, varying the thickness of the scleral flap, and selecting the number and types of sutures used and their relative tensions. The method of conjunctival flap dissection, the decision to excise Tenon's fascia, and the technique for closure of the conjunctival flap are other surgical options. Pre- and postoperatively, a number of medical interventions may be used. No single method suffices in the surgical management of these patients. Therefore, the choices made for a patient should be based on statistical analysis in conjunction with knowledge gained through thoughtful study of previous individual cases.

Glaucoma surgery is a major event in the life of a patient. Successful surgery can achieve glaucoma control, thus permitting a patient to lead a normal life. Alternatively, failure of the first operation reduces the chance for a successful result at subsequent operations. The best chance for success is with the initial surgery, and the patient and family should be fully indoctrinated in advance about the seriousness of the undertaking. A patient's cooperation is thus enhanced preoperatively, operatively, and postoperatively while reducing the chance of a patient's disillusionment and anger about results that are less than ideal.

The theme of the postoperative period has been addressed with increasing importance since the 1960s. At that time, Chandler experimented with various suture techniques in an attempt to provide more resistance to full-thickness filtration procedures, thus avoiding hypotony and its complications. Grant encouraged the use of pharmacologic adjuncts during the postoperative period. He urged the use of cycloplegics postoperatively to tighten the zonular fibers of the crystalline lens, thus deepening the anterior chamber. He advocated the use of phenylephrine to move the pupil and prevent formation of posterior synechiae. He promoted the use of topical steroids to reduce postoperative inflammation. Cycloplegia and the use of topical steroids are considered routine postoperative care today. Currently, laser suture lysis,[2, 50] 5-fluorouracil[3–5] (5-FU), digital pressure,[6] and other techniques are being increasingly used to enhance operative success. The appropriate use of these techniques is essential to an optimal outcome.

PREOPERATIVE ASSESSMENT

A critical part of the preoperative assessment of patients involves determining the intraocular pressure (IOP) and range at which a patient has lost visual field. This information can aid us in determining which surgical technique can optimally produce the desired "target tension." A target tension is a preoperative estimate of the IOP at which progressive glaucomatous optic nerve damage will be halted. Some patients experience optic nerve damage at pressures as high as 35 or 40 mmHg, and reduction of pressure to the high teens or low 20s may slow or halt glaucomatous progression. On the other hand, some patients with extremely vulnerable discs or advanced disease experience progressive visual field loss with pressures in the high teens or low 20s. Chandler stated that lowering IOP to the 8 to 10 mmHg range achieves control in nearly every patient with glaucoma.[7, 8] Some patients experience progressive visual field loss with IOP ordinarily considered normal. Although normal IOP is considered to be between 12 and 21 mmHg, in reality, this number is merely a statistical value derived from a curve of the IOP distribution in the general population. Unfortunately, glaucoma occurs in patients with IOP at all levels, including pressures well within this statistically normal range.[9]

The initial choice concerning glaucoma filtration surgery is whether to perform a full-thickness procedure or a trabeculectomy. It has been argued that full-thickness procedures produce a lower IOP in the long term.[10–12] However, other studies have failed to confirm these findings.[13–15] Either operation effectively reduces IOP for long periods. Complications, including prolonged postoperative hypotony, flat anterior chamber, choroidal effusion, and earlier postoperative cataract formation, are more common in full-thickness procedures.[10, 11, 13] For these reasons, trabeculectomies are more commonly performed today.

1623

Table 143–1. CLINICAL COMPARISON OF LIMBUS- VERSUS FORNIX-BASED TRABECULECTOMY

	1977[16]		1989[17]	
	LB	FB	LB	FB
Preoperative IOP	25	30.5	30	27
Postoperative IOP	10.8	14.3	11	14
Postoperative IOP with digital pressure	8.7	9.4	8	13
% Digital pressure	34%	54%	43%	50%
% Requiring postoperative medication	23%	38%	21%	56%

LB, limbus-based conjunctival flap; FB, fornix-based conjunctival flap.

Trabeculectomies may be performed using a fornix- or limbus-based conjunctival flap.

Limbus-based conjunctival flaps produce a lower postoperative pressure than fornix-based flaps.[16, 17] A comparison of final IOP after limbus- versus fornix-based conjunctival flaps is outlined in Table 143–1. These results were obtained in patients having trabeculectomy with laser suture lysis and adjunctive subconjunctival 5-FU postoperatively.

Both limbus- and fornix-based techniques are useful in glaucoma filtration surgery. The method selected should be based on assessment of the individual case and the target tension that is required postoperatively. In cases of advanced field loss and disc damage, when visual loss has progressed at relatively low IOP, a limbus-based technique is most likely to achieve a lower postoperative IOP. In cases in which Tenon's fascia is thick, such as in young patients, a tenonectomy is more easily performed in a limbus-based approach. When access to the globe is difficult owing to a crowded orbit, a prominent brow ridge, or deeply set eyes, the fornix-based technique permits easier access. In cases in which visual field loss has occurred at a high IOP (e.g., 30 to 40 mmHg) and postoperative IOP reduction to the teens should suffice, a fornix-based flap approach may be satisfactory. When the conjunctiva is scarred, as often occurs as a result of cataract or scleral buckling surgery, attempts to dissect a limbus-based flap are frequently complicated by significant bleeding or accidental perforations of the overlying conjunctiva called *buttonholes*. In this situation, a fornix-based approach is most suitable. Thickened and scarred conjunctiva can be liberated by sharp dissection with the creation of a fornix-based flap, which is then sutured to the perilimbal region (Table 143–2).

Table 143–2. OPERATIVE PROCEDURE BASED ON CLINICAL CHARACTERISTICS

Limbus-Based Conjunctival Flap (Trabeculectomy or Full-Thickness Procedure)
Low postoperative IOP requirement (far advanced glaucoma)
Thick Tenon's fascia
Young patients

Fornix-Based Conjunctival Flap (Trabeculectomy)
Visual field loss at high IOP
Scarred conjunctiva (reoperations)
Deep-set orbit or prominent brow limiting access to globe

PREOPERATIVE PREPARATION

A carefully orchestrated preoperative medical regimen can assist in making the eye optimally responsive to surgical intervention. Topical and some systemic β-blockers induce prolonged suppression of aqueous humor secretion, which may last for 1 to 2 wk.[18] When it is clinically possible, β-blockade can be discontinued 1 to 2 wk preoperatively to reduce postoperative hypotony and maximize postoperative aqueous flow through the bleb (Table 143–3). Propine and epinephrine derivatives can be stopped 1 wk preoperatively to decrease conjunctival injection. Indirect-acting miotics, such as echothiophate iodide (Phospholine Iodide), should be discontinued 2 wk preoperatively to reduce postoperative inflammation and permit maximal postoperative cycloplegia.

In order to compensate for the cessation of these long-acting drugs, pilocarpine 4 percent can be administered every 2 to 3 hr while a patient is awake, for 2 wk before surgery. This regimen often produces adequate pressure control, even in eyes with high IOP, precarious discs, or advanced visual field loss. Pilocarpine has a relatively short half-life. Therefore, frequent administration reduces IOP fluctuation in the preoperative period. Pilocarpine is discontinued at bedtime the night before surgery.

Carbonic anhydrase inhibitors (CAIs) are continued preoperatively in most cases, unless there are contraindications. Many patients are scheduled for filtration surgery, in part, because CAIs are not tolerated. However, average patients in relatively good health can tolerate CAIs for a short time.

Table 143–3. SAMPLE PREOPERATIVE MEDICATION ADJUSTMENT SCHEDULE

*Beta blockers are discontinued 3 to 14 days preoperatively.
*Epinephrine derivatives are discontinued 3 to 7 days preoperatively.
*Pilocarpine 4% is begun every 2–3 hr after β-blockers are discontinued.
*Carbonic anhydrase inhibitors are started (or continued) after β-blockers are discontinued.
 Topical antibiotic is started in both eyes 1 to 3 days preoperatively.
*Topical prednisolone 1% is started q 2 hr 24 hr preoperatively.
All glaucoma medications are discontinued the night before surgery in the operated eye.

*Refers to the operated eye only.

When IOP is high, visual field loss is advanced, and there is concern about reducing medications during this 2-wk period, IOP should be checked frequently, as often as every 2 to 3 days. If the IOP becomes unacceptably high, the medical regimen can be altered or surgery can be performed sooner. Frequent pilocarpine instillation and continued CAI administration may be viewed as an inconvenience, but most patients find it tolerable on a temporary basis.

Antibiotic prophylaxis is begun 1 to 3 days preoperatively to reduce pathogens in the conjunctival flora. Interestingly, when compared with cataract surgery, the occurrence of endophthalmitis is exceedingly rare in the early period after filtration surgery. Perhaps this is because most filtration surgery is primarily extraocular, and only rarely is manipulation of the posterior segment or vitreous cavity necessary.

One day preoperatively, prednisolone acetate 1 percent may be started every 1 to 2 hr while the patient is awake to reduce irritation related to the preoperative topical regimen and to suppress the inflammatory reaction during the postoperative period.

Generally, other systemic medications that a patient may be taking are not altered before filtering surgery. Anticoagulants are an exception. In order to reduce intraoperative bleeding and to decrease the risk of suprachoroidal hemorrhage, aspirin and nonsteroidal antiinflammatory agents should be discontinued 4 to 6 wk before surgery, if possible. If a patient is taking aspirin or coumadin therapy for transient ischemic attacks or myocardial infarction prophylaxis, the patient's internist should be consulted. In many cases, prophylactic anticoagulation therapy can be temporarily suspended during the perioperative period. Anticoagulants can be safely restarted 2 to 4 wk or earlier during the postoperative period in the absence of ongoing hypotony.

OPERATIVE TECHNIQUES (Refer to Figs. 143–1 to 143–32 and Table 143–4)

Trabeculectomy, Limbus-Based Conjunctival Flap

BRIDLE SUTURE PLACEMENT

Superior Rectus

The globe is depressed by placing a muscle hook in the inferior fornix while the assistant gently sweeps the conjunctiva of the superor fornix toward the limbal area

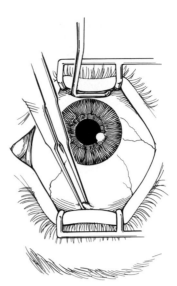

Figure 143–1. The technique of superior rectus bridle suture placement. A muscle hook is applied to the inferior fornix to depress the globe while 0.5-mm forceps are used to grasp the superior rectus muscle tendon at a distance greater than 7.7 mm posterior to the limbus.

with a Weck-cell sponge. The surgeon grasps the tendon of the superior rectus muscle with 0.5-mm forceps at a point posterior to its insertion, approximately 7 to 8 mm posterior to the limbus, and passes a 4–0 silk suture on a tapered needle beneath the superior rectus muscle tendon. The suture arms are gently drawn superiorly and clamped to the drape (Figs. 143–1 to 143–3).

Corneal Bridle Suture

The corneal bridle suture is an excellent alternative to the superior rectus bridle suture. The suture can be placed in clear cornea near the limbus either superiorly or inferiorly. For placement of a superior corneal bridle suture, a 6–0 silk suture on a spatulated needle is passed at midstromal thickness along the superior 2 mm of clear cornea and then advanced for a distance greater than the pupillary axis. If increased surgical exposure is required superiorly, the suture arms can be drawn inferiorly and passed underneath the lid speculum before being clamped to the drape. A disadvantage of the superior corneal bridle suture is inadvertent abrasion of the corneal epithelium, which can delay the postoperative use of adjunctive 5-FU injections. Caution must be exercised while placing the suture to avoid penetrating the cornea and entering the anterior chamber, which may result in a soft globe. Also, corneal distortion can

Table 143–4. NEEDLES AND SUTURES IN FILTRATION SURGERY

Type	Manufacturer	Needle	Suture
Corneal bridle	Ethicon	Spatula	6–0 silk
Superior rectus bridle	Ethicon	Taper	4–0 silk
Limbus-based conjunctival closure	Ethicon	BV75 vascular	10–0 nylon
Fornix-based conjunctival closure	Davis & Geck No. 1573-38	Lancet four wire	10–0 nylon
Scleral flap	Ethicon	Spatula 160–6 Six-wire	10–0 nylon

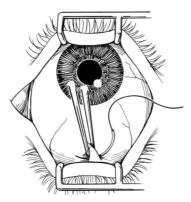

Figure 143–2. A 4–0 silk suture on a taper needle is passed beneath the superior rectus muscle tendon and drawn superiorly.

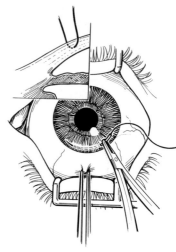

Figure 143–4. The technique of corneal bridle suture placement. The globe is stabilized with 0.5-mm forceps, and a 7–0 silk corneal bridle suture on a spatulated noncutting needle is placed at midstromal depth through the superior peripheral cornea.

interfere with accurate alignment of the trabeculectomy flap. If this occurs, the anterior chamber can be reformed and maintained with intracameral viscoelastic. Alternatively, the corneal bridle suture can be placed at a midstromal level along the inferior junction of clear cornea and sclera then retracted inferiorly, although this method may not provide adequate access to the superior globe. Corneal bridle sutures improve exposure of the surgical field while avoiding conjunctival manipulation adjacent to the filtering site. In many cases, a superior rectus bridle suture may not be necessary (Figs. 143–4 and 143–5).

PARACENTESIS

Filtration surgery requires paracentesis, which is a 1.5- to 2-mm beveled incision made through the peripheral cornea using a Wheeler's knife or a sharply pointed 15-degree blade. Paracentesis permits access to the anterior chamber for chamber deepening with balanced salt solution or viscoelastic. Additionally, while injecting balanced salt solution through the paracentesis, the surgeon is able to observe fluid flow through the sclerostomy and to examine the filtering bleb for leaks at the completion of surgery. It is helpful to carefully select and remember the entry site and direction of the paracentesis. Generally, the paracentesis should be located in the periphery and aligned parallel to the limbus. The knife should be directed toward a specific location (usually 6 o'clock) so that the orientation of the paracentesis can be easily remembered. The internal entry of the paracentesis should be over the iris; otherwise, in a phakic eye, cannulation of a shallow or flat anterior chamber places the crystalline lens in jeopardy. A well-placed beveled paracentesis can be readily located and cannulated as needed. In a soft eye, attempting to cannulate a poorly placed paracentesis is frustrating to the surgeon and traumatic to the eye. A paracentesis is typically self-sealing; however, on occasion, a 10–0 nylon suture may be required for closure (Fig. 143–6).

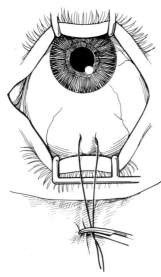

Figure 143–3. The 4–0 silk suture is clamped to the drape superiorly to stabilize the globe and allow wide exposure to the superior fornix.

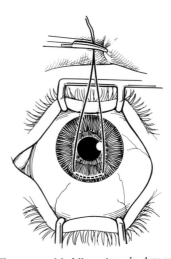

Figure 143–5. The corneal bridle suture is drawn inferiorly, with care taken to minimize corneal epithelial disruption, and is clamped to the drape to stabilize the globe in a depressed position.

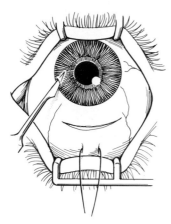

Figure 143–6. A supersharp blade is used to create a beveled paracentesis incision that is located within 3 clock hours of the 12 o'clock meridien. Care is taken to avoid inadvertent trauma to uveal or lenticular tissue.

Limbus-Based Conjunctival Flap

A functional filtering bleb is usually delineated posteriorly by the scar that results from surgical closure of the conjunctiva. Therefore, it is best to enter the subconjunctival space at a site that is far posteriorly (in the fornix) as possible and that still permits access for surgical closure at the end of the procedure. A more posteriorly placed conjunctival wound is associated with less inflammation and reduced tendency to develop wound leaks postoperatively.

The conjunctiva is first grasped 10 to 15 mm posterior to the limbus with nontoothed conjunctival forceps and gently lifted off the surface of the globe. The conjunctival incision is made using sharp-tipped Westcott's scissors in a circumferential orientation for approximately 2 clock hr. The conjunctival flap is bluntly dissected anteriorly above the level fo Tenon's fascia, immediately beneath the conjunctiva. Dissection is carried anteriorly through the insertion of Tenon's fascia to the insertion of the conjunctiva at the limbus, which is typically 0.5 to 1.0 mm over clear cornea. This limbal dissection can be facilitated with a Beaver No. 57 blade.

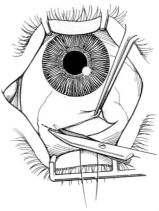

Figure 143–8. The limbus-based conjunctival flap dissection is extended nasally and temporally for an arc length of approximately 14 mm.

Sharp Westcott's scissors can then be used to excise Tenon's fascia overlying the area of the scleral flap. Tenon's fascia is gently retracted and then incised slightly above the surface of the episclera, thus reducing the likelihood of accidentally severing large episcleral vessels. Meticulous hemostasis should be maintained in order to prevent inflammation induced by red blood cell and fibrin deposition. Underwater monopolar diathermy with a fine 0.25-mm tip provides excellent hemostasis with superb control (Figs. 143–7 to 143–11).[19]

Scleral Flap

While the globe is stabilized with 0.12-mm forceps or a cotton-tipped applicator, a diamond blade or other suitably sharp knife is used to create the margins of a 3 × 3-mm rectangular scleral flap. A Beaver No. 57 or No. 64 blade is used to dissect the scleral flap anteriorly. The flap should extend beyond white sclera into clear cornea. The flap should be approximately one-half to three-quarters scleral thickness. Thinner flaps may shred, tear, or even be avulsed during suturing. The size

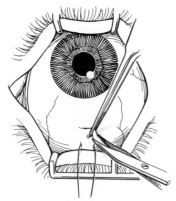

Figure 143–7. The conjunctival flap of the limbus-based trabeculectomy originates 12 to 16 mm posterior to the limbus, with the initial conjunctival incision made anterior to the superior rectus bridle suture.

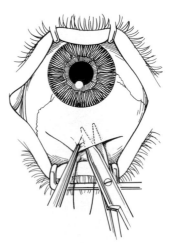

Figure 143–9. A combination of blunt and sharp dissection anteriorly toward the limbus in the plane between the conjunctiva and Tenon's capsule creates a thin conjunctival flap.

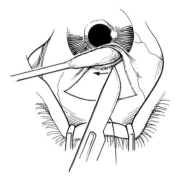

Figure 143–10. Dissection of the limbus-based conjunctival flap continues anteriorly with fine dissection of Tenon's fibers at the limbus, while the assistant gently rolls the conjunctival flap anteriorly with a premoistened cotton-tipped applicator.

of the flap is not as important as the ratio between the flap and the sclerostomy opening. In general, the scleral flap should be twice the size of the inner sclerostomy opening in order to tamponade aqueous flow.

A rectangular or triangular flap can be used. A rectangular flap permits two corner and three side sutures for flap closure, compared with one corner and two side sutures for a triangular flap. If laser suture lysis is planned postoperatively, the rectangular flap provides greater flexibility during suture lysis postoperatively (Figs. 143–12 and 143–13).

SCLEROSTOMY

While the globe is stabilized with 0.12-mm or Pierce-Hoskins forceps, the assistant gently retracts the sclerectomy flap tip with tissue forceps. A diamond blade or other sharp blade is used to enter the anterior chamber at the base of the sclerectomy flap. Using the sharp blade, two radial incisions are made approximately 1 mm apart, joining the initial incision and forming a small flap. The flap is grasped with 0.12-mm forceps and is resected at its base with Vannas scissors, creating a 1 × 1-mm sclerostomy. Alternatively, a Kelly-Descemet punch can be placed through the slit opening at the base of the scleral flap. Two to three punches usually suffice to create a rounded 1 × 1-mm sclerostomy.

Care should be taken to avoid dissection posterior to the scleral spur, because ciliary body bleeding may

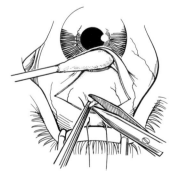

Figure 143–11. A tenonectomy is performed while the assistant gently retracts the conjunctival flap.

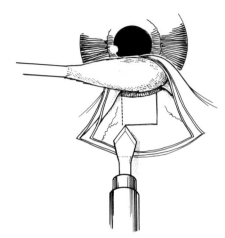

Figure 143–12. The perimeter of a 4 × 3-mm sclerectomy flap is defined by a diamond blade or other sharp blade.

occur. Within a few minutes, uveal bleeding from the iris or ciliary body often stops spontaneously after gentle irrigation and observation. However, blood should not be allowed to accumulate in the eye. If bleeding persists, a drop of 1:100,000 sterile unpreserved epinephrine can be used to provide additional hemostasis. Bleeding may be preempted in some cases by prior application of epinephrine. Underwater monopolar diathermy to the ciliary body or iris root can effectively provide hemostasis as a last resort if performed *under direct visualization.* However, considerable caution is advised when performing cautery in this manner, because accidental cautery of the lens or hyaloid face with resultant cataract formation or vitreous loss can occur (Fig. 143–14).

IRIDECTOMY

The peripheral iridectomy should be broad, basal, and larger than the inner sclerostomy. The surgeon

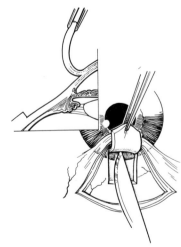

Figure 143–13. The sclerectomy flap of approximately one-half scleral thickness is beveled forward onto 1.5 mm of clear cornea while the assistant gently retracts the apex of the flap with Colibri forceps. Note the depth of the scleral bed and the underlying blue choroid.

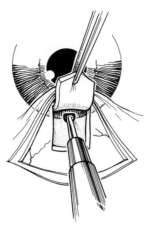

Figure 143–14. A Descemet's punch is used to create a sclerostomy anterior to and including a portion of the scleral spur. Several bites are usually required to achieve an adequate size.

grasps the iris approximately 0.5 mm from its base using 0.12-mm or other fine forceps in order to avoid accidental inclusion of the greater arterial circle of the iris or ciliary body. The iris is then gently retracted through the sclerostomy. Vannas scissors are held in the surgeon's dominant hand, while the iris is drawn to the nondominant hand. The initial incision is created, and aqueous may be released. The jaws of the Vannas scissors are reopened, the iris is drawn to the opposite side, and the iridectomy incision is completed. This technique intentionally creates a wider iridectomy than the inner sclerostomy and thus prevents occlusion of the sclerostomy by uveal tissue. A basal iridectomy should not extend anteriorly near the visual axis, because monocular diplopia can result. A prolapsed iris is gently irrigated and reposited into the anterior chamber with balanced salt solution (Fig. 143–15).

SCLERAL FLAP CLOSURE

Size 10–0 nylon suture on a spatulated needle is used to place interrupted sutures at midscleral thickness through the two corners and three sides of the sclerectomy flap. Four throws of 10–0 nylon allow the surgeon to set the tension of the sutures and titrate aqueous runoff along the sides of the flap. In order to fashion a secure flap, the sutures must be carefully placed. Once

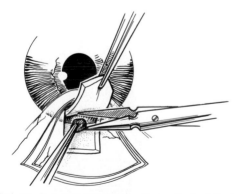

Figure 143–15. A basal iridectomy is created while the iris is gently placed on stretch and drawn into the jaws of the Vannas scissors in a nasal and temporal direction.

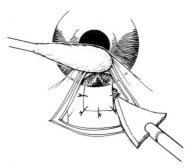

Figure 143–16. The sclerectomy flap is secured with interrupted 10–0 nylon sutures, and aqueous runoff is evaluated by Weck-cell sponge assessment.

they are placed, aqueous runoff can be assessed by infusing balanced salt solution through the paracentesis. By placing a Weck-cell sponge near the scleral flap, the surgeon can gauge the flow rate. If flow is brisk, the eye rapidly softens, or the anterior chamber shallows after balanced salt infusion, more or tighter flap sutures are required. If there is no fluid flow and the eye remains hard, sutures should be loosened. Overall, the flow should be minimal, with good maintenance of the anterior chamber to avoid postoperative hypotony and its complications (Fig. 143–16).

Monopolar (Underwater) Diathermy

Monopolar diathermy is used selectively to cauterize small vessels and permits concise focal application of cautery in a wet surgical field. It can be used throughout the entire operation, including cauterization of fine bleeding vessels during conjunctival closure. Additionally, the tip of the underwater diathermy probe can be placed at the margin of the scleral flap after it is closed to retract the edges, thus increasing fluid flow around the flap, if desired.[19] (Refer to Chapter 135.)

Conjunctival Hydrodissection

Before conjunctival closure, a strong stream of balanced salt solution can be directed beneath the perilimbal conjunctiva to elevate the tissue hydraulically. The insertion of Tenon's fascia is then incised with Westcott's scissors, thus connecting the perilimbal bleb region with the peripheral bleb and the full 360-degree subconjunctival space. This may promote circumlinear filtration of aqueous humor through the bleb postoperatively (Figs. 143–17 and 143–18).

Limbus-Based Conjunctival Flap Closure

Meticulous watertight conjunctival closure is as integral to a successful result as the surgery that precedes it. Conjunctival wound leaks cause hypotony and contribute to formation of localized blebs and surgical

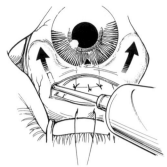

Figure 143–17. Hydrodissection of the conjunctival tissue is achieved by irrigating with a steady stream of balanced salt solution.

failure. Additionally, wound leaks cause delay in the institution of adjuvant 5-FU therapy. As for technique, there is a great deal of variation in suture technique, suture type, and the needle used for conjunctival wound closure. Each surgeon will find a method that produces optimal results in his or her hands.

It is helpful to approximate the anterior and posterior conjunctival wound margins before wound closure. This reduces tension across the surgical wound during closure. It is best to use nontoothed forceps during conjunctival manipulation and wound closure in order to minimize tissue trauma. The conjunctival wound is apposed and bisected or trisected by two or three interrupted 10–0 nylon sutures. These sutures should incorporate the anterior and posterior conjunctival flap. A running mattress closure of a limbus-based conjunctival flap is begun by using 10–0 nylon suture on a four-wire vascular tapered needle (Ethicon BV75) and incorporating a 2:1:1 square knot at the initiation. Six-wire spatulated needles cut openings through the conjunctiva. These openings are larger than the 10–0 nylon suture that follows, and wound leaks can result postoperatively, especially if 5-FU is administered. The needle and its holder are held parallel to the wound, and the conjunctiva is placed on the needle with the Pierse-Hoskins conjunctival forceps or straight nontoothed McPherson tying forceps, alternating successive bites of posterior and anterior conjunctival lips with no more than 0.5 to 1.0 mm between bites. Each 5 mm of conjunctival closure is then reduced to 4 mm by slight contraction of the conjunctival tissue, and a locking suture is placed.

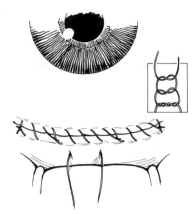

Figure 143–19. The limbus-based conjunctival running closure incorporates locking sutures every 5 mm and square knots at the initiation and end.

The wound closure is usually 15 to 20 mm in length and is secured with a double lock at the distal end. Alternatively, a traditional running-locking or interrupted closure provides adequate wound closure in most cases (Fig. 143–19).

Fornix-Based Conjunctival Flap

The conjunctival opening for a fornix-based trabeculectomy begins with a peritomy along 2 to 3 clock hr at the limbus (usually superiorly).

The conjunctival flap is bluntly and sharply dissected posteriorly, and conjunctival hydrodissection and tunneling are used to create a circumferential bleb. Minimal cautery is applied to prevent scarring. A tenonectomy is difficult to perform because of poor access to the undersurface of the conjunctiva, especially after prior surgery, but can be accomplished in some cases. Creation of a sclerectomy flap, sclerostomy, basal iridectomy, and sclerectomy flap suture closure are the same as previously described for limbus-based trabeculectomy (Fig. 143–20).

The technique for fornix-based conjunctival flap closure varies according to a surgeon's preference. Some place winged nylon or Vicryl sutures at either ends of the conjunctiva to the adjoining corneoscleral junction.

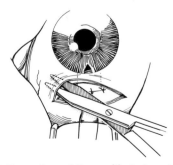

Figure 143–18. Tunneling of the perilimbal conjunctiva through sharp dissection encourages diffuse filtration.

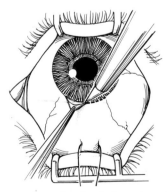

Figure 143–20. Creation of a fornix-based conjunctival flap by peritomy formation at the limbus.

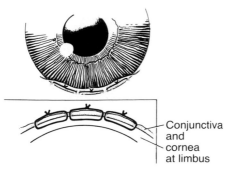

Figure 143–21. A fornix-based trabeculectomy closure with conjunctival-corneal interrupted sutures. A Seidel's test is performed with 2 percent sodium fluorescein to check for leaks at the close of surgery.

Fornix-based conjunctival closure is frequently associated with postoperative wound leaks, which decrease bleb survival. Additionally, wound leaks cause delay in implementing adjuvant 5-FU, laser suture lysis, and digital pressure therapy.

Watertight conjunctival-corneal closure can be enhanced by débriding the superior 1 to 2 mm of corneal epithelium adjacent to the limbus. Gentle abrasion with the back of a rounded surgical blade, such as a Bard-Parker No. 15 or Beaver No. 64 knife, or use of eraser cautery effectively removes the epithelium. The conjunctival flap can be sutured in place using 10–0 nylon on a four-wire spatula-tip needle (e.g., Davis and Geck, Ophthalon). Two to four long circumferential interrupted mattress sutures are placed along the limbal edge (Fig. 143–21). The needle should be passed at the midstromal corneal level. The interrupted suture is passed through conjunctiva, cornea, then conjunctiva and is tied with a 4:1:1 knot. This method of flap closure provides a secure barrier that reduces the incidence of bleb leaks. The sutures typically become buried by conjunctival tissue, causing patients little discomfort. Exposed sutures can be removed after the wound has healed.

Full-Thickness Procedures

Historically, the primary filtering procedure performed for medically uncontrolled glaucoma utilized the creation of an unobstructed opening, a sclerostomy, through the eye wall for aqueous outflow.[20, 21] These procedures include trephination,[22, 23] thermal sclerostomy,[24] and more recently the posterior lip sclerectomy.[25] Similarities far outweigh the differences among these procedures. Proponents feel that postoperative IOP control with full-thickness filtration surgery is superior to that obtained after trabeculectomy.[10, 12] Complications, including prolonged hypotony, shallow or flat anterior chamber, choroidal effusion, choroidal hemorrhage, and cataract formation, reportedly occur more frequently with full-thickness filtration procedures than with trabeculectomy.[10, 11, 13] Full-thickness procedures are currently used only for those patients for whom especially low postoperative IOP is essential (e.g., far ad-

vanced glaucomatous optic nerve damage) or for patients with low-tension glaucoma.

The most commonly performed full-thickness procedure is a posterior lip sclerectomy, in which a knife or a punch is used to create an unguarded sclerostomy.[25] The initial surgical approach is identical to that for a trabeculectomy using a limbus-based conjunctival flap. After the corneal or rectus muscle bridle suture is placed, a paracentesis is made. The conjunctiva is grasped 10 to 15 mm posterior to the limbus with nontoothed forceps, and a 2 clock hr circumlinear incision is made with sharp Westcott's scissors. Blunt dissection is carried out at the plane between the conjunctiva and Tenon's fascia. The insertion of Tenon's fascia is incised, and dissection to the limbal insertion of conjunctiva is made for 1 to 2 clock hr. The back of a No. 15 Bard-Parker blade is used in order to advance the conjunctival insertion maximally. Reflecting the conjunctival flap anteriorly over the cornea and applying gentle traction with a moistened cotton-tipped applicator or cellulose sponge facilitate dissection at the limbus. A tenonectomy is usually performed in the area underlying the conjunctival flap. A diamond blade or 15-degree supersharp blade is used to enter the eye immediately posterior to the conjunctival insertion. If the eye is soft or the anterior chamber is shallow after the paracentesis is created, the anterior chamber should be re-formed before entering the eye at the sclerostomy site. The sclerostomy incision should be 1.5 to 2 mm long. The knife should be advanced far enough to incise the wall of the eye, while taking care to avoid accidental injury to the iris or lens. A Kelly-Descemet punch is then gently inserted through the incision, and a 1- to 1.5-mm opening is created. The iris typically protrudes through the sclerostomy. The iris is grasped with 0.12-mm or other fine forceps, and a broad basal iridectomy is performed as previously described. Flow through the sclerostomy is assessed by injecting balanced salt solution through the paracentesis. Flow should be brisk and unobstructed by the iris, ciliary body, or lens. The conjunctival flap is closed in the fornix-based manner described previously. The bleb is evaluated for leaks using 2 percent sodium fluorescein solution after conjunctival closure is complete. If the anterior chamber collapses or is extremely shallow at the end of surgery, it should be re-formed with viscoelastic (Figs. 143–22 to 143–24).

POSTOPERATIVE MEDICATION AND INSTRUCTION

At the close of surgery, subconjunctival steroids (e.g., dexamethasone phosphate, 1 to 2 mg) can be injected subconjunctivally, opposite the filtering bleb. Routine postoperative injection of subconjunctival antibiotics is unnecessary at the conclusion of filtering surgery. Topical scopolamine 0.25 percent (or atropine 1 percent solution) and antibiotic drops (Tobrex) or ointment (e.g., Polysporin or bacitracin ointment) are administered. The eyelid is gently taped shut, and an eye patch and shield are placed on the eye. Care is taken to avoid

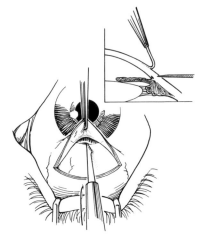

Figure 143–22. A full-thickness limbus-based filter. A supersharp blade creates the anterior boundary of the sclerostomy.

pressure on the eye. In some cases, patching the contralateral eye is helpful to reduce bilateral eye movement during the immediate postoperative period. Patients are usually admitted to the hospital for bed rest for 2 to 3 days to discourage excessive activity. They are instructed to avoid straining, bending, or heavy lifting in the postoperative period. Mild anxiolytics (e.g., diazepam, 2 mg every 4 hr) and nonaspirin-containing pain medications (acetaminophen, 1 g every 4 hr) may be ordered for use, as needed. Excessive activity during this period, especially when hypotony coexists, significantly increases the risk for suprachoroidal hemorrhage, which can be devastating. Mild laxatives should be ordered postoperatively for patients with a history of constipation.

POSTOPERATIVE PERIOD

The postoperative period is crucial to the success of filtration surgery. The goal is to modulate wound healing. The primary concern is to promote healing of the conjunctival wound while maintaining a patent sclerostomy and limiting subconjunctival fibrosis. IOP must be

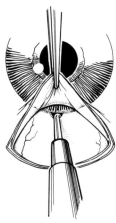

Figure 143–23. A full-thickness limbus-based filter. A full-thickness sclerostomy is created with a Kelly-Descemet punch.

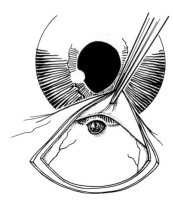

Figure 143–24. A full-thickness limbus-based filter. Iris prolapse develops spontaneously through the patent sclerostomy.

closely monitored throughout the postoperative period. Thorough knowledge regarding the use of topical steroids, cycloplegics, antibiotics, and various adjunctive therapies is essential for successful management of the filter in the postoperative period. Surgeons must keep pace with new adjuncts as they become available.

Early Postoperative Period

At the first postoperative visit, the general filtration pattern is noted. Both eyes are applanated. The corneal status, anterior chamber depth, and status of the posterior segment are assessed. If the IOP is low or the bleb is flat, 2 percent sodium fluorescein solution is instilled in the conjunctival cul-de-sac and the wound is examined for a leak (Seidel's test). In the absence of a bleb leak, topical prednisolone acetate 1 percent or dexamethasone sodium phosphate 0.1 percent suspension is started every 2 to 4 hr, and a steroid ointment can be given at bedtime as well if needed. If a leak is detected, topical steroids should be withheld or given at a reduced rate (e.g., every 4 to 8 hr). Antibiotic prophylaxis in the form of topical sulfacetamide (Bleph 10 percent) or chloramphenical (Chloroptic) should be administered b.i.d. to t.i.d. Alternatively, erythromycin (Ilotycin) or polymyxin-bacitracin ointment can be given at night, and in cases with corneal surface irregularities, ointment can be given more frequently. In order to help maintain anterior chamber depth and to prevent formation of posterior synechiae, scopolamine 0.25 percent or atropine 1 percent is administered b.i.d. to q.i.d. In order to increase dilation of the pupil, phenylephrine 2.5 percent can be used q.i.d. (Table 143–5).

Tapering the Medical Regimen

Topical prednisolone acetate 1 percent administration is continued until the anterior segment is devoid of inflammation and the conjunctiva in the region of the filtering bleb is pale. During the first 3 wk, prednisolone is administered every 1 to 4 hr according to the clinical response. Thereafter, prednisolone is gradually tapered. The frequency is gradually reduced from four times to

Table 143–5. POSTOPERATIVE MEDICAL REGIMEN

Medication	Frequency
Topical antibiotic:	
Drops: sulfa, chloramphenicol	b.i.d.
*Ointment: erythromycin, polymyxin-bacitracin	At bedtime
Cycloplegic:	
Scopolamine 0.25%, atropine 1%	b.i.d.
Steroid:	
Prednisolone acetate 1% suspension	Every 2–4 hr
Dexamethasone phosphate 0.1% suspension	Every 2–4 hr
Dexamethasone phosphate 0.05% ointment	At bedtime
†Phenylephrine 2.5%	q.i.d.

*Used when ocular surface is irregular or for comfort (after drops are given).

†Used when anterior chamber is shallow or pupil is miotic.

once daily, typically allowing 1 wk at each level. If the eye is quiet, steroids can often be discontinued by the eighth postoperative week. The length of time an individual patient will require topical steroids varies from patient to patient. If significant postoperative inflammation persists, betamethasone, 4 to 6 mg (Celestone Soluspan 0.8 ml with 0.2 ml Xylocaine 2 percent solution), can be injected into the sub-Tenon's space 180 degrees from the bleb every 4 days or as needed to control inflammation.

Cycloplegic medications are usually continued for approximately 3 wk postoperatively. Both scopolamine and atropine are long acting. If the anterior chamber is deep and quiet, IOP is greater than 5 mmHg, and there is no choroidal effusion, these medications can be administered once daily after the first postoperative week.

Antibiotics are gradually tapered in conjunction with topical steroids. Long-term prophylaxis with topical sulfa drops or erythromycin ointment given at bedtime is recommended for the lifetime of the patient, especially in the presence of thin, functioning filtration blebs. This suggestion is based on the clinical impression that the treatment may reduce the incidence of late bleb infections and endophthalmitis. Filtration blebs extending into the inferior quadrants may be at greater risk for bleb infection.[26] In these cases, topical tobramycin or trimethoprim-sulfisoxazole may be considered for prophylaxis. Antibiotic solutions should be replaced every 2 to 3 mo. It may be helpful to refrigerate prophylactic medications to reduce the likelihood of bacterial contamination.[27]

CONTRALATERAL EYE

It is extremely important to monitor the IOP in both the operated and unoperated eye during the period after filtration surgery because a small number of patients may evidence significant pressure rises in the unoperated eye. This may be due to discontinuation of CAIs, the crossover effect of topically administered steroids, or confusion about the intended postoperative drug regimen. Postoperative instruction and medication cards that detail the medical regimen help to facilitate patients' compliance. If the contralateral eye reaches unsafe levels

of pressure, CAIs can be reinstituted at low doses on a temporary basis with the risk of reducing aqueous flow through the filtering bleb during the early postoperative period. Although not approved for chronic use, apraclonidine hydrochloride 1 percent (Iopidine 1 percent) b.i.d. or t.i.d. can be administered as a temporary adjunct to reduce IOP. Laser trabeculoplasty may also be a viable option. In the event that pressure control cannot be achieved by medical or laser therapy, filtration surgery is indicated.

POSTOPERATIVE ADJUNCTIVE THERAPIES

Appropriate use of adjunctive therapies following glaucoma filtration surgery can markedly improve overall success. Currently available adjuncts include digital pressure, laser suture lysis, subconjunctival 5-FU injections, pressure patching, and use of the Simmons's shell tamponade technique.

Digital Pressure

By temporarily elevating IOP, digital pressure promotes the flow of aqueous humor through the sclerostomy. Continued use can produce bleb expansion and a gradual decrease in baseline IOP. Digital pressure is measured on a scale of 1 to 10 in terms of strength and duration. In most cases it is not initiated for several days or weeks postoperatively. In selected cases, it can be used as early as postoperative day one. After IOP is obtained by applanation tonometry, the physician administers digital pressure to reduce the IOP to within the target pressure range. Digital pressure is typically performed through the lower eyelid while gaze is directed superiorly. The degree of pressure may vary from light to firm; however, digital pressure should never cause severe discomfort. Digital pressure can be applied as often as hourly or as seldom as weekly. Patients must receive careful instruction about the proper technique and frequency of application. It is essential to observe patients applying digital pressure. Afterward, the IOP is measured in order to evaluate its effectiveness. Repeating both observation and instruction at subsequent visits is necessary to ensure success with this technique. In some cases, incipient bleb failure can be reversed by introduction of digital pressure.[6]

Laser Suture Lysis

An extremely helpful procedure that is being increasingly used after tight suture closure of the scleral flap is laser suture lysis. Developed independently and concurrently by Simmons and associates[2, 50] and Hoskins and Migliazzo,[28] this procedure may permit gradual conversion of a guarded trabeculectomy to a full-thickness filtering procedure with graded IOP reduction. After suture lysis is performed, resistance to aqueous flow through the sclerostomy is reduced in a more controlled manner. This technique promotes early stabilization of the anterior chamber and mobilization of the patient postoperatively while reducing the incidence of hypotony and its attendant complications.

Laser suture lysis is performed using topical anesthesia (proparacaine 0.5 percent). An argon blue-green (or comparable wavelength) laser is used. Laser settings are 50 μm spot size, power of 300 to 900 mW, and duration of 0.05 to 0.2 sec. A Hoskins lens or the flat edge of a four-mirror Zeiss lens is gently used to compress the conjunctiva, facilitating a clear view of the scleral flap sutures. To avoid applying unnecessary stress on the conjunctival wound in limbus-based conjunctival flaps, the lens should be applied to the superior cornea first, then gently advanced posteriorly over the conjunctiva until the scleral flap and sutures are in view. This reduces production of inadvertent conjunctival wound leaks. For fornix-based flaps, the reverse is true. The lens should be placed superior to the limbus-based conjunctival wound and moved anteriorly until the sutures are in view. In order to avoid accidentally producing a hole in the filtering bleb, the beam is retrofocused beneath the suture to decrease energy delivery to overlying conjunctiva. One shot typically lyses the suture. An immediate retraction of the cut ends of the suture is usually seen, often with elevation of the filtering bleb. When subconjunctival hemorrhage partially obscures the view of the scleral sutures, a krypton laser with a 640-nm wavelength or a diode laser using an 805-nm wavelength can be used to penetrate the hemorrhage more effectively. The presence of thick Tenon's tissue can entrap 10–0 nylon sutures, and after laser suture lysis, the suture may stand vertically, potentially causing a bleb leak. The Hoskins lens can be used to flatten these sutures, after which the suture can be cut at its base with the laser, leaving a small segment of inert nylon suture within the bleb.

It is generally advisable to wait until postoperative day 3 before performing laser suture lysis. This delay allows the conjunctival wound to seal before manipulation. Suture lysis is most effective between 3 days and 3 wk postoperatively and is usually of no benefit thereafter. Incorporating five sutures into the scleral flap permits improved titration of aqueous flow; this usually reduces the incidence of acute hypotony following lysis of a single suture. Only one suture usually is lysed per day. If the IOP is still deemed too high 30 to 45 min after suture lysis, digital pressure can be applied cautiously. In addition to laser suture lysis, other postoperative adjuncts, such as 5-FU and sub-Tenon's steroid injections, may be used.

Releasable Suture Technique

If laser equipment is not available or if the presence of conjunctival scarring and thickening is expected to prevent adequate visualization of the sutures postoperatively, a releasable trabecular flap suture can be used.[29] The releasable suture technique permits adjustment of aqueous outflow at the slit lamp during the early postoperative period following filtration surgery. It is applicable to limbus- and fornix-based trabeculectomy and full-thickness procedures, as well as combined cataract extraction and glaucoma filtering procedures.

The primary filtration procedure is performed using either a limbus- or fornix-based approach. A triangular or rectangular sclerectomy flap may be created with interrupted 10–0 nylon sutures tied to secure the sides of the flap. A 10–0 nylon apical suture is placed through the intact sclera posterior to the sclerectomy flap and brought out anteriorly through the apex of the scleral flap. This suture is then passed beneath the conjunctival insertion at the limbus into partial-thickness cornea and out onto the epithelial surface of the cornea. Four throws of the distal end of the suture are passed around the tying forceps before grasping the suture lying on the surface of the scleral flap. This slipknot is closed tightly rather than loosely to reduce aqueous runoff and lessen the risks of hypotony during the immediate postoperative period. The end of the releasable suture exiting onto the corneal epithelial surface is trimmed to permit approximately 2 mm to remain exposed. The conjunctiva is closed in the usual manner appropriate for either the limbus- or fornix-based techniques. After the eye has stabilized during the initial postoperative period, the releasable suture can be removed to increase aqueous flow and effectively convert a partial-thickness to a full-thickness procedure in a more controlled fashion. If postoperative filtration is adequate, removal of the releasable suture can be delayed for a period of 2 to 3 wk or until the eye is fully stabilized (Fig. 143–25).[29]

5-Fluorouracil

The chemotherapeutic agent 5-FU has become an important adjunct to successful filtration surgery.[3–5] 5-FU is a pyrimidine base analog that is incorporated into replicating strands of both messenger RNA and DNA and inhibits fibroblastic proliferation and subsequent scar formation. Subconjunctival scarring is considered the major cause of bleb failure. The original protocol, used only in eyes considered at high risk for surgical failure, called for 5 mg subconjunctival injections b.i.d. for 1 wk, followed by daily injections for a second week, at which time therapy was discontinued. Although this regimen was effective, many side effects were reported. It has become apparent that 5-FU can be effective at lower doses.[30, 31] Deciding which regimen will be most effective without incurring unwanted side effects is a central question in using 5-FU therapy. At the first sign of impending bleb failure, in both high-risk and primary filtration surgery cases, 5-FU administration should be considered. Initial signs of bleb failure include progressive conjunctival vascularization with corkscrew vessels on the surface and internal aspects of the bleb, localization of the bleb, decrease in microcyst formation, and a progressive rise in IOP on successive visits, even if IOP is within an otherwise acceptable range. For example, if IOP rises from 3 mmHg on day 1 to 9 mmHg on day 6, in the presence of increasing bleb injection, serious consideration should be given to instituting 5-FU injections until IOP and bleb appearance improve. 5-FU injections are administered daily or b.i.d. in high-

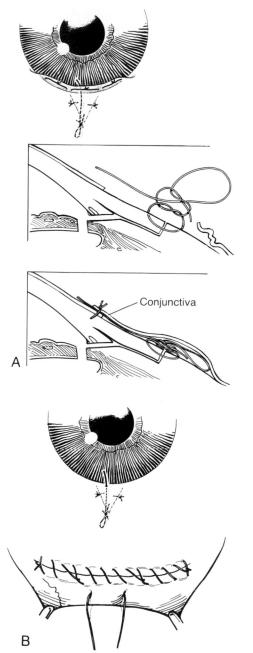

Figure 143–25. The releasable suture technique. (*A*, fornix based; *B*, limbus based).

risk cases, with treatment tailored to the individual patient's response.

5-FU is packaged in 10-ml vials containing 500 mg of 5-FU per vial. Five milligrams of 5-FU is used per injection. 5-FU can be injected undiluted (0.1 ml) or may be diluted with normal saline (e.g., 0.1 ml 5-FU in 0.4 ml normal saline) using a 30-gauge needle on a tuberculin syringe. Before delivery, topical proparacaine 0.5 percent is instilled in the conjunctival cul-de-sac. Phenylephrine 2.5 percent may be used to blanch conjunctival vessels before injection. Additional anesthesia may be achieved by applying a cotton pledget moistened with proparacaine 0.5 percent or cocaine 4 percent at

the site selected for injection. Injecting the 5-FU solution slowly reduces pain. During the early postoperative course, 5-FU is injected 180 degrees away from the bleb to minimize the risk of conjunctival flap disruption. As conjunctival wound stability increases, injections are placed within 3 clock hr of the filtration site but at least 1 clock hr posterior to the sclerostomy. Care is taken to avoid conjunctival vessels. If bleeding occurs, vessels can be tamponaded with topical phenylephrine 2.5 percent applied directly by a cotton-tipped applicator.

Complications related to 5-FU administration are generally mild and self-limited. Bleb leaks may develop at the conjunctival wound margin or at a needle puncture site. If this occurs, 5-FU must be discontinued until the bleb leak closes. A bandage contact lens or collagen shield can serve to promote closure of the leak. 5-FU causes corneal epithelial toxic changes in 100 percent of patients if therapy is continued long enough. The onset of corneal epithelial defects usually starts as superficial punctate keratopathy with tiny erosions that typically resolve spontaneously over a 3- to 4-wk period after 5-FU administration is discontinued. Geographic corneal epithelial defects may develop after only three injections. 5-FU complications increase with the number and frequency of injections. Delayed and staggered administration of 5-FU over a period of weeks or even months may be helpful; however, if the bleb has failed, 5-FU therapy should be stopped. Patients' comfort can be improved by use of erythromycin ointment two or three times a day. Additionally, a bandage contact lens may permit continued administration of 5-FU in the presence of mild punctate epithelial changes. If corneal changes continue to progress, 5-FU injections should be stopped to prevent formation of large corneal defects, which can result in corneal scarring or, rarely, progress to corneal ulceration.[32, 33] Other complications including bleb-related endophthalmitis, suprachoroidal hemorrhage, and retinal detachment have been reported with 5-FU therapy.[5]

Shell Tamponade Technique

Excessive subconjunctival flow after full or guarded filtration procedures can lead to hypotony and shallowing of the anterior chamber. These consequences predispose to choroidal separation and a vicious cycle of decreased aqueous production, low flow through the bleb, flat anterior chamber, cataract formation, peripheral anterior synechiae formation, and occasionally corneal decompensation. This cycle can be avoided by early and judicious application of a Simmons shell, which is a large scleral lens with vent holes. A smooth raised platform (for placement over the sclerostomy) is located on the posterior surface. When placed on the eye, the shell tamponades aqueous flow through the sclerostomy.[34–36]

Proparacaine anesthesia is applied to the cul-de-sac, and viscoelastic or antibiotic ointment is applied to the concave surface of the shell. The shell is grasped by jeweler's forceps through peripheral holes and applied to the conjunctival surface of the eye. The lids are closed, and moistened cotton balls in the form of a torpedo are applied to the upper and lower orbital recesses. One or two eye pads are then placed over the periorbital region, and the eye is firmly patched. 3-M Dermiclear tape appears to be well tolerated by patients. Placing an 8–0 or 9–0 silk tether suture to the shell and anchoring the end to the adjacent skin can help prevent lens rotation.[37] Ideally, patients are reexamined within 1 to 3 hr after the shell is initially inserted, but reexamination at 24 hr is mandatory. Dramatic deepening of the anterior chamber is frequently seen within 30 to 45 min after application. The shell can be left in place for one to several days, as needed, until the anterior chamber stabilizes. Thereafter, patients must be examined at least daily. Topical antibiotic and steroid ointments can be used concurrently.[36]

Pressure Patching

An alternative to using a Simmons shell is pressure (torpedo) patching. Moistened cotton balls are rolled between the hands to make a firm, elongated roll (the "torpedo"). With the patient's eyes closed, one roll is placed in the superior orbital sulcus and the other in the inferior sulcus. One or two eye pads are applied over the torpedos and firmly taped in place. If the pressure patch is not firmly taped, aqueous flow is not adequately slowed. Patients must be monitored in the same manner as patients with a Simmons shell.

FILTRATION REVISION SURGERY

When primary filtration surgery fails, filtration revision is an option for achieving glaucoma control entailing minimal tissue manipulation. The causes of filtration failure can be divided into intraocular, scleral, and extraocular factors.[38] Appropriate management of a failing bleb can be initiated only after the site of resistance has been identified. Prolapse of the lens, iris, vitreous, or ciliary body into the sclerostomy may block filtration. The opening made during filtration surgery should be greater than 1 mm in diameter to avoid inadvertent closure due to accumulation of postoperative inflammatory debris or incorporation of remnants of the iris, sclera, lens, capsule, or Descemet's membrane.[40]

Most filtration failures are caused by fibrovascular proliferation at the episcleral level, which blocks the external aspect of the sclerostomy and may extend peripherally along the filter bleb.[39, 40] Other cases of failed filtration are due to the formation of a Tenon's cyst. This cyst is a domelike elevation of cicatrized conjunctiva that overlies a patent sclerostomy and has outer walls that resist transconjunctival filtration.

Filtration revision is the preferred solution to filtration failure in selected cases because it conserves conjunctiva for future filtration surgery, if needed. Filtration revision surgery is technically less invasive than other forms of surgery and is therefore associated with less inflammation and subsequent fibrosis. In eyes with good visual potential, we recommend continued attempts to establish adequate glaucoma control through primary filtration rather than resorting to transscleral Nd. YAG laser cyclophotocoagulation, cyclocryotherapy, or the placement of setons because of the risk of visual loss related to these latter techniques. We have found that incorporation of postoperative 5-FU therapy and digital pressure techniques has enhanced filtration success.

Risk factors for filtration failure include hemorrhage, inflammation, excessive surgical manipulation, prior ocular surgery, youth, and in some cases darker skin pigmentation.[39]

EVALUATION OF THE FAILING FILTER

Clinical signs of bleb failure can be evaluated by slit-lamp examination. These include lack of conjunctival microcysts, reduced and localized subconjunctival flow, increased conjunctival injection, vascularization, thickening of the bleb wall, and the presence of Tenon's cyst formation. External inspection may provide clues about whether the primary procedure was a guarded trabeculectomy or a full-thickness procedure. The presence of a rectangular flap suggests the former, whereas the latter may or may not show a punched-out sclerostomy beneath thickened conjunctiva, demonstrating a fornix-based closure.

Conjunctival Mobility Test

The conjunctival mobility test is performed to assess the degree and location of bleb scarring and to determine which revision procedure is most suitable. At the slit lamp, proparacaine anesthetic is instilled in the conjunctival cul-de-sac and a sterile, moistened, cotton-tipped applicator is gently applied to the perilimbal and bulbar conjunctiva for 360 degrees. Cicatrized conjunctiva resists movement over underlying Tenon's and episcleral layers. In these situations, external revision with blunt or sharp dissection is usually required. If greater conjunctival mobility is noted preoperatively, the bleb may elevate more easily during surgical revision. These cases lend themselves to revision techniques that do not involve dissection of a conjunctival flap (e.g., internal revision or fistulization of the sclera for glaucoma with thermal cauterization).

Gonioscopy

Gonioscopic examination with a Zeiss or Posner's four-mirror goniolens is essential to evaluate the patency and size of the internal sclerostomy opening. Special notation is made about the relationship of the sclerostomy to the surrounding structures such as the lens, vitreous face, iris, and ciliary body. A sclerostomy may be occluded by lens capsule, Descemet's membrane, vitreous, or iris.

LASER REVISION TECHNIQUES IN SELECTED CASES OF FAILED FILTRATION

Special attention should be paid to membranes overlying the internal or external aspect of the sclerostomy and their degree of pigmentation or lack of it. In selected cases involving full-thickness procedures in which previously adequate filtration has failed owing to the formation of a pigmented membrane overlying the internal sclerostomy opening, argon laser application through a goniolens has successfully restored filtration.[41–43] In selected cases in which nonpigmented membranes such as the posterior lens capsule, vitreous bands, or thin membranes have occluded the internal aspect of the sclerostomy, Nd. YAG laser has been able to vaporize the site of obstruction.[44, 45] In three cases of filtration that failed after full-thickness procedures due to the presence of pigmented membranes occluding the external aspect of the sclerostomy, filtration has been restored through argon laser applied externally with the aid of an Abraham's lens.[46] More recently, Q-switched Nd. YAG laser has successfully restored filtration in seven cases of bleb failure that followed both full-thickness and trabeculectomy procedures.[47, 48] This technique delivers Nd. YAG laser energy transconjunctivally through an Abraham's lens to eliminate sites of episcleral fibrosis overlying a sclerostomy or along the borders of a sclerectomy flap in conjunction with elimination of membranous resistance overlying the internal aspect of the sclerostomy through a gonioscopic approach.

Before it is decided that filter revision surgery is necessary, certain maneuvers can be used to eliminate resistance with the patient at the slit lamp or laser. Some trabeculectomy failures are caused by resistance at the scleral level by the outer scleral flap itself. The surgeon may apply firm, steady digital pressure at an area 180 degrees away from the sclerostomy site, with reestablishment of flow in some cases. If the previous surgery was a trabeculectomy using guard sutures, these should first be released by laser suture lysis. Focal pressure with a muscle hook adjacent to the scleral flap can occasionally reestablish flow.[49] If no change in filtration flow or IOP occurs after these maneuvers, it is appropriate to proceed with filtration revision surgery.

SURGICAL FILTRATION REVISION TECHNIQUES

Three surgical approaches to the revision of filtering blebs are internal revision, fistulization of the sclera for glaucoma with thermocauterization, and external revision.[52]

Internal Revision (Transcameral Approach With a Blunt Cyclodialysis Spatula With or Without Swan's or Similar Needle-Knife)[51]

The internal revision technique developed by Simmons is the simplest approach to revising a failed filter

in the presence of an open sclerostomy with adequate overlying conjunctival mobility. The most appropriate candidates have a history of adequate bleb function for several months preceding failure. Cystic filtering blebs may respond to digital pressure when combined with aggressive topical steroids; however, surgical revision is often necessary to restore adequate bleb function and IOP control.

OPERATIVE TECHNIQUE

Retrobulbar anesthesia is induced using a 50/50 mixture of 2 percent lidocaine (Xylocaine) and 0.75 percent bupivacaine (Marcaine) to which 1:200,000 units of epinephrine and 150 units of hyaluronidase (Wydase) are added. The eye is prepared and draped in the usual sterile fashion. Under microscopic visualization, conjunctival mobility is inspected, and the sclerostomy site is examined using a sterile Zeiss goniolens placed on a cornea premoistened with balanced salt solution. A beveled paracentesis is created in peripheral clear cornea within 4 clock hr of the sclerostomy site. The anterior chamber is deepened with intracameral viscoelastic (Healon), which provides protection against anterior chamber collapse and lenticular injury for phakic patients (Fig. 143–26). Under gonioscopic visualization, a 0.5-mm cyclodialysis spatula is advanced through the paracentesis incision toward the anterior chamber wall to recanalize the sclerostomy (Fig. 143–27). It is maintained on a course tangential with the external scleral wall and advanced subconjunctivally along the base of the failed bleb. When the tip is visualized in the subconjunctival space, the goniolens is removed and Chandler's forceps are used to stabilize the globe by grasping the inferior rectus muscle tendon. The surgeon eliminates episcleral resistance by sweeping the spatula in a forceful, arclike fashion throughout the region of the bleb. Aqueous commonly fills the subconjunctival space spontaneously during this procedure. After external resistance is relieved, balanced salt solution is injected through the sclerostomy to further hydrodissect the region surrounding the bleb. The anterior chamber is redeepened with balanced salt solution, and the bleb is

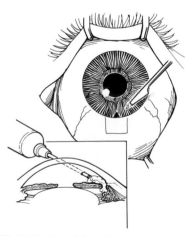

Figure 143–26. Internal revision. Anterior chamber deepening is accomplished when intracameral viscoelastic is introduced through a beveled paracentesis incision.

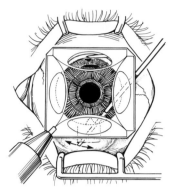

Figure 143–27. Internal revision. Under gonioscopic visualization, a cyclodialysis spatula or needle-knife is guided through the paracentesis incision to recanalize the sclerostomy and free up adhesions at the sclerostomy flap and episcleral level. The "hot-wire" goniodiathermy probe can be similarly positioned and used to cauterize the sclerostomy site.

inspected for leaks after 2 percent sodium fluorescein is placed on the eye (Fig. 143–28). Topical scopolamine 0.25 percent and Tobrex 0.03 percent drops are applied to the cul-de-sac, and sub-Tenon's deposteroid (Celestone Soluspan, 0.8 ml) is placed 180 degrees opposite the sclerostomy site at the close of the procedure.

Fistulization of the Sclera for Glaucoma With Thermocauterization (Transcameral Approach With the Coaxial Endodiathermy Probe; "Hot Wire" Technique)

This technique developed by Simmons is preferred for revision of failed filters that have closed or nonexistent sclerostomy sites in the presence of moderately mobile conjunctiva. Coaxial endodiathermy (Mira) is a 25.5-gauge, 35-degree, angulated endodiathermy probe that allows transcanalization of previously patent sclerostomies by controlled, forceful scleral wall puncture followed by thermal shrinkage of the surrounding tissue. Its angulated design reduces corneal distortion during the transcameral maneuver (Fig. 143–29).

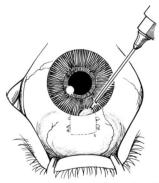

Figure 143–28. Internal revision. Balanced salt solution is introduced intracamerally to promote hydrodissection of the bleb.

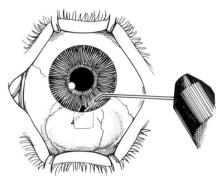

Figure 143–29. Fistulization of the sclera for glaucoma with thermocauterization. The coaxial endodiathermy probe assists in maintaining patency of the sclerostomy site.

OPERATIVE TECHNIQUE

Induction of local anesthesia and surgical steps are performed as for internal revision. These include goniolens-assisted visualization of the sclerostomy site, placement of the beveled paracentesis, introduction of intracameral viscoelastic, recanalization of the sclerostomy transcamerally with a 0.5-mm cyclodialysis spatula, and subconjunctival forceful dissection of scar tissue at the base of the filter bleb. If scleral wall resistance does not permit recanalization of the sclerostomy, then a Swan's or other needle-knife may be used for this purpose. At this juncture, all instruments are withdrawn from the eye and the coaxial endodiathermy probe is tested on the palpebral conjunctival surface. The desired cautery effect (blanching of fine vessels) can be achieved by adjusting the settings on the radio-frequency control box. The coaxial endodiathermy probe is then introduced transcamerally through the beveled paracentesis incision with its tip directed through the sclerostomy on a course tangential with the external scleral wall in the subconjunctival space. In the presence of thickened conjunctiva, the tip of the probe may be difficult to visualize, and using the edge of a goniolens may assist in visualization. Subconjunctival hydrodissection usually occurs spontaneously from the anterior chamber and serves as a desired buffer for thermal distribution and conjunctival protection during the endodiathermy procedure. While the assistant generously applies balanced salt solution to the external aspect of the filtering bleb, the surgeon depresses the endodiathermy foot pedal in short bursts of 3 to 5 sec. The endodiathermy effect is distributed to the base of the bleb and the sclerostomy site in multiple applications. The desired effect is achieved when the sclera and overlying conjunctiva slightly blanch. Care must be taken to avoid excessive application of the endodiathermy, or structural defects can result. As the probe is withdrawn from the sclerostomy, cauterization of the scleral wall continues. The anterior chamber is deepened with balanced salt solution, which causes further elevation of the subconjunctival space. At the close of the procedure, topical scopolamine 0.25 percent and Tobrex 0.03 percent are applied to the cul-de-sac. Sub-Tenon's deposteroid (Celestone Soluspan, 0.8 ml) injections are placed 180 degrees from the filtering bleb.

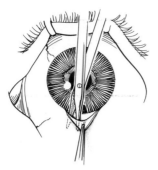

Figure 143–30. External revision. Creation of a fornix-based conjunctival flap overlying the failed filtration region.

External Revision Technique

The technique of external revision requires sharp dissection of a new fornix-based conjunctival flap (Fig. 143–30). This technique is reserved for cases with extensive conjunctival scarring or when more conservative measures, including internal revision, have failed. Other indications include revision of filtration blebs that are not acceptable based on their size, location (interpalpebral fissure), associated corneal defects, or rarely because of unacceptable cosmetic appearance.

A beveled paracentesis is performed outside of the area where the filter revision is to be performed. A conjunctival peritomy 2 to 3 clock hr in length is fashioned at the limbus. The flap is undermined posteriorly by a combination of sharp and blunt dissection. Monopolar diathermy is used to maintain hemostasis. Scar tissue overlying the trabeculectomy or sclerostomy is excised (Fig. 143–31). The anterior chamber can be maintained by introducing balanced salt solution or viscoelastic material through the paracentesis. Once the sclerostomy is recanalized, the trabeculectomy flap is sutured and aqueous humor runoff is titrated by Weck-cell assessment (Fig. 143–32). To encourage adherence of the conjunctival flap, the superior corneal epithelium is débrided. Three to four interrupted conjunctival-

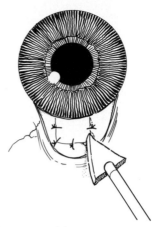

Figure 143–32. External revision. Aqueous flow titration by Weck-cell assessment adjacent to guard sutures in the sclerectomy flap.

corneal sutures usually are placed to anchor the anterior conjunctival flap to clear cornea using 10–0 nylon on a four-wire Lancet's needle (Ophthalon, Davis and Geck). Sutures are brought anteriorly and tied in a 4:1:1 fashion, and the suture tips are trimmed. The conjunctival flap tends to be more fibrotic in revision procedures, and a tight closure helps to prevent early bleb leaks, thus permitting prompt administration of adjunctive therapies including digital pressure, 5-FU, and laser suture lysis. Topical scopolamine 0.25 percent and Tobrex 0.03 percent are applied to the cul-de-sac, and sub-Tenon's deposteroid (Celestone Soluspan, 0.8 ml) is delivered 180 degrees from the filtering bleb. The eyelid is gently taped shut to prevent lid motion from disrupting the flap edge, and an eye pad and Fox's shield are applied.

POSTOPERATIVE CARE

At the close of the three surgical revision procedures described, the operated eye is taped shut and an eye pad and shield are applied. The contralateral eye is patched to reduce bilateral eye movement. Patients are usually admitted to the hospital for hypotony precautions and medication adjustment. Postoperative care is similar to that for primary filtration surgery, with postoperative application of 5-FU and digital pressure. In selected cases of external redissection, the release of guard sutures through laser suture lysis may be applicable.

COMPLICATIONS

Complications after filtration revision surgery are similar to those following primary filtration procedures but may be reduced in incidence and severity because of reduced surgical time, minimal tissue manipulation, and lessened patient morbidity.

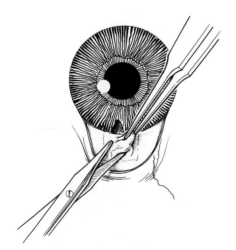

Figure 143–31. External revision. Excision of episcleral tissue overlying the sclerostomy flap allows aqueous flow to be reestablished.

REFERENCES

1. Epstein DL: Chandler and Grant's Glaucoma, 3rd ed. Philadelphia, Lea & Febiger, 1986.
2. Savage JA, Condon GP, Lytle RA, Simmons RJ: Laser suture lysis after trabeculectomy. Ophthalmology 95:1631, 1988.
3. Heuer DK, Parrish RK, Gressel MG, et al: 5-Fluorouracil and glaucoma filtering surgery. II: A pilot study. Ophthalmology 91:384, 1984.
4. Heuer DK, Parrish RK, Gressel MG, et al: 5-Fluorouracil and glaucoma filtering surgery. III: Intermediate followup of a pilot study. Ophthalmology 93:1537, 1986.
5. Rockwood EJ, Parrish RK, Heuer DK, et al: Glaucoma filtering surgery with 5-fluorouracil. Ophthalmology 94:1071, 1987.
6. Cashwell LF, Simmons RJ: Adjunctive techniques to glaucoma filtering surgery. Perspect Ophthalmol 4:115, 1980.
7. Epstein DL: Chandler and Grant's Glaucoma, 3rd ed. Philadelphia, Lea & Febiger, 1986.
8. Abedin S, Simmons RJ, Grant WM: Progressive low tension glaucoma: Treatment to stop glaucomatous cupping and field loss when these progress despite normal intraocular pressure. Ophthalmology 89:1, 1982.
9. Anderson DR: Glaucoma: The damage caused by pressure. XLVI Edward Jackson memorial lecture. Am J Ophthalmol 108:485, 1989.
10. Lamping KA, Bellows AR, Hutchinson BT, et al: Longterm evaluation of initial filtration surgery. Ophthalmology 93:91, 1986.
11. Blondeau P, Phelps CD: Trabeculectomy vs thermosclerostomy: A randomized prospective clinical trial. Arch Ophthalmol 99:810, 1981.
12. Wilson MR: Posterior lip sclerectomy vs trabeculectomy in West Indian blacks. Arch Ophthalmol 107:1604, 1989.
13. Shields MB: Trabeculectomy vs full thickness filtering operations for control of glaucoma. Ophthalmic Surg 11:498, 1980.
14. Spaeth GL, Poryzees E: A comparison between peripheral iridectomy with thermal sclerostomy and trabeculectomy: A controlled study. Br J Ophthalmol 65:783, 1981.
15. Lewis RA, Phelps CD: Trabeculectomy vs thermosclerostomy: A five-year followup. Arch Ophthalmol 102:533, 1984.
16. Thomas JV: Fornix-based vs Limbus-based Conjunctival Flaps in Filtration Surgery: Solving Glaucoma Problems. Boston, Massachusetts Eye and Ear Infirmary, 1988.
17. Simmons RJ, et al: Comparison of limbus-based vs fornix-based flaps in glaucoma filtration surgery. Personal communication, 1989.
18. Brubaker RF, Schlecht LP: The effects of withdrawal of timolol in chronically treated glaucoma patients. 28(Suppl 3) Invest Ophthalmol Vis Sci:377, 1987.
19. Savage JA, Simmons RJ: Coaxial radio frequency (RF) diathermy in anterior segment surgery. Ophthalmic Surg 16:333, 1985.
20. LaGrange F: Iridectomie et sclerectomie combinees dans le traitement du glaucome chronique: Procede nouveau pour l'etablissement de la cicatrice filtrante (1). Arch Ophthalmol Rev Gen 26:481, 1906.
21. Holth S: Sclerectomie avec la pince emporte piece dans le glaucome de preference apres incision a la pique. Ann Ocul 142:1, 1909.
22. Elliot RH: A preliminary note on a new operative procedure for the establishment of a filtering cicatrix in the treatment of glaucoma. Ophthalmoscope 7:804, 1909.
23. Fergus F: Treatment of glaucoma by trephining. Br Med J 2:983, 1909.
24. Scheie HG: Retraction of scleral wound edges as a fistulizing procedure for glaucoma. Am J Ophthalmol 45:220, 1958.
25. Iliff CE, Haas JS: Posterior lip sclerectomy. Am J Ophthalmol 54:688, 1962.
26. Wolner BW, Liebmann JM, Ritch R, et al: Late bleb-related endophthalmitis after trabeculectomy with adjunctive 5-fluorouracil. Ophthalmology 97:125, 1990.
27. Waltz KL, Sherwood MB: Contamination of dropper bottles in a glaucoma clinic. Ophthalmology 97:141, 1990.
28. Hoskins HD Jr, Migliazzo C: Management of failing filtering blebs with the argon laser. Ophthalmic Surg 15:731, 1984.
29. Cohen JS, Osher RH: Releasable suture in filtering and combined surgery. In Shields MB, Pollack IP, Kolker AE (eds): Perspectives in Glaucoma. Transactions of the First Scientific Meeting of the American Glaucoma Society. Thorofare, NJ, Slack, 1988, pp 157-162.
30. Krug JH, Melamed S: Adjunctive use of delayed and adjustable low-dose 5-fluorouracil in refractory glaucoma. Am J Ophthalmol 109:412, 1990.
31. Weinreb RN: Adjusting the dose of 5-fluorouracil after glaucoma filtering surgery to minimize the side effects. Ophthalmology 94:564, 1987.
32. Knapp A, Heuer DK, Stern GA, Driebe WT Jr: Serious corneal complications of glaucoma filtering surgery with postoperative 5-fluorouracil. Am J Ophthalmol 103:183, 1987.
33. Lee DA, Hersh P, Kersten D, Melamed S: Complications of subconjunctival 5-fluorouracil following glaucoma filtering surgery. Ophthalmic Surg 18:187, 1987.
34. Simmons RJ, Kimbrough RL: Shell tamponade in filtering surgery for glaucoma. Ophthalmic Surg 10:17, 1979.
35. Simmons RJ, Singh OS: Shell tamponade technique in glaucoma surgery. In Symposium on Glaucoma: Transactions of the New Orleans Academy of Ophthalmology. St. Louis, CV Mosby, 1981, p 266.
36. Savage JA, Simmons RJ: The shell tamponade technique for glaucoma filtration surgery. Waltham, MA, MIRA, 1988.
37. Joiner DW, Liebmann JM, Ritch R: A modification of the use of the glaucoma tamponade shell. Ophthalmic Surg 20:441, 1989.
38. Maumenee AE: External filtering operations for glaucoma: The mechanism of function and failure. Trans Am Ophthalmol Soc 58:319, 1960.
39. Friedenwald JS: Some problems in the diagnosis and treatment of glaucoma. Am J Ophthalmol 33:1523, 1950.
40. Swan KC: Reopening of nonfunctional filters: Simplified surgical techniques. Trans Am Acad Ophthalmol Otolaryngol 79:OP-342, 1975.
41. Ticho U, Ivry M: Reopening of occluded filtering blebs by argon laser photocoagulation. Am J Ophthalmol 84:413, 1977.
42. Van Buskirk EM: Reopening filtration fistulas with the argon laser. Am J Ophthalmol 94:1, 1982.
43. Budenz DL, Brown SVL, Thomas JV, et al: Laser therapy for internally failing glaucoma filtration surgery. Ophthalmic Laser Therapy 1:169, 1986.
44. Cohn HC, Aron-Rosa D: Reopening blocked trabeculectomy sites with the YAG laser. Am J Ophthalmol 95:293, 1983.
45. Praeger DL: The reopening of closed filtering blebs using the Nd:YAG laser. Ophthalmology 91:373, 1984.
46. Kurata F, Krupin T, Kolker AE: Reopening filtration fistulas with transconjunctival argon laser photocoagulation. Am J Ophthalmol 98:340, 1984.
47. Rankin GA, Latina MA: Transconjunctival Nd:YAG laser revision of failing trabeculectomy. Ophthalmic Surg 21:365, 1990.
48. Latina MA, Rankin GA: Internal and transconjunctival neodymium:YAG laser revision of late failing filters. Ophthalmology 98:215, 1991.
49. Traverso CE, Greenidge KC, Spaeth GL, Wilson RP: Focal pressure: A new method to encourage filtration after trabeculectomy. Ophthalmic Surg 15:62, 1984.
50. Savage JA, Simmons RJ: Staged glaucoma filtration surgery with planned early conversion from scleral flap to full-thickness operation using the argon laser. Ophthalmic Laser Therapy 1:201, 1986.
51. Lytle RA, Simmons RJ: Internal revision in glaucoma filtration surgery. Scientific Poster 79, American Academy of Ophthalmology Annual Meeting, Las Vegas, NV, October 8-12, 1988.
52. Sofinski SJ, et al: Filtration bleb revision techniques. In Thomas JV (ed): Glaucoma Surgery. St. Louis, Mosby–Year Book, 1992 pp 75-82.

Chapter 144

■

Management of Glaucoma and Cataract

B. THOMAS HUTCHINSON

There is an established increased incidence of both cataract and glaucoma as one becomes older; both diseases are among the leading causes of preventable blindness in the United States.[1,2] The presence of glaucoma and cataract in the same patient and same eye is understandable, considering the frequency of the two disease processes. Although either may have the other disease as the principal etiologic factor, most patients with cataract and glaucoma have each disease independent of the other. However, the management of cataract and that of glaucoma are heavily interdependent. The visual deficit associated with the cataract is recoverable, assuming no other ocular disease is present. A delay in treatment/surgery of the patient with a cataract is visually limiting to the patient only by the length of the delay. Appropriate cataract surgery restores vision without regard to the timeliness of the operation. In contrast, the timeliness of glaucoma management, both medically and surgically, is exceedingly important, because vision lost to glaucoma is not recoverable. Therefore, glaucoma management should take precedence over treatment of the cataract.[3,4]

The criterion for successful management of glaucoma associated with a cataract that is not visually compromising is control of the intraocular pressure (IOP) at a level protective to the optic nerve. In eyes in which the immature cataract is not visually significant, we treat chronic open-angle glaucoma with medication as if no cataract were present. The medical management of these patients includes the use of topical β-adrenergic antagonists (e.g., timolol, maleate, betaxolol, hydrochloride, or levobunolol hydrochloride), sympathomimetic topical agents (e.g., epinephrine hydrochloride, propine), parasympathomimetic topical medications (e.g., pilocarpine hydrochloride, carbachol, echothiophate iodide), and systemic carbonic anhydrase inhibitors (e.g., acetazolamide, methazolamide, dichlorphenamide). Because of the potential further decrease in visual acuity with the use of miotics in patients with asymptomatic cataract, we generally begin therapy with topical β-blockers or epinephrine products. As the cataracts become visually significant, miotic therapy may decrease the visual acuity more than the cataract alone. Conversely, a pupil dilated with topical epinephrine drops may expose more of the cataractous lens in the pupil and produce a reduction of visual acuity from light scatter. In patients with cataract visually worsened by miotic drops, one may consider the Ocusert or pilocarpine gel as an alternative form of pilocarpine delivery. Both produce less miosis and may deliver a therapeutically effective pilocarpine dosage. In patients with chronic open-angle glaucoma who are intolerant of miotic therapy and uncontrolled with other medications, we use the laser trabeculoplasty to decrease the IOP before resorting to the carbonic anhydrase inhibitors or invasive surgery. In many cases, the IOP is adequate on medical therapy without miotics after trabeculoplasty (usually one half of the trabecular circumference, followed by the other half if an effect, albeit inadequate, is obtained) and with good visual acuity and a normal pupil. If the IOP is not adequately controlled by nonmiotic therapy and laser, yet responds well to miotic therapy but with significant visual blurring, one might consider a planned extracapsular cataract extraction (ECCE) with placement of a posterior chamber intraocular lens (IOL). In the absence of intraoperative and postoperative complications, the patient with chronic open-angle glaucoma should respond as well to medication following cataract surgery as effectively as preoperatively. Postoperatively, the patient may tolerate miotic therapy well.[4,5]

Cataract extraction in the presence of controlled glaucoma, especially in the older patient, does not require extra techniques because of the glaucoma; one may perform the standard operation and treat the residual glaucoma medically. In patients with marginally controlled, chronic open-angle glaucoma and visually significant cataract or in patients requiring two or three medications for glaucoma control, we often use laser trabeculoplasty preoperatively, because this modality produces more favorable results before cataract surgery than after the cataract and implant procedures. We prefer an adequate time interval to pass between the laser surgery and the cataract extraction to allow the postlaser inflammation to subside and to assess the results of the laser treatment. However, one must not wait too long for laser effect, especially if the IOP is substantially elevated and the optic nerve is severely compromised. If adequate glaucoma control is in question, we perform a combined procedure.

Echothiophate iodide, a cholinesterase-inhibiting miotic, may create mild but significant inflammation in the phakic eye and even contribute to cataract formation. Although we do not use this medication in the phakic eye as often as pilocarpine, carbachol, the Ocusert, or pilocarpine gel, the cholinesterase inhibitors are appropriate for use in the phakic eye if the surgical risks outweigh the potential side effects and complications of the medication. However, the cholinesterase inhibitors are particularly valuable in the management of aphakic and pseudophakic glaucoma. Because all miotics have been implicated in the development of a retinal detachment (as has cataract surgery, with or without intraocular lens implantation), a detailed retinal assessment should be performed before prescribing these medications, especially in eyes that have undergone cataract extraction.

We use the planned ECCE or phacoemulsification with an IOL implant combined with a trabeculectomy in a patient with poorly controlled glaucoma associated with a visually significant cataract. The trabeculectomy does not significantly increase the risk to the eye in either the intraoperative or postoperative interval. Indeed, the combined procedure may protect against a potential IOP elevation immediately postoperatively and also may continue to provide more prolonged glaucoma control with either reduction or elimination of medication possible. Further, the combined procedure of cataract and glaucoma surgery is appropriate in patients with particularly vulnerable optic nerves, even if the glaucoma is well controlled, because an acute IOP elevation after ECCE, and implant surgery may cause permanent visual damage.[7–11]

In relatively young patients with controlled glaucoma and visually significant cataract, a planned ECCE with IOL implantation might be considered for the temporal limbus to preserve the superior conjunctiva and posterior capsule for future pseudophakic filtering surgery. However, one may consider a combined procedure, even in the young patient, especially if the glaucoma requires substantive treatment or has the potential to worsen.

In patients with uncontrolled chronic open-angle glaucoma with medical and laser therapy and those with cataract visually significant only with miotic therapy, filtration surgery rather than cataract or combined surgery is an option, especially if the cataract is stable and the patient is asymptomatic with a normal-sized pupil without miotic therapy. This may be the treatment of choice in eyes that have had previous glaucoma surgery that has failed and in which the vision is adequate. Filtration surgery in the phakic eye has been shown to be more successful for a longer time than the combined procedures in which the cataract is removed at the time of filtration surgery. Thus, not all eyes with glaucoma and cataract require cataract extraction.

The successful treatment of uncontrolled glaucoma must be accomplished either before or concurrent with cataract extraction. Although cataract extraction alone in patients with concurrent chronic open-angle glaucoma and cataract often may render the glaucoma more easily controlled postoperatively, even to the extent that glaucoma therapy may be reduced or eliminated, one cannot rely on this effect if the glaucoma is uncontrolled.[12] (This lowering of the IOP subsequent to cataract surgery may occur in the absence of filtering bleb, cyclodialysis cleft, wound leak, and choroidal detachment.)

We strongly recommend that in patients with uncontrolled chronic open-angle glaucoma and visually significant cataract, the IOP should be controlled by filtration surgery before cataract extraction or by glaucoma surgery simultaneously with cataract extraction and placement of an IOL. Phakic glaucoma surgery and combined procedures are more effective in glaucoma control and are substantially safer and more successful than the same glaucoma procedures performed in aphakia or pseudophakia.[13] The increased use of the ECCE, with or without filtration surgery in patients with glaucoma, not only provides enhanced vision with the IOL implant but also has reduced the complications of wound leak, choroidal detachment, pupillary block, retinal edema, and retinal detachment, as well as "aphakic and pseudophakic glaucoma." These postoperative glaucomas are usually secondary to acquired angle-closure due to wound leak or pupillary block or to chronic inflammation.

In relatively young patients (fifth decade of life and younger) who have uncontrolled glaucoma and visually significant cataract and in patients who have responded poorly to previous combined surgery in the fellow eye, or if extensive disease exists, one might consider a two-stage approach to visual rehabilitation by first performing filtration surgery, and then, after allowing an appropriate interval for the inflammation to subside, performing a planned ECCE with placement of a posterior chamber IOL away from the filtration bleb. Most surgeons make the cataract incision 180 degrees opposite the filtration bleb, although approaches closer to the filtration area are appropriate with phacoemulsification and a small incision lens implantation.[13, 14, 16]

In aphakic or pseudophakic eyes with uncontrolled glaucoma in the presence of maximum medical therapy, we prefer performing the trabeculectomy in virgin or very mobile conjunctiva, with adjunctive therapy (mitomycin-C, 5-fluorouracil) and early suture lysis. With heavily scarred tissue at the surgical limbus, a Molteno tube procedure, cyclodialysis, or a cyclodestructive procedure may be necessary.

GENERAL PRINCIPLES OF GLAUCOMA AND CATARACT SURGICAL MANAGEMENT

Several factors influence the success of the combined procedure and the two-stage procedure, in addition to the surgeon's experience with the operation, the operating time, and other intangible elements. Measurable factors influencing the choice of operative procedure include the patient's age, the need for improved visual acuity by cataract extraction, the corneal endothelial status, and the presence of other ocular pathology including inflammation, as well as the patient's willingness to have one or two operations. In addition, the vision and the experience with the fellow eye as well as long-term considerations (of compliance with medication, infection, and risk), the best method for optical correction helps to determine the most beneficial approach.

In general, the surgical success is influenced by the patient's age (creation of a filtering bleb is generally easier in older patients), the severity of glaucoma, the presence of previous surgical scar tissue, tissue manipulation, the degree of inflammation present, the use of postoperative antiinflammatory medications, and complications.

Operative considerations that influence the success of glaucoma and cataract surgery include the protection of the conjunctiva, controlling bleeding with minimal cautery, and the use of atraumatic needles and sutures. Complete cortical removal with the sclerectomy site free of capsule, cortex, blood, and vitreous in the combined procedures is exceedingly important. The success rate varies depending on the ocular status and on the skill of the surgeon in minimizing tissue manipulation as well as the postoperative management. The relatively new posterior chamber IOL implantation techniques in patients with glaucoma following phacoemulsification or planned ECCE have already proved to be better for both visual rehabilitation and glaucoma control than eyes with aphakia or anterior chamber implants.

Adjunctive therapy, mitomycin-C intraoperatively and 5-fluorouracil postoperatively, may effectively limit fibrosis, scarring, and bleb failure when used in conjunction with steroidal and nonsteroidal antiinflammatory agents. A gradual tapering of postoperative medications is warranted until inflammation completely subsides if successful filtration is to be maintained.[17] The interval for tapering the medications varies but may be as long as several months.

Cataract management in patients who already underwent successful filtration surgery is necessary not only in those glaucoma-cataract patients in whom two operations have been planned but also in those glaucoma patients who have developed cataract subsequent to filtration surgery. In cataract surgery with filtering blebs, we believe that the IOL implantation is safer for visual rehabilitation than contact lens use. In patients who are aphakic in the eye with better visual acuity and who are comfortable visually with aphakic spectacles, we favor a planned ECCE or phacoemulsification from the inferotemporal limbus, away from the filtering bleb, without an IOL implant. Also, in a patient requiring binocularity if the fellow eye has normal vision without a cataract or has an IOL, a secondary IOL implantation may be considered in a patient who is aphakic with a filtering bleb, in either the posterior or anterior chamber. The relative risks are greater in these aphakic eyes than in eyes having IOL implantation surgery at the time of cataract removal and need to be reviewed carefully, with the patient's understanding and consent. We generally do not favor anterior chamber or iris-supported implants in patients with or without glaucoma, because these lenses are often a factor in the development of chronic secondary open-angle glaucoma and chronic angle-closure glaucoma. We have found that posterior chamber IOLs are infrequent factors in secondary open-angle glaucoma or in postoperative angle-closure glaucoma. Similarly, we have not found the posterior chamber implant to adversely affect the control of chronic open-angle glaucoma, whether or not a filtration bleb has been necessary to stabilize the IOP. However, regardless of the surgical technique for cataract extraction chosen for an eye with a functional filtering bleb, we find that the average IOP after the second procedure is usually higher, because some bleb function is often lost. The degree of bleb failure and pressure elevation determines whether or not medication is reinstituted or even if additional surgery is necessary.

In patients who require filtration surgery with the likelihood of later cataract surgery, we prefer the full-thickness sclerectomy over the trabeculectomy, because the full-thickness procedure provides a better precataract extraction bleb and IOP control than does the trabeculectomy.

In cataract extraction after long-term miotic therapy or filtration surgery, the pupil usually dilates poorly and may have posterior synechiae. It is often necessary to enlarge the pupil intraoperatively to remove the nucleus and, with loss of the pigmented layer, the iris becomes atrophic and nonreactive and the pupil becomes distorted, commonly resulting in exposure of the implant edge, positioning holes or the haptics in the pupillary aperture. In cases such as these, we free the posterior synechiae, create an iridotomy, and close the pupillary aperture with a 10–0 Prolene suture after placing a large-diameter (7 mm) posterior chamber optic without positioning holes. In patients with large pupils and atrophic irides and without a sphincterotomy, we often suture the pupil to avoid pupillary capture of the implant optic. In patients who have fully reactive pupils that dilate well for the cataract extraction, we may elect no extra maneuvers for the pupillary aperture, except the use of an intracameral or topical miotic at the time of surgery.

MONITORING GLAUCOMA IN THE PRESENCE OF CATARACT

The assessment of the optic nerve and the visual field may be significantly more difficult with cataract development. Optic disc pallor may be masked by an increase of nuclear sclerosis; the crystalline lens may also blunt the details of the nerve head and its vasculature. Additionally, cataract development may produce an apparent increase in visual field defect that could be erroneously attributed to glaucoma, even with maximum pupillary mydriasis. If the patient is not subjectively visually compromised by cataract, which might occur in the presence of monocular cataract and glaucoma, it is sometimes necessary to remove the cataract and treat the glaucoma concurrently because of the inability to satisfactorily monitor a marginally controlled glaucoma. To appropriately monitor all patients with combined cataract and glaucoma, it is necessary to examine the patient regularly to ensure a continuing stability. It is appropriate to perform follow-up evaluation of a well-controlled glaucomatous eye three to four times annually to monitor the IOP and the effect of antiglaucoma therapy. On one or more visits, it may be appropriate to discontinue miotic therapy to allow maximal mydriasis for the most accurate optic nerve and visual field assessment. More frequent examinations are appropriate if the IOP is not well controlled or if additional parameters are necessary to determine the ocular status.

Patient education is important not only at the initial visit but also on a continuing basis to ensure that the patient fully understands the nature of his or her eye diseases as well as the prognosis and the management of the clinical course. It is vital that the patient and the family be fully informed about the glaucoma and cataract management to better understand the rationale for treatment recommendations. They should understand that glaucoma control takes precedence over the cataract treatment and that both diseases must be considered in the management by medication, laser, and/or conventional surgery. It is valuable for the physician to periodically review with the patient his or her progress and for the professional office staff to complement medical management with information and appropriate counseling. The chronicity of glaucoma and cataract and the potential consequences leading to blindness mandate this important informational interface with the patient.

CATARACT AS THE CAUSE OF GLAUCOMA

Although it is more common for the two diseases to be present independently in a given eye, less commonly glaucoma may be precipitated by the development of a cataract as in the following circumstances: in acute angle-closure glaucoma in which the increasing lens bulk creates angle narrowing that predisposes the eye to pupillary block angle-closure glaucoma; in phacolytic glaucoma, wherein leaking lens material incites a monocyte phagocytic response, which with the free lens protein causes a secondary open-angle glaucoma; and in cases in which lens-induced uveitis promotes either angle-closure glaucoma secondary to posterior synechia and iris bombé or a secondary open-angle glaucoma due to inflammatory debris—phacoanaphylaxis. The literature on the latter secondary open-angle glaucomas is not concise, principally because of new and confusing terminology associated with the diseases based on our more recent understanding of the disorders. Lens dislocation or subluxation may be associated with phacolytic and phacoanaphylactic reactions as well as the cause of angle-closure glaucoma due to pupillary block. Conversely, the crystalline lens, capsule, or cortex may become opacified because of acute glaucoma and ischemic changes of the anterior segment. In addition, medical, laser, and surgical therapies for the glaucoma may be associated with developing cataract. The pathophysiology of both diseases should be considered if optimal management and preservation of vision are to be obtained.

Angle-Closure Glaucoma Associated With Developing Cataract

Advancing cataract may result in sufficient hydration of the lens cortex to cause anterior chamber shallowing and allow pupillary block angle-closure glaucoma to develop in an eye that was not previously susceptible to angle-closure secondary to pupillary mydriasis. In these unilateral "acquired" narrow angles secondary to lens intumescence, a laser iridectomy sometimes relieves the acute angle-closure attack, but the anterior chamber remains shallow. These eyes may remain susceptible to repeat angle-closure, and cataract extraction with an implant, if appropriate, should be performed if the anterior chamber does not significantly deepen upon iridectomy. Gonioscopy of the fellow eye may help to identify this lens-induced pupillary block glaucoma. Miotics, β-blockers, carbonic anhydrase inhibitors, and osmotics may be necessary to lower the IOP before laser iridotomy or surgery; in neglected cases in which synechial closure is evident, a chamber-deepening procedure combined with cataract extraction and implant placement may be warranted (if the angle opens with chamber deepening); combined cataract extraction, trabeculectomy, and IOL placement should be performed if the angle remains closed after a therapeutic chamber deepening. The chamber-deepening technique, described in Chapter 142, is valuable in lysing early synechiae that have not yet become permanent. This technique may be effective in all angle-closure glaucomas secondary to pupillary block with entrapment of aqueous in the posterior chamber, but only if performed after iridectomy and early in the acute phases of the disease. We have found that ECCE with a posterior chamber IOL implant is sufficient without accompanying glaucoma surgery, only if most of the angle has been opened by the earlier therapeutic measures as evidenced by gonioscopy.

Lens-Induced Open-Angle Glaucoma

Phacolytic glaucoma, usually occurring with dense immature or hypermature cataracts, may be manifested by leakage of lens protein into the aqueous circulation, which creates an open-angle glaucoma by proteinaceous debris or macrophages "plugging" the trabecular outflow channels. This acute glaucoma, often with a deep chamber, has a significant inflammatory component that does not respond to antiinflammatory or antiglaucomatous therapy. For best visual rehabilitation, we perform a planned ECCE (and implant a posterior chamber IOL) that usually cures this secondary open-angle glaucoma. Phacolytic open-angle glaucoma also may occur with immature cataracts and is manifest by chronic, low-grade inflammation that usually does not respond to antiinflammatory medications or to medical therapy for the glaucoma.

Patients with retained lens cortex after planned or unplanned ECCE may have sufficient inflammation in the early phases either to cause pupillary block secondary to adhesions or to cause a secondary open-angle glaucoma that is unremitting until the lens material has been absorbed or removed. Phacoanaphylactic endophthalmitis, a more unusual lens-induced inflammation with glaucoma, is thought to be secondary to an immune response to lens protein. In rare circumstances, even the fellow eye may be involved. In cataract secondary to penetrating trauma, phacoanaphylactic reactions have been noted to clinically mimic sympathetic ophthalmia. In cases of lens-induced glaucoma in which there is significant inflammatory response, we use β-blockers, carbonic anhydrase inhibitors, cycloplegia, and topical steroids even though the latter may complicate the glaucoma assessment in steroid-sensitive eyes. When a moderate amount of retained lens material is present, it may be necessary to surgically remove the lens particles if they are not reabsorbed promptly.

Subluxation and Dislocation of the Crystalline Lens

Although subluxation and dislocation of the crystalline lens into the vitreous cavity often are associated with the development of a mature or hypermature cataract, it is not always necessary to remove the lens assuming there is no secondary glaucoma, potential for pupillary block, or posterior vitreous or retinal adhesions. A laser iridotomy may substantially reduce the likelihood of pupillary block in cases in which the lens may potentially occlude the pupil and the forward flow of aqueous from the posterior chamber. If a pupillary block process is sufficient to cause dislocation of the cataract into the anterior chamber, it is better removed than repositioned posteriorly. In eyes with an intracapsular cataract removed owing to dislocation, in the absence of secondary angle-closure glaucoma or angle-recession glaucoma, one might consider an anterior chamber implant. Furthermore, a posterior chamber lens may be sutured into the sulcus of these aphakic eyes. This technique protects the filtration angle from the trauma that is often associated with anterior chamber implants.

This chapter should serve only as a guide for the individual surgeon's preferences in cataract and glaucoma management. There are many variations that are clinically effective in the management of these diseases. Fortunately, today's rapidly evolving technology provides the ophthalmic surgeon with ever-changing materials and methods for the medical and surgical management of glaucoma and cataract. As Robert Henry Elliot noted, "Each surgeon must be guided not only by the environment of his patients but also by his own idiosyncrasies, each case must be considered on its own merits; statistics are wanted of both success and failure. Those who follow us will know what we guess and walk boldly where we grope."

REFERENCES

1. Gifford SR: Lens extraction following filtration operations for glaucoma. Am J Ophthalmol 26:468, 1943.
2. Callahan A: Cataract extraction after glaucoma surgery: Lateroinferior approach following filtering glaucoma operation. Arch Ophthalmol 47:132, 1952.
3. Scheie HG, Muirhead JF: Cataract extraction after filtering operations. Arch Ophthalmol 68:67, 1962.
4. Bigger JF, Becker B: Cataract and primary open-angle glaucoma: The effect of uncomplicated cataract extraction on glaucoma control. Trans Am Acad Ophthalmol Otolaryngol 75:260, 1971.
5. Randolph ME, Maumenee AE, Iliff CE: Cataract extraction in glaucomatous eyes. Am J Ophthalmol 71:328, 1971.
6. Spaeth GL: The management of patients with conjoint cataract and glaucoma. Ophthalmic Surg 11:780, 1980.
7. Spaeth GL: The management of cataract in patients with glaucoma: A comparative study. Trans Ophthalmol Soc UK 100:195, 1980.
8. Kass MA: Cataract extraction in an eye with a filtering bleb. Ophthalmology 89:871, 1982.
9. Shields MB: Combined cataract extraction and glaucoma surgery. Ophthalmology 89:231, 1982.
10. Savage JA, Thomas JV, Belcher CD III, Simmons RJ: Extracapsular cataract extraction and posterior chamber intraocular lens implantation in glaucomatous eyes. Ophthalmology 92:1506, 1985.
11. McGuigan LJB, Gottsch J, Stark WJ, et al: Extracapsular cataract extraction and posterior chamber lens implantation in eyes with preexisting glaucoma. Arch Ophthalmol 104:1301, 1986.
12. Epstein DL: Chandler and Grant's Glaucoma, 3rd ed. St Louis, CV Mosby, 1986.
13. Kooner KS, Dulaney DD, Zimmerman TJ: Intraocular pressure following ECCE and IOL implantation in patients with glaucoma. Ophthalmic Surg 19:570, 1988.
14. Vu MT, Shields MB: The early postoperative pressure course in glaucoma patients following cataract surgery. Ophthalmic Surg 19:467, 1988.
15. Murchison JF Jr, Shields MB: An evaluation of three surgical approaches for coexisting cataract and glaucoma. Ophthalmic Surg 20:393, 1989.
16. Krupin T, Feitl ME, Bishop KI: Postoperative intraocular pressure rise in open-angle glaucoma patients after cataract or combined cataract filtration surgery. Ophthalmology 96:579, 1989.
17. Hoskins HD Jr, Kass MA: Becker-Shaffer's Diagnosis and Therapy of Glaucoma, 6th ed. St Louis, CV Mosby, 1989.
18. Spaeth GL: Ophthalmic Surgery: Principles and Practice. Philadelphia, WB Saunders, 1990.
19. Minckler DS, Van Buskirk EM, Wright KW, Ryan SJ Jr: Color Atlas of Ophthalmic Surgery. Glaucoma. Philadelphia, JB Lippincott, 1992.

Chapter 145

∎

Complications of Filtering Surgery

A. ROBERT BELLOWS

The primary goal of filtration surgery is to establish long-term intraocular pressure (IOP) reduction to preserve all possible visual function. Since the myriad of surgical and postoperative complications can alter the success of filtration operations, medical management for chronic glaucoma is preferred. However, recommendations for earlier surgical intervention have been suggested,[1, 2] and if the incidence and severity of postoperative complications can be diminished, surgical therapy indeed may be advised earlier in the disease state.[3]

A number of important developments have diminished the intraoperative and postoperative complications of filtration surgery. The almost universal use of the operating microscope, combined with the development of microsurgical instruments, has facilitated tissue manipulation and permits highly complex intraocular maneuvers because of better visualization and exact instrumentation. The development of viscoelastic material for use in the anterior chamber and subconjunctival space has enhanced the capacity to maintain tissue and architectural integrity during glaucoma surgery in the anterior chamber and on the globe surface. These materials have also improved the capacity to maintain tissue relationships during the early postoperative period.

Additional technical developments have resulted in less traumatic surgery, and fewer postoperative tissue-related complications because of the use of fine wire needles that are bonded to delicate and strong nylon and absorbable suture material. These exquisite needles in varying shapes allow fastidious wound closure with minimal attendant tissue trauma and diminution of the intraoperative and postoperative problems of wound leak and late wound dehiscence.

The renewed attention to wound healing and tissue restructuring in successful and failed filtering blebs[4, 5] has encouraged the use of pharmacologic substances that alter the fibrovascular proliferation process.[6–8] The inhibition of collagen cross-linking[9] also serves to decrease the scarring process. Adjunctive factors, including laser suture lysis, digital pressure, and devices, such as soft contact lenses, silicone shells, and collagen shields, have expanded the postoperative armamentarium of the surgeon and have enhanced the techniques that can result in successful filtration surgery.

ANTICIPATION OF FILTRATION SURGERY

Careful patient assessment before glaucoma filtering surgery potentially decreases the possibility of significant complications. Discontinuation of medications that en-

hance vascular congestion (phospholine iodide and epinephrine-containing products) decreases vessel engorgement and the chance of operative bleeding. Elimination of aspirin-containing or other medications that alter blood clotting preoperatively is an absolute necessity. Careful lid and lacrimal sac examination may uncover an infectious process that requires treatment before elective surgery. Intraocular or periocular inflammation must be treated preoperatively with topical, local, and, occasionally systemic corticosteroids. In high-risk patients with markedly elevated IOP, administration of preoperative osmotic agents and gradual globe decompression, through a paracentesis site, should be accomplished before proceeding with filtration surgery. In neovascular glaucoma, preoperative panretinal photocoagulation and, if visualization of the retina does not permit laser treatment, transconjunctival cryoablation should be performed 1 to 2 wk before filtration surgery to decrease the fibrovascular proliferative process that is characteristic of this disease.

Careful assessment of the patient's capacity to cooperate during surgery helps in making the decision to use local anesthesia. The preference for monitored intravenous anesthesia allows local anesthesia to be administered and decreases both the systemic risks of general anesthesia and the problems associated with extubation or vomiting postoperatively. General anesthesia is restricted to extremely apprehensive patients and young patients who cannot be expected to cooperate during surgery.

INTRAOPERATIVE COMPLICATIONS

A high index of suspicion, recognition of high-risk eyes, and anticipation of intraoperative complications often minimize or modify intraoperative difficulties.

Bleeding

Every possible effort should be made to minimize intraoperative bleeding, and when it occurs prompt and delicate cautery is the rule. The careful and atraumatic handling of ocular tissues is a requisite during glaucoma surgery. Use of a tapered needle and moderate-sized toothed forceps decreases the chance of tissue trauma and bleeding during the placement of the superior rectus stay suture. The use of smooth or fine cusped forceps decreases the chance of crushing or perforating conjunctival tissue and thus minimizes the release of the factors responsible for postoperative inflammation. Immediate cautery is encouraged to prevent blood entrapment in Tenon's capsule, because blood under the bleb during the postoperative period contributes significantly to inflammation and scarring. The use of unipolar diathermy (MIRA, Boston) has proved to be an extremely important adjunct to surgery. Because the heat energy emitted from the diathermy instrument can be carefully regulated, and a wet field can be maintained, significant tissue denaturation and shrinkage does not occur. The instrument can be used safely within or near the sclerectomy and is often used to treat bleeding of the iris or ciliary body as well as allowing cautery close to the conjunctival flap (Fig. 145–1).

Structures that contribute most to intraoperative bleeding during glaucoma surgery are the vessels on the scleral surface. All efforts to minimize episcleral trauma should be encouraged, because the episcleral vessels are extremely fragile and bleed readily. If bleeding occurs into Tenon's capsule, it cannot be drained effectively, thus excision of the blood in Tenon's capsule often reduces a source of postoperative inflammation. The dissection of the scleral flap, creation of a sclerectomy, or full-thickness sclerectomies often involves a highly vascular area. Cautery beforehand or the use of topical epinephrine 1:000 can be applied directly to the bleeding areas to provide hemostasis. Cautery to the internal lip of the sclera can often be risky and ineffective; topical epinephrine and even cautery to adjacent scleral feeder vessels can stop bleeding.

All efforts should be made to stop any surface bleeding before entering the anterior chamber. When blood is present in the anterior chamber, it can be irrigated through a temporal paracentesis site through the sclerectomy. Care should be taken to minimize the chance of blood remaining under the conjunctival flap. If blood or blood elements block the sclerectomy, injection through the paracentesis clears the obstruction, and the free flow of fluid is reestablished.

Conjunctival Perforation and Leak

Careful manipulation of the conjunctiva is always emphasized and represents one of the most critical steps in filtration surgery. Nontoothed forceps or dampened cellulose sponges should be used whenever tissues on the globe surface are manipulated. It is advisable not to injure or perforate Tenon's capsule, because this tissue is responsible for the release of many of the mediators that promote inflammation. Careful observation of the integrity of the conjunctiva and Tenon's capsule minimizes the likelihood of inadvertent perforation.

When perforation occurs during the dissection of the conjunctival flap, it can be repaired if it is relatively small and distant from the proposed sclerectomy site. The buttonhole opening can be closed with a delicate, tapered needle on a 10–0 nylon suture (Ethicon 2850 BV-75 needle, Ethicon Inc, Somerville, NJ). This suture is invaluable in closing conjunctival perforations, be-

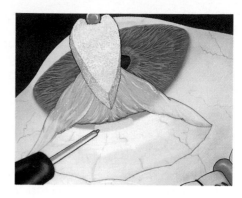

Figure 145–1. Unipolar diathermy (MIRA, Boston) applied to the episcleral region adjacent to the conjunctival flap with minimal shrinkage or tissue scarring. Utilized in the wet field, conjunctival thermal injury is minimal.

cause the fine tapered needle produces a hole that is sealed by the slightly larger suture material and does not create additional leaks. If the conjunctival perforation is large but close to the limbus in the region of the proposed sclerectomy, it is wise to perform the conjunctival dissection and sclerectomy in an adjacent quadrant to minimize the likelihood of a postoperative limbal leak.

The most frequent site for intraoperative wound leaks is at the conjunctival closure area. Some surgeons advocate separate closure of Tenon's capsule and conjunctiva as two layers to create a watertight seal. It is extremely important to ensure wound integrity before completing the procedure. A test of a watertight closure is performed by using the existing temporal paracentesis. Balanced salt solution should be injected into the anterior chamber, while topical 2 percent fluorescein is applied to the surface of the entire bleb. When green fluorescence occurs (indicative of wound leak), conjunctival closure should be done with the recommended 10–0 nylon suture. When fornix-based conjunctival flaps are used, carefully placed wing sutures firmly oppose the cornea and conjunctiva and are often self-sealing. When the use of early digital pressure or postoperative antimetabolite injections are expected, a running corneal-conjunctiva suture, in addition to wing sutures, has proved to be advisable.

SCLERECTOMY COMPLICATIONS

Fraying or amputation of the trabeculectomy flap can occur if the scleral tissue is extremely thin or fragile. A thinly dissected flap or a flap that becomes very thin at the limbus can also be problematic during manipulation. If a perforation exists or if the flap is completely amputated, the residual flap can be sutured to adjacent sclera and can act as a tamponade to the sclerectomy and minimize aqueous flow. Rotation of a partial-thickness flap from the adjacent sclera or use of preserved sclera to cover the defect are other possible repair techniques.

Premature posterior entry over the ciliary body is a

serious complication during the creation of the sclerectomy. Successful filtration does not occur unless an adequate opening can be made into the anterior chamber. Recognition of this complication occurs when the smooth tan ciliary body is distinguished from the normal iris tissue with a radial orientation and iris cripts (Fig. 145–2). When posterior entry occurs, it can often be corrected by dissecting anteriorly into clear cornea. By using a Descemet's punch, or even unipolar diathermy, an adequate anterior chamber opening can be created. Caution is emphasized because the posterior location makes amputation of the ciliary processes and vitreous loss more likely during the creation of an iridectomy.

Recognition of an incomplete sclerectomy can be quite difficult when full-thickness excision of the sclera is not accomplished. Observation of the residual ground-glass membrane is essential, and a Descemet's punch or Vanass scissors should be used to remove the obstructing tissue and create an adequate opening. The possibility of vitreous loss is another complication that can occur at the time of the sclerectomy or iridectomy. Despite the fact that this complication is not common, it can occur in young patients or in traumatized eyes or iatrogenically upon inadvertent violation of the vitreous cavity. All prolapsing vitreous should be removed by utilizing a cellulose sponge or a mechanized vitrectomy instrument. If an adequate vitrectomy cannot be accomplished, an adjacent quadrant should be prepared for a new sclerectomy. Lens injury or perforation can occur at this point in the procedure and can result in cataract formation with associated significant inflammation, necessitating emergency lens extraction.

Obstruction of the Sclerectomy

Hemorrhage and fibrin material can remain within the sclerectomy site and obstruct fluid flow, as can an imperforate iris or an incarcerated iris pillar. A more unusual form of sclerectomy obstruction can occur when the ciliary processes rotate anteriorly and prolapse into the sclerectomy site, resulting in profound obstruction (Fig. 145–3). If this occurs, minimization of the posterior pressure, release of the superior rectus stay suture, and adjustment of the lid speculum can be helpful. Topical

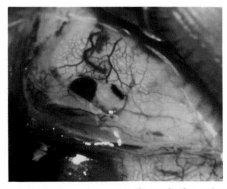

Figure 145–2. The posterior entry through the sclera over the ciliary body during filtration surgery.

cycloplegic (atropine 1 percent) may result in relaxation of the ciliary body and posterior rotation of the ciliary processes. If the processes remain incarcerated within the sclerectomy site, surgical amputation relieves the obstruction and ensures adequate patency (see Fig. 145–3).

Intraoperative Suprachoroidal Effusion or Hemorrhage

When the eye becomes hard and the anterior chamber flattens during glaucoma surgery, one must suspect a possible intraoperative choroidal effusion or suprachoroidal hemorrhage. The clinical picture results when fluid in the suprachoroidal space forces the ciliary processes, the iris, and even the lens into the sclerectomy, producing an obstruction to flow and increased IOP. Patients with prominent episcleral vessels and elevated episcleral venous pressure are particularly likely to develop intraoperative choroidal effusions during filtration surgery.[10] The creation of a sclerotomy before filtration surgery can minimize the collection of suprachoroidal fluid and decrease the postoperative complications. If a sclerectomy has not been prepared, it can be made in the inferonasal quadrant or adjacent to the sclerectomy 3 mm from the visible limbus to release suprachoroidal fluid. Efforts to maintain the ocular integrity by repositioning extruded contents and closing the sclerectomy flap should be accomplished quickly after ocular decompression.

EARLY POSTOPERATIVE COMPLICATIONS

Inflammation and Hemorrhage

The normal postoperative inflammatory process that occurs soon (1 to 3 wk) after glaucoma surgery can be detrimental to the long-term success of the procedure.[5] Multiple treatment opportunities can minimize inflammation and can alter the proliferative scarring process. Immediate postoperative hemorrhage into the bleb, or hemorrhage that migrates from the anterior chamber into the subconjunctival space, can create an inflammatory reaction and can result in fibrosis and scarring. The evidence is accumulating that the long-term use of topical antiglaucoma drugs may be toxic to the conjunctiva and Tenon's capsule and can contribute to the scarring process.[11] Frequently, administered topical corticosteroid drops and ointment and occasionally subconjunctival injection are the mainstay of early antiinflammatory therapy. The introduction of antimetabolites, prescribed for use during the early postoperative period, represents a major contribution to diminishing the postoperative fibrovascular proliferative response.[6, 7, 12, 13] The postoperative injection of 5-fluorouracil (5-FU) clearly has improved the prognosis of difficult glaucoma cases[13]; adjustment of the dose and schedule of 5-FU administration has helped to minimize side effects.[14]

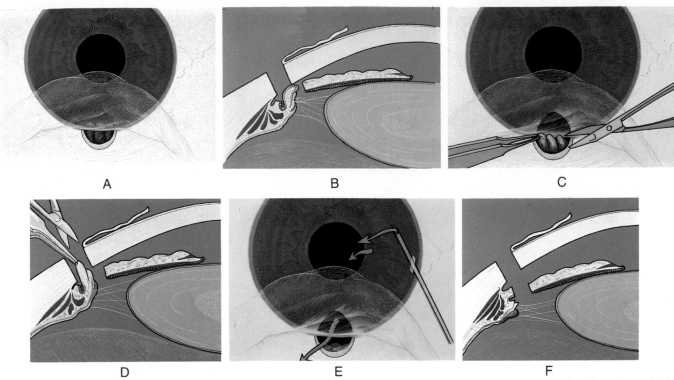

Figure 145–3. *A* and *B*, Front and side view. A ciliary process incarcerated into the sclerectomy, preventing flow through the sclerectomy. *C* and *D*, Excision of the obstructing ciliary processes. *E* and *F*, Amputated ciliary processes and patent sclerectomy permitting adequate aqueous flow from the anterior chamber through the sclerectomy.

5-FU is indicated for use in all problematic glaucomatous eyes following filtering surgery, specifically those with chronic uveitis, iridocorneal endothelial syndromes, neovascular glaucoma, aphakia, or pseudophakia, and in primary filters when early vascularization is expected. This drug is contraindicated in the presence of conjunctival wound leaks or corneal epithelial defects (Fig. 145–4). Corneal toxicity is more likely to occur in patients with previous abrasions or epithelial pathology. Administration of 5-FU is simple, and it should be incorporated into the armamentarium of all surgeons who perform filtration surgery or combined cataract and filtering surgery. A tuberculin syringe with a 30-gauge needle containing 5 mg of undiluted 5-FU is injected into the subconjunctival space 90 degrees from the bleb (Fig.

145–5). The inferonasal quadrant is frequently the selected site after a drop of topical anesthetic on a cotton-tipped pledget has been used to anesthetize the conjunctiva. The injection is usually painless and can be started 1 to 2 days after surgery in the absence of a wound leak or corneal pathology. The dosage schedule is individualized, and an effort is made not to exceed a total dose of 40 mg to minimize toxic effects on the corneal epithelium.

Intraoperative administration of the antimetabolite, mitomycin-C, has been advocated as a simple and effective new modality.[8] A single application (0.25 to 0.5 mg) placed in the episcleral sub-Tenon space during surgery decreases fibrovascular proliferation.[8, 15, 16] A recent prospective study has demonstrated that mitomycin-C is more effective than 5-FU postoperatively and has better lowering of IOP, fewer postoperative complications, and less need for antiglaucoma medication.[17] The role of 5-FU administered postoperatively following intraoperative mitomycin-C has not been clearly established, but it provides another possible way to diminish wound scarring in difficult cases.

Flat or Shallow Anterior Chamber

The development of a shallow or flat anterior chamber following successful filtration surgery presents a common and dreaded complication. Evaluation of the differential diagnosis of a flat anterior chamber is absolutely essen-

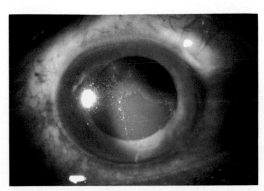

Figure 145–4. Corneal epithelial defect following subconjunctival injections of 5-fluorouracil.

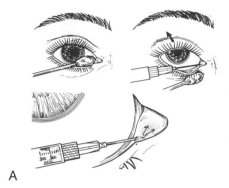

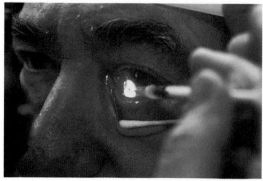

Figure 145–5. *A,* The technique used to inject 5 mg of 5-fluorouracil beneath the semilunar fold after topical anesthetic is applied with a cotton-tipped pledget. *B,* The patient is encouraged to look up and out, exposing the conjunctiva adjacent and beneath the semilunar fold. This technique is most carefully done at the biomicroscope with the patient's head supported.

tial to its management. The surgeon must distinguish among the possibilities of overfiltration, with a large bleb, low IOP, and no wound leak; versus a choroidal detachment, with fluid in the suprachoroidal space, low IOP, and ± wound leak. The other diagnostic possibilities include definitive wound leak, pupillary block, and malignant glaucoma.

Recognizing a wound leak is one of the most important diagnostic steps and is most easily accomplished by applying 2 percent fluorescein to the bleb surface and by visualizing the anterior segment through the biomicroscope using a cobalt blue filter. When a wound leak is present (evident by bright green fluorescence at the leak site), it can be treated with aqueous suppressants (carbonic anhydrase inhibitors and β-blockers) to decrease aqueous flow through the leak, encouraging epithelial cells to migrate and close the defect. The use of topical steroids should be decreased or eliminated to allow more normal epithelial proliferation.

If the wound leak persists and the anterior chamber remains shallow or flat, it is possible to close the leak with a tapered 10–0 nylon suture (Ethicon No. 2850) with a cooperative patient positioned at the biomicroscope using only topical anesthesia (Fig. 145–6). When the exact location of the leak has been identified, the closure is usually accomplished with a single suture. Closure of the leak results in an almost immediate bleb elevation and re-formation of the anterior chamber. Wound leaks that develop close to the limbus are managed efficiently with large, soft contact lenses (18 to 22 mm) applied in conjunction with a firm pressure patch to create a tamponade to the leaking conjunctiva.

Tissue glues can also be effective, particularly when conjunctival suture ends provide scaffolding for the glue adhesion and sealing of the wound. The rigid glaucoma shell is also effective in managing friable conjunctiva with multiple holes.

Choroidal Detachment

Fluid commonly is present in the suprachoroidal space following most glaucoma procedures. When enough fluid collects to cause the anterior chamber to shallow or flatten, it becomes a more significant factor. The collection of suprachoroidal fluid occurs when significant hypotony is responsible for the transudation of fluid from the choroidal vasculature into the suprachoroidal space.[18, 19] The diagnosis of choroidal effusion is usually made when large balloon-like elevations of the choroid are seen through a dilated pupil. B-scan ultrasonography can also be used to establish the diagnosis of choroidal detachment when visualization through the pupil is impossible. Ultrasonography can also be helpful to distinguish between effusion and hemorrhage in the suprachoroidal space.

Choroidal detachment becomes a clinical concern when flattening of the anterior chamber results in lens corneal touch with corneal edema or persistent kissing choroidals resulting in retinal apposition with possible adhesion. Significant suprachoroidal hemorrhage with increased ocular inflammation or a flattening, inflamed bleb are indications to drain the suprachoroidal space and re-form the anterior chamber (Fig. 145–7).[18]

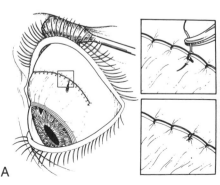

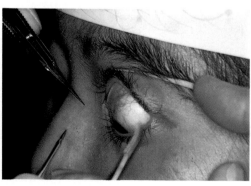

Figure 145–6. *A,* Closure of a conjunctival incision wound leak at the slit lamp with topical anesthesia. *B,* The patient is encouraged to look down while a fine needle holder places the tapered needle (Ethicon No. 2850) with 10–0 nylon at the exact site of the leak. Instrumentation includes forceps (Castroviejo 0.12 mm) and Vanass scissors.

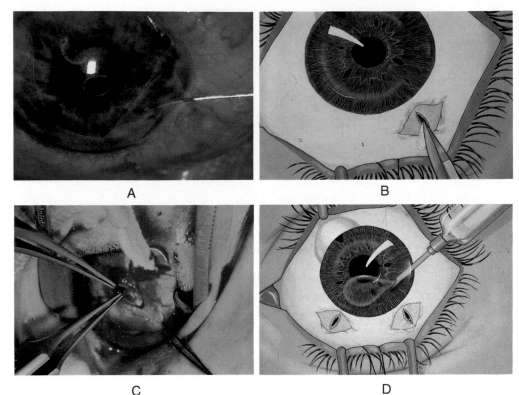

Figure 145–7. *A,* Choroidal tap with re-formation of the anterior chamber using a blunt 30 gauge, non-disposable needle through an anterior chamber paracentesis. *B,* Scleral incision 3.5 mm from the visible limbus with evacuation of suprachoroidal fluid. *C,* Evacuation of suprachoroidal blood following a hemorrhagic choroidal detachment. *D,* Re-formation of the anterior chamber alternating with draining of suprachoroidal fluid from 2 inferior sclerotomies.

Malignant Glaucoma

Malignant glaucoma (aqueous diversion) is also included in the differential diagnosis of flat anterior chamber following filtration surgery, particularly after chronic angle-closure glaucoma. This entity is characterized by a very shallow anterior chamber with a low bleb and high IOP during the postoperative period. It is important to establish a patent peripheral iridectomy, because pupillary block can also cause a flat chamber with elevated IOP.

When malignant glaucoma is diagnosed, medical therapy should be instituted[20]: a topical cycloplegic agent (atropine 1 percent) and an α-agonist (phenylephrine HCl, 10 percent) combined with a topical β-blocker (timolol 0.5 percent) and a carbonic anhydrase inhibitor (acetazolamide, 250 mg). Often, 2 to 3 days of this therapy results in deepening of the anterior chamber and lowering of the IOP. The possibility of using an osmotic agent orally or intravenously in conjunction with the topical regimen is also helpful. If medical therapy is not successful, a surgical approach has been developed.[21] It is postulated that by using a needle or an automated vitrectomy instrument, perforation of the anterior hyaloid face and possibly posterior hyaloid with removal of liquid vitreous can be curative. When malignant glaucoma is present in aphakia or pseudophakia,[22] Nd.YAG laser disruption of the posterior capsule and anterior hyaloid face has resulted in immediate deepening of the anterior chamber and resolution of this complication.[23]

Suprachoroidal Hemorrhage

Localized or diffuse hemorrhage into the suprachoroidal space that occurs postoperatively is heralded by severe pain and can cause shallowing of the anterior chamber with associated elevated IOP.[24–26] This serious complication occurs more frequently in aphakia and pseudophakia, and, when extensive, it should be managed by draining the suprachoroidal space with emphasis on evacuating the hemorrhage, performing a vitrectomy, and creating a choroidal-retinal tamponade with intravitreal gas. Aggressive management of this serious complication can result in the preservation of vision.[27]

Tenon's Cyst

When an adhesion develops between the episclera and Tenon's capsule, aqueous can be entrapped, resulting in functional extension of the anterior chamber (Fig. 145–8).[28] The characteristic appearance of smooth, domed, markedly elevated, cystlike structure at the site of the filtering procedure has been seen more frequently during the last decade.[29] The possibility that chronic antiglaucoma therapy might have an adverse effect on the cell structure and function of the conjunctiva and Tenon's capsule has been reported.[11, 29] When cyst formation is recognized during the early phase following filtration surgery, medical therapy can be instituted,[30] but surgical manipulation may often be necessary.[31, 32]

Active steps in the management following the early recognition of a Tenon cyst can minimize the likelihood

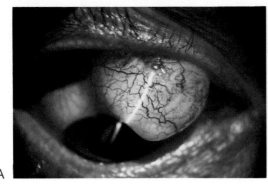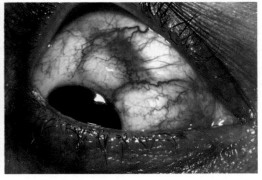

Figure 145–8. *A,* Tenon's cyst. A large overhanging domed lesion. *B,* Localized encapsulated cyst with prominent vascular margin at the site of Tenon's episcleral scarring.

of bleb failure. The timely use of digital pressure that requires the patient to press firmly on the lower lid transfers pressure to the eye and encourages fluid to disrupt the adhesions between Tenon's capsule and the episclera (Fig. 145–9).[32] The possibility of pressing directly on the dome of Tenon's capsule with a cotton-tipped applicator or digital pressure may also disrupt adhesions and deter cyst formation.[28] When the cyst persists and the IOP is elevated while the patient is on medical therapy, needling the cyst has been valuable (Fig. 145–10). When repeated needlings are unsuccessful, surgical bleb revision can result in long-term success (Fig. 145–11).[32]

Failure of the Filtering Bleb

Bleb failure is heralded by a gradual but definite increase in the IOP, with flattening of the bleb occurring

at any time during the postoperative period. When this occurs at an early stage, the inflammatory response with thickening and vascularity of the bleb eventually results in poor control of IOP. There are many ways that a bleb can fail; Tenon's cyst has been described as a stage in bleb failure. The initial stage of fibrovascular proliferative processes occurs early in the postoperative filtering state but can be altered by the use of mitomycin-C intraoperatively and 5-FU postoperatively. The possibility of sclerectomy obstruction must be evaluated any time when bleb failure is anticipated. Careful gonioscopy can reveal the presence of iris or a ciliary process prolapse into the sclerectomy, and laser or surgical removal is necessary.[33] A clear membrane can occasionally be perforated by Nd.YAG laser.[34] A fibrous sheet or membrane can be present within the sclerectomy site and often requires surgical removal.

The most common site of obstruction in the early and late stages of bleb failure is at the episcleral level. A fibrotic proliferative process usually seals the trabecu-

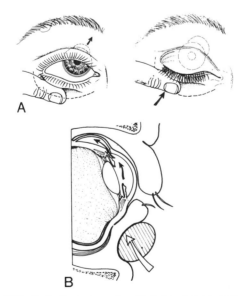

Figure 145–9. *A,* Technique for digital pressure using a finger applied to the lower lid while the patient is instructed to look up and in. Inferior orbital rim is palpated and the globe identified as firm pressure is placed on the lid for 5 to 10 sec, repeated after a 5-sec interval for 5 to 10 applications. This maneuver may be performed from two to six times or more per day. *B,* Mechanism of pressure transferred from the lid to the globe forcing fluid through the sclerectomy and into the bleb, acting to separate the tissue adhesions and enhance filtration.

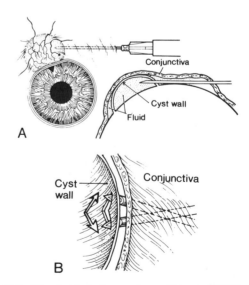

Figure 145–10. *A,* Technique of needling a Tenon cyst with topical anesthesia at the slit lamp. A remote conjunctival perforation is placed and a needle or a Wheeler knife passed in the subconjunctival space to engage and penetrate the cyst. *B,* Radial movements are made with the needle-knife to carefully incise the cyst wall for at least 2 or 3 mm, taking precautions to avoid blood vessels.

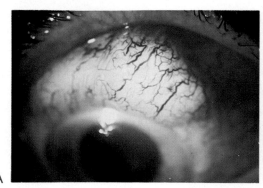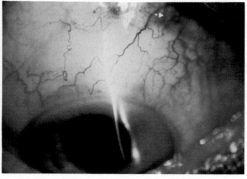

Figure 145–11. *A*, Tenon's cyst with prominent vascularization and elevated intraocular pressure despite medical therapy. *B*, Excellent filtration following surgical revision of a Tenon cyst with excision of a dense fibrovascular cyst wall.

lectomy site or covers the full-thickness opening with nonporous membrane. Laser therapy is occasionally effective in perforating this seal,[35] but often surgical revision is required by internal revision through the sclerectomy or an external approach by taking down the conjunctival flap and surgically opening the sealed sclerectomy.

When a guarded sclerectomy has been performed with a sutured closure, the earliest sign of elevated IOP or bleb failure should prompt immediate laser suture lysis (Fig. 145–12). This is done most effectively through a Hoskins lens using a low-power argon laser with 100-μ spot size for 1/10 of a second, taking precautions to minimize the possibility of conjunctival perforation. One suture at a time should be lysed, and digital pressure should be applied to elevate the scleral flap. This is done most effectively at the slit lamp, while the surgeon monitors the depth of the anterior chamber.

A paradoxical complication of hypotony and choroidal detachment can occur following bleb failure with the introduction of aqueous suppressants.[36, 37] When topical β-blocking agents or carbonic anhydrase inhibitors are used for pressure control, hypotony and choroidal detachment can occur with an alteration of vision. The mechanism of this occurrence is not well established, but cessation of the aqueous suppressant agents often results in resolution of the choroidal detachment. It has been possible to reinstitute topical betaxolol to control IOP without recurrence of the choroidal detachment.[37]

When the bleb fails and no other methods of medical management are available, surgery must be considered. Filtration surgery in a virgin quadrant, utilizing intra-operative mitomycin-C and 5-FU postoperatively, is an option. If the conjunctiva has been violated and the visual acuity is better than 20/200, an anterior chamber drainage device can be inserted. If the vision is compromised and the conjunctiva tissue is not amenable to adequate dissection, cycloablation therapy with Nd.YAG laser can prevent further visual loss.

LATE POSTOPERATIVE COMPLICATIONS

Wound Leak

Wound leak following filtration surgery most frequently occurs with thin walled and cystic blebs. This form of bleb morphology is more common following full-thickness procedures than trabeculectomies but can occur after either operation. Whenever there has been profound lowering of IOP or the patient has persistent tearing, 2 percent fluorescein should be applied to the bleb surface to identify even the most subtle wound leak (Fig. 145–13). Spontaneous closure often occurs and can be enhanced by introducing aqueous suppressants. If the leak persists and the eye is aphakic or pseudophakic, or if there is a high risk for infection, surgical closure should be considered. The possibility of creating a pedicle flap of conjunctiva from the posterior edge of the existing bleb deep into the conjunctival cul-de-sac and advancing it to cover the bleb can effectively seal the leak. The leak can be sealed by excising the bleb and covering it with conjunctiva or sclera, but the result is often bleb failure and IOP elevation. A free conjunctival graft can be considered to close persistent bleb leaks. It is usually possible to perform filtration surgery in an adjacent quadrant and to suture the existing leak.

Infection

Intraocular infection is the most serious threat to vision following successful filtration surgery. Often bleb infection and subsequent endophthalmitis can be prevented by alerting the patient to symptoms of infection and by insisting on immediate examination. It has been

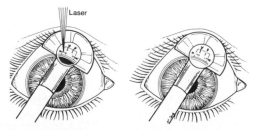

Figure 145–12. Laser suture lysis with a Hoskins lens and argon laser using low power to minimize the chance of conjunctival perforation.

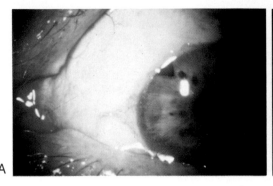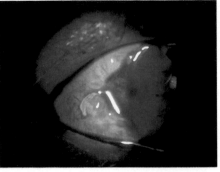

Figure 145–13. *A,* A chronic recurrent bleb leak with hypotony. *B,* The diagnosis is established with 2 percent fluorescein.

recognized that *Streptococcus* species and *Haemophilus influenzae* are the most common pathogens in bleb infection[38]; however, *Staphylococcus epidermidis* and gram-negative organisms may also be implicated. The diagnosis must be established as early as possible, and cultures are obtained from the anterior chamber and vitreous before instituting appropriate antibiotic therapy (Table 145–1). The treatment of endophthalmitis necessitates intraocular, periocular, and often intravenous antibiotics, combined with systemic steroids for 7 to 10 days. Aphakic and pseudophakic eyes are more vulnerable to infection because the absence of the crystalline lens makes pathogen penetration into the vitreous cavity a greater likelihood. If infection reoccurs or is associated with an existing bleb leak and the leak persists, excision of the bleb may be indicated.

Cataract Formation

The development or progression of lens opacification is a frequent complication of filtration surgery. When a preexisting cataract is present, a decrease in visual acuity can be anticipated. The incidence of cataract formation following full-thickness operation is approximately 34 percent; whereas the likelihood of cataract development following trabeculectomy is approximately 21 percent.[39] With the advent of IOL implantation, cataract surgery can result in more effective visual rehabilitation. The principle concern following cataract surgery is to maintain a functioning bleb, which is done most effectively when the cataract operation is performed as far from the bleb as possible.

CONCLUSION

The incidence and severity of complications following filtration surgery have become less catastrophic. However, until the risk of vision-threatening complications can be diminished further, the surgical management of glaucoma remains a significant challenge. If the evidence supporting the success of early surgery is established, the standard use of long-term medications will diminish, and it is expected that the patient's quality of life will improve. With major efforts in the research of wound healing and remodeling, combined with new developments in noninvasive laser filtration procedures, a more effective cure for glaucoma will be forthcoming.

Table 145–1. TREATMENT OF BLEB INFECTION AND ENDOPHTHALMITIS

Infection	Therapy
Bleb involved with the anterior chamber reaction	Topical antibiotics* Topical steroids§ Cycloplegics¶
Bleb involvement with hypopyon	Topical* and systemic† antibiotics Topical steroids§ Cycloplegics¶
Bleb with anterior chamber and vitreous reaction	Topical§ and systemic† antibiotics Intravitreal‡ antibiotics Topical† and systemic ‖ steroids Cycloplegia¶ Pars plana vitrectomy

Antibiotics	
Topical	*Gentamycin 1 gtt q 1 hr Vancomycin (50 mg/ml) 1 gtt q 1 hr Bacitracin-polymyxin ointment q 6 hr
Systemic intravenous	†Vancomycin 500 mg q 8 hr Gentamycin 80 mg q 8 hr
Intravitreous	‡Vancomycin 1 mg Amikacin 400 μg
Steroids (after 12–24 hr)	
Topical	§Prednisone acetate 1 gtt q 1–2 hr
Systemic	‖ Prednisone 40 mg po q 12 hr
Cycloplegics	¶Atropine 1% gtt bid to qid

REFERENCES

1. Watson PG, Grierson I: The place of trabeculectomy in the treatment of glaucoma. Ophthalmology 88:175, 1981.
2. Midgal C, Hitchings R: Control of chronic simple glaucoma with primary medical, surgical, and laser treatment. Trans Ophthalmol Soc UK 105:653, 1986.
3. Wax MB, Addelson A: Indications for early glaucoma surgery. Ophthalmology Clin North Am 1:1175, 1988.
4. Addicks EM, Quigley AJ, Green RW, Robin AL: Histologic characteristics of filtering blebs in glaucomatous eyes. Arch Ophthalmol 101:795, 1983.
5. Skuta GL, Parrish RK: Wound healing in glaucoma filtering surgery. Surv Ophthalmol 32:149, 1987.
6. Heuer DK, Parrish RK, Gressel MG, et al: 5-Fluorouracil in glaucoma filtering surgery. II: A pilot study. Ophthalmology 91:384, 1984.

7. Heuer DK, Parrish RK, Gressel MG, et al: 5-Fluorouracil in glaucoma filtering surgery. III: Intermediate follow-up of a pilot study. Ophthalmology 93:1537, 1986.
8. Chen C-W: Enhanced intraocular pressure controlling effectiveness of trabeculectomy by local application of mitomycin C. Trans Asia-Pacific Acad Ophthalmol 9:172–177, 1983.
9. Moorhead LC: Inhibition of collagen cross-linking: A new approach to ocular scarring. Curr Eye Res 1:77, 1981.
10. Bellows AR, Chylack LT, Epstein DL, Hutchinson BT: Choroidal effusion during glaucoma surgery in patients with prominent episcleral vessels. Arch Ophthalmol 97:593, 1979.
11. Sherwood MB, Grierson I, Millar L, Hutching RA: Long-term morphologic effects of anti-glaucoma drugs on the conjunctiva and Tenon's capsule in glaucomatous patients. Ophthalmology 96:327, 1989.
12. Rockwood EJ, Parrish RK, Heuer DK, et al: Glaucoma filtering surgery with 5-fluorouracil. Ophthalmology 91:831, 1984.
13. Fluorouracil Filtering Surgery Study Group: Fluorouracil filtering surgery follow-up. Am J Ophthalmol 108:625, 1989.
14. Weinreb RN: Adjusting the dose of 5-fluorouracil after filtration surgery to minimize side effects. Ophthalmology 94:564, 1987.
15. Chen C-W, Huang H-T, Chen M: Enhancement of IOP control effect of trabeculectomy by local application of anti-cancer drug. Acta XXV, Concilium Ophthalmologicum (Rome) 2:1487, 1986.
16. Palmer SS: Mitomycin adjacent chemotherapy with trabeculectomy. Ophthalmology 98:317, 1991.
17. Skuta GL, Beeson CC, Higginbotham EJ, et al: Intraoperative mitomycin versus postoperative 5-FU in high risk glaucoma filtering surgery. Ophthalmology 99:438, 1992.
18. Bellows AR, Chylack LT, Hutchinson BT: Choroidal detachment, clinical manifestation, therapy and mechanism of formation. Ophthalmology 88:1107, 1981.
19. Brubaker RF, Pederson JE: Ciliochoroidal detachment. Surv Ophthalmol 27:281, 1983.
20. Chandler PA, Grant WM: Mydriatics cycloplegic treatment in malignant glaucoma. Arch Ophthalmol 62:353, 1962.
21. Chandler PA, Simmons RJ, Grant WM: Malignant glaucoma, medical and surgical treatment. Am J Ophthalmol 66:495, 1968.
22. Schrader CE, Belcher CD, Thomas JV, et al: Pupillary and iridovitreal block in pseudophakic eyes. Ophthalmology 91:831, 1984.
23. Epstein DL, Steinert RF, Puliafito C: Nd:YAG therapy to the anterior hyaloid in aphakic malignant (ciliovitreal block) glaucoma. Am J Ophthalmol 98:137, 1984.
24. Gressel MG, Parrish RK, Heuer DK: Delayed non-expulsive suprachoroidal hemorrhage. Arch Ophthalmol 102:1757, 1984.
25. Ruderman JM, Harbin TS, Campbell DJ: Postoperative suprachoroidal hemorrhage filtration procedures. Arch Ophthalmol 104:201, 1986.
26. Givens K, Shields MB: Suprachoroidal hemorrhage after glaucoma filtering surgery. Am J Ophthalmol 103:689, 1987.
27. Lambrou FH, Meredith TA, Kaplan HG: Secondary surgical management of explosive choroidal hemorrhage. Arch Ophthalmol 105:1195, 1987.
28. VanBuskirk EM: Cyst of Tenon's capsule following filtration surgery. Am J Ophthalmol 94:522, 1982.
29. Richter CU, Shingleton BJ, Bellows AR, et al: The development of encapsulated filtering blebs. Ophthalmology 95:1163, 1988.
30. Scott DR, Quigley AJ: Medical management of apparently encysted blebs after trabeculectomies. Ophthalmology 95:1169, 1988.
31. Pederson JE, Smith SG: Surgical management of encapsulated filtering blebs. Ophthalmology 92:955, 1985.
32. Shingleton BJ, Richter CU, Bellows AR, Hutchinson BT: Management of encapsulated filtration blebs. Ophthalmology 97:63, 1990.
33. VanBuskirk EM: Reopening filtration fistulas with the argon laser. Am J Ophthalmol 94:1, 1982.
34. Dailey RA, Samples JR, VanBuskirk EM: Reopening filtration fistulas with the Nd:YAG laser. Am J Ophthalmol 102:491, 1986.
35. Rankin GA, Latina MA: Transconjunctival Nd:YAG laser revision of failing trabeculectomy. Ophthalmol Surg 21:365, 1990.
36. Vela MA, Campbell DJ: Hypotony and ciliochoroidal detachment following pharmacologic aqueous suppressant therapy in previous filtered patients. Ophthalmology 92:50, 1985.
37. Berke SJ, Bellows AR, Shingleton BJ, et al: Chronic and recurrent choroidal detachment after glaucoma filtration surgery. Ophthalmology 94:154, 1987.
38. Mandelbaum S, Forster RK, Gelender H, Cobertson W: Late onset endophthalmitis associated with filtering blebs. Ophthalmology 92:964, 1985.
39. Lamping K, Bellows AR, Hutchinson BT, et al: Long-term evaluation of initial filtration surgery. Ophthalmology 93:931, 1986.

Chapter 146

■

Setons in Glaucoma Surgery

A. SYDNEY WILLIAMS

Seton, derived from the Latin word *seta,* meaning bristle, is defined as "a whisp of threads, a strip of gauze, a length of wire or other foreign material passed through the subcutaneous tissues or a cyst to form a sinus or a fistula."[1] Glaucoma-filtering surgery provides an alternate drainage route that allows aqueous to escape from the anterior chamber at a lower pressure. The normal healing process causes many of these operations to fail. Beginning early in the 20th century, various materials, including horse hair, silk thread, metals, plastics and iris tissue, were incorporated into limbal wounds to maintain fistula patency.[2-19] Various substances were also placed in the suprachoroidal space through cyclodialysis clefts to maintain filtration.[13]

The era of the true seton has passed. Present filtration devices are implants connected to tubes that enter the anterior chamber and shunt aqueous to the implant, which serves as a reservoir for aqueous dispersal at a site distant from the limbal wound. The most popular of these, the Molteno implant, and other currently available implants are discussed in this chapter. Even though implants generally have been reserved for glaucoma that is refractory to filtration surgery, there has been a trend toward using implants as primary procedures in certain types of glaucoma with which standard filtering surgery is likely to fail.

This chapter presents the theory behind the function of implants in glaucoma surgery, the current indications for their use, and the surgical technique for inserting the Molteno implant.[1] Postoperative management and the intraoperative and postoperative problems encountered with these shunting devices are discussed, as is the histopathology of implants.

HISTORY OF GLAUCOMA SETONS

Glaucoma filtering surgery was pioneered in 1830 by MacKenzie,[20] who realized that in order to relieve elevated ocular tension, separate drainage for egress of "trapped" aqueous humor must be achieved. Various types of fistulizing operations were performed to meet this goal with some success. However, many failed due to dense fibrosis in the episcleral tissues overlying the fistula. The nonphysiologic nature of this surgery was, therefore, appreciated. Because of the persistent failure of the external fistulizing operations, Heine[20] proposed detaching the ciliary body from the scleral spur to provide an internal fistula into the suprachoroidal space and thus lower pressure. However, this operation was also plagued by closure of the internal cleft. The first publications on use of setons in glaucoma surgery in the English literature appeared in 1912 when Zorab[2] and Mayou[3] independently reported using a No. 2 silk suture to produce permanent filtration from the anterior chamber into the subconjunctival space. In 1906, a similar procedure had been reported by Rollet and Moreau[4] in the French literature. Because of the limited success of these early studies, many substances including silk thread were used in the vitreous cavity.[7] Gold wire,[8] devices,[9] horse hair, or iridium-platinum wire,[10, 11] magnesium,[12, 13] tantalum,[14, 15] gelatin film,[16, 17] polyvinyl tubes,[18] silicon,[19] and Teflon[21] were subsequently incorporated into limbal wounds or through cyclodialysis clefts to establish filtration.

Organic materials have also been incarcerated in wounds. Holth developed the well-known procedure iridencleisis in which the iris is pulled into a limbal wound to encourage fistula patency.[20] Makusch[22] in 1939 and Suker[23] in 1931 used iris inclusion combined with cyclodialysis, in what was termed an "aqueodialysis operation," to improve outflow to the suprachoroidal space. Sondermann[24] placed conjunctival tissue through a cyclodialysis wound into the angle to establish a vascular connection with the angle structures and thus lower intraocular pressure. A similar attempt was made using an extraocular vein to drain the anterior chamber.[25-27] Cartilage, lacrimal canaliculus, and sclera have been incorporated into filtration wounds to improve their success.[28-30] Even though the early reports on seton surgery were favorable, these operations never gained widespread acceptance possibly because their long-term success was the same as that of routine trephine or cyclodialysis operations.

Recent microsurgical advances have improved the success of filtering surgery. However, enthusiasm has been tempered by the uniformly poor results seen in high-risk eyes. Patients with aphakia or pseudophakia or neovascularization of the anterior segment, uveitis, conjunctival scarring, and young patients are more likely to have unsuccessful filtration surgery,[31-41] as are members of certain ethnic groups, such as patients of African heritage.[42-46] Failures generally result from excessive episcleral fibrosis that obstructs ocular flow. Table 146–1 summarizes the results of filtration surgery in patients at high risk for failure. Only studies with at least 6 mo of follow-up, pressure lower than 21 mmHg, and no further surgical intervention have been included. One can see that high-risk filtration surgeries fail nearly 50 percent of the time, with some groups failing even more frequently. The introduction of antimetabolite therapy such as 5-fluorouracil has improved the outlook for these patients[47-49]; however, many still have unsuccessful standard filtering operations.

The earliest report of an acrylic type implant was made in 1955 by Qadeer from Pakistan.[50] The implant consisted of a subconjunctival plate at the limbus connected to a tube placed into the anterior chamber. In the late 1960s, Molteno independently furthered this idea using a similar silicone glaucoma implant to help control intraocular pressure in high-risk eyes.[51] His early implants consisted of a silicone tube passed into the anterior chamber and connected to an acrylic reservoir situated at the limbus. In 1973, he began using a modified implant to shunt the aqueous fluid to sub-Tenon's space in the ocular equator away from the limbus,[52] where the fluid was taken up by vessels and lymphatics that formed in the tissue overlying the large

Table 146–1. RESULTS OF FILTRATION SURGERY FOR HIGH-RISK PATIENTS

Risk	Author	No. of Eyes	Success (%)	Comment
Aphakia	Herschler[34]	41	78	Vitrectomy
	Bellow and Johnstone[36]	21	62	
	Heuer et al[35]	92	39	
	Gross et al[37]	15	27	
	5-FU Study Group (1989)[49]	81	48	No 5-FU
	5-FU Study Group (1989)	81	72	With 5-FU
NVG	Herschler and Agness[38]	13	77	Diathermy to ciliary process
	Parrish and Herschler[39]	13	54	Same group with >2-yr follow-up
Youth	Beauchamp and Parks[32]	22	50	Ages 1–20
	Gressel et al[33]	45	54	Ages 10–29
Failed Prior	Kitizawa et al[41]	24	10	

aqueous reservoir. These devices, although not true setons, were designed to shunt aqueous through a tube to a distal reservoir around which a fibrous capsule formed. The purpose of the long tube was to separate the limbus and conjunctival wound from the area of future filtration and to move the plastic shunting device away from the anterior segment of the eye where conjunctival breakdown and discomfort frequently were seen. The aqueous escaped through the capsule wall that formed around the reservoir, thus lowering intraocular pressure. Virtually all modern implants utilize this principle. In the United States, the Molteno implant is still the most widely used filtering device (Fig. 146–1).

Since its introduction, other drainage devices have been developed. In 1976, Krupin and associates experimented with the valve implant,[53] which differed from the Molteno implant in that it provided a unidirectional valve that opened at pressures of approximately 15 mmHg and closed at pressures 2 to 3 mm lower. This valve, which was designed to prevent hypotony (a common problem with the Molteno implant), was fashioned from a closed Silastic tube with horizontal and vertical slits in the sealed end. This implant was smaller in size than the Molteno implant and provided a bleb close to the limbus as seen in more conventional filtration surgery. Because no reservoir plate was incorporated into this device, the tube suffered fibrous encapsulation and resultant pressure elevation. The anterior location of these devices resulted in erosion through the conjunctiva. Ormerod and associates reported that the supramid tubes of these valves also were subject to biodegradability.[54] These problems led to the device's abandonment. The Krupin tube later was revived, using a long tube and a grooved scleral element, with better results and fewer complications, having borrowed principles from the work of Schocket and associates and Molteno.[55, 56]

In 1982, Schocket and associates introduced a tube shunt that connected to an encircling scleral element.[55] This device had the same long tube from the anterior chamber to direct aqueous posteriorly to the ocular equator. The aqueous entered a hollow space created by sewing a grooved scleral element upside down on the ocular surface. The tube passed from the anterior chamber into this space in which it is directed for a short distance. The tube was sutured to the eye to prevent migration. This procedure required placement of a 360-degree encircling band. The large drainage surface area resulted in severe hypotony and a 5 percent incidence of suprachoroidal hemorrhage.[57] Other problems included hyphema and resultant fibrous membrane development in the anterior chamber that blocked the tube internally or pulled the iris over the tube tip. Occlusion of the external end of the tube beneath the buckle also was a problem. In an exhaustive review, Schocket discussed modifications to these problems,[57] including heparinizing the implant tubes to prevent hyphema. Initial work was somewhat successful. Recently, hyphema, although fairly common, has not been associated with a poor outcome.[58]

Hitchings and associates proposed a modification using a valved tube and a variable surface area implant that decreased the severe hypotony and provided excellent pressure control.[59] In addition, a one-piece implant, using the same principle, has been developed by Joseph and associates with promising clinical results.[60] Other glaucoma implants, such as the Drake-Hoskins valve and the Mendez pump shunt implant incorporated a valve mechanism to address the immediate postoperative hypotony or late pressure elevation often seen with other implants.[61, 62] These devices offer promising surgical alternatives for patients who have had unsuccessful conventional glaucoma surgery. However, no prospective controlled clinical study has been performed comparing any of the implants with conventional surgery, either with or without fluorouracil. Lieberman and Ewing published a review of the various filtration devices.[61] Melamed and Fiore published a more limited review covering the Molteno implant.[63]

MOLTENO IMPLANT

The Molteno implant, the prototypical implant after which most tube shunting devices have been fashioned, has evolved during the 20 yr since its introduction. It consists of one or two circular silicone plates, each about 13 mm in diameter, with an elevated lip around the circumference that measures about 1 mm in height from the plate surface. The surfaces are rounded and curved to fit flush against the ocular surface, thus minimizing trauma to tissue. The double plate has a flexible interconnecting tube that is 10 mm long. The implants are available in right- and left-eye versions in which the tube to the anterior chambers leaves the nasal plate. The tube, which is 20 mm long with internal and external diameters of 0.3 mm and 0.64 mm respectively, must be cut to the desired length during surgery, usually providing an entry of 2 to 3 mm into the anterior chamber. The plates each have two suture holes on their anterior aspect to facilitate scleral attachment (see Fig. 146–1).

Adequate functioning of the implant depends on the fibrous capsule surrounding the plate. Histology shows that a dense connective tissue capsule, probably derived from the episclera, envelopes all surfaces of the plate (Fig. 146–2).[64, 65] This tissue shows little or no inflammatory reaction over the plate surface, and there has

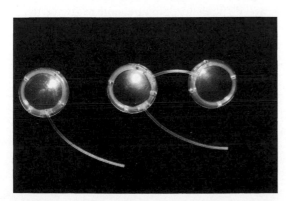

Figure 146–1. Single- and double-plate Molteno implants.

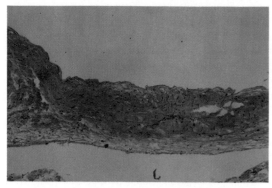

Figure 146–2. Histology of the capsule removed from a marginally functioning implant. Note the scleral appearance. The tissue is more cellular and thicker. The inner lining is not endothelialized, although flattened fibroblasts can occasionally be seen. Typically, the inside surface of the bleb is more loosely organized, and the outer surface is denser. A few lymphocytes are seen.

never been fibrosis adhering to the plate.[66] Rubin and associates reported minimal inflammatory reaction beneath the plate.[64] The tissue in direct contact with aqueous humor shows necrosis and thinning and variable amounts of inflammation. It appears that aqueous may have a tissue-molding property as shown in previous in vitro studies.[67–69] Intraocular pressure is lowered as aqueous passes more readily through this tissue capsule than from the intact anterior chamber. The facility of outflow from the reservoir depends not only on the wall thickness but also on the surface area, vascularity, and lymphatic supply.[70–72] Marker studies by Minckler and associates, which are confirmed by Peiffer and coworkers, showed passive diffusion through the bleb wall with uptake into the vessels.[71, 72] The double-plate implant with a greater surface area is theorized to lower pressure more effectively. Clinically, while surface area appears to play a role in pressure lowering, it is a complex relationship and is not directly related.[70] For instance, even though the Joseph and Schocket devices have a surface area as much as 10 times greater than that of the double-plate Molteno implant, the postoperative pressure that these implants provide is lower, but not correspondingly so. Peiffer and associates recently completed a study comparing the histologic characteristics and the flow pathways of the Joseph and Schocket devices in monkey eyes and found that the devices behaved remarkably similarly.[72] Unfortunately, the effectiveness of the devices was not compared in that study. To date, no study has been undertaken that compares the clinical efficacy of the various filtration devices.

INDICATIONS FOR IMPLANT SURGERY

Initially, implant surgery was reserved for eyes that had undergone multiple unsuccessful conventional surgeries and cyclodestructive procedures. A few years ago, Molteno implants were used only after conventional surgery failed. Today, they are being used increasingly in difficult cases as primary procedures in which failure of conventional surgery or intraoperative complications are likely. This surgery is advantageous in that it is primarily an extraocular procedure in which the eye is opened minimally for a short period of time compared with standard filtration operations. Molteno implants may provide the safest, most rational, and successful drainage method for patients with a tendency to choroidal expansion as seen in dural shunts or Sturge-Weber syndrome.

The Molteno implant may be the current treatment of choice in neovascular glaucoma. Trabeculectomy is likely to successfully lower intraocular pressure in only about 40 percent of patients.[38] Conventional cyclodestructive procedures lower pressure in approximately 50 percent,[73–77] but they are complicated by a high rate of visual morbidity and pain. More than 50 percent of patients lost light perception vision in the series reported by Krupin and associates.[75] This is a rare complication of implant surgery and is more likely to occur from the disease process itself. Newer laser cyclophotocoagulation techniques may have improved the safety and efficacy of the destructive procedures, but they remain potentially dangerous, unpredictable, and painful especially in patients with neovascular glaucoma.[78] A study comparing 5-fluorouracil trabeculectomy with the Molteno implant has not been performed.

RESULTS

Numerous studies on the efficacy of the Molteno and other implants have been completed[78–104]; however, the results are difficult to compare and evaluate because of

Table 146–2. RESULTS OF MOLTENO IMPLANT IN MIXED GLAUCOMA

Author	No. of Eyes	Mean FU	Success by IOP (%)	Definition	FST
Molteno et al[52]	64	18 m	91	<21	+
Molteno et al[83]	20	>3 m	100	<21	—
Downes et al[103]	96	6–87 m	58	<21	—
Hoare Nairne et al[108]	13	14 m	96	<25	+ (4 pts)
Ward and Cooper[88]	28	24 m	64	<25	+
Goldberg[89]	38	6 m	92	<20	+
Minckler	79	20 m	59	<22	—
Egbert and Lieberman[109]	38	18 m	79	<21	—
Feldman	89 (82)	15 m	71	<21	—

Table 146–3. RESULTS OF MOLTENO IMPLANT IN NEOVASCULAR GLAUCOMA

Author	No. of Eyes	FU (mo)	Success (%)	IOP	FST	Implant
Molteno et al[80]	12	13 m	58	<21	+	1 P
Ancker and Molteno[32]	36	15.5 m	83	<20	+	1 S 1 P
Brown and Cairnes[86]	16	14 m	75	<25	+	1 and 2 S 1 P
Molteno and Haddad[105]	24	>6 m	83	<20	?	1 S 2 P
Downes et al[103]	50	29.5 m	60	<25	—	1 S 1 P
Minckler	15	19 m	47	<22	—	1 S 1 and 2 P
Heuer	16	>3 m	58	<22	—	1 or 2 S 1 and 2 P

the various types of glaucomas treated, the different definitions of success, and the postoperative management techniques used. Tables 146–1 to 146–4 list the results of the Molteno implant studies and our work. Even though follow-up, age, implant type, antimetabolite use, and diagnosis vary, the implants appear to be "effective" in approximately 50 to 90 percent of patients.

The visual results for patients who underwent Molteno implant surgery are also difficult to evaluate. The underlying disease process sometimes results in high rates of blindness. Molteno and Haddad, upon assessing the visual results in patients with neovascular glaucoma,[105] compared data from patients who received implants before 1982 (group 1) when they were reserved for advanced cases with data from patients who underwent surgery from 1982 to 1984 (group 2) when the implant was used earlier in the disease process. Seven of 24 eyes (29 percent) lost light perception in group 1. Only four of 24 (16 percent) lost all vision in group 2. Of the group 2 eyes, eight (33 percent) had vision of 6/60 or better; in group 1 only three (12 percent) had visual acuity of 6/60 or better. They believed that earlier intervention resulted in less ischemic retinal damage and a better visual prognosis. At our institution, 61 cases with an average follow-up of 17 mo and a minimum of at least 3 mo were reviewed by Stormogipson.[87] Thirty-seven patients (60 percent) maintained their vision; the remainder lost vision (defined as a loss of at least two lines). Only three patients (5 percent) lost all vision, and two of them had neovascular glaucoma. The other one had only light perception vision preoperatively. Of the 61 patients in this group, 27 had neovascular glaucoma. Melamed and associates reported a 22 percent decrease in vision after implant surgery.[58] Only eight of

41 eyes (19.5) in their study had neovascular glaucoma. There appears to be little serious visual morbidity resulting from implant surgery; however, caution must be exercised in choosing the correct patient. In our experience, the average postoperative pressure level in patients with functioning Molteno implants appears to be higher than in patients with functioning filtering blebs.

To date, no prospective, controlled, and randomized study comparing the effectiveness of the Molteno or other implant with conventional filtration surgery has been performed. In general, filtering implants are reserved for high-risk eyes. The decision to use implants or conventional surgery awaits the outcome of a clinical trial comparing these two methods. Until these data are available, the prudent course is dictated by the surgeon's personal experience with each technique. The surgeon who is unfamiliar with Molteno implants may have more success with conventional filtration procedures. On the other hand, cases may arise in which one may opt for a Molteno implant rather than conventional surgery. Generally, it is preferable to use the implant in eyes with secondary glaucoma, high preoperative pressures, and a relatively well-preserved disc and filtration surgery in patients with advanced cupping or relatively low preoperative pressures.

SURGICAL TECHNIQUE

The surgical technique varies according to the type of glaucoma implant chosen. Because of my experience with the Molteno implant and its current favored status, the discussion herein is limited to this device.

Table 146–4. RESULTS OF MOLTENO IMPLANT IN OTHER HIGH-RISK GROUPS

Glaucoma	Author	No. of Eyes	FU	Success (%)	Criteria	Type
Post PKP	McDonnell et al[92]	17	13m	71	<21	1 P
Post PKP	Beebe et al[91]	25	25m	96	<22	1 S 1 and 2 P
Downgrowth	Fish et al[102]	9	19m	78	<22	1 and 2 S 1 and 2 P

Two Plates or One Plate?

There are two types of Molteno designs: the first has a one-plate drainage reservoir, the second, a two-plate drainage reservoir (see Fig. 146–2). Molteno developed the latter to lower the elevated intraocular pressure that is sometimes associated with the one-plate implant.[70] Before the two-plate implant was available, a second one-plate implant was often used to lower pressure further in the belief that two plates provide greater surface area for aqueous dispersion and, therefore, lower pressure to a greater degree. The recent report by Hever and associates lends support to the greater pressure lowering afforded by the double-plate implant.[104a] The disadvantage of the two-plate implant is that it requires a wider dissection for installation. For infant eyes, an 8-mm–diameter double-plate implant is available.

Two Stage or One Stage?

The early implant operations performed by Molteno and others were complicated by hypotony and flat chambers because of the excess run-off seen before development of a fibrous capsule around the Molteno plate. In 1979, Molteno and associates reported on the two-stage implant procedure[81] in which the plates were placed in the equatorial region of the eye approximately 1 mo or more before the tube was implanted in the anterior chamber, thus allowing time for fibrous capsule formation. The capsule provided sufficient resistance to outflow to maintain the anterior chamber. Until recently, many surgeons preferred the two-stage approach to prevent the hypotony commonly seen with the one-stage insertion. Because intraocular pressure is often difficult to control during the 1-mo waiting period and to avoid a second operation, modifications of the one-stage procedure, consisting of several techniques of temporary tube occlusion, are in vogue. The Vicryl tie technique was reported by Molteno and associates in 1986.[106] A Vicryl suture usually dissolves in from 2 to 6 wk, thus opening the lumen of the silicone tube. However, the variable nature of the release of Vicryl is problematic. A Vicryl suture of 8–0 diameter or less can cut the tube; therefore, 5–0 or 6–0 Vicryl has been recommended. Others have suggested tying a polypropylene suture around the tube in the anterior chamber and releasing it later with a laser.[107] Hoare Nairne and associates, utilizing 3–0 polypropylene,[108] first reported the intraluminal suture occlusion technique in 1988. In 1989, Egbert and Lieberman reported on the same technique in which a suture is placed directly into the lumen of the tube in a retrograde fashion and passed out through the conjunctiva overlying the plates where it is secured in the fornix of the eye for later removal (Fig. 146–3).[109] In their study, the dissolving suture, 4–0 chromic collagen, and the permanent suture, 3–0 polypropylene, provided the best tube occlusion. The latter buries itself in the conjunctiva and is removed by cutting down on it if left for longer than 1 wk. However, the former

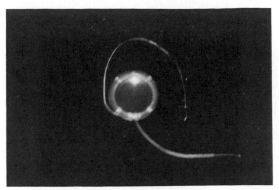

Figure 146–3. A single-plate Molteno implant with 4–0 collagen suture occluding the tube.

occasionally breaks, leaving material embedded in the tube lumen, if removed after 2 wk. Because of swelling, the chromic suture provided better occlusion. Since problems with suture breakage rarely were encountered between 7 and 14 days, the authors recommended that the chromic suture be used and retrieved before 14 days. Indeed, it is rare for a flat chamber to occur if the suture is removed after only 1 wk. However, some surgeons prefer to bury the polypropylene and other nondissolving suture because of the fear of intraocular infection. Either approach provides satisfactory results.

Other methods and sutures have successfully achieved temporary occlusion. Franks and Hitchings used perfluoropropane gas.[110] Rose and associates reported on a large series of patients in which a venting stab wound on the tube surface anterior to a ligature type occluding suture combined to help prevent early high pressure (sometimes requiring surgical release of the suture) and postoperative hypotony.[111] Beebe and associates used a host of various techniques for early suture occlusion, including 6–0 nylon occlusion and laser suture lysis and a slip knot approach with the same suture.[91] Latina reported a combination of internal and external occlusion techniques to introduce a graded release.[112] To the best of my knowledge, there have been no reports of endophthalmitis associated with these techniques. Ball and associates reported several cases of hypopyon associated with the internal occlusion technique using chromic suture; however, none was thought to be infectious.[113] We performed the internal occlusion technique with a chromic suture in children and infants and removed the suture with topical anesthesia in the clinic without complications. Suture occlusion techniques are a promising method of performing the Molteno implant in a single stage with minimal hypotony.

TECHNIQUE

The Molteno implant can be inserted under either general or local anesthesia. With the latter, supraorbital and retrobulbar blocks should be performed because of the excessive manipulation that is often required to pass the double-plate implants underneath the superior rectus muscle.

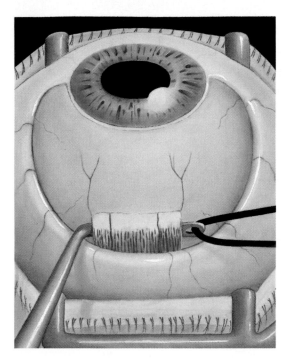

Figure 146–4. Initial stage of the implant operation showing a large peritomy with small relaxing incisions. A 2–0 silk suture is being passed under the superior rectus muscle. The quadrants have been opened far posteriorly by blunt dissection.

No special preoperative preparation is necessary; however, I try to control the pressure medically as well as possible. The pupil is not dilated, and preoperative antibiotics are used if desired. I proceed with the peritomy without using a bridle suture. A large fornix-based flap is dissected carefully from the limbus (Fig. 146–4). The peritomy must be carried out for a full 180 degrees for a double-plate insertion but can be smaller for a single plate. If a relaxing incision is required, it should be made radially or slightly inferiorly, directed away from the plates. Any conjunctival wound too near the rigid plates will heal poorly, setting the stage for a wound dehiscence. I also try to make only one relaxing incision on the side away from the site at which the tube will enter the anterior chamber. Tenon's layer is opened with blunt and sharp dissection. Blunt spreading is carried out posterior to the equator to clear room for the 13-mm plates that must be anchored at least 7 to 8 mm from the limbus. I then pass a 2–0 silk underneath the superior rectus muscle for retraction (see Fig. 146–4). Before inserting the plates, the quadrants are double-checked, and any remaining Tenon's attachments are freed. Check ligaments beneath the belly of the superior rectus muscle are bluntly removed with the muscle hook.

Before mounting the implant, the intraluminal suture should be placed if desired. I generally use a 4–0 chromic suture that is passed in a retrograde fashion from the inside of the plate through the anterior chamber tube (see Fig. 146–3). The needle is passed later on through the conjunctiva overlying the plate. Care should be taken to minimize crimping, which may cause suture weakness and possible breakage.

The conjunctiva should slide freely back to near the rectus muscle insertion. If it does not, a relaxing incision 3 to 5 mm long should be made radially from the limbus at the side of the wound farthest from the anterior chamber tube. The implant can now be passed beneath the superior rectus muscle. Some surgeons prefer to place the implant over the muscle tendon. Technically, this is somewhat easier but can lead to plate migration if they are not sutured securely (Fig. 146–5).

The superior rectus muscle is lifted with two muscle hooks (see Fig. 146–5). A curved mosquito clamp is passed beneath the muscle belly, and the plate is grasped and pulled from the nasal to the temporal quadrant. Care is taken to minimize trauma to Tenon's tissue and the muscle capsule. The implant is then positioned so that the anterior edge of each plate is located at least 8 mm posterior to the limbus. The superior rectus muscle tendon insertion is used as a natural ruler delimiting the anteriormost location. The plates are rotated and positioned to eliminate kinks of sharp bends in the tubing. A 5–0 Dacron suture with a spatula needle is used to anchor the plates firmly to the episclera, generally one suture per plate. Occasionally, two are required to prevent rotation; two should be used if the connecting tube is placed on top of the superior muscle tendon. Slip knots can be tied initially to ensure correct tube and plate alignment. The plate should be rotated so that the tube crosses the limbus at a right angle.

If a two-stage operation is performed, the tube is hidden beneath the plate or the rectus muscle and is sutured to the episclera. Some surgeons then perform a trabeculectomy for temporary pressure control. The conjunctiva is replaced, and the relaxing incision is secured.

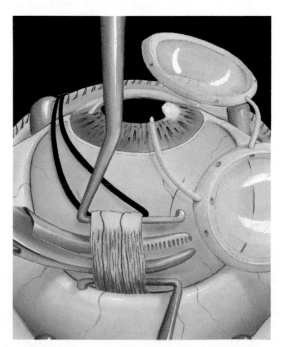

Figure 146–5. Passing the Molteno implant beneath the superior rectus muscle.

We prefer a one-stage suture occlusion technique, which has little risk of hypotony and flat chamber early postoperatively. Once the plate has been positioned, attention is directed to the tube, which must be covered with sclera to prevent possible exposure. Either a tunnel can be fashioned or exogenous sclera can be used. Freedman reported the use of glycerin-preserved sclera in 1987.[114] We have used alcohol-preserved sclera since then. The use of exogenous sclera has simplified the procedure; however, donor tissue is required. In my experience, tube erosion can occur through the thickest tunnels and flaps, but no tube erosion has occurred through donor sclera. This tissue is not rejected. The location chosen for donor sclera must be considered carefully, because there are several areas of natural thinning on the eye. I cut a 5 × 6-mm piece of sclera before surgery and soak it in sterile saline.

A tunnel or flap can also be used. Molteno and associates advocated using a Z-flap in their study of juvenile glaucoma.[83] I prefer a tunneling technique. First, a rectangular 4-mm flap is raised and brought within 1 to 2 mm of the limbus. Clear cornea should not be exposed because this causes a weak seal around the tube entry site, resulting in leakage and hypotony in the immediate postoperative period. A longer cuff of limbal tissue holds the tube more firmly and minimizes leakage. A No. 57 Beaver blade or other rounded or blunt blade is used to dissect the tissue posterior toward the implant in a lamellar plane of sclera. A vertical incision 1 to 2 mm from the plate-tube junction exposes the tunnel. The tube is pulled through the tunnel toward the limbus with a curved blunt forceps. A 5–0 Dacron suture should secure the tube just posterior to its entry into the tunnel. By so doing, upward pressure against the sclera, which may result in the tube erosion and exposure, is minimized. Care must be taken not to obstruct the tube with this permanent suture. If external tube occlusion is used, a 5– or 6–0 Vicryl suture can be placed around the distal tube near the junction with the plate to ligate the tube temporarily. This should be performed before placing the tube in the anterior chamber.

A 23-gauge needle (with or without Healon) is passed into the anterior chamber and oriented in the same direction as the tube crossing the limbus (Fig. 146–6). This is a critical part of the procedure. The needle track should be at a right angle to the limbus and parallel to the iris. Ideally, the needle should engage the sclera about 1 mm posterior to the limbus and should penetrate the angle tissues just posterior to Schwalbe's line. This ensures against permanent contact with the iris and cornea, which may block the tube either directly or by causing endothelialization of the tube orifice. This is especially common in patients with neovascular glaucoma. I generally place the tube without using viscoelastics. If a patient is suspected of being at risk for choroidal detachment, Alvarado has suggested pressurizing the anterior chamber by using a separate infusion cannula.[115] In patients with obliteration of the anterior chamber, the tube can be placed into the posterior chamber through the pars plana, but only in eyes that

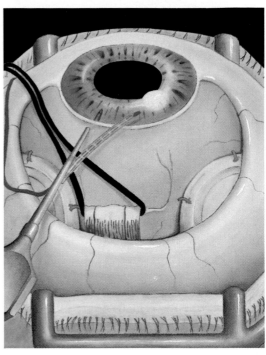

Figure 146–6. With the implant positioned and sutured in place, the 23-gauge needle is passed into the anterior chamber parallel to the surface of the iris. The needle should pierce the sclera about 1 mm posterior to the limbus and enter the anterior chamber just posterior to Schwalbe's line.

have undergone vitrectomy. The tube should be left long enough so that the tip can be observed at the slit lamp through the dilated pupil.

The tube must be covered by either an exogenous graft or closure of the lamellar dissection. An 8–0 Vicryl suture is used on the donor tissue. The scleral graft is trimmed and beveled to minimize sharp edges that could cause conjunctival breakdown or scleral exposure at the limbus. There is no need to sew the material tightly to the eye because the 23-gauge needle leaves a very tight tract. An 8–0 Vicryl or a 10–0 nylon suture can close the lamellar flap if this technique is used.

In the internal occlusion technique, the 4–0 chromic suture is pulled through the conjunctiva as high in the fornix as possible (Fig. 146–7). A 6- to 8-cm segment is left attached to suture the free end superficially to the conjunctiva in the inferior fornix. If polypropylene is used, it is pulled beneath the conjunctiva in the inferior quadrant, where it is cut flush with the surface and remains buried. The conjunctiva is repositioned over the limbus and secured with an absorbable suture. I inject only an antibiotic. Steroids are rarely necessary and can inhibit early capsule formation, resulting in early hypotony.

POSTOPERATIVE MANAGEMENT

Postoperative management of implant surgery is controversial. The three components of greatest concern are the conjunctival wound, hypotony, and bleb perme-

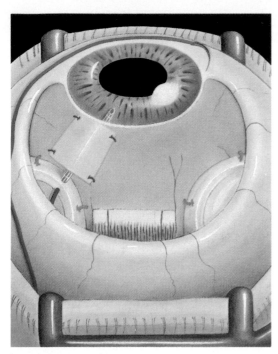

Figure 146–7. The implant is correctly positioned, and the tube is occluded by the 4–0 collagen suture. The tube is cut bevel up to extend 2 to 3 mm into the anterior chamber. The scleral patch is sewn into place overlying the tube. The collagen suture is passed high in the fornix, exiting between the plates and tied loosely to the conjunctiva in the inferior fornix.

ability, the last being the most important long-term pressure control; however, it is the factor about which the least is known. Much controversy exists regarding the benefit of fibrosis-suppressing medications.

Fibrosis Suppression

In 1976, Molteno and associates reported on 64 patients who were treated with a postoperative regimen that included systemic steroids, colchicine, and flufenamic acid and topical dexamethasone, epinephrine, and atropine.[116] After a minimum follow-up period of 18 mo, 58 of the patients were controlled. The authors believed that the patients achieved more favorable results than did those in previous studies, and this regimen was advocated for several years. Molteno and coworkers reported on several series of patients with various glaucomas who used the antifibrosis regimen until 1986.[52, 80–83] More recently, surgeons have abandoned the unprotected, single-stage procedure because of the excessive and sometimes devastating complications due to hypotony. In 1983, Brown and Cairns,[86] in their study of 30 patients, used the antifibrosis regimen in half of the patients. Even though the statistical power of this study is limited, they concluded that the benefits of the regimen were questionable. Other authors found that a high proportion of their patients developed serious adverse systemic effects.[103] In 1986, Molteno and associates reported on 20 eyes in which a Vicryl ligature occlusion

technique was used.[106] Only one patient in this series received systemic inflammatory suppression. The early success rate in these patients was comparable with their previous studies: 80 percent were controlled without medication, and the remainder were controlled with medication. They concluded that the bleb appearance dictated using an antifibrosis regimen such as this.

Clinical experience with the two-stage procedure showed that a very dense fibrous capsule forms in a few weeks around the entire implant. With suture occlusion techniques, it is unusual to encounter flat chambers even when the suture is removed 2 to 5 days postoperatively, suggesting that some capsule provides resistance soon after completion of the first stage of the procedure. The effect of fibrosis suppression on the ultimate permeability of the connective tissue overlying the implant is unclear.

The two-stage approach was designed to allow capsule formation that provides resistance to outflow. Excessive early fibrosis suppression could result in the very hypotony complications that one is trying to avoid. While some advocate the use of 5-fluorouracil for routine postoperative management, others rarely utilize it. The role of 5-fluorouracil in implant surgery currently is undefined.

POSTOPERATIVE HYPOTONY

Hypotony, which can lead to more serious problems such as suprachoroidal hemorrhages, flat chambers, and corneal decompensation or other complications, is among the most important postoperative considerations. Leakage or breakdown of the conjunctival wound can expose the implant and result in severe hypotony. Despite carefully occluding the tube and providing a watertight seal, hypotony may result from leakage either through or around the tube. Hypotony complications due to overfiltration generally are managed conservatively. If anterior chamber re-formation is required for cornea-lens touch, an attempt to obstruct or tie the tube should probably be made, and the suprachoroidal space should be drained. Conservative measures generally include cessation of steroids, intense cycloplegia, and, occasionally, vitreous dehydration.

Although rare, wound leakage can complicate the early postoperative period. Using a 23-gauge needle to enter the anterior chamber usually precludes leakage around the entry site; however, it can occur, especially if a scleral flap is raised and dissected too far anteriorly into clear cornea. Attention to the conjunctival closure usually prevents leakage from becoming problematic. Occasionally, a leak may occur due to a conjunctival tear or buttonhole near the plates, which is a serious complication that may require removing or repositioning the plate. Too much tension is exerted on the tissue for direct closure to be performed. Despite the use of 8–0 silk sutures and conjunctival mobilization, wound breakdown persisted. In most cases, the postoperative management is straightforward and simple. Because most of the procedure is extraocular, there is usually little postoperative inflammation and only a small risk of infection. Topical steroids and cycloplegia are used minimally. Antibiotics are prescribed more frequently if the suture from the anterior chamber is left exposed in the fornix. In these cases, a combination of steroid ointment and antibiotics at bedtime and an aminoglycoside eyedrop three to four times during the day is administered. The suture is generally removed between 7 and 10 days postoperatively so as not to severely inhibit encapsulization of the implant. The conjunctival wound should also be secure by the time when the tube is opened.

INTRAOCULAR PRESSURE

After the opening of the anterior chamber tube shunt, hypotony is the rule, followed by a period in which the pressure returns to near preoperative levels. The blebs look large and distended and similar in appearance to what has been called an encapsulated bleb. Occasionally, they appear inflamed. This hypertensive phase, although not invariable, generally occurs 1 to 2 mo following insertion or opening of the tube and lasts from 1 to 4 mo. This phase seems to occur earlier with internal suture occlusion than with two-stage techniques. Aqueous suppression, epinephrine, and sometimes miotics are used to treat elevated pressure. Molteno maintains that vigorous steroid treatment alone lowers the pressure, but this does not seem to be so. Digital pressure occasionally enhances bleb expansion if it is successful in lowering the pressure in the office. If the blebs appear flat while the pressure is elevated, the tube is presumed to be blocked. If some uncertainty remains regarding tube blockage, the bleb space can be tapped with a fine needle. Once final stability is achieved, the pressure tends to decrease slightly over time. When possible, hypotensive medicines are carefully withdrawn.

COMPLICATIONS

Numerous complications may potentially arise during the intraoperative and postoperative implant periods (Table 146–5).

As we gain more experience with this procedure, the complication rate has decreased. Melamed and associates reported no intraoperative complications with 41 patients.[58] Postoperatively, prolonged hypotony occurred in six (15 percent) patients, despite tube occlusion with a 5–0 Vicryl tie. Because they used a 21-gauge needle to introduce the tube into the anterior chamber, leakage occurred around the tube, resulting in early postoperative hypotony. Four (10 percent) patients (all with neovascular glaucoma) had postoperative hyphema that resolved spontaneously. Malignant glaucoma occurred in two (5 percent) patients and was treated successfully by laser. This complication may also have resulted from shallowing anterior chambers. Sixteen patients (nearly 40 percent) had a peripheral choroidal effusion. One eye suffered a retinal detachment after a

Table 146–5. COMPLICATIONS IN IMPLANT SURGERY

Intraoperative	Conjunctival laceration
	Muscle disinsertion or laceration
	Suprachoroidal hemorrhage
	Cataract
	Cornea edema/scar
	Ocular penetration
	Hyphema
	Vitreous loss
	Choroidal effusion
	Iris damage
Early postoperative	Endophthalmitis
	Pupillary block
	Malignant glaucoma
	Inflammation
	Hyphema
	Severe glaucoma
	Tube obstruction
	Intraluminal suture breakage
	Hypotony
	Suprachoroidal hemorrhage
	Wound leak
	Tube retraction
	Plate shift
	Hypopyon
	Corneal edema
	Graft failure
	Retinal detachment
Late postoperative	Large bleb formation
	Hypotropia, strabismus
	Glaucoma
	Wound leak
	Tube or plate extrusion
	Infection/orbital cellulitis
	Tube blockage
	Cataract formation
	Fibrous ingrowth
	Proptosis
	Phthisis bulbi
	Band keratopathy[117]

choroidal hemorrhage, and two eyes (5 percent) developed vitreous hemorrhage. Many of these problems could have been avoided by using the 23–gauge needle track and Vicryl tie or internal suture occlusion to prevent hypotony. The large number of surgical revisions required earlier in our experience for malfunction or exposure (25 percent in our series) seem to be the exception rather than the rule at this time.[87]

Most complications can be managed routinely, but a discussion of intraluminal suture breakage and poor bleb function is worthwhile, because these problems may require unique surgical intervention.

In suture occlusion techniques, occasionally a suture may break while still occluding the tube. Generally, the break occurs at the junction of the tube, and the plate and the suture inside the tube remain undissolved. By cutting longitudinally into the tube, the surgeon can remove the suture by using either a Sinskey hook or a jeweler's forceps. The tube should then be irrigated with a fine cannula in both directions to ensure patency.

It is unusual to encounter excessive bleb resistance that requires repeat surgical intervention. Time, medication, and digital pressure should be allowed to work. If pressure reduction is not seen by 6 mo it is unlikely to occur. However, one must be certain that the tube is not occluded. If there is any doubt, the blebs can be tapped. It is unlikely that any blockage is present if the blebs are large.

Many procedures have been proposed to treat this condition; however, they almost always fail to achieve adequate pressure decreases. Some surgeons have had limited success with bleb needling procedures; the success is usually short-lived, and the needling must be repeated. I recommend partial or complete removal of the capsule. The dissection is carried out from the limbus posteriorly to the implant. The conjunctiva slides easily over the bleb wall and provides for an easy dissection. Traction is provided inferiorly either by a superior rectus or by a corneal traction suture. The tube is tied with a temporary suture of either chromic or Vicryl. Blunt dissection is carried out over the blebs and posteriorly as far as possible. The bleb walls are grasped with a toothed forceps and excised with sharp dissection. Care is taken not to buttonhole the conjunctiva and also to remove as much of the capsule as possible. The tube is tied loosely with a 6–0 Vicryl suture so that minimal leakage occurs. The conjunctiva is pulled back into place and is sutured at the limbus. Postoperative injections of 5–fluorouracil are recommended, and in some cases systemic steroids can be tried. Ocular inflammation is usually minimal, but any seen over the plates should be treated vigorously.

SUMMARY

Implant surgery has found an important niche in the management of difficult glaucomas. As our experience with this surgery has grown, we can now avoid many of the early complications such as hypotony, tube blockage, and extrusion. The implant devices seem to be well tolerated ocularly, and final pressure levels appear to remain stable for long periods of time. The implant efficacy compared with conventional filtration surgery with or without fibroblast suppression remains to be known. Because the implants rarely can provide the low pressures needed in the presence of severe disc damage, they may best be utilized in secondary glaucomas in which the pressures are high and the disc relatively well preserved and in patients in whom conventional filtration surgery is likely to fail.

REFERENCES

1. Stedman's Medical Dictionary, 25th ed. Baltimore, Williams & Wilkins, 1989, p 1410.
2. Zorab A: The reduction of tension in chronic glaucoma. The Ophthalmoscope 10:258, 1912.
3. Mayou MS: An operation in glaucoma. The Ophthalmoscope 10:254, 1912.
4. Rollet M, Moreau M: Traitement de hypopyon par le drainage capillaire de la cambre antérieure. Rev Gen D'Ophthalmol 25:481, 1906.
5. Wood CA: The sclerocorneal seton in the treatment of glaucoma. Ophthal Rec p 235, April 1915.
6. Wolfe OR, Blaess MJ: Seton operation in glaucoma. Am J Ophthalmol 19:400, 1936.
7. Vail DT: Retained silk-thread of "seton" drainage from the vitreous chamber to Tenon's lymph channel for relief of glaucoma. Ophthal Rec p 184, April 1915.
8. Stefansson J: An operation for glaucoma. Am J Ophthalmol 8:681, 1925.
9. Weekers L: Le drainage permanent du vitre dans le glaucome. Arch d'Ophthalmol 39:279, 1922.
10. Row H: Operation to control glaucoma. Arch Ophthalmol 12:325, 1934.
11. Muldoon WE, Ripple PH, Wilder HC: Platinum implant in glaucoma surgery. Arch Ophthalmol 45:666, 1951.
12. Chiazzaro D: Sur la resorption du magnesium metal dans l'oeil humain: Note préliminaire sur son application dans le glaucome chronique. Ann d'Ocul 167:809, 1936.
13. Troncoso MU: Cyclodialysis with insertion of a metal implant in the treatment of glaucoma. Arch Ophthalmol 23:270, 1940.
14. Bick MW: Use of tantalum for ocular drainage. Arch Ophthalmol 42:373, 1949.
15. Troncoso MU: Use of tantalum implants for inducing a permanent hypotony in rabbits' eyes. Am J Ophthalmol 32:499, 1949.
16. Lehman RN, McCaslin MF: Gelatin film used as a seton in glaucoma. Am J Ophthalmol 47:690, 1959.
17. Antoszyk A, Robinson D, Proia AD, et al: Gelatin implants in glaucoma filtering surgery. Am J Ophthalmol 101:618, 1986.
18. Richards RD, Van Bijsterveld OP: Artificial drainage tubes for glaucoma. Am J Ophthalmol 60:405, 1965.
19. MacDonald RK, Pierce MBE: Silicone setons. Am J Ophthalmol 59:635, 1965.
20. Duke-Elder S: System of Ophthalmology, vol. XI. St. Louis, CV Mosby, 1969, pp 528–533.
21. Pinnas G, Boniuk M: Cyclodialysis with Teflon tube implants. Am J Ophthalmol 68:879, 1969.
22. Makusch H: Ein Vorschlag fur eine neue Glaukomoperation. Ztschr f Augenh 67:313, 1939.
23. Suker GF: The filtration operation of Makusch for chronic glaucoma with preliminary report on twenty-four operations. Am J Ophthalmol 14:732, 1931.
24. Sondermann R: Eine neue Glaukomoperation. Klin Monatsbl Augenheilkd 93:227, 1934.
25. Lee PF, Schepens CL: Aqueous-venous shunt and intraocular pressure: Preliminary report of animal studies. Invest Ophthalmol 5:59, 1966.
26. Strampelli B, Valvo A: Phlebo-goniostomy: A new surgical procedure. Am J Ophthalmol 64:371, 1967.
27. Lee P, Wong W: Aqueous-venous shunt for glaucoma. Ann Ophthalmol 6:1083, 1974.
28. Blumenthal M, Harris SL, Galin MA: Experimental study of cartilage setons. Br J Ophthalmol 54:62, 1979.
29. Gibson G: Transscleral lacrimal-caniculus transplants. Am J Ophthalmol 27:258, 1944.
30. Nhan NT: Subscleral sclerencleisis (technique and results). Paper read at 92nd Annual Congress of the Ophthalmological Society of Japan.
31. Stewart RH, Kimbrough RL, Bach H, et al: Trabeculectomy and modifications of trabeculectomy. Ophthalmic Surg 10:76, 1979.
32. Beauchamp G, Park M: Filtering surgery in children. Trans Am Acad Ophthalmol Otolaryngol 86:170, 1979.
33. Gressel M, Heuer D, Parrish R: Trabeculectomy in young patients. Ophthalmology 91:1242, 1984.
34. Herschler J: The effect of total vitrectomy in aphakic eyes. Ophthalmology 88:229, 1981.
35. Heuer D, Gressel N, Parrish R II, et al: Trabeculectomy in aphakic eyes. Ophthalmology 91:1045, 1984.
36. Bellow A, Johnstone M: Surgical management of glaucoma in aphakia. Ophthalmology 90:807, 1983.
37. Gross RL, Feldman RM, Spaeth GL, et al: Surgical therapy of chronic glaucoma in aphakia and pseudophakia. Ophthalmology 95:1195, 1988.
38. Herschler J, Agness J: A modified filtering operation for neovascular glaucoma. Arch Ophthalmol 97:2329, 1979.
39. Parrish R, Herschler J: Eyes with end stage neovascular glaucoma: Natural history following successful modified filtering operation. Arch Ophthalmol 101:745, 1983.
40. Hoskins D Jr, Hetherington J Jr, Shaffer R: Surgical management of the inflammatory glaucoma. Perspect Ophthalmol 1:173, 1977.

41. Kitizawa Y, Taniguchi T, Nakano Y, et al: 5-Fluorouracil for trabeculectomy in glaucoma. Graefes Arch Clin Exp Ophthalmol 225:403, 1987.

42. Freedman J, Stern E, Ahrems M: Trabeculectomy in a Black American glaucoma population. Br J Ophthalmol 67:573, 1976.

43. Berson D, Zankerman H, Landau L, et al: Filtering operation in Africans. Am J Ophthalmol 67:395, 1969.

44. Ferguson T, MacDonald R Jr: Trabeculectomy in Blacks: A 2 year follow-up. Ophthalmic Surg 8:41, 1977.

45. Welsh N: Failure of filtration surgery in the African. Br J Ophthalmol 54:594, 1970.

46. Miller R, Barker J: Trabeculectomy in Black patients. Ophthalmic Surg 12:46, 1981.

47. Weinreb R: Adjusting the dose of 5-fluorouracil after filtration surgery to minimize side effects. Ophthalmology 94:564, 1987.

48. Ruderman J, Welch D, Smith M, et al: A randomized study of 5 fluorouracil and filtration surgery. Am J Ophthalmol 104:218, 1987.

49. The Fluorouracil Filtering Surgery Study Group: Fluorouracil filtering surgery study one-year follow-up. Am J Ophthalmol 108:625, 1989.

50. Qadeer SA: Acrylic gonio-subconjunctival plates in glaucoma surgery. Br J Ophthalmol 38:353, 1954.

51. Molteno ACB: New implant for drainage in glaucoma. Br J Ophthalmol 53:606, 1969.

52. Molteno ACB, Straughan JL, Ancker A: Long tube implants in the management of glaucoma. South African Med J 50:1062, 1976.

53. Krupin T, Podos SM, Becker B, et al: Valve implants in filtering surgery. Am J Ophthalmol 81:232, 1976.

54. Ormerod LD, Pickford M, Baerveldt G: Biodegradability of the Krupin-Denver valve. Am J Ophthalmol 105:559, 1988.

55. Schocket SS, Lakhanpal V, Richards RD: Anterior chamber tube shunt to an encircling band in the treatment of neovascular glaucoma. Ophthalmology 89:188–194, 1982.

56. Krupin T, Ritch R, Camras C, et al: A long Krupin-Denver valve implant attached to a 180 degree scleral explant for glaucoma surgery. Ophthalmology 95:1174, 1988.

57. Schocket SS: Investigations of the reasons for success and failure in the anterior shunt-to-the-encircling-band procedure in the treatment of refractory glaucoma. Trans Am Ophthalmol Soc 84:743, 1986.

58. Melamed S, Cahane M, Gutman I, Blumenthal M: Postoperative complications after Molteno implant surgery. Am J Ophthalmol 111:319, 1991.

59. Hitchings RA, Joseph NH, Sherwood MB, et al: Use of one-piece valved tube and variable surface area explant for glaucoma drainage surgery. Ophthalmology 94:1079, 1987.

60. Joseph NH, Sherwood MB, Trantas RA, et al: A one-piece drainage system for glaucoma surgery. Trans Ophthalmologic Soc UK 105:657, 1986.

61. Lieberman MF, Ewing RH: Drainage implant surgery for refractory glaucoma. Int Ophthalmol Clin 30:198, 1990.

62. Cameron JD, White TC: Clinico-histopathologic correlation of a successful glaucoma pump-shunt implant. Ophthalmology 95:1189, 1988.

63. Melamed S, Fiore PM: Molteno implant surgery in refractory glaucoma. Surv Ophthalmol 34:441, 1990.

64. Rubin B, Chan C, Burnier M, et al: Histopathologic study of the Molteno glaucoma implant in three patients. Am J Ophthalmol 110:371, 1990.

65. Loeffler KU, Jay JL: Tissue response to aqueous drainage in a functioning Molteno implant. Br J Ophthalmol 72:29, 1988.

66. Baier RE, Meyer AE, Natiella Jr, et al: Surface properties determine bioadhesive outcomes: Methods and results. J Biomed Mater Res 18:337, 1984.

67. Kornbleuth N, Tennenbaum E: The inhibitory effect of aqueous humor in the growth of cells in tissue cultures. Am J Ophthalmol 42:70, 1956.

68. Epstein E: Fibrosing response to aqueous. Br J Ophthalmol 43:641, 1959.

69. Radius R, Herschler J, Claflin A, et al: Aqueous humor changes after experimental filtering surgery. Am J Ophthalmol 89:250, 1980.

70. Molteno ACB: The optimal design of drainage implants for glaucoma. Trans Ophthalmological Soc N Z 33:39, 1981.

71. Minckler D, Shammas A, Wilcox M, et al: Experimental studies of aqueous filtration using the Molteno implant. Trans Am Ophthalmol Soc 85:368, 1987.

72. Peiffer RL, Popovich KS, Nichols DA: Long-term comparative study of the Schocket and Joseph glaucoma tube shunts in monkeys. Ophthalmic Surg 21:55, 1990.

73. Feibel RM, Bigger JF: Rubeosis irides and neovascular glaucoma: Evaluation of cyclocryotherapy. Am J Ophthalmol 74:862, 1972.

74. Shields MB: Cyclodestructive surgery for glaucoma: Past, present and future. Trans Am Ophthalmol Soc 83:285, 1985.

75. Krupin T, Mitchell KB, Becker B: Cyclocryotherapy in neovascular glaucoma. Am J Ophthalmol 86:24, 1978.

76. Bellows AR, Grant WM: Cyclocryotherapy in advanced inadequately controlled glaucoma. Am J Ophthalmol 75:679, 1973.

77. Schuman JS, Puliafito CA: Laser cyclophotocoagulation. Int Ophthalmol Clin 30:111, 1990.

78. Molteno ACB: Uveitis with glaucoma treated by implants. South African Arch Ophthalmol 1:125, 1973.

79. Krupin T, Podos SM, Becker B, et al: Valve implants in filtering surgery. Am J Ophthalmol 81:232, 1976.

80. Molteno ACB, Van Rooyen MB, Bartholomew RS: Implants for draining neovascular glaucoma. Br J Ophthalmol 61:120, 1977.

81. Molteno ACB, Van Biljon G, Ancker E: Two-stage insertion of glaucoma drainage implants. Trans Ophthalmological Soc N Z 31:17, 1979.

82. Ancker E, Molteno ACB: Molteno drainage implant for neovascular glaucoma. Trans Ophthalmological Soc UK 102:122, 1982.

83. Molteno ACB, Ancker E, Van Biljon G: Surgical technique for advanced juvenile glaucoma. Arch Ophthalmol 102:51, 1984.

84. Freedman J: The use of the single stage Molteno long tube seton in treating resistant cases of glaucoma. Ophthalmic Surg 16:480, 1984.

85. Bartholomew RS: Glaucoma implants. Trans Ophthalmological Soc UK 98:482, 1978.

86. Brown RD, Cairns JE: Experience with the Molteno long tube implant. Trans Ophthalmological Soc UK 103:297, 1983.

87. Stormogipson J: The Molteno implant: Our results. Presentation at Stanford University Department of Ophthalmology Residents Day, May 1990.

88. Ward WJ, Cooper RL: Molteno tube implants: Long-term results. Aust N Z J Ophthalmol 15:109, 1987.

89. Goldberg I: Management of uncontrolled glaucoma with the Molteno system. Aust N Z J Ophthalmol 15:97, 1987.

90. Hitchings RA, Lattimer J: How to manage the unresponsive patient. Eye 1:55, 1987.

91. Beebe WE, Starita RJ, Fellman RL, et al: The use of Molteno implant and anterior chamber tube shunt to encircling band for the treatment of glaucoma in keratoplasty patients. Ophthalmology 97:1414, 1990.

92. McDonnell PJ, Robin JB, Schanzlin DJ, et al: Molteno implant for control of glaucoma in eyes after penetrating keratoplasty. Ophthalmology 95:364, 1988.

93. Billson F, Thomas R, Aylward W: The use of two-stage Molteno implants in developmental glaucoma. J Pediatr Ophthalmol Strabismus 26:3, 1989.

94. Sutton GE, Popp JC, Records RE: Krupin-Denver valve and neovascular glaucoma. Trans Ophthalmological Soc UK 102:119, 1982.

95. Stewart RH, Kimbrough RL, Okereke PC: Trabeculectomy with implantation of the Mendez glaucoma seton: early results. Ophthalmic Surg 17:221, 1986.

96. Schocket SS, Nirankari VS, Lakhanpal V, et al: Anterior chamber tube shunt to an encircling band in the treatment of neovascular glaucoma and other refractory glaucomas. Ophthalmology 92:553, 1985.

97. Krupin T, Kaufman P, Mandell AI, et al: Long term results of valve implants in filtering surgery for eyes with neovascular glaucoma. Am J Ophthalmol 95:775, 1983.

98. Krupin T, Kaufman P, Mandell AI, et al: Filtering valve implant surgery for eyes with neovascular glaucoma. Am J Ophthalmol 89:338, 1980.

99. Kuljaca Z, Ljubovjevic V, Momirov D: Draining implant for neovascular glaucoma. Am J Ophthalmol 6:372, 1983.

100. Folberg RT, Hargett NA, Weaver JE, et al: Filtering valve implant for neovascular glaucoma in proliferative diabetic retinopathy. Ophthalmology 89:286, 1982.

101. Davidovski F, Stewart RH, Kimbrough RL: Long-term results with the White glaucoma pump-shunt. Ophthalmic Surg 21:288, 1990.

102. Fish LA, Heuer DK, Baerveldt G, et al: Molteno implantation for secondary glaucomas associated with advanced epithelial ingrowth. Ophthalmology 97:557, 1990.

103. Downes RN, Flanagan DW, Jordan K, et al: The Molteno implant in intractable glaucoma. Eye 2:250, 1988.

104. Billson F, Thomas R, Aylward W: The use of two-stage Molteno implants in developmental glaucoma. J Pediatr Ophthalmol Strabismus 26:3, 1989.

104a. Hever DK, Lloyd M, Abrams DA, et al: A randomized clinical trial of single-plate versus double-plate Molteno implantation for glaucomas in aphakia and pseudophakia. Ophthalmology 99:1512, 1992.

105. Molteno ACB, Haddad PJ: The visual outcome in cases of neovascular glaucoma. Aust N Z J Ophthalmol 13:329, 1985.

106. Molteno ACB, Polkinghorne PJ, Bowbyes JA: The Vicryl tie technique for inserting a draining implant in the treatment of secondary glaucoma. Aust N Z J Ophthalmol 14:343, 1986.

107. Price FW, Whitson WE: Polypropylene ligatures as a means of controlling intraocular pressure with Molteno implants. Ophthalmic Surg 20:781, 1989.

108. Hoare Nairne JEA, Sherwood D, Jacob JSH, et al: Single stage insertion of the Molteno tube for glaucoma and modifications to reduce postoperative hypotony. Br J Ophthalmol 72:846, 1988.

109. Egbert PR, Lieberman MF: Internal suture occlusion of the Molteno glaucoma implant for the prevention of postoperative hypotony. Ophthalmic Surg 20:53, 1989.

110. Franks WA, Hitchings RA: Injection of perfluoropropane gas to prevent hypotony in eyes undergoing tube implant surgery. Ophthalmology 97:899, 1990.

111. Rose GE, Lavin MJ, Hitchings RA: Silicone tubes in glaucoma surgery: The effect of technical modifications on early postoperative intraocular pressures and complications. Eye 3:553, 1989.

112. Latina MA: Single stage Molteno implant with combination internal occlusion and external ligature. Ophthalmic Surg 21:444, 1990.

113. Ball SF, Loftfield K, Scharfenberg J: Molteno rip-cord suture hypopyon. Ophthalmic Surg 21:407, 1990.

114. Freedman J: Scleral patch grafts with Molteno setons. Ophthalmic Surg 18:532, 1987.

115. Alvarado J: Personal communication, 1989.

116. Molteno ACB, Straughan JL, Ancker A: Control of bleb fibrosis after glaucoma surgery by anti-inflammatory agents. South African Med J 50:881, 1976.

117. McClellan KA, Billson FA: Late development of localized band keratopathy in relation to a Molteno tube. Cornea 8:227, 1989.

Chapter 147

▪

Cycloablation*

JOEL S. SCHUMAN

Cyclodestructive procedures lower intraocular pressure (IOP) by decreasing aqueous production. Filtration procedures, in contrast, increase aqueous outflow, which generally is abnormally low in patients with glaucoma. Because filtration surgery treats the underlying problem in glaucoma whereas cycloablation attacks the outcome and because ciliodestructive surgery tends to have more complications than filtering surgery, cycloablation is rarely the primary surgical procedure of choice for glaucoma. Cyclodestruction is frequently reserved for patients with glaucoma refractory to medical or other surgical therapies. Several methods have been used to ablate the ciliary processes.

DIATHERMY TO CYCLOCRYOTHERAPY AND BEYOND

Diathermy was introduced by Weve in 1933,[1] and penetrating diathermy by Vogt in 1936[2] and Stocker in 1945.[3] The technique was gradually abandoned after a report by Walton and Grant in 1970 revealed low success rates and significant hypotony with diathermy,[4] although some investigators have reported success in controlling IOP using nonpenetrating diathermy.[5] Beta irradiation has been reported by Haik and colleagues to cause ciliary body destruction but is cataractogenic.[6] Berens and associates described cycloelectrolysis in 1949,[7] but the technique offered no significant advantage over diathermy and did not gain favor.[8] Bietti first proposed the use of freezing to destroy the ciliary body in 1950.[9] In 1964, Polack and de Roetth[10] and McLean and Lincoff[11] published the first reports of cyclocryotherapy (CCT) in rabbits and in humans. De Roetth later produced data documenting the long-term effectiveness of this treatment modality in lowering IOP.[12, 13]

CCT was generally believed to be less destructive and more predictable than penetrating diathermy, and it slowly replaced the older procedure.[14] Bellows and Grant found the procedure useful in advanced, inadequately controlled glaucoma, especially in aphakic eyes.[15, 16] CCT has been shown to have limited success in treating neovascular glaucoma, although reports in the literature regarding IOP reduction are not consistent.[17, 18] Rates of phthisis vary and may range from 0 to 12 percent or more, with rates of visual loss from none to 67 percent.[15–22] Nissen and colleagues reported on the use of xenon arc panretinal photocoagulation in combination with CCT, describing favorable

---

*Portions of this chapter originally appeared in Schuman JS, Puliafito CA: Laser photocoagulation. Int Ophthalmol Clin 30:111, 1990. Reprinted with permission.

results and no phthisis after 2.5 years, although the investigators did not compare this technique with CCT alone.[23]

Purnell and associates reported in 1964 that ultrasound causes focal ciliary body destruction[24]; Coleman and others found significant pressure lowering with this technique and postulate that ultrasound causes ciliary body destruction, thinning of scleral collagen, and separation of the ciliary body from the sclera.[25-27] These findings have been corroborated by several researchers clinically[28] and in animal models.[29-31] Freyler and Scheimbauer found that partial cyclectomy may control end-stage glaucoma in some cases, with a phthisis rate of 10 to 15 percent.[111]

CYCLOPHOTODESTRUCTION

In 1971, Lee and Pomerantzeff introduced transpupillary cyclophotocoagulation.[32] Shields has only very limited success with this procedure, likely because of the restricted amount of ciliary process that can be seen through the pupil.[14] Shields described better experience with argon laser endocyclophotocoagulation.[14, 33]

Transscleral xenon arc cyclophotocoagulation was proposed by Weekers and coworkers in 1961.[34] Investigation into the destruction of the ciliary processes by light continued despite the fact that no clear advantage to this treatment modality could be demonstrated, and in 1972 Beckman and coauthors described transscleral cyclodestruction with the ruby laser.[35] In 1973, Beckman and others reported on the use of the neodymium laser for this same purpose.[36] Beckman and Waeltermann's 10-year study of 241 patients treated with ruby laser transscleral cyclophotocoagulation found 62 percent with an IOP of 5 to 22 mmHg, with greatest success in aphakic patients and the highest phthisis rates in patients with neovascular glaucoma (10 percent, compared with 7 percent overall and 17 percent incidence of hypotony overall).[37]

Because of the very limited availability of the ruby laser, CCT has until recently remained the treatment of choice in patients with glaucoma refractory to medical and surgical treatment; however, neodymium yttrium-aluminum-garnet (Nd.YAG) and diode laser cyclophotocoagulation have now been shown to be effective means to lower IOP by ciliodestruction. The advantages of Nd.YAG and diode laser cyclophotocoagulation are manifold. Longer wavelengths penetrate sclera better and with less backscatter than shorter wavelengths.[38-40] The Nd.YAG laser emits light at 1064 nm, the longest wavelength of lasers studied for cyclophotocoagulation; the diode laser wavelength is also in the near-infrared range, at 780 to 850 nm. Nd.YAG and diode lasers are more plentiful than ruby lasers, and contact Nd.YAG lasers may be found in many general hospitals, because they have a multitude of uses outside of ophthalmology. Diode lasers have many uses as photocoagulators in addition to transscleral cyclophotocoagulation, including trabeculoplasty,[41-43] iridectomy,[44-46] retinal photocoagulation and endophotocoagulation,[47-56] and transscleral retinopexy.[52] They are compact, lightweight, and portable and are air or electrically cooled and use standard current. Finally, the Nd.YAG and diode lasers offer a less expensive means to perform cyclophotocoagulation than does the ruby laser.

Indications and Case Selection for Transscleral Laser Cyclophotocoagulation

Cyclophotocoagulation by definition *destroys* tissue; it lowers IOP by destruction of the ciliary body, decreasing the amount of aqueous humor produced. A treatment that is too aggressive may result in hypotony, owing to an inadequate amount of remaining functional ciliary body. An insufficient treatment will not satisfactorily reduce IOP. Cyclodestructive procedures have a relatively narrow therapeutic window.

In addition, the possible untoward effects of ciliary body ablation are numerous and serious, including inflammation, pain, chronic hypotony, macular edema, vitreous hemorrhage, and phthisis. Although cyclophotocoagulation may have fewer and less profound side effects than the other forms of cyclodestructive therapy mentioned earlier, these risks persist; they combine to make cyclophotocoagulation a treatment of last resort in the management of advanced glaucoma.

Of course, many patients with uncontrolled IOP despite maximum tolerated medical therapy may benefit from cyclophotocoagulation. The procedure can be used effectively in patients who have not been helped by previous filters and in whom a repeat filtration procedure would be expected to fail. It is useful after failed filtering surgery in patients who are aphakic or who have had prior corneal transplantation or scleral buckling surgery.

The patients for whom glaucoma therapy has traditionally had the least to offer are those with neovascular or inflammatory glaucoma. Cyclophotocoagulation is indicated in these individuals when filtering surgery is expected to fail. A patient who has neovascular glaucoma and in whom abnormal vessels have regressed from the iris and angle may benefit from filtration surgery; the same patient would not be expected to have a successful glaucoma surgical procedure if the neovascularization were active after retinal photocoagulation or cryoablation.

Each patient must be evaluated individually before treatment. A decision to treat with cyclophotocoagulation should mean that the patient has uncontrolled IOP despite maximum tolerated therapy and

1. Has failed prior filtration surgery, is expected to fail further glaucoma surgery, and therefore is to be treated with cyclophotocoagulation or
2. Has a type of glaucoma in which failure is the most likely outcome of filtration surgery (e.g., neovascular, inflammatory, postpenetrating keratoplasty, postscleral buckling) and therefore is to be treated with cyclophotocoagulation or
3. Has lost ambulatory level vision and is being

treated with cyclophotocoagulation for comfort or to prevent further visual loss or

4. Is not a surgical candidate for filtering surgery for general medical reasons and therefore is to be treated with cyclophotocoagulation.

Transscleral Nd.YAG Laser Cyclophotocoagulation

Two methods are used to deliver Nd.YAG laser energy for transscleral cyclophotocoagulation: noncontact and contact.

NONCONTACT

Laboratory Studies

The use of the Nd.YAG laser for transscleral cyclophotocoagulation in rabbits was first reported by Wilensky and coworkers in 1985.[57] The investigators used a noncontact delivery system—that is, the laser energy was delivered through the air. Several reports on the histopathology of the laser lesions[38, 58–60] and the use of the technique in patients soon followed.[61–63]

Transscleral Nd.YAG laser cyclophotocoagulation in rabbits results in destruction of the ciliary epithelium and associated vessels acutely, with atrophy of the ciliary processes 4 to 8 wk after the injury.[38, 58, 59] The ciliary epithelium may regenerate in rabbits, although these cells may not be functional.[30] Although laser effects were seen in pigmented rabbits (e.g., Dutch belted), no histopathologic changes were discerned in albino rabbits[64]; therefore, pigment may be necessary to absorb the laser energy, produce heat, and cause resultant tissue destruction. This observation is relevant in light of the "pigment effect" seen clinically (see the later discussion).

Clinical Studies

Fankhauser and associates clearly demonstrated that it was possible to create a lesion in the ciliary body of a human eye at autopsy using a Nd.YAG laser in the free-running mode (20-msec pulse) at 6 to 7 J, positioned 0.5 to 1 mm posterior to the limbus, with maximum defocusing.[38, 65] Hampton and Shields further refined these studies by histopathologic examination of the lesions in the treated eyes at autopsy.[66] They found that the optimum parameters for treatment based on the location and extent of histopathologic damage were an energy level of 8 J delivered 1.0 to 1.5 mm posterior to the limbus with maximum defocusing. Gross histologic damage to the iris was seen when the beam was directed more anteriorly. No differences were noted for energy delivered tangentially versus perpendicular to the sclera.[66] Shields and colleagues and Simmons and associates found that the use of a specialized contact lens could increase the efficiency and accuracy of laser delivery.[67, 68]

Hampton and Shields consistently found destruction

of the ciliary epithelium with the creation of a blister-like space.[66] There was no coagulative necrosis.[66] Similar findings have been reported just before enucleation in in vivo blind human eyes treated for pain, with the addition of an eosinophilic material in the blister-like space.[69]

Clinical reports have attested to the efficacy of noncontact transscleral Nd.YAG laser cyclophotocoagulation (NCYC). In 1985, Cyrlin and coworkers reported 60 to 70 percent of treated patients with an IOP of 22 mmHg or less and greater than 5 mmHg with a 6- to 12-mo follow-up.[62] They used 32 spots at 8 J for 10 msec.[62] Schwartz and Moster, in 1986, reported 20 of 29 treated eyes (69 percent) with final IOPs of 22 mmHg or less, with one questionable phthisis (IOP ranged 2 to 7 mmHg), with an average 32-week follow-up.[70] Twelve of the 29 eyes (41 percent) in this group required multiple treatments; their parameters were 32 spots at 0.5 to 2.75 J for 20 msec placed 3 mm posterior to the limbus, with maximum defocusing.[70]

Devenyi and colleagues used 40 spots at 1.8 to 3.0 J for 20 msec, placed 2 to 3 mm posterior to the limbus with maximum defocusing. This group found an IOP of 21 mmHg or less in 11 of 24 patients (45.8 percent). The patients with neovascular glaucoma fared somewhat worse and the aphakic patients somewhat better than average in terms of IOP control. Eleven of 24 patients (45.8 percent) required multiple treatments.[63]

In the initial report, no patients were found to have developed phthisis bulbi after 8.8 months average follow-up by Devenyi and coworkers; however, Trope and Ma reported a phthisis rate of 10.7 percent (3 of 28 eyes) and a 30 percent rate (8 of 28 eyes) of loss of some vision in patients monitored for an average of 21.9 mo.[71]

Klapper and coworkers reported that 26 of 30 patients (86 percent) achieved an IOP of 5 to 22 mmHg, with a mean decrease in IOP of 68 percent (average 6 mo follow-up). Six of 30 patients (21 percent) required multiple treatments. The researchers used 32 spots at 3.5 to 4.5 J for 20 msec, placed 2 to 3 mm posterior to the limbus, with maximum defocusing.[72]

Hampton and colleagues amplified the work of Trope and Ma, reporting on 100 NCYC treatments and finding severe pain in 13.5 percent, severe inflammation in 28 percent, a retreatment rate of approximately 25 percent, and visual loss in nearly 50 percent.[73] Wright and associates found that a majority of the 35 eyes that they treated required further intervention or lost all vision if monitored long enough, with 31 percent of eyes losing two or more lines of vision or light perception during the 3-yr follow-up period of their study.[74]

Maus and Katz reported severe hypotony, flat anterior chamber, and serous choroidal detachment after NCYC in three patients, all of whom had had previous filtering surgery and two of whom were black. These complications appeared 1 to 2 wk after treatment and resolved spontaneously in one of the three patients.[75] Fiore and coworkers reported focal scleral thinning after NCYC in one patient.[76] Hardten and Brown described a case of malignant glaucoma after NCYC in one eye.[77] In the laboratory, Blomquist and colleagues have shown that NCYC can damage intraocular lens (IOL) haptics in cadaver eyes if sufficient energy is used; however, the investigators used energies in excess of clinically utilized levels (8.8 J).[78] Lim and colleagues failed to demonstrate any damage to IOL haptics with contact transscleral Nd.YAG laser cyclophotocoagulation (CYC).[79] Although subretinal fibrosis[80] and lens subluxation[81] can occur with CCT, these complications have not been reported after Nd.YAG or diode laser cyclophotocoagulation.

Edward and coauthors described a case of sympathetic ophthalmia associated temporally with Nd.YAG cyclophotocoagulation[82]; however, the patient had undergone two prior filtering operations and had uveal incarceration. In addition, the treatment was directed to the area of the previous surgery. The relationship between the cyclophotocoagulation and the sympathetic ophthalmia is uncertain[83]; however, sympathetic ophthalmia has been described following cyclocryotherapy,[84] as well as after helium ion irradiation followed by CCT.[85]

Operative Technique

A technique for NCYC is summarized in Table 147–1. All glaucoma medications are continued before laser treatment. After written informed consent is obtained, a retrobulbar or peribulbar injection of 2 percent lidocaine without epinephrine is given (because this is not incisional surgery, epinephrine is not needed). Marcaine may be added to the block if desired. The contralateral eye should be patched to prevent the entrance of any stray laser light. The patient is then seated at the slit-lamp delivery system for the laser (Fig. 147–1).

The laser is set to 4 to 8 J energy, 20 msec duration, and maximum offset (9). These settings are for use with the Lasag MR2 (Microruptor 2, Lasag, Thun, Switzerland). The parameters for the Lasag MR3 have not been determined; however, it is likely that a longer *duration* will be used, consistent with that for *contact* cyclophotocoagulation (discussed later). Thirty-two spots (eight applications per quadrant) are applied in a circumferential pattern sparing 3 and 9 o'clock (to avoid the long posterior ciliary arteries) (Fig. 147–2). Spots are placed 1.0 to 1.5 mm posterior to the limbus, because Hampton and Shields have shown that this location is most likely to produce ciliary body destruction (Fig. 147–3).[66] Crymes and Gross similarly reported greater clinical efficacy with treatments 1.5 mm posterior to the limbus than at 3 mm posterior.[92] Measurements are made with calipers or can be performed by keeping the aiming beam in the center of a 3-mm-high slit beam, as demonstrated by Fiore and Latina.[86] Keeping the edge of the 3-mm slit at the limbus, the aiming beam will always be 1.5 mm posterior.

The treatment parameters are documented, and a diagram is made of the areas covered.

Postoperative Care

The eye is patched for 4 to 6 hr postoperatively after instillation of prednisolone acetate 1 percent and atro-

---

Table 147–1. TRANSSCLERAL Nd:YAG LASER CYCLOPHOTOCOAGULATION: TREATMENT TECHNIQUE

1. Continue all preoperative glaucoma medications prior to laser treatment.
2. Obtain informed consent.
3. Confirm satisfactory operation of laser.
4. Administer retrobulbar or peribulbar anesthesia.
5. Seat the patient at the laser slit lamp (noncontact) or lie the patient on a stretcher (contact).
6. Laser settings:

	Noncontact	*Contact*
	Energy: 4–8 J	Power: 7 W
	Duration: 20 msec	Duration: 0.7 sec
	Offset: maximum (9)	

7. Treatment parameters:

	Noncontact	*Contact*
Number of applications:	32	
Treatment pattern:	8 spots per quadrant	
	Spare 3 and 9 o'clock	
Spot location:	1.0–1.5 mm posterior to the limbus. Measure with calipers or use aiming beam in center of 3-mm slit beam. Keeping edge of slit beam at limbus, aiming beam will always be 1.5 mm posterior.[86]	Anterior edge of probe 0.5–1.0 mm posterior to limbus (i.e., center of probe 1.5–2.0 mm posterior to limbus). Measure with calipers. Press gently with probe, keeping handpiece perpendicular to sclera. Maintain contact throughout energy delivery.

Noncontact and Contact:

8. Document total energy delivered, and diagram treatment.
9. Postoperative medications:
   Patch eye postoperatively 4 to 6 hr.
   Atropine 1% b.i.d.; taper as inflammation subsides.
   Prednisolone acetate 1% q.i.d.; taper as inflammation subsides.
   Continue all preoperative glaucoma medications except miotics.
   May resume miotics if needed when inflammation subsides.
10. Check IOP at 1 hr, 1 day, and 1 wk after treatment. Follow-up and medications thereafter depend on the clinical response.
11. Patient may require retreatment if IOP is not adequate at 1-mo check up.

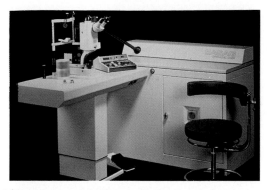

Figure 147–1. Laser and slit-lamp delivery system for noncontact transscleral Nd.YAG cyclophotocoagulation. (Microruptor 2, Lasag, Thun, Switzerland.)

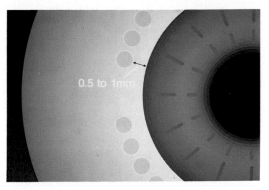

Figure 147–3. Distance of application from limbus for cyclophotocoagulation. Noncontact spots should be centered 1.0 to 1.5 mm posterior to the limbus (not shown). With contact transscleral Nd.YAG cyclophotocoagulation, the anterior edge of the probe should be placed 0.5 to 1.0 mm posterior to the limbus (as illustrated).

pine sulfate 1 percent. Prednisolone acetate 1 percent is applied four times a day, and atropine sulfate 1 percent is given twice a day; both are tapered as the inflammation subsides. All preoperative glaucoma medications are continued, with the exception of miotics. Miotics may be reinstituted, if needed, when the inflammation is reduced.

Areas of treatment with NCYC are usually visible as white conjunctival lesions that fade with time (Fig. 147–4). IOP is checked at 1 hr, 1 day, and 1 wk. Follow-up thereafter depends on a patient's clinical response.

Retreatment

Patients who have an inadequate response to NCYC after 1 to 4 wk may benefit from retreatment. All parameters are the same as for the initial treatment, with the exception that only half the original number of spots should be applied (16 instead of 32). This adjustment may help to decrease the incidence of hypotony and phthisis from this procedure. Patients may be retreated more than once; however, each retreatment increases the possibility of phthisis.

CONTACT

Laboratory Studies

CYC was first suggested by Brancato and coworkers in 1987, when they reported on CYC treatment of

chinchilla rabbits.[87] Lesions in rabbit ciliary bodies using CYC were later reported by Federman and coworkers in 1987,[88] Peyman and colleagues in 1987,[93] Schubert and Federman in 1989,[89, 90] and Latina and coauthors in 1989.[91] Gross examination 1 day after treatment revealed CYC lesions to be 1-mm, white, well-demarcated spots.[87, 91] Thermal damage to the ciliary body stroma was noted, with coagulation necrosis of the ciliary non-pigmented and pigmented epithelia. No significant scleral damage was noted with CYC.[87, 91] Longer follow-up after CYC in rabbits revealed ciliary body atrophy, with flattening, fusion, and shortening of the ciliary processes 4 weeks after treatment.[89, 91] The ciliary processes may be covered by a fibrous membrane.[87] The ciliary epithelium was abnormal, with pigment epithelial proliferation and focal epithelial interruptions.[89, 91] Areas of scleral compression and hypercellularity were seen, but no clear evidence of scleral thermal damage.[89] Van der Zypen and colleagues have shown that ciliary epithelial regeneration is incomplete for at least 8 mo after treatment with CYC or NCYC and that the vascular network also remains atrophic for this period.[94, 95]

Iwach and coauthors described the use of a pulsed contact Nd.YAG laser for transscleral cyclophotocoagulation; however, the effects of this laser were more similar to the explosive tissue damage seen with the

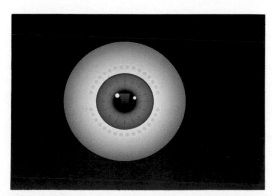

Figure 147–2. Pattern for noncontact or contact cyclophotocoagulation. Note that 3 and 9 o'clock meridians are spared treatment.

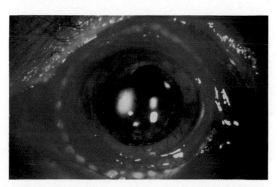

Figure 147–4. Appearance of eye immediately after noncontact cyclophotocoagulation. Note white conjunctival lesions, which fade with time.

noncontact technique than the coagulative effects of continuous wave Nd.YAG laser cyclophotocoagulation.[96] Cyclophotocoagulation is the surgical procedure of choice in veterinary cases in which maximal medical treatment has failed to control IOP.[97]

CYC of human eyes at autopsy resulted in coagulation necrosis of the ciliary body, with ciliary pigmented and nonpigmented epithelial disruption.[98] Allingham and coworkers demonstrated that placement of the probe at the limbus resulted in damage to the peripheral iris and lens, whereas positioning the anterior edge probe 1.5 mm posterior to the limbus resulted in burns of the pars plana. Similarly, 5 W of power produced only minimal coagulative necrosis of the ciliary body, with 11 W causing a striking loss of anatomic integrity of the ciliary processes. The investigators did not note any scleral damage at any power setting. Their recommendations, therefore, were for treatment with the anterior edge of the probe 0.5 to 1.0 mm posterior to the limbus using 5 to 9 W of power for 0.7 sec.[98] Brancato and colleagues, in a study that used human eyes destined for enucleation because of choroidal melanoma, found that only 2 J was needed to create lesions in the ciliary body; placement was identical to that of Allingham and colleagues.[99] Later clinical data reported by Brancato and associates, however, supported the use of the higher energy levels suggested by Allingham and coworkers.[101]

Clinical Studies

In 1990, Schuman and associates reported the results of CYC in 160 treatments of 140 eyes of 136 patients.[100] They found that 71 percent of eyes (97) achieved an average final IOP of 25 mmHg or less, 62 percent (85) 22 mmHg or less, and 49 percent (67) 19 mmHg or less. IOP decreased rapidly, with more than half the patients achieving their final IOP within the first week after treatment (Fig. 147–5). The parameters used were 7 to 9 W of power, 0.7 sec, and 32 to 40 spots; the anterior edge of the contact probe was placed 0.5 to 1.5 mm posterior to the limbus. A pressure of less than 5 mmHg was noted in 5 of 140 eyes; three of the five eyes had a final IOP of 0 mmHg. Eleven percent of eyes (15) required retreatment. More inflammation and pain oc-

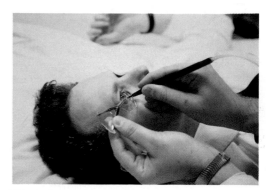

Figure 147–6. Patient is supine for treatment. A lid speculum is placed in the eye to be treated, and the probe is held perpendicular to the sclera. Contact between the probe and the eye is maintained throughout energy delivery.

curred in nonwhite (black, Hispanic, Asian) patients and patients with neovascular glaucoma.[100]

Brancato and coauthors summarized their results with CYC in 23 patients. They used 16 applications of 4 W for 0.5 sec with the anterior edge of the probe approximately 1.5 mm posterior to the limbus. A final IOP of 25 mmHg or less was achieved in 66.6 percent of patients (15); 15 percent (3) of the 23 patients had a final IOP of less than 20 mmHg. Retreatment was required in 57 percent of patients (13), and 21 percent (5 patients) needed three sessions.[101]

Schuman and associates updated their results in 1992 in 116 eyes of 114 patients monitored for a minimum of 1 year after treatment with CYC. IOP control was similar to their earlier report, with three-quarters of eyes achieving an average final IOP of 25 mmHg or less, two-thirds 22 mmHg or less, and more than half of the eyes 19 mmHg or less. Complications were more apparent with longer follow-up, however, with a greater need for retreatments and an increased incidence of hypotony and visual loss. Retreatment was required in 31 eyes (27 percent). IOP in nine eyes fell to less than 3 mmHg, and to 0 mmHg in six. Seventeen of 36 eyes (47 percent) with visual acuity of 20/200 or better lost two or more Snellen's lines. Nineteen eyes, all with initial visual acuity of counting fingers or worse, deteriorated to no light perception.[102]

Operative Technique

A treatment technique for CYC is listed in Table 147–1. As with NCYC, all glaucoma medications are continued before laser treatment. After obtaining written informed consent, retrobulbar or peribulbar anesthesia is administered, as noted earlier for NCYC. A patch is applied to the contralateral eye, and the patient lies supine on a stretcher. A lid speculum is placed in the eye to receive CYC, and the surgeon and assistants don protective eyewear blocking 1064 nm radiation (Fig. 147–6).

The laser is set to deliver 7 W for 0.7 sec (Figs. 147–7 and 147–8). Patients with neovascular glaucoma, and nonwhite patients may develop fewer complications if treated with 5 to 6 W of power instead of 7 W; however,

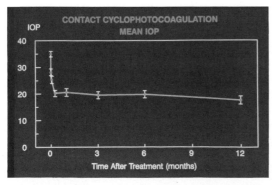

Figure 147–5. Pattern of intraocular pressure lowering after contact transscleral Nd.YAG cyclophotocoagulation. Pressure falls rapidly within the first 1 to 4 wk after treatment.

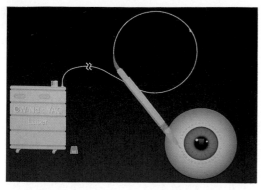

Figure 147–7. Schematic of contact transscleral Nd.YAG cyclophotocoagulation delivery system (Surgical Laser Technologies, Inc., Malvern, PA). Laser unit is portable.

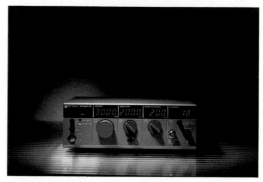

Figure 147–8. Diode laser unit (Oculight SLx, Iris Medical Instruments, Mountain View, CA). Laser is small, lightweight, portable, and air cooled. It uses standard current and can be used for contact cyclophotocoagulation and transscleral retinopexy, adapted to a slit lamp or indirect ophthalmoscope for photocoagulation, or used as an endophotocoagulator.

this has not yet been systematically evaluated. As stated earlier for NCYC, treatment is performed with 32 spots (8 per quadrant), sparing the 3 and 9 o'clock meridians (see Fig. 147–2). Fewer spots may be used, and Schuman and coworkers found no difference in results with 24 versus 32 spots, either for IOP effects or complications.[102] The anterior edge of the probe is 0.5 to 1.0 mm posterior to the limbus (see Fig. 147–3). This distance is measured with calipers. The probe is pressed gently and kept perpendicular to the sclera. Contact with the eye is maintained throughout energy delivery.

Power, duration, number of applications, distance from the limbus, total energy delivered, and treatment pattern are documented.

Postoperative Care

Postoperative care is identical to that for NCYC, described earlier. The treated eye is patched for 4 to 6 hr postoperatively after instillation of prednisolone acetate 1 percent and atropine sulfate 1 percent. Prednisolone acetate 1 percent is applied four times a day, and atropine sulfate 1 percent is given twice a day; both are tapered as the inflammation subsides. All preoperative glaucoma medications are continued, with the exception of miotics. Miotics may be reinstituted, if needed, when the inflammation is reduced.

Unlike NCYC, after CYC the treated eye generally does not show any conjunctival lesions. IOP is checked at 1 hr, 1 day, and 1 wk. Follow-up thereafter depends on a patient's clinical response.

Retreatment

Patients who have an inadequate response to CYC after 1 to 4 wk may benefit from retreatment. All parameters are the same as for the initial treatment, with the exception that only half the original number of spots should be applied (16 instead of 32). This may help to decrease the incidence of hypotony and phthisis from this procedure. Patients may be retreated more than once; however, each retreatment increases the possibility of phthisis.

Transscleral Semiconductor Diode Laser Cyclophotocoagulation

Laboratory Studies

The effects of contact diode laser cyclophotocoagulation (CDC) in rabbits were reported by Schuman and colleagues[103] and Peyman and coworkers in 1990[52] and by Brancato and associates in 1991 (Figs. 147–9 and 147–10).[104] CDC effectively lowered IOP during a 6-wk period. Acute immediate lesions were similar to lesions created by CYC, with thermal damage to the ciliary pigmented and nonpigmented epithelia and stroma.[52, 103, 104] Examination at 6 wk showed discrete lesions with atrophy, fibrosis, and fusion of the ciliary processes. Histopathologic examination revealed ciliary epithelial and stromal focal atrophy and fibrosis, with pigment-laden macrophages in the ciliary body and outflow pathways. Scleral perforation and lens capsule rupture could be seen when excessive power was used.[103]

Effects of CDC in human cadaver eyes included ciliary epithelial coagulation necrosis and thermal coagulation

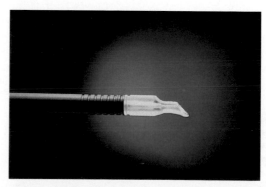

Figure 147–9. Contact cyclophotocoagulation probe (G-Probe, Iris Medical Instruments, Mountain View, CA) for use with diode laser. Offset of center of fiberoptic from limbus is preset at 1.2 mm.

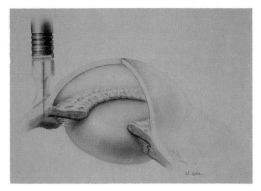

Figure 147-10. Placement of probe on eye for cyclophotocoagulation.

of the ciliary stroma and stromal vasculature. Optimal energy levels were 3 to 5 J.[105] In a study of transscleral noncontact diode laser cyclophotocoagulation (NCDC), Hennis and coauthors demonstrated thermal effects in the ciliary body with as little as 900 mJ. They used a spot size of 100 to 500 μm, placed the beam 0.5 mm posterior to the limbus, and defocused 1 mm posteriorly.[106] In a study of living rabbits, comparing CDC and NCDC using the same laser for both treatments, Shepps and colleagues reported that approximately 50 percent more energy was needed to create the same lesion with NCDC compared with CDC.[107] This observation is consonant with findings on scleral light scattering predicted by Vogel and associates.[108] Assia and coworkers compared NCDC with NCYC and CCT in cadaver eyes and found that all were effective in ciliary body destruction, without damaging the crystalline lens.[109]

Hennis and Stewart reported on the use of NCDC in treating advanced glaucoma in 14 eyes, using 1.2 W for 0.99 sec (1.2 J) with 40 to 45 applications of a 100 μm spot, placed 1 mm posterior to the limbus, defocused 1 mm posteriorly. They found a 30 percent reduction in IOP during a 6-month follow-up period with a single treatment. Complications included conjunctival burns and inflammation.[110] Gaasterland and colleagues, in a study of CDC in 30 eyes of 30 patients, found a 36 percent reduction in IOP with 3 mo of follow-up. They treated with 1.5 to 2.0 W for 2 sec (3 to 4 J), using 16 to 18 spots over 270 degrees, with the fiberoptic centered 1.2 mm posterior to the limbus. There was no significant change in vision, no hypotony, mild transient inflammation, and minimal discomfort.[112] Carassa and colleagues found similar results, 50 percent IOP reduction in 12 eyes of 12 patients, using a contact diode laser with 16 spots over 360 degrees and 2.5 W for 1.5 sec (3.75 J).[113]

CONCLUSIONS

CCT has long been the standard by which other cyclodestructive modalities have been measured. Bellows and Grant demonstrated the effectiveness of CCT in advanced uncontrolled glaucoma, especially in aphakia[15, 16]; however, severe complications, including phthisis bulbi in 0 to 12 percent of patients and visual loss in more than two-thirds of patients, may occur.[15–19] The significant risks associated with CCT make it a treatment of last resort in glaucoma refractory to other therapeutic modalities. Higginbotham and colleagues found that CYC and CCT produced similar levels of IOP reduction in rabbits but that CYC destroyed less tissue than CCT.[114] Suzuki and associates demonstrated that NCYC was as effective as CCT clinically and that NCYC produced fewer complications.[115] In a nonrandomized study, Noureddin and coworkers compared NCYC with drainage tube implantation surgery. They found that both procedures lowered IOP but that serious complications, such as retinal detachment, expulsive hemorrhage, phthisis, and endophthalmitis, were much more common in the tube-treated group. They also found a higher incidence of visual loss among the tube-treated eyes than those treated with NCYC. There was no significant difference in postoperative IOP in the two groups treated.[116]

Transscleral laser cyclophotocoagulation creates new options in the management of advanced glaucoma uncontrolled with medical and surgical therapy. NCYC and CYC, the two delivery systems for transscleral Nd.YAG laser cyclophotocoagulation, differ in several important ways. NCYC is performed with the patient sitting at a slit lamp; CYC is done with the patient supine. The contact laser, which is portable, can be moved as needed to remote locations (e.g., to treat patients in the operating room under general anesthesia). NCYC uses 5 to 8 J of energy delivered over 20 msec (250 to 400 W) in 32 applications[38, 63, 70, 72, 73]; this is more energy and significantly more power than CYC, which is performed using 2 to 6.3 J over 0.5 to 0.7 sec (4 to 9 W) in 16 to 40 applications.[100, 101]

As shown by Hampton and Shields, optimum location for beam placement in NCYC is 1.5 mm posterior to the limbus.[38, 66] Allingham and coworkers found that the anterior edge of the contact probe should be placed 0.5 to 1.0 mm posterior to the limbus in CYC; the 2.2-mm-diameter probe is therefore centered 1.6 to 2.1 mm posterior to the limbus.[98] Schuman and associates did not find any clinical differences in treatments performed with the anterior edge of the probe at 0.5, 1.0, or 1.5 mm posterior to the limbus.[102]

Schubert showed that NCYC and CYC lesions performed 3 mm posterior to the limbus caused lesions in the pars plana.[117] He later found that such lesions resulted in an increase in outflow facility.[118] These results were supported by Pham-Duy, who found that CCT improved outflow facility while transiently reducing aqueous flow; however, this study was limited by blood-aqueous barrier disruption following CCT.[119] In a well-designed study, Higginbotham and associates demonstrated that graded CCT produced graded ciliary epithelial destruction, with proportional effects on IOP and aqueous flow.[120] These workers, however, did not examine outflow in this study. Schmidt and coworkers found that CYC increases uveoscleral outflow in rabbits, perhaps by a prostaglandin-mediated effect; uveoscleral flow returned to nearly baseline levels for 5 to 6 wk after treatment, as IOP returned to normal.[121]

Preexisting glaucoma type appears to be significant in response to cyclophotocoagulation. Of all types of glaucoma studied, patients with neovascular glaucoma react least well to cyclophotocoagulation.[15, 18] These patients tend to develop the most numerous and most severe complications (inflammation, pain, visual loss) and have a trend to a poorer IOP response, although this does not achieve statistical significance.[100, 102]

Aphakic patients with glaucoma were shown by Bellows and Grant to respond better to CCT than phakic patients.[16] This difference did not exist in CYC; however, aphakic patients did have less inflammation than other individuals.[100, 102] Cyclophotocoagulation may be an effective means of IOP control in eyes following penetrating keratoplasty.[100, 122–124]

Darkly pigmented eyes develop more severe side effects and a more profound treatment effect than lighter eyes. De Roetth[13] mentioned this phenomenon in regard to CCT, and Cantor and coworkers[64] found this in comparing NCYC in albino and pigmented rabbits. Schubert and Federman[84, 92] have also noted this phenomenon with regard to cyclophotocoagulation. Coleman and associates reported similar findings in cadaver eyes and in monkeys.[125] This same result was described by Schuman and coauthors in a large clinical study on CYC.[100] Patients with more pigmentation may require less energy for the same level of cyclodestruction than those who are less heavily pigmented; the pigment acts to absorb and distribute the light energy as heat locally, with more resultant tissue damage at the same energy level in eyes with more pigmentation.

Results with both NCYC and CYC have been encouraging in showing these treatments to be effective in reducing IOP in advanced glaucoma refractory to maximum tolerated medical therapy and surgery; however, CYC appears to have several advantages over NCYC. CYC uses a longer exposure time than NCYC, with resultant coagulative necrosis of the ciliary processes with CYC, as opposed to the blister formation noted with NCYC.[66, 67, 89, 98] Anecdotally, there appears to be less inflammation and pain with CYC as opposed to NCYC; this finding may be related to the type of damage seen histopathologically. The CYC unit is portable, can be transported to the operating room, and may be more readily available to the general ophthalmologist (e.g., a small hospital might have a contact Nd.YAG laser for gastrointestinal and plastic surgery; it could be used for cyclophotocoagulation as well). Either technique offers a titratable treatment that is generally well tolerated by carefully selected patients.

The diode laser provides similar results to those of the Nd.YAG laser, with the advantages of small size, light weight, portability, air cooling, use of standard current, and relatively low cost. The diode laser has the theoretical advantage of greater melanin absorption, although slightly less scleral transmission, compared with the Nd.YAG laser.[108] Although still in its infancy, transscleral diode laser cyclophotocoagulation appears to deliver many of the benefits of transscleral Nd.YAG

laser cyclophotocoagulation with greater convenience and economy.

Although still a therapeutic modality restricted to patients with the most advanced glaucoma unresponsive to other medical and surgical treatments, transscleral laser cyclophotocoagulation appears to be the next step in the evolution of cyclodestructive procedures, from cyclodiathermy through CCT to cyclophotocoagulation.

REFERENCES

1. Weve H: Die Zyklodiatermie das Corpus ciliare bei Glaukom. Zentralbl Ophthalmol 29:562, 1933.
2. Vogt A: Versuche zur intraokularen Druckherabsetzung mittels Diatermieschadigung des Corpus cilare (Zyklodiatermiestichelung). Klin Monatsbl Augenheilkd 97:672, 1936.
3. Stocker FW: Response of chronic simple glaucoma to treatment with cyclodiathermy puncture. Arch Ophthalmol 34:181, 1945.
4. Walton DS, Grant WM: Penetrating cyclodiathermy for filtration. Arch Ophthalmol 83:47, 1970.
5. Waked N, Hamard H, Godde JD, et al: Cyclodiathermy: Is it effective in the treatment of glaucoma? J Fr Ophtalmol 13:159, 1990.
6. Haik GM, Breffeilh LA, Barbar A: Beta irradiation as a possible therapeutic agent in glaucoma: An experimental study with the report of a clinical case. Am J Ophthalmol 31:945, 1948.
7. Berens C, Sheppard LB, Duel AB Jr: Cycloelectrolysis for glaucoma. Trans Am Ophthalmol Soc 47:364, 1949.
8. Sheppard LB: Retrociliary cyclodiathermy versus retrociliary cycloelectrolysis: Effects on the normal rabbit eye. Am J Ophthalmol 46:27, 1958.
9. Bietti G: Surgical intervention on the ciliary body: New trends for the relief of glaucoma. JAMA 142:889, 1950.
10. Polack FM, de Roetth A: Effect of freezing on the ciliary body (cyclocryotherapy). Invest Ophthalmol 3:164, 1964.
11. McLean JM, Lincoff HA: Cryosurgery of the ciliary body. Trans Am Ophthalmol Soc 62:385, 1964.
12. de Roetth A: Cryosurgery for the treatment of glaucoma. Trans Am Ophthalmol Soc 63:189, 1965.
13. de Roetth A: Cryosurgery for the treatment of advanced simple glaucoma. Am J Ophthalmol 66:1034, 1968.
14. Shields MB: Cyclodestructive surgery for glaucoma: Past, present, and future. Trans Am Ophthalmol Soc 83:285, 1985.
15. Bellows AR, Grant WM: Cyclocryotherapy in advanced inadequately controlled glaucoma. Am J Ophthalmol 75:679, 1973.
16. Bellows AR, Grant WM: Cyclocryotherapy of chronic openangle glaucoma in aphakic eyes. Am J Ophthalmol 85:615, 1978.
17. Feibel RM, Bigger JF: Rubeosis iridis and neovascular glaucoma: Evaluation of cyclocryotherapy. Am J Ophthalmol 74:862, 1972.
18. Krupin T, Mitchell KB, Becker B: Cyclocryotherapy in neovascular glaucoma. Am J Ophthalmol 86:24, 1978.
19. Brindley G, Shields MB: Values and limitations of cyclocryotherapy. Graefes Arch Clin Exp Ophthalmol 224:545, 1986.
20. Ibid.
21. Benson MT, Nelson ME: Cyclocryotherapy: A review of cases over a 10-year period. Br J Ophthalmol 74:103, 1990.
22. Gross RL, Feldman RM, Spaeth GL, et al: Surgical therapy of chronic glaucoma in aphakia and pseudophakia. Ophthalmology 95:1195, 1988.
23. Nissen OI, Schiodte SN, Kessing SV: Panretinal xenonphotocoagulation combined with cyclocryotherapy in the treatment of severe glaucoma. Acta Ophthalmol (Copenh) 67:652, 1989.
24. Purnell EW, Sokollu A, Torchia R, et al: Focal chorioretinitis produced by ultrasound. Invest Ophthalmol 3:657, 1964.
25. Coleman DJ, Lizzi FL, Driller J, et al: Therapeutic ultrasound in the treatment of glaucoma. I: Experimental model. Ophthalmology 92:339, 1985.
26. Coleman DJ, Lizzi FL, Driller J, et al: Therapeutic ultrasound in the treatment of glaucoma. II: Clinical applications. Ophthalmology 92:347, 1985.
27. Margo CE: Therapeutic ultrasound: Light and electron micro-

scopic findings in an eye treated for glaucoma. Arch Ophthalmol 104:735, 1986.

28. Haut J, Colliac JP, Falque L, Renard Y: Indications and results of Sonocare (ultrasound) in the treatment of ocular hypertension: A preliminary study of 395 cases. Ophtalmologie 4:138, 1990.

29. Finger PT, Moshfeghi DM, Smith PD, Perry HD: Microwave cyclodestruction for glaucoma in a rabbit model. Arch Ophthalmol 109:1001, 1991.

30. Valtot F, Kopel J, Le MY: Principles and histologic effects of the treatment of hypertension with focused high-intensity ultrasound. Ophtalmologie 4:135, 1990.

31. Finger PT, Smith PD, Paglione RW, Perry HD: Transscleral microwave cyclodestruction. Invest Ophthalmol Vis Sci 31:2151, 1990.

32. Lee P-F, Pomerantzeff O: Transpupillary cyclophotocoagulation of rabbit eyes: An experimental approach to glaucoma surgery. Am J Ophthalmol 71:911, 1971.

33. Shields MB: Intraocular cyclophotocoagulation. Trans Ophthalmol Soc UK 105:237, 1986.

34. Weekers R, Lavergne G, Watillion M, et al: Effects of photocoagulation of ciliary body upon ocular tension. Am J Ophthalmol 52:156, 1961.

35. Beckman H, Kinoshita A, Rota AN, et al: Transscleral ruby laser irradiation of the ciliary body in the treatment of intractable glaucoma. Trans Am Acad Ophthalmol Otolaryngol 46:423, 1972.

36. Beckman H, Sugar HS: Neodymium laser cyclocoagulation. Arch Ophthalmol 90:27, 1973.

37. Beckman H, Waelterman J: Transscleral ruby laser cyclocoagulation. Am J Ophthalmol 98:788, 1984.

38. Fankhauser F, van der Zypen E, Kwasniewska S, et al: Transscleral cyclophotocoagulation using a neodymium:YAG laser. Ophthalmic Surg 17:94, 1986.

39. Rol P, Niederer P, Durr P, et al: Experimental investigations on the light scattering properties of the human sclera. Lasers and Light in Ophthalmology 3:201, 1990.

40. Vogel A, Dlugos C, Nuffer R, Birnguber R: Optical properties of human sclera, and their consequences for transscleral laser applications. Lasers Surg Med 11:331, 1991.

41. Schuman JS, Puliafito CA, Allingham RR, et al: A controlled clinical trial of diode versus argon laser trabeculoplasty. Ophthalmology 97(Suppl):143, 1990.

42. Brancato R, Carassa R, Trabucchi G: Diode laser compared with argon laser for trabeculoplasty. Am J Ophthalmol 112:50, 1991.

43. McHugh D, Marshall J, Ffytche JT, et al: Diode laser trabeculoplasty for primary open angle glaucoma and ocular hypertension. Br J Ophthalmol 74:743, 1990.

44. Jacobson JJ, Schuman JS, El-Khoumy H, Puliafito CA: Diode laser peripheral iridectomy. Int Ophthalmol Clin 30:120, 1990.

45. Schuman JS, Jacobson JJ, Puliafito CA: Semiconductor diode laser peripheral iridotomy. Arch Ophthalmol 108:1207, 1990.

46. Emoto I, Okisaka S, Nakajima A: Diode laser iridotomy in rabbit and human eyes. Am J Ophthalmol 113:321, 1992.

47. Balles MW, Puliafito CA, D'Amico DJ, et al: Semiconductor diode laser photocoagulation in retinal vascular disease. Ophthalmology 97:1553, 1990.

48. Brancato R, Pratesi R, Leoni G, et al: Histopathology of diode and argon laser lesions in rabbit retina: A comparative study. Invest Ophthalmol Vis Sci 30:1504, 1989.

49. Duker JS, Federman JL, Schubert H, Talbot C: Semiconductor diode laser endophotocoagulation. Ophthalmic Surg 20:717, 1989.

50. Jennings T, Fuller T, Vukich JA, et al: Transscleral contact retinal photocoagulation with an 810-nm semiconductor diode laser. Ophthalmic Surg 21:492, 1990.

51. McHugh JD, Marshall J, Ffytche TJ, et al: Initial clinical experience using a diode laser in the treatment of retinal vascular disease. Eye 3:516, 1989.

52. Peyman GA, Naguib KS, Gaasterland D: Trans-scleral application of a semiconductor diode laser. Lasers Surg Med 10:569, 1990.

53. Puliafito CA, Deutsch TF, Boll J, To K: Semiconductor laser endophotocoagulation of the retina. Arch Ophthalmol 105:424, 1987.

54. Sato Y, Berkowitz BA, Wilson CA, DeJuan EJ: Blood-retinal barrier breakdown caused by diode vs argon laser endophotocoagulation. Arch Ophthalmol 110:277, 1992.

55. Suh JH, Miki T, Obana A, et al: Effects of indocyanine green dye enhanced diode laser photocoagulation in non-pigmented rabbit eyes. Osaka City Med J 37:89, 1991.

56. Wallow IH, Sponsel WE, Stevens TS: Clinicopathologic correlation of diode laser burns in monkeys. Arch Ophthalmol 109:648, 1991.

57. Wilensky JT, Welch D, Mirolovich M: Transscleral cyclocoagulation using a neodymium:YAG laser. Ophthalmic Surg 16:95, 1985.

58. England C, van der Zypen E, Fankhauser F, et al: Ultrastructure of the rabbit ciliary body following transscleral cyclophotocoagulation with the free-running Nd:YAG laser: Preliminary findings. Lasers Ophthalmol 1:61, 1986.

59. Gross RL, Smith JA, Font RL, et al: Transscleral Nd:YAG laser cycloablation in rabbits [Abstract]. Invest Ophthalmol Vis Sci 27(Suppl):253, 1986.

60. Devenyi RG, Trope GE, Hunter WH: Neodymium-YAG transscleral cyclocoagulation in rabbit eyes. Br J Ophthalmol 71:441, 1987.

61. Moster MR, Schwartz LW, Cantor LB, et al: Treatment of advanced glaucoma with Nd:YAG laser cyclodiathermy [Abstract]. Invest Ophthalmol Vis Sci 27(Suppl):253, 1986.

62. Cyrlin MN, Beckman H, Czedik C: Neodymium:YAG transscleral cyclocoagulation for severe glaucoma [Abstract]. Invest Ophthalmol Vis Sci 26(Suppl):253, 1985.

63. Devenyi RG, Trope GE, Hunter WH, et al: Neodymium:YAG transscleral cyclocoagulation in human eyes. Ophthalmology 94:1519, 1987.

64. Cantor LB, Nichols DA, Katz J, et al: Neodymium-YAG transscleral cyclophotocoagulation: The role of pigmentation. Invest Ophthalmol Vis Sci 30:1834, 1989.

65. Fankhauser F, Kwasniewska S, Van der Zypen E: Experimental and clinical use of the thermal mode neodymium:YAG laser. Klin Monatsbl Augenheilkd 191:169, 1987.

66. Hampton C, Shields MB: Transscleral neodymium-YAG cyclophotocoagulation: A histologic study of human autopsy eyes. Arch Ophthalmol 106:1121, 1988.

67. Shields MB, Blasini M, Simmons R, Erickson PJ: A contact lens for transscleral Nd:YAG cyclophotocoagulation. Am J Ophthalmol 108:457, 1989.

68. Simmons RB, Blasini M, Shields MB, Erickson PJ: Comparison of transscleral neodymium:YAG cyclophotocoagulation with and without a contact lens in human autopsy eyes. Am J Ophthalmol 109:174, 1990.

69. Blasini M, Simmons R, Shields MB: Early tissue response to transscleral neodymium-YAG cyclophotocoagulation [Abstract]. Invest Ophthalmol Vis Sci 31:1114, 1990.

70. Schwartz LW, Moster MR: Neodymium: YAG laser transscleral cyclodiathermy. Ophthalmic Laser Ther 1:135, 1986.

71. Trope GE, Ma S: Mid term effects of Nd:YAG transscleral cyclocoagulation in glaucoma. Ophthalmology 97:73, 1990.

72. Klapper RM, Wandel T, Donnenfeld E, et al: Transscleral neodymium:YAG thermal cyclophotocoagulation in refractory glaucoma: A preliminary report. Ophthalmology 95:719, 1988.

73. Hampton C, Shields MB, Miller KN, et al: Evaluation of a protocol for transscleral cyclophotocoagulation in 100 consecutive patients. Ophthalmology 97:910, 1990.

74. Wright MM, Grajewski AL, Feuer WJ: Nd:YAG cyclophotocoagulation: Outcome of treatment for uncontrolled glaucoma. Ophthalmic Surg 22:279, 1991.

75. Maus M, Katz LJ: Choroidal detachment, flat anterior chamber and hypotony as complications of Nd:YAG laser cyclophotocoagulation. Ophthalmology 97:69, 1990.

76. Fiore PM, Melamed S, Krug JHJ: Focal scleral thinning after transscleral Nd:YAG cyclophotocoagulation. Ophthalmic Surg 20:215, 1989.

77. Hardten DR, Brown JD: Malignant glaucoma after Nd:YAG cyclophotocoagulation [Letter]. Am J Ophthalmol 111:245, 1991.

78. Blomquist PH, Gross RL, Koch DD: Effect of transscleral neodymium:YAG cyclophotocoagulation on intraocular lenses. Ophthalmic Surg 21:223, 1990.

79. Lim ES, Solomon KD, VanMeter WS, Hooper RW: Continuous

wave transscleral Nd:YAG laser: A postmortem study of probe placement and destructive effects on tissue, transscleral sutured lenses and capsular bag fixated lenses. Invest Ophthalmol Vis Sci 33 (Suppl):1268, 1992.

80. Kao SF, Morgan CM, Bergstrom TJ: Subretinal fibrosis following cyclocryotherapy: Case report. Arch Ophthalmol 105:1175, 1987.

81. Pearson PA, Baldwin LB, Smith TJ: Lens subluxation as a complication of cyclocryotherapy. Ophthalmic Surg 20:445, 1989.

82. Edward DP, Brown SVL, Higgenbotham E, et al: Sympathetic ophthalmia following Nd:YAG cyclotherapy. Ophthalmic Surg 20:544, 1989.

83. Minckler DS: Does Nd:YAG cyclotherapy cause sympathetic ophthalmia? Ophthalmic Surg 20:543, 1989.

84. Sabates R: Choroiditis compatible with the histopathologic diagnosis of sympathetic ophthalmia following cyclocryotherapy of neovascular glaucoma. Ophthalmic Surg 19:176, 1988.

85. Fries PD, Char DH, Crawford JB, Waterhouse W: Sympathetic ophthalmia complicating helium ion irradiation of a choroidal melanoma. Arch Ophthalmol 105:1561, 1987.

86. Fiore PM, Latina MA: A technique for precise placement of laser applications in transscleral Nd:YAG cyclophotocoagulation. Am J Ophthalmol 107:292, 1989.

87. Brancato R, Leoni G, Trabucchi E, et al: Transscleral contact cyclophotocoagulation with CW Nd:YAG laser: Experimental study on rabbit eyes. Int J Tissue React 6:493, 1987.

88. Federman JL, Ando F, Schubert HD, et al: Contact laser for transscleral photocoagulation. Ophthalmic Surg 18:183, 1987.

89. Schubert HD, Federman JL: A comparison of CW Nd:YAG contact transscleral cyclophotocoagulation with cyclocryopexy. Invest Ophthalmol Vis Sci 30:536, 1989.

90. Schubert HD, Federman JL: The role of inflammation in CW Nd:YAG contact transscleral photocoagulation and cryopexy. Invest Ophthalmol Vis Sci 30:543, 1989.

91. Latina MA, Patel S, de Kater AW, et al: Transscleral cyclophotocoagulation using a contact laser probe: A histologic and clinical study in rabbits. Lasers Surg Med 9:437, 1989.

92. Crymes BM, Gross RL: Laser placement in noncontact Nd:YAG cyclophotocoagulation. Am J Ophthalmol 110:670, 1990.

93. Peyman GA, Katoh N, Tawakol M, et al: Transscleral and intravitreal contact Nd:YAG laser application: An experimental study. Retina 7:190, 1987.

94. van der Zypen E, England C, Fankhauser F, Kwasniewska S: Cyclophotocoagulation in glaucoma therapy. Int Ophthalmol 13:163, 1989.

95. van der Zypen E, England C, Fankhauser F, Kwasniewska S: The effect of transscleral laser cyclophotocoagulation on rabbit ciliary body vascularization. Graefes Arch Clin Exp Ophthalmol 227:172, 1989.

96. Iwach AG, Drake MV, Hoskins HDJ, et al: A new contact neodymium:YAG laser for cyclophotocoagulation. Ophthalmic Surg 22:345, 1991.

97. Brooks DE: Glaucoma in the dog and cat. Vet Clin North Am Small Anim Pract 20:775, 1990.

98. Allingham RR, de Kater AW, Hsu J, et al: Probe placement and power levels in contact transscleral neodymium:YAG cyclophotocoagulation. Arch Ophthalmol 108:738, 1990.

99. Brancato R, Leoni G, Trabucchi G, Cappellini A: Probe placement and energy levels in continuous wave neodymium-YAG contact transscleral cyclophotocoagulation. Arch Ophthalmol 108:679, 1990.

100. Schuman JS, Puliafito CA, Allingham RR, et al: Contact transscleral Nd:YAG laser cyclophotocoagulation. Ophthalmology 97:571, 1990.

101. Brancato R, Giovanni L, Trabucchi G, et al: Contact transscleral cyclophotocoagulation with Nd:YAG laser in uncontrolled glaucoma. Ophthalmic Surg 20:547, 1989.

102. Schuman JS, Bellows AR, Shingleton BJ, et al: Contact transscleral Nd:YAG laser cyclophotocoagulation: Mid-term results. Ophthalmology 99:1089, 1992.

103. Schuman JS, Jacobson JJ, Puliafito CA, et al: Experimental use of semiconductor diode laser in contact transscleral cyclophotocoagulation in rabbits. Arch Ophthalmol 108:1152, 1990.

104. Brancato R, Leoni G, Trabucchi G, Cappellini A: Histopathology of continuous wave neodymium:yttrium aluminum garnet and diode laser contact transscleral lesions in rabbit ciliary body: A comparative study. Invest Ophthalmol Vis Sci 32:1586, 1991.

105. Schuman JS, Noecker RJ, Puliafito CA, et al: Energy levels and probe placement in contact transscleral semiconductor diode laser cyclophotocoagulation in human cadaver eyes. Arch Ophthalmol 109:1534, 1991.

106. Hennis HL, Assia E, Stewart WC, et al: Transscleral cyclophotocoagulation using a semiconductor diode laser in cadaver eyes. Ophthalmic Surg 22:274, 1991.

107. Shepps GJ, Schuman JS, Wang N, Puliafito CA: Non-contact versus contact semiconductor diode laser transscleral cyclophotocoagulation in rabbits. Invest Ophthalmol Vis Sci 32(Suppl):861, 1991.

108. Vogel A, Dlugos C, Nuffer R, Birngruber R: Optical properties of human sclera, and their consequences for transscleral laser applications. Lasers Surg Med 11:331, 1991.

109. Assia EI, Hennis HL, Stewart WC, et al: A comparison of neodymium: yttrium aluminum garnet and diode laser transscleral cyclophotocoagulation and cyclocryotherapy. Invest Ophthalmol Vis Sci 32:2774, 1991.

110. Hennis HL, Stewart WC: Semiconductor diode laser transscleral cyclophotocoagulation in patients with glaucoma. Am J Ophthalmol 113:81, 1992.

111. Freyler H, Scheimbauer I: Excision of the ciliary body (Sautter procedure) as a last resort in secondary glaucoma. Klin Monatsbl Augenheilkd 179:473, 1981.

112. Gaasterland DE, Abrams DA, Belcher CD, et al: A multicenter study of contact diode laser transscleral cyclophotocoagulation in glaucoma patients. Invest Ophthalmol Vis Sci 33(Suppl):1019, 1992.

113. Carassa RG, Trabucchi G, Bettin P, et al: Contact transscleral cyclophotocoagulation (CTCP) with diode laser: A pilot clinical study. Invest Ophthalmol Vis Sci 33(Suppl): 1019, 1992.

114. Higginbotham EJ, Harrison M, Zou XL: Cyclophotocoagulation with the transscleral contact neodymium:YAG laser versus cyclocryotherapy in rabbits. Ophthalmic Surg 22:27, 1991.

115. Suzuki Y, Araie M, Yumita A, Yamamoto T: Transscleral Nd:YAG laser cyclophotocoagulation versus cyclocryotherapy. Graefes Arch Clin Exp Ophthalmol 229:33, 1991.

116. Noureddin BN, Wilson-Holt N, Lavin M, et al: Advanced uncontrolled glaucoma: Nd:YAG cyclophotocoagulation or tube surgery. Ophthalmology 99:430, 1992.

117. Schubert HD: Noncontact and contact pars plana transscleral neodymium:YAG laser cyclophotocoagulation in postmortem eyes. Ophthalmology 96:1471, 1989.

118. Schubert HD, Agarwala A, Arbizo V: Changes in aqueous outflow after in vitro neodymium:yttrium aluminum garnet laser cyclophotocoagulation. Invest Ophthalmol Vis Sci 31:1834, 1990.

119. Pham-Duy T: Cyclocryotherapy in chronic glaucoma. Fortschr Ophthalmol 86:214, 1989.

120. Higginbotham EJ, Lee DA, Bartels SP, et al: Effects of cyclocryotherapy on aqueous humor dynamics in cats. Arch Ophthalmol 106:396, 1988.

121. Schmidt KG, Lee PY, Bhuyan DK, et al: The role of prostaglandins (PGs) and uveoscleral outflow (Fu) in the reduction of intraocular pressure (IOP) after contact transscleral Nd:YAG laser cyclophotocoagulation (CYC) in pigmented rabbits. Invest Ophthalmol Vis Sci 33(Suppl):1269, 1992.

122. Zaidman GW, Wandel T: Transscleral YAG laser photocoagulation for uncontrollable glaucoma in corneal patients. Cornea 7:112, 1988.

123. Levy NS, Bonney RC: Transscleral YAG cyclocoagulation of the ciliary body for persistently high intraocular pressure following penetrating keratoplasty. Cornea 8:178, 1989.

124. Cohen EJ, Schwartz LW, Luskind RD, et al: Neodymium:YAG laser transscleral cyclophotocoagulation for glaucoma after penetrating keratoplasty. Ophthalmic Surg 20:713, 1989.

125. Coleman AL, Jampel HD, Javitt JC, et al: Transscleral cyclophotocoagulation of human autopsy and monkey eyes. Ophthalmic Surg 22:638, 1991.

Chapter 148

■

New Surgical Techniques in Glaucoma Management

DAVID ANSON LEE

An understanding of the basic mechanisms of glaucoma and the biologic response following surgical therapy is essential to develop effective and safe surgical techniques for glaucoma management. Glaucoma is a diverse group of ocular disorders linked by intraocular pressure (IOP) as a major risk factor and progressive optic neuropathy, which may cause irreversible vision loss if not treated appropriately. Fortunately, effective medical, laser, and surgical therapies exist to prevent blindness from glaucoma, but these treatments are not completely safe and effective. IOP can be reduced either by decreasing aqueous humor production or by increasing aqueous humor drainage out of the eye. All aqueous humor drainage procedures utilize the principles of glaucoma filtration surgery, which creates an opening or fistula (sclerostomy) at the limbal region of the eye to facilitate aqueous humor drainage, bypassing the pathologic blockage in the anterior chamber angle. The aqueous humor enters an artificial reservoir between the conjunctiva and sclera and eventually filters through the conjunctiva into the tear film or is absorbed by the conjunctival and episcleral vasculature. A variety of surgical procedures have been devised to drain the aqueous humor. These procedures are all subject to wound-healing phenomenon, which may influence the ultimate success of the procedure.

Wound healing involves a complex, natural, and normal series of events that occur over a limited period of time and result in scar formation (Fig. 148–1).[1, 2] The process begins with the surgical injury, which results in vascular leakage of cells and proteins, causing inflammation and clot formation. Prostaglandins and leukotrienes are synthesized at the wound, mediate many aspects of inflammation, and have chemotactic effects on leukocytes. Platelets and extravascular procoagulants such as fibrinogen, fibrin, and fibronectin are the major factors that promote rapid clotting of trapped plasma and blood proteins.

Platelets stimulate cellular migration into wounds by releasing platelet derived growth factors (PDGF). Neutrophils, the major function of which is to prevent infection in the injured tissue, are the first cells to enter the wound and are attracted by chemotactic factors secreted by platelets, leukotrienes, and complement. Their proteolytic enzymes digest tissue debris in preparation for phagocytosis by macrophages. Neutrophils achieve their maximum activity acutely by 2 days after wounding and rapidly decrease during the next few days (Fig. 148–2).

Macrophages, which enter the healing site from the surrounding tissue and also differentiate from hematogenous monocytes, phagocytose necrotic tissue and débride the wound to prepare it for fibroblastic proliferation. They also secrete lymphokines and monokines, such as interleukins that promote fibroblast migration and proliferation as well as prepare the immune system against infectious agents. Macrophages are most active at the wound site 3 days after injury, and their activity begins to decrease by the fifth day after an injury (see Fig. 148–2).

Granulation tissue is formed by fibroblastic and vascular endothelial cells that are attracted into the wound by the clot and by growth factors secreted by macrophages and platelets. The fibroblasts originate from mesenchymal cells in the surrounding tissue, which dedifferentiate into fibroblasts and migrate into the wound. Fibronectin, cytokines, and serum proteins stimulate the migratory process. Fibroblasts are the major producers of connective tissue including collagen, elastin, and mucopolysaccharides, all of which are regulated by numerous tissue hormonal factors. Fibroblasts are most active at the wound's site as early as 3 to 5 days after injury; their activity lasts for several months until the wound-healing process is complete (see Fig. 148–2).

Angiogenesis (new capillary formation) immediately follows the migration of fibroblasts into the wound, providing nutrition and oxygen to the metabolically active fibroblasts. Many different cytokines and angiogenic factors have been identified that promote the migration and proliferation of these vascular endothelial cells.

The primary component of scar tissue is collagen, which is synthesized and secreted by the fibroblasts. Type III collagen is the first component to fill the wound and is replaced later by type I collagen as the scar tissue matures and granulation tissue regresses. The degree of collagen cross-linking (not the amount of collagen deposited) determines the strength of scar tissue. Wound closure is ultimately achieved by a combination of epithelialization and contraction of myofibroblasts, which are differentiated fibroblasts resembling smooth muscle cells. Finally, the remodeling phase of wound healing begins as collagen matures and polymerizes. This process lasts for more than 1 yr.

The wound-healing sequence is similar in all species and organ systems and is essential to an organism's survival. This dynamic and complex process, which involves several different cell types and numerous

1678

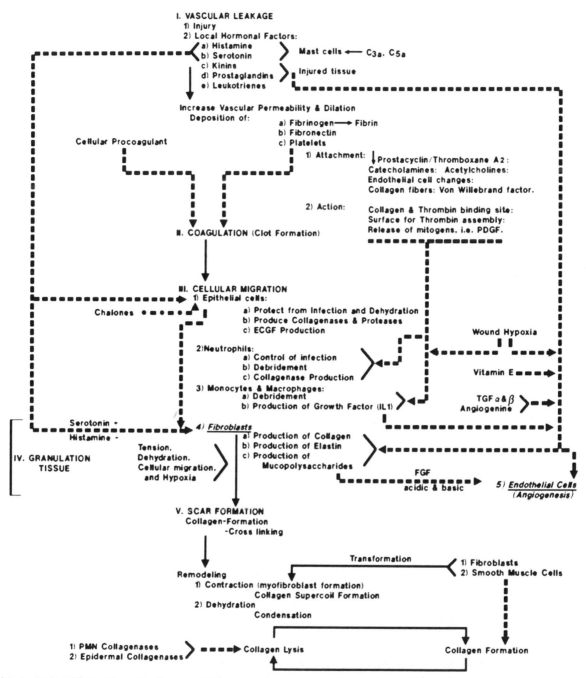

Figure 148–1. A simplified schematic diagram of the complex wound-healing pathways illustrating the overlapping relationships of the different components involved in wound healing. (From Tahery MM, Lee DA: Pharmacologic control of wound healing in glaucoma filtration surgery. J Ocul Pharmacol 5:155, 1989.)

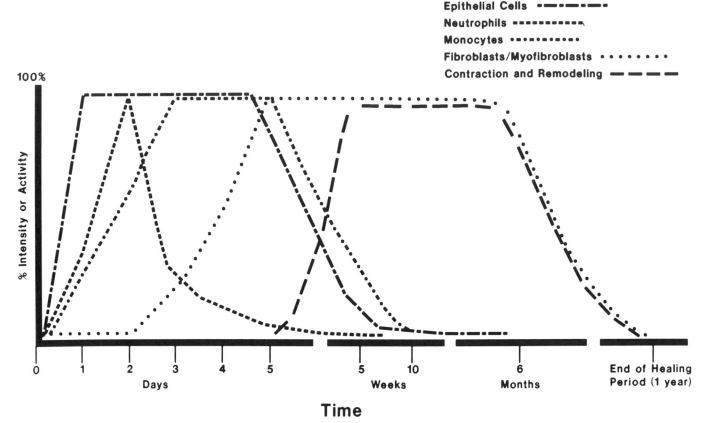

Figure 148–2. A semiquantitative diagram of the chronological sequence of the cellular components involved in the wound healing process. (From Tahery MM, Lee DA: Pharmacologic control of wound healing in glaucoma filtration surgery. J Ocul Pharmacol 5:155, 1989.)

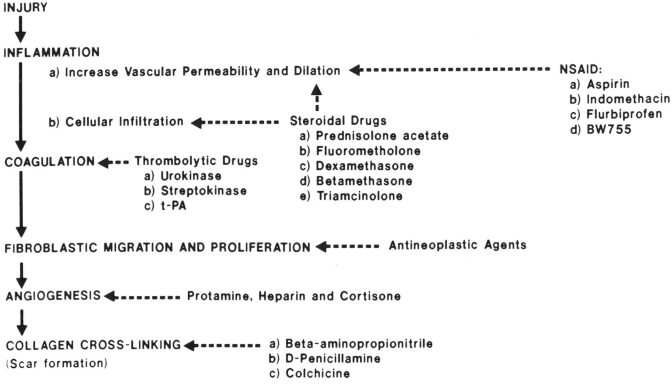

Figure 148–3. A schematic diagram of various drugs used to inhibit ocular wound-healing and their modes of action at different stages of the wound-healing process. (From Tahery MM, Lee DA: Pharmacologic control of wound healing in glaucoma filtration surgery. J Ocul Pharmacol 5:155, 1989.)

growth factors and feedback loops, makes the clinical modulation of the wound-healing process challenging.

Many synthetic and natural compounds may be useful in controlling the wound-healing process to minimize excessive scar tissue formation and maximize the success of glaucoma filtering surgery (Fig. 148–3). Steroidal and nonsteroidal antiinflammatory drugs inhibit prostaglandin synthesis and decrease the initial inflammatory response. Topical steroids significantly improve the success of trabeculectomy.[3] Various thrombolytic agents can minimize fibrin deposition and limit clot formation, thus inhibiting scar formation. Several antineoplastic cancer drugs can nonspecifically inhibit metabolically active cells in the proliferative phase of wound healing.[4-8] Their cytotoxic effects interfere with DNA, RNA, or protein synthesis or cell division to inhibit fibroblast proliferation. The antimetabolites are structural analogs to nucleic acids and interfere with DNA and RNA synthesis. 5-Fluorouracil and cytarabine have been used to inhibit ocular fibroblast proliferation. Unfortunately, they can also inhibit corneal epithelial cell mitosis and cause corneal erosions.[9] Natural plant alkaloids and antibiotic agents such as mitomycin cause mitotic arrest and inhibit DNA-dependent RNA synthesis. These agents can nonspecifically inhibit fibroblast proliferation and decrease scar tissue formation.[10] Agents that inhibit angiogenesis, such as protamine and the combination of heparin and cortisone, may potentially decrease scar formation. Drugs that inhibit collagen formation and cross-linking include colchicine, which interferes with microtubule-mediated intracellular translocation of collagen in fibroblasts; β-aminopropionitrile, which inhibits lysyl oxidase to prevent collagen cross-linking; and D-penicillamine, which chelates copper and interferes with collagen cross-linking.[11, 12] These nonphysiologic and relatively nonspecific wound-healing modifiers have greater potential for adverse side effects than do physiologic and relatively specific modulators such as gamma interferon. Antibodies and immunoconjugates (antibody-toxin conjugates) directed against growth factor receptors or other surface proteins such as transferrin receptors, which are selectively expressed in actively proliferating fibroblasts, may also prevent scar tissue formation with minimal adverse side effects. Other as yet undefined mediators of wound healing in aqueous humor[13] and perigraph seroma[14] potentially may be useful to control ocular scarring.

Various models, including tissue culture and animal models, have been developed to simulate the complex wound-healing process. All are limited in accurately portraying the human ocular wound-healing response. Tissue culture models have the advantage of isolating and quantitatively measuring the individual wound-healing process of fibroblast attachment, migration, proliferation, and extracellular matrix synthesis.[15-19] Unfortunately, the complex immune response and vascular system cannot be simulated accurately in vitro. Therefore, animal models of ocular wound healing are necessary to study the interactions of several simultaneously occurring wound-healing processes. Rabbits[10, 20-22] and monkeys[23, 24] most commonly have been used to study the human ocular wound-healing process primarily be- cause of their convenience and eye size. However, both models are limited because their ocular wound-healing response is much more intense and rapid than that found in humans.

Potential agents first are tested in the tissue culture models to measure their relative potencies and mechanisms of action. Those that seem to be most promising may be tested further in the animal models for safety and efficacy. The substances with the greatest potential for clinical application may be tested further in prospective and controlled human trials (Fig. 148–4).

The most common modes of ocular drug delivery are topical application of eye drops or ointments or injection of medications into the surrounding tissues of the eye, subconjunctiva, or subtenons. Orally or intravenously administered drugs are usually not as effective in achieving high intraocular drug concentrations over extended periods. Topical medications commonly used after glaucoma surgery to control intraocular inflammation, in prophylaxis against infection, and for ocular comfort include steroids (prednisolone acetate and decadron), antibiotics, cycloplegic agents, and sometimes nonsteroidal antiinflammatory agents (ibuprofen). Topical steroids are important in controlling the wound-healing response to ensure optimum surgical success. Subconjunctival injections of steroids (triamcinolone) before surgery may decrease scar formation.[25] The most widely used antimetabolite to limit wound healing following filtering surgery is 5-fluorouracil, which is injected subconjunctivally.[8] Its disadvantages are the necessity for frequent injections and poorly localized drug delivery.

Other methods for delivering antimetabolites in a more localized and sustained manner include the use of liposomes, collagen sponges, and biodegradable polymers. Liposomes are small vesicles that consist of a phospholipid bilayer that contains drugs.[26] These drug-filled liposomes may be injected at the treatment site, thus avoiding more extensive surgical manipulation. Unfortunately, it has been found that these liposomes may release their drugs before the phospholipid bilayer dissolves. The residual phospholipids may create an inflammatory reaction. In the situation in which the liposomes or their delivered drugs are toxic to the eye, it may be difficult to remove the liposomes completely before they spontaneously dissolve.

Biodegradable collagen sponges impregnated with antimetabolites such as 5-fluorouracil and bleomycin have been implanted during glaucoma filtration surgery to prevent scar tissue formation.[27, 28] In preliminary trials, it appears that the delivered drug is depleted before the collagen matrix completely degrades. The duration of drug delivery is only a few days following implantation. The collagen matrix, depleted of drug, may incite an inflammatory reaction at the implantation site and cause further scar tissue formation.

Synthetic biodegradable materials such as polyanhydrides have been used to deliver drugs to prevent excessive wound healing following glaucoma filtering surgery in animals (Fig. 148–5).[20-22, 24] Biodegradable polymers are particularly well suited for this purpose and have advantages over other ocular drug delivery

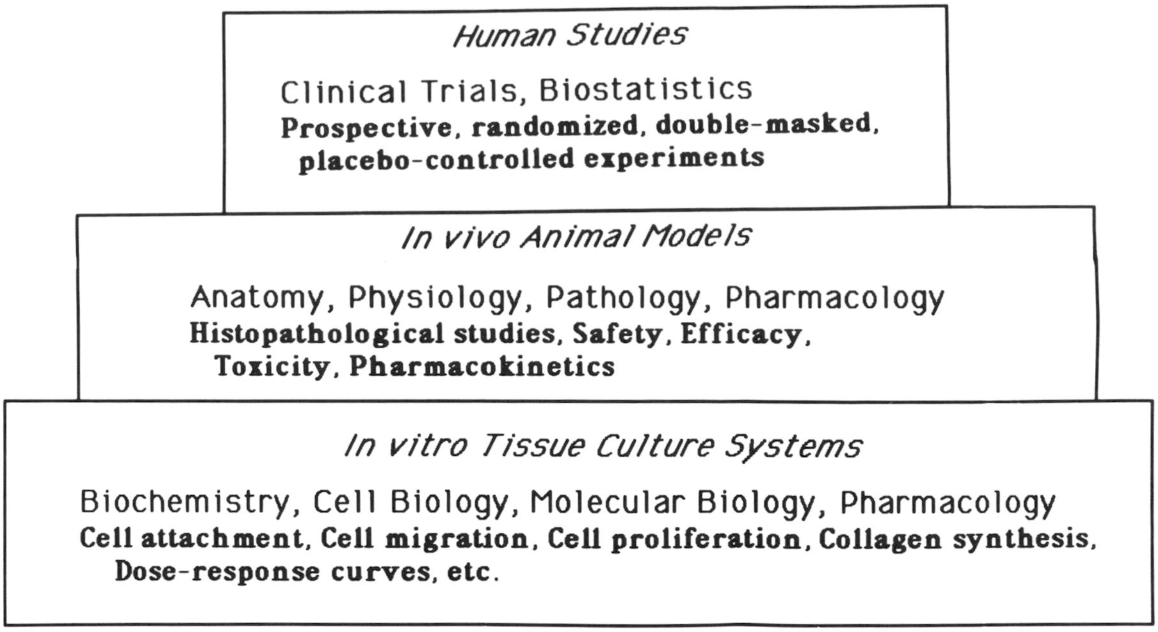

Human Studies
Clinical Trials, Biostatistics
Prospective, randomized, double-masked, placebo-controlled experiments
In vivo Animal Models
Anatomy, Physiology, Pathology, Pharmacology
Histopathological studies, Safety, Efficacy, Toxicity, Pharmacokinetics
In vitro Tissue Culture Systems
Biochemistry, Cell Biology, Molecular Biology, Pharmacology
Cell attachment, Cell migration, Cell proliferation, Collagen synthesis, Dose-response curves, etc.

Figure 148–4. An approach to the scientific investigation of modulating the wound-healing response utilizing tissue culture, animal models and clinical trials.

systems in that they allow localized and sustained release of medication to the intended treatment site. Because the medication can be delivered directly to the treatment site, less drug is necessary, thus decreasing the potential risk of ocular and systemic side effects. When the drug or polymer causes an adverse side effect, the entire solid monolithic biodegradable device can be removed from its implantation site. This drug delivery system has potential mechanical advantages similar to a seton, which supports the opening of a drainage area. The shape of this device can be changed to a disc, cylinder, or sphere that can alter the surface erosion characteristics of the polymer. These biodegradable polymers may be laminated with different types of medication to deliver specific drugs in sequential order to control several different stages of wound healing (Fig. 148–6). Since the biodegradable polymer eventually dissolves, there is less chance of long-term foreign body complications such as infection and extrusion.

A series of experiments were performed in which biodegradable polymers impregnated with 5-fluorouracil[20, 21] and mitomycin[22] were implanted at the time of glaucoma filtering surgery in rabbit eyes. These experiments showed a definite decrease in IOP in the eyes that received the devices. Unfortunately, the IOP lowering effect and wound-healing inhibitory effect were limited, and the drugs were depleted from the polymer matrix before the entire matrix had dissolved. The polymer matrix was noninflammatory and nontoxic, but zero-order drug-release kinetics was not achieved. Future developments in polymer technology may allow drugs to be covalently linked to the polymer matrix so that their delivery is more sustained, and zero-order kinetics is achieved throughout the wound-healing response.

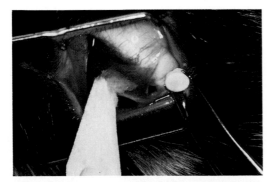

Figure 148–5. A disc-shaped polymer impregnated with experimental drug that is being placed adjacent to the sclerostomy site during glaucoma filtration surgery. (From Lee DA, Leong KW, Panek WC, et al: The use of bioerodible polymers and 5-fluorouracil in glaucoma filtration surgery. Invest Ophthalmol Vis Sci 29:1692, 1988.)

Laminated Biodegradable Polymers
Anti-Inflammatory Drugs
Anti-Proliferative Drugs
Collagen Cross-Linking Inhibitory Drugs

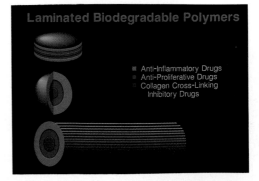

Figure 148–6. Biodegradable polymers of different shapes that release their drugs by surface erosion may be laminated so that they can release different drugs at each of the different stages of healing.

INDICATIONS OF TREATMENT

Patients with glaucoma who are at greatest risk of glaucoma filtering surgery failure due to excessive scar tissue formation include patients who have had previously unsuccessful glaucoma filtering surgery, aphakia or pseudophakia, ocular inflammatory disorders, and neovascularization of the anterior ocular segment.[29-32] In addition, those who are young and black patients may have unsuccessful surgeries.[33-35] Others who may benefit from the use of wound-healing retardants following primary or secondary glaucoma filtering surgery include patients with low-tension glaucoma and patients undergoing combined cataract extraction and glaucoma filtering surgery. In these situations, agents that control the wound-healing process may increase the success rate of glaucoma filtering surgery as well as achieve lower postoperative IOPs. As safer wound-healing inhibitors are discovered, they may be used even more commonly during and after uncomplicated primary filtering surgery.

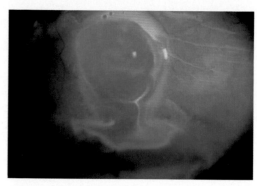

Figure 148–7. Fluorescein staining of a thin cystic bleb with a slow leak in an eye that underwent trabeculectomy with 5-fluorouracil several months earlier.

TECHNIQUE

The field of ocular wound-healing modulation is continually evolving; new agents to specifically control the wound-healing response and new drug delivery systems to control local and sustained release of medications for improved safety, efficacy, and convenience are being developed. Presently, the most common way to inhibit the wound-healing process following glaucoma filtering surgery is by subconjunctival injection of 5-fluorouracil. Briefly, 1 or 2 drops of proparacaine hydrochloride 0.5 percent is used to topically anesthetize the treated eye. A cotton pledget soaked with anesthetic is then applied to the intended injection site for approximately 2 min. A solution of 5-fluorouracil is constituted in a concentration of 10 mg/ml in sterile, normal saline. Five milligrams of 5-fluorouracil in 0.5 ml is injected using a 30-gauge needle subconjunctivally 90 to 180 degrees away from the bleb. These injections are usually given twice a day during the first postoperative week and once a day during the second postoperative week. The injections may be titrated according to the clinical appearance of the postoperative bleb and the cornea.

POSTOPERATIVE MANAGEMENT

The usual topical postoperative medications, including steroids, antibiotics, and cycloplegic agents, may be used during the treatment with 5-fluorouracil. The patient should be examined carefully by slit-lamp biomicroscopy before each injection for evidence of corneal epithelial toxicity and bleb leaks. If these are seen, the injections of 5-fluorouracil should be discontinued; they may be resumed, if necessary, following the resolution of corneal epithelial toxicity and bleb leaks. It has been noted that 5-fluorouracil may create very thin, cystic blebs that may leak several weeks or months after treatment is discontinued (Fig. 148–7). Hypotony usually occurs in the postoperative period, and there may be an increased

risk of suprachoroidal hemorrhaging. Therefore, patients should wear adequate protection over the operated eye; have limited activity (preferably bedrest); and avoid bending, stooping, and straining.

COMMON COMPLICATIONS

Following treatment with 5-fluorouracil, the complications are secondary to its nonspecific antimetabolic effects on dividing cells.[9] The most common complications include corneal epithelial keratopathy and erosions, which are reversible when 5-fluorouracil is discontinued. Filtering bleb leaks, which increase the risk of postoperative endophthalmitis, may occur early and late in the postoperative course and are probably related to conjunctival epithelial toxicity. Profound hypotony and suprachoroidal hemorrhaging may occur. There may be a small risk of hematologic and bone marrow suppression as a systemic side effect from 5-fluorouracil.

CONCLUSION

There are exciting new developments on the horizon for wound-healing modulation to improve our present surgical techniques in management of glaucoma. Many of these developments will probably involve use of more specific, natural, and physiologic modulators to address the different stages of the wound-healing process. In addition, advances will occur in localized, sustained-release, safe, and convenient drug delivery systems to address the various stages of the complex wound-healing process.

Acknowledgment

The author is grateful for the support from NIH grants EYO7701 and EY00331, Research to Prevent Blindness, and the Lucille Ellis Simon Glaucoma Research Fund.

REFERENCES

1. Tahery MM, Lee DA: Pharmacologic control of wound healing in glaucoma filtration surgery. J Ocul Pharmacol 5:155, 1989.
2. Skuta GL, Parrish RK: Wound healing in glaucoma filtering surgery. Surv Ophthalmol 32:149, 1987.

3. Starita RJ, Fellman RL, Spaeth GL, et al: Short and long term effects of postoperative corticosteroids and trabeculectomy. Ophthalmology 92:938, 1985.

4. Gressel MG, Parrish RK, Folberg R: 5-Fluorouracil and glaucoma filtering surgery. I: An animal model. Ophthalmology 91:378, 1984.

5. Heuer DK, Parrish RK, Gressel MG, et al: 5-Fluorouracil and glaucoma filtering surgery. II: A pilot study. Ophthalmology 91:384, 1984.

6. Heuer DK, Parrish RK, Gressel MG, et al: 5-Fluorouracil and glaucoma filtering surgery. III: Intermediate follow-up of a pilot study. Ophthalmology 93:1537, 1986.

7. Heuer DK, Gressel MG, Parrish RK, et al: Topical fluorouracil. II: Postoperative administration in an animal model of glaucoma filtering surgery. Arch Ophthalmol 104:132, 1986.

8. The Fluorouracil Filtering Surgery Study Group: Fluorouracil filtering study one year follow-up. Am J Ophthalmol 108:625, 1989.

9. Lee DA, Hersh P, Kersten D, Melamed S: Complications of subconjunctival 5-fluorouracil following glaucoma filtration surgery. Ophthalmic Surg 18:187, 1987.

10. Wilson MR, Lee DA, Baker RS, et al: The effects of topical mitomycin on glaucoma filtration surgery in rabbits. J Ocul Pharmacol 7:1, 1991.

11. Moorhead LC, Smith J, Stewart R, Kimbrough R: Effects of beta-aminopropionitrile after glaucoma filtration surgery: Pilot human trial. Ann Ophthalmol 19:223, 1987.

12. McGuigan LJB, Cook DJ, Yablonski ME: Dexamethasone, D-penicillamine, and glaucoma filtering surgery in rabbits. Invest Ophthalmol Vis Sci 27:1755, 1986.

13. Kornbleuth W, Tenebaum E: The inhibitory effect of aqueous humor on the growth of cells in tissue cultures. Am J Ophthalmol 42:70, 1956.

14. Ahn SS, Machleder HI, Gupta R, Moore WS: Perigraft seroma: Clinical, histological, and serologic correlates. Am J Surg 154:173, 1987.

15. Givens KT, Lee DA, Rothschiller J, et al: Antiproliferative drugs and human ocular fibroblasts: Colorimetric vs. cell counting assays. Curr Eye Res 9:599, 1990.

16. Givens KT, Kitada S, Chen AK, et al: Proliferation of human ocular fibroblasts: An assessment of in vitro colorimetric assays. Invest Ophthalmol Vis Sci 31:1856, 1990.

17. Lee DA, Tehrani SS, Kitada S: The effect of 5-fluorouracil and cytarabine on human fibroblasts from Tenon's capsule. Invest Ophthalmol Vis Sci 31:1848, 1990.

18. Lee DA, Lee TC, Cortez AE, Kitada S: Effects of mithramycin, mitomycin, daunorubicin, and bleomycin on human subconjunctival fibroblast attachment and proliferation. Invest Ophthalmol Vis Sci 31:2136, 1990.

19. Wong VKW, Tehrani SS, Kitada S, et al: Inhibition of rabbit ocular fibroblast proliferation by 5-fluorouracil and cytosine arabinoside. J Ocul Pharmacol 7:27, 1991.

20. Lee DA, Flores RA, Anderson PJ, et al: Glaucoma filtration surgery in rabbits using bioerodible polymers and 5-fluorouracil. Ophthalmology 94:1523, 1987.

21. Lee DA, Leong KW, Panek WC, et al: The use of bioerodible polymers and 5-fluorouracil in glaucoma filtration surgery. Invest Ophthalmol Vis Sci 29:1692, 1988.

22. Charles JB, Ganthier R, Wilson MR, et al: The use of bioerodible polymers impregnated with mitomycin in glaucoma filtration surgery in rabbits. Ophthalmology 98:503, 1991.

23. Jampel HD, McGuigan LJB, Dunkelberger GR, et al: Cellular proliferation after experimental glaucoma filtration surgery. Arch Ophthalmol 106:89, 1988.

24. Jampel HD, Leong KW, Dunkelberger GR, Quigley HA: Glaucoma filtration surgery in monkeys using 5-fluorouridine in polyanhydride disks. Arch Ophthalmol 108:430, 1990.

25. Giangiacomo J, Dueker DK, Adelstein E: The effect of preoperative subconjunctival triamcinolone administration on glaucoma filtration. I: Trabeculectomy following subconjunctival triamcinolone. Arch Ophthalmol 104:838, 1986.

26. Assil KK, Lane J, Weinreb RN: Sustained release of antimetabolite 5-fluorouridine-5'-monophosphate by multivesicular liposomes. Ophthalmic Surg 19:408, 1988.

27. Kay JS, Litin BS, Jones MA, et al: Delivery of antifibroblast agents as adjuncts to filtration surgery. Part II: Delivery of 5-fluorouracil and bleomycin in a collagen implant: Pilot study in the rabbit. Ophthalmic Surg 17:796, 1986.

28. Herschler J, Kay JS, Litin BS, Chvapil M: Drug delivery of antimetabolites as adjuncts to glaucoma filtration surgery: Preliminary clinical experience. In Krieglstein GK (ed): Glaucoma Update III. Heidelberg, Springer-Verlag, 1987, pp 215–219.

29. Bellows AR, Johnstone MA: Surgical management of chronic glaucoma in aphakia. Ophthalmology 90:807, 1983.

30. Heuer DK, Gressel MG, Parrish RK, et al: Trabeculectomy in aphakic eyes. Ophthalmology 91:1045, 1984.

31. Jampel HD, Jabs DA, Quigley HA: Trabeculectomy with 5-fluorouracil for adult inflammatory glaucoma. Am J Ophthalmol 109:168, 1990.

32. Parrish RK, Herschler J: Eyes with end-staging neovascular glaucoma: Natural history following successful modified filtering operation. Arch Ophthalmol 101:745, 1983.

33. Beauchamp GR, Parks MM: Filtering surgery in children: Barriers to success. Ophthalmology 86:170, 1979.

34. Gressel MG, Heuer DK, Parrish RK: Trabeculectomy in young patients. Ophthalmology 91:1242, 1984.

35. Miller RD, Barber JC: Trabeculectomy in black patients. Ophthalmic Surg 12:46, 1981.

SECTION VIII

Lids

Edited by
JOHN J. WOOG and FREDERICK A. JAKOBIEC

Chapter 149

■

Eyelid Disorders: Overview and Clinical Examination

JOHN J. WOOG

OVERVIEW

The eyelids play an important role in the maintenance of the normal structure and function of the eye and visual system.[1] The eyelids, eyelashes, and eyebrow, in conjunction with the bone orbit, constitute the primary source of mechanical protection of the globe from noxious environmental influences. From the physiologic perspective, voluntary and involuntary eyelid movement comprise one level of regulation of the entry of light into the eye and visual pathways. In addition, the phenomenon of spontaneous blinking is important in the continuous resurfacing and replenishment of the precorneal tear film, components of which are secreted by aqueous, sebaceous, and mucinous glands contained within the eyelids and adjacent conjunctiva.[2] It is thus clear that abnormalities of the eyelids may compromise visual function and the structural integrity of the globe.

Numerous disorders listed in Table 149–1 may affect the eyelids, and these disorders are discussed in detail in the chapters that follow. In anticipation of this discussion, we conclude this introductory chapter with a brief review of the clinical examination of the patient with an eyelid disorder.

CLINICAL EXAMINATION

Important features of the examination of the patient with an eyelid abnormality are summarized in Table 149–2 and are described below.

Ophthalmic Examination

Eyelid abnormalities may be associated with changes in virtually every aspect of the eye examination. Tri-

Table 149–1. EYELID DISORDERS

Congenital anomalies
Infectious disorders
Benign epithelial tumors
Basal cell carcinoma
Premalignant lesions and squamous cell carcinoma
Sebaceous gland tumors
Sweat gland and hair tumors
Pigmented eyelid lesions
Other inflammatory and neoplastic eyelid lesions
Upper eyelid malpositions: ptosis and retraction
Lower eyelid malpositions: entropion and ectropion
Disorders of the eyebrows and eyelashes
Eyelid manifestations of systemic disease

chiasis, for example, may result in superficial punctate keratitis noted on slit-lamp examination and secondary decrease in visual acuity. Congenital ptosis may be associated with limitation of upgaze on motility testing. Similarly, eyelid retraction may be encountered with proptosis in the setting of dysthyroid orbitopathy. Other examples of important associations between eyelid abnormalities and ocular disease include the findings of eyelid thickening, contour abnormalities, and ipsilateral glaucoma in patients with neurofibromatosis, as well as the occasional presence of widespread conjunctival and corneal involvement in patients with sebaceous cell carcinoma of the eyelid. A complete eye examination is thus an important component of the evaluation of the patient with an eyelid disorder.

Dermatologic Examination

Examination of the facial skin may reveal evidence of primary dermatoses such as acne rosacea or psoriasis, which may be important in the pathogenesis of inflammatory eyelid disease and various secondary eyelid malpositions.

Eyelid Examination

PALPEBRAL FISSURE MEASUREMENTS
(Fig. 149–1)

Assessment should be made of the size and shape of the palpebral fissure. Useful measurements of size include (1) the vertical palpebral fissure height (VPF), or distance between the upper and lower eyelid margins; (2) the palpebral fissure width (HPF), or distance between the medial and lateral commissures; and (3) the margin-reflex distance (MRD), or distance between the

Table 149–2. CLINICAL EXAMINATION

Ophthalmic examination
Dermatologic examination
Eyelid examination
　　Palpebral fissure measurements
　　Eyelid and eyebrow malpositions
　　Canthal tendon laxity
　　Eyelid muscle function
　　Eyelid skin
　　Eyelid lesions
　　Cilia

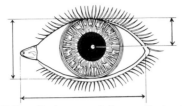

Figure 149–1. Tall vertical arrows define vertical palpebral fissure (VPF), whereas short vertical arrows delineate margin-reflex distance (MRD). Horizontal arrows denote horizontal palpebral fissure (HPF).

pupillary light reflex and the upper eyelid margin in the primary position of gaze.[3] Normal values for the MRD and VPF may vary with age but are generally considered to be 3.5 to 4.5 mm and 9 to 10 mm, respectively.[4–6] The normal HPF is approximately 28 to 30 mm in the adult patient.[7] The lower eyelid is normally at the level of the inferior limbus, although variation in lower eyelid position may occur with age.[8] The upper eyelid crease is made by subcutaneous insertion of fibers from the levator aponeurosis and is usually 8 to 11 mm from the eyelid margin.[9]

EYELID MALPOSITION

Inspection may reveal various malpositions of the eyelid margin such as ectropion, entropion, blepharoptosis, and lower eyelid retraction, as discussed in Chapters 150, 160, 161, and 162.

CANTHAL TENDON LAXITY

Assessment of medial and lateral canthal tendon laxity is important in the evaluation of patients with lower eyelid malposition, as noted in Chapter 162.

EYELID MUSCLE FUNCTION

Measurement of levator function is particularly important in the initial evaluation of patients presenting with blepharoptosis and in the planning of subsequent surgical correction. Normal levator function has approximately 12 to 17 mm.[10] Orbicularis and frontalis function should be assessed in casual and forced eyelid closure and in brow elevation, respectively.

EYELID SKIN

The coloration and integrity of the eyelid skin should be noted. Changes in texture and consistency may reflect underlying dermatologic or systemic disease.

EYELID LESIONS

Measurements are made, and photographs are taken to document the size and location of eyelid lesions. Comment may be made in terms of clinical characteristics of the lesion including mobility, nodularity, ulceration, and associated findings such as erythema, warmth, and tenderness. Various eyelid lesions are described in Chapters 151 to 159.

CILIA

Various abnormalities of the eyelid and eyebrow cilia may be observed, as described in Chapter 163.

We continue our review of eyelid disorders with a discussion of eyelid anatomy in Chapter 150.

REFERENCES

1. Moses RA: The Eyelids. *In* Moses RA: Adler's The Physiology of the Eye, 5th ed. St. Louis, CV Mosby, 1970, pp 1–16.
2. Warwick R: Wolff's Anatomy of the Eye and Orbit, 7th ed. Philadelphia, WB Saunders, 1976, p 181.
3. Putterman AM, Urist MJ: Mueller muscle-conjunctiva resection. Arch Ophthalmol 93:619–623, 1975.
4. Frueh BR: Graves' eye disease: Orbital compliance and other clinical measurements. Trans Am Ophthalmol Soc 82:493–598, 1984.
5. Sarver BL, Putterman AM: Margin limbal distance to determine amount of levator resection. Arch Ophthalmol 103:354–356, 1985.
6. Small RG, Sebates NR, Burrows D: The measurement and definition of ptosis. Ophth Plast Reconstr Surg 5:171–175, 1989.
7. Lemke BN: Anatomy of the ocular adnexa and orbit. *In* Smith BC, Della Rocca RC, Nesi FA, Lisman RD (eds): Ophthalmic Plastic and Reconstructive Surgery. St. Louis, CV Mosby, 1987, pp 1–77.
8. Shore JW: Changes in lower eyelid resting position, movement, tone with age. Am J Ophthalmol 99:415–423, 1985.
9. Doxanas MT, Anderson RL: Clinical Orbital Anatomy. Baltimore, Williams & Wilkins, 1984, p 82.
10. Beard C: Ptosis, 3rd ed. St. Louis, CV Mosby, 1981, p 28.

Chapter 150

∎

Basic Eyelid Anatomy

MARLON MAUS

The importance of the lids in the visual system cannot be overstated. Neither the anterior segment specialist nor the retina surgeon can expect successful results from their interventions without the presence of good lid function. The lids protect the eye both physically and physiologically. They provide the moisture that is required for clear vision, which in our aquatic ancestors was simply obtained from their environment. They create the complex tear film that nourishes, protects from infection, lubricates, and cleans the ocular surface of accumulated debris. They also actively excrete the tears via the lacrimal pump. An understanding of lid anatomy is therefore essential for all ophthalmologists.

The actual extent of the lids as viewed externally is easily demarcated when they are swollen. The skin of the eyelids is much thinner than surrounding skin and has a base of loose connective tissue. The upper lid has its superior border at the orbital rim, whereas the lower lid extends onto the upper portion of the malar eminence. In older individuals, it is demarcated by the malar sulcus and the nasojugal sulcus.

The surface of the eyelids is divided into two portions by a horizontal crease. The superior palpebral sulcus divides the upper lid into orbital and tarsal parts. It is 8 to 11 mm above the eyelid margin and is formed by the attachment of levator aponeurosis fibers to the skin. The crease of the lower lid is much less obvious and is formed by thin connections between the skin and the orbicular muscle of the eye.

The eyelids come together at the medial and lateral canthi. The interpalpebral fissure measures 10 to 12 mm in the adult. The lateral canthal angle is about 60 degrees and attaches laterally 2 mm higher than does the medial angle.

There are several differences between the eyelid in Asian individuals and that in white or black individuals. The Asian interpalpebral fissure is widest at the midway point; that in the occidental eyelid is widest at its medial third. The lateral canthus of the eyelid in Asians attaches 5 mm higher than does the medial canthus. The medial angle has a fold of skin called the epicanthus. There are several types described, depending on the origin and termination of the fold. The orbital septum inserts on a lower position in the Asian eyelid, resulting in the protrusion of orbital fat onto a larger area of the levator aponeurosis. This can be significant enough that the lid crease is obliterated. On primary gaze, only the upper margin of the cornea is covered by the open lid. The lower lid abuts the limbus inferiorly.

The eyelid margin is 2 mm thick and about 30 mm long. It is divided into two parts: the lateral five-sixths, or ciliary portion, and the medial sixth, or lacrimal portion. The lateral part is square, whereas the medial portion is rounded. Five millimeters from the medial angle is the punctum lacrimale, sitting on the top of the papilla lacrimalis. This mound marks the border of the medial and lateral portions of the lid. On the medial angle there is a triangular structure, the caruncle, and next to it, laterally, lies the plica semilunaris, which is of vestigial origin. This area serves as a place in which tears accumulate and is called the lacus lacrimalis (Fig. 150–1).

The eyelashes, or cilia, are modified short, thick hairs originating at the lid margins. They curve away from the globe. The upper cilia are longer and are arranged in double or triple rows. There are approximately 150 cilia in the upper lid and 75 cilia in the lower lid. The roots form the pilosebaceous units that lie within dense connective tissue anterior to the tarsus. The sebaceous glands of Zeis open into the hair follicles. Posterior to the cilia, in front of the lid margin, are the excretory ducts of the tarsal glands, or meibomian glands. They mark the border of skin and conjunctiva. Between this junction and the cilia, a gray line (sulcus of Graefe) can sometimes be seen, which is the anatomic position of a continuation of the orbicular muscle of the eye known as the muscle of Riolan. It is important as a surgical landmark (Fig. 150–2).

The eyelids have six layers, which are present at different distances from the lid margin. From superficial to deep we find (1) skin, (2) subcutaneous tissue, (3)

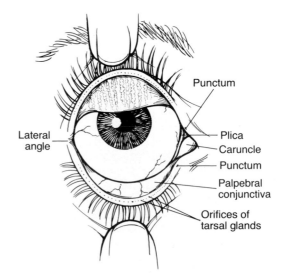

Figure 150–1. Right upper lid is everted and lower lid is pulled downward to demonstrate gross anatomy.

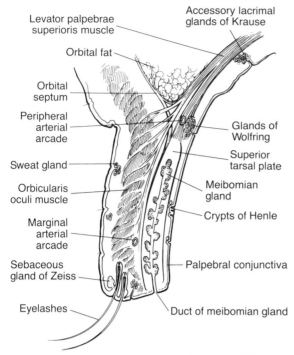

Figure 150–2. Cross section of upper eyelid.

striated orbicular muscle of the eye, (4) septum and tarsal plate, (5) smooth muscle of Müller, and (6) conjunctiva.

Depending on the level of cross section of the upper lid, the insertion of the levator muscle may also be present. At the margin, only skin, orbicular muscle, tarsus, and conjunctiva are present. Further up, the levator aponeurosis starts its insertion into the anterior border of tarsus. At the upper border of tarsus, we find the insertion of Müller's muscle. At the level of the septum, there is a fat sandwich representing the pre-aponeurotic fat pad.

The skin of the eyelids is extremely thin, only three to four cells thick. It contains numerous, fine hair follicles, with their associated sweat and sebaceous glands. Melanocytes are found in the epidermis. The dermis becomes thicker as it reaches the lid margin. Sweat glands are associated with the cilia; they are called the glands of Moll. The subcutaneous tissue, particularly in the pretarsal region, is devoid of fat.

The orbicular muscle of the eye is a striated muscle that surrounds the orbit and lids. It has several portions: the orbital portion, the preseptal portion (overlying the eyelids), and the pretarsal portion (over the tarsus)(Fig. 150–3). The pretarsal and preseptal portions form the palpebral orbicular muscle. It is innervated by branches from the facial nerve and serves to close the lids. It has several complicated relationships with the surrounding muscles. Superiorly, it interdigitates with the procerus, corrugator supercilii, and frontalis muscles. Laterally, it abuts the temporalis and masseter muscles. Inferiorly, it extends as far down as the levator muscle of the upper eyelid.

The origins of the orbital portion are, medially, from the orbital margin, the maxillary process of the frontal bone, the medial canthal tendon, and the frontal process of the maxilla. Laterally, it extends onto the temporal region and cheek. The preseptal portion continues from its medial origin at the medial canthal ligament and the lacrimal fascia around the lacrimal crest and diaphragm to the lateral canthal raphe. The pretarsal muscles form a lateral canthal ligament that inserts at the lateral orbital tubercle (of Whitnall) formed by the zygomatic bone. It is not very defined anatomically but helps support the lateral borders of the tarsal plates. Superficial to it can be found the lateral palpebral raphe, which is formed by the interdigitation of the lateral fibers of the palpebral orbicular muscle of the eye.

The medial canthal ligament divides around the lacrimal sac to merge with its fascia and attach to the posterior lacrimal crest and the frontal process of the maxillary bone. The anterior portion, which is more defined than the posterior portion, is formed by the ligaments of the orbicular muscles of the upper and lower lids (Fig. 150–4). It has, in addition, an extension to the frontal bone, which further anchors and supports the medial canthal structures. The canalicular system and lacrimal sac lie under the anterior portion of the medial canthal ligament.

The levator muscle of the upper eyelid is a striated muscle that has no counterpart in the lower lid. It is the main eyelid retractor, causing the upper lid to open through its much greater excursion than that of the lower lid. It originates outside the annulus of Zinn at the apex of the orbit and follows closely the anterior course of the superior rectus muscle of the eye, under the periorbita of the orbital roof. It changes direction 15 to 20 mm from the upper border of tarsus through the effect of the superior transverse ligament of Whitnall. This ligament is a condensation of the muscular fascia that spans the entire width of the orbit. Medially, the fibers attach to the trochlea and to the bone around the supraorbital notch. Laterally, it joins the lacrimal

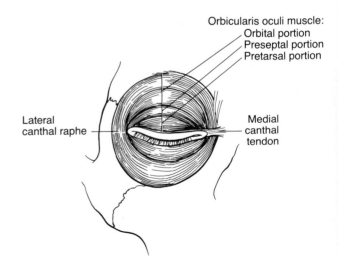

Figure 150–3. Frontal view of orbicularis oculi muscle.

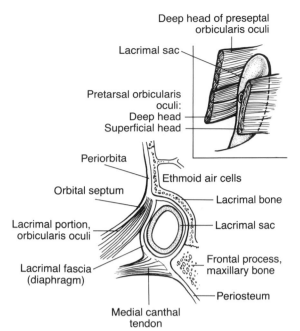

Figure 150–4. Cross-sectional view of lacrimal portion of orbicularis oculi muscle.

gland fascia to ultimately gain the support of the supralateral orbital wall. It contributes to the stability of the lacrimal gland.

Ten to 12 mm above the upper border of tarsus, the levator muscle becomes the levator aponeurosis. It has attachments in both the vertical and horizontal directions. Horizontally, it has two horns; the medial horn attaches to the medial orbital wall and the medial canthal ligament and the lateral horn divides the lacrimal gland into the palpebral and orbital lobes before attaching to the lateral orbital tubercle.

In the vertical direction, after its origin in the muscle, the levator aponeurosis fuses with the orbital septum around the preaponeurotic fat pad. It then becomes a large number of separate fibers, which attach anteriorly to the orbicular muscle and to the skin. This contributes significantly to the formation of the upper eyelid crease. The posterior fibers attach to the anterior border of tarsus and are most firmly anchored 3 mm from the lid margin.

At the origin of the levator aponeurosis is the upper insertion of the smooth superior tarsal muscle of Müller. This upper lid retractor, which is under sympathetic control, follows inferiorly on the underside of the levator aponeurosis. It is covered on the posterior aspect by conjunctiva. Its insertion is on the upper border of tarsus; however, the analogous structure of the lower lid has a much less defined insertion.

There are other differences between the upper and lower eyelids. Since there is no separate muscle serving as the eyelid retractor in the lower lid, the capsulopalpebral fascia serves this purpose. This fascia originates from the muscular fascia of the inferior rectus muscle and forms part of the suspensory system of the globe, or Lockwood's ligament. Posterior to Lockwood's ligament, it courses around the inferior oblique muscle. It

then inserts on the lower border of tarsus. Fibers from the capsulopalpebral fascia are also found in Tenon's fascia on the globe, in the area of the lower fornix, and in the orbital septum with which it fuses before inserting on tarsus.

Another difference is the height of the tarsal plates of the upper and lower lids. The upper lid tarsus is 11 mm, and the lower lid tarsus is 3.5 to 4 mm. They are composed of dense connective tissue, not cartilage, and are 29 mm in length and 1 mm thick.

The palpebral conjunctiva is a mucous membrane covered by nonkeratinized epithelium. It covers the fornices and merges with the bulbar conjunctiva. It is a very vascular structure and contains an important part of the immune system of the eye. The substantia propria of the adult is profusely infiltrated with lymphocytes, mast cells, and histiocytes. There are also lymph nodules that give rise to follicular reactions. Mucus-secreting goblet cells are found within the conjunctival epithelium but disappear near the lid margin. Serous glands, the accessory lacrimal glands (approximately 50 of them), are also contained in the conjunctiva: the glands of Krause at the fornix level, the glands of Henle overlying the tarsus on both lids, and the glands of Wolfring on the upper border of tarsus.

The eyelids contain other glands, which have been mentioned previously. The sebaceous meibomian glands are contained within the tarsal plates and do not normally have an associated hair follicle. They consist of a central canal surrounded by 10 to 15 acini. The ducts are lined by stratified squamous epithelium near their openings. There are 30 glands in the upper lid and 20 glands in the lower lid. They secrete through the ducts at the eyelid margin and help form the lipid layer of the tear film.

The glands of Zeiss are also sebaceous and are associated with the cilia. The glands of Moll, in contrast, are apocrine sweat glands and are associated with the cilia, from which they secrete either into the ducts of the glands of Zeiss or directly into their own ducts. Eccrine sweat glands are smaller than the glands of Moll and are found throughout the skin of the lids.

The arterial supply of the eyelids is via the medial and lateral palpebral arteries. The lateral palpebral arteries are derived from the lacrimal artery, a branch of the ophthalmic artery. The medial palpebral arteries arise directly from the ophthalmic artery at the level of the trochlea. They enter the lids as superior and inferior branches. The superior branch then subdivides into two arcades. These are the marginal and the peripheral arcades of the upper lid (Fig. 150–5).

In the upper lid, the marginal arcade is just anterior to tarsus, 4 mm from the lid margin. The single marginal arcade of the lower lid is 2 mm from the margin. There is a pretarsal and a posttarsal plexus of small arteries. Many anastomoses exist between the medial system and the lateral palpebral arteries—the superficial temporal, transverse facial, angular, and infraorbital arteries. Thus the rich vascular supply of the lids is actually derived from both the external and internal carotid systems.

The venous system of the lids, which is much more diffuse than is the arterial system, drains medially into

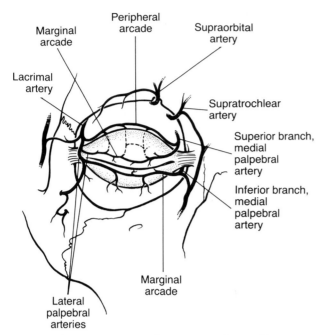

Figure 150–5. Arterial supply to the eyelids.

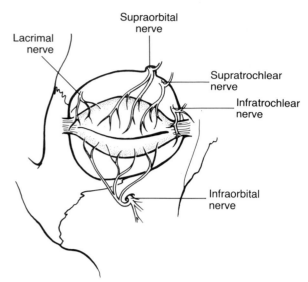

Figure 150–7. Innervation of the eyelids.

the ophthalmic and angular veins and laterally into the superficial temporal vein. This provides an important connection between the facial and orbital venous systems, leading directly from the lids to the cavernous sinus. The angular vein is the largest one draining the lids and is located 8 mm from the inner canthus. It is somewhat lateral and more superficial than the angular artery. Other structures that connect to the angular vein are the frontal, supraorbital, and anterior facial veins.

The lymphatics of the lids are also divided into a pre- and posttarsal plexus. They drain, respectively, the skin and orbicularis and the tarsal plate and conjunctiva. Part of the lower lid and the medial canthal area drain into the submandibular lymph nodes. The upper lid and lateral canthal area drain into the parotid and preauricular lymph nodes (Fig. 150–6).

The sensory supply of the upper lid is provided by branches of the ophthalmic division of the trigeminal nerve (cranial nerve V), including the infratrochlear, supratrochlear, supraorbital, and lacrimal nerves. The lower lid is supplied medially by the infratrochlear branch of the ophthalmic division of cranial nerve V. Laterally, the infraorbital nerve, a branch of the maxillary division of cranial nerve V, provides sensory innervation (Fig. 150–7).

The excretory lacrimal system is described in *Principles and Practice of Ophthalmology: Basic Sciences*, Chapters 27 to 31; however, the lacrimal "pump" mechanism is an integral part of the lids and their function. The lacrimal pump has three main components: the superficial and deep heads of the pretarsal orbicular muscle of the eye, the deep head of the preseptal muscle, and the lacrimal diaphragm. The lacrimal diaphragm is a fascial condensation on the lateral wall of the lacrimal sac. Tension applied in this area causes a vacuum in the lacrimal sac. As the lids close, the lacrimal ampullae in the proximal portion of the canalicular system are compressed by the contraction of the pretarsal muscles. The preseptal muscle pulls on the lacrimal diaphragm, and tears get pulled into the vacuum thus created. As the lids open, the lacrimal ampulla relaxes and expands, pulling tears from the lacrimal lake. The lacrimal sac also relaxes, causing the tears contained in it to drain, mostly by gravity, into the nasolacrimal duct. Other theories have been postulated for the lacrimal drainage system. Further research will determine the accuracy of the models presented.

BIBLIOGRAPHY

American Academy of Ophthalmology: Basic and Clinical Science Course, vol. 1. San Francisco, American Academy of Ophthalmology, 1990.

Doxanas MT, Anderson RL: Clinical Orbital Anatomy. Baltimore, Williams & Wilkins, 1984.

Duke-Elder S, Wybar KC: The anatomy of the visual system. *In* Duke-Elder S (ed): System of Ophthalmology. St. Louis, CV Mosby, 1961.

Snell RS, Lemp MA: Clinical Anatomy of the Eye. Cambridge, Blackwell Scientific Publications, 1989.

Zide BM, Jelks GW: Surgical Anatomy of the Orbit. New York, Raven Press, 1985.

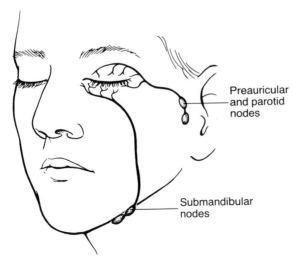

Figure 150–6. Lymphatics of the eyelids.

Chapter 151

·

Congenital Eyelid Anomalies

M. RONAN CONLON and FRANCIS C. SUTULA

Congenital anomalies of the eyelid are a diverse group of disorders with a wide spectrum of clinical presentations. An understanding of the surgical anatomy, natural history, and management options is fundamental to the successful treatment of these often difficult cases. The purpose of this chapter is to review the pertinent historical, clinical, and current therapeutic options available to help facilitate ophthalmologists in accurate diagnosis and management of these anomalies. The surgical procedures are outlined in principle, and readers are referred to the appropriate references for more detailed accounts. Congenital ptosis merits special consideration and is discussed in detail in Chapter 228.

For ophthalmologists dealing with these problems, it is important to realize that many of these abnormalities are associated with systemic problems. Assessment of these patients should include a thorough physical examination by an ophthalmologist, possibly in conjunction with a pediatrician. When appropriate, genetic counseling should be made available to the parents so they can make informed decisions about the risk to potential future offspring.

We cannot overemphasize the importance of instituting simple ocular protective measures such as lubrication and moisture chambers to prevent corneal decompensation in conditions with exposure keratopathy.

An understanding of the natural history of these anomalies is essential because some resolve spontaneously. The timing of surgery needs to take into account a child's maturity and emotional state. In most instances, it is preferable to perform surgery before the child enters school, and indeed in many circumstances it is possible to perform surgery much earlier.

EMBRYOLOGY OF THE EYELIDS

In order to understand the pathogenesis and anatomic variations that characterize these anomalies, a basic knowledge of normal eyelid development is required. The following section reviews the basic derivation of the eyelid structures with reference to developmental abnormalities as a background for more detailed discussion in the following sections.

Eyelid development represents a complex "inductive interaction" between mesoderm- and ectoderm-derived tissues. The first sign of eyelid development is the appearance of the lid fold at the seventh week of gestation. The upper lid is formed by fusion of the medial and lateral aspect of the frontonasal processes, and the lower lid is formed by the maxillary process. Complete or partial failure of lid fold development is believed to be responsible for a number of congenital eyelid anomalies including cryptophthalmos, ablepharon, and microblepharon.

The next key step in eyelid development is fusion of the lids at 9 weeks of gestation. It is while the lids are fused that differentiation of the eyelid margin occurs. Inward migration of ectodermal cords of cells gives rise to the meibomian glands, sweat glands, and cilia. At the same time, condensation of the mesenchymal tissue forms the tarsus around the immature meibomian glands. Failure of fusion of the eyelid margin is one of the proposed causes of colobomas of the eyelid margin. The secretion of sebum by the meibomian glands at the fifth month of gestation may help initiate the separation of the lids in the sixth month of gestation. Keratinization of the eyelid margin and contraction of the lower lid retractors have also been proposed as possible additional factors in eyelid separation. Incomplete separation of the lids may result in ankyloblepharon or ankyloblepharon filiforme adnatum. Included in defects of the eyelid margin differentiation are the palpebral aperture anomalies: euryblepharon, blepharophimosis, and congenital lid folds (epicanthus).

ANOMALIES OF LID FOLD DEVELOPMENT

Cryptophthalmos

Cryptophthalmos is an unusual condition in which the globe and the deeper ocular structures are covered by a fold of skin that extends from the brow to the cheek. Zehender initially described the condition in 1872 in a 4-month-old girl with bilateral cryptophthalmos, and Manz in the same year characterized the histopathologic features.[1] The most likely mode of inheritance is autosomal recessive.[2-4] The condition typically occurs in association with other congenital anomalies, the most frequent being syndactyly, urogenital defects, and dysencephaly.

Three morphologic variations of cryptophthalmos are generally recognized: complete cryptophthalmos, partial cryptophthalmos, and congenital symblepharon.[5] In complete cryptophthalmos, the most common type, a skin fold extends from the brow to the cheek, completely covering the globe. In partial (incomplete) cryptophthalmos a skin fold covers the medial aspect of the palpebral aperture, with the lateral lid structures being normal. In congenital symblepharon, the upper lid is fused to the superior aspect of the globe with sparing of the inferior portion of the globe and lower lid.[1]

The pathogenesis of cryptophthalmos has not been fully elucidated, although investigators have suggested that a deficiency in vitamin A and retinoids during gestation may be a causative factor. This observation is based on the earlier work of Warkany and Schraffenberger,[6] who were able to develop an animal model of cryptophthalmos through maternal deprivation of vitamin A. Studies have now demonstrated that adequate levels of vitamin A and retinoids are necessary for normal cellular differentiation, which is probably related to gene modification by retinoids.[7-9] Although local factors such as amniotic bands and inflammation have been proposed as possible pathogenic factors, the syndromic nature of cryptophthalmos points to a genetically induced abnormality, capable of causing widespread changes, as being the more likely pathogenic mechanism.

Histopathologic examination has shown the underlying globe to be usually microphthalmic; the anterior segment is markedly disorganized, and the posterior segment is usually better preserved.[5, 10, 11] The main pathologic features are anterior stromal scarring, anterior segment dysgenesis with hypoplasia or absence of the anterior segment, trabecular meshwork, Schelmm's canal, dislocated or absent lens, and atrophy of the iris and ciliary body. The retina and choroid have often been found to have a high degree of differentiation. The orbicularis muscle and levator are generally well preserved, but the tarsus is generally absent.[3, 12]

Treatment of this condition is very difficult and is often unsuccessful.[2, 11] Cases of successful surgical treatment of partial cryptophthalmos have been reported.[13, 14] The demonstration of normal retinal function through ancillary tests in some cases of complete cryptophthalmos has led to attempts to reconstruct the lids and anterior segment, but results have been poor.[11, 15, 16]

Microblepharon and Ablepharon

Microblepharon is an unusual deformity of the lid characterized by a shortening in the vertical direction. The clinical presentation can vary from mild vertical shortening to almost complete colobomatous absence of the lid with only a rudimentary integument forming the lid margin. Ablepharon, complete failure of lid development, is an even rarer occurrence, and it tends to be associated with more severe ocular and systemic abnormalities.[1]

Proposed pathogenetic mechanisms include primary failure of lid fold development, possibly related to defective migration of neural crest cells, resulting in an ectodermal-mesodermal induction defect.[17, 18] Other proposed mechanisms include mechanical local factors such as inflammation, amniotic bands, or reabsorption processes. Bosniak and colleagues pointed out that local factors are less likely given the frequency with which other syndromic anomalies have been reported with the condition.[19] It is possible that the underlying defect in the pathogenesis of ablepharon/microblepharon and cryptophthalmos may be closely related. It has been

noted in cryptophthalmia that the contralateral eye may demonstrate various degrees of ablepharon/microphthalmia.[3, 20, 21] Hence, it is possible that the proposed secondary metaplasia of the corneal and conjunctival epithelium into a smooth epithelial covering believed to occur in cryptophthalmos does not occur in ablepharon/microphthalmia, for reasons not fully understood.

Reconstruction of these deformities is dependent on the degree of involvement of the lid structures and the integrity of the underlying ocular structures. In the presence of a normal globe, treatment is directed at preserving the ocular surface. In milder cases, ocular lubrication may be sufficient. In more severe cases, reconstruction of the anterior lamellae of the lid may be necessary. Pedicle rotation flaps from the cheek or brow, eyelid sharing, and full-thickness skin grafts are some ways to accomplish this.[22, 23] When the underlying globe is abnormal, multiple procedures may be necessary to create a socket in which a prosthesis can be maintained. Management of this problem can be further complicated by abnormal development of the bony orbit. The use of subperisoteal orbital expanders may be helpful in this circumstance.

Colobomas

A coloboma of the eyelid can be either a partial- or full-thickness defect of the lid margin. The majority of these lesions occur as an isolated finding in the upper eyelid. Colobomas of the upper lid typically occur at the junction of the inner and middle thirds and are not associated with other systemic anomalies (Fig. 151–1). In the lower lid, they tend to occur at the junction of the middle and lateral third of the lid and are often associated with systemic anomalies, most notably the autosomal dominant condition mandibulofacial dysostosis (Treacher Collins syndrome) (Fig. 151–2).[24-26] Twenty per cent of these cases are bilateral. Defects in the upper lid tend to be full thickness, with the adjacent lid margin normal. In the lower lid, partial-thickness defects with adjacent margin abnormalities are more

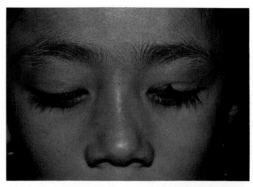

Figure 151–1. Typical eyelid coloboma occurring at the junction of the medial third and lateral two-thirds of the left upper eyelid. (Courtesy of Dr. L. H. Allen.)

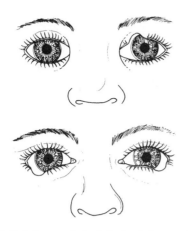

Figure 151–2. Coloboma. *A,* Isolated coloboma of the upper lid. *B,* Bilateral colobomatous defects of the lower eyelid, typically seen in association with Treacher Collins syndrome.

common. Morphologically, these defects vary from small divots in the lid margin to large triangular or quadrilateral defects involving the entire lid margin.

A number of theories have been postulated about the pathogenesis of these defects. Poswillo[24] proposed local mechanical influences (e.g., hematoma in colobomas associated with Goldenhar's syndrome), which would account for the marked asymmetry seen in this condition. A more central defect, such as a defect in the migration of neural crest cells, must be postulated in mandibulofacial dysostosis, which is characterized by symmetric lower lid defects.[24] Other proposed causes include amniotic bands, failure of fusion of the lid folds, inflammation, excess vitamin A, and decreased placental circulation.[1, 24, 27]

Management is determined by the size of the defect and the state of the corneal epithelium.[28] Initially it is possible to manage most defects with conservative measures such as topical lubricants, bandage contact lenses, and moisture chambers. The size of defect that can exist before the cornea is compromised in children is often surprising.[23, 26, 28] In general, colobomas of the lower lid are better tolerated than those of the upper lid.[23] Trichiasis is more frequently associated with colobomas of the lower lid and is often the precipitating factor in the decision to operate. Before or during surgery, the integrity of the lacrimal drainage system should be evaluated because lacrimal anomalies can be common. It is also important to assess the state of the adjacent eyelid tissues and the visual status of the child, especially when considering a lid-sharing procedure in an age group in which the risk of occlusion amblyopia still exists.

When surgical intervention is mandated, a number of surgical options exist. Small defects (less 30 per cent) can be repaired by direct layered closure after freshening up the skin edges. Moderate defects (50 to 60 per cent) of the upper and lower lid should be converted in a pentagonal lid defect by freshening the margins, and then closed with or without a lateral cantholysis and semicircular flap as described by Tenzel. Larger defects (greater than 50 per cent) are better repaired in the pediatric age group using procedures that do not require

bridging flaps that can induce amblyopia. Options include a myocutaneous skin flap or a full-thickness lid rotation flap from the upper lid to the lower lid.[23, 25, 28, 29]

ANOMALIES OF THE EYELID MARGIN

Ankyloblepharon

Congenital fusion between the upper and lower lid, known as *ankyloblepharon*, was originally described by von Ammon in 1841.[1] The most common site for this fusion of the lid is at the lateral canthus (external ankyloblepharon), followed by the inner canthus (internal ankyloblepharon). It is usually inherited in an autosomal dominant fashion with incomplete penetrance; however, sporadic cases are well recognized.[30, 31] A rarer variant in which either single or multiple bands of tissue pass between the lids (ankyloblepharon filiforme adnatum) is discussed in the next section.

It is believed that this condition is related to a primary growth arrest of the canthal area at the time of development of the lid fold.[1] The occasional association of anophthalmos and microphthalmia has implicated a lack of mechanical stimulus in some cases. The resultant fusion of the lid at the lateral or medial canthus can give rise to pseudoextropia or pseudoesotropia, respectively.

The treatment is primarily surgical. In external ankyloblepharon, a lateral canthoplasty can be performed at age 3 to 4 years, with care taken to leave an overlying edge of conjunctiva to avoid keratinization of the lid margin and secondary corneal irritation. The normal fissure is 25 mm long, so the incision should not be extended beyond this length. Burns and Cahill have emphasized that in internal ankyloblepharon, the medial canaliculus and punctum may be involved, and any repair in this area should involve careful identification of these structures.[32] The use of a punctoplasty with silicone intubation of the canalicular system to reestablish patency of the drainage system may be required. It is not uncommon for there to be a significant amount of symblepharon formation in these patients, requiring lysis or conjunctival grafting in more severe cases.[31]

Ankyloblepharon Filiforme Adnatum

Ankyleblepharon filiforme adnatum is characterized by the presence of isolated strands of extensile tissue passing between the upper and lower lid margins. This aberrant tissue attaches to the lid margin between the cilia and meibomian gland orifices and can involve one or both lids to various degrees (Fig. 151–3). Depending on the extent of lid involvement, it is sometimes possible to separate the lids fully; however, this condition often results in shortening of the vertical palpebral aperture.

This abnormality has been reported in isolation, with other abnormalities, and in association with other syn-

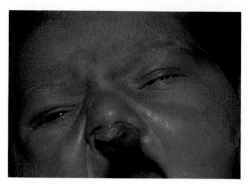

Figure 151–3. Ankyloblepharon filiforme adnatum. Extensile strands of tissue extending between the lid margins. Note the presence of a cleft lip, an abnormality frequently associated with this condition. (Courtesy of Dr. L. H. Allen.)

dromes.[33–38] Rosenman and colleagues[36] proposed classifying this disorder into four types based on their review of the literature and reported cases. In types 1 and 2, the inheritance is sporadic. The latter has been associated with central nervous system or cardiac defects, and the former is not associated with any other anomalies. In types 3 and 4, the inheritance is autosomal dominant with variable expression. Type 3 is associated with ectodermal syndromes such as the popliteal pterygium syndrome, which is characterized by cleft lip or palate, popliteal pterygia, and genitourinary abnormalities, whereas type 4 is associated with cleft lip or palate alone. The occurrence of various systemic abnormalities with this condition underscores the importance of a pediatric assessment and genetic counseling for these patients.

Pathologically, these bands have been shown to be composed of an outer layer of epithelial tissue covering a fibrovascular core.[35] The pathogenesis of this condition remains unclear. It has been proposed that a relative arrest of epithelial growth allows a more rapid proliferation of mesodermal tissue to bridge the future lid fissure. The subsequent separation of the lid fold stretches these bands and contributes to their sometimes elongated appearance.[1, 30]

The recommended treatment is simply dividing the bands with scissors or a muscle hook if the bands are thin. Bleeding is generally minimal, and the resultant skin tags regress with time.

Euryblepharon

Euryblepharon was first described in 1854 by Desmarres and is characterized by a primary symmetric enlargement of the horizontal palpebral fissure.[1] Other features that present in variable amounts include downward and anterior displacement of the lateral canthus, ectropion of the lateral third of the lid, and tightness of the lids.

Clinically, the increased length of the lower lid leads to a loss of the normal snug apposition of the lower lid to the globe, and an intervening gutter is evident on examination (Fig. 151–4). The condition usually presents as an isolated clinical finding; however, other associated ocular anomalies include ptosis, a double row of meibomian glands, lateral displacement of the inferior punctum, strabismus, and telecanthus.[39, 40] The majority of cases do not manifest an inheritance pattern, but isolated case reports of autosomal dominant inheritance have been reported.[39, 41–43] It is important when examining these patients to rule out secondary causes of enlargement of the palpebral fissure such as globe enlargement and craniofacial dysostosis.

The exact cause of congenital euryblepharon is unknown, but proposed mechanisms include abnormal separation of the lid fissure, abnormal displacement of the lateral canthus, abnormal pull of the platysma muscle, and hypoplasia of the orbicularis muscle or the tarsal plate.[1, 40, 44] It is probable that a combination of these factors is the cause of this condition, given the wide clinical spectrum of its appearance.

The treatment in mild cases is observation, because the tendency is for this condition to improve with age.[40] In more severe cases, with a marked degree of ectropion with vertical lid shortening and secondary exposure keratopathy, then lateral tarsorrhaphies are required. It is important to accurately identify the underlying defect in these patients, because this to a degree dictates the surgical approach used in the repair. If downward displacement of the lateral canthus is significant, a lateral canthoplasty is indicated, with reattachment of the lower limb of the lateral canthal tendon to a more superior and posterior position on the orbital rim. This procedure can be combined with shortening of the lower lid if a redundancy of the lower lid is noted at the time of repair.[40, 45]

Epicanthal Folds

Epicanthal folds are vertical skin folds in the medial canthal area; they can cover the caruncular structures (Fig. 151–5). Four types of epicanthus are now recognized, depending on the position of the skin fold: epicanthus palpebralis, epicanthus tarsalis, epicanthus

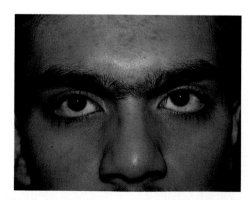

Figure 151–4. Euryblepharon. Symmetric enlargement of the palpebral apertures with anterior and downward displacement of the lateral canthal tendons. Note the loss of apposition of the lower eyelid margin to the globe. (Courtesy of Dr. L. H. Allen.)

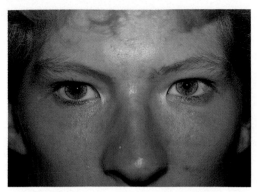

Figure 151–5. Bilateral epicanthal folds. (Courtesy of Dr. L. H. Allen.)

superciliaris, and epicanthus inversus.[1] According to Duke-Elder,[1] this condition was originally described by Schon (1828), and von Ammon (1831) is credited for introducing the term *epicanthus* and describing the first three variations. Axenfeld and Brons (1912) later described epicanthus inversus.[1, 46]

In epicanthus superciliaris, the fold of skin arises from above the brow and extends downward to the lateral aspect of the nose. Epicanthus palpebralis, the most common type of epicanthal fold, is characterized by a fold of skin that begins medially and is symmetrically distributed between the upper and lower lid. Epicanthus tarsalis is most frequently encountered in Asians and consists of a skin fold originating from the lateral aspect of the upper lid and extending to the medial canthal area before dissipating. Epicanthus inversus (see Blepharophimosis) is usually associated with other lid anomalies and consists of a fold of skin originating in the lower lid and extending upward to the medial canthal area (Fig. 151–6).

Studies of fetal development have shown epicanthus to be present at the 3- to 6-month stage in all humans; however, at birth it is rarely apparent.[1, 47] During the first 2 years of life, epicanthus becomes more apparent, with a reported incidence of 20 per cent by the second year.[47] With growth and development of the nasal bridge, it is common to see a diminution in the size of skin fold; by school age, the problem resolves itself in the majority of children. Although this is particularly true of epicanthus superciliaris and palpebralis, the same cannot be said about epicanthus inversus, which does not have the same tendency to resolve with growth and may eventually require surgical correction.[46] In Asians, epicanthus tarsalis often persists throughout life, and anatomic studies have suggested it may be related to the lower insertion of the orbital septum on the anterior surface of the tarsal plate.

The cause of epicanthus remains unclear. Proposed mechanisms include arrested fetal development, hypoplasia of the nasal bones, and an excess or deficiency of skin in the medial canthal area relative to bone development. In some cases, a hereditary component is apparent, and this is especially true of the dominantly inherited blepharophimosis syndrome.

Many techniques have been described to repair epicanthal folds, and it is beyond the scope of this chapter to discuss each method in detail. In considering surgery, clinicians should remember that in most cases surgical correction is not necessary and development of the nasal bridge in the preschool years diminishes the cosmetic detraction. Procedures currently advocated include Spaeth's epicanthus operation, Verwey's Y to V operation, Mustarde's technique (an opposite double Z-plasty combined with a Y to V), and Roveda's technique. In general, Spaeth's procedure is reserved for less severe cases of epicanthal folds, whereas the Y to V procedure, Mustarde's technique, multiple Z-plasties, and Roveda's procedure are reserved for more severe cases. Mustarde's technique, which combines a double opposing Z-plasty with a YV procedure, has been criticized by some surgeons as posing technical difficulties of aligning the flaps and requiring multiple sutures in a small area, leading to excess scarring.[48] What is common to all these techniques is the rotation of skin from areas of relative excess to areas of relative deficiency.

Despite the number of procedures advocated to repair this deformity, certain common surgical principles apply to all methods of repair. It is important to carefully dissect the orbicularis from the transposition flap in order to flatten the medial canthal area. Carefully sutured apposition of the skin edges is needed to reduce postoperative scarring. Even with meticulous attention to detail, an intense wound reaction is not unusual in the postoperative period. It may be ameliorated with topical steroids, although there is some tendency for these folds to re-form to some extent.[46]

Epiblepharon

Epiblepharon is characterized by a medial redundancy of eyelid skin causing the eyelashes to assume a vertical

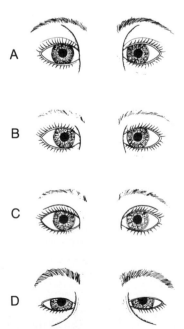

Figure 151–6. Epicanthal folds. *A*, Epicanthus superciliaris. *B*, Epicanthus palpebralis. *C*, Epicanthus tarsalis. *D*, Epicanthus inversus.

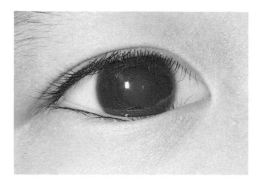

Figure 151–7. Epiblepharon. An excess of eyelid skin nasally, causing a vertical orientation of the lashes. (Courtesy of Dr. L. H. Allen.)

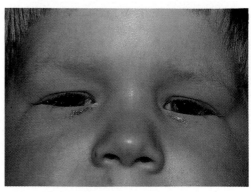

Figure 151–8. Congenital entropion. Complete inturning of the eyelid margin with secondary corneal irritation. (Courtesy of Dr. L. H. Allen.)

orientation (Fig. 151–7). It can involve either the upper or lower eyelid, although involvement of the lower eyelid is far more common. It occurs most frequently in the Asian population and is often bilateral. Epiblepharon often resolves spontaneously in the first few years of life, with growth of the nasal bridge. Important in the initial assessment of these patients is distinguishing this condition from congenital entropion, marked by an actual turning inward of the eyelid margin (discussed later). Initial therapy is conservative, with the use of topical lubricants and attention to the ocular surface. If irritation of the ocular surface necessitates surgical correction, simple excision of the excess skin and orbicularis with primary closure of the wound has proved to be effective. Another option is the placement of Quickert-Rathburn eyelid creases sutures.[49, 50]

Congenital Entropion

Congenital entropion is a rare eyelid anomaly that is often confused clinically with the more common condition epiblepharon. It usually presents as a primary condition with turning inward of the lid margin toward the globe and by definition is not associated with other abnormalities (Fig. 151–8).[51–53] Congenital entropion does infrequently occur secondary to other anomalies of the lid and globe such as microphthalmos, epiblepharon, and anophthalmos.[1]

It was generally accepted that congenital entropion was due to a combination hypertrophy/spasm of the orbicularis muscle until Tse and coworkers failed to demonstrate histopathologic evidence of orbicularis hypertrophy and suggested disinsertion of the lower lid retractors as a causative factor.[54]

Clinically, it is important to distinguish between congenital entropion and epiblepharon because the approach to each anomaly is different. The following are important differentiating features between congenital entropion and epiblepharon (Fig. 151–9):

1. Congenital entropion tends to worsen with time, whereas epiblepharon often spontaneously improves.

2. The cilia are directed toward the globe in congenital entropion, whereas in epiblepharon they are orientated vertically.

The urgency of surgery is dictated by the state of the underlying cornea. If the corneal epithelium is compromised, then urgent treatment is required. In cases in which the corneal epithelium is in good condition, surgery is elective. The state of the cornea must be monitored closely. The recommended treatment is to remove a horizontal strip of skin and orbicularis below the eyelid margin and reattach the lower lid retractors to the tarsal plate to cause eversion of the lower lid.[54]

A variant of congenital entropion is congenital horizontal tarsal kink. In this condition, a vertical kink develops in the tarsal plate of the upper lid in utero, resulting in direct apposition of the lid margin to the globe. This condition requires immediate attention, because corneal scarring and infection are early complications.[19, 55] It has been postulated that this anomaly is a result of mechanical factors causing bending of the immature and malleable collagen fibers in the tarsal plate.[19]

A number of surgical procedures have been proposed to correct tarsal kink syndrome. Excision of the tarsal kink and eversion of the eyelid with mattress sutures is effective, but some investigators have expressed concern about possible vertical lid shortening with this approach.[19, 55] The use of a transverse blepharotomy at

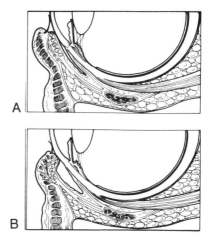

Figure 151–9. A, Epiblepharon. B, Congenital entropion.

the level of the kink combined with marginal rotation of the lower lid has been reported as successful.[55–57] Bosniak and coworkers[19] have suggested using a nonincisional approach by passing three interrupted 6–0 black silk everting sutures from the conjunctiva to the skin and tying them over bolsters without the use of a blepharotomy. Regardless of the method of repair chosen to treat this condition, the potential emergency must be recognized and treatment instituted without delay.

Congenital Ectropion

Primary congenital ectropion is a rare condition in isolation and is usually encountered in association with blepharophimosis syndrome or Down's syndrome.[1, 58] Other secondary disorders in which congenital ectropion has been reported include microphthalmia, buphthalmos, euryblepharon, and cysts.[1] The treatment depends on the underlying cause. If excess horizontal lid laxity is found, then a horizontal lid-shortening procedure can be corrective. Ectropion associated with blepharophimosis is due to insufficient vertical lid skin and can be corrected with a retroauricular skin graft.

A variant of congenital ectropion is total bilateral eversion of the upper lids in newborns, originally described by Adams in 1896.[1] The cause is uncertain, and it is thought that the eyelids become everted secondary to venous obstruction during delivery.[1] Marked chemosis and prolapse of the conjunctiva result. It is generally accepted that this condition can be treated conservatively, and many investigators report success without surgical intervention.[59, 60] The goal of management is to prevent desiccation of the exposed conjunctiva and allow spontaneous inversion of the lid. This can generally be achieved conservatively by use of lubrication and a moisture chamber.

ANOMALIES OF THE FISSURE

Blepharophimosis

Blepharophimosis is shortening of the palpebral fissure. Kohn and Romano in 1971 recognized the occurrence of this anomaly with blepharoptosis, epicanthus inversus, and telecanthus in a distinctive entity now referred to as the *congenital tetrad syndrome*.[61] The four anomalies are inherited in an autosomal dominant fashion with a high degree of penetrance.[1, 61] Other associated features include hypoplasia of the tarsal plate, generalized tightness of lid skin (often producing lower eyelid ectropion), prominent vertical brow hair often extending across the nasal bridge, and a flat brow (Fig. 151–10). Affected individuals are usually of normal intelligence. Females may be infertile owing to hypogonadism and specific hormonal deficiencies.[62] Females with features of the congenital tetrad syndrome should be monitored for menstrual irregularity and infertility.

Clinically, the diagnosis is readily apparent when other affected family members are introduced to the

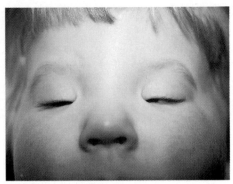

Figure 151–10. Congenital tetrad syndrome. Blepharophimosis, blepharoptosis, epicanthus inversus, and telecanthus.

examiner. However, in cases in which a clear family history is unavailable, Older[63] has pointed out that other syndromes in which shortening of the palpebral fissure, telecanthus, and epicanthus can occur need to be considered. Such syndromes include Waardenburg's syndrome, Williams's syndrome, fetal alcohol syndrome, Dubowitz's syndrome, trisomy 18, and cerebro-oculo-facial-digital syndrome.

Three different variations of congenital tetrad syndrome are recognized. Type 1 most closely resembles the classic tetrad, with ptosis, telecanthus, and epicanthus inversus being the prominent features. Patients with type 2 have ptosis, telecanthus, and lower lid ectropion (due to a relative sparsity of eyelid skin). Type 3 resembles type 2 except for having associated hypertelorism.

Surgical correction of this deformity is generally deferred until the preschool years to allow for some growth of the nasal bridge, which often helps reduce the extent of the epicanthal folds and also allows the tissues to enlarge enough to make surgical correction easier. The operation is usually carried out in a staged fashion, with the medial canthoplasty being performed before the ptosis surgery. A perfect cosmetic result is not possible, and it is important that this be understood before any surgical repair is undertaken.[61, 63, 64]

Type 1 repair is directed at correcting the medial canthus deformity and the ptosis. Some investigators have described using Mustarde's quadrilateral flaps to repair the epicanthus inversus, but a YV-plasty is gaining increased popularity owing to the minimal scarring.[30] Kohn has suggested modifying the incision used in a YV-plasty to a C shape to have the incision conform to Langer's skin folds and further reduce the amount of scarring postoperatively.[30] Both of these procedures can be combined with direct resection of the medial canthal tendon, with suturing to the periosteum or transnasal wiring to address the telecanthus. In transnasal wiring, the medial canthal tendons are attached to each other by a No. 21 wire, which is passed between osteotomies in the lacrimal bone.

Affected children usually have minimal levator function, and blepharoptosis is repaired using either internal or external suspensions.[30, 63, 64] Readers are referred to Chapter 160 for a detailed description of this procedure.

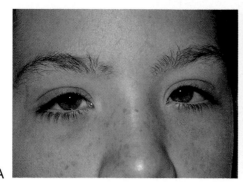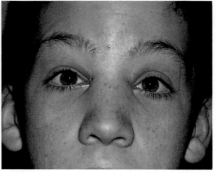

A

B

Figure 151–11. Telecanthus. A, Preoperative appearance. B, Postoperative appearance after transnasal wiring.

When insufficient lid skin is present, it may be necessary to use a full-thickness skin graft to relieve the tension and help increase the vertical length of the lid.

ABNORMALITIES OF THE CANTHAL TENDONS

Telecanthus

Telecanthus is caused by an increase in length of the medial canthal tendons, resulting in an increased distance between the medial canthi (Fig. 151–11). This is in distinction to hypertelorism, in which the distance between the medial walls of the orbit is increased, resulting in an increased distance between the globes. Hypertelorism is often associated with ocular abnormalities such as exotropia, optic atrophy, microcornea, and microophthalmia. Telecanthus most frequently occurs in association with the dominantly inherited congenital tetrad syndrome, blepharophimosis, blepharoptosis, epicanthus inversus, and telecanthus. The natural course of this anomaly is to remain unchanged, and cosmetic improvement requires surgical intervention. Correction of telecanthus often requires transnasal wiring to shorten the distance between the canthi, combined with excision of redundant skin in the medial canthal area.

Medial Canthal Dystopia

Abnormal formation of the medial canthal tendon may occur in isolation or in association with other syndromes.[65] Medial canthal dystopia is frequently encountered in the setting of Waardenburg's syndrome.[66] This autosomal dominant inherited condition is manifested by medial ankyloblepharon, telecanthus, lateralization of the puncti, prominence of the root of the nose, hyperplasia of the medial part of the brow, heterochromia iridis, a median white forelock, and deafness. Few reports in the literature address the surgical management of patients with Waardenburg's syndrome, and procedures described have been adopted from techniques for repair of other distinct anomalies, such as epicanthus and blepharophimosis. It has been our experience (FCS) that after identification of the canalicular system, direct excision of the aberrant skin, conjunctiva, and fibrous tissue between the canaliculi, followed by reapproximation of the conjunctiva-cutaneous epithelial junction with interrupted sutures, resulted in a satisfactory eyelid contour (Fig. 151–12).[67]

Congenital malposition of the medial canthal tendon in association with ipsilateral nasal deformities is a rare disorder manifested by inferior displacement and attachment of the medial canthal tendon.[65] Instead of inserting just posterior to the posterior lacrimal crest, the medial canthal tendon inserts lower down at the junction of the medial and lateral walls of the orbit. This condition is believed to result from an arrest at 2 mo of embryonic development, because this is the crucial time period for normal development of canthal structures and the external nose. Successful repair is contingent on reestablishing the normal insertion of the medial canthal tendon. This may be achieved by directly suturing the medial canthal tendon to the medial wall of the orbit. If adequate suture placement cannot be obtained, then

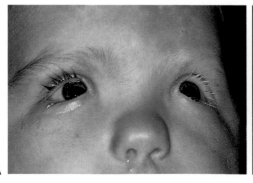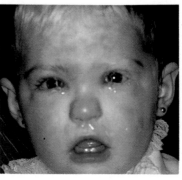

A

B

Figure 151–12. A, Medial canthal dystopia. An infant with Waardenburg's syndrome manifesting blepharophimosis, telecanthus, and medial ankyloblepharon. B, Postoperative appearance following reconstruction of the medial canthus and silicone intubation.

transnasal wiring may be necessary to re-form the canthal angle. Any coexistent lacrimal drainage abnormalities and nasal defects also need to be addressed at the time of repair.

REFERENCES

1. Duke-Elder S: Congenital anomalies of the ocular adnexa. *In* Duke-Elder S (ed): System of Ophthalmology. London, Henry Kimpton, 1964.
2. Thomas IT, Frias JL, Felix V, et al: Isolated and syndromic cryptophthalmos. Am J Med Genet 25:85, 1986.
3. Sugar HS: The cryptophthalmos-syndactyly syndrome. Am J Ophthalmol 66:897, 1968.
4. Codere F, Brownstein S, Chen MF: Cryptophthalmos syndrome with bilateral renal agenesis. Am J Ophthalmol 91:737, 1981.
5. Francois J: Syndrome malformatif avec cryptophtalmie. Acta Genet Med Gemellol 18:18, 1969.
6. Warkany J, Schraffenberger E: Congenital malformations of the eyes of rats by maternal vitamin A deficiency. Arch Ophthalmol 35:150, 1946.
7. Fuchs E, Green H: Regulation of terminal differentiation of cultured human keratinocytes by vitamin A. Cell 25:617, 1981.
8. Goodman DS: Vitamin A and retinoids in health and disease. N Engl J Med 310:1023, 1984.
9. Hall JG: Vitamin A: A newly recognized teratogen. Harbinger of things to come? J Pediatr 105:583, 1984.
10. Pe'er J, BenEzra D, Sela M, et al: Cryptophthalmos syndrome: Clinical and histopathological findings. Ophthalmic Paediatr Genet 8:177, 1987.
11. Hing S, Wilson HN, Kriss A, et al: Complete cryptophthalmos: Case report with normal flash-VEP and ERG. J Pediatr Ophthalmol Strabismus 27:133, 1990.
12. Waring GO, Shields JA: Partial unilateral cryptophthalmos with syndactyly, brachycephaly, and renal anomalies. Am J Ophthalmol 79:437, 1975.
13. Brazier DJ, Hardman LSJ, Collin JR: Cryptophthalmos: Surgical treatment of the congenital symblepharon variant. Br J Ophthalmol 70:391, 1986.
14. Morax S, Herdan M: Reconstruction orbito-palpebral au cours de deux cas de cryptophthalmos partielle. Ann Chir Plast Esthet 32:319, 1987.
15. Levine RS, Powers T, Rosenberg HK, et al: The cryptophthalmos syndrome. Am J Roentgenol 143:375, 1984.
16. Brodsky I, Waddy G: Cryptophthalmos of ablepharia: A survey of the condition with a review of the literature and the presentation of a case. Med J Aust 1:894, 1949.
17. Noden DM: Periocular mesenchyme, neural crest and mesodermal interactions. *In* Duane TD, Jaeger EA (eds): Biochemical Foundations of Ophthalmology. New York, Harper & Row, 1982.
18. Edwards W: Facial and orbital dysplastic syndrome. *In* Duane TD, Jaeger EA (eds): Biochemical Foundations of Ophthalmology. New York, Harper & Row, 1982.
19. Bosniak S, Hornblass A, Smith B: Re-examining the tarsal kink syndrome: Considerations of its etiology and treatment. Ophthalmic Surg 16:437, 1985.
20. McCarthy GT, West CM: Ablepharon macrostomia syndrome. Dev Med Child Neurol 19:659, 1977.
21. Francois J: Malformative syndrome with cryptophthalmia. Int Ophthalmol Clin 8:817, 1968.
22. Baylis HI, Bartlett RE, Cies WA: Reconstruction of the lower lid in congenital microphthalmos and anophthalmos. Ophthalmic Surg 6:36, 1975.
23. Patipa M, Wilkins RB, Guelzow KW: Surgical management of congenital eyelid coloboma. Ophthalmic Surg 13:212, 1982.
24. Poswillo D: Pathogenesis of craniofacial syndromes exhibiting colobomata. Trans Ophthalmol Soc UK 96:69, 1976.
25. Casey TA: Congenital colobomata of the eyelids. Trans Ophthalmol Soc UK 96:65, 1976.
26. Mann I: Developmental Abnormalities of the Eye. Philadelphia, JB Lippincott, 1957.
27. Roper-Hall MJ: Congenital colobomata of the lids. Trans Ophthalmol Soc UK 88:557, 1969.
28. Kidwell ED, Tenzel RR: Repair of congenital colobomas of the lids. Arch Ophthalmol 97:1931, 1979.
29. Bullock JD: Eyelid coloboma. *In* Fraunfelder FT, Roy FH (eds): Current Ocular Therapy, 3rd ed. Philadelphia, WB Saunders, 1990.
30. Kohn R: Congenital anomalies of the eyelid and socket. *In* Hornblass A (ed): Oculoplastic, Orbital, and Reconstructive Surgery. St Louis, CV Mosby, 1988.
31. Vastine DW, Stamper RL: Ankyloblepharon. *In* Fraunfelder FT, Roy FH (eds): Current Ocular Therapy, 3rd ed, Philadelphia, WB Saunders, 1990.
32. Burns JA, Cahill KV: Congenital eyelid anomalies. *In* Waltman SR, Keates RH, Hoyt CS, et al (eds): Surgery of the Eye, vol 1. New York, Churchill Livingstone, 1988.
33. Akkermans CH, Stern LM: Ankyloblepharon filiforme adnatum. Br J Ophthalmol 63:129, 1979.
34. Yamaguchi C, Kimura R: Ankyloblepharon filiforme adnatum. Jpn J Ophthalmol 26:37, 1982.
35. Kazarian EL, Goldstein P: Ankyloblepharon filiforme adnatum with hydrocephalus, meningomyelocele, and imperforate anus. Am J Ophthalmol 84:355, 1977.
36. Rosenman Y, Ronen S, Eidelman AL, et al: Ankyloblepharon filiforme adnatum: Congenital eyelid-band syndromes. Am J Dis Child 134:751, 1980.
37. Hay RJ, Wells RS: The syndrome of ankyloblepharon, ectodermal defects and cleft lip and palate: An autosomal dominant condition. Br J Dermatol 94:277, 1976.
38. Ehlers N, Jensen IK: Ankyloblepharon filiforme congenitum associated with harelip and cleft-palate. Acta Ophthalmol (Copenh) 48:465, 1970.
39. Gupta AK, Saxena P: Euryblepharon with associated ocular anomalies. J Pediatr Ophthalmol 13:163, 1976.
40. McCord CDJ, Chappell J, Pollard ZF: Congenital euryblepharon. Ann Ophthalmol 11:1217, 1979.
41. Shannon GM: Disorders of the lids. *In* Harley RD (ed): Pediatric Ophthalmology. Philadelphia, WB Saunders, 1975.
42. Waardenburg PJ, Franceschetti A, Klein D: Genetics and Ophthalmology. London, Oxford University Press, 1961.
43. Gupta AK, Ramanurthy S, Shukan KM: Euryblepharon: A case report. J Pediatr Ophthalmol 9:175, 1972.
44. Feldman E, Bowen SFJ, Morgan SS: Euryblepharon: A case report with photographs documenting the condition from infancy to adulthood. J Pediatr Ophthalmol Strabismus 17:307, 1980.
45. Keipert JA: Euryblepharon. Br J Ophthalmol 59:57, 1975.
46. Johnson CC: Epicanthus and epiblepharon. Arch Ophthalmol 96:1030, 1978.
47. Goldberger E: Epicanthus and its variants among caucasians. Arch Ophthalmol 16:506, 1936.
48. Dailey R: Epicanthus. *In* Fraunfelder FT, Roy FH (eds): Current Ocular Therapy, 3rd ed. Philadelphia, WB Saunders, 1990.
49. Quickert MH, Rathburn E: Suture repair of entropion. Arch Ophthalmol 85:778, 1971.
50. Quickert MH, Wilkes TD, Dryden RM: Nonincisional correction of epiblepharon and congenital entropion. Arch Ophthalmol 101:778, 1983.
51. Zak TA: Congenital primary upper eyelid entropion. J Pediatr Ophthalmol Strabismus 21:69, 1984.
52. Fox SA: Primary congenital entropion repair. Arch Ophthalmol 56:839, 1956.
53. Levitt JM: Epiblepharon and congenital entropion. Am J Ophthalmol 44:112, 1957.
54. Tse DT, Anderson RL, Fratkin JD: Aponeurosis disinsertion in congenital entropion. Ophthalmology 436, 1983.
55. Biglan AW, Buerger GFJ: Congenital horizontal tarsal kink. Am J Ophthalmol 89:522, 1980.
56. Wies IL: Spastic entropion. Trans Am Acad Ophthalmol Otolaryngol 59:503, 1955.
57. Ballen PH: A simple procedure for the relief of trichiasis and entropion of the upper lid. Arch Ophthalmol 72:239, 1964.
58. Young RJ: Congenital ectropion of the upper lids. Arch Dis Child 29:97, 1954.
59. Stern EN, Campbell CH, Faulkner HW, et al: Conservative management of congenital eversion of the eyelids. Am J Ophthalmol 75:319, 1973.
60. Forbes D: Congenital eversion of the eyelids. 18:180, 1965.

61. Kohn R, Romano PE: Blepharoptosis, blepharophimosis, epicanthus inversus, and telecanthus—A syndrome with no name. Am J Ophthalmol 72:625, 1971.
62. Zlotogora J, Sagi M, Cohen T: The blepharophimosis, ptosis, and epicanthus inversus syndrome: Delineation of two types. Am J Hum Genet 35:1020, 1983.
63. Older JJ: Blepharophimosis. *In* Fraunfelder FT, Roy FH (eds): Current Ocular Therapy, 3rd ed. Philadelphia, WB Saunders, 1990.
64. Callahan MA, Callahan A: Ophthalmic Plastic and Orbital Surgery. Birmingham, Aesculapius, 1979.
65. Carroll RP, Wilkins RB, Fredricks S, et al: Congenital medial canthal tendon malposition. Ann Ophthalmol 10:665, 1978.
66. DiGeorge AM, Olmstead RW, Harley RD, et al: Waardenburg's syndrome. Trans Am Acad Ophthalmol Otolaryngol 64:816, 1960.
67. Sutula FC, Fant EL: Repair of medial canthal dystopia. Ophthalmic Surg 17:570, 1986.

Chapter 152

■

Eyelid Infections

A. TYRONE GLOVER

The eyelids are subject to a variety of infectious diseases. Essentially any organism that infects the skin can also infect the eyelids. The eyelids may be the primary site of infection or they may be part of a larger multisystem infectious disease.

With the frequency and ease of worldwide travel and the increased emigration of individuals from less developed countries, the American physician is more likely than ever to encounter unusual infections. Many of these diseases may go unsuspected if they are not indigenous to one's practice locale.

Despite improvements in living conditions and health education, diseases such as tuberculosis and syphilis are on the rise. Immunocompromised patients, including those with AIDS, are susceptible to a number of opportunistic infections, e.g., candidiasis, aspergillosis, herpes zoster infection, and tuberculosis.

Early diagnosis and prompt treatment of eyelid infections are essential in decreasing ocular morbidity.

BACTERIAL INFECTIONS

Angular Blepharitis

Angular blepharitis is characterized by maceration, fissuring, scaling, and redness at the lateral or medial canthus, or both (Fig. 152–1). Frequently, there is an associated follicular conjunctivitis, moderate mucopurulent discharge, and adherent exudate. Classically, the causative organism is *Moraxella lacunata,* a gram-negative diplobacillus. *Staphylococcus aureus* may also be found, especially in colder climates. Previously, bacterial proteases were felt to be the reason for the localized angular maceration, although this has been refuted by Thygeson and Kimura[2] and van Bijsterveld.[3] Localization of the infection to the canthi probably is a result of the predilection of *Moraxella* exudate to accumulate at the canthal angles.[3] Maceration is related to the quantity and position of coherent exudate rather than to the proteolytic ability of the bacterial strains.[2] Localized

recurrent blepharitis may be caused by herpes simplex virus and should be included in the differential diagnosis.[4] Treatment consists of lid scrubs; massage; warm, moist compresses; and topical bacitracin or erythromycin. Oral tetracycline, doxycycline, or erythromycin should be prescribed for resistant cases.

Impetigo

Impetigo of the eyelids is frequently associated with infections of the face. This superficial skin infection is caused by group A *Streptococcus* or *S. aureus*. The lesions begin as small, 1- to 2-mm, erythematous macules that develop into vesicles and bullae. They rapidly progress and rupture, forming a thin, varnish-like crust in cases of staphylococcal (bullous) impetigo.[1] The crusts are thick and honey-colored in cases of *Streptococcus* alone or in mixed infections of streptococci and staphylococci.[1, 5, 51] The infection can be spread by fingers, towels, or household utensils, forming satellite lesions.

Impetigo occurs most frequently in children.[1, 5, 6] In a study of 37 children, Dajani and coworkers[5] recovered group A streptococci alone from 21 percent of lesions,

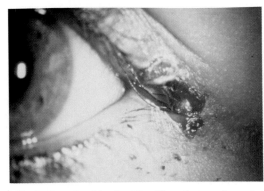

Figure 152–1. Angular blepharitis. Fissuring and exudate from the left lateral canthus. (Courtesy of MB Moore, M.D.)

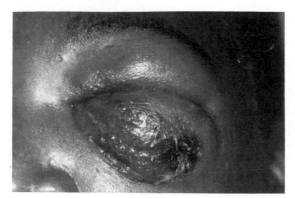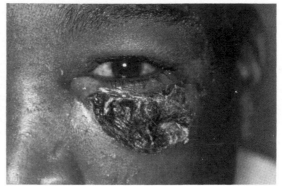

Figure 152–2. Anthrax of left lower lid. Black eschar occurs when lid edema resolves. (From Yorston D, Foster A: Cutaneous anthrax leading to corneal scarring from cicatricial ectropion. Br J Ophthalmol 73:809–811, 1989.)

S. aureus alone from 5 percent of lesions, and mixtures of streptococci and staphylococci from 61 percent of lesions.

Group A hemolytic streptococcal skin infections can lead to acute glomerulonephritis in 2 to 5 percent of cases.[6] In 150 children studied over a 2-yr period, however, impetigo contagiosum was associated with glomerulonephritis in only one instance.[7]

The disease can be diagnosed by its characteristic clinical appearance. Specimens should be obtained for culture and sensitivity testing to guide the antimicrobial therapy. The disease is highly contagious, thus precautions should be taken to prevent transmission.

Treatment consists of gentle washing of the affected area, followed by the application of bacitracin or erythromycin ointment. Oral administration of erythromycin for 7 to 10 days is effective treatment for bullous impetigo caused by *S. aureus,* and oral penicillin is best initially for group A streptococcal infections.[8]

Anthrax

Bacillus anthracis was the first organism proved to be the specific cause of an infectious disease.[9] Anthrax is primarily a disease of cattle, goats, and sheep, but humans can be infected by contact with contaminated animal hides. The average number of cases of anthrax reported annually in the United States has declined from 127 (1916 to 1925) to 0.7 (1977 to 1986).[10]

The disease, which is most prevalent in wool sorters, livestock workers, tanners, butchers, and cattlemen, occurs through injured skin, or more rarely the spores may be directly inhaled. The organisms proliferate at the site of inoculation, causing an inflammatory papule surrounded by bullae and intense edema. The papule progresses to a vesicle, then a pustule, and finally to a necrotic ulcer, forming a black eschar (Fig. 152–2). Progressive lid edema may lead to sloughing of the skin of the eyelid and ectropion with corneal exposure.[11]

The anthrax bacillus is readily recovered from the skin lesions. The drug of choice for cutaneous anthrax is oral potassium penicillin V. For extensive lesions, aqueous procaine penicillin G should be prescribed for

5 to 7 days.[10] Tetracycline, erythromycin, and sulfadiazine are also effective. Cicatricial eyelid deformities may require full-thickness skin grafts.

Malakoplakia

Only two cases of malakoplakia involving the eyelid have been described[12, 13] since its original description by Michaelis and Gutmann in 1902.[13a] This is a rare disorder that is unfamiliar to most ophthalmologists. Histologically, it is characterized by lesions containing peculiar, laminated basophilic structures within foamy histiocytes (von Hansemann histiocytes). The peculiar inclusions are called Michaelis-Gutmann bodies. The genitourinary, musculoskeletal, and gastrointestinal systems may be involved. Skin lesions are uncommon (Fig. 152–3). The disease occurs more often in immunosuppressed patients or in those with debilitating illnesses such as carcinoma, lymphoma, leukemia, or tuberculosis.[12, 13] Others have immunologic or inflammatory diseases such as sarcoidosis, ulcerative colitis, or rheumatoid arthritis.

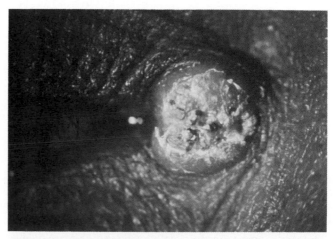

Figure 152–3. Clinical appearance of cutaneous malakoplakia showing a hyperkeratotic, dome-shaped, umbilicated mass on the right medial canthal region. (From Font RL, Bersani T, Eagle RC Jr: Malakoplakia of the eyelid. Published courtesy of Ophthalmology 95:61–68, 1988.)

It is difficult to diagnose this lesion clinically because there have been so few case reports.[12, 13] A medical history of predisposing factors may be helpful in making a diagnosis. Fortunately, excisional biopsy is generally both diagnostic and curative.[12, 13]

Syphilis

Syphilis is a contagious venereal disease caused by *Treponema pallidum*. The chancre of primary syphilis rarely occurs on the eyelid.[14] After an average incubation period of 21 days, the typical chancre begins as a single, painless, small, firm, red papule or a crusted superficial erosion. The lesion rapidly erodes, leaving a smooth base and indurated borders that have a characteristically cartilaginous consistency when palpated. Regional lymphadenopathy is common. Extragenital chancres may be more painful and follow a more chronic course than do genital chancres.[15] Spontaneous healing usually occurs within 3 to 6 wk.

Darkfield examination is the most specific and sensitive method for verifying the clinical diagnosis of primary syphilis. The fluorescent treponemal antibody absorption (FTA-ABS) and the micro-hemagglutination-*T. pallidum* (MHA-TP) test are positive in approximately 90 percent of such cases. In secondary syphilis, the Venereal Disease Research Laboratory (VDRL) test is always reactive. Once positive, the FTA-ABS and MHA-TP tests appear to remain so for life. These tests are usually positive in secondary, latent, and tertiary disease.

A maculopapular, papulosquamous, pustular, follicular, or nodular lesion can occur in secondary syphilis. The eyelid manifestations of late benign syphilis include the typical granulomatous lesion known as the gumma. Tarsitis or lid abscess may be found in cases of tertiary syphilis.[14]

Parenteral penicillin is the treatment of choice for all stages of acquired syphilis. Early syphilis is treated with benzathine penicillin G: 2.4 million units total (1.2 million units in each buttock) by intramuscular injection. Late syphilis is treated with benzathine penicillin G: 7.2 million units total (2.4 million units [1.2 million in each buttock]) intramuscularly weekly for 3 successive wk.[15, 16]

VIRAL INFECTIONS

Primary Herpes Simplex

An estimated 20,000 new cases of ocular herpes simplex virus infection occur yearly in the United States; 400,000 to 500,000 individuals are affected nationally.[17, 18] Liesegang[19] found a mean age of onset of 37 yr; the greatest incidence occurred among middle-aged individuals.[18] The primary infection is generally mild and frequently is clinically silent. For this reason, many cases go undiagnosed. Following infection, the virus becomes latent in the ganglionic cells of sensory neurons.

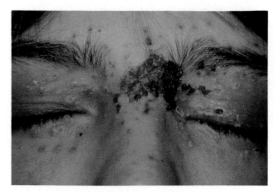

Figure 152–4. Herpes simplex infection, showing large number of periorbital and lid skin papules and vesicles. Note crusting of glabellar area as lesions heal. (Courtesy of MJ Mannis, M.D.)

The primary infection may involve the eyelids, with a crop of pinhead-sized vesicles that at first contain a clear fluid that later becomes seropurulent. The rupture of these vesicles leads to crusting (Fig. 152–4); they heal without scarring in about 7 days. The eyelid lesions may masquerade as edema or as a black eschar.[20] An erosive blepharitis may also occur[21] in primary or recurrent disease. A follicular or papillary conjunctivitis with or without keratitis may accompany the skin lesions. Corneal involvement is most commonly seen as a punctate epithelial keratitis but may appear as a dendrite or geographic ulcer.

Generally the diagnosis can be made clinically. Indirect immunofluorescent staining is a quick and reliable technique in confirming the diagnosis.[21] Topical antiviral agents are often reserved for cases with corneal involvement,[22] although many authors recommend their use prophylactically in all cases of herpetic blepharoconjunctivitis.[23]

Eczema Herpeticum (Kaposi's Varicelliform Eruption)

Patients with atopic eczema, severe seborrheic dermatitis, impetigo, scabies, Darier's disease, pemphigus, T-cell lymphoma, severe acne, or thermal burns may experience severe herpes simplex virus infection of diseased skin areas. Hundreds of nongrouped umbilicated vesicles may erupt. Fever and regional lymphadenopathy are common. The lesions rapidly become pustular and desiccate, leaving considerable scarring.

Herpes Zoster

Herpes zoster represents reactivation of latent varicella-zoster virus. This previously latent virus is activated by some change or depression in cell-mediated immunity. Precipitating factors include iatrogenic immunosuppression, chronic lymphocytic leukemia, Hodgkins' disease, or AIDS.[28]

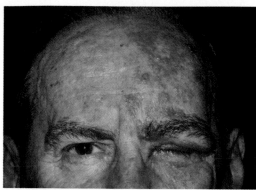

Figure 152–5. Herpes zoster ophthalmicus. Maculopapular and vesicular skin eruption in dermatomal distribution of the ophthalmic division of the trigeminal nerve. (Courtesy of MJ Mannis, M.D.)

In ophthalmic herpes zoster, the activated virus moves down the first division of cranial nerve V to cause an erythematous or maculopapular skin eruption, followed by vesiculoulcerative lesions in a dermatomal distribution (Fig. 152–5). The skin of the eyelids shows grouped vesicles on an erythematous base. The vesicles soon pustulate, ulcerate, and scar.

Although the histopathologic features of lesions in herpes zoster are similar to those in varicella, scarring may occur because of the deeper involvement of the dermis in herpes zoster. Cicatrization leads to lid margin abnormalities such as entropion, ectropion, lash loss, aberrant lashes, trichiasis, punctal and canalicular stenosis, lid retraction, and frank necrosis with subsequent exposure keratitis. Nasociliary branch involvement is heralded by Hutchinson's sign (vesicles on the side of the midportion of the nose).

Herpes zoster is more common in elderly persons and affects 300,000 individuals annually. The usual prodrome consists of headache, fever, malaise, nausea, burning, tingling, and paresthesias.

Treatment of eyelid lesions generally consists of topical or systemic antibiotics, or both, to decrease bacterial superinfection as well as cool saline or Domeboro compresses.[28] Bucci and coworkers described the successful management of postherpetic neuralgia with Zostrix, a topical analgesic cream containing 0.025 percent capsaicin.[29] Oral acyclovir should be administered early to decrease viral shedding and hasten the resolution of lesions and decrease the incidence of postherpetic neuralgia.[30] Immunosuppressed patients should be treated with intravenous acyclovir. The role of systemic steroids remains controversial.

Varicella

Chickenpox, or varicella, which usually occurs in children, is caused by the varicella-zoster virus. Although uncommon, lid involvement is characterized by nongrouped vesicular lesions resting on an erythematous base. An occasional lesion may become superinfected with bacteria, but most heal within 2 wk without treatment or scarring. Eyelid lesions should be treated with topical antibiotic ointment to prevent bacterial superinfection. Immunocompromised patients are treated with acyclovir within 3 days of the onset of disease.

Individuals with lid vesicles should be examined for conjunctival or corneal lesions and anterior uveitis. The conjunctival lesions consist of small limbal or perilimbal pocklike elevations or tarsal and bulbar conjunctival ulceration that heals without sequelae.[25, 26] The cornea may show superficial punctate keratitis, disciform keratitis, or dendritic figures.[25, 27] Treatment with topical steroids remains controversial.[25] Further guidelines for the management of herpes zoster keratouveitis are outlined in Chapter 6.

Molluscum Contagiosum

Molluscum is a double-stranded DNA poxvirus that causes multiple, round, waxy umbilicated skin papules (Fig. 152–6). The characteristic skin papules may be associated with a toxic follicular conjunctivitis with superior pannus and keratitis simulating trachoma. Severe disseminated disease may occur in patients with AIDS.[32, 33] The diagnosis is based upon recognition of the characteristic lesions. Incision with a No. 11 Bard-Parker scalpel, followed by expression of the viral bead using a chalazion curette is curative.[34, 35]

Vaccinia

Inoculation with vaccinia virus may lead to ocular complications such as infection of the eyelid or conjunctiva (Fig. 152–7). The cornea is involved in some patients. Vaccinia is primarily a disease of individuals who have been vaccinated against smallpox; the majority are preschool children. The virus is spread from the primary inoculation site by the hands or clothing. Eyelid involvement may cause scarring and permanent eyelash loss;[35] however, most lesions heal without scarring.[36] Lid disease is manifested by ulcerating pustules covered by a dirty gray membrane.[36] Preauricular adenopathy is common.

Most patients have no underlying predisposing con-

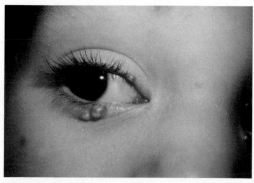

Figure 152–6. Molluscum contagiosum. Multiple, dome-shaped, waxy papules are situated along the lid margin.

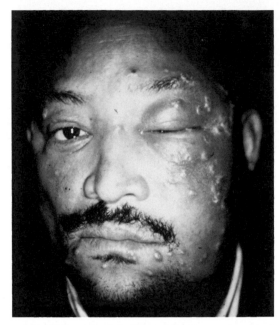

Figure 152–7. Vaccinia infection of the face, characterized by marked edema and erythema with crops of vesicles and pustules. The patient was accidentally infected by a recently vaccinated child. (Courtesy of A. P. Ferry, M.D.)

ditions; however, several conditions are known to predispose to the spread of vaccinia—eczema, hypogammaglobulinemia, steroid therapy, and AIDS.[35, 37]

In May 1990, the World Health Organization declared the world free of smallpox. Because of the virtual impossibility of contracting smallpox, the production of smallpox vaccine for general use was discontinued in 1982.[38] Smallpox vaccine continues to be administered to certain military populations worldwide and to laboratory workers exposed to orthopox viruses.[37, 38]

Treatment consists of topical vidarabine or rifampin administration.[36]

FUNGAL INFECTIONS

Blastomycosis

The causative agent of blastomycosis is *Blastomyces dermatitidis,* a yeastlike, dimorphic fungus that dwells in the soil as a saprophyte worldwide. It is most prevalent in the southeastern United States and the Ohio and Mississippi River basins. The fungus is found in endemic proportions in Kentucky.[39] Attempts to isolate the saprophytic source from which humans and others acquire *B. dermatitidis* have been essentially unsuccessful. Primary, but often subclinical, pulmonary infection occurs following inhalation of the conidia. The fungus then spreads hematogenously to involve various organs, but most frequently skin, bone, and the internal genitalia are involved. Skin involvement is marked by small, painless, nonpruritic, nondistinctive macules or papules that gradually enlarge, becoming raised, verrucous, reddened, and alternately weeping and crusted (Fig. 152–8).[39, 40] Facial lesions may spread to involve the eyelids.

The diagnosis is established by microscopic examination of potassium hydroxide–treated preparations of drainage from skin lesions.

Blastomycosis is effectively treated with amphotericin B, ketoconazole, or hydroxystilbamidine isethionate. The latter drug should be reserved for patients with nonprogressive cutaneous disease.[40]

Coccidioidomycosis

Coccidioides immitis is a dimorphic fungus found principally in the soil of the San Joaquin Valley of southeastern California and other dry regions of the southwestern United States. Pulmonary involvement, which may be subclinical, occurs during the summer and fall, the dry and dusty months of the year. Spread of infection to other organs occurs rarely. Lid involvement usually occurs as a consequence of disseminated disease and appears to take two forms: granulomatous fungating lesions from which organisms can be demonstrated or lid edema (Fig. 152–9).

Coccidioidin skin testing and serologic testing (tube precipitin or complement fixation) are valuable in establishing the diagnosis.[41] In addition, the diagnosis can be confirmed by demonstrating the organisms in culture or in tissue biopsy specimens.

Amphotericin B is the treatment of choice for severe disseminated or meningeal infections. Oral ketoconazole administration is of value in suppressing chronic progressive pulmonary, skeletal, or soft tissue infections.[42]

Cryptococcosis

Cryptococcosis is caused by *Cryptococcus neoformans,* a yeastlike, globose, budding fungus. There are two varieties: *C. neoformans neoformans* and *C. neoformans gattii.* Each variety has two serotypes; serotype A and D for *C. neoformans neoformans* and serotype B and C for *C. neoformans gattii.*[43] Serotype A is respon-

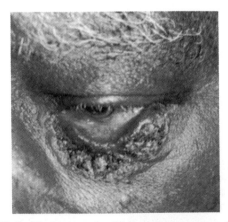

Figure 152–8. Blastomycosis. Clinical appearance of left lower lid. Note ectropion and blackish discoloration of papillomatous lesion. (From Barr C, Gamel JW: Blastomycosis of the eyelid. Arch Ophthalmol 104:96–97, 1986. Copyright 1986, American Medical Association.)

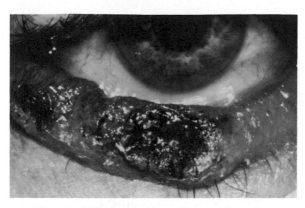

Figure 152–9. Coccidioidomycosis of the eyelid. The lateral two thirds of the right lower lid is thickened, reddened, and indurated with areas of ulceration and crusting. (From Font RL: Eyelids and lacrimal drainage system. *In* Spencer WA [ed]: Ophthalmic Pathology, 3rd ed. Philadelphia, WB Saunders, 1986, pp 2141–2336.

sible for disease worldwide and accounts for most infections in the United States; types B and C are uncommon as causes of cryptococcosis; however, type B has been isolated in southern California and southeastern Oklahoma. Serotype D causes most disease in Europe.[44] The organism lives freely in the soil; however, its association with avian feces, especially pigeons, has received the most notoriety. Human infections occur through inhalation of particles containing live *C. neoformans*.

Multiple organ systems can be infected, including the bone marrow, skin, liver, kidneys, lymph glands, and prostate gland. Involvement of the central nervous system is the most common form of cryptococcal infection and is particularly common in patients with AIDS. Skin lesions most commonly affect the face and scalp as erythematous papules, nodules, acneiform pustules, or subcutaneous abscesses that sometimes break down to form ulcers.

Confirmation of the clinical diagnosis is based upon culture of the organism from skin lesions, cerebrospinal fluid, blood, or urine. Of the available serodiagnostic tests that can indicate the presence of cryptococcal infections, the latex agglutination test is the most valuable.[45] The optimum therapeutic regimen for cryptococcal meningitis has yet to be established. Four agents are effective: amphotericin B, flucytosine, fluconazole, and ketoconazole. Oral ketoconazole may be effective in less severe infection of skin, lung, or bone.[42]

Sporotrichosis

Sporotrichosis is caused by the fungus *Sporothrix* (formerly called *Sporotrichum*) *schenckii*. This diphasic fungus thrives on living or dead vegetation. Although worldwide in distribution, it is found most often in central and South America.[42] Three forms occur, the cutaneous-lymphatic form, the pulmonary form, and the disseminated form. Cutaneous inoculation usually occurs from a thorn or splinter in a finger or hand. Horticulturists are particularly at risk.

The eyelid may be primarily affected; firm, painless, moveable subcutaneous nodules form.[9] Sometime following inoculation, a small, gradually enlarging subcutaneous nodule culminates in indurated, inflamed areas with overlying indolent ulceration. Subsequent lymphatic spread results in multiple subcutaneous nodules along the course of the draining lymphatics.[10] The nodules may ulcerate, releasing pus. The cutaneous lymphatic form can generally be diagnosed by its classic appearance. Unequivocal diagnosis is established by culture and identification of the organism. The treatment of choice for lymphocutaneous sporotrichosis is a saturated solution of oral potassium iodide. Alternate treatment is with oral ketoconazole.[42]

Mycetoma (Pseudallescheriasis)

Mycetoma is a slowly progressive, local, chronic infection of the skin, bone, and subcutaneous tissues. It can be caused by species of *Nocardia* or *Streptomyces*. The most common sites of infection are the feet (Madura foot) or legs. Lid involvement is rare.[9] Mycetomas usually begin as small, indurated, painless subcutaneous nodules that later break down to form sinus tracts that drain granule-containing pus. The disease is further characterized by grotesque and disfiguring swelling. Mycetoma occurs worldwide and has been isolated frequently from soil in the eastern, central, and northern portions of the United States. The most common cause in the United States is *Pseudallescheria boydii*.[42] Immunocompromised or debilitated individuals are most susceptible.

Mycetomas may be diagnosed by their characteristic clinical appearance. The diagnosis is confirmed by finding granules in pus or tissue samples. The treatment of choice is intravenous miconazole. Alternate treatment is with intravenous amphotericin B or oral ketoconazole.[42]

Aspergillosis

Aspergillosis refers to a variety of conditions ranging from colonization of previously damaged respiratory tissues (aspergillar bronchitis, extrinsic allergic alveolitis) to invasion of the lung or other loci, e.g., eyes, paranasal sinuses, burn wounds, and prosthetic heart valves.[44] Invasive aspergillosis is a significant cause of morbidity and mortality in immunocompromised patients. As an opportunistic mycosis in immunocompromised individuals, it is second only to *Candida*. Infection of the lids is rare, but chronic granulomatous lesions have been reported.[9] Aspergillar keratomycosis or endophthalmitis may occur following trauma or surgery, and orbital involvement occasionally occurs in immunosuppressed patients. The diagnosis is secured by the demonstration of the organism in cultures and smears. Amphotericin B remains the drug of choice for disseminated or pulmonary disease.[41]

Candidiasis

Candida is a saprophytic, yeastlike dimorphic fungus. Primary eyelid infection with *Candida* is rare; it usually occurs as a secondary infection, with the mouth being the primary site of infection. It is the most common opportunistic fungus occurring in children and debilitated or immunocompromised adults. There is a white, slightly adherent, membranous deposit on a reddened base in the mouth. On the lids, milder cases show scaly, gray or reddish, definitely marginated lesions, whereas in more severe cases, vesicles develop and rupture, leaving oozing areas and small, whitish yellow pustules enclosed by undermined epidermis.[9, 36]

Diagnosis is established by scrapings and culture of the lesion. Treatment consists of topical nystatin, clotrimazole, or miconazole and correction of underlying causes, such as control of diabetes mellitus or cessation of the administration of systemic corticosteroids. Patients with chronic mucocutaneous or disseminated disease should receive oral ketoconazole or intravenous amphotericin B, or both.[42]

MYCOBACTERIAL INFECTIONS

Tuberculosis

Primary infection of the eyelid with *Mycobacterium tuberculosis* is rare. The earliest lesion is a brownish red, soft papule that develops into an indurated nodule or plaque that may ulcerate. There is prominent regional lymphadenopathy. Tuberculous tarsitis may appear as a result of direct spread from the overlying lid skin or as a metastatic process.[36, 45] The diagnosis is established through tuberculin skin testing, stains for acid-fast organisms, and cultures. The currently recommended regimen for treatment of active tuberculosis is isoniazid, rifampin, and pyrazinamide for 2 mo, followed by isoniazid and rifampin daily or biweekly for 4 mo.[46] If isoniazid resistance is suspected, ethambutol should be included in the initial phase. Longer courses of treatment are prescribed for HIV-infected persons.

Nontuberculous (Atypical) Mycobacterial Infections

Atypical mycobacteria may cause granulomatous infection and abscess of the eyelid skin. In the United States, the major cause for disease in humans is *M. avium* complex followed by *M. kansasii* and *M. fortuitum–M. chelonei.*[47] *M. fortuitum* may cause cutaneous infections after inoculation through penetrating wounds or traumatized tissues. *M. fortuitum–M. chelonei* infections are rare but have been reported as a cause of dacryocystitis, orbital granuloma, and keratitis.[48–51] The *M. fortuitum–M. chelonei* group of atypical mycobacteria are quite resistant to all available antimycobacterial drugs. Treatment is guided by antimicrobial susceptibility testing of the mycobacterial isolate. Large doses of erythromycin, doxycycline, amikacin, or sulfamethizole

have appeared helpful in isolated cases.[46] Débridement, incision, and drainage should be employed as well. Cryotherapy proved to be effective treatment in one case.[48]

Leprosy

Leprosy is a chronic infectious disease caused by *M. leprae,* a pleomorphic, acid-fast bacillus. It most commonly affects the skin, nerves, and lymphoreticular system.

The diagnosis of leprosy is based on the typical skin findings and peripheral nerve involvement. Skin scrapings or biopsy will show the typical noncaseating tuberculoid granuloma or acid-fast bacilli (scant in tuberculoid variant) and a positive result on a lepromin skin test result.[45] The fluorescent leprosy antigen absorption test is also effective.

Four variants of the disease are recognized: indeterminate, tuberculoid, borderline, and lepromatous. The variants probably reflect differences in host cell-mediated immunity.[45, 52] The tuberculoid variant (good cell-mediated immunity) is characterized by few skin lesions and early neural involvement of cranials nerves V and VII. The skin lesion classically appears as a large erythematous plaque with well-defined borders that are elevated and slope down to a central shallow ulcer.

Lepromatous leprosy (poor cell-mediated immunity) is marked by a macular skin rash that quickly develops into nodular dermal lesions (lepromas). The progressive thickening and wrinkling of the skin of the nose, forehead, and cheeks produces the characteristic "leonine facies."

In borderline leprosy, only the skin and nerves are involved. The indeterminate type is short-lived and will evolve into the other types or resolve completely.

In both tuberculoid and lepromatous leprosy, involvement of the eyelid gives rise to a number of secondary changes. Common findings include loss of eyebrows and eyelashes, misdirected lashes, lagophthalmos and exposure keratitis, paralytic ectropion with secondary punctal eversion, and reduction of the blinking rate.[52–54] These cicatricial and paralytic eyelid changes can lead to corneal ulceration, perforation, and ultimately loss of the eye.

Because primary and secondary resistance to dapsone has been increasing, multiple-drug therapy has been recommended. For combined chemotherapy, dapsone, rifampin, and clofazimine should be prescribed. Ethionamide can be substituted for clofazimine when the latter is unacceptable.[46]

Surgical efforts should be directed toward reducing exposure of the cornea. Tarsorrhaphy or lateral tarsal strip procedures, or both, are often necessary.[52, 53]

PARASITIC INFECTIONS

Demodex

Demodex folliculorum is found most commonly in hair follicles of the nasolabial folds, the nose, and the eyelids.[55] Despite the frequent presence of *Demodex* in eyelid hair follicles, their exact role in causing blepharitis remains unclear.[55, 56] An assiduous examination will reveal the organism in most patients; however, most are asymptomatic. In examining 100 biopsy specimens of eyelid skin, Roth found mites in 84 percent of all cases and in 100 percent of patients older than age 70 yr.[56] Symptoms of itching, pain, and burning are common with significant infestations. Diagnosis is established by the clinical findings of a semitransparent, almost plastic, thin, tubelike crusting of the skin around the lashes. Histologic section by English and Nutting showed that the bulk of these cuffs consists of keratin; they proposed that excess keratin may be the result of the abrasive action of the mites' sharp claws.[57] Examination of epilated lashes by light microscopy will confirm the diagnosis.[58] Treatment consists of lid scrubs followed by the application of bacitracin, erythromycin, or sulfacetamide ointment.

Phthiriasis

The crab louse, *Phthirus pubis,* is usually found in the hairs of the genital region; however, infestation of the axilla, beard, eyebrows, and eyelashes may occur. Transmission is by direct contact with infested individuals and occasionally by contact with infested personal articles (towels, clothing). Children may be infested through close personal contact such as sleeping with an infested parent.

Eyelid involvement frequently causes blepharoconjunctivitis. The usual symptoms are itching and burning. Examination of the affected eyelid shows tiny, pearly white nits (eggs or egg cases) attached to the lashes (Fig. 152–10). The nits are easily visualized; however, the transparent adult lice may be impossible to see without slit-lamp magnification. Preauricular lymphadenopathy and secondary infection at the site of the lice bites may occur.[60]

The ideal treatment for *Phthirus pubis* palpebrarum has yet to be established.[61, 62] Mechanical removal of the nits with forceps is tedious and time-consuming; general anesthesia may be required in small children. A thick

occlusive application of ophthalmic ointment smothers the ectoparasite but does not kill the nits. The application of 1 percent γ-benzene hexachloride is effective but may cause ocular irritation, and reapplication in 5 to 6 days is necessary to eliminate the newly hatched nits. Physostigmine eye ointment is often recommended but causes miosis and ciliary spasm and is ineffective against the nits. The application of a smothering coat of antibiotic ointment or physostigmine ointment would have to be continued for up to 14 days to kill the lice emerging from the eggs. Awan has described the use of both cryotherapy and argon laser phototherapy as effective treatments.[63, 64] These modalities have not enjoyed widespread use. Mathew and coworkers found treatment with one or two drops of 20 percent fluorescein on the lid margin to be very effective.[62]

Further management of phthiriasis requires treatment of all contacts and delousing of all clothing, bedding, and personal items. Disinfection can be accomplished by machine washing in hot water and drying using the hot cycle of the dryer or dry cleaning.[16] Any other affected body areas should be treated with permethrin (1 percent) cream (Nix) or Lindane 1 percent shampoo (γ-benzene hexachloride). Patients should be reevaluated after 1 wk; retreatment may be necessary if lice or eggs are found.[16]

Myiasis

The infestation of living vertebrate animal tissues by fly larvae (maggots) is known as myiasis. Ophthalmomyiasis refers specifically to infestations that involve the eye and ocular adnexa. Less than 5 percent of human myiasis cases involve the eye.[66] Eyelid margin involvement is unusual. Classification of ophthalmomyiasis is based on the portion of the eye and ocular adnexa affected. External myiasis occurs when the lids and conjunctivae are infested, and internal myiasis takes place when the larvae are within the globe.[66–69] Orbital myiasis can also occur but is very rare.[66]

The disease is most prevalent in Mexico, Central and South America, tropical Africa, and the southwestern United States. In the United States, conjunctival-external myiasis is usually caused by the cattle botfly (*Hypoderma bovis*). *Estrus ovis* (the sheep botfly) is responsible for most cases of ophthalmomyiasis interna.[69] Human cutaneous myiasis is caused by fly larvae of the following species: *Cochliomyia hominivorax, Dermatobia hominis* (Fig. 152–11A), *Wohlfahrtia vigil, W. magnifica* and *Cordylobia anthropophaga*.[71]

Myiasis of the eyelid has been reported from *Cuterebra larva*[70] and *D. hominis*.[68] Some of these varieties puncture the skin and extrude the ova beneath the surface, whereas others deposit their eggs on open wounds or ulcers. Myiatic maggots produce furuncular, boil-like lesions that periodically drain serosanguineous fluid.[68, 71] Secondary bacterial infections can occur.

Treatment consists of surgical removal of the maggots (Fig. 152–11B). Following the injection of local anesthetic, a small incision is made and the larva is grasped

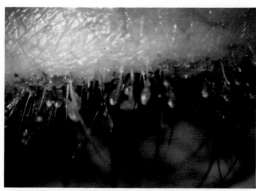

Figure 152–10. Phthiriasis. Eggs and egg cases adhering to base of eyelashes. (Courtesy of ML Mannis, M.D.)

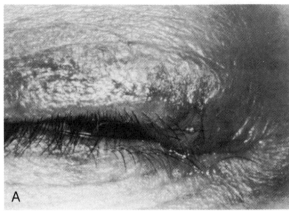

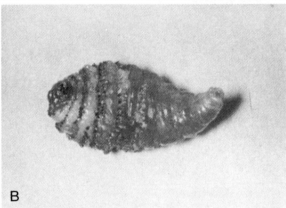

Figure 152–11. *A,* Myiasis. Eyelid cellulitis with a small sore through which the caudal end of a maggot intermittently appeared. *B,* Late-stage *Dermatobia hominis* larva, 15 mm in length, removed from eyelid lesion. Note black spines on anterior segments. (Reprinted with permission from The American Journal of Ophthalmology. Copyright by the Ophthalmic Publishing Company. Wilhemus KR: Myiasis palpebrarum. Am J Ophthalmol 101:496–498, 1986.)

and removed with a small hemostat. The wound is then packed open and antibiotics are prescribed as needed.[72] Ten percent ethyl ether in vegetable oil applied to the opening of the wound before surgical removal may be useful in slightly anesthetizing the maggots.[71]

Leishmaniasis

Leishmaniasis is caused by various morphologically indistinguishable species of *Leishmania*. The protozoa are transmitted by sandflies of the genus *Phlebotomus.* Cutaneous leishmaniasis (oriental sore) is caused by *L. tropica* (Old World leishmaniasis) and *L. brasiliensis, L. mexicana,* or *L. peruviana* (New World leishmaniasis).[73] It occurs in nearly all countries bordering the Mediterranean, the Near and Middle East, parts of India, and on the West Coast of Africa. American mucocutaneous leishmaniasis is found in southern Mexico to northern Argentina, Brazil, and Peru and is caused by *L. brasiliensis.*[74] The nasal mucosa, hard and soft palate, and nasal septum may be invaded and destroyed.[74] Death usually results from secondary infection.[75] Kala-azar or visceral leishmaniasis is prevalent in India, in China north of the Yangtze River, in the former Soviet Union, in countries bordering the Mediterranean, the Sudan, and Kenya and is widely scattered in parts of South America.[75] The reticuloendothelial system, liver, and spleen are invaded. Death usually results from secondary infection.

Sandflies transmit the organism to humans after taking a blood meal from several reservoir hosts that vary according to region; they are usually wild rodents, including rats, mice, agoutis, and pacas.[74] The protozoa live intracellularly as Leishman-Donovan bodies. After an extremely variable incubation period (2 wk to 3 yr), an erythematous pruritic papule occurs at the site of inoculation. The papule may then become scaled, crusted, and finally ulcerated (Fig. 152–12). Characteristically, the sore has a raised circular border. Most lesions heal spontaneously, leaving a depressed and depigmented scar.[75] Secondary bacterial infection occurs frequently and leads to regional lymphadenopathy and scarring. The most common site of involvement is the face, followed by the arms and legs.

Eyelid involvement occurs in 2 to 5 percent of cases of cutaneous leishmaniasis.[9, 76] The first case described in the English literature was by Morgan in 1965. Eyelid lesions may occur if infected material reaches the lid from nasal mucosal lesions via the nasolacrimal duct.[76] The typical lesion has a raised, circular border.

The diagnosis is established by demonstrating the organisms in fluid aspirated from the ulcer bed[75] or by finding the organisms in stained slit-skin smears taken from nonulcerated parts of the lesion.[77] Leishman-Donovan bodies are best seen with Giemsa or Wright stain.[78] The intradermal injection of a killed suspension of leptomonads (Montenegro test) produces positive results in a high percentage of *L. tropica* infections and in more than 95 percent of *L. brasiliensis* infections.[75]

Although the cutaneous lesions are self-limited, the resultant scarring can be disfiguring. Treatment of some eyelid lesions should be instituted to shorten the duration of infection and to prevent scarring and tissue destruction. There are many modes of therapy, but generally the treatment of choice in the United States is systemic sodium stibogluconate (Pentostam); however, this agent has been associated with a number of side effects, including nausea, vomiting, skin rashes, elevated liver enzyme levels, nephropathy, and cardiac arrhythmias.[79, 80] Intralesional sodium stibogluconate[79]

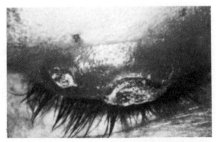

Figure 152–12. Leishmaniasis. Right upper lid ulcers with large primary lesion and satellite lesion temporally. (From Chu FC, Rodriques MM, Cogan DG, et al: Leishmaniasis affecting the eyelid. Arch Ophthalmol 101:84–91, 1983.

and local ultrasound-induced hyperthermia[80] have been suggested as alternative modes of treatment.

Dirofilariasis

Dirofilariasis is a zoonosis caused by several species of *Dirofilaria*. Infections in humans have been sporadically reported from the Mediterranean basin, South America, and Africa,[81] and more than half of case reports have originated in the United States (Florida, Louisiana, Texas).[82, 83] Infections are transmitted to humans by mosquitoes.

D. tenuis, a natural parasite of the racoon, is the most common species acquired in the United States. Both *D. tenuis* and *D. conjunctivae* are found in the subcutaneous tissues (Fig. 152–13); subconjunctival involvement is uncommon.[81–83] *D. immitis,* the dog heartworm, may cause pulmonary infarction and solitary pulmonary nodules ("coin lesions").[81, 82]

The typical lesion is an inflamed subcutaneous lid mass.[83] The diagnosis is confirmed by demonstrating the worm in the excised lid tissues. The worms may be dead or alive. The infection is terminated by removing them.

Cysticercosis

The larval form of the adult pork tapeworm is known as *Cysticercus cellulosae*. The life cycle of *Taenia solium* commonly involves humans as definitive hosts and swine as the natural intermediate hosts, but in some circumstances humans act in this role. Intestinal cestodiasis is acquired by humans through the ingestion of raw or insufficiently cooked pork. In contrast, cysticercosis takes place by the ingestion of soil, water, or food contaminated with eggs, or by reverse peristalsis of eggs or proglottides to the upper portions of the duodenum or stomach.[84] After hatching in the small bowel or stomach, the oncospheres penetrate directly into the intestinal wall. Cysticerci may then invade the brain, striated muscle, eye, heart, and lung.

Although subconjunctival, subretinal-vitreous, and orbital cysticercosis occurs relatively frequently, cysticerci are rarely found in the subcutaneous tissues of the lid.[85, 86] Eyelid involvement was reported in only 1 patient in a series of 452 patients with ocular cysticer-cosis.[87] Patients typically present with a painless, usually stationary, subcutaneous mass.

The diagnosis is made by surgical removal of the subcutaneous mass and demonstration of the cysticercus. If found, an exhaustive search for cysticerci in the central nervous system should be carried out because the continuing shower of eggs may lead to death from massive involvement of the brain.[85]

REFERENCES

1. Oster HB: Blepharitis. *In* Tasman W, Jaeger EA (eds): Duanes Clinical Ophthalmology, vol. 4. Philadelphia, JB Lippincott, 1989, pp 1–7.
2. Thygeson P, Kimura SJ: Chronic conjunctivitis. Trans Am Acad Ophthalmol Otolaryngol 67:494, 1963.
3. Van Bijsterveld OP: Bacterial proteases in *Moraxella* angular conjunctivitis. Am J Ophthalmol 72:181–184, 1971.
4. Jakobiec FA, Srinivasan BD, Gamboa ET: Recurrent herpetic blepharitis in an adult. Am J Ophthalmol 88:744–747, 1979.
5. Dajani AS, Ferrieri P, Wannamaker LW: Natural history of impetigo. J Clin Invest 51:2863–2871, 1972.
6. Domonkos AN: Bacterial infections. *In* Arnold HL Jr, Odom RB, James WD: Andrews' Diseases of the Skin, 6th ed. Philadelphia, WB Saunders, 1971, pp 272–319.
7. Hall WD, Blumber RW, Moody MD: Studies in children with impetigo: Bacteriology, serology and incidence of glomerulonephritis. Am J Dis Child 125:800–806, 1973.
8. Dillon HC: Topical and systemic therapy for pyodermas. Int J Dermatol 19:443–451, 1980.
9. Duke Elder S, MacFaul PA: The ocular adnexa: Diseases of the eyelid. Duke-Elder System of Ophthalmology, vol. 13, part 1. St. Louis, CV Mosby, 1974, pp 81–249.
10. Brachman PS: Anthrax. *In* Hoeprich PD, Jordan MC (eds): Infectious Diseases, 4th ed. Philadelphia, JB Lippincott, 1989, pp 1007–1013.
11. Yorston D, Foster A: Cutaneous anthrax leading to corneal scarring from cicatricial ectropion. Br J Ophthalmol 731:809–811, 1989.
12. Addison DJ: Malakoplakia of the eyelid. Ophthalmology 93:1064–1067, 1986.
13. Font RL, Bersani TA, Eagle RC: Malakoplakia of the eyelid. Ophthalmology 95:61–68, 1988.
13a. Michaelis L, Gutmann C: Über Einschlüsse Blasentumoren. Z Klin Med 47:208–215, 1902.
14. Jegakumar W, Chithra A, Shanmugasundararaj A: Primary syphilis of the eyelid; case report. Genitourin Med 3:192–193, 1989.
15. Rudolph AH: Syphilis. *In* Hoeprich PD, Jordan MC (eds): Infectious Diseases, 4th ed. Philadelphia, JB Lippincott, 1989, pp 666–684.
16. Centers for Disease Control: 1989 Sexually Transmitted Diseases Treatment Guidelines. MMWR 38:7–14, 1989.
17. Liesegang TJ, Melton JM, Daly PJ, et al: Epidemiology of ocular herpes simplex. Arch Ophthalmol 107:1155–1159, 1989.
18. National Institutes of Health: Workshop on the treatment and prevention of herpes simplex virus infections. J Infect Dis 127:117–119, 1973.
19. Liesegang TJ: Epidemiology of ocular herpes simplex. Arch Ophthalmol 107:1160–1165, 1989.
20. Nauheim JS, Sussman W: Herpes simplex of the lids and adjacent areas. Trans Am Acad Ophthalmol Otolaryngol 75:1236–1241, 1971.
21. Egerer I, Stary A: Erosive-ulcerative herpes simplex blepharitis. Arch Ophthalmol 98:1760–1763, 1980.
22. Simon JW, Longo F, Smith RS: Spontaneous resolution of herpes simplex blepharoconjunctivitis in children. Am J Ophthalmol 102:598–600, 1986.
23. Cykiert RC: Spontaneous resolution of herpes simplex blepharoconjunctivitis in children. [Letter] Am J Ophthalmol 103:340, 1987.
24. Chu W, Pavan-Langston D: Ocular surface manifestations of the major viruses. Int Ophthalmol Clin 2:135, 1979.
25. Jordan DR, Leon-Paul N, Clarke WN: Ocular involvement in varicella. Clin Pediatr 23:434–436, 1984.

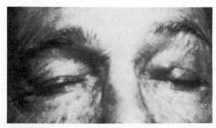

Figure 152–13. Subcutaneous dirofiliariasis. Inflammatory nodule involving left upper lid of 69-year-old man. Nodule had been present for 2 mo. (From Font RL, Neafie RC, Perry HD: Subcutaneous dirofilariasis of the eyelid and ocular adnexa, report of six cases. Arch Ophthalmol 98:1079–1082, 1980. Copyright 1980, American Medical Association.)

26. Edwards TS: Ophthalmic complications from varicella. J Pediatr Ophthalmol 2:37, 1965.
27. Easty DL: Ocular disease in varicella zoster infections. *In* Easty DL: Virus Disease of the Eye. Chicago, Year Book Medical Publishers, 1985, pp 228–252.
28. Liesegang TJ: The varicella-zoster virus: Systemic and ocular features. J Am Acad Dermatol 11:165–191, 1984.
29. Bucci FA, Gabriels CF, Krohel GB: Successful treatment of postherpetic neuralgia with capsaicin. Am J Ophthalmol 106:758–759, 1988.
30. Cobo ML, Foulks GN, Liesegang T, et al: Oral acyclovir in the therapy of acute herpes zoster ophthalmicus. Ophthalmology 92:1574–1583, 1985.
31. Cobbold RJC, MacDonald A: Molluscum contagiosum as a sexually transmitted disease. Practitioner 204:416–419, 1970.
32. Kohn SR: Molluscum contagiosum in patients with acquired immunodeficiency syndrome. Arch Ophthalmol 105:458, 1987.
33. Katzman M, Carey JT, Elmets CA, et al: Molluscum contagiosum and the acquired immunodeficiency syndrome: Clinical and immunological details of two cases. Br J Dermatol 116:131–138, 1987.
34. Gonnering RS, Kronish JW: Treatment of periorbital molluscum contagiosum by incision and curettage. Ophthalmic Surg 19:325–327, 1988.
35. Ruben FL, Lane JM: Ocular vaccinia. Arch Ophthalmol 84:45–48, 1970.
36. Smolin G, Tabbara K, Whitcher J: Lids. *In* Smolin G: Infectious Diseases of the Eye. Baltimore, Williams & Wilkins, 1984, pp 24–53.
37. Wright DC, James WD, Jones TS, et al: Disseminated vaccinia in a military recruit with human immunodeficiency virus (HIV) disease. N Engl J Med 316:673–676, 1987.
38. Centers for Disease Control: Smallpox vaccine no longer available for civilians—United States. MMWR 32:387, 1983.
39. Barr CC, Gamel JW: Blastomycosis of the eyelid. Arch Ophthalmol 104:96–99, 1986.
40. Utz JP: Blastomycosis. *In* Hoeprich AD, Jordan MC (eds): Infectious Diseases, 4th ed. Philadelphia, JB Lippincott, 1989, pp 510–516.
41. Rodenbiker HT, Ganley JP: Ocular coccidiomycosis. Surv Ophthalmol 24:263–290, 1980.
42. American Medical Association: Drugs used for systemic mycoses. *In* Drug Evaluations Annual 1991, 7th ed. Milwaukee, 1990, pp 1479–1492.
43. Kwon-Chung KJ, Polacheck I, Bennett JE: Improved diagnostic medium for separation of *Cryptococcus neoformans* var. neoformans (serotype A and D) and *Cryptococcus neoformans* var. gattii (serotype B and C). J Clin Microbiol 15:535–537, 1982.
44. Hoeprich PD: Crytococcosis. *In* Hoeprich PD, Jordan MC (eds): Infectious Diseases, 4th ed. Philadelphia, JB Lippincott, 1989, pp 1131–1141.
45. Starr MB: Infections and hypersensitivity of the eyelids. *In* Smith BC, Della Rocca RC, Nesi FA, et al (eds): Ophthalmic Plastic and Reconstructive Surgery, vol. 1. St Louis, CV Mosby, 1987, pp 283–308.
46. American Medical Association: Antimycobacterial drugs. *In* Drug Evaluations Annual, 7th ed, 1991. Milwaukee, 1990, pp 1447–1475.
47. Obrien RJ, Geiter LJ, Snider DE Jr: Epidemiology of nontuberculous mycobacterial diseases in the United States: Results from a national survey. Am Rev Respir Dis 135:1007–1014, 1987.
48. Katowitz JA, Kropp TM: *Mycobacterium fortuitum* as a cause for nasolacrimal obstruction and granulomatous eyelid disease. Ophthalmic Surg 18:97–99, 1987.
49. Centers for Disease Control: *Mycobacterium* infections following eye surgery—Texas. MMWR 32:591–597, 1983.
50. Meisler DM, Friedlander MH, Okumoto M: *Mycobacterium chelonei* keratitis. Am J Ophthalmol 94:398–401, 1982.
51. Smith RE, Salz JJ, Moors R, et al: *Mycobacterium chelonei* and orbital granuloma after tear duct probing. Am J Ophthalmol 89:139–141, 1980.
52. Schwab IR: Ocular leprosy. *In* Tabbara KF, Hyndiuk RA (eds): Infections of the Eye. Boston, Little, Brown, 1986, pp 613–623.
53. Choyce DP: Diagnosis and management of ocular leprosy. Br J Ophthalmol 53:217–223, 1969.
54. Holmes JW: Leprosy of the eye. Trans Am Ophthalmol Soc 55:145, 1957.
55. Ruffi T, Mumcuoglu Y: The hair follicle mites *Demodex folliculorum* and *Demodex brevis:* Biology and medical importance: A review. Dermatologica 162:1–11, 1987.
56. Roth AM: *Demodex folliculorum* in hair follicles of eyelid skin. Ann Ophthalmol 11:37–40, 1979.
57. English FP, Nutting WB: Demodicosis of ophthalmic concern. Am J Ophthalmol 91:362–372, 1981.
58. Coston TO: *Demodex folliculorum* blepharitis. Trans Am Ophthalmol Soc 65:361–392, 1967.
59. English FP: Demodex: A cause of blepharitis in Australia. Med J Aust 28:1359–1360, 1969.
60. Couch JM, Green WR, Hirst LW, et al: Diagnosing and treating *Phthirus pubis palpebrarum*. Surv Ophthalmol 26:219–225, 1982.
61. Burns DA: The treatment of *Phthirus pubis* infestation of the eyelashes. Br J Ophthalmol 117:741–743, 1987.
62. Mathew M, D'Souza P, Methta DK: A new treatment of phthiriasis palpebrarum. Ann Ophthalmol 14:439–441, 1982.
63. Awan KJ: Cryotherapy in phthiriasis palpebrarum. Am J Ophthalmol 83:906–907, 1977.
64. Awan KJ: Argon laser phototherapy of phthiriasis palpebrarum. Ophthalmic Surg 17:813–814, 1986.
65. Kersten RC, Shoukiey NM, Tabbara KF: Orbital myiasis. Ophthalmology 93:1228–1232, 1986.
66. Ziemianski MC, Lee KY, Sabates FN: Ophthalmomyiasis interna. Arch Ophthalmol 98:1588–1589, 1986.
67. Savino DF, Margo CE, McCoy ED, et al: Dermal myiasis of the eyelid. Ophthalmology 93:1225–1227, 1986.
68. Hennessy DJ, Sherrill JW, Binder PS: External ophthalmomyiasis caused by *Estrus ovis*. Am J Ophthalmol 84:802–805, 1977.
69. Rodrigues MM, Weis MD, Muncy DW: Ophthalmomyiasis of the eyelid caused by *Cutebra larva*. Am J Ophthalmol 78:1024–1026, 1974.
70. Trpis M: Cutaneous myiasis. *In* Hoeprich PD, Jordan MC (eds): Infectious Diseases, 4th ed. Philadelphia, JB Lippincott, 1989, pp 1084–1086.
71. Wilhelmus KR: Myiasis palpebrarum. Am J Ophthalmol 101:496–498, 1986.
72. Kenney RL, Baker FJ: Botfly (*Dermatobia hominis*) myiasis. Int J Dermatol 23:676–677, 1984.
73. American Medical Association: Antiprotozoal Drugs. *In* Drug Evaluations Annual 1991, 7th ed. Milwaukee, 1990, pp 1493–1531.
74. Roizenblait J: Interstitial keratitis caused by (mucocutaneous) leishmaniasis. Am J Ophthalmol 87:175–179, 1979.
75. Markell EK, Voge M: Other blood and tissue dwelling protozoa. *In* Markell EK, Voge M: Medical Parasitology, 3rd ed. Philadelphia, WB Saunders, 1971, pp 113–149.
76. Morgan G: Case of cutaneous leishmaniasis of the lid. Br J Ophthalmol 49:542–545, 1965.
77. Ferry AP: Cutaneous leishmaniasis (oriental sore) of the eyelid. Am J Ophthalmol 84:349–353, 1977.
78. Chu FC, Rodriques MM, Cogan DG, et al: Leishmaniasis affecting the eyelid. Arch Ophthalmol 101:84–91, 1983.
79. Sharquie KE, Al-Talib K, Chu AC: Intralesional therapy of cutaneous leishmaniasis with sodium stibogluconate antimony. Br J Dermatol 119:53–57, 1988.
80. Aram H, Leibovici V: Ultrasound-induced hyperthermia in treatment of cutaneous leishmaniasis. Cutis 40:350–353, 1987.
81. Marsden PD: Dirofilariasis. *In* Wyngaarden JB, Smith LH Jr (eds): Cecil Textbook of Medicine, 17th ed. Philadelphia, WB Saunders, 1982, p 1777.
82. Markell EK, Voge M: The blood and tissue-dwelling nematodes. *In* Markell EK, Voge M: Medical Parasitology, 3rd ed. Philadelphia, WB Saunders 1971, pp 243–274.
83. Font RL, Neafie RC, Perry HD: Subcutaneous dirofilariasis of the eyelid and ocular adnexa, report of six cases. Arch Ophthalmol 98:1079–1082, 1980.
84. Markell EK, Voge M: The cestodes. *In* Markell EK, Voge M: Medical Parasitology, 3rd ed. Philadelphia, WB Saunders 1971, pp 187–215.
85. Perry HD, Font RL: Cysticercosis of the eyelid. Arch Ophthalmol 96:1255–1257, 1978.
86. Jampol LM, Caldwell JBH, Albert DM: *Cysticercus cellulosae* in the eyelid. Arch Ophthalmol 8:319–320, 1973.
87. Malik SRK, Gupta AK, Choundhry S: Ocular cysticercosis. Am J Ophthalmol 66:1168–1171, 1968.

Chapter 153

■

Benign Epithelial Tumors

CRAIG E. GEIST

Numerous benign and malignant tumors occur on the lids. In Iowa, in a study spanning a 38-year period between 1932 and 1969, 892 lid lesions were processed through the pathology laboratory.[1] Of these lesions, 76 per cent were benign; the most common tumors were seborrheic keratosis (23.8 per cent), benign epithelial cyst (21.9 per cent), chalazion (16 per cent), inflammatory dermatosis and nevus (each about 12 per cent), and xanthelasma (4.4 per cent). Among the malignant tumors, the vast majority (80.4 per cent) were basal cell carcinoma.

It is important when evaluating lid lesions to bear in mind that malignancies can mimic a host of benign conditions. Early diagnosis requires an accurately taken history, a high index of suspicion, and even more important, a biopsy when the diagnosis is uncertain.

CYSTIC LESIONS

Hidrocystoma

APOCRINE HIDROCYSTOMA

Apocrine hidrocystoma is a common cystic nodule[2-5] that is small and frequently found on the face, often involving the lids (Fig. 153–1).[6] The apocrine hidrocystoma is a multiloculated solitary and occasionally multiple translucent lesion that often has a blue tint.[7, 8] In addition to its location on the face, this benign cyst is occasionally found on the ears, chest, shoulders, orbit,[9-11] and even the prepuce.[12] It typically occurs in adults, but four patients of pediatric age were reported to have an apocrine hidrocystoma in a series at the Wilmer Eye Institute.[13]

The size of this cyst is quite variable but generally ranges between 1 and 11 mm.[8] A cyst as large as 7 × 5 cm has been observed on the trunk.[10] In the lid, it arises

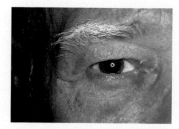

Figure 153–1. Apocrine hidrocystoma of the right lower lid.

from the blocked Moll's gland and thus appears generally at the lid margin.[6]

One study revealed an equal sex distribution and an average age of 55 yr.[7] These painless lesions were removed either for cosmetic reasons or to rule out malignancy. All but two of them were located in the head and neck region. The skin overlying the lesion was found to be smooth and glistening, particularly at the apex. In cases in which color characteristics had been noted, 64 per cent were clear, 13 per cent were pearly, and 20 per cent were blue tinged.[7] These lesions were slightly firmer than adjacent tissue, and the edges were well defined. In this study, the correct clinical diagnosis was made in only 1 of 42 cases.[7]

The clinical distinction between hidrocystomas (eccrine) and apocrine hidrocystomas is often difficult, but the latter are characteristically larger, darker, and not as frequently seen in the periorbital skin. Unlike the eccrine hidrocystoma, the apocrine hidrocystoma usually occurs as a solitary lesion[7, 14]; however, a case of multiple apocrine cysts of the eyelids has been reported.[15]

The histologic appearance of this lesion is that of several cystic spaces in the dermis with papillary projections and a lining of two layers of secretory cells. In the periphery, the lesion is lined by myocardial cells.[16] The inner layer is composed of columnar cells that contain eosinophilic cytoplasm and bulbous expansions of cells undergoing decapitation secretion. Apocrine hidrocystomas are regarded as a type of papillary cystadenoma because experimental evidence suggests this tumor is proliferative and not a retention cyst due to dilatation of ducts, which occurs with eccrine cysts.[17, 18] The term *apocrine hydrocystoma* is still used in the literature.[19, 20]

Unlike eccrine hidrocystomas, apocrine hidrocystomas do not change or become symptomatic in hot climates.[7] Two shades of blue have been observed in hidrocystomas. Deep blue-black is thought to be secondary to the dark-colored fluid in the cysts. These are thought to be due to the nonmelanin, nonhemosiderin secretory granules found in apocrine hidrocystomas.[17] It has been observed that most hidrocystomas that are superficially located may appear blue, but when their fluid content is examined, it is usually clear. The lesion's color is believed to be due to Tyndall's effect (a phenomenon caused by the scattering and polarization of light passing through a system of particles).[7]

This tumor is best treated by surgical excision. Simple drainage leaving the wall intact may result in cyst recurrence. This tumor frequently occurs near the punctum, and care is required in its removal.[21]

1713

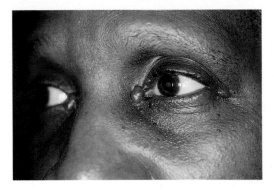

Figure 153–2. Multiple eccrine hidrocystomas on both eyes.

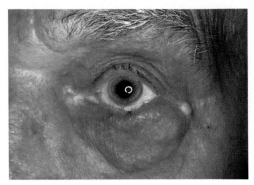

Figure 153–3. Epithelial inclusion cyst in the lateral canthal region.

ECCRINE HIDROCYSTOMA

Eccrine hidrocystoma occurs on the face, where it is commonly found on the eyelids (Fig. 153–2) The classic description of eccrine hidrocystomas by Robinson in 1893[14] held that these were multiple lesions that occurred on the faces of middle-aged women, especially cooks and washerwomen working in hot and moist environments. More current literature has challenged this concept, and in one series, more than 80 per cent of these lesions were solitary and 93 per cent of patients had four or fewer lesions. Additionally, 40 per cent of the patients were male, and the average age was 50.[7] In patients with fewer than four lesions, more than 87 per cent occurred in the periorbital region, and a large percentage of these cysts were present on the eyelid skin. The skin overlying these elevated nodules was smooth and shiny. These cysts were often translucent, and several of the patients had lesions that appeared clear or pearly.[7]

These are considered ductal retention cysts and clinically resemble the appearance of apocrine hidrocystomas. Only one cystic cavity is noted histologically in the dermis, and this is often partially collapsed and does not contain papillary infolding.[18] Two layers of small cuboidal epithelial cells line the cyst. Sometimes only one layer is found. No myoepithelial cells are seen.[18] The eccrine glands are made up of a large cyst, which may spread throughout the dermis. It is lined by two rows of flat epithelial cells, and a dilated sweat duct leads into it, but there is no exiting duct.[19]

The differential diagnosis includes cystic basal cell carcinoma, milia, apocrine hidrocystoma, and sebaceous, mucoid, or epidermoid cysts. A mucoid cyst tends to have a more viscous, although clear, fluid.[5] An apocrine hidrocystoma is usually darker blue or bluish-black, compared with an eccrine hidrocystoma. Sebaceous and epidermal inclusion cysts may possess an enlarged follicle, and the contents may consist of an opaque, white or yellow, thick, and foul-smelling material.[5] Milia contain yellow opaque material.[5] Treatment is by surgical excision of the entire lesion. The cystic structure collapses if traumatized or surgically incised, and a dilute transparent liquid is usually obtained.[5]

Epidermal Inclusion Cyst

Epidermal inclusion cysts are slowly progressive, firm subepithelial lesions. They tend to be solitary cysts and commonly occur on the face, scalp, neck, and trunk. These lesions are frequently found on the upper eyelid,[13] where they occur on either the conjunctival or the skin surface (Figs. 153–3 and 153–4).[21] Epidermal cysts are freely movable lesions that possess a layer of epidermis. They may vary in size from 1 to 5 cm in diameter.[18] Epidermal cysts generally occur during adolescence through late adulthood. These cysts contain a cheesy material that consists of keratin produced by the inner lining of squamous epithelium. The wall arises from proliferation of surface epidermis, and the absence of communication with the surface and production of keratin create the cyst.[22]

Epidermal cysts are thought to originate from occluded pilosebaceous follicles or surface epidermis.[23] They may occur at the time of birth and are then referred to as *congenital epidermoid cysts*. When secondary to trauma or prior surgery, these lesions are termed *epidermal inclusion cysts*. Histologically, both lesions are identical.[24] Trauma, however, is not commonly associated with lesions that occur on the eyelids.[25, 26]

Multiple adjacent superficial small cysts (ranging from 0.4 to 0.7 mm) have been described, occurring predominantly on the eyelids. In each of these lesions, the cyst wall was connected with a hair follicle.[27] It was thought that these lesions represented a retention epidermoid cyst that formed secondary to trauma involving the uppermost part of the follicle; a cyst is formed, and the

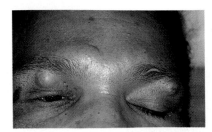

Figure 153–4. Epithelial inclusion cysts on both upper lids.

hair shaft becomes deflected.[27] Differential diagnosis of this lesion includes steatocystoma multiplex, lipomas, dermoid cysts, sebaceous cysts, and neurofibromas.[28, 29]

Rupture of the cyst wall may cause a foreign body granulomatous reaction in surrounding tissues. Complications associated with epidermal inclusion cysts include infection, cyst rupture with secondary granulomatous reaction,[25] and malignant transformation.[30]

If an epidermal cyst becomes infected, an abscess may form; it must be surgically drained. The most common organisms present are *Staphylococcus aureus* and *Streptococcus pyogenes*.[31] In a study of 192 patients with infected epidermal cysts, only two cysts were ocular.[22] This study demonstrated the prevalence of anaerobic bacteria in infected cysts. As stated, surgical drainage is the treatment of choice, and antimicrobial agents are required in severe cases. The antibiotic chosen should demonstrate effectiveness against *S. aureus* and anaerobic bacteria.[22]

Epidermal cysts may be found in large numbers in patients with Torre's syndrome or Gardner's syndrome. Torre's syndrome is associated with multiple sebaceous gland tumors, other cutaneous tumors, and visceral carcinomas, especially of the colon.[32] The other skin lesions may consist of epidermal hyperplasias, keratoacanthomas, and squamous cell carcinomas. Gardner's syndrome is associated with intestinal polyposis, multiple osteomas of facial bones, fibromas and epidermal inclusion cysts of the skin, and fibromatosis (desmoid tumors) of the abdominal wall, mesentery, and breast.[33]

Treatment of choice is surgical excision. This eyelid and orbital lesion commonly afflicts children.[34–36, 117] Various surgical techniques have been described for removing these cysts, depending on their location. These include direct incisions over the mass,[37, 38] brow incision,[39–41] and periorbital incisions such as Lynch's superomedial incision,[39] transmarginal eyelid-splitting incision,[42] lateral canthotomy,[42] or incision through the upper eyelid crease.[39, 40, 43]

Direct incisions over the mass and brow may lead to significant scarring. Lynch's incision is effective for lesions in the superomedial orbit, but the lateral canthotomy approach often is inadequate for approaching most of these lesions. Direct incision over the eyelid crease provides surgical access to most of these lesions, good exposure, and familiar anatomic landmarks in the lid. Simple closure may be performed with minimal cosmetic deformity.[39, 43, 44] Surgical techniques for obliterating the dead space remaining after excision of a large epidermoid cyst have been described.[45]

Sebaceous (Pilar) Cyst

Sebaceous cyst is a common benign disorder frequently noted in elderly patients. Sebaceous cysts clinically resemble epidermal inclusion cysts,[46] but they tend to be less common. They are found in locations with many hair follicles, particularly in the brow region and inner canthus.[47] Nearly 90 per cent of pilar cysts are found on the scalp.[48]

Sebaceous cysts are smooth, elevated yellow subcutaneous tumors that often contain a waxy comedo plug in the center.[6] These cysts may occur secondary to obstruction of Zeiss's gland, meibomian glands, or sebaceous glands associated with hair follicles of the lid or brow region.[21] Unlike an epidermal inclusion cyst filled with horny keratin material, a sebaceous cyst contains eosinophilic material composed of degraded epithelial cells, keratin, fats, and cholesterol crystals.[6] These cysts have a broad base and may be found among the cilia at the lid margin or elsewhere on the lid.[4]

Histologically, the epithelial cells that line the cysts have no intercellular bridges and possess palisading nuclei in the periphery. The nuclei are lost in these desquamating epithelial cells, and the cells demonstrate a swollen cytoplasm with indistinct cell boundaries. The cells then are released into the lumen, and the cyst exhibits homogeneous eosinophilic staining.[18]

Sebaceous cysts may either remain dormant for extended periods or gradually grow to a significant size over time. Inflammation may develop after trauma,[6] and calcification can be seen in some of these cysts. After rupture of the cyst wall, a granulomatous foreign body reaction may occur.[49] Meibomian gland cysts are true retention cysts that often occur as a secondary response to inflammation or lid margin neoplasms. They may occasionally arise spontaneously with preexisting conditions. They may also be associated with the presence of a chalazion.

The differential diagnosis includes fibroma, epidermal inclusion cyst, and xanthelasma.[4] Treatment is complete excision. Simply removing the contents is not adequate, because recurrence is common when the lining epithelium is not excised.[6] The skin incision should be somewhat longer than the length of the cyst, following the natural skin creases. Blunt dissection may be used to separate the cyst from surrounding tissues. The cyst is entirely removed through this incision. Excess skin is excised, and the wound is closed.[21] If infection exists, systemic antibiotics must be given.

Milia

Milia are umbilicated, multiple firm lesions ranging from 1 to 3 mm in diameter. Milia are found on the face, lids, malar region, and nose (Fig. 153–5). They

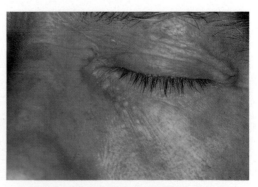

Figure 153–5. Milia of the lower lid.

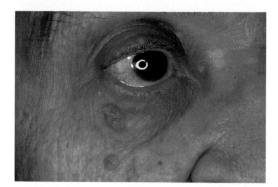

Figure 153–6. Papilloma of the lower lid.

occur as well-delineated, elevated round white tumors about the size of a pinhead.[6] These lesions may occur spontaneously or may arise after trauma,[50] radiation, or herpes zoster infection. They may also accompany bullous diseases such as epidermolysis bullosa.[6] Love and Montgomery suggested that these tumors arose from a pilosebaceous follicle.[51] Milia are believed to be retention follicular cysts caused by blockage of the pilosebaceous unit. Microscopically, the lesions are found to have a dilated hair follicle filled with layered accumulation of keratin. The adjacent sebaceous glands demonstrate various degrees of atrophy.[18] The pore of the cystic follicle has been shown to open to the skin surface.[18]

Surgical excision is the treatment of choice. Other methods of removal include diathermy and electrolysis.[6]

NONCYSTIC LESIONS

Squamous Papilloma

Squamous papilloma is a nonspecific term used for several lesions that display a benign hyperplasia of squamous epithelium. Squamous papillomas are the most common benign lesions of the eyelid[4] and may be sessile or pedunculated (Figs. 153–6 and 153–7). They are found in middle-aged and elderly individuals.[4] Usually found as solitary lesions, papillomas may be multiple and involve the lid margin, especially near the medial canthus. Growth tends to be slow. Their appearance is

generally that of small, firm, pedunculated lesions with a nodular or cerebriform convoluted surface.[4] Their color approximates that of the surrounding skin, and they may also be keratinized. Less frequently, the tumor may have a broad base, and the surface may be smooth. The differential diagnosis may thus include nevus, fibroma, epithelioma,[4] actinic keratosis,[24] verruca vulgaris, and seborrheic keratosis.[24]

Histologically, squamous papillomas are composed of papillae with vascularized connective tissue covered by acanthotic epithelium. Papillomas differ from the infective warts, which consist of inflammatory hypertrophy of papillae with viral inclusions.[52] Papillomas consist of epithelial acanthosis and hyperkeratosis surrounding a central fibrous core.[6] Squamous papillomas tend to occur in groups and to develop gradually rather than suddenly. There is no tendency for spontaneous recovery or acute enlargement.[6]

Treatment is generally by surgical excision of the lesion. Carbon dioxide laser ablation of this lesion has been used, with effective control of incision and hemostasis.[53]

Seborrheic Keratosis (Basal Cell Papilloma, Seborrheic Wart, or Senile Verruca)

Seborrheic keratosis is a common lesion found on the eyelids and face of middle-aged and elderly persons. It is a well-circumscribed growth that is friable and has a stuck-on appearance (Fig 153–8). This lesion is superficially located and, unless attended by infection or inflammation, does not involve the dermis.[51] It is often pigmented and has a soft consistency.[6] In Caucasians, the lesions are light to dark brown and consist of discrete, lobulated raised lesions with a frond appearance.

A variant of seborrheic keratosis is dermatosis papulosa nigra, which is a heavily pigmented lesion found in blacks, particularly on the malar region (Fig. 153–9).[54–56] These lesions generally occur at puberty and may be seen on the torso as well as the face.[57]

Seborrheic keratosis lesions may be multiple and occur over large areas of the face, lids, trunk, and arms.[6]

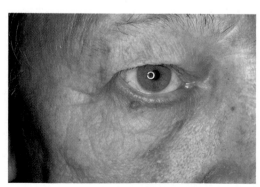

Figure 153–7. Pigmented papilloma of the lower lid.

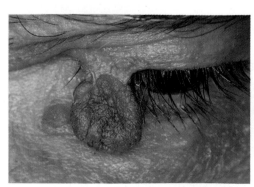

Figure 153–8. Pendulous seborrheic keratosis of the upper lid.

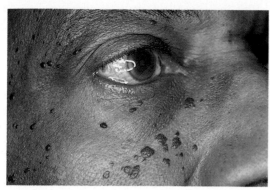

Figure 153–9. Dermatosis papulosa nigra.

Their size is variable, ranging from a few millimeters to more than 1 cm in diameter.[58]

Microscopically, three forms are noted: hyperkeratotic, acanthotic, and adenoid.[59] Most lesions share components of all three forms. The acanthotic form may contain cystic lesions filled with keratin. They are referred to as *horn cysts* when occurring within the mass and as *pseudohorn cysts* if they are simply invaginations of the surface keratin. Hyperkeratotic forms demonstrate more papillomatosis than does the acanthotic type.[18] The adenoid form demonstrates less keratinization and possesses branching epithelial strands with a double row of basal cells. Melanin may be abundant in keratinocytes, especially in the adenoid and acanthotic forms.[18]

Irritation is frequent in seborrheic keratoses, and the swelling of these lesions may be mistaken for basal cell carcinoma or malignant melanoma. An associated dermal inflammation by chronic inflammatory cells may be noted along with squamous cell proliferation. The lesion may thus resemble a squamous cell carcinoma.[60] The pathology resembles an inverted follicular keratosis, and differentiating between these lesions is difficult.[18]

Curettage may be adequate for a smaller flat lesion. However, pedunculated lesions of any size should be excised.[6] Carbon dioxide laser vaporization has also apparently produced good results.[53]

Keratoacanthoma

Keratoacanthoma was first described by Hutchinson in 1889,[61] and in 1950, the term *keratoacanthoma* was applied to this benign lesion afflicting middle-aged and elderly individuals.[62, 63] This elevated, dome-shaped tumor is commonly found on sun-exposed areas of the skin, such as the hands, scalp, and face, including the eyelids. It tends to occur on the lower lid and is commonly a solitary lesion.[6]

Keratoacanthoma is a rapidly growing tumor, sometimes developing within a period of weeks or months, at which time it may achieve a maximum growth of 0.5 to 3 cm in diameter. In one series, 36 of 44 cases of keratoacanthoma had arisen within less than 2 mo.[64] The tumor may thereafter remain unchanged for several

months and ultimately involute to leave a pitted scar.[6, 65] If these lesions involve the lid margin, they may lead to destruction of the margin structures. It has been postulated that the abundant Langerhans' cells in an inflamed keratoacanthoma may have a role in its ability to regress.[66]

This lesion characteristically has a crater-like appearance with a central keratin-filled pit. Telangiectasia may be found on the tumor, and it may often be confused with a basal cell or squamous cell carcinoma.[64, 67] Keratoacanthoma is benign and may represent an inflammatory reaction. A viral cause was long postulated,[68, 69] and human papillomavirus has now been identified in keratoacanthomas by the use of in situ DNA hybridization.[70–72]

Keratoacanthomas have been reported in immunocompromised patients, such as renal transplant recipients[73, 74] and patients with leukemia[75, 76] and leprosy.[77, 78] This lesion may also be seen in cases of radiodermatitis and at graft donor sites.[79] It is rare for a patient to have more than one lesion at a time, although several lesions may develop over the course of a few years.[80–82] Multiple recurrences of keratoacanthomas in surgically treated areas and their formation at donor and host graft sites suggest an infectious cause.[83]

Keratoacanthomas are not believed to be genetically transmitted, although lesions in several family members have been reported.[84] Multiple lesions are noted in the Ferguson-Smith syndrome[85] and with Grzybowski's type,[86] Witten's and Zak's types,[87] and giant or confluent keratoacanthomas.[88] Others have arisen in psoriatic patches after treatment with tar[89]; some are associated with cell-mediated immune deficiency[90]; and finally, others are found in the Muir-Torre syndrome.[91]

The most common of the multiple keratoacanthoma syndromes is Ferguson-Smith syndrome, which was first described in 1934.[92] Several members of the same family can have multiple lesions, suggesting an autosomal dominant mode of inheritance.[93–96] This type is commonly found in adolescence or early adulthood.[95] These tumors generally have a duration of several months and in younger individuals may resolve spontaneously.[97] The appearance of new lesions contributes to widespread keratoacanthomas.[98] These tumors are deeper than the nonfamilial form and tend to leave scars after regression.[99] The keratoacanthomas may measure up to 5 cm in diameter and number from several to more than 90 lesions on one individual.[100] They tend to occur on sun-exposed areas, and subungual lesions have been reported. Multiple keratoacanthomas may not regress entirely and sometimes prove resistant to standard therapy. One method of treatment that has been described is surgical excision combined with 13-*cis*-retinoic acid.[101]

Another multiple form, Grzybowski's type, is referred to as *eruptive keratoacanthoma* and is found in older individuals.[86] These pruritic lesions are small and occur in larger numbers than in the Ferguson-Smith syndrome. The entire skin surface may be involved, including the palms and the soles of the feet. Keratoacanthomas can also develop on the oral mucosa or larynx. Lesions may last several months and later heal with scar formation.[102]

Multiple keratoacanthomas of Witten's and Zak's types have a variable size and occur over most of the body. The lesions appear at different stages of the disease, and their characteristics are classified as the following types: small, conical, pinhead-sized papules; split pea–sized verrucous nodules; or cherry-sized tumors.[87] In one report, two lesions that developed on the lower lids were described as similar to molluscum contagiosum. The most common symptom was pruritus.[87]

A variant of multiple keratoacanthomas is the group of giant or confluent keratoacanthomas. Any lesion longer than 2 cm is considered a giant keratoacanthoma.[103] It has been stated that giant keratoacanthomas may be caused by proliferative change occurring simultaneously in hair follicles over a wide area.[88] They also may be the result of coalescence of many closely spaced keratoacanthomas or a combination of the two earlier processes. A variant of giant keratoacanthoma is keratoacanthoma centrifugum marginatum, which demonstrates spreading borders, central scar formation, and commonly destruction of the surrounding structures.[104]

Keratoacanthomas, as well as sebaceous lesions, are considered signs of the Muir-Torre syndrome. This syndrome consists of multiple internal neoplasms, sebaceous proliferations, and keratoacanthomas.[32, 91, 105] The number of systemic neoplasms may be significant in Torre's syndrome, but prolonged survival is characteristic of the condition. Other reports have described recurrent sebaceous lesions that have invaded bone and soft tissue.[105–107]

Individuals with multiple keratoacanthomas and systemic malignancies without sebaceous lesions have been identified.[108, 109] This presentation is believed to represent a variant of the Muir-Torre syndrome.

The cutaneous lesions of the Muir-Torre syndrome are not considered an inheritable condition, but evidence suggests that they may be markers for the cancer family syndrome, which is autosomal dominant.[110] In both of these syndromes, multiple primary malignancies are present at an early age but survival may not be affected.[110] At least one investigator believed that the Muir-Torre syndrome is inheritable.[111] It has been recommended that all individuals with multiple sebaceous lesions or keratoacanthomas be screened for systemic malignancy and that other family members be questioned about skin tumors and history of cancer.[111]

Histologically, the lesion may have a cuplike nodular elevation and thickening of the epidermis surrounding a central area of keratin. The base of the lesion may be well demarcated from the surrounding dermis by an area of moderate inflammation. Microabscesses of neutrophils may be found within some of the islands of epithelium.[18]

Microscopic differentiation of well-differentiated squamous cell carcinoma and keratoacanthoma is often difficult.[112–116] Islands of proliferating squamous epithelium may extend onto orbicularis muscle and occasionally involve cutaneous nerves without clear-cut evidence of perineural or lymphatic involvement, thus explaining the frequent misdiagnosis of squamous cell carcinoma. The differential diagnosis includes actinic keratosis, inverted follicular keratosis, isolated dyskeratosis follicularis, syringocystadenoma papilliferum, and adenoid squamous cell carcinoma.[18]

A history of accelerated tumor growth is suggestive of keratoacanthoma, but the growth rate of squamous cell carcinoma and keratoacanthoma is recognized as variable.[56, 65] A tumor present for longer than 6 months should be considered a squamous cell carcinoma and not a keratoacanthoma.[65] It is sometimes imperative that a complete excisional biopsy sample be obtained.[21]

A wealth of literature describes the misdiagnosis of squamous cell carcinoma as keratoacanthoma.[61, 62, 64, 65] There are no reliable immunohistochemical markers available to differentiate these two tumors.[117–122] A retrospective analysis of paraffin-embedded keratoacanthomas and squamous cell carcinomas was performed using ploidy analysis or proliferative index by flow cytometry, which showed no significant differences between these two tumors.[123]

It has been suggested by some investigators that keratoacanthoma should be reclassified as a low-grade squamous cell carcinoma rather than a benign lesion.[123, 131] Transition of keratoacanthomas into squamous cell carcinoma in instances of immunosuppression has been reported.[124, 125] Immunohistochemical studies of malignant tumors and various epidermal benign lesions have demonstrated full loss of the B2M site in basal cell carcinoma and complete to partial loss in squamous cell carcinoma as well as in Bowen's disease, compared with seborrheic keratoses and keratoacanthoma.[126] However, in each group a large quantitative difference in staining was noted, and the differences between normally staining keratoacanthoma and the minimal stain of squamous cell carcinoma were qualitative and not definite.[76]

Treatment of these lesions has varied in the past, and because this is generally a self-healing lesion, conservative management has been advocated. Various methods have been used, including podophyllin, curettage, cauterization, cryosurgery, irradiation, and steroids.[6, 127] However, histologic differentiation is important to rule out malignancy in some of these lesions, and thus, an excisional biopsy is the treatment of choice.[128] This is especially true for rapidly growing tumors, which may eventually become too large for management. In such cases, cosmetic and functional surgery will become more difficult.

A case of basal cell carcinoma underlying a keratoacanthoma has been reported.[129] Lesion recurrence has been reported after incomplete excision or other conservative methods of treatment.[130, 131] Some of these lesions are particularly aggressive or destructive and may involve functionally and cosmetically important structures. In these cases, they should be treated as soon as possible.

In other circumstances, keratoacanthomas may lie in areas where extensive resection is indicated, and their excision may cause severe cosmetic or functional deformity. In such cases, surgical excision is not the most desirable mode of treatment and more conservative treatment is indicated.

Therapy for multiple keratoacanthomas is diverse, and response is variable. Surgery, cryosurgery, electrodesiccation,[65] topical and systemic chemotherapy,[99, 131] and intramuscular bismuth have been recommended.[132] Retinoids have been successfully used in the treatment of keratoacanthomas. Several investigators have reported successfully treating multiple keratoacanthomas with oral isotretinoin.[133, 134] Reports have also described successful treatment of multiple keratoacanthomas with oral etretinate.[135, 136] It should be noted that a maintenance dose of etretinate was needed in all cases described. Successful treatment of multiple keratoacanthomas has also been reported with applications of 5-fluorouracil ointment or injections of 5-fluorouracil in the base of the lesion.[137–139] Radiotherapy has reportedly been useful for treating destructive or aggressive keratoacanthomas[140]; however, other reports suggest that this mode of treatment may not be adequate in the aggressive form of this lesion.[79] Two cases of destructive keratoacanthomas rapidly responded to intramuscular injections of methotrexate.[141] Multiple keratoacanthomas have responded to methotrexate[99] and bleomycin.[142]

Pseudoepitheliomatous (Pseudocarcinomatous) Hyperplasia

Pseudoepitheliomatous hyperplasia is a benign condition occurring in areas of cryosurgery or surgical wounds as well as in patients with chronic proliferative disorders and chronic ulcers.[24, 143, 144]

Pseudoepitheliomatous hyperplasia has been clinically and pathologically mistaken for various malignant tumors.[145] The lesion is generally elevated and has an uneven surface that is either ulcerated or crusty, giving it the appearance of a squamous cell carcinoma or a basal cell carcinoma. It is frequently found on the eyelid, develops rapidly over weeks, and may last from weeks to months. This lesion represents a disorder of the epidermis with active proliferation of epidermoid or squamous cells that develop into a hyperkeratotic nodule on the skin surface. It is commonly associated with chronic inflammation usually due to mycotic infections (blastomycosis[146, 147] and chromoblastomycosis[148]), gumma of tertiary syphilis,[147] cutaneous tuberculosis, granuloma inguinale,[147] insect bites, medications (bromoderma,[145] iododerma[149]), burns, and radiation therapy.[18] Pseudoepitheliomatous hyperplasia may also be seen on the periphery of malignancies such as basal cell carcinoma,[150] squamous cell carcinoma[151] (or following Mohs' micrographic surgery for the latter[152]), and metastatic breast carcinoma.[153]

Microscopically, acanthosis may be seen with interconnecting islands of squamous epithelium and, at times, microabscesses. A mild inflammatory reaction may be noted at the base of the lesion, with multinucleated giant cells and eosinophils. The inflammation may involve the sweat glands. These lesions can demonstrate epithelial changes that resemble low-grade squamous cell carcinoma. Clinical analysis and repeated biopsies may be required to establish the correct diagnosis.[18]

Inverted Follicular Keratosis (Basosquamous Cell Epidermal Tumor, Basosquamous Cell Acanthoma, Irritated Seborrheic Keratosis)

Inverted follicular keratosis is a benign lesion that has a wartlike or nodular appearance. It tends to occur in middle-aged and older individuals and resembles malignancies such as squamous cell carcinoma or, if pigmented, melanoma. Forty-three percent of lesions in one study were found at the lid margin.[154] Five of these had a cutaneous horn, and 50 percent had an onset of less than 3 months' duration.

Inverted follicular keratosis is a small, usually solitary lesion found predominantly on the face of males.[1, 6, 154] It presents clinically as a circumscribed keratotic growth on the skin surface or lid margin, with a nodular, papillomatous, verrucous, or cystic appearance (Fig. 153–10). The lesion may develop quickly over months and is believed to have a viral cause.[154] Rarely, follicular keratosis appears as a cutaneous horn or is pigmented.[6]

This lesion infrequently recurs unless the excision is incomplete; this nonrecurrence may account for the fact that it has been confused with squamous cell carcinoma. In one study, all skin lesions between 1966 and 1976 were reviewed and 17 lesions diagnosed as follicular keratosis in 17 patients were reviewed.[155] The median age was 69 years (46 to 93 years of age). Lesions were found on both upper and lower lids. The median duration before excision was 6 months. Clinical diagnoses were verruca in four, skin lesion in three, cutaneous horn in two, granuloma in one, senile keratosis in one, carcinoma in one, and malignant melanoma in five.[155] All tumors had a papillomatous appearance. These growths were found four times more frequently in males. In one series, 34 of 40 inverted follicular keratoses occurred predominantly on the face, although only 2 lesions appeared on the eyelids or eyebrows.[156]

Microscopically, the epithelium demonstrates lobular acanthosis, and proliferation of both basal and squamous cell elements is noted. In 1954, Helwig introduced the term *inverted follicular keratosis* to describe the pathology of a keratotic lesion relating to a hair follicle.[157] The histologic description was of a cup-shaped inverted lesion containing a central mass with a depression. Helwig

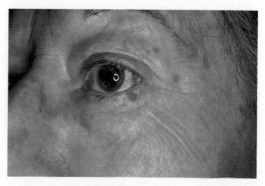

Figure 153–10. Inverted follicular keratosis of the lower lid.

considered the lesion to be derived from a pilosebaceous unit. Duperrat and Mascaro were the first to suggest that this lesion arose from the infundibulum of the hair follicle.[158] However, subsequent histologic studies demonstrate no relationship to hair follicles. Boniuk and Zimmerman reported 64 cases of inverted follicular keratoses occurring on the eyelid and eyebrows; they noted that a large number of these lesions had no inverted cup-shaped architecture.[154] Furthermore, they found no evidence that this lesion was derived from a follicle. Although the term *inverted follicular keratosis* has prevailed, others have described this lesion as a basosquamous cell acanthoma.[159] It is now believed that inverted follicular keratosis represents a type of irritated seborrheic keratosis[160–162] or a variant of a seborrheic wart.[163]

When this lesion is on the face, it is more prone to irritation and trauma than when it is elsewhere on the body. Desquamation of abnormal epithelium may cause a scab and lead to bleeding, burning, or itching. For cosmetic reasons, it should be completely excised when small.[6, 162]

PYOGENIC GRANULOMA

Pyogenic granuloma is a common vascular lesion of the eyelid that often occurs after trauma or surgery (Fig. 153–11).[18] Clinically, it is a fast-growing pinkish mass with occasional superficial ulceration of the epithelium.[164, 165] The term *granuloma pyogenicum* was first used in 1904 by Hartzell. Although this lesion is considered to be a hemangioma of granulation tissue,[18, 166] the name *pyogenic granuloma* has persisted.

This sessile or pedunculated growth ranges from a few millimeters to greater than 3 cm in diameter.[165] It may afflict all ages and both sexes. The most frequent sites of occurrence are the hand, foot, lip, cheek, chin, shoulder, back, and umbilicus.[54] Because of its vascularity, pyogenic granuloma easily bleeds after trauma.

Microscopically, this lesion contains granulation tissue with prominent radiating capillaries that spread from the base of the lesion toward the surface. Local excision is the treatment of choice.[18]

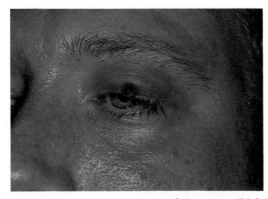

Figure 153–11. Pyogenic granuloma of the upper lid following chalazion removal.

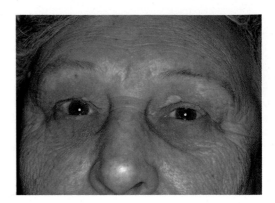

Figure 153–12. Xanthelasma of both upper lids.

XANTHELASMA

Xanthelasma is a term used to describe the form of xanthomas found on the eyelids. These commonly occurring lesions are usually found on the inner canthus (Fig. 153–12).[16] Clinically, they are seen as multiple soft, yellow, elevated plaques.[165] Xanthelasmas are more commonly seen in females of middle age or older.[165]

Many studies have investigated the relationship of xanthelasma to cholesterol and lipid levels in the population. The majority of patients with these lesions have no lipid metabolism abnormalities, but xanthelasma may accompany all the subtypes of hyperlipidemia.[18, 167] Various reports have placed the incidence of elevated cholesterol or triglyceride levels at between 30 and 40 per cent in patients with xanthelasma.[168]

In one controlled study of both sexes, a higher level of low-density lipoprotein cholesterol and apoprotein B was noted in patients with xanthelasma, but the total and subfraction 2 high-density lipoprotein (HDL) cholesterol levels were lower.[169] In another study, a large number of patients were found to have low levels of HDL-C (94 per cent of the reference population).[170] HDL-C has been shown to have an inverse relationship to cardiovascular disease.

These tumors are always superficial and rarely occur in the subcutaneous region.[6] Histologically, xanthelasmas contain foamy histiocytes (xanthoma cells), which are found about the vessels and adnexa of the papillary and reticular dermis.[6] These lesions are generally excised for cosmetic reasons. Treatment consists of full-thickness excision, and large lesions may require advancement flaps or grafts. An alternative surgical treatment for large xanthelasmas is excision of a portion of the tumor. The wound is then allowed to heal before the remainder of the lesion is excised.[21]

The carbon dioxide laser has also been used to treat these lesions. The tumor is vaporized while surrounding tissues are preserved.[171] The color and texture of this lesion allow the surgeon to determine when all the xanthelasma has been removed by the laser. Because this tumor is generally found in the reticular dermis, the laser vaporization should not cause scar formation if the treatment extends no deeper than the involved tissue.

REFERENCES

1. Aurora AL, Blodi FC: Lesions of the eyelids: A clinicopathological study. Surv Ophthalmol 15:94, 1970.
2. Luckasen JR, Goltz RW: Clinical Dermatology, vol. 4, Unit 22–1. Hagerstown, Harper & Row 1979, p 1.
3. Reese AB: Discussion of "common tumors of the eyelids." JAMA 107:933, 1936.
4. O'Brien CS, Braley AE: Common tumors of the eyelids. JAMA 107:933, 1936.
5. Smith JD, Chernosky ME: Hidrocystomas. Arch Dermatol 108:676, 1973.
6. Duke-Elder S, MacFaul PA: The ocular adnexa. In Duke-Elder S (ed): XIII. System of Ophthalmology. St. Louis, CV Mosby, 1974.
7. Smith JD, Chernosky ME: Apocrine hidrocystoma (cystadenoma). Arch Dermatol 109:700, 1974.
8. Kruse TV, Khan MA, Hassan MO: Multiple apocrine cystadenomas. Br J Dermatol 100:675, 1979.
9. Benisch B, Peison B: Apocrine hidrocystoma of the shoulder. Arch Dermatol 113:71, 1977.
10. Holder WR, Smith JD, Mocega EE: Giant apocrine hidrocystoma. Arch Dermatol 104:522, 1971.
11. Saunders JF: Congenital sudoriferous cyst of the orbit. Arch Ophthalmol 89:205, 1973.
12. Ahmed A, Jones AW: Apocrine cystoadenoma: A report of two cases occurring on the prepuce. Br J Dermatol 80:899, 1969.
13. Doxanos MT, Green WR, Arentsen JJ, et al: Lid lesions of childhood: A histopathologic survey at the Wilmer Institute (1923–1974). J Pediatr Ophthalmol 13:7, 1976.
14. Robinson AR: Hidrocystoma. J Cutan Gen Urin Dis 11:292, 1893.
15. Sacks E, Jakobiec FA, McMillan R, et al: Multiple bilateral apocrine cystadenomas of the lower eyelids. Light and Electron Microscopic Studies 94:1:65, 1987.
16. von Michel J: Klinische beitrage zur kenntniss seltener krankheiten der lidhaut und bindehaut. Arch Augenheilkd 42:1, 1900.
17. Mehregan AH: Apocrine cystadenoma: A clinicopathologic study with special reference to the pigmented variety. Arch Dermatol 90:274, 1964.
18. Font RL: Cystic lesions. Eyelids and lacrimal drainage system. In Spencer WH (ed): Ophthalmic Pathology. An Atlas and Textbook, vol. 3. Philadelphia, WB Saunders, 1986.
19. Hashimoto K, Lever WF: Tumors of skin appendages. In Fitzpatrick TB, Eisen AZ, Wolff K, et al (eds): Dermatology in General Medicine, 3rd ed. New York, McGraw-Hill, 1987.
20. Gross BG: The fine structure of apocrine hidrocystoma. Arch Dermatol 92:706, 1965.
21. Older JJ: Eyelid Tumors. Clinical Diagnosis and Surgical Treatment. New York, Raven Press, 1987.
22. Brook I: Microbiology of infected epidermal cysts. Arch Dermatol 125:1658, 1989.
23. Cavo WA, Bronstein BR: Tumors of the skin. In Moschella SL, Hurley HJ (eds): Dermatology. Philadelphia, WB Saunders, 1985.
24. Yanoff M, Fine BS: Ocular Pathology: A Text and Atlas, 3rd ed. Philadelphia, JB Lippincott, 1987.
25. Aurora AL, Blodi FC: Benign epithelial cysts of the eyelids. In Blodi FC (ed): Current Concepts in Ophthalmology. St. Louis, CV Mosby, 1972.
26. McGavran MH, Binnington B: Keratinous cysts of the skin. Arch Dermatol 94:499, 1966.
27. Aloi FG, Tomasini CF: Hair shafts in epidermoid cysts. Dermatologica 179:29, 1989.
28. Kronish JW, Sneed SR, Tse DT: Epidermal cysts of the eyelid. Arch Ophthalmol 106:270, 1988.
29. Traboulsi EI, Azar DT, Khattar J, et al: A-scan ultrasonography in the diagnosis of orbital dermoid cysts. Ann Ophthalmol 20:229, 1988.
30. Bauer BS, Lewis VL: Carcinoma arising in sebaceous and epidermoid cysts. Ann Plast Surg 5:222, 1980.
31. Marks MI: Common bacterial infection in infancy and children: A skin and wound infection. Drugs 16:202, 1978.
32. Torre D: Multiple sebaceous tumors. Arch Dermatol 98:549, 1968.
33. Gardner EJ: Follow-up study of family group exhibiting dominant inheritance for syndrome including intestinal polyps, osteomas, fibromas and epidermal cysts. Am J Hum Genet 14:376, 1962.
34. Nicholson DH, Green WR: Tumors of the eye, lids and orbit in children. In Harley RD (ed): Pediatric Ophthalmology. Philadelphia, WB Saunders, 1983.
35. Iliff WJ, Green WR: Orbital tumors in children. In Jakobiec FA (ed): Ocular and Adnexal Tumors. Birmingham, Aesculapius Publishing, 1978.
36. Shields JA, Bakewell B, Augsburger JJ, et al: Space-occupying orbital masses in children. Ophthalmology 93:379, 1986.
37. Grove AS, McCord CD Jr: Orbital disorders: Diagnosis and management. In McCord C Jr, Tanenbaum M (eds): Oculoplastic Surgery. New York, Raven Press, 1987.
38. Henderson JW: Orbital Tumors. Philadelphia, WB Saunders, 1973.
39. Leone CR Jr: Surgical approaches to the orbit. Ophthalmology 86:930, 1979.
40. Wright JE: Surgical exploration of the orbit. In Stewart WB (ed): Ophthalmic Plastic and Reconstructive Surgery. San Francisco, American Academy of Ophthalmology, 309, 1984.
41. Howard GM: Cystic tumors. In Jones IS, Jakobiec FA (eds): Diseases of the Orbit. New York, Harper & Row, 1979.
42. Smith B: The anterior surgical approach to orbital tumors. Ophthalmology 70:607, 1966.
43. Wolfley DE: The lid crease approach to the superomedial orbit. Ophthalmic Surg 16:652, 1985.
44. Kronish JW, Dortzbach RK: Upper eyelid crease surgical approach to dermoid and epidermoid cysts in children. Arch Ophthalmol 106:1625, 1988.
45. Ocampo J, Camps A: The application of the tie-down suture to the excision of cutaneous tumors. J Dermatol Surg Oncol 14:12, 1988.
46. Kudoh K, Hosokawa M, Miyazawa T, et al: Giant solitary sebaceous gland hyperplasia clinically simulating epidermoid cyst. J Cutan Pathol 15:396, 1988.
47. Daicker von B: Zur kenntnis des xanthogranuloma juvenile der lidhaut. Ophthalmologica 152:267, 1966.
48. McGavran MH, Binnington B: Keratinous cysts of the skin. Arch Dermatol 94:499, 1966.
49. Sternberg C: Verkalktes atherom des augenlides. Zentralbl Allg Pathol Pathol Anat 15:988, 1904.
50. Cohen BH: Prevention of postdermabrasion milia. J Dermatol Surg Oncol 14:1301, 1988.
51. Love WR, Montgomery H: Epithelial cyst. Arch Dermatol Syphilol 47:185, 1943.
52. Apple DJ, Rabb MJ: Ocular Pathology. Clinical Applications and Self-Assessment. St. Louis, CV Mosby, 1985.
53. Beckman H, Fuller TA, Boyman R, et al: Carbon dioxide laser surgery of the eye and adnexa. Ophthalmology 87:990, 1980.
54. Montgomery H: Dermatopathology, vol. 2. New York, Harper & Row, 1967.
55. Lever WF: Histopathology of the Skin, 3rd ed. Philadelphia, JB Lippincott, 1961.
56. Allington HV, Allington JH: Eyelid tumors. Arch Dermatol 97:50, 1968.
57. Hairston MA Jr, Reed RJ, Derbes VJ: Dermatosis papulosa nigra. Arch Dermatol 89:655, 1964.
58. Miki T: Two cases of benign lid tumors clinically suspected as malignant. Folia Ophthalmol Jpn 23:421, 1972.
59. Braun-Falco O, Kint A: Zur histogenese der verruca seborrhoica. Arch Klin Exp Dermatol 216:615, 1963.
60. Rowe L: Seborrheic keratoses. I: "Pseudo-epitheliomatous hyperplasia" (Weidman). J Invest Dermatol 29:165, 1957.
61. Hutchinson J: The "crateriform ulcer of the face," a form of acute epithelial cancer. Transactions of the Pathological Society of London, 40:275, 1889.
62. Rook A, Whimster IW: Le Keratoacanthome. Arch Belg Dermatol Syphilol 6:137, 1950.
63. Musso L, Gordon H: Spontaneous resolution of a molluscum sebaceum. Proc R Soc Med 43:838, 1950.
64. Boniuk M, Zimmerman LE: Eyelid tumors with reference to

lesions confused with squamous cell carcinoma. III: Kerato-acanthoma. Arch Ophthalmol 77:29, 1967.

65. Graham R: What is a keratoacanthoma? Practitioner 233:1594, 1989.

66. Korenberg R, Penneys NS, Kowalczyk A, Nadji M: Quantitation of S100 protein-positive cells in inflamed and noninflamed kera-toacanthoma and squamous cell carcinoma. J Cutan Pathol 15:104, 1988.

67. Kwitko ML, Boniuk M, Zimmerman LE: Eyelid tumors with reference to lesions confused with squamous cell carcinoma. Arch Ophthalmol 69:693, 1963.

68. Ereaux LP, Schopflocher P, Fournier CJ: Keratoacanthoma. Arch Dermatol 71:73, 1955.

69. Zelickson AS, Lynch FW: Electron microscopy of virus-like particles in a keratoacanthoma. J Invest Dermatol 37:79, 1961.

70. Pfrister H, Gassenmaier A, Fuchs PG: Demonstration of human papilloma virus DNA in two keratoacanthomas. Arch Dermatol Res 48:820, 1986.

71. Scheurlen W, Gissman L, Gross G, et al: Molecular cloning of two new HPV types (HPV37 and HPV38) from a keratoacan-thoma and a malignant melanoma. Int J Cancer 37:505, 1986.

72. Brigati DJ, Myerson D, Leary JJ, et al: Detection of viral genomes in cultured cells and paraffin-embedded tissue sections using biotin labeled hybridization probes. Virology 126:32, 1983.

73. Walder BK, Robertson MR, Jeremy D: Skin cancer and immu-nosuppression. Lancet ii:1282, 1971.

74. Stewart WB, Nicholson DH, Hamilton G, et al: Eyelid tumors and renal transplantation. Arch Ophthalmol 98:1771, 1980.

75. Degos R, Bernard J, Delort J, et al: Kératoacanthomes centri-fuges disséminés. Bull Soc Fr Dermatol Syphiligr 74:417, 1967.

76. Weber G, Stetter H, Pliess G, et al: Vorkommen von eruptiven Keratoacanthomen, Tubencarcinom und paramyeloblasten Leu-kamie. Arch Klin Exp Deramatol 238:107, 1970.

77. Job C: Keratoacanthoma associated with leprosy. Indian J Pathol Bacteriol 6:160, 1963.

78. Sebra-Santos H, Martins RC: Queratoacanthoma em doente de lepra. A proposite de um caso clinico. Rovisco Pais 7:3, 1968.

79. Kopf AW, Bart RS, Andrade R: Atlas of Tumors of the Skin. Philadelphia, WB Saunders, 1978.

80. Degos R, Cottenot F, Civatte J: Kératoacanthome reformé après abrasion. Bull Soc Fr Dermatol Syphiligr 65:122, 1958.

81. Rook A, Kerdel-Vegas F, Young T: Recurrences in kerato-acanthoma. Med Cutan 11:17, 1967.

82. Stevanovic DV: Récidives du kératoacanthome. Ann Dermatol Syphiligr 96:415, 1969.

83. Pellicano R, Giuseppe F, Cerimele D: Multiple keratoacantho-mas and junctional epidermolysis bullosa: A therapeutic conun-drum. Arch Dermatol 126:305, 1990.

84. Baer RL, Kopf AW: Keratoacanthoma. Year Book of Derma-tology, 1962–1963 Series. Chicago, Year Book Medical Publish-ers, 1962–1963, p 7.

85. Smith JF: A case of multiple primary squamous cell carcinomata of the skin in a young man with spontaneous healing. Br J Dermatol 46:267, 1934.

86. Grzybowski M: Case of peculiar generalized epithelial tumors of the skin. Br J Dermatol 62:310, 1950.

87. Witten VH, Zak FG: Multiple, primary, self-healing prickle-cell epithelioma of the skin. Cancer 5:539, 1952.

88. Webb AJ, Ghadially FN: Massive or giant keratoacanthoma. J Pathol Bacteriol 91:505, 1966.

89. Vickers CFH, Ghadially FN: Keratoacanthomata associated with psoriasis. Br J Dermatol 73:120, 1961.

90. Claudy A, Thivolet J: Multiple keratoacanthomas: Association with deficient cell-mediated immunity. Br J Dermatol 93:593, 1975.

91. Fahmy A, Burgdorf WHC, Schosser RH, et al: Muir-Torre syndrome: Report of a case and reevaluation of the dermato-pathologic features. Cancer 49:1898, 1982.

92. Lever WF, Schaumburg-Lever G: Histopathology of the Skin, 5th ed. Philadelphia, JB Lippincott, 1975.

93. Sommerville J, Milne JA: Familial primary self-healing squamous epithelioma of the skin. Br J Dermatol 62:485, 1950.

94. Currie AR, Ferguson Smith J: Multiple primary spontaneous-healing squamous-cell carcinomata of the skin. J Pathol Bacteriol 64:827, 1952.

95. Epstein NN, Biskind GR, Pollack RS: Multiple primary self-healing squamous-cell epitheliomas of the skin: Generalized keratoacanthomas. Arch Dermatol 75:210, 1957.

96. Degos R, Civatte J, Touraine B, et al: Spontan heilende Epithe-liome Ferguson-Smith und multiple familiare Keratoacanthome. Hautarzt 15:7, 1964.

97. Charteris AA: Self-healing epithelioma of the skin. Am J Roent-genol 65:459, 1951.

98. Schnitzler L, Schubert B, Verret JL, et al: Epithéliomatose familiale de Ferguson-Smith, à propos de 2 cas familiaux. Ann Dermatol Venereol 104:206, 1977.

99. Tarnowski WM: Multiple keratoacanthomata: Response of a case to systemic chemotherapy. Arch Dermatol 94:74, 1966.

100. Ferguson Smith MA, Wallace DC, James ZH, et al: Multiple Self-Healing Squamous Epitheliomas. The Clinical Delineation of Birth Defects. XII. Skin, Hair and Nails. Baltimore, Williams & Wilkins, 1971.

101. Haydey RP, Reed ML, Dzubow LM, et al: Treatment of keratoacanthomas with oral 13-cis-retinoic acid. N Engl J Med 303:560, 1980.

102. Lo JS, Bergfeld WF, Taylor JS, et al: Multiple erythematous plaques with infiltrated borders on the forearms. Arch Dermatol 126:101, 1990.

103. Kopf AW, Bart RS: Giant keratoacanthoma. J Dermatol Surg Oncol 4:444, 1978.

104. Heid E: Keratoacanthoma centrifugum marginatum. Ann Der-matol Venereol 106:367, 1979.

105. Muir EG, Yates Bell AJ, Barlow KA: Multiple primary carci-nomata of the colon, duodenum, and larynx associated with keratoacanthomata of the face. Br J Surg 54:191, 1967.

106. Tschang TP, Poulos E, and Ho CK: Multiple sebaceous adenoma and internal malignant disease: A case report with chromosomal analysis. Hum Pathol 7:589, 1976.

107. Schwartz RA, Flieger DM, Saied NK: The Torre syndrome with gastrointestinal polyposis. Arch Dermatol 116:312, 1980.

108. Poleksic S: Keratoacanthoma and multiple carcinomas. Br J Dermatol 91:461, 1974.

109. Stewart W-M, Lauret P, Hemet J, et al: Kératoacanthomes multiples et carcinomes viscéraux: Syndrome de Torre. Ann Dermatol Venereol 104:622, 1977.

110. Lynch HT, Lynch PM, Pester J: The cancer family syndrome: Rare cutaneous phenotypic linkage of Torre's syndrome. Arch Intern Med 141:607, 1981.

111. Anderson DE: An inherited form of large bowel cancer (Muir's syndrome). Cancer 45:1103, 1980.

112. Goldenhersh MA, Olsen TG: Invasive squamous cell carcinoma initially diagnosed as giant keratoacanthoma. J Am Acad Der-matol 10:372, 1984.

113. Jackson IT: Diagnostic problem of keratoacanthoma. Lancet 1:490, 1969.

114. Kern WH, McCray MK: The histopathologic differentiation of keratoacanthoma and squamous cell carcinoma of the skin. J Cutan Pathol 7:318, 1980.

115. Peterkin GAG, McMillan JB, McLain S: Pseudo-carcinoma of the skin: A follow-up of cases of keratoacanthoma seen in the years 1951–1960. Scott Med J 7:27, 1962.

116. Schnur PL, Bozzo P: Metastasizing keratoacanthomas? The difficulties in differentiating keratoacanthomas from squamous cell carcinomas. Plast Reconstr Surg 62:258, 1978.

117. Graham RM, MacFarlane AW, Curley RK, et al: B2 microglob-ulin expression in keratoacanthoma and squamous cell carci-noma. J Dermatol 117:441, 1987.

118. Klein-Szanto AJP, Barr RJ, Reiners JJ, et al: Filaggrin distri-bution in keratoacanthoma and squamous cell carcinoma of the skin. Arch Pathol Lab Med 108:888, 1984.

119. Kute TE, Gregory B, Galleshaw J, et al: How reproducible are flow cytometry data from paraffin-embedded blocks? Cytometry 9:494, 1988.

120. Kvedar JC, Fewkes J, Baden HP: Immunologic detection of markers of keratinocyte differentiation. Arch Pathol Lab Med 110:183, 1986.

121. Murphy GF, Flynn TC, Rice RH, et al: Involucrin expression in normal and neoplastic human skin: A marker for keratinocyte differentiation. J Invest Dermatol 82:453, 1984.

122. Said JW, Sassoon AF, Shintaku IP, et al: Involucrin in squamous

and basal cell carcinoma of the skin: An immunohistochemical study. J Invest Dermatol 82:449, 1984.

123. Randall MB, Geisinger KR, Kute TE, et al: DNA content and proliferative index in cutaneous squamous cell carcinoma and keratoacanthoma. J Cutan Pathol 93:259, 1990.

124. Sullivan JJ, Colditz GA: Keratoacanthoma in a subtropical climate. Aust J Dermatol 20:34, 1979.

125. Poleksic S, Yeung KY: Rapid development of keratoacanthoma and accelerated transformation into squamous cell carcinoma of the skin. Cancer 41:12, 1978.

126. Markey AC, Churchill LJ, MacDonald DM: Altered expression of major histocompatibility complex (MHC) antigens by epidermal tumours. J Cutan Pathol 17:65, 1990.

127. Crawford JB: Keratoacanthoma. In Fraunfelder FT, Roy FH (eds): Current Ocular Therapy 2, Philadelphia, WB Saunders, 1985.

128. Iverson RE, Vistnes LM: Keratoacanthoma is frequently a dangerous diagnosis. Am J Surg 126:359, 1973.

129. Einaugler RB, Henkind P, de Oliveira LE, et al: Keratoacanthoma with basal cell carcinoma. Am J Ophthalmol 65:922, 1968.

130. Belisario JC: Brief review of keratoacanthomas and description of keratoacanthoma centrifugum marginatum, another variety of keratoacanthoma. Aust J Dermatol 8:65, 1965.

131. Requena L, Romero E, Sanchez M, et al: Aggressive keratoacanthoma of the eyelid: "Malignant" keratoacanthoma or squamous cell carcinoma? J Dermatol Surg Oncol 16:564, 1990.

132. Ephraim AJ, Kaufman JJ: Multiple keratoacanthoma. Arch Dermatol 77:191, 1958.

133. Shaw JC, White CR Jr: Treatment of keratoacanthoma with oral isotretinoin. J Am Acad Dermatol 15:1079, 1986.

134. Haydey RP, Reed ML, Dzubow LM, et al: Treatment of keratoacanthomas with oral 13-cis-retinoic acid. N Engl J Med 303:560, 1980.

135. Benoldi D, Alinovi A: Multiple persistent keratoacanthomas: Treatment with oral etretinate. J Am Acad Dermatol 10:1035, 1984.

136. Yoshikawa K, Hirano S, Kato T, et al: A case of eruptive keratoacanthoma treated by oral etretinate. Br J Dermatol 112:579, 1985.

137. Ebner H, Mischer P: Lokalbehandlung des keratoakanthoms mit 5-Fluoruracil. Hautartz 26:585, 1975.

138. Odom RB, Goette DK: Treatment for keratoacanthomas with intralesional fluorouracil. Arch Dermatol 114:1779, 1978.

139. Klein E, Helm F: Keratoacanthoma: Local effect of 5-fluorouracil. Skin 1:153, 1982.

140. Farina AT, Leider M, Newall J, et al: Radiotherapy for aggressive and destructive keratoacanthomas. J Dermatol Surg Oncol 3:177, 1977.

141. Kestel JL Jr, Blair S: Keratoacanthoma treated with methotrexate. Arch Dermatol 108:723, 1973.

142. Sayama S, Iagami H: Treatment of keratoacanthoma with intralesional bleomycin. Br J Dermatol 109:449, 1983.

143. Elton RF: Complications of cutaneous cryosurgery. J Am Acad Dermatol 8:513, 1983.

144. Wingfield DL, Fraunfelder FT: Possible complications secondary to cryotherapy. Ophthalmic Surg 10:47, 1979.

145. Sommerville J: Pseudoepitheliomatous hyperplasia. Acta Dermatol Venereol 33:236, 1953.

146. Stone OJ: Hyperinflammatory proliferative (blastomycosis-like) pyodermas: Review, mechanisms, and therapy. J Dermatol Surg Oncol 12:271, 1986.

147. Su WPD, Duncan SC, Perry HO: Blastomycosis-like pyoderma. Arch Dermatol 115:170, 1979.

148. Uribe-JF, Zuluaga AI, Leon W, et al: Histopathology of chromoblastomycosis. Mycopathologia 105:1, 1989.

149. Kincaid MC, Green WR, Hoover RE, Farmer ER: Iododerma of the conjunctiva and skin. Ophthalmology 88:1216, 1981.

150. Freeman RG: On the pathogenesis of pseudoepitheliomatous hyperplasia. J Cutan Pathol 1:231, 1974.

151. Giunti A, Laus M: Malignant tumors in chronic osteomyelitis: A report of thirty-nine cases, twenty-six with long term follow up. Ital J Orthop Traumatol 4:171, 1978.

152. Weber PJ, Johnson BL, Dzubow LM: Pseudoepitheliomatous hyperplasia following Mohs micrographic surgery. J Dermatol Surg Oncol 15:557, 1989.

153. Haim N, Krugliak P, Cohen Y, et al: Esophageal metastasis from breast carcinoma associated with pseudoepitheliomatous hyperplasia: An unusual endoscopic diagnosis. J Surg Oncol 41:278, 1989.

154. Boniuk M, Zimmerman LE: Eyelid tumors with reference to lesions confused with squamous cell carcinoma. II: Inverted follicular keratosis. Arch Ophthalmol 69:698, 1963.

155. Sassani JW, Yanoff M: Inverted follicular keratosis. Am J Ophthalmol 87:810, 1979.

156. Mehregan AH: Inverted follicular keratosis. Arch Dermatol 89:229, 1964.

157. Helwig EB: Seminar on the skin: Neoplasms and dermatoses. Proceedings of the 20th Seminar, American Society of Clinical Pathologists, International Congress of Clinical Pathology, Washington DC, 1954. Published by American Society of Clinical Pathologists, 1955.

158. Duperrat B, Mascaro JM: Une tumeur benigne developpee auz depens de l'acrotrichium ou partie intraepidermique du follicule pilaire. Porome follicularie. Dermatologica 126:291, 1963.

159. Lund HZ: Tumors of the skin. In Atlas of Tumor Pathology. Section I, Fascicle 2. Washington DC, Armed Forces Institute of Pathology, 1957.

160. Morales A, Hu F: Seborrheic verruca and intraepidermal basal cell epithelioma of Jadassohn. Arch Dermatol 91:342, 1960.

161. Mevorah B, Mishima Y: Cellular response of seborrheic keratosis following croton oil irritation and surgical trauma. Dermatologica 131:452, 1965.

162. Lever WF: Tumors and cysts of the epidermis. In Lever WF (ed): Histopathology of the Skin, 4th ed. Philadelphia, JB Lippincott, 1967.

163. Sim-Davis D, Marks R, Wilson-Jones E: The inverted follicular keratosis: A surprising variant of seborrheic wart. Acta Dermatovenereol 56:337, 1976.

164. Malik SRK, Sood GC, Aurora AL: Granuloma pyogenicum. Br J Ophthalmol 48:502, 1964.

165. Lucas DR: The eyelids. In Greer's Ocular Pathology, 4th ed. Boston, Blackwell Scientific, 1989.

166. Knoth W, Ehlers G: Zur frage der existenz des granuloma pyogenicum teleangiectaticum unter besonderer berucksichtigung seiner beziehungen zum hamangiom und hamangio-endotheliom. Arch Klin Exp Dermatol 214:394, 1962.

167. Fredrickson DS, Lees RS: A system for phenotyping hyperlipoproteinemia. Circulation 31:321, 1965.

168. Allander E, Bjornsson OJ, Kolbeinsson A, et al: Incidence of xanthelasma in the general population. Int J Epidemiol 1:211, 1972.

169. Pinto X, Ribera M, Fiol C, et al: Dyslipoproteinemia in patients with xanthelasma. Arch Dermatol 125:1281, 1989.

170. Bates MC, Stafford GW: Xanthelasma: Clinical indicator of decreased levels of high-density lipoprotein cholesterol. South Med J 82:570, 1989.

171. Gladstone GJ, Beckman H, Elson LM: CO_2 laser excision of xanthelasma lesions. Arch Ophthalmol 103:440, 1985.

Chapter 154

∎

Basal Cell Carcinoma

CHARLES K. BEYER-MACHULE and KLAUS G. RIEDEL

EPIDEMIOLOGY AND PATHOGENESIS

Basal cell carcinomas are the most frequent malignant lid lesions. In the periocular region, they represent more than 90 percent of all malignant tumors (Table 154–1). As in many other skin tumors, basal cell carcinomas display a considerable diversity of appearances, both clinically and microscopically. Their distribution favors the lower lid to approximately 70 percent, whereas the medial canthus, the upper lid, and the lateral canthus follow in frequency.[1–6]

Synonymous with basal cell carcinoma are rodent ulcer, basalioma, and basal cell epithelioma. The term basal cell epithelioma is particularly emphasized by some authors because of its development from basal cells of the epidermis and the external root sheath of hair follicles, its relationship to benign adnexal tumors, and the hypothesis that it does not arise from malignant transformation of preexisting mature structures.[6, 7] To date, the term basal cell epithelioma is not generally accepted, and most clinicians and pathologists prefer the name of basal cell carcinoma, thus appreciating the locally invasive and destructive growth of this tumor.

The malignant cells arise from the so-called basal or germinal cells of the epidermis. This layer lies above the basement membrane and separates the dermis from the epidermis. Tumor enlargement arises from the change in the basal cells that increase in size and reach into the dermis and form, in most cases, a nodular tumor. The margin enhances in substance as its center suffers a diminution of blood supply that then breaks down to produce a crusted, umbilicated center. The latter central crust may loosen and give rise to episodes of bleeding. It is often this feature that initiates the patient's visit to his or her physician.

Although basal cell carcinomas may be seen in children and young individuals,[8–10] the upper middle-aged patient typifies the average case which appears in relation to exposure to actinic radiation. The latter factor appears to play an increasing role in the development of basal cell and other epidermal tumors. Most lesions occur in fair skinned individuals, e.g. the "fair" Irish or Scandinavians, compared with those who have a more pigmented skin, although basal cell carcinomas have been reported in blacks.[11] The length of actinic exposure plays a direct role in the frequency of the tumor occurrence. Thus, basal cell carcinomas are seen more often in the "outdoor" types of individuals (e.g., cowboys, fishermen, golfers, sailors) compared with the so-called "indoor" or sedentary professions.

Certain varieties of basal cell carcinoma demonstrate a propensity to recur.[12–18] Morphea or sclerosing lesions in the area of the canthi display a particular tendency towards invasion of the deeper structures of the orbit and the nasal sinuses.[19–21] Death from cerebral invasion of a basal cell carcinoma is possible.[1, 2] The mortality rate of basal cell carcinoma is reported from 2 percent to as high as 4.5 percent.[22] In severe orbital involvement, an exenteration of the involved orbit represents the only potential treatment and a possible cure. Recurrent basal cell carcinomas in the canthal regions present severe problems of management for the patient and his or her physician.[9, 18, 20, 21]

Basal cell carcinomas, as a rule, do not metastasize; however, in 0.02 to 0.1 percent such tumor spread is reported.[6, 23–28] In most patients with metastases the primary tumors usually presented as very large, often multifocal, and deeply infiltrative lesions with a history of multiple recurrences. Although some authors found that the basosquamous type of basal cell carcinoma metastasized more frequently, others saw no evidence for a specific type of basal cell carcinoma showing a more frequent metastasizing than others.[26, 28–30] Metastatic spread in basal cell carcinomas may occur both via hematogenic and lymphogenic avenues.[27, 31]

CLINICAL APPEARANCE AND HISTOPATHOLOGY

Basal cell carcinomas may be divided into (1) a localized form (nodular, ulcerative, cystic); (2) a diffuse form (morpheaform, sclerosing); (3) a superficial form (multifocal); and (4) the fibroepitheliomatous basal cell carcinoma of Pinkus. Additionally, three clinical syndromes are associated with the presence of basal cell carcinomas: (1) the nevoid basal cell carcinoma syndrome; (2) the linear unilateral basal cell nevus; and (3) the Bazex syndrome.[6, 32–34]

Table 154–1. FIVE MOST COMMON EYELID TUMORS SUBMITTED BETWEEN 1955 AND 1980 (MASSACHUSETTS EYE AND EAR INFIRMARY, BOSTON, HARVARD MEDICAL SCHOOL)

	Total	% of Total
Basal cell carcinoma	1427	92.5
Squamous cell carcinoma	71	4.6
Sebaceous cell carcinoma	23	1.5
Melanoma	16	1.1
Lymphosarcoma	6	0.3
Total	1543	100.0

Noduloulcerative Basal Cell Carcinoma

The localized nodular and noduloulcerative subtype is, with approximately 75 percent of all basal cell carcinomas, the most common mode of presentation. It usually begins as small translucent papules with a pearly appearance and with some telangiectatic vessels. The epidermis is markedly thinned over the surface of the tumor (Fig. 154–1A–C). With increasing growth, there appears central umbilication, erosion, or ulceration leading to the typically sharply demarked lesion with a central ulcer and a pearly, rolled margin (so-called rodent ulcer; Fig. 154–2A–C).

The skin color determines the amount of pigment in basal cell carcinomas; however, in some noduloulcerative types a marked hyperpigmentation may be found (Fig. 154–3A and B). These pigmented basal cell carcinomas may clinically be misdiagnosed as malignant melanomas.[35, 36]

Histologically, nodular and noduloulcerative basal cell carcinomas consist of large, well-defined basaloid lobules of varying shape and form. The usually loose surrounding stroma shows shrinkage at tissue fixation with characteristic separation of the tumor lobules from their neighboring stroma (Fig. 154–4). Noduloulcerative basal cell carcinomas consist of small, hyperchromatic cells of uniform size with oval nuclei and inconspicuous nucleoli. The cytoplasm is scanty, resulting in a large ratio of nucleus to cytoplasm. The mitotic activity is variable, with 0 to 10 division figures per high-power field. Abnormal mitoses are rare. Characteristically, tumor cells show a parallel alignment at the periphery of the lobules, forming the so-called peripheral palisading. Within the center tumor, cells may be arranged in strands or bundles and often lack any alignment.

A common feature of the noduloulcerative basal cell carcinoma is a cystic, keratotic, and adenoid differentiation, whereas a squamous, sebaceous, and eccrine definition is rare (Fig. 154–5A–C). Central cavitation is associated with degenerative changes. The extensive cystic characteristic in basal cell carcinoma may be confused with an epithelial inclusion cyst and prominent hyperkeratosis may lead to the misdiagnosis of keratotic papilloma, seborrheic keratosis, or familial trichoepithelioma.[6, 37, 38] The combination of a reticulate tumor cell pattern with an amorphous, granular, or colloid-like stroma represents the adenoid or glandular basal cell carcinoma. The retention of peripheral nuclear palisading and the presence of stromal retraction help to distinguish this growth mode from true glandular tumors.

Uncommon histologic variants of basal cell carcinomas include an adenomatoid type, a granular type, a basosebaceous type, a clear cell type, and a type with matricial differentiation.[6, 34] A sixth variety, the basosquamous or metatypical basal cell carcinoma, is often referred to as being an intermediate mode between basal cell carcinoma and squamous cell carcinoma. These tumors contain both typical basaloid cells and cells with an abundant eosinophilic cytoplasm and with larger nuclei that are arranged in a concentric pearl-like configuration. In correlation with these features, these tumors present a more aggressive and deeply infiltrating growth pattern and tend to metastasize more frequently.[39, 40]

Morpheaform Basal Cell Carcinoma

The diffusely growing morpheaform or sclerosing form accounts for approximately 15 percent of all basal cell carcinomas. Consisting of a flat or slightly depressed indurated plaque of white-pink to yellow color, this lesion is associated with a poorly demarked clinical margin. The overlying epidermis remains intact for a long time and there is no obvious translucency as in the noduloulcerative form (Fig. 154–6A–C). Because of these features, morpheaform basal cell carcinomas are difficult to treat as they notoriously exceed the clinically visible tumor range. Additionally, morpheaform basal cell carcinoma is characterized by its deep invasion into

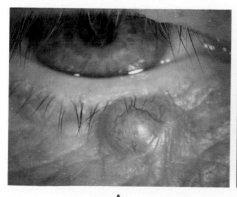 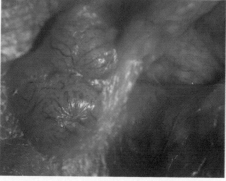 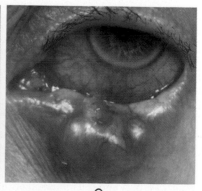

A   B   C

Figure 154–1. A–C, Nodular basal cell carcinoma. Clinical appearance, showing three different cases with firm, pearly nodules; telangiectatic vessels; and markedly thinned epidermis at the surface of the tumor.

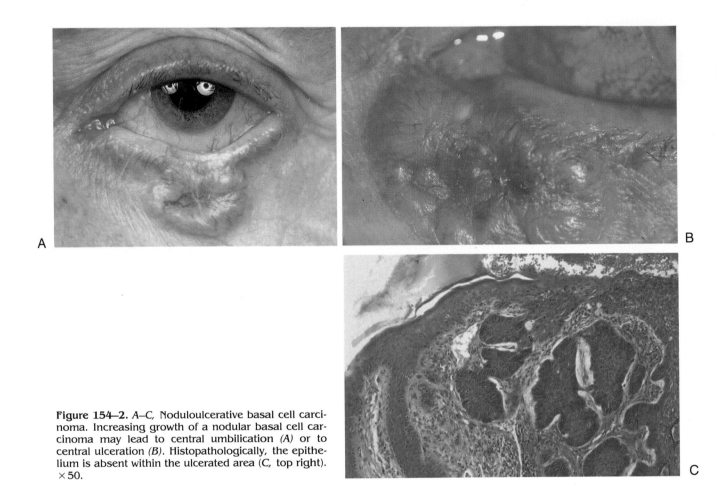

Figure 154–2. *A–C,* Noduloulcerative basal cell carcinoma. Increasing growth of a nodular basal cell carcinoma may lead to central umbilication *(A)* or to central ulceration *(B).* Histopathologically, the epithelium is absent within the ulcerated area (*C,* top right). ×50.

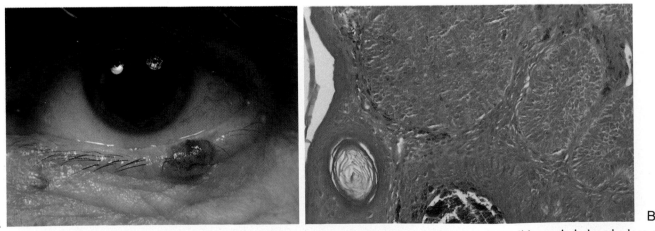

Figure 154–3. *A* and *B,* Pigmented basal cell carcinoma. The nodular growth pattern of this tumor at the lid margin induced a loss of lid lashes at the tumor site. Histopathology reveals a marked amount of pigment. ×100.

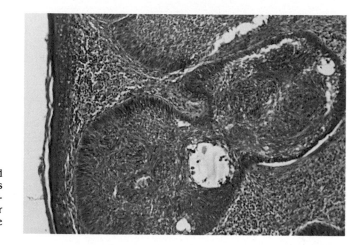

Figure 154–4. Nodular basal cell carcinoma. Nodular or solid basal cell carcinomas present as well-defined masses of various shapes and sizes, consisting of small hyperchromatic cells. Characteristically, they show parallel alignment of peripheral tumor cells (palisading) and separation of tumor lobules from the neighboring stroma following tissue fixation. ×50.

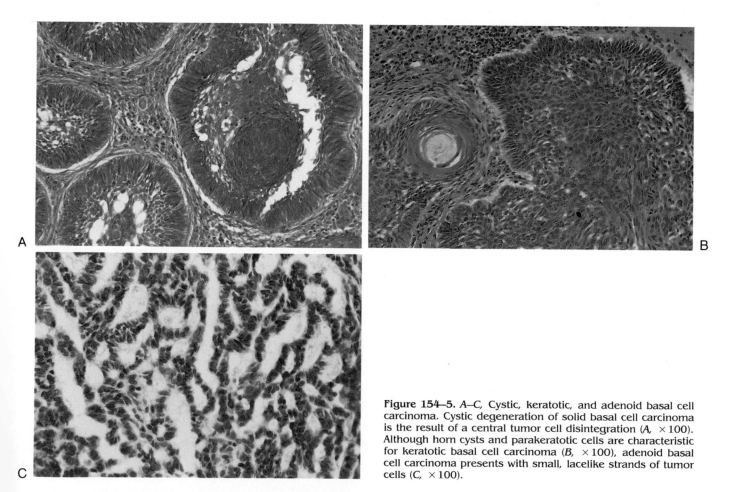

Figure 154–5. A–C, Cystic, keratotic, and adenoid basal cell carcinoma. Cystic degeneration of solid basal cell carcinoma is the result of a central tumor cell disintegration (A, ×100). Although horn cysts and parakeratotic cells are characteristic for keratotic basal cell carcinoma (B, ×100), adenoid basal cell carcinoma presents with small, lacelike strands of tumor cells (C, ×100).

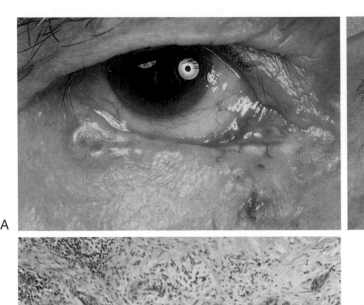

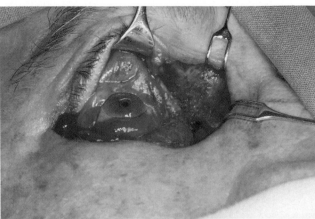

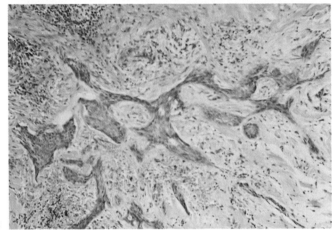

Figure 154–6. *A–C,* Morpheaform basal cell carcinoma. Clinically, this growth pattern leads to flat, pale, and indurated plaques. In the patient shown, tumor reaches from the inner canthal region along the entire lower lid to the lateral lid angle, leading to a total loss of lid lashes at the lower lid *(A).* The defect following microscopic–controlled tumor removal discloses the full extent of this lesion *(B).* Numerous groups of tumor cells, arranged in small nests or strands, are embedded in a dense fibrous stroma (*C,* ×50).

the dermis and even the subcutis. Such morpheic eyelid tumors may invade the orbit and the paranasal sinuses.

Histologically, the morphea or sclerosing growth pattern is characterized by its intense stromal fibrous proliferation. Tumor cells are divided in numerous branches of narrow cords and strands that often consist of only one to two cell layers. Peripheral palisading is usually nonexistent. Occasionally, focal connections of the tumor cells with the overlying epidermis can only be demonstrated by serial sections.

Superficial Basal Cell Carcinoma

Superficial basal cell carcinomas are seen almost exclusively on the trunk. They are multifocal in a high percentage of cases and present as slowly growing scaly red patches. The erythematous appearance may be misleading and suggest a diagnosis of psoriasis. However, both the peripheral translucent rolled border and the central epidermal atrophy provide the correct diagnosis.[41]

Fibroepitheliomatous Basal Cell Carcinoma of Pinkus

Fibroepitheliomatous basal cell carcinoma of Pinkus occurs mainly on the trunk.[7] Being a nodular plaque or

a firm polypoid lesion, these tumors present with an erythematous or skin-colored appearance resembling a fibroma. Translucency may be present and leads to the true nature of this lesion. Histopathologically, they are characterized by elongated strands of basaloid cells, which are connected to the epidermis and contain horn cysts.[42]

Nevoid Basal Cell Carcinoma Syndrome (Gorlin-Goltz-Syndrome)

The nevoid basal cell syndrome is an autosomal dominant form of basal cell carcinoma that demonstrates a high penetrance with a variable degree of expressivity. The basal cell carcinomas usually develop in adolescence; however, they are also seen in early childhood.[43] The eyelids were involved in 21.6 to 25 percent of cases.[44, 45] Histologically these tumors are usually superficial and indistinguishable from the noninherited form of basal cell carcinoma.[46, 47]

Clinically, one sees small nodules on the face and the trunk before the subsequent increase in size and number occurs. The "nevoid" stage reveals nodules that appear to enlarge and also increase in number. In the neoplastic and "cavernous" stage, these lesions become destructive and invasive in areas of the orbit or brain. Fifty percent of the adult patients with the nevoid basal cell carcinoma syndrome demonstrate numerous areas of dyskeratosis or pitting at the palms and soles, which develop in the first 2 decades of life.[48, 49] Widespread involvement including dystrophia canthorum, hypertelorism, congenital blindness, cataract, glaucoma, colobomas of the choroid and optic nerve, skeletal abnormalities, hypogonadism, ovarian fibromas, and central nervous system tumors are associated with this syndrome.[48, 50]

Linear Unilateral Basal Cell Nevus

The linear unilateral basal cell nevus is rare and is characterized by a unilateral linear eruption consisting of nodular basal cell carcinomas, striaelike areas of atrophy, and multiple comedones.[6, 51, 52] These types of abnormalities neither increase with aging nor do they enlarge.

Bazex Syndrome

The autosomal dominantly inherited Bazex syndrome is characterized by multiple basal cell carcinomas on the face, developing between late childhood and adolescence.[53] This syndrome also displays "ice-pick marks" on the extremities caused by atrophic dermal follicular changes. Congenital and permanent hypotrichosis, including scalp, body hair, eyebrows, and eyelashes as well as multiple milia and hypohidrosis, are also noted.[6, 53–55]

THERAPY

All types of therapy for basal cell carcinomas have their advocates, and every form of treatment has its advantages and disadvantages. Superficial basal cell carcinomas are likely to be more effectively treated with relative ease; however, the deep presence of the morpheic, sclerosing, or multicentric basal cell carcinoma signifies problems. They need to be treated aggressively and thoroughly to avoid recurrences or potential invasion of orbital or lacrimal tissues, or even death with cerebral involvement. In those cases, the interests of the patient are best represented by full information of all complications and a synergistic approach for the benefit and best results of therapy. In some cases with orbital invasion by basal cell carcinomas, exenterations are essential. Reexaminations at regular intervals of patients after initial surgery or after other forms of treatment are imperative. Basal cell carcinomas may require years to recur, and morpheaform basal cell carcinomas may present only in a thickened, waxy, yellow plaquelike manner, a form of appearance that is easily overlooked.

The following discussion describes the presently applied principal forms of therapy of basal cell carcinoma.

Micrographic (Mohs') Surgery

The application of the fresh tissue micrographic surgical approach supplies the best data in anticipated tumor removal. Its principle has been well established. The continous histologic control of margins ensures a very low recurrence rate. The latter is reported as 1.9 percent for 318 primary lesions without prior treatment and 6.4 percent for 313 previously treated lesions.[56] The micrographic method has the advantage over frozen section surgery, because it provides a three-dimensional view of the tumor through histologic drawings and markings. In this manner, only areas that demonstrate evidence of tumor are excised, which brings about an often less-extensive surgical removal of tissue and therefore, provides most likely a better functional reconstructive result. The fresh tissue micrographic surgical approach is considered to be, at this time, the best treatment method for periocular basal cell carcinomas. The tumor removal method by Mohs' surgery is time consuming. In many institutes, this portion of the procedure is carried out by dermatologists trained in micrographic surgery with subsequent referral of the patients to reconstructive surgeons, rather than allowing granulation to take place with later reconstructive surgery. The latter was done in the past and is generally not recommended in the periorbital region, with the possible exception of canthal defects. Therefore, a combination of micrographic surgery for removal of basal cell carcinoma followed by direct reconstruction ensures the best method of predictable tumor removal and the most functional and cosmetically acceptable reconstructive results.[21, 56–65]

Frozen Section or Permanent Section Control

Removal of basal cell carcinoma without histologic diagnosis and histologic control of tissue margin results in the highest recurrence rates. A micrographic control of the surgical margins at the time of surgical excision of a basal cell carcinoma brings about the lowest recurrence rate. The latter principle of Mohs' is a more cumbersome method that is not always available in all operating rooms. In our own experience, when the micrographic surgical control was not available, we have applied frozen section control of tissue margins during surgery and had a most acceptable cure rate by using this approach. Our own data of more than 500 tumors treated with frozen section controls revealed a recurrence rate of 3 percent over 5 yr. We hasten to add that we strongly believe that the micrographic principle of tumor removal is superior and specifically must be used when at all possible in the region of the medial or lateral canthal cancers. The morpheaform type of basal cell carcinoma with its high recurrence rates often requires a very thorough approach to ensure its complete removal at surgery. In those cases, when a "Mohs' surgeon" was not on hand, we have also applied a two-staged principle of treatment. This involves the removal of the tumor with numerous marginal sections being subjected to permanent paraffin-embedded biopsies. Only after these were reported as being free of tumor was the second stage of reconstruction begun.[4, 32, 66–70]

Radiotherapy and Electron Beam Therapy

Radiotherapy may be useful for treatment of basal cell carcinoma. Although most skin cancers can be treated with orthovoltage superficial x-rays, low-energy electrons have been used in such tumor therapy to minimize the radiation to structures adjacent to the tumor. The somewhat lower surface dose of electron beam therapy reduces the known side effects of radiation (e.g., telangiectasia, atrophy of the skin, keratinization of the conjunctiva, corneal damage, or dryness of the lacrimal gland). In effect, all side effects of radiation therapy are reduced with protraction of treatment and use of smaller doses per fraction as well as appropriate skin shielding. Well-standardized x-ray therapy of basal cell carcinoma in the periocular area usually involves doses in the total range of 35 Gy given in fractionated doses every 2 days for three initial doses in 1 wk and then application of the remaining two doses in the following week. Meticulous shielding of the eye is essential. Cure rates reach 96 percent.[71] In morpheaform basal cell carcinoma, radiotherapy was less effective compared with the other types.[19] The recurrence rate after x-ray therapy is listed between 6 and 8 percent. Loss of lashes, ectropion, and obstruction of the tear ducts, may occur following therapy. No cataracts were observed with shielding material. Tissue sampling is done at appropriate intervals.[71–76]

Chemotherapy

Systemic and local chemotherapy has been used on patients with basal and squamous cell carcinomas. This form of treatment was administered in patients with invasive basal cell carcinomas and squamous cell carcinomas, who refused extensive surgery or were medically unfit to undergo surgery. Local application, whenever indicated, of cisplatin and doxorubicin was accomplished by iontophoresis. Such therapy potentially widens the scope of available methods for treatment of extensive basal cell carcinomas in selected cases. The contraindications to systemic chemotherapy are renal failure, uncompensated heart failure, neutrocytopenia, and thrombocytopenia.[77–81]

Cryotherapy

Cryosurgery for skin tumors has gained in popularity because of its proposed cure rates, its good cosmetic results, its relative ease of application, and its reported low rate of complications.[22, 82–88]

Most forms of cryotherapy result in a recurrence rate for a treated skin tumor well below 10 percent. The 5-yr recurrence rate for basal cell carcinoma after cryotherapy of the eyelids with liquid nitrogen is reported as 4.6 percent.[89] The question of the more cumbersome and time-consuming Mohs' micrographic surgery in comparison with the easily applied cryotherapy would tempt many physicians to choose the latter method. The treatment involves a rapid freezing and a slow thawing of the treated tissues. A tissue temperature of $-40°C$ is aimed for with a freezing temperature of $100°C/min$ and a thawing temperature of $10°C/min$. Administration of a local anesthetic with added vasoconstrictors promotes a slow thawing temperature and lends itself toward improving the required slow thawing time. Two to three freeze: thaw cycles follow each other. N_2O (nitrous oxide) does not appear to be suitable for treatment of basal cell carcinoma, whereas liquid nitrogen affords great efficiency with appropriate instruments. The latter is of significance. Concentration of the beam of the spray of the liquid nitrogen is technically more difficult to apply in lid lesions, and surrounding normal tissue is often treated and involved in the breakdown after therapy. The treating temperature is in the range of $-160°C$ to $-180°C$, depending on the instruments utilized. The tissue shows early edema and then a breakdown and ulceration after 2 days, with slow granulation and long contractile scarring. Depigmentation is noted and also loss of lashes. The slow process of healing after cryotherapy compares with that following x-ray therapy or photodynamic therapy. The lack of histologic monitoring remains a significant disadvantage for all three of these treatment modalities.

Photodynamic Therapy

During the last 10 yr photodynamic therapy, using hematoporphyrin-derivative (HpD) has gained in significance for the treatment of superficial malignant tumors. The method consists of intravenous injection of HpD 48 hr prior to application of laser light (630 nm) of an argon-pumped dye laser system. Such laser light is applied to the superficial tumor, covering an area of 2 cm beyond the tumor margin, with the total dose of 100 J/cm^2 at a power of 100 mW/cm^2. The patient remains in an artificially illuminated room after the HpD injection and stays out of sunlight for at least 4 wk. The tumor site breaks down and is allowed to epithelialize. Biopsies taken 2 mo after treatment confirm the effective result, with retreatability in case of rare recurrences. HpD is an effective principle of treatment of superficial cancers.[90–95]

Carbon-Dioxide Laser Treatment

Capillary hemangiomas, port-wine stains, papillomas, and other tumors and also basal cell carcinomas have been treated effectively with CO_2 lasers. There is an advantage with the use of such a system because it coagulates small blood vessels; however, large vessels may bleed during application of CO_2 laser treatment. Carbon dioxide lasers raise the tissue temperature to approximately 100°C, which vaporizes the cells under treatment. An area of coagulation ulcers develops, and the affected region is permitted to granulate.[96–98] Scarring is minimal. Obviously, the lesions under treatment must be superficial. The CO_2 laser treatment prevents dissemination of tumor cells during treatment. Contrary to cryotherapy, it does not produce depigmentation. This technique, like cryotherapy and radiation therapy, does not allow for histologic confirmation of tumor eradication.

DELIBERATIONS

In our own experience cryosurgery has been successfully applied for superficial basal cell carcinomas in the periorbital area, using liquid nitrogen and thermocouple temperature control mechanisms. However, our experience has not warranted cryotherapy as the primary treatment vehicle in deep lid tumors or in canthal lesions. The latter are particularly likely to recur. We have not advocated any form of treatment in the canthal area other than histologically controlled excisions. The absence of histologic specimens with radiation or cryotherapy have been deterrents for these methods. The Mohs' micrographic surgery provides the best results in this regard. The synergistic approach between a "Mohs' surgeon" and an ophthalmic plastic reconstructive surgeon has allowed the time-consuming histologically assured excision of the tumor with appropriately suitable reconstruction. If a Mohs' laboratory is not available, detailed frozen section control of the lesion is recommended.

With regard to radiation therapy, its success rate resembles that of other forms of therapy in its effectiveness, with the exception of excision with frozen sections or micrographic Mohs' surgery. Although radiation is one of the oldest forms of treatment of the basal cell tumors, the need for fractionated therapy and the known complications after such surgery (e.g., loss of cilia, thinning of the skin, and telangiectasia) should be considered. We have applied this form of therapy in cases only when the medical status of the patients made the risk involved with the use of anesthesia too high or when the patient's old age or simple refusal of surgery dictated this therapeutic alternative. In any case, we do not recommend radiation therapy again after a recurrence has been proved, and the same reservation applies to cryotherapy. In these cases we favor a surgical approach, with histologic evaluations as our second mode of treatment.

Other modalities of therapy were listed earlier. The photodynamic approach or possibly even an immunotherapeutic approach is an exciting new avenue toward successful treatment. Thus, basal cell carcinomas remain a challenge as far as treatment principles are concerned. Many patients and physicians are lulled into a sense of tranquility, because of the low rate of metastases; however, such situations can occur and in some cases a basal cell carcinoma can kill. The observant and knowledgeable eyes of a properly trained physician or surgeon are required to diagnose, treat, and follow patients with basal cell carcinoma.

REFERENCES

1. Payne JW, Duke JR, Butner R, et al: Basal cell carcinoma of the eyelids. Arch Ophthalmol 81:553, 1969.
2. Aurora AL, Blody FC: Reappraisal of basal cell carcinomas of the eyelids. Am J Ophthalmol 70:329, 1970.
3. Henkind P, Friedman A: Cancer of the lids and ocular adnexa. *In* Andrade R, Gumport S, Popkin G, et al (eds): Cancer of the Skin. Philadelphia, WB Saunders, 1976, 1345.
4. Beard C: Observations on the treatment of basal cell carcinomas of the eyelids. Trans Am Acad Ophthalmol 79:664, 1975.
5. Schubert H: Häufigkeit und Lokalisation von Basaliomen im Kopf-Hals-Bereich. Dermatol Monatsschr 170:453, 1984.
6. Lever WF, Schaumburg-Lever G: Histopathology of the Skin, 7th ed. Philadelphia, JB Lippincott, 1990.
7. Pinkus H: Epithelial and fibroepithelial tumors. Bull NY Acad Med 42:176, 1965.
8. Lahbari H, Mehregan AH: Basal cell epithelioma (carcinoma) in children and teenagers. Cancer 49:350, 1982.
9. Keramidas DC, Anagnostou D: Basal-cell carcinoma of the lower lid in a child 27-month-old. Zeitschr für Kinderchir 42:250, 1987.
10. Nerad JA, Whitaker DC: Periocular basal cell carcinoma in adults 35 years of age and younger. Am J Ophthalmol 106:723, 1988.
11. Mora RG: Surgical and aesthetic considerations of cancer of the skin in the black American. J Dermatol Surg Oncol 12:24, 1986.
12. Gooding CA, White G, Yatsuhashi M: Significance of marginal extension in excised basal cell carcinoma. N Engl J Med 273:923, 1965.
13. Einaugler RB, Henkind B: Basal cell epithelioma of the eyelid: Apparent incomplete removal. Am J Ophthalmol 67:413, 1969.
14. Taylor GA, Barrisoni D: Ten-years experience and surgical treatment of basal-cell carcinoma: A study of factors associated with recurrence. Br J Surg 60:522, 1973.
15. Raskofsky SI: The adequacy of surgical excision of basal cell carcinoma. Ann Ophthalmol 5:596, 1973.
16. Blodi FC: Treatment of malignant lid tumors. JAMA 241:1396, 1979.
17. Schubert H, Wolfram G, Göldner G: Basaliomrezidive nach Behandlung. Dermatol Monatsschr 165:89, 1979.
18. Wiggs EO: Incompletely excised basal cell carcinoma of the ocular adnexa. Ophthalmol Surg 12:891, 1981.
19. Wiggs EO: Morpheaform basal cell carcinomas of the canthi. Trans Am Acad Ophthalmol Otol 79:649, 1975.
20. Beard C, Char DH: Prospective views in the treatment of eyelid and adnexal malignancies. Ophthalmol Surg 9:67, 1978.
21. Beard C: Management of malignancy of the eyelids. Am J Ophthalmol 92:1, 1981.
22. Anderson RL: A warning on cryosurgery for eyelid malignancies. Arch Ophthalmol 96:1289, 1978.
23. Costran RS: Metastasizing basal cell carcinomas. Cancer 14:1036, 1961.
24. Paver K, Poyzen K, Burry N, et al: The incidence of basal cell carcinoma and their metastases in Australia and New Zealand. Aust J Dermatol 14:53, 1973.
25. Weedon D, Wall D: Metastatic basal cell carcinoma. Med J Aust 2:177, 1975.
26. Farmer ER, Helwig EB: Metastatic basal cell carcinoma: A clinical pathologic study of 17 cases. Cancer 46:748, 1980.
27. Von Domarus H, Stevens TJ: Metastatic basal cell carcinoma: Report of 5 cases in review of 170 cases in the literature. J Am Acad Dermatol 10:1043, 1984.
28. Soffer D, Kaplan H, Weshler Z: Meningeal carcinomatosis due to basal cell carcinoma. Human Pathol 16:530, 1985.
29. Assor D: Basal cell carcinoma with metastasis to bone. Cancer 20:2125, 1967.
30. Wermuth BM, Fajardo LF: Metastatic basal cell carcinoma. Arch Pathol 90:458, 1970.

31. Safei B, Good RA: Basal cell carcinoma with metastasis. Arch Pathol 101:327, 1977.
32. Doxanas MT, Green WR, Iliff CE: Factors in the successful management of basal cell carcinoma of the eyelids. Am J Ophthalmol 91:726, 1981.
33. Font RL: Eyelids and lacrimal drainage system. In Spencer WH (ed): Ophthalmic Pathology, 3rd ed. Philadelphia, WB Saunders, 1986.
34. Wick MR: Malignant tumors of the epidermis. In Farmer ER, Hood AF (eds): Pathology of the Skin. East Norwalk, CT, Prentice Hall, 1990.
35. Hornblass A, Stefano JA: Pigmented basal cell carcinomas of the eyelids. Am J Ophthalmol 92:193, 1981.
36. Resnick KI, Sadun A, Albert DM: Basal cell epithelioma: An unusual case. Ophthalmology 88:1182, 1981.
37. Petersen RA, Aaberg TM, Smith TR: Solid vs. cystic basal cell epitheliomas of the eyelids: Correlation of clinical and pathological diagnoses. Arch Ophthalmol 79:31, 1968.
38. Sandbank M: Basal cell carcinoma at the base of a cutaneous horn (cornu cutaneum). Arch Dermatol 104:97, 1971.
39. Borel DM: Cutaneous basosquamous carcinoma: Review of the literature and report of 35 cases. Arch Pathol 95:293, 1973.
40. DeFarina JL: Basal cell carcinoma of the skin with areas of squamous cell carcinoma: A basosquamous cell carcinoma? Clin Pathol 38:1273, 1985.
41. Mehregan AH: Acantholysis in basal cell epithelioma. J Cutan Pathol 6:280, 1979.
42. McGibbon DH: Malignant epidermal tumors. J Cutan Pathol 12:224, 1985.
43. Gorlin RJ, Goltz RW: Multiple nevoid basal cell epithelioma, jaw cysts and bifid rib: A syndrome. N Engl J Med 262:908, 1960.
44. Zackheim HS, Loud AV, Howell AB: Nevoid basal cell carcinoma syndrome: Some histologic observations on the cutaneous lesions. Arch Dermatol 93:317, 1966.
45. Hammani H, Faggioni R, Streiff EB, Daiker B: Le syndrome d'épitheliomatose naevobasocellulaire multiple. Ophthalmologica 172:382, 1976.
46. Mason JK, Helwig EB, Graham JH: Pathology of the nevoid basal cell carcinoma syndrome. Arch Pathol 79:401, 1965.
47. Lindeberg H, Jepsen FL: The nevoid basal cell carcinoma syndrome: Histopathology of the basal cell tumors. J Cutan Pathol 10:68, 1983.
48. Howell JB, Freeman RG: Structure and significance of the pits with their tumors in the nevoid basal cell carcinoma syndrome. J Am Acad Dermatol 2:224, 1980.
49. Gorlin RJ: Nevoid basal cell carcinoma syndrome. Med Baltimore 66:98, 1987.
50. Geeraets WJ (ed): Ocular Syndromes, 3rd ed. Philadelphia, Lea & Febiger, 1976, p 199.
51. Anderson TE, Best PV: Linear basal cell nevus. Br J Dermatol 74:20, 1962.
52. Horio T, Komura J: Linear unilateral basal cell nevus with comedo-like lesions. Arch Dermatol 114:95, 1978.
53. Bazex A, Dopré A, Christol B: Atrophodermie folliculaire, proliférationce basocellulaires et hypotrichoses. Ann Dermatol Syph 93:241, 1966.
54. Viksnins P, Berlin A: Follicular atrophoderma and basal cell carcinomas. Arch Dermatol 113:948, 1977.
55. Polosila N, Keestala R, Neame KM: The Bazex syndrome: Follicular atrophoderma with multiple basal cell carcinoma, hypotrichoses and hypohidroses. Clin Exp Dermatol 6:31, 1981.
56. Robins P, Rodriguez-Sains R, Rabinovitz H, et al: Mohs' surgery for periocular basal cell carcinomas. Dermatol Surg Oncol 11:1203, 1985.
57. Baylis HI, Cies WA: Indications of Mohs' chemosurgical excision of eyelid and canthal tumors. Am J Ophthalmol 80:116, 1975.
58. Kopf AW, Bart RS: Recurrent basal cell carcinoma following Mohs' surgery. J Dermatol Surg Oncol 1:13, 1975.
59. Mohs FE: Microscopically controlled excision of medial canthal carcinomas. Ann Plast Surg 7:308, 1981.
60. Robbins P: Chemosurgery: My 15 years of experience. J Dermatol Surg Oncol 7:779, 1981.
61. Anderson RL: Results in eyelid malignancies treated with the Mohs fresh-tissue technique. In Trans New Orleans Acad Ophthalmol, St. Louis, CV Mosby, 1982, p. 380.
62. Mohs FE: Micrographic surgery for the microscopically controlled excision of eyelid cancers. Arch Ophthalmol 104:901, 1986.
63. Callahan MA, Monheit G, Callahan A: Five years' experience with the Mohs-Tromovitch technique of skin cancer removal. Int Ophthalmol Clin 29:247, 1989.
64. Monheit GD, Callahan MA, Callahan A: Mohs' micrographic surgery for the periorbital skin cancer. Dermatol Clin 7:677, 1989.
65. Downes RN, Walker NPJ, Collin JRO: Micrographic (Mohs') surgery in the management of periocular basal cell epitheliomas. Eye 4:160, 1990.
66. Older JJ, Quickert MM, Beard C: Surgical removal of basal cell carcinoma of the eyelids using frozen section control. Trans Am Acad Ophthalmol 79:658, 1975.
67. Collin JRO: Basal cell carcinoma in the eyelid region. Br J Ophthalmol 60:806, 1976.
68. Grove AS: Staged excision and reconstruction of extensive facial-orbital tumors. Ophthalmic Surg 8:91, 1977.
69. Chalfin J, Putterman AM: Frozen section control in the surgery of basal cell carcinoma of the eyelid. Am J Ophthalmol 87:802, 1979.
70. Frank HJ: Frozen section control of excision of eyelid basal cell carcinomas: 8½ years' experience. Br J Ophthalmol 73:328, 1989.
71. Gladstein AH: Efficacy, simplicity and safety of x-ray therapy of basal cell carcinomas on periocular skin. J Dermatol Surg Oncol 4:586, 1978.
72. Lederman M: Radiation treatment of cancer of the eyelids. Br J Ophthalmol 60:794, 1976.
73. Fitzpatrick PJ, Thompson GA, Easterbrook WM, et al: Basal and squamous cell carcinoma of the eyelids and their treatment by radiotherapy. Int J Radiat Oncol Biol Phys 10:449, 1984.
74. Sinese C, McNeese M, Peters LJ, et al: Electron beam therapy for eyelid carcinomas. Head Neck Surg 10:31, 1987.
75. Rodriguez-Sains R, Robins P, Smith B, et al: Radiotherapy of periocular basal cell carcinomas: Recurrence rates and treatment with special attention to the medial canthus. Br J Ophthalmol 72:134, 1988.
76. Gladstein AH, Kopf AW, Bart RS: Radiotherapy of cutaneous malignancies. In Goldschmidt H (ed): Physical Modalities in Dermatologic Therapy. New York, Springer Verlag, (in press)
77. Vizel M, Oster MW: Ocular side effects of cancer chemotherapy. Cancer 49:1999, 1982.
78. Wiesman TJ, Shively EH, Woodcock TM: Responsiveness of metastatic basal-cell carcinoma to chemotherapy: A case report. Cancer 52:1583, 1983.
79. Daly NJ, De Lafontan B, Combes PF: Results of the treatment of 165 lid carcinomas by iridium wire implant. Int J Radiat Oncol Biol Phys 10:455, 1984.
80. Guthrie TH Jr, McElveen LJ, Porubsky ES, Harmon JD: Cisplatin and doxorubicin; an effective chemotherapy combination in the treatment of advanced basal cell and squamous carcinoma of the skin. Cancer 55:1629, 1985.
81. Luxenberg MN, Guthrie TH: Chemotherapy of basal cell and squamous cell carcinoma of the eyelids and periorbital tissues. Ophthalmology 93:504, 1986.
82. Beard C, Sullivan JH: Cryosurgery of eyelid disorders including malignant tumors. In Zacarian SA (ed): Cryosurgical Advances in Dermatology and Tumors of the Head and Neck. Springfield, IL, Charles C Thomas, 1977.
83. Jacobiec FA, Iwamoto J: Cryotherapy for intraepithelial conjunctival melanoma proliferations. Arch Ophthalmol 101:904, 1983.
84. Zacarian SA: Cryosurgery of cutaneous carcinomas: An 18-year study of 3,022 patients with 4,228 carcinomas. J Am Acad Dermatol 9:947, 1983.
85. Fraunfelder FT, Zacarian SA, Wingfield DL, Limmer BL: Results of cryotherapy for eyelid malignancies. Am J Ophthalmol 97:184, 1984.
86. Zacarian SA: Cryosurgery for skin cancer and cutaneous disorders. St. Louis, CV Mosby, 1985.
87. Buschmann W, Linnert D: Bisherige Ergebnisse der Stickstoff-Kryotherapie bei Lidbasaliomen. Klin Monatsbl Augenheilkd 189:278, 1986.
88. Prskavec FH: Indikation und Ergebnisse der Kryotherapie von Lidtumoren. Wiener Klin Wochensch 98:279, 1986.
89. Matthäus W: 15jährige Erfahrung mit Kryotherapie von Lid-, Gesichts- und Bindehauttumoren in 2745 Fällen. Fortschr Ophthalmol 84:568, 1987.

90. Andreoni A, Cubeddu R: Fluorescence properties of HpD and its components. Chem Phys Lett 100:503, 1983.
91. Dahlman A, Wile AG, Burns RG, et al: Laser photoradiation therapy of cancer. Cancer Res 43:430, 1983.
92. Berns MW, Wile AG: Hematoporphyrin phototherapy of cancer. Radiother Oncol 7:233, 1986.
93. Grossweiner LI: Optical dosimetry in photodynamic therapy. Laser Med Surg 6:462, 1986.
94. Sery TW, Shields JA, Augsburger JJ, et al: Photodynamic therapy of human ocular cancer. Ophthal Surg 18:413, 1987.
95. Feyh J, Goetz A, Martin F, et al: Photodynamische Lasertumor-therapie mit Hematoporphyrin-Derevat (HpD) eines spinozellulären Karzinoms der Ohrmuschel. Laryngo Rhino Otol 68:563, 1989.
96. Adams EL, Price NM: Treatment of basal cell carcinomas with a carbon dioxide laser. J Dermatol Surg Oncol 5:803, 1979.
97. Beckman H, Fuller TA, Boyman R, et al: Carbon dioxide laser surgery of the eye and adnexa. Am Acad Ophthalmol 87:990, 1980.
98. Chopdar A: Carbon-dioxide laser treatment of eyelid lesions. Trans Ophthalmol Soc UK 104:176, 1985.

Chapter 155

■

Premalignant Lesions and Squamous Cell Carcinoma

KEVIN R. SCOTT and JAN W. KRONISH

Primary epithelial carcinomas of the skin are the most common malignancies in the United States.[1] The majority of these tumors develop in sun-exposed areas of the body in fair-skinned adults. Periocular skin lesions require early diagnosis and treatment due to their proximity to the globe, nose, paranasal sinuses, and brain. Benign, precancerous, and malignant cutaneous tumors are frequently difficult to distinguish from one another based on clinical appearance; therefore, a biopsy of all suspicious lesions of the ocular adnexa is mandatory to provide a histologic diagnosis.[2–5]

Squamous cell carcinoma of the eyelids is a potentially lethal tumor that can invade the orbit and periorbital structures, spread to regional lymph nodes, as well as metastasize to distant sites. Actinic keratoses, Bowen's disease, and radiation dermatoses may behave as precursors to this invasive neoplasm. Patients with the autosomal recessive disorder of xeroderma pigmentosa are predisposed to all forms of malignant epithelial tumors.[6] The clinical features, etiologic factors, histopathology, and treatment of each of these conditions are reviewed in this chapter.

ETIOLOGY

Sun exposure is by far the most important factor in the development of squamous cell carcinoma of the skin.[7–11] The ultraviolet (UV) radiation reaching the earth's surface is primarily UVA (315 to 400 nm) with a small percentage in the UVB (280 to 315 nm) range.[12] It is well established that UVB radiation is primarily responsible for the carcinogenic effect of the sun's radiation[7, 13–16]; however, experimental studies indicate that UVA may also have carcinogenic effects on the skin, but to a lesser degree.[12, 17] An increase of two- to threefold in the incidence of squamous cell carcinoma in the past 3 decades has been attributed to greater volitional exposure to the sun's UV radiation and possibly greater nonvolitional exposure secondary to atmospheric ozone depletion.[11] UV radiation is believed to induce skin cancer by direct damage to the DNA of the skin and through alterations in cellular immunity resulting from injury to Langerhans cells within the epidermis.[18–21]

The earliest report of chemical carcinogenesis dates back to 1775, when Pott reported an association between exposure to chimney soot and the development of scrotal cancer.[22] Subsequently, many carcinogens have been associated with the development of squamous cell carcinoma, including arsenic,[23, 24] tar,[25] and various hydrocarbons derived from coal and oils.[26] Other risk factors include human papilloma virus,[7, 27–29] exposure to ionizing radiation,[30, 32] UVA photochemotherapy (PUVA) for psoriasis,[33, 34] burn scars,[7, 35, 36] immunosuppression,[37–40] and chronic inflammatory conditions such as osteolytic sinusitis, osteomyelitic foci, and discoid lupus.[41–45] Xeroderma pigmentosum,[6, 18, 46–48] albinism,[49, 50] and familial acne conglobata[51] are heritable conditions that have also been associated with an increased incidence of developing cutaneous carcinomas.

PREMALIGNANT LESIONS

Squamous cell carcinoma may occur in previously normal-appearing skin (de novo) or, more commonly, arises from a preexisting lesion.[52] In the context of this chapter, a premalignant lesion is defined as a skin condition that has the potential to progress to an invasive squamous cell carcinoma. Actinic (solar, senile) keratosis, Bowen's disease (intraepithelial carcinoma), skin damaged by ionizing radiation, and xeroderma pigmentosum are well-established premalignant dermatoses.[46, 47, 52–54] Although thermal injuries to the skin and various chronic inflammatory conditions as listed earlier have been associated with the development of squamous cell carcinoma, these conditions are typically considered to be risk factors and not precancerous dermatoses.[8]

Actinic Keratoses

Actinic (solar, senile) keratosis is the most common precancerous skin lesion. As has been noted with squamous cell carcinoma, exposure to UV radiation is fundamental to the development of this dermatosis. These lesions exhibit a constant state of flux on the skin surface because of their inherent instability.[53, 55] For example, Marks and associates[55] reported that 25 percent of actinic keratoses observed over 12 mo spontaneously resolved, whereas during the same observation period, there was a generalized increase in the total number of actinic keratoses caused by the formation of new lesions.[55] The risk of malignant transformation has been reported to range as high as 20 percent.[52, 56, 57] In a prospective study, though, the risk of squamous cell carcinoma transformation from a single actinic keratosis lesion was calculated to be less than 0.1 percent per year.[53] It is also important to emphasize that squamous cell carcinoma arising from an actinic keratosis is generally considered to be less aggressive with a lower metastatic potential than one arising de novo.[45, 47, 52, 58]

CLINICAL PRESENTATION

Actinic keratoses most often occur in the sun-exposed areas of fair-complexioned, middle-aged individuals. They are more common in males, increase in number with age, and most often develop on the face, dorsum of the hands, forearms, and scalp.[47, 52, 59] Solar keratoses may take on a variety of clinical appearances but are typically rounded, flat, scaly, keratotic lesions with an erythematous base (Fig. 155–1). The keratotic plaque is centrally adherent with irregular edges, and the lesions generally measure only a few millimeters in diameter. Actinic keratoses occasionally have a nodular, horny, or even a wartlike configuration.[47, 52, 59] These lesions may be confused with a multitude of other similar-appearing benign and malignant tumors.[52]

HISTOPATHOLOGY

Microscopically, actinic keratoses are characterized by hyperkeratosis, irregular acanthosis, focal parakeratosis, dyskeratosis, focal atrophy, and atypical keratinocytes partially replacing the normal epidermal maturation or polarity. The atypical keratinocytes may show hyperchromatic nuclei, mitotic figures, vacuolated cells, multinucleated cells, prominent nucleoli, and loss of the intercellular bridges resulting in acantholysis. Focal areas of parakeratosis overlie areas of dysplastic keratinocytes and are frequently bordered by regions of normal keratin maturation (orthokeratosis) surrounding the follicular ostia (Fig. 155–2). The normal rete ridges are altered by the proliferation of small buds or wide,

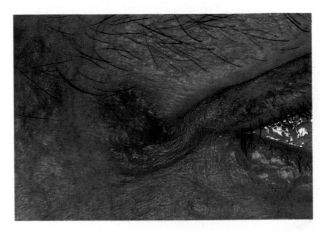

Figure 155–1. Actinic keratosis of the lateral canthal region showing a rounded erythematous lesion with a central keratotic plaque.

broadened rete ridges that extend down into the dermis. The dermoepidermal basement membrane remains intact, and the underlying dermis may show a variable inflammatory response consisting of lymphocytes and plasma cells. Actinic keratoses may occasionally show prominent papillomatosis or verrucous acanthosis.[52]

TREATMENT

Treatment of solar keratoses should be based on size, location, clinical symptoms, and an understanding of their malignant potential. Small flat lesions that do not involve the eyelids or the immediate periocular area may be observed. Within the periocular region, the development of all new potentially malignant growths demands a histologic diagnosis in the form of an incisional or excisional biopsy. The choice of biopsy technique is determined by the anatomic location, patient's age, and laxity of the surrounding skin. Once the diagnosis of actinic keratosis is confirmed, any residual component of the lesion can be surgically excised or treated with cryotherapy.

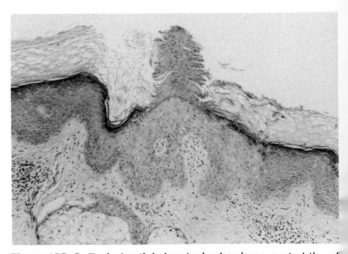

Figure 155–2. Typical actinic keratosis showing a central tier of parakeratosis surmounting a focus of abnormal keratinocytic maturation. H&E, ×120.

Bowen's Disease

Bowen's disease of the skin was previously believed to be a marker for the development of internal malignancies.[60-62] There have been several reports refuting this claim based on several methodologic flaws identified in the early studies including (1) lack of adequate control groups; (2) inclusion of individuals with known internal malignancies when Bowen's disease was diagnosed; and (3) lack of life-table analysis comparing cancer incidence rates over time.[54, 63, 64] It is now generally accepted that Bowen's disease is synonymous with squamous cell carcinoma in situ and that there is no conclusive evidence to correlate this condition with the subsequent development of primary internal carcinomas.[54, 63-65] A variety of factors have been associated with Bowen's disease and are similar to those linked with the development of squamous cell carcinoma.[47, 65]

CLINICAL PRESENTATION

Bowen's disease characteristically occurs in the sun-exposed areas of middle-aged or elderly fair-skinned individuals. The face, neck, and hands are the most commonly affected areas; however, Bowen's disease may also involve the oral mucosa, nail beds, conjunctiva, and urogenital area.[65, 66] In the periocular region, Bowen's disease normally presents as an isolated erythematous, scaly, crusty, pigmented keratotic plaque.[47, 52, 59, 65] The lesions are free of hair and have well-demarcated borders. The average diameter of Bowen's disease at

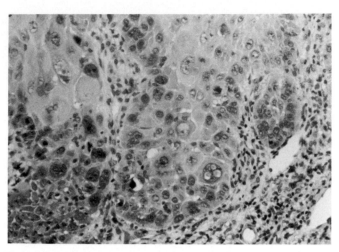

Figure 155–4. Same case as in Figure 155–3 demonstrating extreme cellular atypia with hyperchromatic nuclei, multinucleated giant cells, vacuolated cells, and dyskeratosis. H&E, ×240.

the time of biopsy is 1.3 cm, which is much larger than a typical actinic keratosis.[52]

HISTOPATHOLOGY

Bowen's disease shares some of the microscopic features of actinic keratosis, including hyperkeratosis, parakeratosis, dyskeratosis, hypogranulosis, an intact dermoepidermal basement membrane, and an inflammatory reaction in the superficial dermis.[47, 52, 59] In Bowen's disease, though, the epidermis is replaced with full-thickness cellular atypia and with complete loss of maturation (squamous cell carcinoma in situ) (Fig. 155–3). The atypical cells frequently exhibit bizarre mitotic figures, hyperchromatic nuclei, multinucleated giant cells, vacuolated cells, plaquelike acanthosis, and acantholysis with cleft formation (Fig 155–4). Also, unlike actinic keratoses, the hair follicles and sebaceous glands are not spared.[47]

TREATMENT

All lesions resulting from Bowen's disease should be treated, because at least 5 percent harbor an invasive squamous cell carcinoma.[52] Surgical excision is the treatment of choice in Bowen's disease involving the periocular area. If there are multiple large lesions or if the individual is a poor surgical candidate, radiation therapy or cryotherapy is an effective alternative treatment modality.[65, 67]

Radiation Dermatosis

In the past, ionizing radiation was commonly used to treat a variety of facial skin conditions, such as acne, psoriasis, eczema, and hirsutism. The harmful effects of irradiation were eventually appreciated after the long-term results of these treatments were reported. The link between ionizing radiation and the development of

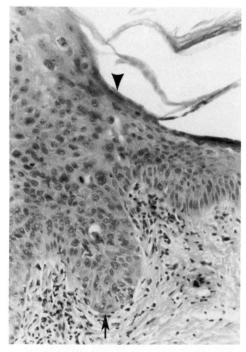

Figure 155–3. Bowen's disease showing the abrupt transition (*arrowhead*) from normal epithelium on the right to the markedly acanthotic epithelium on the left. There is full thickness cellular atypia with loss of maturation, yet the dermoepidermal basement membrane (*arrow*) remains intact (carcinoma in situ). H&E, ×180.

squamous cell carcinoma, basal cell carcinoma, and mesenchymal sarcomas is now well recognized.[32, 59] Dosages of ionizing radiation are now more accurately quantified, and the result has been a significant reduction in the total radiation exposure for a given individual. Additionally, radiotherapy is now reserved almost exclusively for treatment of malignant conditions.

CLINICAL PRESENTATION

Ionizing radiation induces numerous adverse cutaneous effects that can be divided into early or late changes. During the first few days after radiation exposure, the skin develops generalized erythema and becomes edematous secondary to the accumulation of both intracellular and extracellular fluid within the epidermis and superficial dermis.[47] Within a few weeks, stimulated dendritic melanocytes may result in hyperpigmentation in addition to desquamation of keratin. Late periocular changes that can occur over subsequent months to years include the loss of eyelashes, skin atrophy, lid necrosis, mottled pigmentation, telangiectasias of the skin and conjunctiva, conjunctivitis, conjunctival keratinization, ectropion, entropion, punctal or canalicular stenosis, and the late development of radiation-induced tumors.[1, 32, 47, 59, 68, 69] Keratitis, cataract formation, and retinopathy are some of the more serious potential ocular side effects.

HISTOPATHOLOGY

The late histopathologic changes of the epithelium following irradiation are similar to those induced by extensive actinic solar damage. Ionizing radiation, however, also damages the deeper dermal layers and results in marked atrophy, homogenization of the collagen, vascular thrombosis, and the development of large isolated atypical fibroblasts within the dermis. Characteristic changes of the eyelids include squamous cell metaplasia or atrophy of the meibomian glands and keratinization of the palpebral conjunctiva and canaliculi.[32, 47, 68]

TREATMENT

The ocular surface changes resulting from exposure to ionizing radiation can usually be managed with frequent applications of lubricating drops or ointment. Keratinization of the conjunctiva generally improves over time; however, symptoms of ocular irritation may be relieved with a topical retinoid or, in severe cases, require mucous membrane grafting. The development of punctal or canalicular obstruction is not uncommon following radiation to the medial canthal area.[70] Prior to initiating radiation therapy in high doses (>2500 cGy) to the eyelids or orbit, we recommend prophylactic intubation of the lacrimal drainage system with a silicone stent in order to limit the cicatrizing and keratinizing effects of irradiation on the puncta and canaliculi.[71] The treatment of radiation-induced tumors is dictated by the biologic behavior of the malignancy and by its location in the periocular region.

Xeroderma Pigmentosum

Xeroderma pigmentosum is a rare autosomal recessive disorder in which the repair of UV light-induced damage to the DNA of epidermal cells is defective.[6, 18, 46] This extreme sensitivity to UV light has been demonstrated in cell cultures of epithelial cells from skin and conjunctiva from affected patients as well as their dermal fibroblasts and peripheral blood lymphocytes.[46] Individuals with this condition have a marked predisposition to develop squamous cell carcinomas, basal cell carcinomas, and malignant melanomas over their entire skin surface. The vast majority of these malignant tumors, though, occur in the areas of maximal sun exposure, including the head and neck regions.[6] Families of affected individuals often have a history of consanguinity.[6, 46, 47] This disorder has been reported in all races and afflicts males and females equally.[6, 46–48]

CLINICAL PRESENTATION

The cutaneous changes associated with xeroderma pigmentosum pass through three stages.[47] Sun sensitivity in the first stage is manifested by erythema, scaling, and numerous freckles during the first 2 yr of life.[6, 47] During the second stage, the skin exhibits mottled pigmentation, diffuse telangiectasias, and areas of atrophy.[46, 47] Malignant tumors of the skin develop in the third stage, including squamous cell carcinoma, basal cell carcinoma, and malignant melanoma, as well as various sarcomas.[47] Correspondingly, there is a marked reduction in life expectancy in individuals with xeroderma pigmentosum attributed to the development of metastatic carcinomas.[48]

The ophthalmic manifestations of xeroderma pigmentosum can involve any tissues exposed to UV light such as the eyelids, conjunctiva, and cornea. In addition to a loss of lashes and ectropion, the eyelid skin can progress through the three stages previously described.[6] The conjunctival and corneal changes can be extensive with the development of inflammation, conjunctival neoplasms, exposure keratitis, corneal clouding, and vascularization.[46] In addition to the cutaneous and ocular changes, neurologic abnormalities have been documented, including progressive mental deterioration, abnormal reflexes, impaired hearing, and retarded growth and sexual development.[46, 47]

HISTOPATHOLOGY

The nonmalignant histologic alterations associated with xeroderma pigmentosum are similar to the actinic changes previously described; however, these alterations occur at a markedly accelerated pace.[47]

TREATMENT

Individuals with xeroderma pigmentosum constantly develop new cutaneous and ocular surface tumors. Suspicious lesions in the periocular region require a biopsy to confirm the diagnosis; the exact treatment is based on the biologic behavior of that specific lesion. Studies have reported limited success in treating multiple skin tumors in patients with xeroderma pigmentosum using a variety of topical and systemic chemotherapies.[72–78] At present, these treatments should be viewed as adjuvant therapeutic modalities for advanced cases and cannot be broadly recommended for all patients with this disorder.

SQUAMOUS CELL CARCINOMA

Squamous cell carcinoma is the second most common malignancy of the eyelids and represents 9 percent of periocular cutaneous cancers.[79] Basal cell carcinoma had previously been reported to occur 40 times more frequently than squamous cell carcinomas,[2] but a ratio of approximately 12:1 is consistent with more recent studies.[79–81] They may develop de novo, but more commonly squamous cell carcinomas arise from a precancerous dermatosis. Early diagnosis and definitive treatment are of paramount importance in the management of squamous cell carcinoma due to its metastatic potential.[41, 56, 79, 82, 83]

Clinical Presentation

Squamous cell carcinoma of the skin occurs primarily in elderly individuals with fair complexions and a history of chronic sun exposure.[41, 79, 84, 85] Men are affected more commonly than women in a ratio of approximately 2:1,[11, 41] and the risk of developing this cutaneous neoplasm rises with increasing proximity to the equator.[86] Squamous cell carcinoma may occur anywhere on the body, although most lesions occur in sun-exposed areas. In the periocular region, the lower eyelid is more commonly affected than the upper eyelid, with a ratio of 1.4:1, and there is a propensity for lesions to involve the lid margin.[47, 79] These tumors also frequently arise in the canthal areas, particularly the medial canthus.[79] Most cutaneous squamous cell carcinomas arise from preexisting lesions such as actinic keratoses, Bowen's disease, radiation dermatoses, burn scars, or chronic inflammatory lesions, yet de novo lesions are not uncommon.[7, 52, 56]

Squamous cell carcinoma in the periocular area has no pathognomonic features to allow the clinician to easily differentiate it from other cutaneous lesions. These tumors vary in presentation, although most often appear as painless nodular or plaquelike lesions with irregular rolled edges, chronic scaling, fissuring of the skin, pearly borders, telangiectasias, and early central ulceration (Figs. 155–5 and 155–6). Occasionally, they may initially present as papillomatous growths, cutaneous horns, or cystic lesions along the lid margin.[87, 88] Individuals with squamous cell carcinoma of the periocular region frequently have additional actinic-related lesions on the face, neck, scalp, and dorsum of the hands (Fig. 155–7). A thorough inspection of these sun-exposed areas is important to identify any additional suspicious lesions.

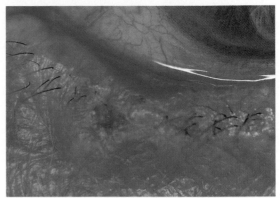

Figure 155–5. Clinical appearance of an early nodular squamous cell carcinoma of the lower lid with central ulceration, anterior displacement of the mucoepidermal junction, and madarosis.

The differential diagnosis of squamous cell carcinoma is extensive because of the diverse clinical appearance of this tumor. Lesions that may mimic squamous cell carcinoma include basal cell carcinoma, keratoacanthoma, actinic keratosis, Bowen's disease, sebaceous cell carcinoma, inverted follicular keratosis, seborrheic keratosis, pseudoepitheliomatous hyperplasia, papilloma or verruca, nevus, tricholemmoma, and deep fungal infections.[2–5, 7, 41, 56] A biopsy is mandatory in all suspicious eyelid lesions to accurately distinguish squamous cell carcinoma from these other benign and malignant conditions.

Patterns of Invasion and Metastasis

Squamous cell carcinoma of the eyelids and periocular area, unlike basal cell carcinoma and precancerous dermatoses, exhibits an invasive pattern of spread with the potential for regional lymph node and distant metastasis. These tumors also tend to proliferate more rapidly than

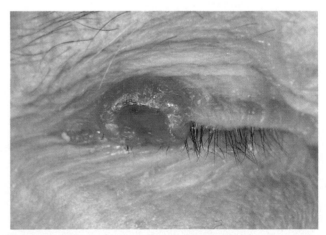

Figure 155–6. An erythematous nodular squamous cell carcinoma with rolled edges and central ulceration involving the upper lid margin.

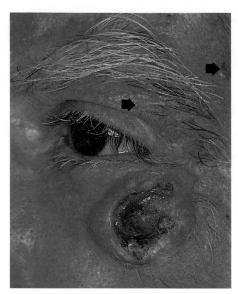

Figure 155–7. A large squamous cell carcinoma of the lower lid and cheek. In addition, note the actinic changes on the lateral aspect of the upper lid and forehead (*arrows*).

basal cell carcinomas, with a mean duration from the onset to the time of diagnosis of approximately 9 mo to 1 yr.[89, 90] Invasion of the thin dermis in the eyelids often results in extension into the superficial orbicularis muscle. Deeper penetration may result in spread of the tumor along both fascial and embryologic fusion planes, periosteum, lymphatic vessels, blood vessels, and nerve sheaths (Fig. 155–8).[79, 82, 83, 87, 91, 92]

The likelihood that a given squamous cell carcinoma will metastasize is related to the following clinical and histologic features: degree of differentiation, etiology, tumor size, and depth of dermal invasion.[7, 41, 42, 56, 87, 88, 93] Broders' classification for the microscopic grading of squamous cell carcinoma divides tumors into four different grades based on the proportion of differentiated cells within the tumor.[93] In grade I, most cells are well differentiated, whereas in grade IV, most cells are undifferentiated or anaplastic. It is generally accepted that the more anaplastic the tumor, the more likely it is to both metastasize or to recur locally after treatment.[7, 41, 91]

The incidence of metastasis from squamous cell carcinomas arising from actinic keratoses is low and is frequently reported to be less than 2 percent.[7, 42, 56, 89, 94–96] Lesions that arise de novo, however, behave more aggressively and are more likely to metastasize.[45, 47, 57, 97, 98] Cutaneous squamous cell carcinoma arising in areas of previous ionizing radiation, burn scars, chronic inflammatory conditions (osteomyelitic foci, discoid lupus), and in immunosuppressed patients exhibit more invasive patterns of spread.[32, 38, 42, 43, 94] Finally, reports have suggested a correlation between the overall size and depth of tumor invasion with the risk of metastatic spread.[99, 100]

Regional lymph node involvement has been reported to range from 1.3 to 21.4 percent in patients with squamous cell carcinoma of the eyelids. Metastases to the lymphatic chain usually develop late in the more advanced cases.[79] Lymphatic spread follows the normal anatomic channels with preauricular lymph node drainage of the outer two thirds of the upper lid, outer one third of the lower lid, and lateral canthus, and submandibular lymph node drainage of the inner one third of the upper lid, inner two thirds of the lower lid, and medial canthus.[47, 79]

Squamous cell carcinoma is the most common secondary orbital tumor, but, the vast majority of these originate in the sinuses.[101] Direct extension into the orbital tissues from cutaneous squamous cell carcinoma is generally associated with lesions that have been chronically neglected, irradiated, or have had multiple local recurrences after treatment.[79, 90, 101] Tumors that reach the periorbita may travel along its surface or may directly invade the underlying bone (Fig. 155–9A and B).[79, 91]

Perineural infiltration of squamous cell carcinoma of the eyelids is another mode of spread into the orbit, intracranial cavity, and periorbital structures along distal branches of the trigeminal nerve, the extraocular motor nerves, and the facial nerve.[41, 56, 82, 83, 92] Initial involvement of the trigeminal nerve occurs painlessly; however, with time, the nerve may become dysfunctional and may cause constant or intermittent dysesthesias, such as burning, tingling, numbness, and aching.[83, 92, 102] These symptoms may become so severe as to cause the clinician to misdiagnose this condition as tic douloureux.[82] Extraocular motor nerve and facial nerve involvement are rarely encountered, yet ocular motility and orbicularis function should be carefully assessed in all cases of periocular squamous cell carcinoma. Although it has been documented that there is a high percentage of false-negative examination results, computed tomography scans should be performed on all patients who have large or suspicious tumors in order to survey for orbital extension and bone involvement.[83, 102, 103]

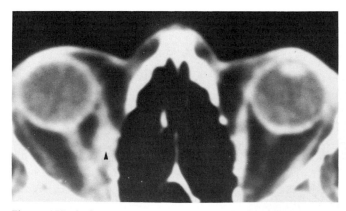

Figure 155–8. Computer tomography scan demonstrates a mass adjacent to the medial wall of the right orbit (*arrow*) in a patient who had a squamous cell carcinoma previously resected from the right lower lid. The orbital lesion was biopsied and found to represent a squamous cell carcinoma with perineural infiltration of the orbit.

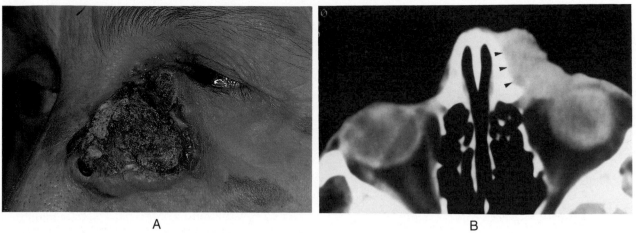

Figure 155–9. *A,* Clinical appearance of a large squamous cell carcinoma involving the lower lid, medial canthus, and nasal bridge. *B,* Computed tomography scan of the same patient demonstrates the nasal bone involvement (*arrowheads*) with early orbital extension. This lesion was removed by exenteration with en bloc excision of the involved bone.

Histopathology

Squamous cell carcinoma arises from the prickle-squamous cell layer of the epidermis. Its hallmark feature is extension of the tumor beyond the level of the dermoepidermal basement membrane into the underlying dermis.[52] The superficial epithelial changes are generally an exaggeration of the actinic changes previously described for actinic keratosis and Bowen's disease. The downward growth of cells proceeds as irregular masses or nests of cells extending into the dermis. These masses often appear to be discrete, yet they are interconnected as finger-like extensions or "claws" extending down from the surface.[87] A surrounding chronic inflammatory reaction composed of lymphocytes and plasma cells is frequently noted in all forms of squamous cell carcinoma.[87, 88, 104]

The histologic appearance of squamous cell carcinoma varies greatly from well-differentiated tumors with obvious keratinization to poorly differentiated anaplastic spindle cell tumors resembling sarcomas. Well-differentiated tumors are characterized by eosinophilic cytoplasm, keratin pearl formation with nesting of cells, intercellular bridges, and mild pleomorphism (Figs. 155–10 and 155–11).[47, 88, 105] Poorly differentiated tumors may exhibit little or no signs of keratinization or intercellular bridging, making these lesions difficult to interpret histologically. Immunoperoxidase stains for prekeratin, cytokeratin, and involucrin may be needed to clearly establish the diagnosis in these acantholytic or spindle cell variants.[106–111] The detection of cytoplasmic tonofilaments by electron microscopy may also assist in verifying the squamous cell origin of these tumors.[7] Perineural infiltration is another histopathologic feature of squamous cell carcinoma that can have important prognostic implications (Fig. 155–12).

Adenoid squamous cell carcinoma is another variant of squamous cell carcinoma that exhibits marked acantholysis and a pseudoglandular configuration.[47, 96, 104] Within the tumor mass are distinct lobules defined by a single layer of cuboidal epithelial cells around the periphery and acantholytic dyskeratotic cells forming lumina centrally.[96, 104] These lesions are believed to arise from actinic keratoses with acantholysis.[96, 104] The biologic behavior of this tumor is similar to that of squamous cell carcinoma arising from actinic skin damage and has a low risk of metastasis.[96, 104]

Treatment

Management of patients with cutaneous lesions in the periocular region that appear suspicious for squamous cell carcinoma should include making a rapid diagnosis, providing definitive treatment for tumor eradication, and restoring the function and cosmesis of the affected structures. An incisional biopsy should be performed on all suspicious lesions to confirm the diagnosis. The

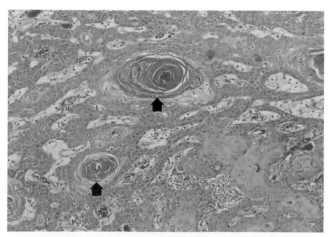

Figure 155–10. A moderately well-differentiated squamous cell carcinoma exhibiting mild pleomorphism and extensive interconnecting cords of tumor cells with keratin pearl formation (*arrows*). The brightly eosinophilic cytoplasm results from abnormal intracellular keratin production. H&E, ×160.

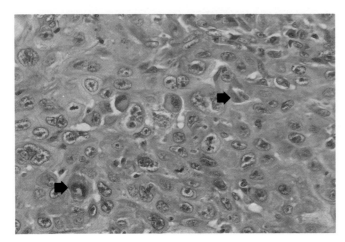

Figure 155–11. Squamous cell carcinoma showing dyskeratosis (*arrowheads*), moderate pleomorphism, and numerous mitotic figures (*arrows*). H&E, ×360.

preferred mode of treatment for primary squamous cell carcinoma in the periocular region is surgical excision with microscopically controlled margins.[56, 79, 82, 112–117] Radiation and cryotherapy are alternative methods of treatment for management of patients who are poor surgical candidates.[67, 69, 113, 117–124] Topical and systemic chemotherapy have limited applications and are best reserved as adjuvant therapies in advanced cases or in individuals with multiple recurrent skin cancers related to xeroderma pigmentosum.[41, 73–78, 125, 126] Curettage and electrodesiccation, although used successfully elsewhere on the body, have no role in the treatment of squamous cell carcinoma in the periocular region.[113, 127]

Prior to the selection of any treatment option, a careful search for deep orbital invasion and metastatic spread is essential, particularly in patients with advanced lesions. Orbital ultrasound and computed tomography are useful to identify extension of tumor into the orbital soft tissues and secondary bone changes. The limitations in the resolution of these imaging studies must be appreciated; for example, perineural orbital extension may initially occur without significant cranial nerve enlargement and may only be detectable at the time of surgery.[82, 83, 103] The preauricular or submandibular lymph nodes are the most common sites for regional metastasis, mandating a thorough examination for even subtle changes.[7, 41, 90]

SURGERY

Microscopically controlled surgical excision utilizing either frozen section control or Mohs' micrographic technique offers one main advantage over all alternative treatments in that these allow for the detection of occult extensions of tumor cells beyond the apparent clinical margins. A wider excision than that for other lid neoplasms is recommended regardless of the technique used because of the potential of metastasis and mortality. We prefer Mohs' microsurgery, performed by a trained dermatologist, over excisions utilizing frozen section

control because it offers the following advantages: (1) an unbiased surgical excision; (2) maximal conservation of normal tissue; (3) reduced operating time for the reconstructive surgeon; (4) additional time to plan the reconstructive approach; and (5) greater scheduling flexibility. The surgical reconstruction following Mohs' surgery may be performed the same day but can be delayed for 24 to 48 hr if necessary. Mohs' microsurgical excision of both primary and recurrent periocular squamous cell carcinoma results in 5-yr cure rates of 90 to 95 percent,[112, 128–131] which is slightly less than the 5-yr cure rate of 95 to 98 percent for basal cell carcinomas treated with the same technique.[112, 129–133]

When surgical excision is performed using frozen section control methods, the pathologist must be skilled in this technique, and the orientation of the tissue must be clearly marked to avoid errors in interpretation and to maximize the procedure's efficacy. Utilizing this technique, immediate reconstruction usually follows once the margins are clear. Both microsurgical techniques become unreliable once the orbital septum is violated and a tumor is identified in the orbital fat.[130] Additionally, these techniques cannot be used to obtain clear surgical margins if bone is involved, which can be recognized intraoperatively by pitting, dehiscences, and frank bone destruction. When possible, squamous cell carcinoma involvement of bone should be treated with en bloc surgical excision, which almost always necessitates orbital exenteration to obtain adequate margins. Squamous cell carcinoma with bone involvement responds poorly to radiotherapy and therefore radiotherapy should not be used as the main form of treatment.[69, 82, 90, 103]

Orbital exenteration with microscopic analysis of the apical margins is the treatment of choice when a tumor extends directly into the orbital fat or when perineural orbital involvement is detected. The addition of radiotherapy has been advocated in cases of deep orbital invasion by either direct or perineural spread of tumor or obvious central nervous system extension detected

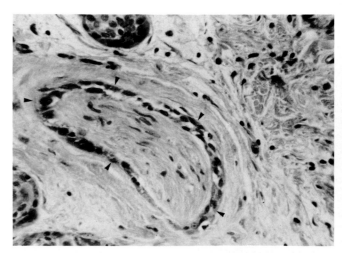

Figure 155–12. A branch of the trigeminal nerve containing perineural tumor infiltration by squamous cell carcinoma (*arrowheads*). H&E, ×240.

preoperatively by computed tomography.[82, 90] The prognosis in cases with intracranial extension is poor, and radiation is used principally as palliative therapy.[82]

Regional metastases may present as palpable, enlarged preauricular and submandibular lymph nodes. Chronically ulcerated or secondarily infected squamous cell carcinomas may induce a secondary inflammatory lymphadenopathy; therefore, an open biopsy is required to exclude the possibility of metastasis. In addition to the primary surgical excision, radical neck dissection is recommended when malignant extension to the regional lymph nodes is detected and there is no evidence of distant metastases. The routine use of neck dissection in the treatment of periocular squamous cell carcinoma is not recommended because of its mutilating effects and the low probability of subclinical lymph node involvement at the time of initial therapy.[134]

RADIOTHERAPY

Radiotherapy is an alternative primary treatment for patients with squamous cell carcinoma of the eyelids who either have contraindications to surgery or refuse surgical excision and reconstruction. It may also provide palliative treatment of advanced tumors with orbital extension in patients with known distant metastases. Squamous cell carcinoma is more resistant to ionizing radiation than basal cell carcinomas. Consequently, treatment with radiotherapy necessitates the use of significantly higher dosages of radiation to obtain an adequate tumoricidal effect.[90] Careful planning by the radiation oncologist to maximally shield the globe reduces both the immediate and late ocular side effects.

Radiotherapy generally results in a cure rate of 90 to 95 percent, with good functional results if the tumor is well localized and the globe is carefully protected.[69, 135] Despite these encouraging statistics, though, numerous disadvantages of this treatment modality exist. First, radiation therapy lacks histologic control in the management of cutaneous lesions, and, as a result, the tumor margins may extend beyond the field of treatment. Second, postradiation complications of the periocular tissues and globe can be severe and pose a potential threat to vision, such as lid necrosis, keratitis, cataract formation, retinopathy, and optic atrophy.[69, 135] Third, the patient must commit to daily visits to the treatment facility for a period of weeks until the total dosage is administered.

Numerous conditions also exist that are specific contraindications or limitations of this form of treatment. For example, radiotherapy should be avoided in areas previously treated with radiation and for tumors that involve the central aspect of the upper eyelid where palpebral conjunctival keratinization may have devastating corneal side effects.[69] Squamous cell carcinoma involving bone is more radioresistant than are tumors limited to soft tissues. Also, this form of treatment, as a rule, should be avoided in patients less than 40 yr of age and in individuals with xeroderma pigmentosum because of its carcinogenic potential.[136, 137] In addition, the surgical excision of recurrent tumors and reconstruc-

tion utilizing tissues previously irradiated may be compromised because of radiation-induced atrophy and vascular damage.[32, 113]

CRYOTHERAPY

Cryotherapy for squamous cell carcinoma and basal cell carcinoma located in the periocular area is slowly gaining acceptance as an alternative to surgery or radiation.[67, 113, 119, 120, 122-124, 138] This modality offers several advantages over radiation, such as lower cost, greater convenience for the patient with only one treatment visit, absence of a cataractogenic potential, and the ability to treat an area repeatedly if necessary. There are several important clinical features, though, that have been associated with a reduced cure rate for cryotherapy. These include tumors that are fixed to the periosteum, located in the medial canthus, greater than 10 mm in diameter, and lesions that have indistinct margins or extend into the conjunctival fornix.[67, 119, 120, 122]

Treatment is applied in the form of a liquid nitrogen spray utilizing a double freeze-thaw technique while protecting the globe with a styrofoam shield or Jaeger lid retractor.[118, 119, 122, 123, 138] This form of therapy is ideally suited for individuals who refuse surgery or are poor surgical candidates and in whom the tumor is small (less than 10 mm), well demarcated, and does not involve the conjunctival fornix, medial canthus, or bone.[67, 119, 120, 122] Depigmentation, loss of lashes, hypertrophy of previously healed surgical scars, lid notching, ectropion, epiphora, and pseudoepitheliomatous hyperplasia are some of the more common periocular side effects following cryotherapy. Darkly pigmented individuals and patients with cold intolerance (e.g., cryoglobulinemia or cold urticaria) are poor candidates for this form of treatment.[67, 120]

CHEMOTHERAPY

There have been a number of encouraging reports on the efficacy of topical and systemic chemotherapy for advanced or multiple squamous cell carcinomas. The leading drugs that have been shown to yield partial or complete regression of cutaneous squamous cell carcinoma include cisplatin alone or in combination with doxorubicin, bleomycin, isotretinoin, and α-interferon.[41, 73-78, 125, 126, 139-141] There is even some evidence to support that isotretinoin taken orally may act to both treat and prevent the development of cutaneous malignancies.[72, 74, 125, 142, 143] These chemotherapeutic agents, though, have potential serious side effects and are generally recommended as adjuvant therapy for advanced squamous cell carcinoma or multiple periocular tumors when the standard protocols of surgery or radiation have either been refused or would not be curative.[73, 74, 125] Patients with xeroderma pigmentosum who have multiple advanced cutaneous and conjunctival tumors and patients with regional or distant metastases from squamous cell carcinoma represent those who are most likely to benefit from these chemotherapeutic agents.[73-75, 125, 126]

Prevention

The recent increase in incidence of cutaneous squamous cell carcinoma has been attributed to the popularity of sunbathing and outdoor activities and the associated exposure to UV radiation.[11, 84] Squamous cell carcinoma is best prevented, therefore, by a lifelong commitment to shield the skin from the harmful effects of solar radiation. Patients especially with actinic skin damage or cutaneous malignant tumors should be counseled to adhere to the following measures:

1. Apply sunscreen with a sun protection factor (SPF) of 15 or greater to the face and below the eyelids every day. A very light application of sunscreen to the upper lids and forehead is recommended to minimize potential ocular irritation.

2. Wear protective clothing when outdoors, such as a wide-brimmed hat and dark clothing with a nonreflective surface.

3. Avoid exposure to the sun, particularly between 10:00 A.M. and 3:00 P.M. when the sun's rays are most intense.

The importance of these preventative measures cannot be overemphasized. Some have speculated that regular use of protective sunscreen for the first 18 yr of life reduces the lifetime incidence of both squamous cell and basal cell carcinomas by 78 percent.[13] Furthermore, a diminishing ozone layer leading to an increase of harmful rays reaching the earth's surface underscores the need for such preventative measures.[14, 15] New measures of prevention are being studied, especially for individuals who are susceptible to actinic skin damage. For example, an ongoing study has demonstrated a protective effect of oral isotretinoin for the prevention of development of various lesions, such as actinic keratoses, keratoacanthoma, and Bowen's disease.[142, 143]

REFERENCES

1. Hornblass A: Clinical evaluation of tumors of the eyelid and ocular adnexa. In Hornblass A (ed): Oculoplastic, Orbital and Reconstructive Surgery, Vol 1. Baltimore, Williams & Wilkins, p 193, 1988.
2. Kwitko ML, Boniuk M, Zimmerman LE: Eyelid tumors with reference to lesions confused with squamous cell carcinoma. I: Incidence and errors in diagnosis. Arch Ophthalmol 69:693–697, 1963.
3. Kwitko ML, Boniuk M, Zimmerman LE: Eyelid tumors with reference to lesions confused with squamous cell carcinoma. II: Inverted follicular keratosis. Arch Ophthalmol 69:698–707, 1963.
4. Kwitko ML, Boniuk M, Zimmerman LE: Eyelid tumors with reference to lesions confused with squamous cell carcinoma. III: Keratoacanthoma. Arch Ophthalmol 77:29–40, 1967.
5. Welch RB, Duke JR: Lesions of the lids: A statistical note. Am J Ophthalmol 45:415–416, 1958.
6. Kraemer KH, Lee MM, Scotto J: Xeroderma pigmentosum: Cutaneous, ocular, and neurologic abnormalities in 830 published cases. Arch Dermatol 123:241–250, 1987.
7. Arnold HL Jr, Odom RB, James WD (eds): Andrews' Diseases of the Skin: Clinical Dermatology, 8th ed. Philadelphia, WB Saunders, 1990, p 745.
8. Aubry F, MacGibbon B: Risk factors of squamous cell carcinoma of the skin: A case-control study in the Montreal region. Cancer 55:907–911, 1985.
9. Stetson CG, Schulz MD: Carcinoma of the eyelid. N Engl J Med 241:725–732, 1949.
10. Fry RJM, Ley RD: Ultraviolet radiation-induced skin cancer. Carcinog Compr Surv 11:321–337, 1989.
11. Glass AG, Hoover RN: The emerging epidemic of melanoma and squamous cell skin cancer. JAMA 262:2097–2100, 1989.
12. Strickland PT: Photocarcinogenesis by near-ultraviolet (UVA) radiation in Sencar mice. J Invest Dermatol 87:272–275, 1986.
13. Stern RS, Weinstein MC, Baker SG: Risk reduction for nonmelanoma skin cancer with childhood sunscreen use. Arch Dermatol 122:537–545, 1986.
14. Kripke ML: Impact of ozone depletion on skin cancers. J Dermatol Surg Oncol 14:853–857, 1988.
15. Fears TR, Scotto J: Estimating increases in skin cancer morbidity due to increases in ultraviolet radiation exposure. Cancer Invest 1:119–126, 1983.
16. Engel A, Johnson ML, Haynes SG: Health effects of sunlight exposure in the United States. Results from the first National Health and Nutrition Examination Survey, 1971–1974. Arch Dermatol 124:72–79, 1988.
17. Stagerg B, Wulf HC, Klemp P, et al: The carcinogenic effect of UVA irradiation. J Invest Dermatol 81:517–519, 1983.
18. Robbins JH, Moshell AN: DNA repair processes protect human beings from premature solar skin damage: Evidence from studies on xeroderma pigmentosum. J Invest Dermatol 73:102–107, 1979.
19. Hersey P, Hasic E, Edwards A, et al: Immunological effects of solarium exposure. Lancet 1:545–548, 1983.
20. Aberer W, Schuler G, Stingl G, et al: Ultraviolet light depletes surface markers of Langerhans cells. J Invest Dermatol 76:202–210, 1981.
21. Kripke ML: Immunological unresponsiveness induced by ultraviolet radiation. Immunol Rev 80:87–102, 1984.
22. Pott P: Cancer Scroti, vol 5. In Hawes L, Clarke W, Collins R: Chirurgical Works. London, Longmans, Green & Co., 1775, p 63.
23. Tseng W: Effects and dose-response relationships of skin cancer and blackfoot disease with arsenic. Environ Health Perspect 19:109–119, 1977.
24. Neubauer O: Arsenical cancer: A review. Br J Cancer 1:192–251, 1947.
25. Moy LS, Chalet M, Lowe NJ: Scrotal squamous cell carcinoma in a psoriatic patient treated with coal tar. J Am Acad Dermatol 14:518–519, 1986.
26. Hueper WC: Chemically induced skin cancers in man. NCI Monogr 10:377–391, 1963.
27. Lynch PJ: Viral oncogenesis in cutaneous malignancy. In Friedman RJ, Rigel DS, Kopf AW, et al (eds): Cancer of the Skin. Philadelphia, WB Saunders, 1991, p 85.
28. Syrjanen KJ: Human papillomavirus (HPV) infections and their associations with squamous cell neoplasia. Archiv Geschwulstforsch 57:417–443, 1987.
29. McDonnell JM, McDonnell PJ, Stout WC, Martin WJ: Human papillomavirus DNA in a recurrent squamous carcinoma of the eyelid. Arch Ophthalmol 107:1631–1634, 1989.
30. Traenkle HL: X-ray induces skin cancer in man. NCI Monogr 10:423–432, 1963.
31. Sadamori N, Mine M, Hori M: Skin cancer among atom bomb survivors. Lancet 1:1267, 1989.
32. Martin H, Strong E, Spiro RH: Radiation-induced skin cancer of the head and neck. Cancer 25:61–71, 1970.
33. Stern RS, Laird N, Melski J, et al: Cutaneous squamous-cell carcinoma in patients treated with PUVA. N Engl J Med 310:1156–1161, 1984.
34. Stern RS, Lange R: Non-melanoma skin cancer occurring in patients treated with PUVA five to ten years after treatment. J Invest Dermatol 91:120–124, 1988.
35. Mora RG, Perniciaro C: Cancer of the skin in blacks. I: A review of 163 black patients with cutaneous squamous cell carcinoma. J Am Acad Dermatol 5:535–543, 1981.
36. Mosborg DA, Crane RT, Tami TA, Parker GS: Burn scar carcinoma of the head and neck. Arch Otolaryngol Head Neck Surg 114:1038–1040, 1988.
37. Rao NA, Dunn SA, Romero JL, Stout W: Bilateral carcinomas of the eyelid. Am J Ophthalmol 101:480–482, 1986.
38. Hoxtell EO, Mandel JS, Murray SS, et al: Incidence of skin carcinoma after renal transplantation. Arch Dermatol 113:436–438, 1977.

39. Gupta AK, Cardella CJ, Haberman HF: Cutaneous malignant neoplasms in patients with renal transplants. Arch Dermatol 122:1288–1293, 1986.

40. Hardie IR, Strong RW, Hartley LCJ, et al: Skin cancer in Caucasian renal allograft recipients living in a subtropical climate Surgery 87:177–183, 1980.

41. Dzubow L, Grossman D: Squamous cell carcinoma and verrucous carcinoma. *In* Friedman RJ, Rigel DS, Kopf AW, et al (eds): Cancer of the Skin. Philadelphia, WB Saunders, 1991, p 74.

42. Moller R, Reymann F, Hou-Jensen K: Metastases in dermatological patients with squamous cell carcinoma. Arch Dermatol 115:703–705, 1979.

43. Sedlin ED, Fleming JL: Epidermoid carcinoma arising in chronic osteomyelitic foci. J Bone Joint Surg 45:827–838, 1963.

44. Presser SE, Taylor JR: Squamous cell carcinoma in blacks with discoid lupus erythematosus. J Am Acad Dermatol 4:667–669, 1981.

45. Morgan RJ: Metastases from squamous cell epitheliomas of the skin. *In* Epstein E: Controversies in Dermatology. Philadelphia, WB Saunders, 1984, p 134.

46. Gaasterland DE, Rodrigues MM, Moshell AN: Ocular involvement in xeroderma pigmentosum. Ophthalmology 89:980–986, 1982.

47. Font RL: Eyelids and lacrimal drainage system. *In* Spencer WH (ed): Ophthalmic Pathology: An Atlas and Textbook, Vol 3. Philadelphia, WB Saunders, 1986, p 2141.

48. Cleaver JE: Defective repair replication of DNA in xeroderma pigmentosum. Nature 218:652–656, 1968.

49. Mohle J, Nickoloff BJ: Fatal cutaneous squamous cell carcinoma in a forty-three-year-old male. J Dermatol Surg Oncol 12:276–279, 1985.

50. Okoro AN: Albinism in Nigeria: A clinical and social study. Br J Dermatol 92:485–492, 1975.

51. Quintal D, Jackson R: Aggressive squamous cell carcinoma arising in familial acne conglobata. J Am Acad Dermatol 14:207–214, 1986.

52. Graham JH, Helwig EB: Premalignant cutaneous and mucocutaneous diseases. *In* Graham JH, Johnson WC, Helwig EB (eds): Dermal Pathology. Hagerstown, Harper & Row, 1972, p 561.

53. Marks R, Rennie G, Selwood TS: Malignant transformation of solar keratoses to squamous cell carcinoma. Lancet 1:795–797, 1988.

54. Reymann F, Ravnborg L, Schou G, et al: Bowen's disease and internal malignant diseases: A study of 581 patients. Arch Dermatol 124:677–679, 1988.

55. Marks R, Foley P, Goodman G, et al: Spontaneous remission of solar keratoses: The case for conservative management. Br J Dermatol 115:649–655, 1986.

56. Doxanas MT, Iliff WJ, Iliff NT, Green WR: Squamous cell carcinoma of the eyelids. Ophthalmology 94:538–541, 1987.

57. Fukamizu H, Inoue K, Matsumoto K, et al: Metastatic squamous-cell carcinomas derived from solar keratosis. J Dermatol Surg Oncol 11:518–522, 1985.

58. Jansen T: Clinical Recognition of Skin Neoplasms. Chicago, Year Book Medical Publishers, 1976, p 57.

59. Yanoff M, Fine BS: Ocular Pathology: A Text and Atlas, 3rd ed. Philadelphia, JB Lippincott, 1989, p 163.

60. Graham JH, Helwig EB: Bowen's disease and its relationship to systemic cancer. Arch Dermatol 83:738–758, 1961.

61. Peterka ES, Lynch FW, Goltz RW: An association between Bowen's disease and internal cancer. Arch Dermatol 84:623–629, 1961.

62. Hugo NE, Conway H: Bowen's disease: Its malignant potential and relationship to systemic cancer. Plast Reconstr Surg 39:190–194, 1967.

63. Callen JP: Bowen's disease and internal malignant disease. Arch Dermatol 124:675–676, 1988.

64. Arbesman H, Ransohoff DF: Is Bowen's disease a predictor for the development of internal malignancy? A methodological critique of the literature. JAMA 257:516–518, 1987.

65. Lee MM, Wick MM: Bowen's disease. CA 40:237–242, 1990.

66. Thestrup-Pedersen K, Ravnborg L, Reymann F: Morbus Bowen: A description of the disease in 617 patients. Acta Dermatol Venereol 68:236–239, 1988.

67. Fraunfelder FT, Zacarian SA, Limmer BL, Wingfield D: Cryo-

68. Char D: Clinical Ocular Oncology. New York, Churchill Livingstone, 1989, p 21.

69. Lederman M: Radiation treatment of cancer of the eyelids. Br J Ophthalmol 60:794–805, 1976.

70. Fayos JV, Wildermuth O: Carcinoma of the skin of the eyelids. Arch Ophthalmol 67:298–302, 1962.

71. Jordan DR, Nerad JA, Tse DT: The pigtail probe, revisited. Ophthalmology 97:512–519, 1990.

72. Kraemer KH, DiGiovanna JJ, Moshell AN, et al: Prevention of skin cancer in xeroderma pigmentosum with the use of oral isotretinoin. N Engl J Med 318:1633–1637, 1988.

73. Luxenberg MN, Guthrie TH Jr: Chemotherapy of basal cell and squamous cell carcinoma of the eyelids and the periorbital tissues. Ophthalmology 93:504–510, 1986.

74. Lippman SM, Shimm DS, Meyskens FL Jr: Nonsurgical treatments for skin cancer: Retinoids and alpha-interferon. J Dermatol Surg Oncol 14:862–869, 1988.

75. Guthrie TH, McElveen LJ, Porubsky ES, Harmon JD: Cisplatin and doxorubicin: An effective chemotherapy combination in the treatment of advanced basal cell and squamous carcinoma of the skin. Cancer 55:1629–1632, 1985.

76. Halnan KE, Brewin TB, Bleehen NM, et al: Bleomycin in advanced squamous cell carcinoma: A random controlled trial. Br Med J 1:188–190, 1976.

77. Lippman SM, Meyskens FL Jr: Treatment of advanced squamous cell carcinoma of the skin with isotretinoin. Ann Intern Med 107:499–501, 1987.

78. Lippman SM, Kessler JF, Al-Sarraf M, et al: Treatment of advanced squamous cell carcinoma of the head and neck with isotretinoin: A phase II randomized trial. Invest New Drugs 6:51–56, 1988.

79. Reifler DM, Hornblass A: Squamous cell carcinoma of the eyelid. Surv Ophthalmol 30:349–365, 1986.

80. Aurora A, Blodi FC: Lesions of the eyelids: A clinicopathological study. Surv Ophthalmol 15:94–104, 1970.

81. Shulman J: Treatment of malignant tumours of the eyelids by plastic surgery. Br J Plast Surg 15:37–47, 1962.

82. Trobe JD, Hood I, Parsons JT, Quisling RG: Intracranial spread of squamous carcinoma along the trigeminal nerve. Arch Ophthalmol 100:608–611, 1982.

83. Cottel WI: Perineural invasion by squamous-cell carcinoma. J Dermatol Surg Oncol 8:589–600, 1982.

84. Weinstock MA: The epidemic of squamous cell carcinoma. [Editorial] JAMA 262:2138–2139, 1989.

85. Rodriguez-Sains RS, Jakobiec FA: Eyelid and conjunctival neoplasms. *In* Smith BC, Della Rocca RC, Nesi FA, Lisman RD (eds): Ophthalmic Plastic and Reconstructive Surgery, Vol 2. St. Louis, CV Mosby, 1987, p 759.

86. Scotto J, Fears TR, Fraumini JF: Incidence of nonmelanoma skin cancer in the United States. US Dept Health and Human Services, Bethesda, MD, Publication (NIH) no. 83–2433, 1983.

87. Duke-Elder S, MacFaul PA: The ocular adnexa. *In* Duke-Elder S (ed): System of Ophthalmology. St Louis, CV Mosby, 1974, p 423.

88. Lucas DR: Greer's Ocular Pathology, 4th ed. Oxford, Blackwell Scientific Publications, 1989, p 81.

89. Epstein E, Epstein NN, Bragg K, Linden G: Metastases from squamous cell carcinomas of the skin. Arch Dermatol 97:245–251, 1968.

90. Rootman J, Robertson WD: Tumors. *In* Rootman J: Diseases of the Orbit. Philadelphia, JB Lippincott, 1988, p 281.

91. Mohs FE, Lathrop TG: Modes of spread of cancer of skin. Arch Dermatol Syphilol 66:427–439, 1952.

92. Dodd GD, Dolan PA, Ballantyne AJ, et al: The dissemination of tumors of the head and neck via the cranial nerves. Rad Clin North Am 8:445–461, 1970.

93. Broders AC: Practical points on the microscopic grading of carcinoma. N Y J Med 32:667–671, 1932.

94. Lund HZ: How often does squamous cell carcinoma of the skin metastasize? Arch Dermatol 92:635–637, 1965.

95. Katz AD, Urbach F, Lilienfeld AM: The frequency and risk of metastases in squamous-cell carcinoma of the skin. Cancer 6:1162–1166, 1957.

96. Johnson WC, Helwig EB: Adenoid squamous cell carcinoma

(adenoacanthoma): A clinicopathologic study of 155 patients. Cancer 11:1639–1650, 1966.

97. Graham JH, Bendl BJ, Johnson WC: Solar keratosis with squamous cell carcinoma: A new biology concept. Am J Pathol 55:26A, 1969.

98. Freeman RG, Knox JM, Heaton CL: The treatment of skin cancer: A statistical study of 1341 skin tumors comparing results obtained with irradiation, surgery, and curettage followed by electrodesiccation. Cancer 17:535–538, 1964.

99. Immerman SC, Scanlon EF, Christ M, Knox KL: Recurrent squamous cell carcinoma of the skin. Cancer 51:1537–1540, 1983.

100. Friedman HI, Cooper PH, Wanebo HJ: Prognostic and therapeutic use of microstaging of cutaneous squamous cell carcinoma of the trunk and extremities. Cancer 56:1099–1105, 1985.

101. Shields JA: Diagnosis and Management of Orbital Tumors. Philadelphia, WB Saunders, 1989, p 341.

102. Csaky KG, Custer P: Perineural invasion of the orbit by squamous cell carcinoma. Ophthalmol Surg 21:218–220, 1990.

103. Glover AT, Grove AS: Orbital invasion by malignant eyelid tumors. Ophthal Plast Reconstr Surg 5:1–12, 1989.

104. Caya JG, Hidayat AA, Weiner JM: A clinicopathologic study of 21 cases of adenoid squamous cell carcinoma of the eyelid and periorbital region. Am J Ophthalmol 99:291–297, 1985.

105. Hogan MJ, Zimmerman LE (eds): Ophthalmic Pathology: An Atlas and Textbook, 2nd ed. Philadelphia, WB Saunders, 1962, p 168.

106. Penneys NS: Immunoperoxidase methods and advances in skin biology. J Am Acad Dermatol 11:284–290, 1984.

107. Kahn H, Baumal R, From L: Role of immunohistochemistry in the diagnosis of undifferentiated tumors involving the skin. J Am Acad Dermatol 14:1063–1072, 1986.

108. Smoller BR, Kwan TH, Said JW, Banks-Schlegel S: Keratoacanthoma and squamous cell carcinoma of the skin: Immunohistochemical localization of involucrin and keratin proteins. J Am Acad Dermatol 14:226–234, 1986.

109. Cooper D, Schermer A, Sun TT: Classification of human epithelia and their neoplasms using monoclonal antibodies to keratins: Strategies, applications, and limitations. Lab Invest 52:243–256, 1985.

110. Murphy GF, Flynn TC, Rice RH, Pinkus GS: Involucrin expression in normal and neoplastic human skin: A marker for keratinocyte differentiation. J Invest Dermatol 82:453–457, 1984.

111. Said JW, Sassoon AF, Shintaku IP, Banks-Schlegel S: Involucrin in squamous and basal cell carcinoma of the skin: An immunohistochemical study. J Invest Dermatol 82:449–452, 1984.

112. Anderson RL, Ceilley RI: A multispecialty approach to the excision and reconstruction of eyelid tumors. Ophthalmology 85:1150–1163, 1978.

113. Beard C: Management of malignancy of the eyelids. Am J Ophthalmol 92:1–6, 1981.

114. Mohs FE: Chemosurgical treatment of cancer of the eyelid: A microscopically controlled method of excision. Arch Ophthalmol 39:43–59, 1948.

115. Grove AS Jr, McCord CD Jr, Tanenbaum M: Eyelid tumors: Diagnosis and management. In McCord CD Jr, Tanenbaum M (eds): Oculoplastic Surgery. New York, Raven Press, 1987, p 197.

116. Robins P: Mohs' surgery. In Smith BC, Della Rocca RC, Nesi FA, Lisman RD (eds): Ophthalmic Plastic and Reconstructive Surgery, Vol 2. St. Louis, CV Mosby, 1987, p 841.

117. Loeffler M, Hornblass A: Characteristics and behavior of eyelid carcinoma (basal cell, squamous cell, sebaceous gland, and malignant melanoma). Ophthalmic Surg 21:513–518, 1990.

118. Zacarian SA: Cancer of the eyelid: A cryosurgical approach. Ann Ophthalmol 4:473–480, 1972.

119. Kuflik EG: Cryosurgery for carcinoma of the eyelids: A 12-year experience. J Dermatol Surg Oncol 11:243–246, 1985.

120. Fraunfelder FT, Zacarian SA, Wingfield DL, Limmer BL: Results of cryotherapy for eyelid malignancies. Am J Ophthalmol 97:184–188, 1984.

121. Halnan KE, Britten MJA: Late functional and cosmetic results of treatment of eyelid tumour. Br J Ophthalmol 52:43–53, 1968.

122. Fraunfelder FT, Wallace TR, Farris HE, et al: The role of cryosurgery in external ocular and periocular disease. Trans Am Acad Ophthalmol Otolaryngol 83:713–724, 1977.

123. Kuflik EG: Cryosurgery for basal-cell carcinomas on and around eyelids. J Dermatol Surg Oncol 4:911–913, 1978.

124. Zacarian SA: The cryogenic approach to treatment of lid tumors. Ann Ophthalmol 2:706–713, 1970.

125. Levine N, Miller RC, Meyskens FL Jr: Oral isotretinoin therapy: Use in a patient with multiple cutaneous squamous cell carcinomas and keratoacanthomas. Arch Dermatol 120:1215–1217, 1984.

126. Loeffler JS, Larson DA, Clark JR, et al: Treatment of perineural metastasis from squamous carcinoma of the skin with aggressive combination chemotherapy and irradiation. J Surg Oncol 29:181–183, 1985.

127. Crissey JT: Curettage and electrodesiccation as a method of treatment for epitheliomas of the skin. J Surg Oncol 3:287–290, 1971.

128. Mohs FE: Chemosurgery for facial neoplasms. Arch Otolaryngol 95:62–67, 1972.

129. Mohs FE: Chemosurgery for skin cancer: Fixed tissue and fresh tissue techniques. Arch Dermatol 112:211–215, 1976.

130. Anderson RL: Results in eyelid malignancies treated with the Mohs' fresh-tissue technique. In Symposium on Diseases and Surgery of the Eyelids, Lacrimal Apparatus, and Orbit. St. Louis, CV Mosby, 1982, p 380.

131. Riefkohl R, Pollack S, Georgiade GS: A rationale for the treatment of difficult basal cell and squamous cell carcinomas of the skin. Ann Plast Surg 15:99–104, 1985.

132. Robins P: Chemosurgery: My 15 years of experience. J Dermatol Surg Oncol 7:779–789, 1981.

133. Robins P: Mohs' surgery (microscopically controlled excision) for the removal of cancer in the periorbital area. In Aston SJ, Hornblass A, Meltzer MA, Rees TD (eds): Third International Symposium of Plastic and Reconstructive Surgery of the Eye and Adnexa. Baltimore, Williams & Wilkins, 1982, p 147.

134. Shiu MH, Chu F, Fortner JG: Treatment of regionally advanced epidermoid carcinoma of the extremity and trunk. Surg Gynecol Obstet 150:558–562, 1980.

135. Fitzpatrick PJ, Thompson GA, Easterbrook WM, et al: Basal and squamous cell carcinoma of the eyelids and their treatment by radiotherapy. J Radiat Oncol Biol Phys 10:449–454, 1984.

136. Goldschmidt H: Radiotherapy of skin cancer: Modern indications and techniques. Cutis 171:253–261, 1976.

137. Hornblass A: Tumors of the Ocular Adnexa and Orbit. St. Louis, CV Mosby, 1979, p 1.

138. Fraunfelder FT: The indications and contraindications of cryosurgery. Arch Ophthalmol 96:729, 1978.

139. Kingston T, Gaskell S, Marks R: The effects of a novel potent oral retinoid (Rol3-6298) in the treatment of multiple solar keratoses and squamous cell epithelioma. Eur J Cancer Clin Oncol 19:1201–1205, 1983.

140. Luxenberg MN, Guthrie TH Jr: Chemotherapy of eyelid and periorbital tumors. Trans Am Ophthalmol Soc 83:162–180, 1985.

141. Takehiko T, Endo H: A case of squamous cell carcinoma treated by intralesional injection of oil bleomycin. Dermatologica 170:302–305, 1985.

142. Lippman SM, Kessler JF, Meyskens FL Jr: Retinoids as preventive and therapeutic anticancer agents, Part I. Cancer Treat Rep 71:391–405, 1987.

143. Lippman SM, Kessler JF, Meyskens FL Jr: Retinoids as preventive and therapeutic anticancer agents, Part II. Cancer Treat Rep 71:493–515, 1987.

Chapter 156

∎

Sebaceous Tumors of the Ocular Adnexa*

FREDERICK A. JAKOBIEC

Sebaceous tumors have long been known to arise preferentially in the eyelids owing to the abundant distribution of sebaceous glands within the tough fibrous tarsus of the eyelids (meibomian glands) and in association with the eyelashes (the Zeis glands).[1-3] The caruncle is also endowed with sebaceous glands attached to the fine lanugo or vellus hairs of this structure, and sebaceous glands are associated with the strong hairs of the eyebrow region. All of these sites are therefore capable of spawning both benign and malignant sebaceous tumors. The least common site of origin for well-documented sebaceous carcinoma is the lacrimal gland.[4] There is debate regarding whether malignant sebaceous tumors can develop primarily in metaplastic-neoplastic conjunctival epithelium,[5,6] but this author has discovered unequivocally benign tumors with sebaceous differentiation taking origin from the upper tarsal epithelium. It is important to underscore that sebaceous carcinoma of noneyelid skin is extremely rare[7] and that it therefore behooves ophthalmologists to become extremely familiar with the characteristics of this neoplasm.

From the embryologic point of view, it should not be entirely unexpected that sebaceous tumors might arise in unusual sites such as the lacrimal gland and conjunctival epithelium.[8] The sebaceous glands of the caruncle are evaginations from the embryonic surface conjunctival epithelium and, therefore, it might be possible during neoplastic transformation for conjunctival cells to once again reexpress this potential. Similarly, the lacrimal gland is a tuboloracemose outpouching of the embryonic conjunctival epithelium. The lacrimal gland has been likened to an accessory salivary gland, and it has been well established that sebaceous carcinoma, adenomas, and sebaceous differentiation within a Warthin's tumor may all be seen in the parotid gland. As further proof of conjunctival epithelial plasticity and multipotentiality, there is a report of an acquired dacryoadenoma of the epibulbar surface epithelium that manifested ectopic lacrimal metaplastic differentiation that invaginated as incomplete glandlike structures into the substantia propria.[9]

By light microscopy, sebaceous glands are composed of lobules or alveoli with an outer rim of nonmyoepitheliomatous germinal basal cell delimited by a basement membrane; the latter cells quickly become lipidized centrally. In sections stained with hematoxylin and eosin, the highly differentiated central sebaceous cells are beset with myriad cytoplasmic vacuoles. Their lipid content is dissolved out in the course of tissue processing for light microscopy. The presence of lipid within sebaceous cells can be demonstrated by employing the oil-red-O stain on fresh frozen sections. Many clinicians and pathologists fail to realize that formalin-fixed wet tissue that has not been stored for a long time can be prepared for frozen sections and also stained with oil-red-O. Although the amount of lipid will be less prominent in such specimens and will depend upon how long the specimen has been stored in formalin or another fixative, the presence of lipid can nonetheless be clearly demonstrated and thus help to secure the diagnosis of a sebaceous tumor.

Sebaceous cells produce sebum, which is composed of fat, free fatty acids, and cholesterol. These moieties become incorporated in the trilaminar precorneal tear film and are also distributed throughout the conjunctival sac. In the tear film, the sebum is the outermost layer; the middle layer is contributed by the aqueous of the lacrimal secretion, and the innermost mucoid layer adhering to the epithelium is derived from the goblet cells of the conjunctiva. The external layer of lipid retards tear evaporation and may also help stabilize the precorneal tear film. Unlike the eccrine glands, which are scattered throughout most of the eyelid skin and produce a clear secretion, and the apocrine glands, which contribute the apical part of their secretory cells (decapitation secretion) to a turbid and odoriferous secretion, the sebaceous gland cells create their secretions through the mechanism of holocrine cell extinction. The whole cell in the central alveolus or lobule undergoes dissolution and, therefore, both the lipidic vacuolar contents and the cytoplasmic detritus constitute the essence of the secretion as delivered through the ducts. Even in sebaceous carcinoma, a burlesque of this holocrine-type secretion can be seen in the form of central necrosis within some tumor lobules (comedo pattern).

The majority of this chapter is devoted to malignant tumors of sebaceous glands, namely, *sebaceous carcinomas*. It is preferable to use this generic term instead of *meibomian gland carcinoma*, which is appropriate only for those lesions arising within the tarsus. The next important family of tumors is represented by the benign sebaceous adenomas. It is particularly important that these be accurately diagnosed because they have been discovered to be associated with internal malignancy (notably carcinoma of the proximal or ascending colon) in the Muir-Torre syndrome.[10-12] Finally, sebaceous car-

*Portions of this chapter were included in the Zimmerman Lecture, American Academy of Ophthalmology, Atlanta, GA, November 1, 1990.

cinoma of the lacrimal gland should be recognized by ophthalmologists and oncologists, since it is one of the most malignant epithelial neoplasms of this structure.[4]

One must distinguish the rare primary sebaceous carcinoma of the lacrimal gland from a primary eyelid tumor that secondarily extends directly into the orbit. Sometimes clinicians and pathologists refer to the orbital involvement as a "metastasis" from the eyelid. This is not correct because there are no lymphatic connections between the eyelid (or the conjunctiva for that matter) and the orbital soft tissues, which on a normal embryologic and anatomic basis are bereft of such structures. Only the lacrimal gland possesses true endothelial-lined lymphatic spaces within its parenchyma, a reflection of the fact that it is embryologically an outgrowth from the primitive conjunctival epithelium and, therefore, lymphatic channels of the substantia propria are pulled along with the epithelial buds into the lacrimal gland itself.

True metastases do occur from adnexal sebaceous carcinomas to the regional preauricular, parotid, and cervical lymph nodes. The lymphatic drainage of the outer two thirds of the upper eyelid and the outer one third of the lower eyelid is to the preauricular and intraparotid lymph nodes, whereas the drainage from the medial one third of the upper eyelid and the inner two thirds of the lower eyelid is to the submandibular complex of lymph nodes. All patients with sebaceous carcinoma of the ocular adnexa should be routinely examined for any evidence of preauricular, submandibular, or cervical lymphadenopathy, both at the time of initial presentation and on follow-up visits after surgical therapy has been undertaken.

SEBACEOUS CARCINOMA OF THE EYELIDS

General Features

Sebaceous carcinoma was identified in the ocular adnexa as long ago as the late nineteenth century,[2]

Table 156–1. SEBACEOUS CARCINOMA: SEX AND AGE DISTRIBUTION

Reference	No. of Females/ No. of Males (Ratio)	Age Range in Yr (Mean Age in Yr)
Straatsma[13]	11/4 (2.8:1)	20–84 (57)
Sweebe and Cogan[14]	5/3 (1.7:1)	41–79 (58)
Callahan and Callahan[15]	4/5 (0.8:1)	45–82 (65)
Khalil and Lorenzetti[16]	—	71–86 (77)
Harvey and Anderson[17]	6/3 (2.0:1)	59–88 (72)
Martin and Rogers[18]	4/2 (2.0:1)	55–80 (70)
Ni et al (Boston)[19]	18/5 (3.6:1)	49–80 (67)
Ni et al (Shanghai)[19]	103/53(1.9:1)	16–82 (57)
Rao et al[20]*	61/43(1.4:1)	32–93 (65)
Epstein and Putterman[21]	8/3 (2.7:1)	43–83 (64)
Doxanas and Green[22]	17/23(0.7:1)	39–88 (68)
Wolfe et al[23]	31/12(2.6:1)	28–82 (62)

From Kass LG, Hornblass A: Sebaceous carcinoma of the ocular adnexa. Surv Ophthalmol 33:477–490, 1989.
*Two earlier reports from the Armed Forces Institute of Pathology were excluded because of the possibility of data repetition.

although precise histopathologic criteria distinguishing benign from malignant sebaceous lesions have not always been well delineated. In 1956, Straatsma[13] assembled the first series of 16 patients seen at the Institute of Ophthalmology of the Presbyterian Medical Center. The series from the Armed Forces Institute of Pathology reported by Boniuk and Zimmerman[1] went a long way toward educating ophthalmologists about the clinical presentations of sebaceous carcinoma; these workers discovered that up to 1968 there were 88 cases on file at the Armed Forces Institute of Pathology, with a 30 percent 5-yr fatality rate. Kass and Hornblass[2] tabulated the salient clinical findings of sebaceous carcinoma as established in 13 published series;[13-23] Tables 156–1 and 156–2 are taken from their review article, which is also an excellent source for a comprehensive bibliography on the subject. Khan and associates[24] published a series of 20 cases around the time that this review article appeared.

In surveying the literature on eyelid tumors in general, Kass and Hornblass[2] noted an incidence of sebaceous carcinoma of 0.2 to 0.7 percent among all eyelid tumors

Table 156–2. SEBACEOUS CARCINOMA: TOPOGRAPHIC DISTRIBUTION

Reference	Total No. of Cases Reporting Location	Upper Lid	Lower Lid	Upper and Lower Lid (Diffuse)	Caruncle	Other
Straatsma[13]	16	9	7	—	—	—
Sweebe and Cogan[14]	8	6	2	—	—	—
Callahan and Callahan[15]	9	6	2	—	—	1
Khalil and Lorenzetti[16]	5	4	—	—	—	1
Harvey and Anderson[17]	9	4	2	2	1	—
Martin and Rogers[18]	6	4	2	—	—	—
Ni et al (Boston)[19]	23	15	6	2	—	—
Ni et al (Shanghai)[19]	154	108	38	2	1	5
Rao et al[20]*	98	60	25	6	7	—
Epstein and Putterman[21]	11	6	5	—	—	—
Doxanas and Green[22]	39	19	9	7	2	2
Wolfe et al[23]	41	24	16	1	—	—
Totals (%)	419	265 (63%)	114 (27%)	20 (5%)	11 (3%)	9 (2%)

From Kass LG, Hornblass A: Sebaceous carcinoma of the ocular adnexa. Surv Ophthalmol 33:477–490, 1989.
*Two earlier reports from the Armed Forces Institute of Pathology were excluded because of the possibility of data repetition.

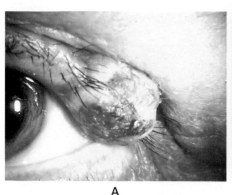 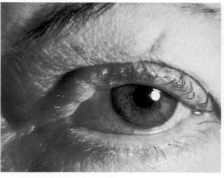 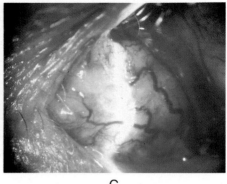

Figure 156–1. *A,* A sebaceous carcinoma at the eyelid margin arising from a gland of Zeis. There is a yellow hue in addition to the superficial ulceration at the surface of the lesion. (Courtesy of Jerry Shields, M.D.) *B,* Another sebaceous carcinoma of the eyelid margin, which has caused loss of eyelashes. (Courtesy of Lorenz E. Zimmerman, M.D.) *C,* A yellow-appearing sebaceous carcinoma arising in the sebaceous glands of the caruncle. (Courtesy of Robert Folberg, M.D. and Pathology of the Eye: An Interactive Videodisc Program, copyright Department of Ophthalmology, University of Iowa, 1991, 1992.)

and 1 to 5.5 percent among only eyelid malignancies. A startling feature of the series reported by Ni and associates[19] from Shanghai was a 33 percent incidence of sebaceous carcinoma among eyelid malignancies in this Chinese population.

Curiously, sebaceous carcinoma afflicts women more than men (between 57 and 77 percent of patients have been women in the various series in the literature). The average age is 60 to 69 yr at the time of presentation, although patients may be symptomatic for several years, thus reducing the patient's age at the time of the tumor's inception. Boniuk and Zimmerman[1] first established that younger individuals who received radiation therapy for bilateral inherited retinoblastoma can acquire sebaceous carcinoma as a secondary tumor. They reported a 13-year-old girl and a 12-year-old boy with this neoplasm; in one case the condition was bilateral. It has also been recognized from the earliest reports that the upper eyelid is involved about twice as often as is the lower and that "multicentric" masses can be encountered in 2 to 18 percent of cases;[22, 23] some authors refer to such cases as "diffuse."

Clinical Presentations

Although considerable progress has been made in improving surgery for sebaceous carcinoma, which has brought down the fatality rate over the last 20 yr, prolonged delays in diagnosis, often measured in years, are still far too common. Only by being alert to the full range of clinical features can the ophthalmologist reduce morbidity and surgical challenges through earlier diagnosis. Once suspicion has been raised, it is probably wisest to proceed with a biopsy rather than to follow the patient.

The clinical appearance of a sebaceous carcinoma depends upon which class of gland it arises from and the manner in which the tumor spreads. For instance, a tumor of the gland of Zeis will create a nodule at the eyelid margin and may destroy the marginal cilia in the region of involvement (Fig. 156–1*A* and *B*). Such lesions frequently invite the mistaken diagnosis of basal cell carcinoma, but a variably intense yellow appearance

should suggest the correct diagnosis; most basal cell carcinomas are white or translucent when observed at the eyelid margin. Likewise in the caruncle, a sebaceous carcinoma should also have a yellow cast (Fig. 156–1*C*) because of the transparency of the overlying nonkeratinizing squamous epithelium. In contrast, lesions of the brow are deeply situated and appear to be "wens" or nondescript dermal nodules. Exceptionally, a sebaceous carcinoma of the eyelid margin (and presumably of the gland of Zeis) can present as a cutaneous horn.[1, 25]

The most frequent origin for a sebaceous carcinoma is within the meibomian glands of the upper eyelids, followed by those of the lower eyelids. Because of the deep location of the carcinoma within the tarsus, the distinctive yellow coloration will not initially be discerned (Fig. 156–2*A*), but it may be detected later as the tumor approaches the epidermis (Fig. 156–2*B*). Instead, one encounters a variably diffuse swelling with a very firm to "rock-hard" texture on palpation. A common clinical impression is a chalazion, and the frequency of various mistaken clinical impressions has not changed much over a 20-yr period (Tables 156–3 to 156–5), thus implying the need for more education of

Table 156–3. SEBACEOUS CARCINOMA: CLINICAL DIAGNOSES* IN 1968 SERIES

Diagnosis	No. of Cases
Chalazion	19
Carcinoma, malignancy, or epithelioma	10
Basal cell carcinoma	7
Meibomitis, blepharoconjunctivitis, or keratoconjunctivitis	5
Tumor	3
Granuloma	3
Meibomian carcinoma	2
Lacrimal gland tumor	2
Nevus	1
Total	52†

From Boniuk M, Zimmerman LE: Sebaceous carcinoma of the eyelid, eyebrow, caruncle, and orbit. Trans Am Acad Ophthalmol Otolaryngol 72:619–641, 1968.

*At the time of biopsy in 48 cases of sebaceous carcinoma of the eyelid.

†Some clinicians considered several clinical possibilities; the total therefore exceeds 48.

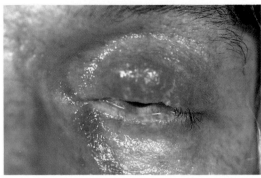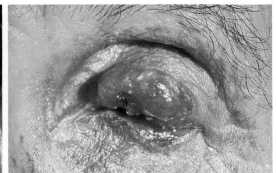

Figure 156–2. *A,* A sebaceous carcinoma of the upper eyelid meibomian glands has diffusely infiltrated the lid. Note the loss of eyelashes in both the upper and lower eyelids. *B,* This tumor has eroded through to the epidermis and has a yellow coloration. (*B,* courtesy of Lorenz E. Zimmerman, M.D.)

ophthalmologists. It is unusual for chalazions to arise later in life without a prior history, and the texture of a chalazion is more rubbery with less diffuse spread throughout the eyelid; also, the eyelashes are usually spared with a chalazion.

Loss of eyelashes may also attend sebaceous carcinoma arising within the meibomian glands, owing to the location of their germinal bulbs, which are embedded in the anterior lamellae of the tarsal collagen. These bulbs will therefore be destroyed early on by meibomian sebaceous carcinoma that extends outward to permeate the orbicular muscle and dermis of the eyelid. Until sebaceous carcinoma erupts out of the tarsus, the skin is generally movable over the lesion (which helps to distinguish it from a squamous cell or a basal cell carcinoma, which moves with the skin). The eyelid should be everted to detect any protrusion beneath the tarsal conjunctiva (Fig. 156–3). As a meibomian carcinoma extends superficially, all the layers of the eyelid become fused into one mass. The smoothness of the taut lid skin should also be serviceable in helping to distinguish the more deeply originating meibomian carcinoma from the more superficial and epidermally arising basal cell and squamous cell carcinomas, which frequently have ulcerations or surface irregularities and hyperkeratoses.

"Multicentric" sebaceous carcinoma of the upper and lower eyelids has been described in 2 to 18 percent of cases (see Table 156–2). Such cases generally represent advanced disease; the issue as to whether these tumors are truly multicentric in origin or represent multifocal nodules arising through the spread of disease from one lid to the other within the conjunctival epithelium is discussed further on in the section on Pathogenetic Considerations. Clinical support for this latter idea is supplied in the series of 43 sebaceous carcinomas reported from the Mayo Clinic by Wolfe and coworkers.[23] They reported only one patient with involvement of the upper and lower eyelids at the time of initial presentation, but in 3 of 24 patients presenting initially with upper eyelid lesions, there was the later development of a lower eyelid lesion.

A most important form of clinical presentation, which frequently leads to a prolonged delay in diagnosis, is unilateral "blepharoconjunctivitis" (masquerade syndrome), with or without the presence of a clinically obvious eyelid mass (Fig. 156–4). A superior limbic keratoconjunctivitis may also be simulated closely.[26] When these findings are found in an older individual who has absolutely no evidence of inflammation in the contralateral eyelids or conjunctival sac, a high index of suspicion must point to the presumptive diagnosis of a sebaceous carcinoma, with appropriate biopsy confirmation. The blepharoconjunctivitis picture predominates in 20 to 50 percent of patients;[24, 27] it is due to

Table 156–4. SEBACEOUS CARCINOMA: FREQUENCY OF CLINICAL DIAGNOSES IN 1985 SERIES

Diagnosis*	No. of Times Recorded
Carcinoma, malignant lesion, or epithelioma	24
Tumor	9
Chalazion	16
Blepharoconjunctivitis	12
Basal cell carcinoma	10
Sebaceous carcinoma	8
Keratosis	1
Squamous cell carcinoma	1
Molluscum contagiosum	1
Benign papilloma	1

From Yeatts RP, Waller RR: Sebaceous carcinoma of the eyelid: Pitfalls in diagnosis. Ophthalmic Plast Reconstr Surg 1:35–42, 1985.
*Mean number of diagnoses per patient was 2.2.

Table 156–5. SEBACEOUS CARCINOMA: CLINICAL DIAGNOSES IN 1989 SERIES

Diagnosis	No.
Blepharoconjunctivitis	9
Chalazion	4
Basal cell carcinoma	3
Tumor	1
Sebaceous cyst	1
Keratosis	1
No diagnosis	1
Sebaceous carcinoma	0

From Khan JA, Grove AS Jr, Joseph MP, Goodman M: Sebaceous carcinoma: Diuretic use, lacrimal system spread, and surgical margins. Ophthalmic Plast Reconstr Surg 5:227–234, 1989.

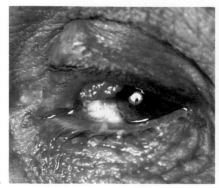
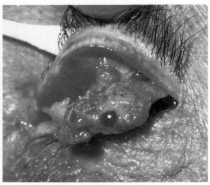

Figure 156–3. *A*, An upper eyelid sebaceous carcinoma visible beneath the eyelid skin has a pendulous component dropping beyond the eyelid margin from the conjunctival surface. *B*, On everting the upper eyelid, a faintly yellow and highly vascularized mass protrudes from beneath the tarsal conjunctiva. (Courtesy of Lorenz E. Zimmerman, M.D.)

infiltration of the sebaceous carcinoma cells within the conjunctival epithelium, including across the corneal epithelium, with a resultant underlying neoplastic pannus formation (Fig. 156–5).[3, 20] Symblepharons can be seen in the fornices. Careful examination of the everted tarsal surface, comparing it with that of the uninvolved contralateral eyelid, reveals a fine telangiectasia and sometimes a flat or erythematous or milky papillary pattern, intimating the truly neoplastic basis for the clinical "irritation" (Fig. 156–6). The intraepithelial spread of the neoplastic cells leads to underlying telangiectasia of the conjunctival vessels and a variably intense lymphocytic and plasmacytic infiltrate within the substantia propria. Although sebaceous carcinoma must be uppermost in the differential diagnosis of a unilateral cryptogenic blepharoconjunctivitis in an older person, there are other possible causes of a uniocular "red eye" (Table 156–6). Conditions such as atopy and rosacea are bilateral, even if asymmetrically so.

Finally, meibomian sebaceous carcinoma that has never been previously operated on can present misleadingly as an anterior orbital or lacrimal gland tumor (Fig. 156–7A and B).[28] In this subset of cases, the likelihood is that the tumor arose in the superior or inferior pole of the tarsal glands and unidirectionally spread into the orbit, including the lacrimal gland. Careful clinical examination with palpation of the involved eyelid will reveal a nodule in the tarsus; eversion of the eyelid is also mandatory in these cases. A fistula can form between the anterior orbital component and the fornix (see Fig. 156–7B). These eyelid lesions must be distinguished from primary sebaceous carcinoma of the lacrimal gland; imaging studies disclosing an epicenter of the mass in the lacrimal fossa are helpful in establishing a lacrimal gland origin.[4] It is rare today, but it is still possible in neglected cases, to see total orbital replacement as the presenting appearance, as in the elderly nursing home patient with Alzheimer's disease shown in Figure 156–7C. This patient already had regional metastases to the parotid gland and neck nodes.

Pathologic Features

INFILTRATING NODULES

Whether arising within the alveoli of the meibomian glands of the tarsus or from the glands of Zeis associated with the eyelashes, the neoplastic cells usually breach the delimiting glandular basement membranes to create intratarsal or dermal nodules. These are unencapsulated masses with "crabgrass" infiltrating margins. The basa-

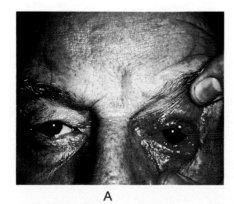
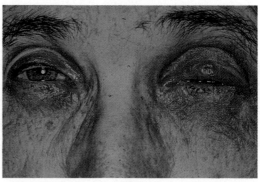

Figure 156–4. *A*, A strictly uniocular reddened eye (blepharoconjunctivitis or masquerade syndrome) is accompanied by nodules of both the upper and the lower eyelids. *B*, A diffuse sebaceous carcinoma with some thickening of the upper eyelid, as well as total loss of lashes of the upper eyelid and some of the lower eyelid. In this case, there is a weeping or eczematous appearance to the eyelid margin, without the dramatic erythema displayed in *A*. (*A* and *B*, Courtesy of Lorenz E. Zimmerman, M.D.)

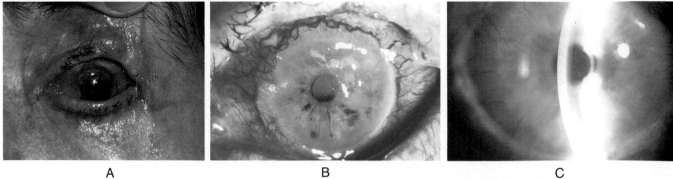

Figure 156–5. *A,* A uniocular, chronically reddened eye with a nodule in the upper eyelid and corneal epithelial irregularity. *B,* There is an opalescence of the corneal epithelium from the spread of sebaceous carcinoma cells within this layer. *C,* Corneal epithelial involvement with sebaceous carcinoma, causing an underlying neoplastic pannus. (*A–C,* courtesy of John W. Shore, M.D.)

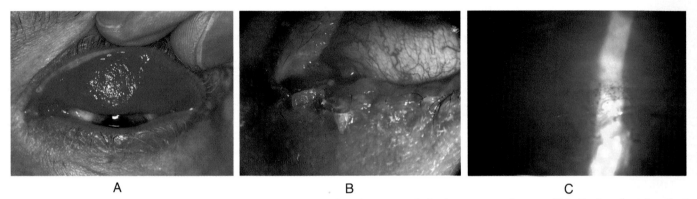

Figure 156–6. *A,* A diffusely reddened and irregular palpebral surface from spread of sebaceous carcinoma within the tarsal conjunctival epithelium. (Courtesy of John W. Shore, M.D.) *B,* An irregular lower eyelid margin with partial loss of eyelashes due to sebaceous carcinoma spread within the epithelium and glands of the eyelid margin. *C,* On everting the lower eyelid, the tarsal epithelium is thickened and beset with numerous tumor-associated curlicue or hairpin vessels, as indicated within the slit beam as well as on either side of it.

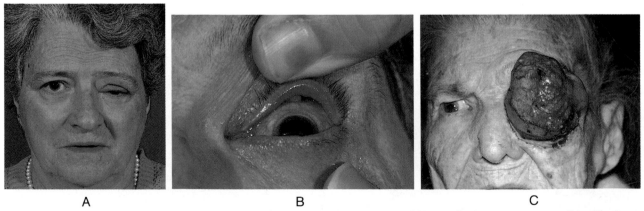

Figure 156–7. *A,* A long-standing left unilateral blepharoconjunctivitis eventuated in swelling of the upper eyelid with downward displacement of the globe. *B,* It was difficult to evert the upper eyelid, but with some effort, a papillary excrescence of tumor tissue was identified along with a fistula communicating with an anterior orbital mass that was readily palpable through the upper lid. The patient had a sebaceous carcinoma of the eyelid that had infiltrated into the anterosuperior orbital tissues. An exenteration was performed. *C,* Massive orbital replacement by sebaceous carcinoma of the eyelid in a neglected patient. (*C,* courtesy of John W. Shore, M.D.)

Table 156–6. CONDITIONS OTHER THAN DIFFUSE SEBACEOUS CARCINOMA TO BE CONSIDERED IN THE DIFFERENTIAL DIAGNOSIS OF CHRONIC UNILATERAL "BLEPHAROCONJUNCTIVITIS"*

Diffuse squamous carcinoma (with or without globe invasion)	Uniocular cicatricial pemphigoid
Diffuse squamous papilloma	Old chemical burn
Kaposi's sarcoma	Radiation damage
Diffuse lymphoid tumor (salmon patch)	Discoid lupus
Diffuse amelanotic melanoma	Chronic follicular conjunctivitis (e.g., with molluscum contagiosum)
Superior limbic keratoconjunctivitis	Giant papillary conjunctivitis (from contact lens or prosthesis wear)
Diffuse lymphangioma and Leber's hemorrhagic telangiectasia	Sarcoidosis
Floppy eyelid (eversion) syndrome	Scleritis-episcleritis
Canaliculitis	Vasculitis
Dacryocystitis	Orbital inflammatory pseudotumor
Chronic fungal infection	Graves' disease
Parasitic infestation	Carotid-cavernous sinus fistula
Retained foreign body	Amyloidosis with hemorrhage
Cilium entrapped in punctum	Conjunctivitis medicamentosa
Globe exposure (entropion, ectropion, lid retraction)	Allergic contact blepharoconjunctivitis
	Munchausen's syndrome (self-inflicted trauma)

Prepared with the assistance of John W. Shore, M.D.
*When in doubt, biopsy.

loid tumor cells may be aggregated in solid lobules, cords, and occasionally disposed in a single-file pattern; clear-cut lumenal units are typically lacking (Fig. 156–8). The stroma is usually not sclerotic but may occasionally be so. Mimicking holocrine secretion, some of the lobules display central necrosis (comedo pattern).

It is the distinctive cytologic features that establish the diagnosis of sebaceous carcinoma.[3, 20] One searches for individual cells or cellular clusters with a finely vacuolated, frothy cytoplasm (Fig. 156–9A and B). When large amounts of lipid are synthesized by the tumor cells and released extracellularly, an interstitial xanthomatous and granulomatous reaction next to the tumor cells may be engendered (see Fig. 156–9C). Another mechanism for a granulomatous reaction is the production of a chalazion if the tumor obstructs the ducts of the uninvolved meibomian glands (see Fig. 156–9D). In the less differentiated neoplasms, these areas of frank sebaceous differentiation may be exiguous, requiring multiple-step sections to detect partially vacuolated cells, whereas this feature will be conspicuously evidenced in more differentiated tumors. Mitotic activity tends to be very high, there is pronounced nuclear pleomorphism, and the nuclei tend to have a finely

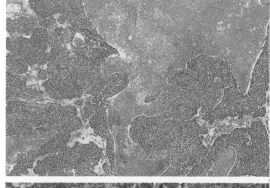

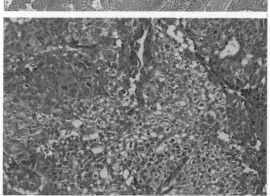

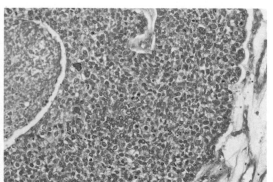

Figure 156–8. *A*, Interconnecting tracts of basaloid cells are separated by an eosinophilic holocrine-type degeneration of the tumor. H&E. *B*, In this lobule of tumor cells, there is a central necrotic zone on the left, referred to as a comedo pattern. Although the tumor cells are basaloid in nature, they do sport cytoplasmic vacuoles. Notice the nuclear pleomorphism toward the upper left border of the central necrotic focus. H&E. *C*, More advanced vacuolization of the tumor cells shown in the center and toward the right. H&E.

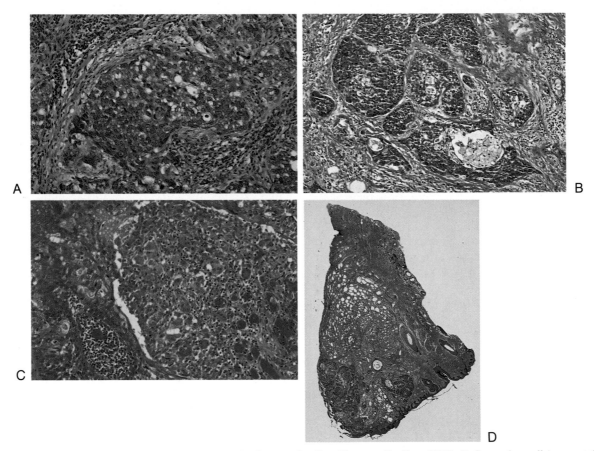

Figure 156–9. *A,* Zone of anaplastic cells with randomly dispersed cells with vacuolization. H&E. *B,* Several small tumor cell islands possess highly vacuolated and frothy cells in their centers, shown particularly well toward the bottom right of the figure. H&E. (Courtesy of Lorenz E. Zimmerman, M.D.) *C,* An interstitial giant cell granulomatous response to the release of sebum-type material synthesized by tumor cells on the left. Note the eosinophilic, frothy, extracellular material toward the upper left of the figure. H&E. *D,* Full-thickness section of an upper eyelid with a sebaceous carcinoma below, presumably arising in a gland of Zeis, which has caused a lipogranulomatous chalazion reaction in the middle and upper portions of the lid. H&E. (Courtesy of Lorenz E. Zimmerman, M.D.)

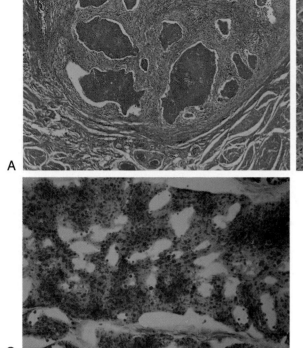

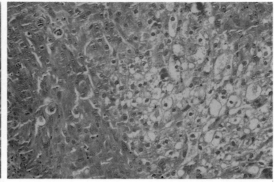

Figure 156–10. *A,* Focus of infiltrating sebaceous carcinoma suggestive of squamous cell carcinoma by virtue of the more eosinophilic staining properties of cytoplasm in the tumor lobules. H&E. *B,* Squamous-type cells on the left with abundant eosinophilic cytoplasm quickly transform into the vacuolated sebaceous cells on the right. H&E. *C,* Either fresh frozen tissue or recently retrieved wet formalin-fixed tissue can be frozen-sectioned and stained with oil-red-O to determine if cytoplasmic lipid is present. Formalin-fixed wet tissue, oil-red-O.

dispersed chromatinic pattern with small nucleoli. Approximately 10 percent of sebaceous carcinomas may show fields that are highly reminiscent of squamous cell carcinoma (Fig. 156–10*A* and *B*), having more eosinophilic cytoplasm and manifesting nuclei with more prominent nucleoli. Sometimes horn cysts can be found in these foci. It should be remembered that the draining ducts of the normal sebaceous glands are composed of a nonkeratinizing squamous epithelium and that the entire pilosebaceous unit is embryologically derived from the epidermis. Therefore, foci of outright squamous differentiation ought to be expected in some sebaceous tumors. Either fresh tissue or recently retrieved formalin-fixed wet tissue, processed by frozen sections, can be stained with oil-red-O (Fig. 156–10*C*) to bring out the focal lipid cytoplasmic droplets of the tumor cells if there is any ambiguity about the cytologic details. A recently discovered, exceptional property of sebaceous carcinoma that can be potentially confounding is that some tumors may rarely show biphasic secretion of lipid in some cells and mucin in others (unpublished data, Ahmed Hidayat, M.D.).

CONJUNCTIVAL INTRAEPITHELIAL SPREAD OF SEBACEOUS CARCINOMA.

The ability of sebaceous carcinoma cells to spread within the conjunctival epithelium has been appreciated from the earliest clinicopathologic series. The most commonly held belief as to how the conjunctival epithelium becomes involved with sebaceous carcinoma is that tumor cells spread down the ducts of the primarily involved Zeis or meibomian glands and thereafter spread superficially within the epidermis or toward the tarsal conjunctival epithelium, with progressive intraepithelial extension farther afield. Another possibility is that infiltrating tumor cells, upon encountering either the conjunctival epithelium or the epidermis, invade these tissue planes and grow radially within them (epidermotropism). Intraepithelial conjunctival extension has been reported in the literature to be as low as 44 percent and as high as 80 percent.[20, 23] In a review of 52 exenterations of orbital contents with sebaceous carcinoma, this author found 100 percent involvement of some segment of the conjunctival epithelium in association with infiltrating sebaceous carcinoma of one of the eyelids (unpublished data, Frederick A. Jakobiec, M.D., 1990 Zimmerman Lecture, American Academy of Ophthalmology). Furthermore, the sebaceous cells can migrate from the conjunctival epithelium or epidermis up the lacrimal gland ducts to the lacrimal acini, down the canaliculus to the lacrimal sac, and across the lid margin into the eccrine and apocrine glands of the dermis.

Three patterns can be exhibited by intraepithelial conjunctival sebaceous carcinoma spread. The most typical is that of a full-thickness replacement of the involved segments of epithelium by polyhedral and variably vacuolated cells that are highly mitotically active and that simulate a carcinoma in situ pattern of indigenous squamous cell carcinoma (Fig. 156–11). A much less common pattern within the conjunctival epithelium, but more likely to be encountered in the epidermal layer of the eyelid, is pagetoid extension (Fig. 156–12*A–D*). This is a specific morphologic variant of intraepithelial spread created by individual cells or small

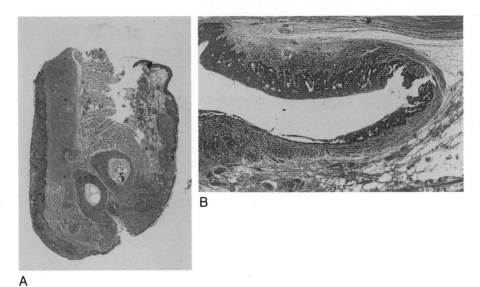

Figure 156–11. *A,* Extensive intraepithelial spread in a carcinoma in situ pattern of sebaceous carcinoma. The tarsal conjunctival epithelium is shown on the left; the tumor cells have not invaded the underlying atrophic tarsus. Tumor cells have crept around the eyelid margin and have invaded two pilar canals. Note the expansion and replacement of the epidermis shown on the right of the figure, with an abrupt transition to normal epidermis shown on the upper right. H&E. *B,* A portion of the conjunctival fornix in an exenteration specimen displays a carcinoma in situ pattern of intraepithelial sebaceous carcinoma cells. Note the subjacent lymphocytic infiltrate in the substantia propria and the desquamation of some of the epithelial cells shown toward the bottom left of the figure. H&E.

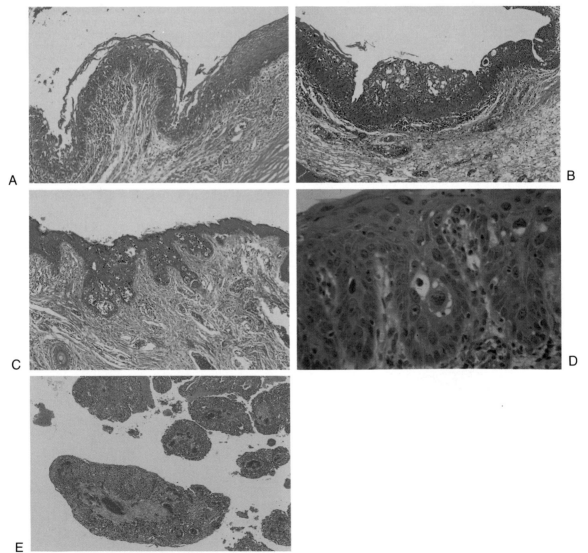

Figure 156–12. *A,* A portion of hyperkeratotic and acanthotic epibulbar conjunctival epithelium with a pagetoid pattern of intraepithelial sebaceous cell spread. The tumor cells percolate individually and in small clusters through all levels of the epithelium. H&E. *B,* In another acanthotic region of forniceal epithelium, small clusters of intraepithelial pagetoid sebaceous carcinoma cells are easily observed. H&E. *C,* Intraepidermal pagetoid spread of sebaceous carcinoma in a segment of eyelid skin. H&E. *D,* Pagetoid intraepidermal pleomorphic sebaceous cells with prominent vacuolization of the cytoplasm. H&E. (Courtesy of Miguel Burnier, M.D.) *E,* A papillary pattern of conjunctival intraepithelial sebaceous carcinoma. H&E.

1754

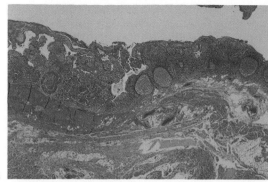

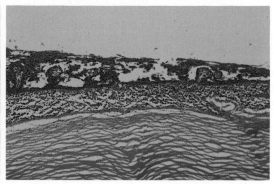

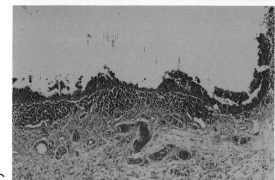

Figure 156–13. *A,* Conjunctival intraepithelial sebaceous spread with an underlying lymphocytic response that is organized into follicles. This intense type of inflammatory response is unusual in squamous lesions. H&E. *B,* Dyscohesive intraepithelial sebaceous carcinoma cells are supplied by stubby papillary units growing across the cornea. Neoplastic epithelium is friable and breaking apart. Notice there is an inflamed and vascularized pannus beneath the tumor cells, with an intact Bowman's membrane. Uninvolved corneal stroma is shown below. H&E. *C,* A desquamative and exfoliative tendency of intraepithelial sebaceous carcinoma cells with "tombstoning" of the remaining cells. H&E.

nests of sebaceous carcinoma cells percolating among recognizable preexistent squamous epithelial elements of the conjunctiva or epidermis. Finally, a papillary pattern can be observed in which the covering cells generally resemble carcinoma in situ (Fig. 156–12*E*).

Other features of intraepithelial sebaceous carcinoma spread within the conjunctival sac include an intense underlying inflammation, sometimes with follicle formation in the substantia propria (which is usually light to moderate if present with squamous lesions) (Fig. 156–13*A*; see also Fig. 156–11*B*); subadjacent pannus formation when the corneal epithelium begins to be replaced (Fig. 156–13*B*); and a friability and tendency toward desquamation with an eosinophilic coating on the surface of the proliferation, acantholysis and schisis cavity formation, or a complete denudation of the epithelium from the underlying connective tissue (Fig. 156–13*B* and *C*; see also Fig. 156–11*B*). The latter phenomenon can lead to problems in diagnosis if fragments of conjunctiva are removed for diagnostic purposes. One should repeat biopsies when no epithelium is found in suspected cases of sebaceous carcinoma with conjunctival extension, and the biopsy should be performed delicately without pre- or intraoperative swabbing of the surface epithelium.

In the interpretation of frozen sections, care should be taken not to be misled by large intracytoplasmic shrinkage vacuoles in either the conjunctival epithelium or epidermis as evidence of sebaceous carcinoma, especially when evaluating surgical margins. These artifactitious vacuoles are large and single, rather than finely reticulated as seen in bonafide sebaceous tumor cells.

Prognostic Features

Numerous features have been found to worsen the prognosis for sebaceous carcinoma and to presage metastasis.[20] From the clinical point of view, a delay in diagnosis greater than 6 mo and a tumor diameter greater than 1 cm appear to be statistically significant ominous portents. Rao and associates[20] reported that patients whose duration of symptoms was less than 6 mo had a 14 percent mortality rate, whereas those with symptoms longer than 6 mo had a 38 percent mortality rate. With respect to size, nodules less than 1 cm in greatest diameter carried an 18 percent mortality rate, whereas nodules greater than 2 cm carried a 60 percent mortality rate. Involvement of both the upper and lower eyelids with nodules resulted in an 83 percent fatality rate, whereas involvement of both the meibomian and Zeis glands manifested a 58 percent mortality rate. It is noteworthy that tumors of the glands of Zeis and tumors located exclusively in the lower eyelid were not associated with metastasis; conversely, tumors of the caruncle generated a 14 percent mortality rate.

The pathologic features[20] that are indicative of a poor prognosis are shown in Table 156–7. As would be expected, either vascular or lymphatic invasion worsens the prognosis; orbital invasion, lower levels of cytologic differentiation, and a highly infiltrative growth pattern are poor auguries. The discovery of a pagetoid intraepithelial pattern of growth also worsens the prognosis. This correlation was not discovered, however, in the series of Doxanas and Green[22] and of Wolfe and associates.[23] It should be emphasized that the pagetoid

Table 156–7. SEBACEOUS CARCINOMA: PATHOLOGIC FEATURES INDICATIVE OF BAD PROGNOSIS IN SEBACEOUS CARCINOMAS OF OCULAR ADNEXA

Clinicopathologic Features	Total No. of Cases	No. of Fatal Outcomes	Percentage Mortality
Vascular invasion	3	3	100
Lymphatic invasion	6	5	83
Upper and lower lid involvement	6	5	83
Orbital invasion	17	13	76
Poor differentiation	10	6	60
Pagetoid invasion	17	10	59
Tumors larger than 10 mm	17	9	53
Highly infiltrative pattern	11	5	45
Multicentric origin	12	5	42

From Rao NA, McLean JW, Zimmerman LE: Sebaceous carcinomas of the ocular adnexa: A clinicopathologic study of 104 cases with five year follow-up data. Hum Pathol 13:113–122, 1982.

pattern is highly specific and is not synonymous with the carcinoma in situ pattern, as mentioned previously. It is easier to recognize the pagetoid pattern at the eyelid margin or in the epidermis of the skin; the conjunctival epithelium is more delicate and more easily replaced by the invasive sebaceous carcinoma cells. In the conjunctival epithelium, a true pagetoid pattern is most apt to be seen at the leading margin of intraepithelial involvement. An interesting parallel exists with primary acquired melanosis associated with invasive nodules of conjunctival melanoma: An enhanced potential for metastasis has been found when the primary acquired melanosis displays a pagetoid pattern of the atypical intraepithelial melanocytic proliferation.[29, 30]

Pathogenetic Considerations

The usual cause of sebaceous carcinoma of the eyelids and caruncle has not been established. Many of the patients are older and may have associated carcinomas of the skin or internal organs (Tables 156–8 and 156–9), but it is not clear whether, in comparison with age-matched controls, this lends any credence to an inherited

Table 156–8. SEBACEOUS CARCINOMA: ASSOCIATED MALIGNANT LESIONS OR EXPOSURE TO IRRADIATION IN 1985 SERIES

	Patients		
		No.	%
Association present		11	26
Exposure to irradiation		5	12
Malignant lesion		10	23
Skin	7		
Breast	5		
Colon	1		
Kaposi's sarcoma	1		
Retinoblastoma	1		
Chondrosarcoma	1		

From Yeatts RP, Waller RR: Sebaceous carcinoma of the eyelid: Pitfalls in diagnosis. Ophthalmic Plast Reconstr Surg 1:35–42, 1985.

Table 156–9. SEBACEOUS CARCINOMA: ASSOCIATED MALIGNANCIES, IRRADIATION, AND DRUG USE IN 1989 SERIES

	Patients	
	No.	Percent
Malignancies	3	15
Bladder	1	5
Leukemia	1	5
Basal cell	1	5
Irradiation	2	10
Diuretics	8	40
Prednisone	1	5

From Khan JA, Grove AS Jr, Joseph MP, Goodman M: Sebaceous carcinoma: Diuretic use, lacrimal system spread, and surgical margins. Ophthalmic Plast Reconstr Surg 5:227–234, 1989.

predisposition to cancer.[24, 27] Although probably one of many possible causes, some patients have received prior head and neck radiotherapy, either for retinoblastoma or for other tumors (Tables 156–8 and 156–9).[1, 24, 31–33] Kahn and coworkers[24] found that 8 of their 20 patients with sebaceous carcinomas were taking diuretic medications and wondered whether this might be contributory to the development of their patients' tumors. Some diuretic medicines have been known to be associated with brain tumors in neonates whose mothers took the medicine and with renal carcinoma in patients taking the medicine themselves. Further epidemiologic work is required in order to establish the relevancy of these observations, as well as that of any other heretofore overlooked factors.

Two other pathogenetic issues need to be further explored. The first has to do with the true multicentric origin of upper and lower eyelid tumors. Because of the extensive spread of conjunctival intraepithelial sebaceous carcinoma (see Fig. 156–11A and B), a ready-made mechanism obviously exists for extension of the process from an initial site in one eyelid to the other, most typically from the upper to the lower eyelid. For this to be proved, the ability of intraepithelial conjunctival sebaceous carcinoma to reinvade the underlying connective tissues of either the conjunctiva or the eyelid would have to be established. In a review of 52 orbital exenteration specimens, this author observed second nodule formation in 30 percent of cases, but remarkably only in areas devoid of preexisting sebaceous glands, such as on the epibulbar surface, in the fornix, or with infiltration of the corneoscleral tissues (Fig. 156–14A and B). The tarsus (see Fig. 156–11A) appears to be a relatively resistant barrier to reinvasion from the palpebral epithelium, whereas the fornices are a favored area for second nodule formation—perhaps because of earlier replacement of the accessory lacrimal glands of Krause and the delicacy and yielding quality of the forniceal connective tissue. Another 30 percent of specimens displayed early microinvasion of the underlying connective tissues (Fig. 156–15A–D) without clear tumefaction (unpublished data, Frederick A. Jakobiec, M.D., 1990 Zimmerman Lecture, American Academy of Ophthalmology). Doxanas and Green[22] and Margo and coworkers[6] have reported cases with an epibulbar focus of invasive sebaceous carcinoma arising from over-

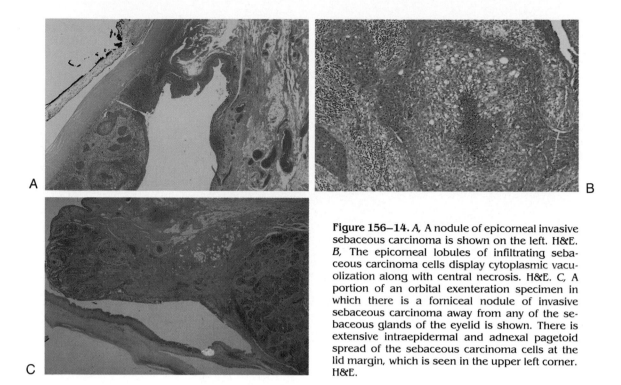

Figure 156–14. *A,* A nodule of epicorneal invasive sebaceous carcinoma is shown on the left. H&E. *B,* The epicorneal lobules of infiltrating sebaceous carcinoma cells display cytoplasmic vacuolization along with central necrosis. H&E. *C,* A portion of an orbital exenteration specimen in which there is a forniceal nodule of invasive sebaceous carcinoma away from any of the sebaceous glands of the eyelid is shown. There is extensive intraepidermal and adnexal pagetoid spread of the sebaceous carcinoma cells at the lid margin, which is seen in the upper left corner. H&E.

lying conjunctival intraepithelial spread, and this author has clinically observed a similar case (Fig. 156–15*E*).

Sebaceous carcinoma cells spread not only within the epithelium of the conjunctiva but also down the canaliculi (see Fig. 156–15*D*) to the lacrimal sac (in one case down the nasolacrimal duct to the lower turbinate of the nose) (Fig. 156–16*A* and *B*),[24] and in the other direction as well, namely, up the ducts of the lacrimal gland into the lobules (Fig. 156–16*C* and *D*). Sebaceous carcinoma cells have been observed to replace extensive numbers of pilosebaceous units (Fig. 156–17*A* and *B*; see also Fig. 156–11*A*) along with the apocrine and eccrine glands of the eyelid skin in association with overlying epidermal pagetoid spread.[1] It seems improbable that all of these different glands and sites would have undergone simultaneous independent neoplastic transformations. Therefore, a more plausible mechanism for multiple or independently arising tumors is reinvasion of the underlying connective tissues or glands from the spread of intraepithelial, intraepidermal, or intraglandular tumor cells.

The favored explanation up until now for multifocal tumors is that either the conjunctival epithelium or the multiplicity of eyelid sebaceous and other glands, or both, undergo a simultaneous neoplastic transformation resulting from an external or internal carcinogen, producing "a field effect."[1, 20, 22, 23, 34] Indeed, this mechanism may be operational in some cases but need not be invoked for all. Other workers have also considered that the shedding of sebaceous carcinoma cells into the tears (oncorrhea) may lead to their reimplantation within the conjunctival sac, their ascent up the lacrimal gland ducts, and their descent into the nasolacrimal drainage apparatus (Fig. 156–17*C*), thus setting the stage for multifocal

nodules, including those in the nasal mucosa (see Fig. 156–16*A*).[24]

A second pathogenetic consideration is the question of whether the conjunctival epithelium itself can be responsible for the development of primary sebaceous carcinoma.[5] This author has seen two cases of papillomas of the tarsal conjunctival epithelium with focal sebaceous differentiation (Fig. 156–18) and has reported with other colleagues a patient with the Muir-Torre syndrome who had a palpebral conjunctival tumor with sebaceous differentiation that invaded the tarsus.[12] These cases would seem to support the contention that the conjunctival squamous epithelium can undergo neoplastic metaplasia with sebaceous differentiation. Also in favor of this possibility is this author's observation in a review of more than 150 biopsy specimens and exenterated orbital specimens that approximately 5 percent of patients with "blepharoconjunctivitis" caused by conjunctival intraepithelial spread of sebaceous carcinoma are not discovered to have a clinically detectable eyelid nodule (Frederick A. Jakobiec, M.D., unpublished data, 1990 Zimmerman Lecture). These lesions typically come to attention because of superior tarsal injection and epithelial surface irregularities; there can be progression throughout the conjunctival sac over a 3- to 10-yr period (Fig. 156–19).

Furthermore, an infiltrating mass may not be discovered on histopathologic evaluation of excised eyelid tissues.[6] In such cases, there is usually scarring of the underlying tarsus, and upon extensive sectioning of the excised eyelid specimen, small foci of sebaceous carcinoma can be discovered,[26] sometimes in a pattern suggesting survival within a remnant of the preexisting Zeis or meibomian gland unit (unpublished data, Dr. Lorenz

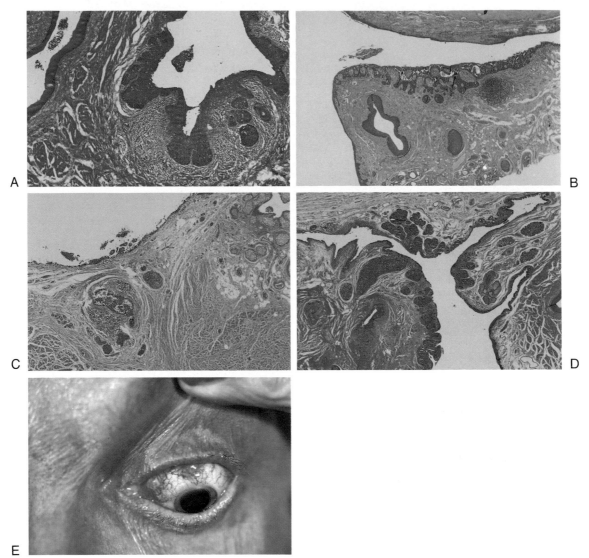

Figure 156–15. *A,* Intraepithelial sebaceous carcinoma proliferation in the medial canthal region. On the left is a portion of uninvolved canaliculus, whereas toward the bottom right there are microinvasive units of sebaceous carcinoma. Note the new stroma associated with these microinvasive nodules. H&E. *B,* In another exenteration specimen, there is microinvasion of the medial canthal skin by intraepithelial sebaceous carcinoma cells. An uninvolved segment of a canaliculus is again shown toward the left. H&E. *C,* Microinvasive sebaceous carcinoma in the fornix. Note the desquamative character of the overlying intraepithelial spread, as well as the presence of some sebaceous glands of the tarsus toward the upper right. The formation of forniceal nodules may occur after replacement of accessory lacrimal glands of Krause, one of which is shown toward the bottom left. H&E. *D,* Microinvasion of sebaceous carcinoma from the conjunctival epithelium of the medial canthus. The canaliculus shown on the left has been totally replaced by tumor cells at its origin, whereas the lumen appears partially patent below and to the left, at which point there is less advanced replacement. H&E. *E,* Two epibulbar nodules of invasive sebaceous carcinoma are shown, one in the 12 o'clock meridian and the other immediately next to the plica. Note the loss of eyelashes in the upper eyelid.

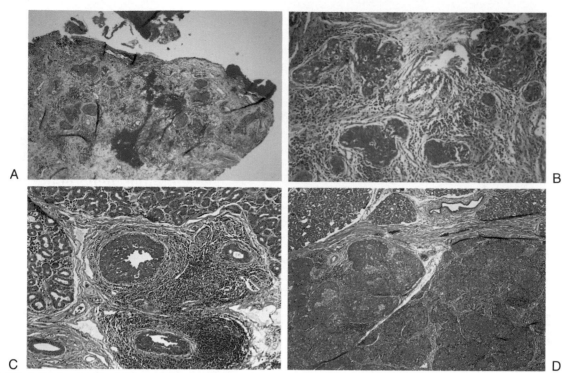

Figure 156–16. *A,* Nests of sebaceous carcinoma cells have infiltrated the nasal mucosa resulting from spread down the nasolacrimal duct. H&E. *B,* Higher power showing the sebaceous carcinoma nests and accessory salivary glands. One of the latter is present in the upper right of the figure. H&E. (*A* and *B,* Courtesy of Max Goodman, M.D.) *C,* Two ductules of the lacrimal gland are partially replaced by sebaceous carcinoma cells. Note the surrounding inflammation of the connective tissue. H&E. *D,* Infiltrating sebaceous carcinoma within the parenchyma of the lacrimal gland, which has been obliterated below but is undisturbed above.

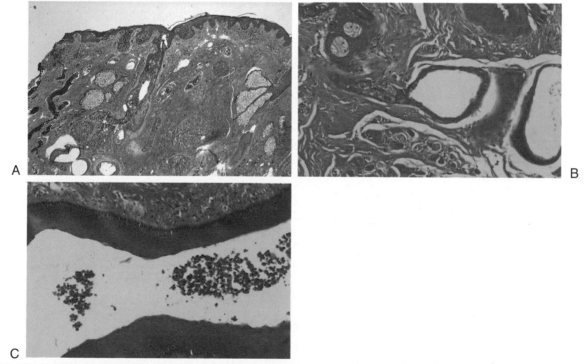

Figure 156–17. *A,* There is intraepidermal pagetoid spread of sebaceous carcinoma cells, which have also extended down the hair canal, shown centrally. There is further involvement of the apocrine and eccrine glands toward the left and bottom right of the figure. H&E. *B,* Two lumina of an apocrine gland are shown, with the constricted tail of the lumen on the left replaced by sebaceous carcinoma cells. H&E. *C,* Necrotic sebaceous carcinoma cells are present within the lumen of a canaliculus. Such tumor shedding into the tears has been referred to as *oncorrhea* and has been proposed as an explanation for some forms tumor spread of sebaceous carcinoma within the conjunctival sac and nasolacrimal drainage apparatus. H&E.

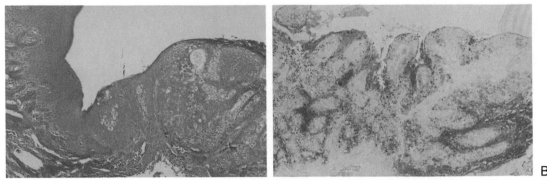

Figure 156–18. *A,* The transition of acanthotic and nonkeratinizing squamous epithelium of the tarsal conjunctiva on the left into a proliferation on the right featuring dispersed clear-staining sebaceous cells. This patient had the Muir-Torre syndrome with bowel cancer. H&E. *B,* Frozen section stained with oil-red-O reveals the presence of lipid within the clear cells.

E. Zimmerman, M.D.). It seems virtually impossible, however, to prove whether the tumor began within the conjunctival epithelium (typically upper tarsal) with subsequent involvement at the eyelid margin of the sebaceous glands through their ducts or whether the reverse occurred, namely, an origin within the meibomian or Zeis gland units with spread down their ducts and subsequent spread within the tarsal epithelium and elsewhere thereafter throughout the conjunctival epithelium.

There are, nonetheless, important prognostic and management features to this ambiguous but intriguing subset of sebaceous carcinoma cases. Without a signifi-

cant tumor burden infiltrating the lids, these cases can have an excellent prognosis regarding metastases, because the overwhelming majority of the tumor cells are restrained either within preexisting glandular sebaceous units or within the conjunctival epithelium. The underlying host response of lymphocytes and plasma cells within the conjunctival substantia propria may be partially responsible for limiting the infiltration of such intraepithelial cells. These patients are frequently uncomfortable and may have some loss of vision from corneal epithelial replacement by tumor cells and pannus formation. The management of these patients is particularly challenging. If the involved eye is the more sighted

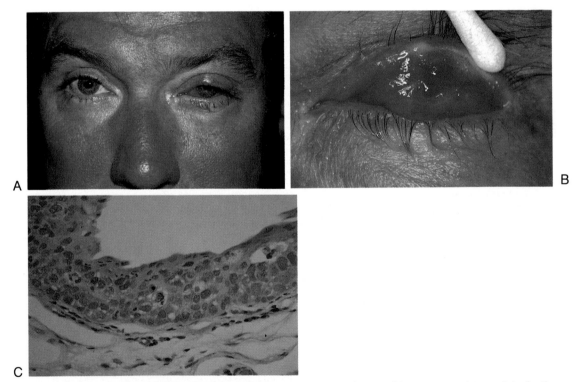

Figure 156–19. *A,* This patient had a several-year history of an irritated left eye without a palpable nodule in the upper or lower eyelids. *B,* Upon everting the upper eyelid, there is thickening and irregularity of the tarsal surface. Note the yellow-white eyelid margin lesion in the middle, which on pathologic examination was established to represent a focus of sebaceous carcinoma cells within a Zeis gland but without infiltration into the surrounding connective tissues. (*A* and *B,* Courtesy of John W. Shore, M.D.) *C,* Map biopsies of the upper tarsal conjunctiva, superior fornix, and all four epibulbar quadrants revealed extensive intraepithelial spread of sebaceous carcinoma cells with vacuolated cytoplasm, as shown here. The patient underwent exenteration. H&E.

one, one should follow the patient every 3 mo to detect any nodule formation. Cryotherapy and radiotherapy might be attempted to partially control the disease or retard progression, but ocular surface problems will undoubtedly ensue. In other patients with severe discomfort, a modified and subtotal exenteration may have to be performed.

Differential Diagnosis

CLINICAL FEATURES

Chalazion is one of the most frequently offered diagnoses in patients with sebaceous carcinoma. The problem is also compounded both clinically and histopathologically by the fact that an infiltrating sebaceous carcinoma can obstruct the ducts of intact meibomian glands, leading to secondary chalazion formation (see Fig. 156–9D). The lack of both a datable history and the typical conjunctival erythema or pyogenic granuloma formation on the tarsal surface militate against the diagnosis of a chalazion, whereas the "rock-hard" feeling of the lesion in the deep tarsus should lead to suspicion of the correct diagnosis. Both squamous cell carcinoma and basal cell carcinoma are highly likely to produce surface epidermal disturbances; in their early stages, they are movable upon the tarsus until they infiltrate more deeply. Other erroneous clinical diagnoses are listed in Tables 156–4 and 156–5. Conversely, Table 156–6 offers an extensive list of causes for unilateral chronic "blepharoconjunctivitis" other than sebaceous carcinoma.

PATHOLOGIC CONSIDERATIONS

Squamous cell carcinoma and basal cell carcinoma are common misdiagnoses for sebaceous carcinoma (Tables 156–10 and 156–11). Squamous cell carcinoma tends to be well differentiated in the eyelid skin and will show

Table 156–10. SEBACEOUS CARCINOMA: PATHOLOGIC DIAGNOSES IN 1968 SERIES

Diagnosis	No.
Sebaceous or meibomian carcinoma	35
Basal cell carcinoma (of skin appendages, 2; with squamoid differentiation, 1)	7
Squamous cell carcinoma	7
Undifferentiated carcinoma	6
Adenocarcinoma	4
Sebaceous adenoma	3
Bowen's disease or carcinoma in situ	2
Mucocarcinoma	1
Amelanotic melanoma	1
Cylindroma	1
Adnexal carcinoma	1
Papilloma	1
Granulomatous inflammation	1
Total	70

From Boniuk M, Zimmerman LE: Sebaceous carcinoma of the eyelid, eyebrow, caruncle, and orbit. Trans Am Acad Ophthalmol Otolaryngol 72:619–641, 1968.

Table 156–11. SEBACEOUS CARCINOMA: FREQUENCY OF PATHOLOGIC DIAGNOSES IN 1985 SERIES

Diagnosis	No. of Times Recorded
Sebaceous carcinoma	31
Squamous cell carcinoma	20
Carcinoma in situ	6
Basal cell carcinoma	4
Adenocarcinoma	4
Carcinoma or malignant lesion, type unspecified	3
Undifferentiated carcinoma	2
Retinoblastoma	1
Transition cell carcinoma	1
Not stated	2

From Yeatts RP, Waller RR: Sebaceous carcinoma of the eyelid: Pitfalls in diagnosis. Ophthalmic Plast Reconstr Surg 1:35–42, 1985.
In 12 cases, sebaceous carcinoma was correctly diagnosed on current review.
Mean number of diagnoses/patient was 1.7.

evidence of squamous eddy formation, pearls, and horn cysts of keratin. The cells are endowed with more abundant eosinophilic cytoplasm, and the nuclei tend to be large with prominent nucleoli. It is possible, however, for foci of sebaceous carcinoma to show evidence of squamous differentiation, in which case one must search in other areas for the vacuolated cells indicative of sebaceous carcinoma. Squamous cell carcinoma should display an origin from the overlying epidermis, as well as evidence of intraepithelial dysplasia or carcinoma in situ without a pagetoid growth pattern.

In basal cell carcinoma, there is much less nuclear pleomorphism, a lower mitotic rate, more sclerosis of the tumor-associated stroma, peripheral cellular palisading within the tumor lobules, and a frequent clefting artifact as the peripheral cells in the lobules pull away from the stroma. There are, however, unusual cases of eyelid basal cell carcinoma with sebaceous differentiation. In the latter instances, the sebaceous cells are scattered as small islands of highly differentiated elements within an otherwise typical basal cell carcinoma pattern. The term *sebaceous epithelioma* is employed by some pathologists to characterize some lesions with a more haphazard admixture of sebaceous elements within a basosquamous proliferation. The problem with this term is that it does not clearly communicate the comparative benignity or malignancy of the lesion.

Mucoepidermoid carcinoma can arise in the conjunctival sac, including from the tarsal epithelium.[35] The clear mucinous cells may simulate sebaceous cells, except that the alcian blue and mucicarmine stains will produce positive results in the former.

DIFFERENTIAL CONSIDERATIONS OF CONJUNCTIVAL INTRAEPITHELIAL SEBACEOUS SPREAD

Probably the most vexing contemporary histopathologic diagnostic problem pertains to the interpretation of conjunctival biopsy specimens in patients who may or may not be suspected of harboring an infiltrating sebaceous carcinoma of the eyelids. There is a more spindled appearance to the cells of many lesions of intraepithelial squamous dysplasia, and in leukoplakic lesions there is definite surface keratinization, which is missing in the typical sebaceous carcinoma. Bilateral diffuse squamous cell dysplasia and carcinoma in situ of the tarsal, epibulbar, and corneal epithelium have recently been reported in association with human papilloma virus, type 16.[36]

Electron microscopy can be a definite aid in evaluating the atypical cells in a conjunctival epithelial lesion (Fig. 156–20). Sebaceous carcinoma cells have a paucity of cytoplasmic tonofilaments, form few intercellular desmosomes, contain polyribosomes, and possess homogeneous cytoplasmic lipidic inclusions that may only survive as peripheral rims in vacuoles. The fibrillogranular inclusions of mucus-producing Paget's cells associated with adnexal carcinomas of other sites in the body (breast, anogenital region) or in primary conjunctival mucoepidermoid carcinoma[31] are lacking in ocular adnexal sebaceous carcinoma cells. Conjunctival intraepithelial spread of sebaceous carcinoma leads to a friability of the epithelium, and such specimens may show evidence of total epithelial denudation. This feature results from the poor desmosome and hemidesmosome formation and should alert the pathologist, who should suggest a rebiopsy with a delicate approach that avoids intense swabbing of the involved conjunctival surface before the biopsy specimen is taken. A full-thickness lid biopsy has been recommended.[37] Squamous cell dysplasia and carcinoma in situ of the conjunctiva tend to be cohesive within the epithelium and to adhere to the underlying stroma; they are also less likely to show the intense underlying chronic inflammation incited by sebaceous carcinoma within the tarsal or epibulbar connective tissues.

The distinction between conjunctival intraepithelial sebaceous carcinoma and in situ squamous cell carcinoma can be aided by immunohistochemistry in that the latter will be more strongly positive for cytoplasmic cytokeratin. With respect to primary acquired melanosis of the conjunctiva exhibiting a pagetoid pattern, melanocytes are S100 protein- and vimentin-positive,[30] whereas these reactions will be negative in sebaceous carcinoma cells. Epithelial membrane antigen will be present in both sebaceous and squamous epithelial cells, whereas it will be lacking in the melanocytes composing primary acquired melanosis.

Management

Doxanas and Green[22] found a 24 percent fatality rate among their patients treated prior to 1970, but there was no tumor-related mortality in patients treated after

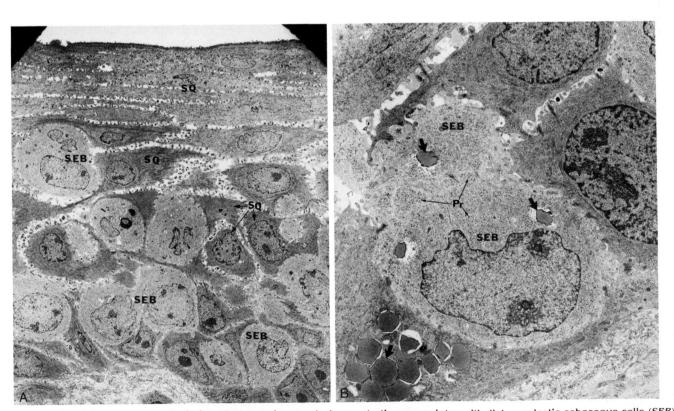

Figure 156–20. *A,* Low-power transmission electron micrograph demonstrating many intraepithelial neoplastic sebaceous cells (*SEB*) interspersed among preexistent squamous epithelium (*SQ*). The sebaceous tumor cells have more electron-lucent cytoplasm because of the sparcity of tonofilaments, which are more prominent in the neighboring squamous epithelial cells. ×3500. *B,* Two intraepithelial sebaceous cells (*SEB*) have homogeneously staining cytoplasmic lipid vacuoles (*arrows*). Their cytoplasm is endowed mostly with polyribosomes (*Pr*). In comparison with the neighboring squamous epithelial cells, the sebaceous tumor cells make a paucity of desmosomal contacts with each other and with the neighboring squamous cells. This feature helps to explain tumor cell shedding, dyscohesiveness, and schisis cavity formation within the epithelium. ×18,500.

1970. This advance is probably attributable to the increased awareness of clinicians of the need to perform wide local excision of sebaceous carcinoma[38] with frozen section control of the margins. The margins ought to extend well beyond the palpable tumor because of the diffusely infiltrating character of the neoplasm and should be more generous than those taken for a nodular basal cell carcinoma. The adequacy of this estimate should be established by frozen section monitoring or the Mohs' chemosurgical technique. Both methods, however, can lead to errors; permanent microscopic evaluation of the margins provides the most reliable confirmation of the adequacy of excision.[39] Intraepithelial spread of sebaceous carcinoma can be difficult to detect in the suboptimal detail provided by frozen sections. What many ophthalmic plastic and reconstructive surgeons are now doing is excising all of the infiltrating and intraepithelial conjunctival disease they can under frozen section control; they then await confirmation of uninvolved margins in permanent microscopic sections before proceeding to a second-stage reconstruction a day or two later.

It must be repeatedly emphasized that, in addition to reliance on frozen sections for nodule resection, one has to take into account any conjunctival intraepithelial spread of sebaceous carcinoma in the overall management strategy. Before undertaking any definitive surgery, experts now recommend performing conjunctival map biopsies in advance on all patients with a suspected or biopsy-proven infiltrating sebaceous carcinoma of the eyelid, whether or not the classic blepharoconjunctivitis clinical picture is seen.[40] All quadrants of the surface of the globe, the fornices, and the tarsal surfaces should be sampled; the biopsy specimens (they can number from 10 to 20 without the need for sutures) ought to be placed in separate bottles of formalin accompanied by a map (Fig. 156–21A). The pathologist can then report in permanent microscopic sections the locations of any evidence of conjunctival intraepithelial spread. The cytologic subtleties of sebaceous intraepithelial spread enforce reliance on the best tissue preparations. Determination of the extent of this spread assists the clinician in deciding how wide the excision of conjunctiva has to be, particularly if reconstructive procedures borrowing tissue from the supposedly uninvolved ipsilateral lid are contemplated.

If several quadrants of the surface of the globe are involved with intraepithelial sebaceous spread, the question arises as to how to treat this involvement. Doxanas and Green[22] recommended excision of the nodular component of sebaceous carcinoma, while leaving behind any flat intraepithelial residua of sebaceous carcinoma within the conjunctival sac. This position has generated some debate.[40–44] Not all ophthalmic plastic surgeons are comfortable with this approach, but others contend that there can occasionally be spontaneous regression of the intraepithelial component.[22, 43] Some workers have attempted to treat residual conjunctival intraepithelial disease with adjunctive cryotherapy (Fig. 156–21B–E).[42] If several quadrants of the conjunctival epibulbar epithelium are simultaneously involved, this treatment can lead to severe complications such as dry eye and delayed corneal healing (Fig. 156–21F). Details of the cryotherapy regimen can be found in the article by Lisman and colleagues.[43] Elderly patients can be affected by some retardation of healing; therefore, there may be wisdom in carefully following these patients without any therapy, as recommended by Doxanas and Green. For those patients in whom there is no nodule of sebaceous carcinoma in one of the eyelids and who have extensive (probably primary) conjunctival sebaceous spread, a similar management logic pertains, as was discussed in the section on Pathogenetic Considerations.

Nonetheless, if there is only minimal epibulbar conjunctival intraepithelial spread of sebaceous carcinoma, this author recommends either excision or cryotherapy, particularly in view of the possibility that the cells can continue to grow onto and within the corneal epithelium, with subsequent loss of vision from pannus formation. If the observations presented earlier regarding the capacity of conjunctival intraepithelial sebaceous carcinoma to reinvade the underlying connective tissues are accepted, this makes it even more imperative to try to extirpate any remaining conjunctival intraepithelial disease. An attempt at complete eradication should be more aggressively pursued in younger patients who, during their remaining decades, would otherwise experience a debilitating progression of disease.

Radiotherapy is not a reliable modality in the treatment of infiltrating sebaceous carcinoma, but it has been employed when patients have been too ill for surgery or have refused to undergo adequate local radical surgery.[46–48] With respect to treating intraepithelial conjunctival disease with radiotherapy, there is a high probability that a dry eye will develop with doses of 5000 to 6000 Gy. This author has shared in the follow-up of a patient whose intraepithelial disease was treated with radiotherapy and who remarkably retained 20/20 vision with a contact lens. Sequential biopsies over a 7-yr period after the initial radiotherapy of the conjunctival intraepithelial component have revealed persistent dysplasia; electron microscopy has suggested that some of the atypical intraepithelial cells may be persistent sebaceous carcinoma cells, whereas others are squamous cells with radiation-induced cytopathologic changes. In more recent follow-up, the patient was discovered to have multifocal elevated leukoplakic lesions, which on histopathologic evaluation have been shown to be hyperkeratotic surface foci surmounting a markedly dysplastic epithelium without invasion of the underlying connective tissue. This patient will be followed very carefully for any evidence of emerging invasive disease.

Exenteration is the only definitive form of therapy when there is orbital invasion (Fig. 156–22A–C). Exenteration is probably also required in bulky lesions of the caruncle because of orbital invasion, although wide local excision of the medial orbit with frozen section monitoring might be attempted if imaging studies reveal only superficial orbital invasion. For diffuse or bulky lesions of the upper and lower eyelids in late disease in neglected cases, exenteration is the only method for local control, but such patients already have a high risk of metastases developing regionally and distantly (Table 156–12), and exenteration will not avoid this risk. When

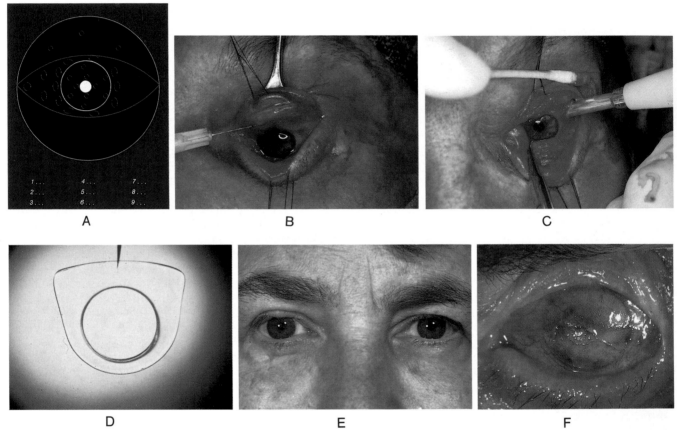

Figure 156–21. *A,* Before proceeding with any definitive form of surgery for an ocular adnexal sebaceous carcinoma, it is now routine to obtain permanent microscopic evaluations of multiple map biopsies of the conjunctival sac. Each biopsy specimen should be placed in its own bottle with a clear label. This permits the pathologist to report normal and abnormal areas precisely. Any opalescence of the corneal epithelium should lead to cytologic scraping, with independent reports of the different corneal epithelial zones. (Courtesy of John W Shore, M.D.) *B,* Cryotherapy has been used to treat residual intraepithelial sebaceous carcinoma of the conjunctival sac. After a Cutler-Beard first-stage procedure has been performed, the superior forniceal and epibulbar conjunctiva is ballooned up with lidocaine (Xylocaine). *C,* A double freeze-thaw application of cryotherapy is administered to the involved zones. Once the cryoprobe cannot be moved from side to side, it is an indication that the iceball has fused to the sclera and the treatment should be stopped. *D,* After the completion of the cryotherapy session, a conformer is placed in the conjunctival sac. Note the widened superior flange shape of the conformer, which is designed to deepen and broaden the superior fornix and prevent contraction from scarification. *E,* An acceptable postsurgical and adjunctive cryotherapy result in the right eye. *F,* An unsuccessful postsurgical and adjunctive cryotherapy result caused by persistent dry eye with delayed corneal healing and vascularization. Most of the epibulbar surface was treated. (*B–D,* from Lisman RD, Jakobiec FA, Small P: Sebaceous carcinoma of the eyelids: The role of adjunctive cryotherapy in the management of conjunctival pagetoid spread. Published courtesy of Ophthalmology 96:1021–1026, 1989.)

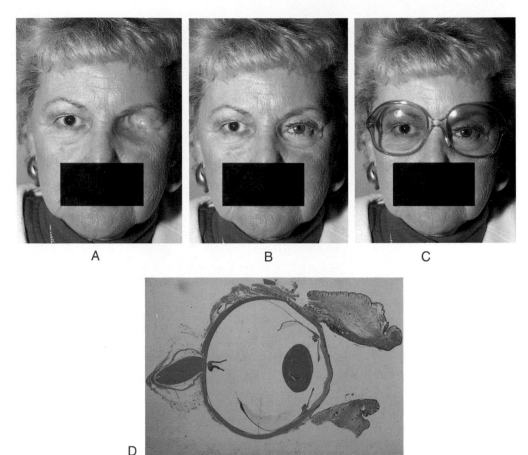

Figure 156–22. *A,* Appearance of the socket after it has healed by spontaneous granulation in a patient who had diffuse sebaceous carcinoma with an upper eyelid nodule and lower eyelid intraepithelial sebaceous spread. All of the epibulbar surface was involved. The deep orbital fat and periorbital membrane were spared. *B,* Appearance of the patient after placement of a prosthesis. *C,* An excellent cosmetic appearance is obtained when the patient further camouflages the prosthesis with slightly tinted glasses. *D,* An orbital exenteration specimen with sparing of the deep orbital connective tissues. Note that the eyelid skin has been taken because of the possibility of intraepidermal spread of sebaceous carcinoma. (*D,* courtesy of Miguel Bernier, M.D.)

exenteration is performed, the periorbital membrane and the deeper orbital tissues do not have to be taken (Fig. 156–21*D*) in view of the lack of lymphatic channels in the orbit. The extent of the orbital exenteration is governed by the depth of invasion of the orbital component. For lesions confined to the preseptal eyelids, most of the retrobulbar tissues can be left behind. Exenteration has been recommended when there is extensive disease of the upper and lower eyelids with intraepithelial sebaceous spread. In view of the possibility that one can have extensive intraepithelial conjunctival disease without clinically significant nodule formation in the eyelids, it might be prudent to follow elderly patients very carefully for any evidence of invasion of the underlying connective tissues.

Table 156–12. SEBACEOUS CARCINOMA: SECONDARY SPREAD AND METASTATIC SITES IN 1985 SERIES

Site	No.
Regional lymph nodes	12
Orbit	6
Skull	1
Brain	1
Bone*	1
Liver	1
Lung	0

From Yeatts RP, Waller RR: Sebaceous carcinoma of the eyelid: Pitfalls in diagnosis. Ophthalmic Plast Reconstr Surg 1:35–42, 1985.
*Other than skull; included ribs, scapula.

A final consideration in the management of sebaceous carcinoma is that attention must be paid to the lacrimal secretory and excretory systems.[24] The extensive intraepithelial spread of sebaceous carcinoma within the conjunctival sac is conducive to extension up the ducts of the lacrimal gland to its parenchyma (see Fig. 156–16*B* and *C*), as well as down the canaliculi via the puncta into the lacrimal sac and nasolacrimal duct (see Figs. 156–15*D* and 156–17*C*). In performing radical surgery, care must be taken to entirely remove the lacrimal gland to prevent a lateral canthal recurrence, as well as the lacrimal sac to prevent a medial recurrence. Furthermore, the nasolacrimal duct should be obliterated. This can be accomplished by using a periosteal elevator or by placing a probe or a stint in the nasolacrimal duct and applying electrocautery to the walls of the duct by moving the probe from side to side in order to coagulate the epithelial lining. The nose in the region of the inferior turbinate, which is the location at which the nasolacrimal duct empties, should be biopsied and treated if it is found to be abnormal (see Fig. 156–16*A*).[24]

SEBACEOUS ADENOMA

Any of the previously described sites of involvement of sebaceous carcinoma can also be the site of a benign sebaceous tumor, namely, a sebaceous adenoma. Because these lesions are highly differentiated, they have

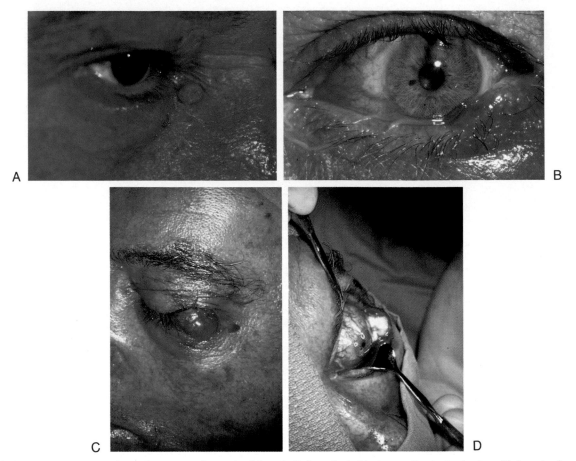

Figure 156–23. *A,* Yellow-appearing sebaceous adenoma of the medial canthal skin in a patient who had multiple colonic carcinomas (Muir-Torre syndrome). *B,* The lid skin has been stretched over a benign sebaceous tumor that originated in the conjunctival epithelium. *C,* After an incomplete excision of the lesion shown in *B,* a massive and explosive growth occurred over a 1-wk period. *D,* At the time of definitive surgery, a whitened inferior palpebral surface indicates an origin from the tarsal epithelium. Incompletely removed sebaceous adenomas can recur rapidly with a pseudoepitheliomatous hyperplasia featuring mostly squamous cells. (*D,* From Jakobiec FA, Zimmerman LE, La Piana F, et al: Unusual eyelid tumors with sebaceous differentiation in the Muir-Torre syndrome: Rapid clinical regrowth and frank squamous transformation after biopsy. Published courtesy of Ophthalmology 95:1543–1548, 1988.)

a yellow appearance if they arise in the skin (Fig. 156–23A), glands of Zeis, or caruncle. Papillomas of the tarsal conjunctiva have also been discovered with sebaceous differentiation; there is a report of a dramatic case of a tumor with randomly admixed squamous and sebaceous elements that invaded the tarsus from an origin in the palpebral conjunctival epithelium (Fig. 156–23B–D).[12]

It is important to be cognizant of the fact that such sebaceous adenomas have a 50 percent chance of being associated with internal malignancy, particularly of the proximal bowel (stomach and duodenum) or the ascending colon, even when they occur in a solitary form.[10–12] Other internal malignancies have also been described in this setting, and they tend to develop at an earlier age than would be otherwise expected. This syndrome of sebaceous adenoma and internal malignancy has been referred to as the Muir-Torre syndrome and is inherited as an autosomal dominant trait. Patients may have a sebaceous adenoma as their first symptom or the sebaceous adenoma may develop after a bowel cancer has been diagnosed and treated. Even in such cases, it is important to segregate these patients from those with more conventional bowel carcinomas, because their tu-

mors are apt to be multicentric and take origin from preexisting multiple adenomatous polyps of the bowel. Patients have been known to have two or three colonic carcinomas in locations from the rectosigmoid to other parts of the colon. Repeated follow-up bowel studies are therefore required even after successful therapy for an initial bowel cancer. When patients experience metastases to the liver, they may still have prolonged survival rates.[10] In addition to sebaceous adenoma, this syndrome also includes multiple eruptive keratoacanthomas, which may or may not involve the eyelid skin.

Pathologically, classic sebaceous adenomas are well-circumscribed lesions that have a lobular growth pattern composed of an outer one or two layers of germinal basal cells that quickly differentiate centrally into highly vacuolated cells (Fig. 156–24A). Sometimes the tumors can grow from the surface epithelium or epidermis and display a retiform or cordlike growth pattern with regularly interspersed pale-staining sebaceous cells but without a lobular architecture (Fig. 156–24B and C). If incompletely excised, these lesions will recur. They can recur quite rapidly and ominously in the eyelid skin, evincing an explosive growth with mass formation over 1 or 2 wk (Fig. 156–23B–D). In the excised recurrence,

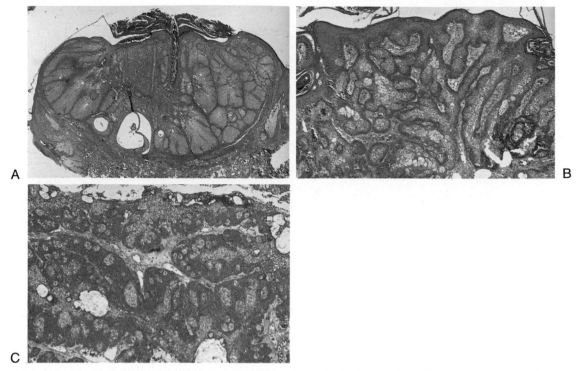

Figure 156–24. *A,* Classic sebaceous adenoma of the cheek in a patient who had an eyelid lesion and a colonic carcinoma in the Muir-Torre syndrome. Note the unencapsulated but highly circumscribed nature of the dermal proliferation. Each lobule has an outer basal germinal cell layer, which quickly becomes lipidized centrally. Note the surface hyperkeratosis and parakeratosis. H&E. *B,* A nonlobular sebaceous adenoma taking origin in cords from the surface epidermis in the patient shown in Figure 156–23A. H&E. (*B,* from Jakobiec FA, Zimmerman LE, La Piana F, et al: Unusual eyelid tumors with sebaceous differentiation in the Muir-Torre syndrome: Rapid clinical regrowth and frank squamous transformation after biopsy. Published courtesy of Ophthalmology 95:1543–1548, 1988). *C,* The palpebral epithelial lesion shown in Figure 156–23*B* features interconnecting units of basaloid cells with scattered nests of highly differentiated, pale-staining sebaceous cells. H&E.

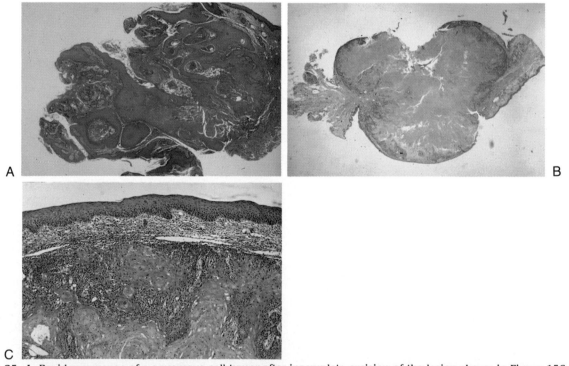

Figure 156–25. *A,* Rapid recurrence of a squamous cell tumor after incomplete excision of the lesion shown in Figure 156–23A. The lesion is essentially a pseudoepitheliomatous hyperplasia of highly differentiated squamous elements. Small vestiges of the preexisting sebaceous adenoma are shown at the pole of the lesion on the left. H&E. *B,* A full-thickness lid excision of the lesion shown in Figure 156–23 *C* and *D* reveals a massively necrotic squamous proliferation, with only an outer rim of surviving tumor cells. H&E. *C,* The proliferation took origin from the conjunctival surface, as witnessed by the fact that the epidermis is uninvolved and the tumor approximates but does not make contact with this tissue plane. Note the highly differentiated nature of the squamous proliferation. H&E. (From Jakobiec FA, Zimmerman LE, La Piana F, et al: Unusual eyelid tumors with sebaceous differentiation in the Muir-Torre syndrome: Rapid clinical regrowth and frank squamous transformation after biopsy. Published courtesy of Ophthalmology 95:1543–1548, 1988.)

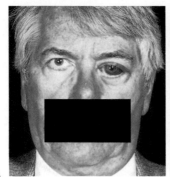 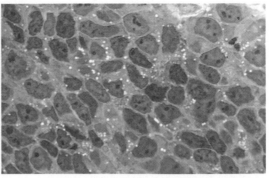

Figure 156–26. A, This patient presented with multiple left recurrent subconjunctival hemorrhages before it became apparent that there was a mass in the lacrimal fossa region that had caused proptosis as well as downward and inward displacement of the eyeball. B, The tumor was composed of islands and lobules of highly undifferentiated cells, which failed to form clear-cut lumina or to secrete mucinous materials. However, 1-µ plastic sections obtained preparatory to electron microscopy revealed that most of the tumor cells possessed myriad cytoplasmic vacuoles. Methylene blue. (From Rodgers IR, Jakobiec FA, Gingold MP, et al: Anaplastic carcinoma of the lacrimal gland presenting with recurrent subconjunctival hemorrhages and displaying incipient sebaceous differentiation. Ophthalmic Plast Reconstr Surg 7:229–237, 1991.)

one can see evidence of a squamous metaplasia mimicking a squamous cell carcinoma, with only minimal surviving elements of the initial sebaceous adenoma (Fig. 156–25).

Sebaceous adenoma must be distinguished from senile pseudoadenomatous (adenomatoid) hyperplasia of preexistent sebaceous glands. Rhinophyma of the nose is an example of such adenomatoid hyperplasia of the sebaceous glands; one can frequently observe benign lobular masses of the caruncle bilaterally representing the same process in older individuals. Because of their differentiation, these lesions have a deep yellow appearance, in contradistinction to the rusty appearance of caruncular oncocytomas of accessory lacrimal origin, which can also develop in the caruncle in older individuals. The major architectural feature of pseudoadenomatous or adenomatoid hyperplasia is that the preexisting lobules of the sebaceous glands enlarge through hyperplasia, but they preserve their orderly structure surrounding a central duct without overwhelming the preexisting unit. Hairs may project out of these enlarged units in the caruncle. It is important to distinguish this entity from true sebaceous adenoma because, as with sebaceous carcinoma of the eyelids and caruncle, it is not associated with an increased incidence of internal malignancy.

SEBACEOUS CARCINOMA OF THE LACRIMAL GLAND

It was not until 10 yr ago that it was appreciated that sebaceous carcinoma could be a primary neoplasm of the lacrimal gland, and four cases have now been reported (Fig. 156–26).[4, 49, 50] This event must be distinguished from a primary tumor of the eyelids that secon-

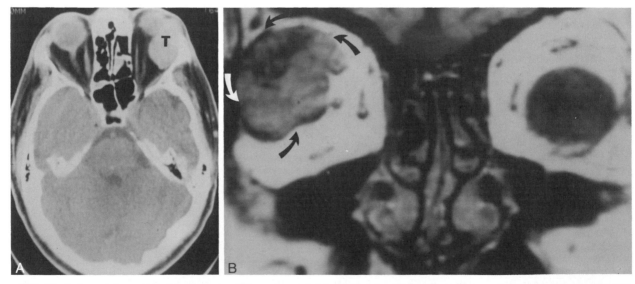

Figure 156–27. A, An axial computed tomogram of the primary lacrimal gland sebaceous carcinoma depicted in Figure 156–26. Note the overall rounded or globular outline of the tumor (T) in the lacrimal fossa region. B, A T_1-weighted coronal image from a magnetic resonance scan shows the tumor outline (arrows), which has more signal intensity than do most primary orbital tumors in T_1-phase images. Lipid, mucus, melanin, and blood breakdown products may all display increased signal intensity in T_1-weighted images. (From Rodgers IR, Jakobiec FA, Gingold MP, et al: Anaplastic carcinoma of the lacrimal gland presenting with recurrent subconjunctival hemorrhages and displaying incipient sebaceous differentiation. Ophthalmic Plast Reconstr Surg 7:229–237, 1991.)

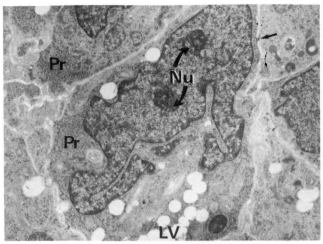

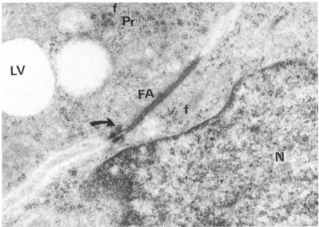

Figure 156–28. *Top,* The upper transmission electron micrograph of lacrimal gland primary sebaceous carcinoma discloses an irregularly shaped tumor cell nucleus with prominent nucleoli (*arrows* and *Nu*). The cytoplasm is endowed with abundant polyribosomes (*Pr*) and dissolved-out lipid vacuoles (*LV*). A primitive desmosomal contact is highlighted by the arrow. × 10,700. *Bottom,* An intercellular fascia adherens (*FA*) with an associated desmosome featuring inserting tonofilaments (*arrow*) unites two adjacent tumor cells. The cytoplasm features scant filaments (*f*), polyribosomes (*Pr*), and dissolved out lipid vacuoles (*LV*). N, tumor cell nucleus. × 38,700. (From Rodgers IR, Jakobiec FA, Gingold MP, et al: Anaplastic carcinoma of the lacrimal gland presenting with recurrent subconjunctival hemorrhages and displaying incipient sebaceous differentiation. Ophthalmic Plast Reconstr Surg 7:229–237, 1991.)

mixed tumor (a malignant mixed tumor or carcinoma ex pleomorphic adenoma).[49] In either of these settings, the sebaceous differentiation tends to be less evident than that in primary neoplasms of the tarsal meibomian glands. As a matter of fact, any highly differentiated sebaceous carcinoma of the orbit or lacrimal region should be suspected of being a secondary invader from the eyelid. One-micron plastic sections (see Fig. 156–26B) preparatory for electron microscopy, and electron microscopy itself (Fig. 156–28), may be helpful in the less well differentiated neoplasms by demonstrating the easily overlooked small cytoplasmic lipid vacuoles.

Sebaceous carcinoma of the lacrimal gland is probably unrivaled in its lethal potential among epithelial malignancies of this structure. Like other adenocarcinomas, it is capable of metastasizing within the lymphatic channels of the lacrimal gland to the intraparotid and cervical lymph nodes. Adenocarcinomas of the lacrimal gland tend to spread in this fashion soon after their clinical presentation; this contrasts with the behavior of adenoid cystic carcinoma, which spreads backward into the orbit perineurally rather than lymphogenously to the cervical lymph nodes. When a sebaceous carcinoma of the lacrimal gland has been discovered early clinically and accurately diagnosed histopathologically, consideration should be given to concurrent parotidectomy and cervical lymphadenectomy. All reported patients experienced local recurrences, sometimes with brain invasion, or else hematogenous dissemination to the lungs and other organs of the body, and have died of this tumor.

REFERENCES

1. Boniuk M, Zimmerman LE: Sebaceous carcinoma of the eyelid, eyebrow, caruncle, and orbit. Trans Am Acad Ophthalmol Otolaryngol 72:619–641, 1968.
2. Kass LG, Hornblass A: Sebaceous carcinoma of the ocular adnexa. Surv Ophthalmol 33:477–490, 1989.
3. Rao NA, McLean JW, Zimmerman LE: Sebaceous carcinoma of the eyelid and caruncle: Correlation of clinicopathologic features with prognosis. *In* Jakobiec FA (ed): Ocular and Adnexal Tumors. Birmingham, Aesculapius, 1978, pp 461–476.
4. Rodgers IR, Jakobiec FA, Gingold MP, et al: Anaplastic carcinoma of the lacrimal gland presenting with recurrent subconjunctival hemorrhages and displaying incipient sebaceous differentiation. Ophthalmic Plast Reconstr Surg 7:229–237, 1991.
5. Freeman LN, Iliff WG, Iliff NT, Green WR: Extramammary Paget's disease/pagetoid change of the conjunctiva without underlying sebaceous gland carcinoma. Invest Ophthalmol Vis Sci 29(Suppl):321, 1988.
6. Margo CE, Lessner A, Stern GA: Intraepithelial sebaceous carcinoma of the conjunctiva and skin of the eyelid. Ophthalmology 99:227–231, 1992.
7. Wick MR, Goellner JR, Wolfe JT III, et al: Adnexal carcinoma of the skin. II: Extraocular sebaceous carcinomas. Cancer 56:1163–1172, 1985.
8. Ozanics V, Jakobiec FA: Prenatal development of the eye and its adnexa. *In* Jakobiec FA (ed): Ocular Anatomy, Embryology and Teratology. Philadelphia, Harper & Row, 1982, pp 11–96.
9. Jakobiec FA, Perry HD, Harrison W, Krebs W: Dacryoadenoma. A unique tumor of the conjunctival epithelium. Ophthalmology 96:1014–1020, 1989.
10. Jakobiec FA: Sebaceous adenoma of the eyelid and visceral malignancy. Am J Ophthalmol 78:952–960, 1974.
11. Tillawi I, Katz R, Pellettiere EV: Solitary tumors of meibomian gland origin and Torre's syndrome. Am J Ophthalmol 104:179–182, 1987.
12. Jakobiec FA, Zimmerman LE, La Piana F, et al: Unusual eyelid

darily invades the orbit or the lacrimal gland region. The primary tumors are situated in the lacrimal fossa region, present rapidly over a 3- to 6-mo period, cause proptosis and globe displacement with or without bone destruction, and have an overall rounded or globular soft tissue appearance in coronal and axial magnetic resonance imaging and computed tomography scans (Fig. 156–27A). Sebaceous carcinoma may have bright signals comparable to fat in T_1-weighted magnetic resonance images (most tumors have low signal intensity in T_1-weighted images) because of the lipid content (Fig. 156–27B); mucoepidermoid carcinoma also has bright T_1-weighted images. The sebaceous tumors may arise de novo (one recent case was associated with recurrent subconjunctival hemorrhages) (see Fig. 156–26A)[4] or as the malignant clone arising out of a preexistent benign tumors with sebaceous differentiation in the Muir-Torre syndrome: Rapid clinical regrowth and frank squamous transformation after biopsy. Ophthalmology 95:1543–1548, 1988.

13. Straatsma BR: Meibomian gland tumors. Arch Ophthalmol 56:71–93, 1956.

14. Sweebe EC, Cogan DG: Adenocarcinoma of the meibomian gland. Arch Ophthalmol 61:282–290, 1959.

15. Callahan MA, Callahan A: Sebaceous carcinoma of the eyelids. *In* Jakobiec FA (ed): Ocular and Adnexal Tumors. Birmingham, Aesculapuis, 1978, pp 477–483.

16. Khalil MK, Lorenzetti DWC: Sebaceous gland carcinoma of the lid. Can J Ophthalmol 15:117–121, 1980.

17. Harvey JT, Anderson RL: Management of meibomian gland carcinoma. Ophthalmic Surg 13:56–61, 1982.

18. Martin PA, Rogers PA: Adenocarcinoma of the meibomian gland. Aust J Ophthalmol 10:63–67, 1982.

19. Ni C, Searl SS, Kuo PK, et al: Sebaceous cell carcinomas of the ocular adnexa. Int Ophthalmol Clin 22:23–61, 1982.

20. Rao NA, McLean JW, Zimmerman LE: Sebaceous carcinomas of the ocular adnexa: A clinicopathologic study of 104 cases with five year follow-up data. Hum Pathol 13:113–122, 1982.

21. Epstein GA, Putterman AM: Sebaceous adenocarcinoma of the eyelid. Ophthalmic Surg 14:935–940, 1983.

22. Doxanas MT, Green WR: Sebaceous gland carcinoma: Review of 40 cases. Arch Ophthalmol 102:245–249, 1984.

23. Wolfe JT III, Yeatts RP, Wick MR, et al: Sebaceous carcinoma of the eyelid: Errors in clinical and pathologic diagnosis. Am J Surg Pathol 8:597–606, 1984.

24. Khan JA, Grove AS Jr, Joseph MP, Goodman M: Sebaceous carcinoma: Diuretic use, lacrimal system spread, and surgical margins. Ophthalmic Plast Reconstr Surg 5:227–234, 1989.

25. Brauninger GE, Hood CI, Worthen DM: Sebaceous carcinoma of lid margin masquerading as cutaneous horn. Arch Ophthalmol 90:380, 1973.

26. Condon GP, Brownstein S, Codere F: Sebaceous carcinoma of the eyelid masquerading as superior limbic keratoconjunctivitis. Arch Ophthalmol 103:1525–1529, 1985.

27. Yeatts RP, Waller RR: Sebaceous carcinoma of the eyelid: Pitfalls in diagnosis. Ophthalmic Plast Reconstr Surg 1:35–42, 1985.

28. Shields JA, Font RL: Meibomian gland carcinoma presenting as a lacrimal gland tumor. Arch Ophthalmol 92:304–306, 1974.

29. Folberg R, McLean IW, Zimmerman LE: Malignant melanoma of the conjunctiva. Hum Pathol 16:136, 1985.

30. Jakobiec FA, Folberg R, Iwamoto T: Clinicopathologic characteristics of premalignant and malignant melanocytic lesions of the conjunctiva. Ophthalmology 96:147, 1989.

31. Justi RA: Sebaceous carcinoma: Report of case developing in area of radiodermatitis. Arch Dermatol 77:195–200, 1958.

32. Schlernitzauer DA, Font RI: Sebaceous gland carcinoma of the eyelid following radiation therapy for cavernous hemangioma of the face. Arch Ophthalmol 94:1523–1525, 1976.

33. Lemos LB, Santa Cruz DJ, Baba N: Sebaceous carcinoma of the eyelid following radiation therapy. Am J Pathol 2:305–311, 1978.

34. Cavanagh HD, Green WR, Goldberg HD: Multicentric sebaceous adenocarcinoma of the meibomian gland. Am J Ophthalmol 77:326–332, 1974.

35. Herschorn BJ, Jakobiec FA, Hornblass A, et al: Mucoepidermoid carcinoma of the palpebral mucocutaneous junction: A clinical, light microscopic and electron microscopic study of an unusual tubular variant. Ophthalmology 90:1437–1446, 1983.

36. Odrich MG, Jakobiec FA, Lancaster WD, et al: A spectrum of bilateral squamous conjunctival tumors associated with human papillomavirus type 16. Ophthalmology 98:623–635, 1991.

37. Leibsohn J, Bullock J, Waller R: Full-thickness eyelid biopsy for presumed carcinoma-in-situ of the palpebral conjunctiva. Ophthalmic Surg 13:840–842, 1982.

38. Tenzel RR, Stewart WB, Boynton JR, Zbar M: Sebaceous adenocarcinoma of the eyelid: Definition of surgical margins. Arch Ophthalmol 95:2203–2204, 1977.

39. Folberg R, Whitaker BC, Tse DT, Neard JA: Recurrent and residual sebaceous carcinoma after Moh's excision of the primary lesion. Am J Ophthalmol 103:817–823, 1987.

40. Putterman AM: Conjunctiva map biopsy to determine pagetoid spread. Am J Ophthalmol 102:87–90, 1986.

41. Boynton JR, Searl SS: Sebaceous gland carcinoma. [Letter] Arch Ophthalmol 103:175, 179, 1985.

42. Green WR, Doxanas MT: Sebaceous gland carcinoma. [Letter] Arch Ophthalmol 103:175, 179, 1985.

43. Lisman RD, Jakobiec FA, Small P: Sebaceous carcinoma of the eyelids: The role of adjunctive cryotherapy in the management of conjunctival pagetoid spread. Ophthalmology 96:1021–1026, 1989.

44. Kass LG: Role of cryotherapy in treating sebaceous carcinoma of the eyelid. [Letter] Ophthalmology 97:2–3, 1990.

45. Lisman RD, Jakobiec FA, Small P: Role of cryotherapy in treating sebaceous carcinoma of the eyelid. [Letter] Ophthalmology 97:3–4, 1990.

46. Ide CH, Ridings GR, Yamashita T, Buesseler JA: Radiotherapy for a recurrent adenocarcinoma of the meibomian gland. Arch Ophthalmol 79:540–544, 1968.

47. Hendley RL, Rieser JC, Cavanagh HD, et al: Primary radiation therapy for meibomian gland carcinoma. Am J Ophthalmol 87:206–209, 1979.

48. Nunery WR, Welsh MG, McCord CD: Recurrence of sebaceous carcinoma of the eyelid after radiation therapy. Am J Ophthalmol 96:10–15, 1983.

49. Witschel H, Zimmerman LE: Malignant mixed tumor of the lacrimal gland: A clinicopathologic report of two unusual cases. Graefes Arch Clin Exp Ophthalmol 216:327–337, 1981.

50. Konrad EA, Thiel HJ: Adenocarcinoma of the lacrimal gland with sebaceous differentiation: A clinical study using light and electron microscopy. Graefes Arch Clin Exp Ophthalmol 221:81–85, 1983.

Chapter 157

■

Eyelid Tumors of Apocrine, Eccrine, and Pilar Origins

I. RAND RODGERS, FREDERICK A. JAKOBIEC, and AHMED A. HIDAYAT

Skin appendages or the adnexa include apocrine and eccrine sweat glands, hair follicles, and sebaceous glands. Each of these structures contributes to the integrity of the integument; each may rarely undergo tumefaction. This chapter describes sweat gland and hair follicle tumors that affect the eyelids, brows, and temples (Table 157–1). Sebaceous gland tumors have been extensively reviewed previously.

Table 157–1. ADNEXAL TUMORS

Apocrine Tumors
Cystadenoma
Nevus sebaceus of Jadassohn
Syringocystadenoma papilliferum
Hidradenoma papilliferum
Papillary oncocytoma
Adenoma
Cylindroma
Adenocarcinoma

Eccrine Tumors
Hidrocystoma
Syringoma
Chondroid syringoma (mixed tumor)
Acrospiroma
Spiradenoma
Primary mucinous carcinoma
Primary infiltrating signet ring carcinoma
Sclerosing sweat duct carcinoma

Pilar Tumors
Pilomatrixoma
Tricholemmoma
Trichofolliculoma
Trichoepithelioma

Lesions Simulating Primary Adnexal Tumors
Metastatic carcinoma
Merkel cell tumor
Phakomatous choristoma

The vast majority of the conditions discussed in this chapter are fortunately benign. This contrasts with sebaceous tumors, among which sebaceous carcinoma far outstrips sebaceous adenoma in the ocular adnexa (but not in other parts of the skin). With respect to cystic conditions of both the eccrine and apocrine glands, these may occasionally undergo a proliferation in their walls with the appearance of solid or adenomatous units, but malignant degeneration is virtually unknown.

It must be admitted, however, that the distinctions between certain adenomas of eccrine and apocrine origins and low-grade carcinomas can be difficult. Adenomas are generally nonencapsulated lesions in the dermis, although they, for the most part, have circumscribed borders. Nonetheless, individual units and cords of cells can occasionally infiltrate beyond the main mass without necessarily signifying malignant transformation. Particularly in apocrine tumors, there may be moderate pleomorphism of the nuclei that, in the absence of mitotic activity, does not militate for a carcinomatous diagnosis. The major criteria that pertain to all carcinomas should be applied to cutaneous lesions: high mitotic activity, frank pleomorphism of the nuclei, diffusely infiltrating borders, and necrosis.

The cells comprising eccrine proliferations tend to be moderately sized, polygonal or cuboidal, and either clear or somewhat eosinophilic, whereas the cells comprising apocrine proliferations are capacious, often columnar with papillary formations, and intensely eosinophilic, glassy, or opaque. Apocrine lesions characteristically have apical decapitation secretion, but this feature may also be observed sometimes in tumors considered to be of eccrine origin. Eccrine or apocrine carcinomas would be suggested if the luminal units consist of a pile-up of cells with a cribriform pattern, whereas the benign lesions tend to consist of an orderly single or double layer.

Some eccrine and apocrine tumors may be so undifferentiated that single cells are dispersed in a sclerotic matrix that simulates a metastatic scirrhous carcinoma of breast or bowel. It should be pointed out that both eccrine and apocrine carcinomas of the eyelids are capable of metastasis, which occurs to the regional parotid and cervical lymph nodes before distant metastasis eventuates, but overall they have a better prognosis than do similar tumors situated elsewhere. This may have to do with their smaller size at the time of initial detection compared with tumors in other parts of the integument. In any case, these malignancies are rare in the eyelids.

Tumors of hair origin are quite variegated but are almost always benign. Encountering multiple trichilemmomas should bring to mind Cowden's syndrome or Lhermitte-Duclos syndrome. Trichoepithelioma may rarely transform into a basal cell carcinoma in the eyelids.

NORMAL APOCRINE APPARATUS

Apocrine glands in the eyelid are modified sweat glands. Referred to as the glands of Moll, these structures lie near the eyelid margin and consist of a secretory coil, an intradermal duct, and an intraepithelial duct. The secretory coil consists of a single layer of secretory cells surrounded by myoepithelial cells. The cytoplasm of the secretory cells is eosinophilic and contains periodic acid-Schiff (PAS)–positive and diastase-resistant granules; these cells may also stain positively for iron. Through a process called decapitation secretion, secretory cells project their apical cytoplasm into the secretory coil's lumen. Secretion occurs as small quantities of cytoplasm are released into the ducts.

The intradermal and intraepithelial apocrine gland ducts consist of a double cuboidal cell layer. Those cuboidal cells facing the duct are lined by a periluminal eosinophilic cuticle. The intradermal apocrine duct contains a basement membrane and a thin connective tissue sheath. In contrast to the spiral configuration of the intraepithelial eccrine duct, the intraepithelial apocrine duct is straight. These apocrine gland structures are associated with cilia and empty their secretions into pilar canals at or near the lid margin[1]; sometimes the ducts empty directly through the epidermis.

Electron microscopic studies of normal apocrine glands of the eyelid reveal a layer of inner secretory cells with apical villi projecting into the lumens. The secretory cells contain both light- and dark-colored granules in their cytoplasm. The light granules are derived from mitochondria and contain cristae and a double-layered membrane. The dark granules are lysosomes containing protein, lipid, iron, and myelin. The myoepithelial cells, possessing filaments and fusiform densities, are found only in the secretory region and not among the ductal cells.[2] Enzyme histochemical studies reveal the presence of acid phosphatase, B-glucuroni-

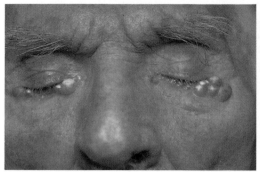
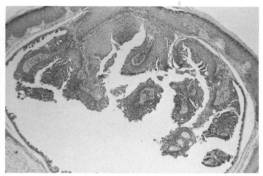

Figure 157–1. Apocrine cystadenoma. *A*, The superior border of these cystic lesions arises from the lash line and contains yellowish-white lipoidal material. The lesions have confluent margins and may affect multiple eyelids. *B*, The excised specimen is well circumscribed and contains numerous fronds projecting into a central cavity (H&E). (*A*, from Sacks E, Jakobiec FA, McMillan R: Multiple bilateral apocrine cystadenomas of the eyelid: Light and electron microscopic studies. Published courtesy of Ophthalmology 94:65–71, 1987.)

dase, and indoxyl esterase.[3] The myoepithelial cells stain positively for alkaline phosphatase. The immunohistochemistry of mature apocrine glands discloses gross cystic disease fluid protein 15 (GCDFP-15) and glycoprotein carcinoembryonic antigen (CEA). GCDFP-15 is found in some apocrine cells but not in eccrine cells,[4, 5] whereas CEA is found in both types of sweat glands.[6]

BENIGN TUMORS OF APOCRINE ORIGIN

Cystadenomas

Apocrine cysts are benign lesions that are typically asymptomatic and solitary.[7] A variety of terms have been used to describe this tumor including apocrine hidrocystoma,[1] apocrine cystadenoma,[8] black hidrocystoma,[9] apocrine retention cyst,[10] sudoriferous cyst, and Moll cyst.[11] The term apocrine cystadenoma is preferable, because evidence suggests that this condition is proliferative and is not a retention cyst secondary to ductal dilatation.[7, 8, 12] Apocrine cystadenomas vary in size from 3 to 5 mm, although a case of a giant cyst measuring 7 × 5 × 5 cm has been reported.[13] Approximately one half of apocrine cystadenomas are blue to light brown. The skin overlying the cysts is smooth and

shiny, with the tumors freely mobile and their walls translucent but thickened. Spontaneous rupture rarely occurs. Multiple, bilateral apocrine cystadenomas of the eyelids have been reported (Fig. 157–1).[14, 15] These lesions are restricted to the lid margin and contain yellow material in the cyst's apices; the color is presumed secondary to the light-density, lipid-rich cellular debris of decapitation secretion. They are distinct from milia, white pilosebaceous retention cysts, which are not limited to the eyelid margin (Fig. 157–2).

By light microscopy, apocrine cystadenomas consist of a cyst wall and papillary projections. These projections are lined by a double row of cuboidal to high columnar secretory epithelial cells displaying decapitation secretion. PAS-positive, diastase-resistant granules are present. Electron microscopy discloses abundant, moderately dense secretory granules within the inner secretory cells; normal mitochondria with increased material density; and decapitation secretion.[16] Some of the cells contain iron in the cytoplasm.

Apocrine cystadenomas may be associated with ectodermal dysplasia. Characterized by bilateral apocrine cystadenomas, hypodontia, palmar-plantar hyperkeratosis, and onychodystrophy, the ectodermal dysplasia syndrome is familial with a presumed autosomal recessive inheritance (Fig. 157–3). In the reported cases, all four eyelids were involved.[17–19]

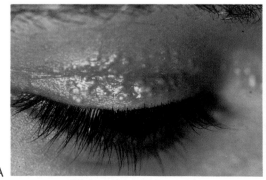
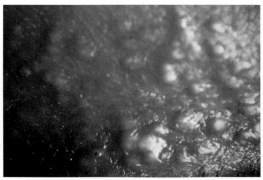

Figure 157–2. Milia. *A*, These retention cysts of pilosebaceous origin may be confused with apocrine cystadenomas. Milia, although multiple and lightly colored, arise from the eyelid and facial skin. *B*, Milia also have umbilicated centers. (*A* and *B*, Courtesy of C. Matta, M.D.)

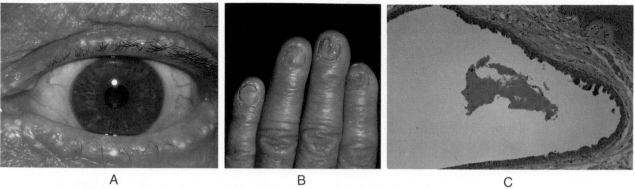

Figure 157–3. Apocrine cystadenoma and ectodermal dysplasia. *A,* Multiple 1- to 2-mm cystic lesions are found along the eyelid margin. *B,* Affected patients have dystrophic fingernails with thickened nail plates, onycholysis, and gray discoloration. *C,* Decapitation secretion occurs from a double cuboidal epithelial lined cyst (H&E). (*A* to *C,* from Font RL, Stone MS, Schanzer C: Apocrine hidrocystomas of the lids, hypodontia, palmar-plantar hyperkeratosis, and onychodystrophy: A new variant of ectodermal dysplasia. Arch Ophthalmol 104:1811–1813, 1986. Copyright 1986, American Medical Association.)

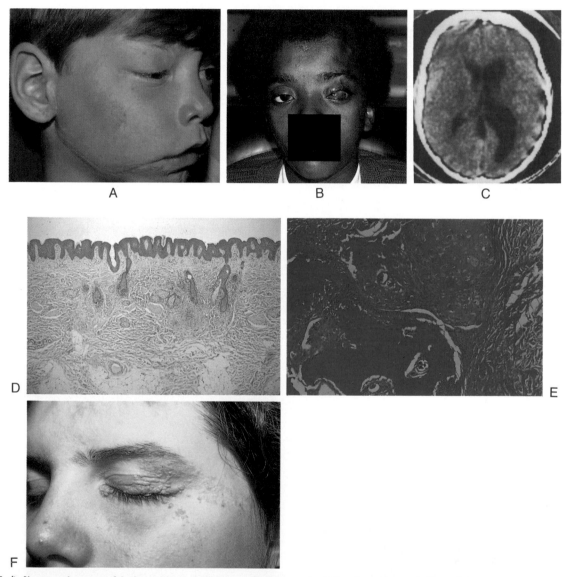

Figure 157–4. Nevus sebaceus of Jadassohn. *A,* This complex phakomatosis involves pigmentation of the cheek and temple. *B,* Ocular manifestations include a complex choristoma of ectopic lacrimal tissue, intrascleral cartilage and bone, and optic nerve colobomas. *C,* Cranial vault involvement may encompass a distended lateral ventricle and localized cerebral hemispheric atrophy. *D,* A thin layer of keratin overlies surface papillations. Dermal hair follicles may be scant in number; the sebaceous glands may be hypertrophied and their cell membranes disrupted; and apocrine glands may be found. H&E. *E,* Sclera containing cartilage and bone. H&E. *F,* The clinical differential diagnosis includes linear nevus: a verrucous-appearing lesion devoid of apocrine glands. (*A,* courtesy of J. Shore, M.D.; *B* and *C,* courtesy of R. J. Campbell; *D,* courtesy of J. B. Crawford, M.D.)

Nevus Sebaceus of Jadassohn

The nevus sebaceus cyst is an organoid malformation not only of sebaceus glands but also of apocrine glands, hair follicles, and the epidermal layer.[20] Apocrine gland involvement occurs in approximately 50 per cent of cases, with the lower dermis infiltrated by hamartomatous apocrine tissue. These glands may become more prominent at puberty. Abortive or rudimentary hair follicle structures may be present, and the epidermis is often hyperplastic or papillomatous. Patients with nevus sebaceus (Fig. 157–4A to E) may demonstrate systemic malformations including epilepsy, mental retardation, and skeletal deformities. Ophthalmic findings include corneoscleral limbal choristomas,[21] intrascleral cartilage and bone, retinal detachment, optic nerve colobomas,[22] and microphthalmos.[23]

The malformation is typically found on the face or scalp and is present from early childhood. Clinically it is a well-defined lesion, recognized by its characteristic yellow to orange color and its waxy, pebbly, or papillomatous surface. It typically enlarges during adolescence, with the dermis featuring abnormalities of adnexal structures. Enlargement during adulthood may signify the development of a secondary tumor such as basal cell carcinoma, squamous cell carcinoma, syringocystadenoma papilliferum, or nodular hidradenoma.[24, 25]

Nevus sebaceus of Jadassohn and linear nevus are often confused clinically as well as histologically. The latter tends to be linear, flesh colored, and slightly raised (see Fig. 157–4F). Its histologic findings are limited to the epidermis.[23]

Syringocystadenoma Papilliferum

Syringocystadenoma papilliferum is a benign tumor derived from apocrine glands. In approximately 75 percent of cases, syringocystadenoma papilliferum arises during puberty from a nevus sebaceus of Jadassohn. In Helwig and Hackney's[26] review of 100 cases, 55 were located on the scalp, 11 on the forehead and temple, five on the face, but none on the eyelids. A basal cell carcinoma secondarily developed in 9 percent of cases. The lesions were typically papular and had a gray, erythematous surface (Fig. 157–5A and B). Jakobiec and coworkers[27] in 1981 reported two cases of eyelid involvement. The patients, aged 34 and 41, presented with slowly enlarging papillated and hyperkeratotic lesions of the eyelid margin. One patient presented with a pinpoint vesicle-like inclusion. In a review of 55 cases of sweat gland tumors evaluated between 1959 and 1980 at the Howe Laboratory of the Massachusetts Eye and Ear Infirmary,[28] there were five cases of syringocystadenoma papilliferum; patients who were affected ranged from 17 to 55 yr of age.

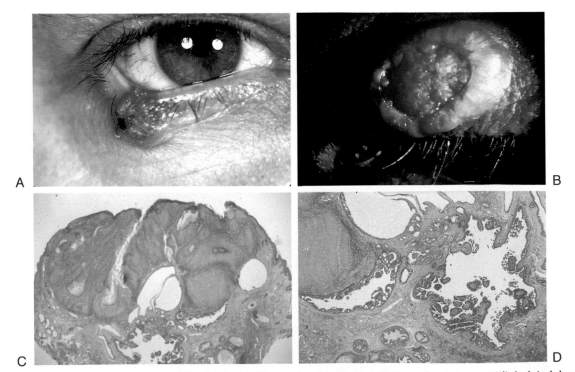

Figure 157–5. Syringocystadenoma papilliferum. A, The eyelid margin and skin have been replaced by a multilobulated, hyperkeratotic lesion. B, A discrete nodule with a central corrugated surface and multiple poral openings. C, This low-power photomicrograph reveals a cup-shaped lesion containing a central keratin core and dilated apocrine cysts. The epidermis displays acanthosis. H&E. D, On higher power, papillae project into a luminal space. Plasma cells are apparent within the papillary cores. H&E. (A, from Jakobiec FA, Streeten BW, Iwamoto T: Syringocystadenoma papilliferum of the eyelid. Ophthalmology 88:1175–1181, 1981; B, courtesy of M. Tso, M.D., and R. Urban, M.D.; C and D, courtesy of R. Eagle, M.D.)

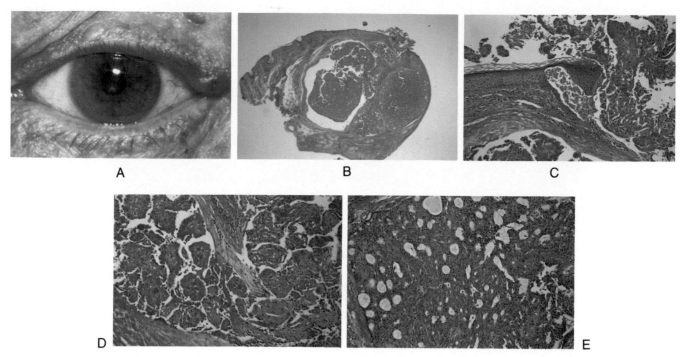

Figure 157–6. Hidradenoma papilliferum. *A,* Hidradenoma papilliferum typically presents as a dermal nodule with a poral opening. This umbilication may represent an ectasia of the apocrine secretion-rich pilar canal or may be the result of burrowing of tumor cells. *B,* Histologically, this well-circumscribed lesion consisting of tumor lobules is present as is a poral connection to the epidermis. H&E. *C,* High-power photomicrograph of the poral opening through which tumor cells are extruding. H&E. *D,* The characteristic papillary configuration of the tumor cells covering fibrovascular cores. H&E. *E,* These lesions consist of solid areas of spindle-like tumor cells and tubular or glandular structures, the lumen of which contains faintly eosinophilic secretory material. H&E. (From Netland PA, Townsend DJ, Albert DM, Jakobiec FA: Hidradenoma papilliferum of the upper eyelid arising from the apocrine gland of Moll. Published courtesy of Ophthalmology 97:1593–1598, 1990.)

On the light microscopic level, syringocystadenoma papilliferum are characterized by keratinized ductlike epithelial lined cystic spaces that open onto the surface epithelium (see Fig. 157–5C). Papillary configurations, often bullous in configuration, protrude into cystic invaginations and have features of a fibrovascular core. Decapitation secretions may occur. One histologic hallmark of syringocystadenoma papilliferum is a stroma infiltrated by plasma cells (see Fig. 157–5D).[29] Electron microscopic studies reveal ductal channels lined by two cell types. Although both cell types contain mitochondria, endoplasmic reticulum, and microvilli, one is cuboidal and the other is flat.

Treatment is directed toward complete surgical excision of the lesion. Radiation is ineffective.

Hidradenoma Papilliferum

Hidradenoma papilliferum is another benign tumor of apocrine gland origin. This lesion occurs almost exclusively in females, with the perineal, perianal, and vulvar regions sites of predilection.[29] Rarely the breasts, external auditory canal, or the eyelids may be involved.[30, 31] Hidradenoma papilliferum is a solitary tumor; on palpation it is a firm, freely mobile nodule millimeters in size. There may be a surface umbilication or poral opening (Fig. 157–6A). Occasionally, bleeding, ulceration, discharge, and itching may occur. Microscopically, this encapsulated tumor arises within the dermis. There

may be a histologic connection to the epidermis (see Fig. 157–6B and C). The tumor consists of interconnecting, well-circumscribed lobules. Both papillary and tubular or glandular patterns may coexist (see Fig. 157–6D and E). In papillary predominated regions, projections composed of a double layer of cells line a lumen. The innermost cells are columnar in shape and display apocrine decapitation secretion. There are no interstitial plasma cells. Histochemical studies reveal apocrine enzymes and PAS-positive diastase-resistant granules.[32] Electron microscopic studies parallel the finding of apocrine cystadenoma. Malignant degeneration of a perianal hidradenoma with metastatic spread has been reported.[33]

Papillary Oncocytoma

Oncocytomas are rare tumors arising within the ductal cell lining of apocrine glandular structures. Oncocytic tumors may arise within salivary, thyroid, parathyroid, and thyroid glands as well as the buccal mucosa, breast, kidney, pharynx, and larynx.[34] In the ocular adnexa, oncocytomas may develop within the caruncle, lacrimal sac, lacrimal gland, and accessory lacrimal glands of the conjunctiva.[35, 36] Recently, an oncocytoma arising within a dermal apocrine gland of the upper eyelid was reported.[37] The patient was a 72-year-old male with a slowly enlarging blue cyst of the upper lid margin (Fig. 157–7A). The tumor was confined to the dermis. His-

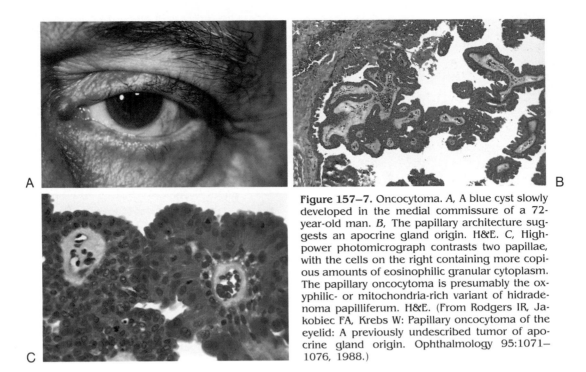

Figure 157–7. Oncocytoma. *A,* A blue cyst slowly developed in the medial commissure of a 72-year-old man. *B,* The papillary architecture suggests an apocrine gland origin. H&E. *C,* High-power photomicrograph contrasts two papillae, with the cells on the right containing more copious amounts of eosinophilic granular cytoplasm. The papillary oncocytoma is presumably the oxyphilic- or mitochondria-rich variant of hidradenoma papilliferum. H&E. (From Rodgers IR, Jakobiec FA, Krebs W: Papillary oncocytoma of the eyelid: A previously undescribed tumor of apocrine gland origin. Ophthalmology 95:1071–1076, 1988.)

tologic examination disclosed a well-circumscribed cystic and papillary tumor. The papillary units were covered by a double layer of regimented epithelium with a granular cytoplasm and occasional apical apocrine type snouts (see Fig. 157–7B). Solid regions with slitlike glandular structures contained cells with richly eosinophilic cytoplasm (see Fig. 157–7C). This histologic picture is somewhat similar to that of apocrine papillary cystadenomas or hidradenoma papilliferum. Electron microscopy, however, showed the densely packed mi-

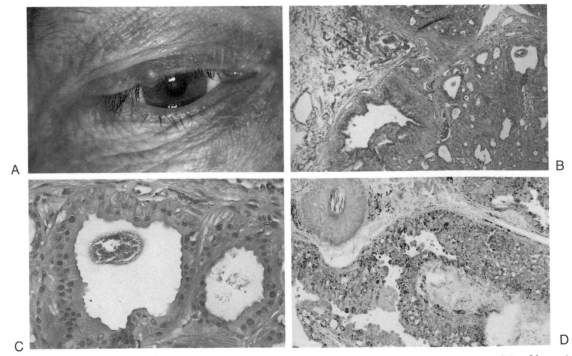

Figure 157–8. Apocrine adenoma. *A,* Flesh-colored nodule arising along the lid margin. *B,* The tumor consists of irregular glandular structures lined by a double layer of eosinophilic staining cuboidal cells. H&E. *C,* Areas of decapitation secretion are readily visible. The individual cells have a normal size and shape. H&E. *D,* Approximately one third of these tumors contain iron-positive intracellular granules (Perl's stain) (A, courtesy of D. Townsend, M.D.)

tochondria of varying sizes and shapes characteristic of oncocytes, and thus distinguished this lesion from papillary cystadenomas and hidradenoma papilliferum.

Apocrine Adenomas

Adenomas are distinctly uncommon lesions originating presumably from the secretory coil. They lack clinical features that would enable the clinician to suspect the diagnosis preoperatively. Apocrine adenomas present as longstanding red or reddish-brown nodules, which are firm and solid but occasionally cystic (Fig. 157–8A).[38] Histologically, the tumor is confined to the dermis. The most prominent features are large glandular lumina lined by a double layer of epithelial cells: an inner columnar cell layer exhibiting decapitation secretions and an outer layer of myoepithelium (see Fig. 157–8B and C). Scattered lymphocytes may be found within the stroma. One third of these tumors contain iron-positive granules (see Fig. 157–8D). Case reports exist of unusual apocrine adenomas composed almost exclusively of tubular structures. These adenomas appear limited to the scalp and are associated with the nevus sebaceus of Jadassohn.[39] Histochemical and electron microscopic data support the apocrine gland origin of these tumors.[40]

Cylindroma

A cylindroma frequently presents as a solitary, slowly growing pink or red dermal nodule involving the head, neck, and scalp. They may occur on the eyelids or the brow.[28] The benign, rubbery tumor varies in size from a few millimeters to several centimeters.[41] Multiple cylindromas are inherited as an autosomal dominant trait and cover the entire scalp similar to a turban (turban tumors).[42] The inherited form appears in adolescence and is characterized by slow tumor growth. Multiple cylindromas have been associated with trichoepitheliomas and eccrine spiradenomas. Cylindromas have been rarely reported to undergo malignant degeneration[43]; their neoplastic counterparts are highly aggressive and capable of local invasion as well as distant hematogenous dissemination.

Histologically, the tumor consists of multiple small epithelial lobules interposed in a jig-saw or mosaic pattern (Fig. 157–9). These lobules are surrounded by an eosinophilic basement membrane and consist of peripheral small cells with scant cytoplasm and larger, more centrally located cells with pale-staining cytoplasm. There is a resemblance to eccrine spiradenoma.

Cylindromas are now presumed to be of apocrine gland origin, although histochemical and electron microscopic investigations have not fully resolved this issue.

Treatment is by surgical excision or electrosurgery.

APOCRINE SWEAT GLAND CARCINOMA

Adenocarcinoma of the Gland of Moll

Apocrine gland carcinoma, unrelated to Paget's disease, is rare (Fig. 157–10A). Approximately 40 cases have been reported, with the eyelid comprising a small subgroup. Many presumed cases have actually proved to be sebaceous cell carcinomas. Hagedoorn,[44] Whorton and Patterson,[45] and Knaver and Whorton[46] have each reported one case of Moll carcinoma, but the pathology in each case has been disputed. Stout and Cooley's[47] case has been accepted by some experts but has been questioned by others.

Aurora and Luxenberg[48] reported the first uncontested case of adenocarcinoma of the gland of Moll. Their patient, a 58-year-old man, reported a 6- to 7-yr history of a left upper eyelid lesion. The tumor was red, irregular, and raised. Wide surgical excision was performed and no recurrence was noted over a 4-mo follow-up. Ni, Wagoner, Kieval, and Albert[49] reported two cases of Moll gland adenocarcinoma. Their first patient was a 66-year-old Chinese man with a chalazion-like left upper eyelid mass of 6-mo duration. One year following excision the tumor recurred, and preauricular and submandibular nodes were apparent. The patient eventually underwent an exenteration and lymph node dissection.

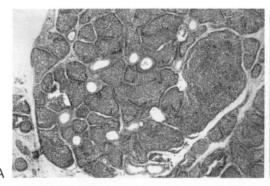
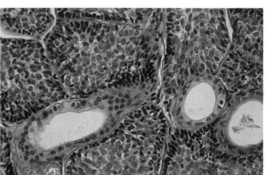

Figure 157–9. Cylindroma. A, This tumor is located in the dermis, is not connected to the overlying epithelium, and is not encapsulated. H&E. B, The tumor cell lobules are interposed in a "jig-saw" or mosaic pattern. A basement membrane surrounds the lobules that contain ductal lumina. H&E.

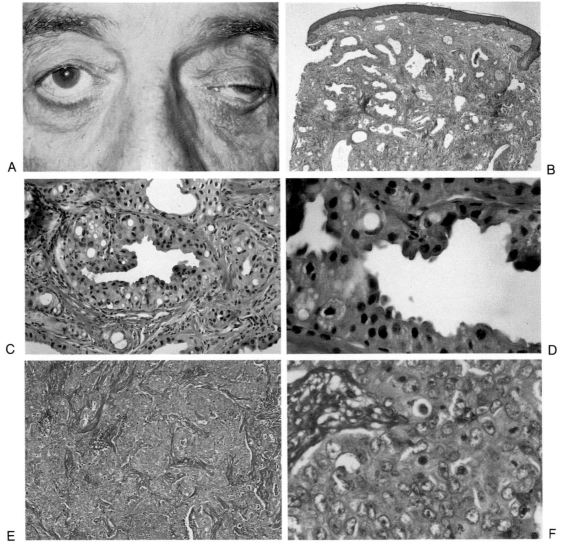

Figure 157–10. Adenocarcinoma of the gland of Moll. *A*, Chalazion-like lesion on the left lower eyelid of this male was locally excised after a biopsy proved that it was an adenocarcinoma. The lesion recurred within 1 yr. *B*, The tumor consisted of adenoid tissue arranged in tubules that deeply infiltrated the dermis. H&E. *C*, In contradistinction to the double layer of cuboidal cells found in benign apocrine tumors, adenocarcinoma is characterized by an irregular cellular proliferation; this "pile-up" of cells may obliterate the lumina. H&E. *D*, The individual cells are pleomorphic. Decapitation secretion is present. H&E. *E*, Poorly differentiated tumors may be characterized by solid epithelial growth patterns. Papillary projections and disorganized tubular structures may not be present. H&E. *F*, This high-power photomicrograph depicts nuclear atypia, mitotic figures, and an opaque cytoplasm. H&E. (*A* to *D*, courtesy of T. Dryja, M.D.)

He died 1 yr later of intracranial extension. Their second case was a 50-year-old man who presented with a left lower lid mass and 7 mm of exophthalmos. Preauricular and submandibular nodes were palpable. The patient underwent an exenteration after having received preoperative radiation therapy. After 49 mo and a radical neck dissection, the patient was lost to follow-up.

In 1989 Thomson and Tanner[50] reported the case of a 66-year-old white man with a documented 9-mo history of a right lower eyelid lesion. At surgery the patient was found to have extensive Moll adenocarcinoma infiltrating the periorbital fat. An exenteration was performed, and 15 mo later there was no evidence of local or metastatic recurrence.

In summary, of the four accepted cases of adenocarcinoma of the gland of Moll, three cases were of short duration whereas one was present for 7 yr. All cases were locally aggressive. The histopathology was characterized by an invasive adenocarcinoma that contained glandlike structures consisting of eosinophilic or opaque glassy cells forming irregularly shaped lumina of varying sizes (see Fig. 157–10B to F). Areas of decapitation secretion were present. A search for a possible other primary site was fruitless in each case.

NORMAL ECCRINE APPARATUS

The normal eccrine gland consists of a secretory coil, an intradermal duct, and an intraepithelial sweat duct unit.[1] The secretory coil consists of a single layer of secretory cells. There are two types of cells: clear cells containing glycogen and dark cells containing PAS-positive, diastase-resistant mucopolysaccharides. Scattered myoepithelial cells are located around the tubular array of secretory cells. Encircling the secretory coil is a basement membrane and an adjacent well-vascularized stroma rich in mucopolysaccharides.

The intradermal eccrine duct consists of two layers of cuboidal epithelial cells. The lumen of the duct is lined with a PAS-positive, diastase-resistant eosinophilic cuticle. The outer cell layer is surrounded by a thin connective tissue sheath and a basement membrane. The intraepithelial duct unit (acrosyringium) consists of one luminal cell layer and three outer cell layers. Keratohyaline granules are formed by the outer cells.

Electron microscopy reveals numerous convolutions in the plasma membrane of secretory coil clear cells. Intercellular canaliculi are present between adjacent clear cells; the canaliculi are opened and closed by tight junctions and empty into the lumen of the secretory coil. The myoepithelial cells are rich in tonofilaments.[2] Enzyme histochemical studies disclose the presence of succinic dehydrogenase, amylophosphorylase, and leucine aminopeptidase. The immunohistochemical analysis of mature eccrine glands reveals cross-reactivity with α-lactalbumin, S100 protein, keratins, and carcinoembryonic antigen.[51]

BENIGN TUMORS OF ECCRINE ORIGIN

Eccrine Hidrocystoma

Eccrine hidrocystomas represent a pseudoadenomatous proliferation of the intradermal eccrine sweat gland (Fig. 157–11).[52] Microscopically, a single cystic cavity or multiple chambers are lined by a double layer of cuboidal epithelial cells. In contrast to apocrine cystadenomas, these eccrine-derived lesions do not display decapitation secretion nor do they possess myoepithelial cells in the periphery of the cyst wall. Eccrine hidrocystomas presumably represent cystic dilatations of previously normal dermal sweat ducts.

Clinically, this luminal structure presents as a translucent papule approximately 1 to 3 mm and may be singular or multiple. They occasionally have a bluish tint and are more common in women. Eccrine cysts enlarge during periods of warm weather and diminish during cold periods. They may be confused with dacryops or canaliculops. The former, an ectasia of the palpebral lobe of the lacrimal gland, is typically blue and waxes and wanes in size, but does not arise on a cutaneous surface.[53] Canaliculops, an ectasia of a canaliculus, may mimic a hidrocystoma but is found along the tear duct passageway and is blue.[54]

Treatment for hidrocystoma, if desired, is surgical excision. Topically applied anticholinergic ointment has been reported to cause tumor regression.[55]

Syringoma

These eccrine tumors frequently present in a symmetric pattern on the lower eyelids or upper cheeks. They classically occur in adolescent females and Japanese women (Fig. 157–12A). Syringomas consist of small papules 1 to 3 mm in diameter, firm in texture, and yellow to light brown in color.[56] They develop slowly and persist indefinitely without symptoms. Unusual variants include the eruptive, plaque, and lichen-planus forms. These variants may be found on the neck, chest, distal extremities, and scalp.[57] Syringomas have been associated with Down's syndrome,[58] Marfan's syndrome, Ehlers-Danlos syndrome,[59] and Hailey-Hailey disease.[60]

Histologically, syringomas consist of numerous small solid nests and cords of faintly eosinophilic epithelial cells and ducts embedded in a dense fibrous stroma (see Fig. 157–12B). A clear cell variant is recognized (see Fig. 157–12C). The ducts are lined by a double layer of flattened cuboidal cells and frequently contain an amorphous, basophilic, or eosinophilic material. The classic tadpole appearance refers to the comma-shaped tails of ducts in continuity with small solid cords due to compression by the sclerotic stroma. Some syringomas undergo cystic dilatation of the ducts; foreign body giant

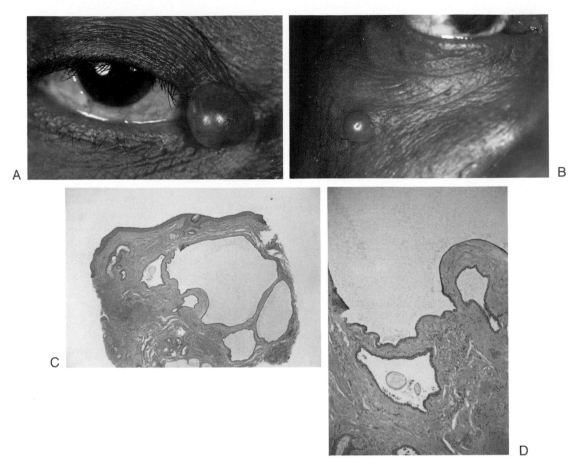

Figure 157–11. Eccrine hidrocystoma. *A,* Translucent cystic-appearing lesion arising in the medial canthus. *B,* Eccrine hidrocystomas are not limited to the eyelid margin but occur wherever eccrine glands are found. *C,* Multiple cystic spaces are lined by a double layer of cuboidal epithelial cells. H&E. *D,* Decapitation secretion is not a feature of eccrine gland lesions. A fibrillary material may be found within the ductals. H&E. (*B,* courtesy of S. Salasche, M.D.)

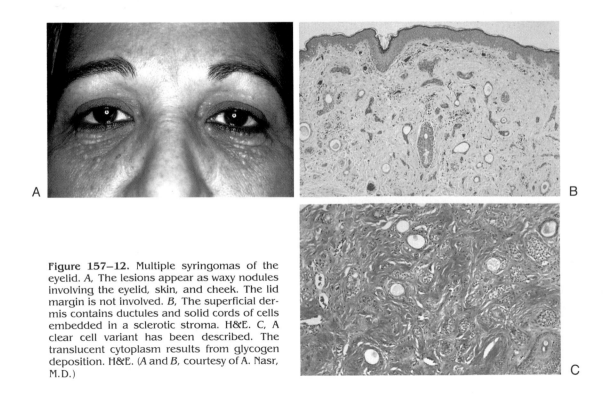

Figure 157–12. Multiple syringomas of the eyelid. *A,* The lesions appear as waxy nodules involving the eyelid, skin, and cheek. The lid margin is not involved. *B,* The superficial dermis contains ductules and solid cords of cells embedded in a sclerotic stroma. H&E. *C,* A clear cell variant has been described. The translucent cytoplasm results from glycogen deposition. H&E. (*A* and *B,* courtesy of A. Nasr, M.D.)

reaction and calcium deposition occurs when these cysts become filled with keratin and rupture.

Enzyme histochemical and electron microscopic studies have established syringomas to be of eccrine origin. The tumor contains eccrine enzymes including succinic dehydrogenase, phosphorylase, and leucine aminopeptidase.[56] The histologic differential diagnosis includes desmoplastic trichoepithelioma and microcystic adnexal carcinoma. These tumors are discussed later in this chapter.

Chondroid Syringoma (Mixed Tumor)

In 1859 Billroth[61] described a group of salivary gland tumors containing mucoid as well as cartilaginous material. Virchow named these benign lesions "mixed tumors."[62] In 1952 Lennox and others reported 52 such cases arising within the skin.[63] Nine years later, Hirsch and Helwig[64] reported 188 cases from the Armed Forces Institute of Pathology (AFIP) files and chose the terminology chondroid syringoma. Syringoma was chosen to describe the invariable mixing of sweat gland elements and an associated cartilaginous component.

Chondroid syringomas rarely affect the ocular adnexa. Of Hirsch and Helwig's 188 cases, seven involved the eyebrows and one occurred on the eyelids. In Ni and coworkers' review of 55 cases of sweat gland tumors evaluated over a 21-yr period at the Howe Laboratory of the Massachusetts Eye and Ear Infirmary,[28] six chondroid syringomas were reported. Clinically, chondroid syringomas appear as asymptomatic nodules that range in size from 0.5 to 3 cm. The overlying skin is often discolored but is intact.

Histologically, chondroid syringomas are virtually identical to pleomorphic adenoma rising in the lacrimal gland. The latter can arise in the palpebral or orbital lobe of the lacrimal gland or in accessory glands found in the fornices (gland of Krause), at the superior tarsal border (gland of Wolfring), or in the caruncle, and therefore are not situated in the dermis of the skin. Chondroid syringomas consist of nests of cuboidal or polygonal epithelial cells that have given rise to tuboalveolar and ductal structures. The ducts are lined by an inner layer of secretory cells producing mucopolysaccharides and an outer myoepithelial cell layer. The stroma that presumably is produced by the myoepithelial cells may be undergoing fibrous, myxoid, or chondrodial metaplastic changes (Fig. 157–13). Electron microscopic studies suggest tumor differentiation toward secretory and intraepidermal ductal eccrine sweat gland structures.[65]

Malignant counterparts of chondroid syringomas occur. Hirsch and Helwig reported such a malignancy arising on the face of a 50-year-old woman.[64] The most malignant chondroid syringomas occur on the extremities and back, are painful, and spread to regional lymph nodes and hematogenously to the lungs.[66] Histologically, the malignant lesions may contain areas that appear benign, which suggests that the former arises from the latter.

Acrospiroma (Clear Cell Hidradenoma)

A wide variety of terms has been used to describe this benign tumor of the eccrine duct and secretory coil. Hidradenoma, cystic hidradenoma, nodular hidradenoma, clear cell hidradenoma, eccrine sweat gland adenoma, adenoma of the clear cell type, porosyringoma, and eccrine acrospiroma are some of the synonyms. On the basis of histochemical studies, Winkelmann and Wolff[67] prefer the name cystic hidradenoma, whereas Johnson and Helwig prefer the name eccrine acrospiroma.[68]

The eccrine acrospiroma characteristically presents as a solid or cystic cutaneous nodule measuring 5 to 30 mm in diameter (Fig. 157–14A). The flesh- to red-colored lesion may be multilobulated, and the overlying skin can be ulcerated.[68] Pressure applied to the nodule produces pain in approximately 20 percent of patients. Acrospiromas are frequently located on the head but may occur anywhere on the body. Middle-aged individuals are affected, and women outnumber men. Eyelid involvement has been reported by Boniuk and Halpert,[69] Ferry and Haddad,[70] Grossniklaus and Knight,[71] Liu,[72] Ni and coworkers,[28] and others.

Histologically, the tumor is well circumscribed and located in the dermis (see Fig. 157–14B to D). It consists of numerous epithelial cell lobules, tubular lumina, and cystic spaces. Two cell types are present. One type is large, cuboidal, or polyhedral with a clear, glycogen-rich cytoplasm surrounded by a distinct membrane. The second cell type is fusiform or polyhedral and has a round nucleus and a basophilic cytoplasm. Degeneration of either cell type results in cystic spaces. A characteristic tumor trait is the presence of small ductal lumina lined by a prominent eosinophilic cuticle, resembling that seen in eccrine sweat ducts. Enzyme histochemical and electron microscopic studies document an eccrine origin.[73]

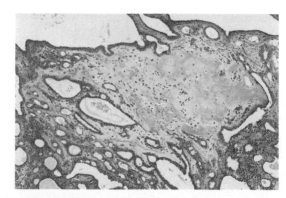

Figure 157–13. Chondroid syringoma (mixed tumor). The epithelial component consists of nests of anastomosing epithelial cords and tubuloalveolar and ductal structures located in the dermis of the lid. The stroma is usually fibrous, or myxoid, or chondroid as shown here. H&E.

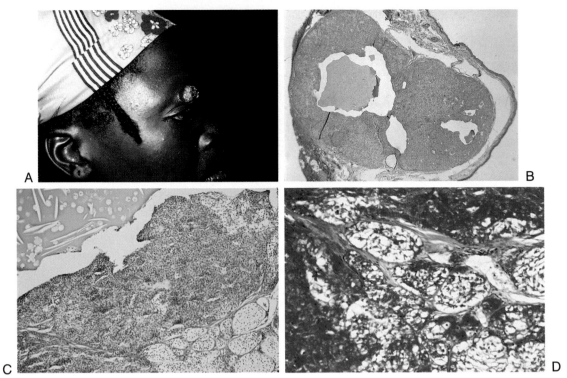

Figure 157–14. Acrospiroma. *A*, A dermal tumor has caused surface hyperkeratosis. *B*, Histologically acrospiromas are well-circumscribed dermal lesions that contain cystic spaces and solid foci of tumefaction. H&E. *C*, Small basophilic cells border an area of degenerative cystic material toward the upper left; while clear cells are present toward the bottom right. Sometimes, but not always, there may be interspersed small lumens. H&E. *D*, An abundance of periodic acid-Schiff (PAS)-positive material is found within the tumor cells, often within the clear cell regions. This material is usually glycogen and is sensitive to diastase predigestion (PAS reaction).

Hernandez-Perez and Cestoni-Parducci[74] have reported a malignant acrospiroma (hidradenocarcinoma) of the eyelid. This adenocarcinoma occurred in a 63-year-old male. The tumor was locally excised, and the patient remained disease-free 4 yr later. Cooper[75] and coworkers have reported two patients with facial hidradenocarcinomas. Both lesions had locally infiltrative appearances, and one involved the subcutaneous fat. Both were completely resected. Data have been collated on approximately 50 malignant acrospiromas described in the literature.[76] Fifty percent recurred one or more times, and sixty percent metastasized to viscera lymph nodes and bone.

Spiradenomas

First described by Kersting and Helwig in 1956, eccrine spiradenomas[77] are typically solitary, deep-seated nodules, covered by normal-appearing skin. Small nodules arising in a zosteriform pattern and large nodules in a linear distribution have also been reported. An unusual symptom is pain occurring in paroxysms. Spiradenomas are exceedingly uncommon. They are the rarest of eyelid adnexal lesions.

Eccrine spiradenomas generally appear between ages 15 and 35. Their course is benign. The chest and face are the most commonly affected sites. Ahluwalia and associates[78] reported a spiradenoma of the left upper eyelid; to our knowledge, this is the only reported case affecting the ocular adnexa. Malignant transformation of spiradenomas may rarely occur, as Cooper and others have reported.[79, 80] Spiradenomas may also coexist in the same lesion with cylindromas.[81]

Histopathologically, a connective tissue capsule frequently surrounds a lobular to multilobular lesion. The lobules consist of basophilic cells arranged in rosettes. Cells with dark nuclei and cells with larger, lighter staining nuclei are present. Hashimoto and Kanzaki[82] have concluded on the basis of ultrastructural studies that the differentiation of spiradenoma is toward the eccrine secretory coil.

ECCRINE SWEAT GLAND CARCINOMAS

Primary Mucinous Carcinoma (Adenocystic)

The uncommon mucinous adenocarcinoma of the eccrine glands was first described in detail by Wolfe and Segerberg in 1954.[83] Berg and McDivitt[84] described additional cases, and Mendoza and Helwig[85] established diagnostic criteria. In 1979 Wright and Font[86] reported 21 cases of eyelid involvement on file at the AFIP, including two cases previously reported.[84, 87] The term adenocystic carcinoma has been used to describe this entity but has fallen into disfavor because it is easily confused with a totally different entity: adenoid cystic carcinoma of salivary and lacrimal glands.

Clinically, mucinous adenocarcinoma of eccrine origin presents as a skin-colored but occasionally tan, gray, red, or blue nodule. The tumor is generally firm to hard but may be soft and spongy. Its contour has been described as papillomatous, pedunculated, and fungating. Transillumination is a frequent finding. Affected patients range in age from 8 to 84 yr, and most present between 50 to 70 yr of age. Males outnumber females, and blacks are frequently affected (Fig. 157–15A to C).

On gross examination, the tumor is lobulated and glistening. Light microscopic evaluation demonstrates tubules, cords, papillae, and solid lobules of epithelial cells found in large pools of mucin. The tumor cells are cuboidal to polygonal and contain moderate amounts of eosinophilic cytoplasm; intracellular mucin can be brought out with the alcian blue and mucicarmine stains. The nucleus is vesicular and isomorphic, and the cytoplasm is homogeneous or slightly vacuolated. Light- and dark-colored cells may be found at the nodule's periphery and core, respectively (see Fig. 157–15D to H). A cribriform or adenocystic configuration is conferred by the arrangement of ductal structures and glandlike lumina.

Most mucinous adenocarcinomas consist of lobules that grow in an expansile fashion. Invasive growth patterns may also be found. The tumors do not exhibit areas of necrosis (except on recurrence) and do not invade blood vessels. The rarity of mitotic figures and the abundant mucin secretion are evidence of the high degree of cellular differentiation. The malignant nature of these tumors is based on evidence of recurrence and metastatic spread (see Fig. 157–15I to J).

Histochemistry reveals that the mucinous pools are rich in sialomucin. This material is PAS-positive and diastase-resistant and stains for mucicarine, colloidal iron, aldehyde fuchsin, and alcian blue at pH 2.5. Sialomucin is hyaluronidase resistant and sialidase labile. An eccrine origin is borne out by the work of Headington,[95] who notes a strong reaction for oxidative enzymes, succinic dehydrogenase, lactic dehydrogenase, and isocitric dehydrogenase. Adenosine triphosphatase, acid phosphatase, and nonspecific esterase are weakly positive. With electron microscopy, the dark cells seen on hematoxylin and eosin stain contain thin filaments, membrane-bound dense granules, and numerous secretory vacuoles that coalesce to form large subplasmalemmal vacuoles. Mucin is presumably contained within these vacuoles. The light cells have a paucity of organelles and contain small whorls of cytoplasmic filaments and rough endoplasmic reticulum.

The histologic differential diagnosis includes metastatic mucinous carcinoma arising from the gastrointestinal tract, breast, or ovary. The mucin histochemistry of metastatic lesions is, however, distinct from most primary mucinous lid lesions.[96] Also included in the differential diagnosis is a basal cell carcinoma containing large areas of mucinous material. When stained with alcian blue, this mucin is hyaluronidase sensitive and sialidase resistant (the reverse of mucinous adenocarci-

noma). Numerous apoptotic cells are also found in basal cell carcinoma. Finally, mucinous adenocarcinomas with solid patterns may resemble acrospiromas or, less likely, spiradenoma.

Mucinous adenocarcinoma of the lid may infiltrate the local tissues and extend into the orbit. Cohen, Peiffer, and Lipper[88] reported the case of a 62-year-old woman who presented with a recurrent medial canthal lesion. The skin overlying the tumor was freely movable, but the mass was fixed to underlying bone. At surgery the mucinous adenocarcinoma hugged the medial wall, extending half way to the orbital apex. Khalil and associates[93] describe a 70-year-old man whose tumor invaded the orbit, optic nerve, sclera, and ethmoid sinus over a 25-yr period.

Long-term follow-up information suggests that mucinous adenocarcinoma has a better prognosis than other sweat gland carcinomas. In Wright and Font's series of 21 patients, follow-up data were available in 20 cases. Twelve patients were alive and free of disease. Eight patients had one or more local recurrences, and only one patient developed submandibular node metastases. Long-term follow-up of other eyelid cases is summarized in Table 157–2. El-Domeiri[97] reported 63 patients who had mucinous adenocarcinoma affecting various parts of the body and who were monitored for 5 yr or more. Regional lymph node metastases developed in 43 percent of patients, and 38 per cent developed widespread metastatic disease. Thus, the eyelid lesions have a better prognosis.

Optimal management consists of wide en-bloc resection of the tumor with frozen section control. Regional lymph node dissection may be indicated for clinically involved nodes. Long-term follow-up is necessary.

Primary Infiltrating Signet Ring Carcinoma

Another unusual adnexal neoplasm with a propensity for eyelid involvement is the infiltrating, poorly differentiated signet ring adenocarcinoma. Four cases have been reported in the literature,[98–101] with a fifth to date unpublished (Table 157–3).[102] All five patients were otherwise healthy, middle-aged, or elderly men, with diffusely thickened, erythematous lower lids and canthi (Fig. 157–16A). The tumor progresses slowly, can involve the other ipsilateral lid, recurs after inadequate excision, and occasionally results in regional and distant metastases. Orbital involvement occurred in two patients.

Histologically, primary signet ring carcinoma consists of compact cords of atypical epithelial cells capable of diffusely infiltrating the dermis, striated muscle, and subcutaneous tissues (see Fig. 157–16B). At high power, some of the cells have a wavy appearance with comma-shaped nuclei suggestive of a neurofibroma. Mitotic figures are absent. The cellular infiltrate consists in part of cells growing diffusely in small cords or in an Indian file in a fibrotic stroma. The cells possess cytoplasmic

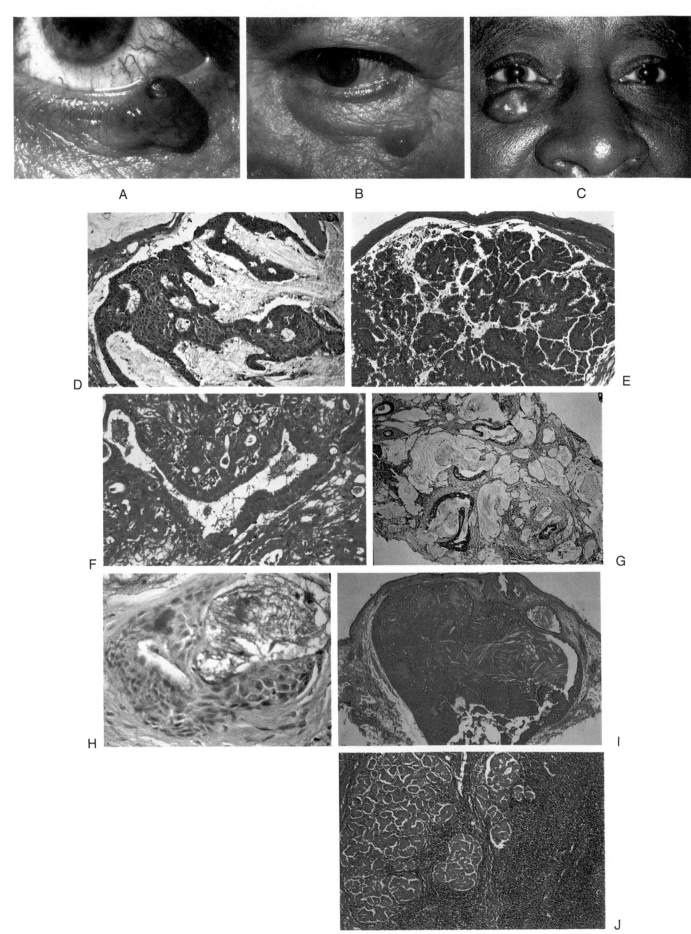

Figure 157–15 *See legend on opposite page*

Table 157–2. LONG-TERM FOLLOW-UP OF PATIENTS WITH MUCINOUS ADENOCARCINOMA

	No. of Cases	Eyelid Location	Median Age	No. of Patients with Tumor Recurrence	No. of Patients with Lymph Node Metastases	No. of Patients with Orbital Involvement	Follow-Up Months
Wright and Font (included case of Mendoza and Rodriguez)[86]	20	All lids	60	8	1*	0	0
Cohen, Peiffer, and Lipper[88]	1	Left medial canthus	60	1	0	1	0
Gardner and O'Grady[89]	1	LLL†	52	0	0	1	24
Shuster, Maskin, and Leone[90]	1	RLL‡	76	0	0	0	42
Boi, DeConcini, and Detassis[91]	1	Right inner canthus	77	0	0	0	36
Liszauer, Brownstein, and Codere[92]	1	LUL§	73	1	0	0	41
Kahil, Brownstein, Codere, and Nicolle[93]	1	RUL‖	70	0	0	1	41
Werber, Hevia, and Gretzula[94]	1	LUL	58	1	0	0	144

*This patient died of his disease.
†LLL, Left lower lid.
‡RLL, Right lower lid.
‖LUL, Left upper lid.
§RUL, Right upper lid.

vacuoles and an eccentrically deformed nucleus resembling a signet ring (see Fig. 157–16C).

Granular cell myoblastoma, neurilemoma, an inflammatory infiltrate comprised of histiocytes, and histocytoid mammary carcinoma metastatic to the eyelid have been mistakenly confused as primary signet ring carcinoma. The finding of mucin production within the cytoplasm of these signet-shaped cells by application of PAS, mucicarmine, and alcian blue stains rules out all the histologic differentials, except for metastatic mucin-producing adenocarcinoma. A clinical evaluation must then be undertaken to exclude a primary neoplasm elsewhere.

Ultrastructural studies reveal intracytoplasmic lumina with villi, abundant smooth and rough endoplasmic reticulum, lipid droplets, and filamentous granular cytoplasmic inclusions. Jakobiec and associates[101] believe in an apocrine gland origin for this tumor but concede that both apocrine and eccrine glands are capable of spawning such a neoplasm. Rosen has proposed an eccrine origin, based on the ultrastructural findings of light and dark cells.[98]

Long-term follow-up of these five cases suggests that, apart from radical exenteration, radiation therapy may be beneficial.

Sclerosing Sweat Duct Carcinoma (Microcystic Adnexal Carcinoma)

Sclerosing sweat duct carcinoma, microcystic adnexal carcinoma, and syringomatous carcinoma are used interchangeably to describe a rare variant of sweat gland carcinoma with a microscopic appearance mimicking that of a benign syringoma (Fig. 157–17A). Histologically, this malignant tumor is distinguished from its benign counterpart by virtue of the former's diffuse subcutaneous involvement, skeletal muscle invasion, and perineural infiltration. Locally aggressive, sclerosing sweat duct carcinoma has a clear-cut predilection for the upper lip, nasolabial region, and periorbita.

In 1982, Goldstein and associates reported six cases

Figure 157–15. Mucinous adenocarcinoma. A to C, These illustrations demonstrate the variable clinical appearance of this eccrine gland neoplasm. The tumor can arise along the eyelid margin or from the eyelid skin. Its coloration ranges from yellow to violaceous to flesh tone. D, This dermal nodule contains epithelial islands and cords. The clear areas contain mucin. H&E. E, A papillary configuration may be present. F, A tubular pattern may predominate. H&E. G, The tumor cells are separated by abundant amounts of mucin. H&E. H, Mucin is found both intracellularly and extracellularly (mucicarmine). I, Degenerative changes including cholesterol clefts are found in tumor recurrences. H&E. J, This low-power photomicrograph shows a submandibular gland infiltrated by metastatic mucinous adenocarcinoma. H&E. (A, courtesy of R. B. O'Grady, M.D.; B, from Wright JD, Font RL: Mucinous adenocarcinoma of the eyelids: A clinicopathologic study of 21 cases with histochemical and electron microscopic observations. Cancer 44:1757–1768, 1979); C, E to H, courtesy of R. L. Font, M.D.)

Table 157–3. LONG-TERM FOLLOW-UP OF PATIENTS WITH SIGNET RING CARCINOMA

Case Report	Patient's Sex	Age at Diagnosis	Initial Site	Treatment	Follow-Up
Jakobiec, Austin, and Iwamoto[101]	M	59	RUL*	3500 Rads	6 yr—invasion of anterior orbit
Rosen, Kim, and Yermakov[98]	M	47	RLL†		5 yr—local recurrence
Grizzard, Torczynski, and Edwards[99]	M	59	LLL‡	5000 Rads	10 yr—local recurrence; orbital invasion; preauricular nodes. Patient subsequently committed suicide; subclinical liver metastases at autopsy
Thomas, Fu, and Levine[100]	M	78	RUL		6 yr—local recurrence; preauricular and submandibular nodes; pulmonary metastases
Grove[102]	M	58	RLL	6500 Rads	6 yr—local recurrence; orbital involvement. Patient presumably died of metastatic prostate carcinoma, no autopsy

*RUL, Right upper lid.
†RLL, Right lower lid.
‡LLL, Left lower lid.

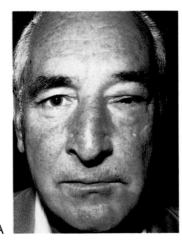

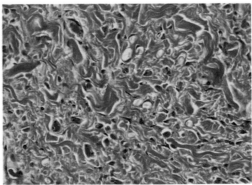

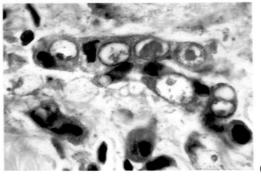

Figure 157–16. Infiltrating signet ring carcinoma. A, The lower eyelid is involved by a diffusely infiltrating process. The vertical palpebral fissure is narrowed owing to upper eyelid involvement as well. B, Fibrotic collagenous stroma separates faintly staining epithelial cells that have invaded the deep dermis. H&E. C, The tumor cells are arranged in "Indian file," and they contain a foamy cytoplasm. A signet ring configuration is visible in cells containing a single vacuole. (A, from Jakobiec FA, Austin P, Iwamoto T, et al: Primary infiltrating signet ring carcinoma of the eyelids. Ophthalmology 90:291–299, 1983; B, courtesy of I. McLean, M.D.)

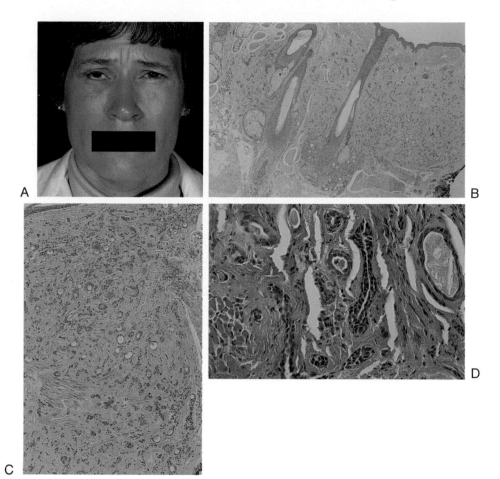

Figure 157–17. Sclerosing sweat duct carcinoma. *A,* This woman has an indurated left lower eyelid. *B,* This low-power photomicrograph reveals a deeply infiltrative lesion composed of solid epithelial strands and microacini formed by small basaloid cells with scant cytoplasm. H&E. *C,* Small keratinous cysts with well-developed lamellar keratin alternate with the glandular lumina. H&E. *D,* Striated muscle is infiltrated by this neoplasia. H&E.

of an unusual adnexal tumor affecting the upper lip of women.[103] He coined the term microcystic adnexal carcinoma in the belief that the cell of origin was a pluripotential adnexal epithelial germ cell capable of both sweat gland and follicular differentiation. Clinically, the lesions grew slowly and had been present for at least 1 yr. In two patients the tumor recurred after surgical excision, but no documented metastases occurred.

Cooper and coworkers[104] reviewed histologic sections of approximately 2000 carcinomas of all types involving the lip, nose, and periorbital area from the University of Virginia Medical Center between 1950 and 1980. Twenty cases of sclerosing cutaneous adnexal carcinoma mimicking benign syringomas were reported, with one quarter of the cases arising in the lid, canthus, eyebrow, or temple. These five patients ranged from 20 to 64 yr of age; three were male and two were female. Clinically the lesions were either ill-defined indurations, firm to hard plaques, discrete nodules, or cystlike growths with a smooth or crusted epidermal surface. The tumors grew slowly and recurred frequently (2 of 5 patients). Documented metastatic disease did not occur. A sixth patient, a 51-year-old woman, presented with tumor infiltrating the upper lip, nose, and cheek.[105] Despite aggressive surgical resection of half the nose, medial cheek, medial half of malar bone, the gingiva of the upper incisors, and a portion of alveolar ridge, the tumor recurred 2¼

yr later and produced infraorbital pain and diplopia. Radiologic imaging revealed orbital involvement. The patient eventually underwent additional surgery and a second recurrence. At the last reported follow-up, 4 yr after initial therapy, she was alive and had tumor infiltrating the orbit but without metastases.

Histologically, these tumors are characterized by solid strands of epithelial cells with scant eosinophilic cytoplasm embedded in a sclerotic stroma. The epithelial cells frequently develop small lumina and calcification. Invasion of neural structures is common. Cellular atypia and mitotic figures are rare (see Fig. 157–17*B* to *D*). Cellular atypia and mitotic figures are rare. Based on the differentiation toward sweat ducts and the accompanying abundant sclerotic stroma, some authors prefer the term sclerosing sweat duct carcinoma in place of microcystic adnexal carcinoma.

Histochemistry reveals that some tumor nests contain small amounts of collagen. The ductal lumen contain eosinophilic PAS-positive material that stains with alcian blue and aldehyde fuchsin. The stroma shows moderate amounts of alcian blue positive material. Cytoplasmic keratin is present with frequent cuticular differentiation. Carcinoembryonic antigen has been detected around the ductal portion of the carcinoma but is absent around keratocytes.

Additional cases of sclerosing sweat duct carcinoma affecting the eyelids have been reported.[106, 107] Grove treated an 89-year-old woman with complete ptosis and external ophthalmoplegia as well as facial numbness.[108] The lower lid was fixed to the orbital rim. Computed tomography (CT) imaging disclosed a soft tissue mass in the inferomedial orbit extending from the orbital rim to the apex. Biopsy of the lid and orbit revealed sclerosing sweat duct carcinoma. One of us (FAJ) has collected several similar cases. The patients all shared in common a protracted clinical course from stromal sclerosis, tumor infiltrating the orbit along perineural planes, and the absence of lymph node metastases.

TUMORS OF PILAR ORIGIN

Pilomatrixoma (Calcified Epithelioma of Malherbe)

The pilomatrixoma is an uncommon tumor with differentiation toward hair cortex cells. It typically presents as a firm, freely mobile, subcutaneous nodule covered by normal-appearing skin (Fig. 157–18 A and B). Occasionally the tumor is superficially located, creating a blue to red skin discoloration; spontaneous fistula for-

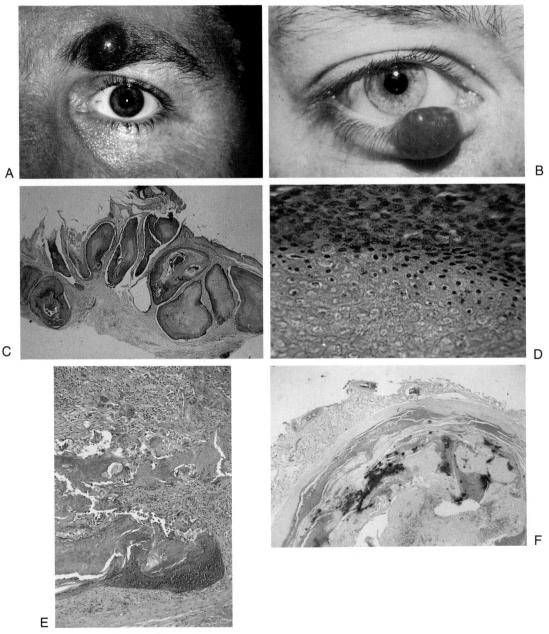

Figure 157–18. Pilomatrixoma. *A*, This young man had a freely mobile, subcutaneous mass of the left brow. Note the characteristic redish-pink color. *B*, This 24 year old had a firm nodule distorting the lower eyelid. *C*, The excised specimen consists of several lobules limited to the dermis. Basophilic cells are found at the periphery of the lobules, and foci of calcification are present. H&E. *D*, Transition zone from basophilic cells to the more centrally located shadow cells. Intensely eosinophilic staining results following the degeneration of shadow cell nuclei. H&E. *E*, The necrotic debris stimulates a granulomatous foreign body reaction. H&E. The presence of multinucleated giant cells and keratin debris can lead to confusion with dermoid cysts of the eyelid and brow. *F*, Dystrophic calcification begins as the shadow cells degenerate (Alizarin red).

mation may occur. More than 50 percent of the reported pilomatrixomas affect the head and neck; of those cases involving the ocular adnexa, the upper lid margin and brow are sites of predilection.[109, 110] Pilomatrixomas vary in size from 0.5 to 3 cm but may be as large as 5 cm.[111] The lesion is usually solitary, but multiple lesions occur in 6 percent of patients. The tumors arise in persons of any age, but 40 percent of the lesions are noted in children younger than 10 yr of age, and 60 percent in patients younger than 20 yr of age.[112] A brow lesion in a young patient may be confused with a dermoid cyst.

Pilomatrixomas occur in patients with myotonic muscular dystrophy; these patients also have frontoparietal baldness and Raynaud's phenomenon.[113] Pilomatrixomas may be seen within certain families. Reports exist of pilomatrixoma-like changes in epidermal cysts in patients with Gardner's syndrome.[114]

Histologically, the tumor is encircled by a fibrous pseudocapsule and is located in the lower dermis and subcutaneous tissues. It is characterized by irregularly shaped islands of epithelial cells embedded in a cellular stroma (see Fig. 157–18C). Peripheral basophilic cells and central shadow cells are present. The former possess round or elongated, deeply basophilic nuclei and scant cytoplasm. Their cellular borders are often indistinct. In early lesions the basophilic cells undergo considerable mitotic activity, which is a normal finding consistent with an origin from the primordial epithelium of the hair matrix or bulb. As the tumor matures, the basaloid matrical cells transform into centrally located shadow or ghost cells. Such cells are characterized by abundant eosinophilic cytoplasm and small, hyperchromatic nuclei (see Fig. 157–18D). These nuclei are eventually lost, resulting in sheets of intensely eosinophilic, keratinous material. There is frequently an associated foreign body giant cell reaction to the keratin (see Fig. 157–18E). Calcification (see Fig. 157–18F) present in approximately 75 percent of cases, and ossification occurs in 15 to 20 percent.[111]

Histochemical studies disclose a hair matrix cell origin for pilomatrixomas. The PAS stain for the sulfhydryl or disulfide group is strongly positive and this is an indication of keratinization.[115] Further evidence of keratinization is provided by the birefringence in polarized light of the shadow cells. Electron microscopic evaluation reveals a striking resemblance between the basophilic cells undergoing transition into shadow cells with the cells in the keratogenous zone of normal hair; both demonstrate thick keratin fibrils arranged concentrically around a faintly visible nucleus.[116]

Simple excision of the lesion is the preferred treatment, although curettage has been performed. Local recurrence occurs in approximately 2 percent of cases. Malignant degeneration (matrical carcinoma) has been reported.[117–119] Malignant lesions exhibit infiltrating features at the edge of the tumor and anaplastic cytologic characteristics.

Trichilemmoma

Trichilemmoma was first described by Headington and French in 1961; it is a benign epithelioma arising from the outer sheath of hair follicles.[120] Clinically, a trichilemmoma is a solitary lesion, small (1 to 8 mm in diameter), and nodular and sometimes has irregular, rough surfaces (Fig. 157–19A and B). The lesion has an insidious onset, affects males and females equally, and almost always involves the head and neck.[121] It is frequently misdiagnosed as a cutaneous horn, papilloma, or basal cell carcinoma. A trichilemmoma may arise within a preexisting nevus sebaceus.

Hidayat and Font[122] reviewed 31 trichilemmomas of the eyelid and eyebrow from material on file at the AFIP. Their patients ranged from 22 to 88 yr of age with a mean age of 56 yr. All except three lesions occurred on the eyelids, with eyelid margin involvement being especially rare. All lesions were asymptomatic and solitary. They were clinically described as papules or nodules resembling verruca and cutaneous horns.

Multiple trichilemmomas can also occur and represent a cutaneous marker for the autosomal dominantly inherited condition known as Cowden's syndrome.[123] Oral mucosal papules, acral keratotic papules, adenomatous and nodular thyroid goiters, lipomas, gastrointestinal polyps, and fibrocystic breast disease represent the benign tumors that develop in patients with Cowden's disease. Breast carcinoma and thyroid carcinoma are among the malignancies associated with this syndrome.[124] Recently cerebellar hamartomas (Lhermitte-Duclos disease) were reported to coexist with Cowden's disease (see Fig. 157–19C and D).[125–127]

Microscopically, trichilemmoma is characterized by a proliferation of the outer root sheath resulting in a small solid lobule or a group of closely set lobules (see Fig. 157–19E to H). The tumor consists of a uniform population of relatively small cells with round or oval vesicular nuclei, clear cytoplasm, and a significant glycogen content (diastase sensitive, PAS positive). There is peripheral palisading of nuclei and an encircling dense eosinophilic hyaline sheath. Hyperkeratosis, acanthosis, and squamous eddies may be present. In pursuit of the possibility that these lesions are verruca, papillomavirus common antigen has been searched for but has not been found. The pathologist must be aware that trichilemmomas may histologically resemble basal cell carcinoma, squamous cell carcinoma, adnexal carcinoma, and seborrheic keratosis.

Treatment is directed toward complete surgical excision of the tumor.[128] Alternate treatment modalities include topical medications (e.g., fluorouracil and tretinoin), superficial curettement, and electrocoagulation.

Trichofolliculoma

Trichofolliculoma is a solitary, dome-shaped nodule commonly found on the face, scalp, or neck.[129, 130] It almost always contains a central depression or pore, through which wisps of white, wooly, lanugo hairs protrude (Fig. 157–20A). The lesion grows slowly and is small. In the eyelids, there is a predilection for the eyelid margin. Intermittent drainage of sebum-like material may occur. Preoperatively, the lesion may be confused with a sebaceous cyst, nevus, or basal cell carcinoma.

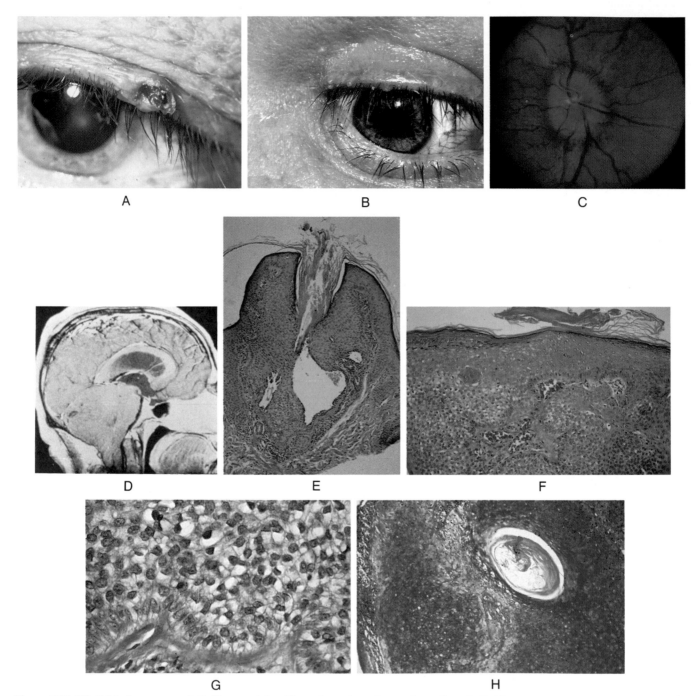

Figure 157–19. Tricholemmoma. *A,* Solitary nodule with surface ulceration and crusting. *B,* Multiple flesh-colored papules resembling verrucae. *C,* Multiple tricholemmomas are associated with Cowden's syndrome. Such patients may develop breast or thyroid carcinoma. This patient suffered from papilledema. *D,* The increased intracranial pressure resulted from the cerebellar mass that characterizes the phakomatosis called Lhermite-Duclose disease. *E,* The skin tumor displays marked acanthosis with palisading of columnar epithelial cells at the periphery. Hyalinization is shown in the center. H&E. *F,* A thickened cuticular membrane encloses the tumor lobule's periphery. A squamous eddy and glycogen-rich clear cells are demonstrated. H&E. *G,* This high-power photomicrograph shows a relatively uniform set of small cells with round nuclei and clear cytoplasm. *H,* This periodic acid-Schiff stain demonstrates the presence of glycogen intracellularly. (*A,* courtesy of R. Eagle, M.D.; *C* and *D,* courtesy of S. Lessell, M.D., and S. Hamilton, M.D.)

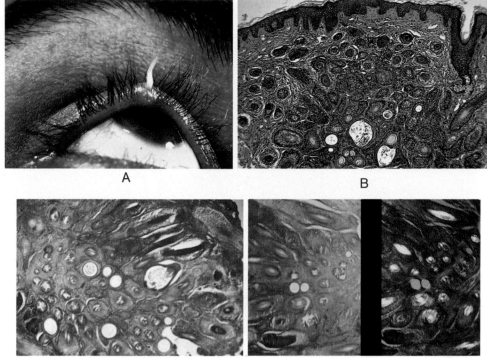

Figure 157–20. Trichofolliculoma. *A,* White wisp of lanugo hairs. *B,* Several cystic spaces representing dilated hair follicles containing keratin. Attempts at hair follicle differentiation are seen radiating from these primary follicles. H&E. *C,* Differing levels of hair follicle differentiation. H&E. *D,* Polarized light depicts several small birefringent hair shafts in the lumens of the follicle. H&E. (The polarized light is on the right; the nonpolarized light is on the left.) (*A,* Courtesy of N. Charles, M.D.)

Histologically, the tumor consists of a dilated follicular orifice that contains keratin material and hair (see Fig. 157–20B). The duct is lined by keratinized stratified squamous epithelium and is continuous with the epidermis. The central hair follicle structure exhibits radial branching into secondary follicular epithelial structures with bulblike modifications or hair roots with highly mature differentiation (see Fig. 157–20C and D). The lesion shows an abundant connective tissue stroma sharply demarcated from the adjacent dermis. Histochemically, glycogen is present in the walls of the abortive hair follicles.[131]

The benign nature of the tumor indicates that simple removal such as an excisional biopsy or fulguration is sufficient.

Multiple Trichoepitheliomas

Multiple trichoepitheliomas are inherited in an autosomal dominant manner with incomplete penetration (Fig. 157–21A).[132] The lesions appear at puberty; involve the face (particularly the nasolabial folds), scalp, neck, and upper trunk; and over time they increase in size and number. Clinically, they are skin-colored or slightly pink, firm nodules 2 to 8 mm in size. Large lesions may have telangiectatic vessels on their surface and may thus be confused with basal cell carcinoma. Trichoepitheliomas tend to remain small and hardly ever ulcerate. In contrast, lesions of the basal cell nevus syndrome may enlarge, ulcerate deeply, and display an invasive character. Multiple trichoepitheliomas, also known as Brooke's tumor or adenoid cystic epithelioma, may occur with cylindromas in some kindreds. Transforma-

tion of a trichoepithelioma into a basal cell carcinoma is infrequent.[133, 134]

The characteristic histologic finding is the presence of multiple horn cysts containing concentrically laminated keratin or a less structured hyaline material (see Fig. 157–21B to D). The cysts lie within the epidermis and dermis and are surrounded by a mantle of basophilic cells similar to those seen in basal cell carcinoma or seborrheic keratosis. These basophilic cells display palisading of nuclei and have a high nuclear:cytoplasmic ratio. There is also a frequent tendency to form anastamosing retiform strands of basaloid epithelium in a cribriform or lacelike pattern. Hair matrix-like differentiation accompanied by hair papilla-like formation of the connective tissue matrix may be identified. Foci of foreign body reaction and calcification can sometimes be identified. Histochemically, this tumor may be confused with other keratinizing neoplasms, and thus the clinical history and an experienced pathologist are helpful in making the proper diagnosis.

Solitary Trichoepithelioma

A trichoepithelioma may occur as a sporadic and solitary lesion. Such lesions are asymptomatic and flesh-colored and grow to 5 mm. They present at any age but occur more commonly in young females. These lesions sometimes have a morphea-like appearance (sclerosing trichoepithelioma) and thus can be confused with basal cell carcinoma, except that the latter is inexorably progressive whereas the former can attain a relatively stationary character.

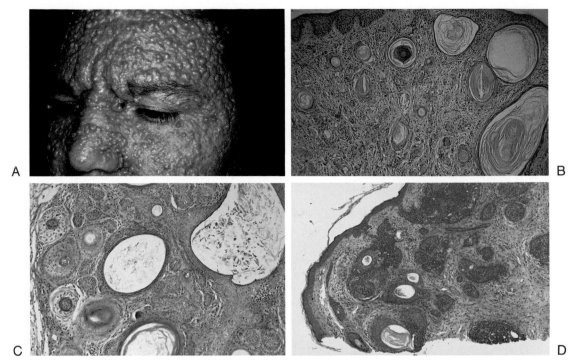

Figure 157–21. Trichoepithelioma (Brooke's tumor). *A,* Multiple trichoepitheliomas involving the entire face. The left medial canthal region was an ulceration that proved to be a basal cell carcinoma. *B,* Extensive replacement of the dermis with numerous keratin-filled cysts. H&E. *C,* Basophilic cells with peripheral palisading surround multiple horn cysts. This lesion may be histologically difficult to differentiate from keratinizing cutaneous neoplasias. *D,* A desmoplastic variant with a thickened, sclerotic stroma. This pattern is similar to sclerosing basal cell epithelioma, except for the abundance of horn cysts. (*A,* courtesy of Lewis Shapiro, M.D.)

Other Tumors Simulating Primary Adnexal Tumors

The clinical and histologic differential diagnoses of primary adnexal tumors include metastatic lesions, Merkel cell carcinoma, and phakomatous choristoma of the lid.

Metastatic Eyelid Tumors

Patients with carcinoma may develop metastases to the ocular adnexa (Fig. 157–22*A* and *B*).[135] In particular, metastatic breast carcinoma to the eyelids and orbit may present with pseudoinflammatory signs and symptoms similar to primary signet ring carcinoma.[136] Findings include lid swelling, erythema, and induration (see Fig. 157–22*D* and *D*). Histologically, this variant of metastatic breast carcinoma does not grow in lobules but rather in an "Indian file" pattern or as dispersed individual tumor cells. It has a peculiar "histiocytoid" appearance,[137] and individual cells contain bland, round to oval nuclei, a distinct nuclear membrane, and uniform chromatin. The cytoplasm has a ground-glass appearance and contains small and large vacuoles resembling signet rings. Histochemical stains for mucopolysaccharides reveal that the vacuoles contain hyaluronidase-resistant alcian blue-positive material that also stains with PAS and mucicarmine techniques. The presence of mucin excludes the diagnosis of granular cell myoblastoma, neurogenic tumors, xanthoma, xanthelasma, or an inflammatory lesion.

Merkel Cell Tumor

Merkel cell tumor is a neoplasm of the amino precursor uptake and decarboxylation (APUD) system. It has a predilection for the head and neck, a high recurrence rate following excision, and a propensity to spread through lymphatic channels.[138] Clinically, Merkel cell tumors present as vascularized violaceous cutaneous nodules (Fig. 157–23).[139] On light microscopic evaluation, the tumor cells contain uniform sized nuclei and scant cytoplasm and are arranged in sheets or in a trabecular pattern. The histologic differential diagnosis includes that of a poorly differentiated cutaneous neoplasm, malignant lymphoma, metastatic oat cell carcinoma, and amelanotic melanoma. An ultrastructural examination of Merkel cell tumors reveals membrane-bound granules, perineural microfilaments, desmosomes, and actin-containing filaments.[140] Immunohistochemistry demonstrates the presence of peptides including metenkephalin, calcitonin, somatostatin, ACTH, and neuron-specific enolase.

Merkel cell lesions may clinically resemble the glomus tumor, a benign vascular hamartoma. Glomus tumors may be solitary or multiple, are tender to touch, and only rarely affect the face and eyelid. An autosomal dominant inheritance pattern has been reported. His-

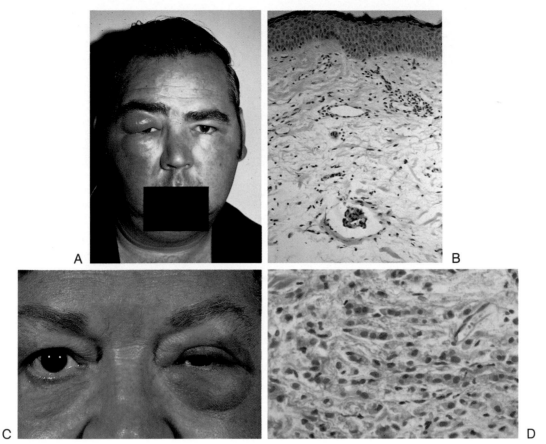

Figure 157–22. Metastatic carcinoma to the eyelids. *A*, A 54-year-old man with chemotic eyelids. The skin has a peau d'orange appearance. *B*, Carcinomatous cells within the eyelid lymphatics. The primary tumor was presumed to be of gastrointestinal origin. H&E. *C*, Painless swelling and pseudoinflammatory nodular induration of the left eyelids in a 56-year-old woman. *D*, The pseudoinflammatory clinical picture resulted from metastatic breast carcinoma. Collagen fibers separate tumor cells that contain abundant cytoplasmic lumina and that are arranged in an Indian file. The "histiocytoid" tumor cells contain one large intracytoplasm vacuole (signet ring cell) rather than myriad ones of true histiocytes. H&E.

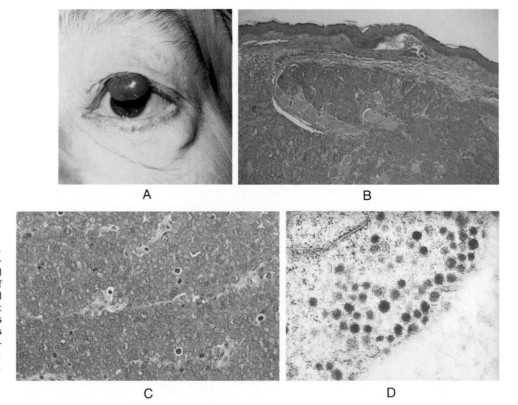

Figure 157–23. Merkel cell tumor. *A*, Red-violaceous lid margin tumor. *B*, Trabecular pattern limited to the dermis. H&E. *C*, Sheets of tumor cells with uniform nuclei and scant cytoplasm. Numerous mitotic figures are present. H&E. *D*, This electron micrograph discloses dense secretory granules that contain catecholamine products. (*A*, Courtesy of Prof. O. A. Jensen; *D*, Courtesy of G. Klintworth, M.D.)

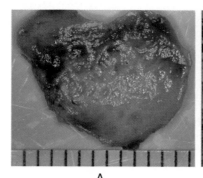
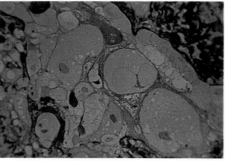
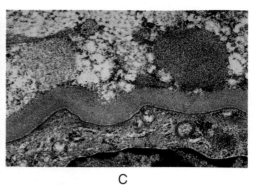

A B C

Figure 157–24. Phakomatous choristoma. *A*, Transverse sectioning of gross specimen details a lobulated white-gray surface. *B*, Swollen cells resemble the "bladder cells" of human cataractous lenses. The positive basement membrane is thickened, irregular, and stains for periodic acid-Schiff. *C*, This electron micrograph reveals that the epithelial cells are surrounded by a thickened, homogeneous basement membrane. (*A* and *C*, from Eustis HS, Karcioglu ZA, Dharma S: Phakomatous choristoma: Clinical, histolopathological and ultrastructural findings in a 4-month-old boy. J Pediatr Ophthalmol Strabismus 27:208–211, 1990; *B*, courtesy of R. T. McMahon, M.D.)

tologic evaluation discloses large, dilated vascular channels lined by glomus cells.

Phakomatous Choristoma

These choristomas involve the nasal aspect of the lower eyelid.[141-146] In each reported case, initial presentation is at birth or within the first 6 mo of life. The mass is located within the dermis, has firm or rubbery consistency, and enlarges slowly.[142] Microscopic evaluation reveals plump, cuboidal epithelial cells that resemble the "bladder cells" of the human lens. The cells are surrounded by a thickened basement membrane and dense collagenous tissue (Fig. 157–24). Zimmerman,[143] McMahon and coworkers,[144] and Tripathi and associates[145] have proposed an aberrant developmental scheme to explain the numerous findings. They believed that surface ectodermal cells that normally form the lens plate and vesicle remain outside the optic vesicle as the embryonic tissue closes. These cells migrate into the inferonasal lid, multiply, and undergo rudimentary differentiation to form this phakomatous choristoma.

REFERENCES

1. Yanoff M, Fine BS: Ocular Pathology: A Text and Atlas Edition. Philadelphia, Harper & Row, 1983.
2. Jakobiec FA, Iwamoto T: Ocular adnexae: Introduction to lids, conjunctiva, and orbit. *In* Jakobiec FA (ed): Ocular Anatomy, Embryology, and Teratology. Philadelphia, Harper & Row, 1982.
3. Johnson WC: Histochemistry of cutaneous adnexas and selected adnexal neoplasms. J Cutan Pathol 11:352, 1984.
4. Mazoujian G, Margolis R: Immunohistochemistry of gross cystic disease fluid protein in 65 benign sweat gland tumors of the skin. Am J Dermatopathol 10(1):28, 1988.
5. Mazoujian G: Immunohistochemistry of GCDFP-24 and zinc alpha-two glycoprotein in benign sweat gland tumors. Am J Dermatopathol 12:452, 1990.
6. Wick MR, Coffin CM: Sweat gland and pilar carcinoma. *In* Wick MR (ed): Pathology of Unusual Malignant Cutaneous Tumors. New York, Marcel Dekker, 1985.
7. Smith JD, Chernosky ME: Hidrocystomas. Arch Dermatol 108:676, 1973.
8. Krause TV, Khan MA, Hassan MO: Multiple apocrine cystadenomas. Br J Dermatol 100:675, 1979.
9. Monfort J: Les hidrocystomes noirs. Semin Hop Paris 8:328, 1962.
10. Shelly WB, Levy EJ, Weidman FD: Apocrine sweat retention in man. III: Apocrine retention cysts. Arch Dermatol 72:171, 1955.
11. Duke-Elder S, MacFaul P: System of Ophthalmology. XIII: The Ocular Adnexa, Part 1. St. Louis, CV Mosby, 1974.
12. Smith JD, Chernosky ME: Apocrine hidrocystoma (cystadenoma). Arch Dermatol 109:700, 1974.
13. Holder WR, Smith JD, Mocega EE: Giant apocrine hidrocystoma. Arch Dermatol 104:522, 1971.
14. Sacks E, Jakobiec FA, McMillan R, et al: Multiple bilateral apocrine cystadenomas of the lower eyelids. Ophthalmology 94:65, 1987.
15. Langer K, Konrad K, Smolle J: Multiple apocrine hidrocystomas on the eyelids. Am J Dermatopathol 11:570, 1989.
16. Gross BG: The fine structure of apocrine hidrocystoma. Arch Dermatol 92:706, 1965.
17. Font RL, Stone MS, Schanzer MC, Lewis RA: Apocrine hidrocystomas of the lids, hypodontia, palmar-plantar hyperkeratosis, and onychodystrophy. Arch Ophthalmol 104:1811, 1986.
18. Schopf E, Schulz H-J, Passarge E: Syndrome of cystic eyelids, palmoplantar keratosis, hypodontia and hypotrichosis as a possible autosomal recessive trait. Birth Defects 8:219, 1971.
19. Burket JM, Burket BJ, Burket DA: Eyelid cysts, hypodontia and hypotrichosis. J Am Acad Dermatol 10:922, 1984.
20. Mehregan AH, Pinkus H: Life history of organoid nevi: Special reference to nevus sebaceus of Jadassohn. Arch Dermatol 91:577, 1965.
21. Pokorny KS, Hyman BM, Jakobiec FA, et al: Epibulbar choristomas containing lacrimal tissue: Clinical distinction from dermoids and histologic evidence of an origin from palpebral lobe. Ophthalmology 94:1249, 1987.
22. Wilkes SR, Campbell RJ, Walker RR: Ocular malformations in association with ipsilateral facial nevus of Jadassohn. Am J Ophthalmol 92:344, 1981.
23. Diven DG, Solomon AR, McNelly MC, Font RL: Nevus sebaceus associated with major ophthalmic abnormalities. Arch Dermatol 123:383, 1987.
24. Wilson-Jones E, Heyl T: Naevus sebaceus: A report of 140 cases with special regard to the development of secondary malignant tumors. Br J Dermatol 82:99, 1970.
25. Domingo J, Helwig EB: Malignant neoplasms associated with nevus sebaceus of Jadassohn. J Am Acad Dermatol 1:545, 1979.
26. Helwig EB, Hackney VC: Syringocystadenoma papilliferum lesions with and without naevus sebaceus and basal cell carcinoma. Arch Dermatol 71:361, 1955.
27. Jakobiec FA, Streeten BW, Iwamoto T, et al: Syringocystadenoma papilliferum of the eyelid. Ophthalmology 88:1175, 1981.
28. Ni C, Dryja TP, Albert DM: Sweat gland tumor in the eyelids: A clinicopathological analysis of 55 cases. Int Clin Ophthalmol 23:1–22, 1981.
29. Warkel RL: Selected apocrine neoplasms. J Cutan Pathol 11:437, 1984.

30. Santa Cruz DJ, Prioleau PG, Smith ME: Hidradenoma papilliferum of the eyelid. Arch Dermatol 117:55, 1981.
31. Netland PA, Townsend DJ, Albert DM, Jakobiec FA: Hidradenoma papilliferum of the upper eyelid arising from the apocrine gland of Moll. Ophthalmology 97:1593, 1990.
32. Tappeiner J, Wolff K: Hidradenoma papilliferum: Eine enzymhistochemische und elektronenmikroskopische studie. Hautarzt 19:101, 1969.
33. Shenoy YMV: Malignant perianal papillary hidradenoma. Arch Dermatol 83:965, 1961.
34. Eneroth CM: Onococytoma of major salivary glands. J Laryngol Otol 79:1064, 1965.
35. Luthra CL, Doxanas MT, Green WR: Lesions of the caruncle: A clinicopathologic study. Surv Ophthalmol 23:183, 1978.
36. Lamping KA, Albert DM, Ni C, Fournier G: Oxyphil cell adenoma: Three case reports. Arch Ophthalmol 102:263, 1984.
37. Rodgers IR, Jakobiec FA, Krebs W, et al: Papillary oncocytoma of the eyelid. Ophthalmology 95:1071, 1988.
38. Warkel RL, Helwig EB: Apocrine gland adenoma and adenocarcinoma of the axilla. Arch Dermatol 114:198, 1978.
39. Landry M, Winkelman RK: An unusual tubular adenoma: Histochemical and ultrastructural study. Arch Dermatol 105:869, 1976.
40. Umbert P, Winkelmann RK: Tubular apocrine adenoma. J Cutan Pathol 3:75, 1976.
41. Brownstein MH: The genodermatopathology of adnexal tumors. J Cutan Pathol 11:457, 1984.
42. Baum EW: Cylindroma. Arch Dermatol 118:692, 1982.
43. Urbanski SJ: Metamorphosis of dermal cylindroma. J Am Acad Dermatol 12:188, 1985.
44. Hagedoorn A: Paget's disease of the eyelid associated with carcinoma. Br J Ophthalmol 21:234, 1937.
45. Whorton CM, Patterson JB: Carcinoma of Moll's glands with extramammary Paget's disease of the eyelid. Cancer 8:1009, 1955.
46. Knauer WJ, Whorton CM: Extramammary Paget's disease originating in Moll's glands of the lids. Tr Am Acad Ophthalmol Otol 67:892, 1963.
47. Stout AP, Cooley SGE: Carcinoma of sweat glands. Cancer 4:521, 1951.
48. Aurora AL, Luxenberg MN: Case report of adenocarcinoma of glands of Moll. Am J Ophthalmol 70:984, 1970.
49. Ni C, Wagoner M, Kieval S, Albert DM: Tumors of the Moll's glands. Br J Ophthalmol 68:502, 1984.
50. Thomson SJ, Tanner NSB: Carcinoma of the apocrine glands at the base of eyelashes: A case report and discussion of histological diagnostic criteria. Br J Plast Surg 42:598, 1989.
51. Pennys NS: Immunohistochemistry of adnexal neoplasms. J Cutan Pathol 11:357, 1984.
52. Hassam MO, Khan MA: Ultrastructure of eccrine cystadenoma: A case report. Arch Dermatol 115:1217, 1979.
53. Stern K, Jakobiec FA, Harrison WG: Caruncular dacryops with extravasated secretory globoid bodies. Ophthalmology 90:1447, 1983.
54. Sacks E, Jakobiec FA, Dodick J: Canaliculops. Ophthalmol 94:78, 1987.
55. Sperling LC, Sakas EL: Eccrine hidrocystomas. J Am Acad Dermatol 7:763, 1982.
56. Hashimoto K, Gross BG, Lever WF: Syringoma. J Invest Dermatol 46:150, 1966.
57. Kikuchi I, Idemori M, Okazaki M: Plaque type syringoma. J Dermatol 6:329, 1979.
58. Urban CD, Cannon JR, Cole RD: Eruptive syringomas in Down's syndrome. Arch Dermatol 117:374, 1981.
59. Dupre A, Bonafe JL: Syringomas, mongolism, Marfan's disease and Ehlers-Danlos disease. Ann Dermatol Venereol 104:224, 1977.
60. King DT, Hirose FM, King LA: Simultaneous occurrence of familial benign chronic pemphigus (Hailey-Hailey disease) and syringoma of the vulva. Arch Dermatol 114:801, 1978.
61. Billroth T: Beobachturgen: Uber Geschwulste der Speicheldrusen. Virchows Arch Path Anat 17:357, 1859.
62. Virchow R: Die Krankhaften Geschwulste. Hirschwald 1:481, 1983.
63. Lennox B, Pearse AGE, Richards HGH: Mucin secreting tumors of the skin: With special reference to the so-called mixed salivary gland tumor of the skin and its relation to hidradenoma. J Pathol Bact 64:865, 1952.
64. Hirsch P, Helwig EB: Chondroid syringoma. Arch Dermatol 84:177, 1961.
65. Varela-Durah J, Diaz-Flores L, Varela-Nunez R: Ultrastructure of chondroid syringoma. Cancer 44:148, 1979.
66. Ishlmura E, Iwamoto H, Kobushi Y, et al: Malignant chondroid syringoma: Report of a case with widespread metastases and review of pertinent literature. Cancer 52:1966, 1983.
67. Winkelmann RK, Wolff R: Solid-cystic hidradenoma of the skin. Arch Dermatol 97:651, 1968.
68. Johnson BL, Helwig EB: Eccrine acrospiroma. Cancer 23:641, 1967.
69. Boniuk M, Halpert B: Clear cell hidradenoma or myoepithelioma of the eyelid. Arch Ophthalmol 72:59, 1964.
70. Ferry AP, Haddad HM: Eccrine acrospiroma (porosyringoma) of the eyelid. Arch Ophthalmol 83:591, 1970.
71. Grossniklaus HE, Knight SH: Eccrine acrospiroma (clear cell hidradenoma) of the eyelid: Immunohistochemical and ultrastructural features. Ophthalmology 98:347, 1991.
72. Liu Y: Histogenesis of clear cell papillary carcinoma of skin. Am J Pathol 25:691, 1949.
73. Hashimoto K, DiBella RJ, Lever WF: Clear cell hidradenoma: Histologic, histochemical, and electron microscopic study. Arch Dermatol 96:18, 1967.
74. Hernandez-Perez E, Cestoni-Parducci R: Nodular hidradenoma and hidradenocarcinoma: A 10 year review. J Am Acad Dermatol 12:15, 1985.
75. Cooper PH, Robinson LR, Green KE: Low grade clear cell eccrine carcinoma. Arch Dermatol 120:1076, 1984.
76. Cooper PH: Carcinomas of sweat glands. In Rosen PP, Fechne RE (eds): Pathology Annual, part 1, vol. 22. Norwalk, CT, Appleton-Century Crofts, 1987.
77. Kersting DW, Helwig ED: Eccrine spiradenoma. Arch Dermatol 73:199, 1956.
78. Ahluwalia BK, Khurana AK, Chugh AP, Mehtani VG: Eccrine spiradenoma of eyelid: Case report. Br J Ophthalmol 70:580, 1986.
79. Cooper PH, Frierson HF, Morrison AG: Malignant transformation of eccrine spiradenoma. Arch Dermatol 121:1445, 1985.
80. Evans HL, Daniel Su WP, Smith JL, et al: Carcinoma arising in eccrine spiradenoma. Cancer 43:1881, 1979.
81. Goette DK, McConnell MA, Fowler VR: Cylindroma and eccrine spiradenoma coexist in the same lesion. Arch Dermatol 118:273, 1982.
82. Hashimoto K, Kanzaki T: Appendage tumors of the skin: Histogenesis and ultrastructure. J Cutan Pathol 11:365, 1984.
83. Wolfe JJ, Segerberg LH: Metastasizing sweat gland carcinoma of the scalp involving the transverse sinus. Am J Surg 88:849, 1954.
84. Berg JW, McDivitt RW: Pathology of sweat gland carcinoma. Pathol Annu 3:123, 1968.
85. Mendoza SB, Helwig EB: Mucinous (adenocystic) carcinoma of the skin. Arch Dermatol 103:68, 1971.
86. Wright SD, Font RL: Mucinous sweat gland adenocarcinoma of eyelid: A clinicopathologic study of 21 cases with histochemical and electron microscopic observations. Cancer 44:1757, 1979.
87. Rodriguez MM, Lubowitz RM, Shannon GM: Mucinous (adenocystic) carcinoma of the eyelid. Arch Ophthalmol 89:493, 1973.
88. Cohen KL, Peiffer RL, Lipper S: Mucinous sweat gland adenocarcinoma of the eyelid. Am J Ophthalmol 92:183, 1981.
89. Gardner TW, O'Grady RB: Mucinous adenocarcinoma of the eyelid. Arch Ophthalmol 102:912, 1984.
90. Shuster AR, Maskin SL, Leone CR: Primary mucinous sweat gland carcinoma of the eyelid. Ophthalmic Surg 20:808, 1989.
91. Boi S, DeConcini M, Detassis C: Mucinous sweat gland adenocarcinoma of the inner canthus: A case report. Ann Ophthalmol 20:189, 1988.
92. Liszauer AD, Brownstein S, Codere F: Mucinous eccrine sweat gland adenocarcinoma of the eyelid. Can J Ophthalmol 23:17, 1988.
93. Khalil M, Brownstein S, Codere F, Nicolle D: Eccrine sweat gland carcinoma of the eyelid with orbital involvement. Arch Ophthalmol 98:2210, 1980.

94. Werber PJ, Hevia OH, Gretzula JC: Primary mucinous carcinoma. J Dermatol Surg Oncol 14:170, 1988.
95. Headington JT: Primary mucinous carcinoma of skin: Histochemistry and electron microscopy. Cancer 39:1055, 1977.
96. Filipe MI: Mucins in the human gastrointestinal epithelium: A review. Invest Cell Pathol 2:195, 1979.
97. El-Domeiri AA, Brasfield RD, Huvos AV, et al: Sweat gland carcinoma: A clinicopathologic study of 83 patients. Ann Surg 173:270, 1971.
98. Rosen Y, Kim B, Yermakov VA: Eccrine sweat gland tumor of clear cell origin involving the eyelids. Cancer 36:1034, 1975.
99. Grizzard WS, Torczynski E, Edwards WC: Adenocarcinoma of eccrine sweat glands. Arch Ophthalmol 94:2119, 1976.
100. Thomas JW, Fu YS, Levine MR: Primary mucinous sweat gland carcinoma of the eyelid simulating metastatic carcinoma. Am J Ophthalmol 87:29, 1979.
101. Jakobiec FA, Austin P, Iwamoto T: Primary infiltrating signet ring carcinoma of the eyelids. Ophthalmology 90:291, 1983.
102. Grove AS Jr: Personal correspondence.
103. Goldstein DJ, Barr RJ, Santa Cruz DJ: Microcystic adnexal carcinoma: A distinct clinicopathologic entity. Cancer 50:566, 1982.
104. Cooper PH, Mills SE, Leonard DD, et al: Sclerosing sweat duct (syringomatos) carcinoma. Am J Surg Pathol 9:422, 1985.
105. Cooper PH, Mills SE: Microcystic adnexal carcinoma. J Am Acad Dermatol 10:908, 1984.
106. Mayer MH, Winton GB, Smith AC: Microcystic adnexal carcinoma (sclerosing sweat duct carcinoma). Plast Reconstr Surg 84:970, 1989.
107. Glatt HJ, Proia AD, Tsoy EA: Malignant syringoma of the eyelid. Ophthalmology 91:987, 1987.
108. Grove AS: Personal correspondence.
109. Boniuk M, Zimmerman LE: Pilomatrixoma (benign calcifying epithelioma) of the eyelid and eyebrow. Arch Ophthalmol 70:399, 1963.
110. Ni C, Kimball GP, Craft SL, et al: Calcifying epithelioma. A clinicopathological analysis of 69 cases with ultrastructural studies of 2 cases. Int Ophthalmol Clin 22:63, 1982.
111. Forbis R, Helwig EB: Pilomatrixoma (calcifying epithelioma). Arch Dermatol 83:608, 1961.
112. Mohlenbeck FW: Pilomatrixoma (calcifying epithelioma). Arch Dermatol 108:532, 1973.
113. Chiaramonti A, Gilgor RS: Pilomatricomas associated with myotonic dystrophy. Arch Dermatol 114:1363, 1978.
114. Cooper PH: Pilomatricoma-like changes in the epidermal cyst of Gardner's syndrome. J Am Acad Dermatol 8:639, 1983.
115. Hashimoto K, Nelson RG, Lever WF: Calcified epithelioma of Malberbe: Histochemical and electron microscopic findings. J Invest Dermatol 46:391, 1966.
116. Hashimoto K: Calcified epithelioma of Malherbe: An electron microscopic study. J Appl Physiol 36:2607, 1965.
117. Wood MG, Purhizzai B, Beerman H: Malignant pilomatrixoma. Arch Dermatol 120:770, 1987.
118. Weedon D, Bell J, Mayze J: Matrical carcinoma of the skin. J Cutan Pathol 7:39, 1980.
119. Lopansri S, Mihm MC: Pilomatrix carcinoma or calcifying epitheliocarcinoma of Malherbe. Cancer 45:2368, 1980.
120. Headington JT, French AJ: Primary neoplasms of the hair follicle. Arch Dermatol 86:430, 1962.
121. Brownstein MH, Shapiro L: Tricholemmoma: Analysis of 40 new cases. Arch Dermatol 107:866, 1973.
122. Hidayat AA, Font RL: Trichilemmoma of the eyelid and eyebrow: A clinicopathologic review of 31 cases. Arch Ophthalmol 98:844, 1980.
123. Starink TM: Cowden's disease. J Am Acad Dermatol 11:1127, 1987.
124. Bardenstein DS, McLean IW, Nerney J, Boatwright RS: Cowden's disease. Ophthalmology 95:1038, 1988.
125. Milbouw G, Born JD, Martin D: Clinical presentation of 32 cases of Lhermitte-Duclos disease. Neurosurgery 22:124, 1988.
126. Starink TM: The Cowden syndrome: A clinical and genetic study in 21 patients. Clin Genet 29:222, 1986.
127. Padberg GW, Schot JD, Vielvoye GJ, et al: Lhermitte-Duclos disease and Cowden's disease: A single phakomatosis. Ann Neurol 29:517, 1991.
128. Reifler DM, Ballitch HA, Kessler DL, et al: Tricholemmoma of the eyelid. Ophthalmology 94:1272, 1987.
129. Schwartz JL: Trichofolliculoma. Arch Dermatol 121:262, 1985.
130. Pinkus H, Sutton RL: Trichofolliculoma. Arch Dermatol 91:46, 1965.
131. Gray HR, Helwig EB: Trichofolliculoma. Arch Dermatol 86:619, 1962.
132. Gaul LE: Heredity of multiple benign cystic epithelioma. Arch Dermatol 68:517, 1953.
133. Wolken SH, Spivey BE, Blodi F: Hereditary adenoid cystic epithelioma (Brooke's tumor). Am J Ophthalmol 68:26, 1968.
134. Sternberg I, Buckman G, Levine MR, Sterin W: Hereditary trichoepithelioma with basal cell carcinoma. Ophthalmology 93:531, 1986.
135. Mansour AM, Hidayat AA: Metastatic eyelid disease. Ophthalmology 94:667, 1987.
136. Mottow-Lippa L, Jakobiec FA, Iwamoto T: Pseudoinflammatory metastatic breast carcinoma of the orbits and lids. Ophthalmology 88:575, 1981.
137. Hood CI, Font RL, Zimmerman LE: Metastatic mammary carcinoma in the eyelid with histiocytoid appearance. Cancer 31:793, 1973.
138. Kivela T, Tarkkanen A: The Merkel cell and associated neoplasms in the eyelids and periocular regions. Surv Ophthalmol 35:171, 1990.
139. Beyer CK, Goodman M, Dickensin GR: Merkel cell tumor of the eyelid: A clinicopathologic case report. Arch Ophthalmol 101:1098, 1983.
140. Wick MR, Millns JL, Sibley RK, et al: Secondary neuroendocrine carcinomas of the skin: An immunohistochemical comparison with primary neuroendocrine carcinoma of the skin ("Merkel cell" carcinoma). J Am Acad Dermatol 13:134, 1985.
141. Eustis HS, Karcioglu ZA, Dharma S, Hoda S: Phakomatous choristoma: Clinical, histopathologic, and ultrastructural findings in a 4-month-old boy. J Pediatr Ophthalmol Strabismus 27:208, 1990.
142. Mansour AM, Barber JC, Reinecke RD, Wang FM: Ocular choristomas. Surv Ophthalmol 33:339, 1989.
143. Zimmerman LE: Phakomatous choristoma of the eyelid: A tumor of lenticular anlage. Am J Ophthalmol 71:169, 1971.
144. McMahon RT, Font RL, McLean IW: Phakomatous choristoma of eyelid: Electron microscopical confirmation of lenticular derivation. Arch Ophthalmol 94:1778, 1976.
145. Tripathi RC, Tripathi B, Ringus J: Phakomatous choristoma of the lower eyelid with psammoma body formation: A light and electron microscopic study. Ophthalmology 88:1198, 1981.
146. Rosenbaum PS, Kress Y, Slamovits TL, Font RL: Phakomatous choristoma of the eyelid: Immunohistochemical and electron microscopic observations. Ophthalmology 99:1779, 1992.

Chapter 158

▪

Pigmented Lesions of the Eyelid

CURTIS E. MARGO

Normal eyelid color in humans is caused by the effects of cutaneous carotenoids and melanin and also by the ratio of oxygenated to reduced hemoglobin in capillaries and venules. The amount and distribution of melanin influence the color of human skin more than any other single factor. This chapter confines its discussion to pigmented eyelid lesions caused by abnormalities of cutaneous melanocyte development, function, and proliferation.

BIOLOGY OF MELANIN

Skin color depends primarily on the number, size, and distribution of melanosomes, which are the cytoplasmic organelles devoted to the production of melanin. Melanin is a complex biopolymer formed by the oxidation and polymerization of tyrosine.[1, 2] The melanin molecule consists of loosely held, alternating single and double bonds that absorb broadly in the 200- to 2400-nm range of the electromagnetic spectrum. This broad absorption gives melanin its black color. The implicit function of melanin in humans is for protection against the effects of ultraviolet radiation. It mitigates carcinogenicity and also retards the effects of aging caused by exposure to the sun. Melanin is synthesized in melanosomes of epidermal melanocytes and is transferred to neighboring keratinocytes in a complex series of steps. Melanosomes are stored in keratinocytes in membrane-bound vesicles. When vesicles contain two or more melanosomes, they are referred to as melanosome complexes. Melanocytes are derived from the neural crest, and by the time of birth melanocytes take permanent residence in the basal layer of the epidermis.

The number of melanocytes varies among individuals according to anatomic location. There are approximately 2000 melanocytes per square millimeter of facial skin.[2] The density is slightly less on the eyelids than on the rest of the face. Each melanocyte is associated with approximately 35 keratinocytes. Variations in racial skin color are attributable to qualitative and quantitative differences of melanin within keratinocytes. Surprisingly, there is little difference in the density of epidermal melanocytes among the races in any given anatomic location. Keratinocytes in whites and mongoloids contain melanosome complexes filled with small melanosomes.[3] This arrangement contrasts with the arrangement in blacks, in whom melanosomes are larger and packaged individually. The size and type of vesicular packaging of melanosomes are genetically inherited traits, yet skin color can be modified by exposure to ultraviolet light and by certain hormones. The number of melanocytes in persons of all races decreases dramatically with age.

Ultraviolet light induces a small increase in the number of melanocytes as well as an increase in the production of melanin. Tanning is an expression of increased storage of melanin within keratinocytes.

The mechanism of transfer of melanosomes to keratinocytes is not fully understood. Following full melaninization, the melanosome moves from its location in the cell body to a dendritic process, where it is prepared for transfer to an adjacent keratinocyte. The investment of melanosomes in membranes occurs at the cell surface, where in whites and orientals two or more melanosomes are packaged together.

Melanosomes disintegrate in melanocytes, dermal macrophages, and keratinocytes. Melanin is durable and relatively resistant to most types of enzymatic digestion.[4] The factors that lead to the destruction of melanosomes are poorly understood.

Melanocytes of the eyelids are modified and affected by the same types of environmental factors as other cutaneous melanocytes. A general classification of primary melanocytic lesions of the skin and eyelids is presented in Table 158–1.

There are a variety of nonmelanocytic lesions of the eyelids that can become secondarily pigmented. The behavior of pigmented basal cell and squamous cell

Table 158–1. CLASSIFICATION OF CUTANEOUS MELANOCYTIC DISORDERS

Melanocytic overactivity
  Generalized: (associated with systemic disease)
  Focal: Ephelis (freckle)
Benign epithelial melanocytic hyperplasia
  Lentigo simplex
  Solar lentigo
Atypical melanocytic hyperplasia (lentigo maligna)
Melanocytic nevi
  Acquired
    Junctional
    Compound
    Dermal
    Halo
    Spitz (epithelioid/spindle cell)
    Dysplastic
    Blue nevus
    Cellular blue nevus
  Congenital (similar varieties as acquired nevi)
Malignant melanoma
  De novo
  Arising within
    Dysplastic nevus
    Lentigo maligna
    Congenital nevus

carcinomas and seborrheic keratosis is the same as that of their nonpigmented counterparts. Clinically, these lesions must be distinguished from primary melanocytic tumors, particularly cutaneous melanoma.

GENERALIZED DISTURBANCES IN SKIN PIGMENTATION

The eyelids are affected by several conditions characterized by generalized hypermelanosis of the skin. These disorders may be difficult to detect clinically in a dimly lit room or in persons whose skin is normally deeply pigmented. Patients may bring attention to the problem by complaining of a summer tan that fails to fade. Early changes in skin color generally begin at mucocutaneous junctions and in deep skin creases, particularly on the palms.

Disorders associated with generalized hypermelanosis can be classified in a variety of ways. Most diseases fall into one of several major categories: endocrine disease, nutritional disorder, toxin ingestion, and metabolic defect.[5] Diffuse hypermelanosis caused by increased secretion of β-melanocyte-stimulating hormone is the hallmark of Addison's disease. Skin color ranges from light to dark brown; pigmentary changes are enhanced by exposure to the sun. Darkening of preexisting nevi and scars also occurs.

Pellagra is characterized by generalized thickening of the skin, scaliness, and hyperpigmentation, especially of sun-exposed surfaces. The dermatosis is preceded by nonspecific symptoms. The diagnosis of pellagra is difficult to establish in the absence of skin changes because symptoms are protean.[5] Treatment with niacin resolves constitutional symptoms and improves skin changes.

Chronic exposure to inorganic arsenic results in a generalized bronze discoloration of the skin caused by increased deposition of melanin in keratinocytes.[6] Involvement of the gastrointestinal tract, bone marrow, liver, and central nervous system causes a variety of symptoms. Lead arsenate is the most frequently implicated source of poisoning. Most cases occur in rural areas; lead arsenate is used in insecticide sprays and in powders for extermination of boll weevils. Treatment includes elimination of toxic exposure and chelation with British antilewisite.

MELASMA

Melasma, or symmetric hypermelanosis of the face, is usually associated with pregnancy or with the use of oral contraceptives. An idiopathic variety also exists. The eyelids, particularly the lower eyelids, are often involved. Histologically, basal melanocytes are normal and mildly hyperplastic.[7] Keratinocytes contain an increased amount of melanin. The condition is aggravated by sunlight but is usually reversible once the offending hormonal stimulus is removed.

EPHELIS

The common freckle, or ephelid, consists of a discrete area of melanocytic overactivity. Junctional melanocytes occur in normal concentrations, but individual cells are slightly larger than normal. Neighboring keratinocytes contain more melanin than surrounding cells, which accounts for the freckle's light tan color. Freckles are more common in persons with a fair complexion. They appear on sun-exposed skin during childhood, often as early as 18 mo of age, and range in diameter from one to several millimeters. Freckles have no propensity to undergo malignant transformation.

LENTIGO SIMPLEX

Lentigo simplex is a congenital or acquired brown macule that occurs either as an isolated lesion on the skin or as part of a systemic syndrome characterized by multiple lentigines (Peutz-Jeghers syndrome, LAMB syndrome, and leopard syndrome) (Fig. 158–1).[8–10] Isolated lesions are difficult to distinguish clinically from junctional nevi, because both are small, discrete, and flat. Histologically, lentigo simplex is characterized by an increase in basal melanocytes and by mild elongation of rete ridges. Melanocytes are morphologically normal; keratinocytes contain increased amounts of melanin due to increased melanocytic activity. Nevus cells are not a feature of lentigo simplex, thus the histologic distinction with a junctional nevus is straightforward. The lentigo simplex macule is smaller and darker than a typical café-au-lait spot.

Isolated lesions need no treatment. Multiple lentigines suggest the possibility of a systemic developmental disorder.[8–10]

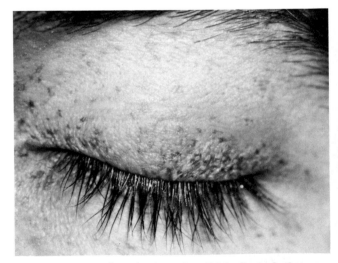

Figure 158–1. Lentigo simplex of eyelid in Peutz-Jeghers syndrome. (From Traboulsi EI, Maumenee I: Periocular pigmentation in the Peutz-Jeghers syndrome. Am J Ophthalmol 102:126, 1986. Published with permission from the American Journal of Ophthalmology. Copyright by the Ophthalmic Publishing Company.)

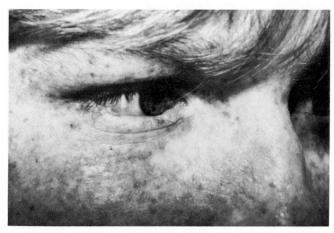

Figure 158–2. Multiple solar lentigines in a young patient with xeroderma pigmentosum. The small irregular tan macules are beginning to coalesce. The absence of lashes in the lower eyelid is due to an infiltrating basal cell carcinoma. (Courtesy of Charles Stoer, M.D.)

SOLAR LENTIGO

Solar lentigines are circumscribed tan macules induced by ultraviolet radiation, both natural and artificial. Found on the sun-exposed surfaces of the skin including the eyelids, solar lentigines consist of increased epidermal growth associated with a concomitant proliferation of melanocytes.[11] This benign proliferation differs from that found in lentigo simplex, because of the greater degree of rete ridges elongation with budlike extensions and branches. Melanocytes display no tendency to nest.

Clinically, individual lesions range in size from one to several millimeters. Upon close inspection, solar lentigines have irregular borders. In heavily sun-damaged skin, they often become confluent. Solar lentigines vary in color from tan to dark black, although most are light brown. Multiple solar lentigines may be found in patients with xeroderma pigmentosum (Fig. 158–2).

Because solar lentigines tend to occur in elderly persons, they were initially referred to as "senile" lentigines. This title has been largely abandoned because solar lentigines are known to occur in young adults as a consequence of prolonged exposure to the sun. The vast majority of all solar lentigines are biologically benign. In xeroderma pigmentosum, solar lentigines develop during the first decade of life; some evolve into lentigo maligna and lentigo maligna melanoma.

Solar lentigines, in general, require no therapy except possibly for cosmetic reasons. Prevention of solar lentigines by the use of sunscreens or blocking agents is effective, especially if initiated during childhood and continued throughout life.

MELANOCYTIC NEVI

Common Acquired Nevi

Common acquired melanocytic nevi are characterized by the presence of a modified melanocyte referred to as a nevocellular nevus cell (which is usually shortened to "nevus cell"). Unlike the normal dendritic melanocyte of the basal epidermis, nevus cells are round to polygonal with abundant cytoplasm. They display a strong tendency to nest with other nevus cells.[12, 13]

Common melanocytic nevi have been subdivided traditionally into three groups based on the location of nevus cells within the skin: *junctional nevus* when cells reside entirely within the epidermis; *dermal nevus* when cells reside entirely within the dermal adventitia; and *compound nevus* when cells are found in both locations. The use of this nomenclature tends to reinforce certain concepts regarding presumed developmental biology.[14]

In brief, the prototypic sequence begins between the ages of 5 and 20 with a small, 1- to 2-mm tan macule. Nevus cells are present only in the epidermis at this nascent stage of evolution. Thus, junctional nevi begin as flat macules. Pinpoint macules gradually enlarge up to 4 to 6 mm. As radial growth ceases during the first few decades of life, nevus cells begin to migrate into the papillary dermis, at which time the lesion is referred to as a compound nevus. Clinically, compound nevi are elevated above normal surrounding skin. They have discrete margins and palpable edges, and they are usually homogeneous tan to brown (Fig. 158–3). As the migration of cells continues into the reticular dermis, nevi become more dome shaped and less pigmented. With time, nevus cells in the epidermis eventually disappear, resulting in a dermal nevus (Fig. 158–4). By this stage of evolution, some dermal nevi are nonpigmented.

Nevus cells in the dermis induce fibroplasia. As nevus cells age, they show morphologic similarities to neural tissue. Neuronization is the beginning of obsolescence (Fig. 158–5).[14] So-called mature nevus cells resemble lymphocytes or histiocytes because they lose their cytoplasm and their tendency to nest. Nevus cells become partitioned by collagen and reticulin fibers and are replaced by a matrix that is usually indistinguishable from that found in the normal dermis. Clinically, skin returns to normal. Thus the cycle ends, giving rise to the dermatologic adage that most persons enter and leave life without clinically detectable nevi.

It is not clear, however, if all dermal melanocytes are

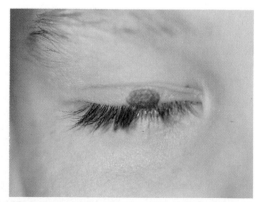

Figure 158–3. Compound nevus on the upper eyelid of a young woman. The discrete pigmented nodule encroaches on the superior lash margin.

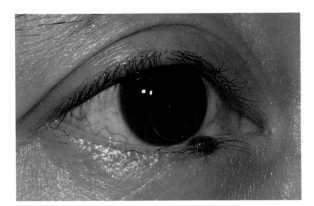

Figure 158–4. Dermal nevus of the eyelid margin. Lashes project from the surface of the pigmented nodule, which has not changed in appearance for many years.

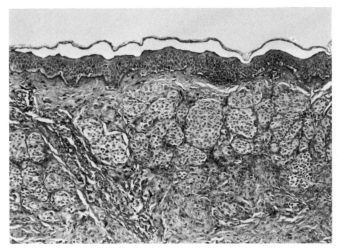

Figure 158–6. Nevocellular nevus. Well-organized nests of uniform cells fill the papillary dermis. Nuclei are centrally located, and cellular cytoplasm is abundant.

derived from junctional nevus cells according to the theory just proposed. There is some evidence to suggest that nevus cells may be derived from Schwann cells of cutaneous nerves or that possibly dermal nevus cells are simply embryogenically misdirected.

The tendency of junctional nevus cells to crowd together differs from the behavior of normal epidermal melanocytes that have their own "territory." Histologically, nuclei of nevus cells are ovoid or round and often contain a plainly visible nucleolus (Fig. 158–6). Chromatin is finely dispersed, and mitotic activity is rarely observed except in lesions from infants or young children. The amount of melanin within nevus cells is highly variable. In general, cells lose melanin during their descent into the dermis. Nevus cells are also characterized by several negative morphologic attributes: They have no intercellular connections and do not contain other visible cytoplasmic granulations or fibers.

There are several compelling reasons to believe that common nevi spawn malignant melanoma. First, melanomas have been reported to arise at the site of a nevus. Second, residual nevus cells can often be found adjacent

to melanomas in histologic section. Despite this evidence, the risks of malignant transformation must be exceptionally low. Simple calculations, based on the prevalence of common nevi (the average young adult has approximately 15) and of cutaneous melanoma,[15] indicate that one in every 150,000 nevi undergoes malignant transformation. It is generally accepted that only junctional nevus cells have the capacity to undergo malignant transformation.[16]

Common acquired nevi usually do not require treatment. Nevi can be excised if they cause mechanical irritation or are cosmetically unacceptable to the patient.

Halo Nevus

A halo nevus is an otherwise typical compound or dermal nevus surrounded by a rim of depigmentation (Fig. 158–7). Among the 108 halo nevi reported by

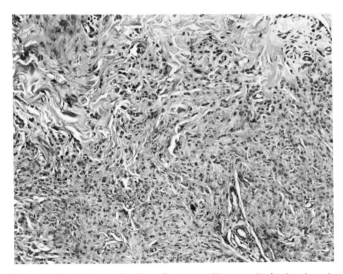

Figure 158–5. Neuronization of a nevus. Nevus cells in the dermis are becoming spindle shaped and have ill-defined boundaries.

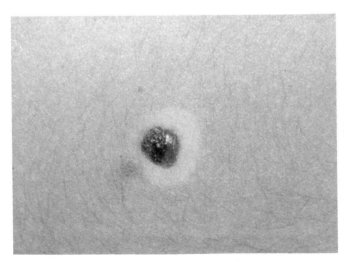

Figure 158–7. Halo nevus surrounded by a rim of nonpigmented skin. This lesion should raise the possibility of an occult melanoma. (Courtesy of Frank Flowers, M.D.)

Wayte and Helwig,[17] three were located on or near the eyelids. The importance of recognizing the halo nevus as a distinct clinicopathologic entity is due to its association with remote cutaneous melanoma.[18] Histologically, nevus cells in the upper dermis are admixed with a dense infiltrate of lymphocytes and histiocytes. Melanin is absent in the peripheral halo. Numerous immune mechanisms have been proposed for the halo phenomenon, which suggests spontaneous, but incomplete nevus regression. Because of the association of cutaneous melanoma and halo nevi, patients with a halo nevus of the eyelid or periorbital skin should be referred for evaluation of a possible occult melanoma. Occasionally, an otherwise typical cutaneous melanoma is surrounded by a rim of depigmentation.

SPITZ NEVUS

The Spitz nevus is a compound nevus composed of large spindle and epithelioid cells. The degree of melanocytic atypia in a Spitz nevus can be more pronounced than in some malignant melanomas. Its striking histologic appearance (and thus potential to be mistaken for a malignant melanoma) as well as its propensity to occur in young persons are the reasons why the Spitz nevus was initially referred to as a juvenile melanoma, which is an unfortunate term that has caused considerable confusion.

The Spitz, or spindle-epithelioid cell nevus, occurs in children and adults.[19] They are typically nonpigmented or orange-red nodules with a smooth or papillomatous surface (Fig. 158–8). Spitz nevi rarely measure more than 9 mm; most occur on the face or extremities. Despite their degree of cellular atypia, Spitz nevi are biologically benign.

Histologically, nests of large atypical spindle or epithelioid cells may be scattered at all levels of the epidermis as well as in the dermis. The axes of spindle-shaped cells are oriented perpendicular or horizontal to

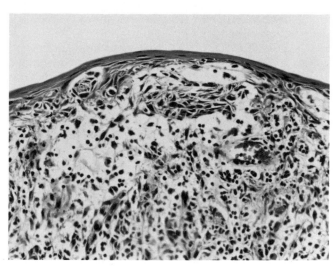

Figure 158–9. Histopathologic appearance of a Spitz nevus in a 9-year-old child shows loosely cohesive, round and spindle-shaped cells in the basal epithelium and upper dermis. Ill-defined nests of melanocytes are present at the dermal-epidermal junction.

the skin surface (Fig. 158–9). Nevus cells can be seen individually at the epidermal-dermal border, but individual atypical melanocytes (pagetoid cells) are rarely found in the suprabasilar epidermis. Horizontal spread of individual atypical melanocytes beyond the most peripheral nest occurs infrequently. Maturation of melanocytes as they descend into the dermis is an important differential feature of the Spitz nevus. Mitotic figures, particularly in younger persons, can be found, but they are rarely seen near the base of the lesion. The dermis usually contains large numbers of lymphocytes and melanophages.

A variant of the Spitz nevus, known as spindle cell nevus, is characterized by its heavy pigmentation and preponderance of spindle cells at the dermal-epidermal junction and papillary dermis.[20]

The histologic distinction between a Spitz nevus and malignant melanoma may be exceptionally difficult to make. Clinicians should consider the possibility of a Spitz nevus whenever a histopathologic diagnosis of malignant melanoma does not correlate with the clinical impression of a benign compound nevus, particularly in children.

DERMAL MELANOCYTIC LESIONS

The mongolian spot, oculodermal melanocytosis (nevus of Ota), blue nevus, and cellular blue nevus are characterized by the presence of dermal melanocytes. The ultraviolet illumination from a Wood's lamp enhances the visibility of dermal melanin, making subtle lesions easier to detect. The histogenesis of the nevus of Ota is placed into better perspective by having some knowledge of the biology of the mongolian spot.

The presence of dermal melanocytes in the skin of the lower back is a common human attribute that is clinically inapparent in most white infants and children.

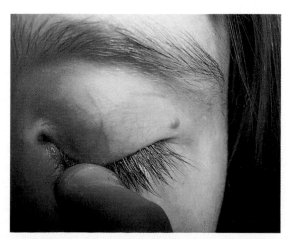

Figure 158–8. Spindle and epithelioid cell nevus (Spitz nevus) of the upper eyelid. The small flesh-colored nodule cannot be distinguished from a common nevus clinically. The diagnosis of Spitz nevus was established by excisional biopsy. (Courtesy of Kenneth Burwell, M.D.)

When dermal melanocytes are present in a threshold concentration that allows visualization over the sacrococcygeal region, they form the typical mongolian spot. It appears at birth as a uniformly blue discoloration and usually disappears within 3 to 4 yr.[21] The mongolian spot is found commonly in oriental and black infants and in 2 to 4 percent of white infants. Dermal melanocytes first appear in this region between the tenth and eleventh week of gestation. Most disappear by birth. The blue color of the mongolian spot is due to differential scattering of light by dermal melanocytes, with shorter wavelengths being preferentially scattered back to the skin surface.[22]

The mongolian spot consists of dermal dendritic melanocytes that are two to three times larger than epidermal melanocytes. They are widely scattered throughout the lower reticular dermis, usually lying parallel to dermal collagen. The lesion is benign. Persistent mongolian spots are associated with the nevus of Ota. Large, persistent mongolian spots have been reported with bilateral nevus of Ota.[23]

Nevus of Ota

The nevus of Ota, or oculodermal melanocytosis, is a unilateral light tan macule that occurs in the distribution of the first and second divisions of the trigeminal nerve (Fig. 158–10). Approximately 10 percent are bilateral. It is frequently associated with ipsilateral melanocytosis of the sclera, conjunctiva, cornea, and uveal tract. Clinically occult melanosis of the orbit and leptomeninges has been documented in patients with the nevus of Ota who have developed primary orbital and intracranial melanomas in these locations.[24, 25]

Although there are certain similarities between the nevus of Ota and the mongolian spot, they differ in several respects. First, the nevus of Ota usually lacks the uniform color of the mongolian spot. Oculodermal melanocytosis tends to have a blue, speckled appearance with irregular edges. The nevus of Ota may be present at birth, but many lesions become noticeable during the first year of life or rarely during adolescence or childhood. The edges of the macule are more irregular than the mongolian spot, and focal nodules, often having a deeper blue or tan color, may rise above the surface.

Histologically, the nevus of Ota consists of fusiform dendritic melanocytes. They tend to be more numerous and more superficial than melanocytes in the mongolian spot.[26] Slightly raised papules correspond to focal clusters of dendritic melanocytes that are histologically similar in appearance to a blue nevus.

The nevus of Ota is a benign condition that usually does not disappear with age. Several cases of malignant melanoma arising within the cutaneous component have been reported; however, the risk of cutaneous malignant transformation is exceedingly low.[26, 27] There are, nonetheless, a number of case reports of malignant melanoma of the choroid, iris, and ciliary body in patients with oculodermal melanocytosis.[28, 29] The plethora of these reports suggests an increased risk of malignant transformation, particularly in white people. Some authorities believe that the incidence of malignant transformation of uveal melanocytosis has been overestimated.[30] Nevertheless, it seems prudent, based on available information, to recommend periodic ophthalmologic examination of the uveal tract.

Blue Nevus

Blue nevi are acquired, solitary papules that range in size from 1 to 10 mm. They occur anywhere, although lesions are most common on the back of the hands and dorsa of the feet, and vary in color from blue-gray to blue.[26] The color of blue nevi, like that of the mongolian spot, is due to the reflection of shorter blue wavelengths of light by dermal melanin.

Clinically, blue nevi can be confused with a variety of skin disorders, including sclerosing hemangioma, pyogenic granuloma, dermatofibroma, and bacillary angiomatosis.

Histologically, the elongated bipolar dermal melanocytes in blue nevi lie parallel to dermal collagen. There is often excessive production of fibrous connective tissue that may extend into the reticular dermis or as deep as the subcutis. The epidermis is normal. A hybrid lesion, referred to as a combined nevus, is characterized by the mixture of a typical blue nevus and a junctional or compound nevocellular nevus.

Most blue nevi remain unchanged throughout life. Blue nevi require no therapy unless they undergo some change in their clinical appearance.

CELLULAR BLUE NEVUS

Cellular blue nevi are usually acquired, solitary lesions with a blue to blue-gray color. They are papular and usually 1 to 3 cm in diameter. They are found on all skin surfaces, but almost half occur on the lower back or buttock.[31] Occasionally, cellular blue nevi occur congenitally (Fig. 158–11).

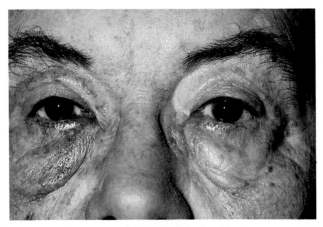

Figure 158–10. Nevus of Ota characterized by large, gray-blue discoloration of the right lower eyelid. The lesion is flat and associated with gray episcleral discoloration.

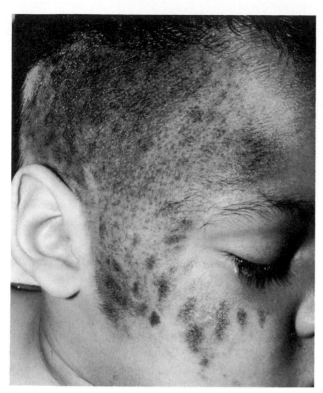

Figure 158–11. Diffuse congenital nevus of the right side of the face and scalp. Focal areas of cellular blue nevus corresponded with dark nodules within the lesion. At other sites, the tumor displayed patterns of a blue nevus and a combined nevus.

Histologically, they are biphasic lesions consisting of deeply pigmented dendritic melanocytes and clusters of pale-staining spindle cells. The pale-staining spindle cells are melanocytes containing little or no melanin and large amounts of cytoplasm. They are morphologically similar to typical nevocellular nevus cells with circular to oval nuclei and finely dispersed chromatin.

Cellular blue nevi may give rise to malignant melanoma, although the exact incidence of malignant transformation is not known.[32] The term malignant blue nevus is used to describe a cellular blue nevus, demonstrating cellular atypia and pleomorphism. Malignant blue nevi usually contain mitotic figures and areas of necrosis. The distinction between a malignant blue nevus and cutaneous metastatic melanoma may be difficult to make.

PRECURSORS TO MALIGNANT MELANOMA

The association between certain preexisting nevi, known as dysplastic nevi, and certain congenital nevi with the development of cutaneous malignant melanoma is clearly established.[33] Malignant melanoma may also arise within a macule of lentigo maligna. Identification of these precursors to cutaneous malignant melanoma is important, because their removal could substantially reduce the incidence of and mortality from melanoma.

Dysplastic Nevus

Dysplastic nevi conceptually occupy a middle ground between common nevi and malignant melanoma. Although they appear to represent a distinct clinicopathologic entity, dysplastic nevi display a spectrum of clinical and pathologic change that overlaps common nevi and early melanoma.[34–36] The concept of dysplastic nevi began with the observation that certain persons with a family history of melanoma had unusually large numbers of cutaneous nevi.[37] Careful inspection of family members revealed that their nevi were clinically atypical. The dysplastic nevus syndrome is used to describe persons with clinically dysplastic nevi and a family history of melanoma, although this definition is not universally agreed upon.[33, 36]

Dysplastic nevi tend to occur in greater numbers than common nevi. Normal young adults have an average of 12 to 20 nevi, compared with persons with dysplastic nevi who may have more than 100 lesions.[34] Like common nevi, dysplastic nevi begin to appear between the ages of 5 and 20; they are not present at birth. Large numbers of normal-appearing nevi in a child between the ages of 5 and 8 may be an early sign of the dysplastic nevus syndrome. Dysplastic nevi are usually, but not invariably, larger than common nevi. They are irregularly shaped and have indistinct borders with a pebbly surface and variable pigmentation (Fig. 158–12). The clinical spectrum is broad and overlaps both common nevi and malignant melanoma. Dysplastic nevi occur in the same general distribution as common nevi, but their frequent occurrence on the buttocks, breast, and scalp differs from the distribution associated with common nevi. Dysplastic nevi also increase in number throughout adult life rather than decline in prevalence as do common nevi.

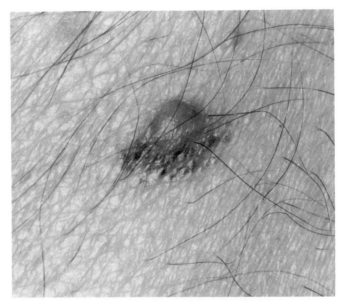

Figure 158–12. Dysplastic nevus of the skin. A tan nodule is situated eccentrically in an irregularly shaped dark macule. (Courtesy of Frank Flowers, M.D.)

The histologic diagnosis of dysplastic nevi is more subjective than the clinical diagnosis. There is disagreement concerning the ability of pathologists to delineate clearly dysplastic nevi from other nevi based solely on morphologic criteria.[38–40] The typical histologic findings are superimposed on those of a junctional or compound nevus. The microscopic findings in dysplastic nevi may occur only focally. Basilar melanocytes are increased in number and show signs of cytologic atypia. Cells often have a spindled or epithelioid appearance.[38] Nests vary in size and may fuse with one another by bridging rete ridges. Spindle-shaped melanocytes may be arranged horizontally within theques. Fibroplasia and patchy or diffuse lymphocyte infiltrates are commonly found in the dermis. Nevus cells do not undergo neuronization, and mitotic figures may be observed. Atypical melanocytes can also be found in the papillary dermis.

Dysplastic nevi, as defined clinically and confirmed pathologically, are a precursor to cutaneous melanoma. They occur both sporadically and in persons with a family history of melanoma. The reported prevalence of dysplastic nevi in the general population has been estimated between 2 and 8 percent.[34, 39] Familial dysplastic nevi are most often inherited as an autosomal dominant trait.[35, 41]

The risk of developing a cutaneous malignant melanoma among white people in the United States is approximately 0.6 percent. Among black Americans, the risk is less than 0.1 percent. In comparison, the overall risk in persons with dysplastic nevi is estimated to be 10 percent. The relative lifetime risk of developing a cutaneous melanoma may approach 100 percent in some melanoma-prone families with dysplastic nevi.[41] The importance of recognizing the clinical features of dysplastic nevi cannot be overemphasized. Early diagnosis and surgical removal before malignant transformation occurs is appropriate prophylaxis.

The nomenclature used to describe the dysplastic nevus syndrome is not ideal and has created confusion regarding central concepts about the disorder. The dysplastic nevus syndrome, as defined by the Consensus Conference on Precursors to Malignant Melanoma, is "the presence of multiple dysplastic nevi in two or more family members."[33] This definition does not fully satisfy the criterion of a syndrome, and it complicates the distinction between familial and sporadic dysplastic nevi.[40] The term "dysplastic nevus" itself is also somewhat ambiguous, because histologically it can refer to any lesion displaying cytologic atypia and abnormal maturation of melanocytes. It is argued that these histologic findings are ubiquitous in the general population and are not a specific marker of a syndrome.[39, 40] Dysplasia may in fact represent an active phase of radial growth in banal nevi.[39] Some authorities claim that the current nomenclature is inappropriate because it fails to consider the variable genotypic expression and heterogeneity of dysplastic nevi.[40] The term "familial atypical multiple mole syndrome" is synonymous with the dysplastic nevus syndrome, and its use has been advocated on the basis of being more fully descriptive.[35, 40]

Currently, the terms dysplastic nevus and dysplastic nevus syndrome are firmly entrenched in the medical vernacular. They refer to clinicopathologic entities characterized by clinically and histologically atypical melanocytic nevi. Dysplastic nevi are considered to be markers for cutaneous melanoma. Their association, if any, with uveal melanoma remains controversial.[42]

Congenital Melanocytic Nevus

Certain congenital melanocytic nevi are precursors to cutaneous melanoma.[33, 43, 44] There are dozens of reports in the literature describing malignant melanoma arising within a large congenital melanocytic nevus, many of them in children. It is unlikely that these reported cases can be logically attributed to coincidence. Based on the incidence of large congenital melanocytic nevi and the incidence of cutaneous malignant melanoma in children, it is estimated that the chances of these two lesions occurring together as random events are about 1 in 400 million.[45]

Nearly a third of all prepubertal cutaneous melanomas have been associated with large congenital melanocytic nevi, which is more than 50,000 times greater than anticipated if the association were due to chance alone.[46] Thus, there is compelling evidence that large congenital melanocytic nevi are precursors to cutaneous melanoma. Unfortunately, there is no universally accepted definition of "large." The distinction between small, medium, and large congenital nevi is unclear.[43, 47] The definition of a "large" congenital nevus on the head or neck has differed from that used to describe lesions on the trunk or extremities.[48] The reasoning behind the differences in definition is not entirely clear. Most of the information about the behavior of congenital periocular melanocytic nevi is inferred from data based on lesions located below the neck.

Many authorities use 2 cm or less as the cut-off point for small congenital nevi[47]; however, this does not necessarily imply that anything larger than 2 cm is a "large" nevus. A study from the Danish Health Service defined a "large" nevus on the face as being equal to or larger than the surface area of the affected patient's palm.[48] This definition has merit since it is a relative measure of total skin area, and size in this sense is minimally influenced by surface area changes due to growth.

Using this definition, almost 20 percent of 151 large congenital melanocytic nevi occurring in persons born in Denmark over a 60-yr period were on the head and neck, and many involved the eyelids.[48]

Congenital melanocytic nevi can become gigantic, involving more than half of the total skin surface of some newborns. Garment nevus describes the clothing-like distribution that many of these nevi assume. For the purposes of this discussion, the term "large" refers to a congenital nevus 4 cm or larger in adults or equal to the surface area of a patient's palm as described by the Danish Health Service.[48]

The risk of malignant transformation of a large congenital melanocytic nevus reported in the literature has ranged from 4.6 to 41 percent.[49] Most of these estimates,

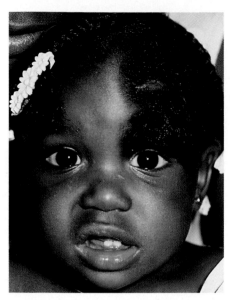

Figure 158–13. A large congenital nevus involving the upper eyelid and extending into the scalp. The nevus is elevated, indurated, and covered with hair. (From Margo CE, Habal MB: Large congenital melanocytic nevus: Light and electron microscopic findings. Published courtesy of Ophthalmology 94:960, 1987.)

however, are biased because they have been based on data collected at referral centers that tend to accumulate difficult cases. Perhaps the most reliable data come from the Danish Health Service, which keeps medical records on all its citizens.[48] In their 60-yr study of 151 patients, they found that the risk of malignant transformation was between 4 and 6 percent.

Clinically, large congenital nevi are obvious at birth. They are heavily pigmented and have raised surfaces with irregular borders (Fig. 158–13). Many congenital nevi are covered with hair. When located on both the upper and lower eyelids, congenital nevi often line up at the same position of both eyelid margins (so-called kissing nevi), indicating that they initially formed when the eyelids were fused. All races are affected, including blacks.

Histologically, congenital melanocytic nevi display a variety of morphologic patterns, including compound nevus, dermal nevus, blue nevus, cellular blue nevus, spindle cell nevus, and epithelioid cell nevus. Often several of these morphologic patterns are found in a single lesion. Congenital nevi may contain areas resembling neurofibroma or schwannoma or display foci of heterotopic tissue such as bone or cartilage.[50] The diagnosis of congenital nevus may often be anticipated histologically by identifying melanocytes in the deep reticular dermis or subcutis, which is an unusual location for cells in common acquired nevi.[51]

Malignant melanomas have been reported in congenital melanocytic nevi of all histologic varieties, including dermal nevus.[49, 50, 52] The prognosis once malignant transformation has occurred is especially grave. Mortality approaches 100 percent and most deaths occur within 2 yr.[53] It is not entirely clear why patients with melanomas arising in congenital nevi do so poorly. One possibility

is the difficulty of early clinical detection. Because congenital nevi are typically heavily pigmented and have rough irregular surfaces, early malignant changes are difficult to identify. Also, unlike common acquired nevi that supposedly undergo malignant transformation at the epidermal-dermal junction, malignant transformation in congenital nevi can occur within the dermis.[51] In such a situation, the tumor may have to attain considerable size before it is clinically detectable.

The histopathologic interpretation of malignant transformation is also fraught with difficulty (Fig. 158–14). The histologic criteria for cutaneous melanoma in prepubertal children is not absolutely clear. Benign nevi in infants and children normally display some degree of cytologic atypia. Mitotic figures, multinucleated giant cells, and individually disposed suprabasilar melanocytes can also be found.

The management of large congenital melanocytic nevi must be individualized, based on the perceived risk of future malignant transformation and the difficulty of surgical excision.[49] If large congenital melanocytic nevi are precursors to cutaneous melanoma, their complete removal should prevent malignant transformation. Periocular congenital nevi also are a cosmetic problem. These considerations must be weighed against the difficulty of surgical extirpation. Some lesions involve the entire thickness of both of the eyelids, making total removal of these lesions impossible (Fig. 158–15). Because there is some reason to believe that the risk of malignant transformation may be proportional to the absolute size of congenital nevi, it can be logically argued that partial removal would reduce the risk of future malignancy equivalent to the proportion excised. This reasoning may have a role in cases in which vital structures such as lid margin need to be preserved. Ophthalmologists should work with dermatologists in advising patients and families about the perceived risks

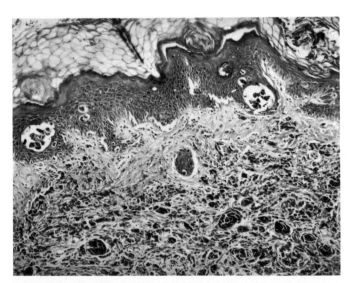

Figure 158–14. Histopathologic appearance of a congenital nevus that displays considerable cellular atypia. Atypical melanocytes are found in nests and are also found individually in the epidermis. The dermis contains heavily pigmented nevus cells.

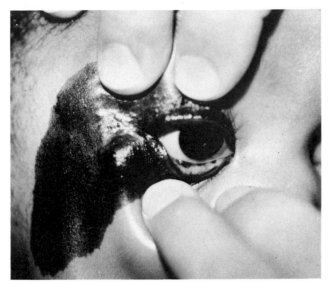

Figure 158–15. A large congenital nevus involving both eyelids. The jet-black lesion, which for the most part is flat, contains numerous firm nodules. The conjunctiva is also involved. (From Margo CE, Habal MB, Rabinowitz M: Periocular congenital melanocytic nevi. J Pediatr Ophthalmol Strab 23:222, 1986.)

of malignancy. Close and continued follow-up is necessary for any patient who does not desire surgical removal of these nevi.

The natural history of small congenital nevi, particularly their potential for malignant transformation, is not entirely clear (Fig. 158–16).[54] Although small congenital nevi are less difficult to excise, optimal management of these lesions is still controversial.[55]

Lentigo Maligna

Lentigo maligna is a variably pigmented macule consisting of a proliferation of cytologically atypical intraepidermal melanocytes found on sun-damaged skin.[56] Some semantic confusion exists concerning the exact classification of lentigo maligna. The controversy revolves around whether it is a form of in situ malignant melanoma or a type of melanocytic dysplasia. In either situation, there is agreement that lentigo maligna is a premalignant condition that has the potential to evolve into a fully invasive malignant melanoma.[57–63] Approximately 30 percent of untreated lesions develop nodules indicative of dermal invasion.[64]

The association of lentigo maligna and malignant melanoma was first described by Hutchinson in 1892. Although lentigo maligna occurs most commonly on the cheek, the first case reported by Hutchinson involved the eyelid.[63] The lesion has been referred to by a variety of names; two of the most popular synonyms are Hutchinson's freckle and precancerous melanosis. Malignant melanoma, arising within a lentigo maligna, is known as a lentigo maligna melanoma.

Lentigo maligna is a relatively common cutaneous condition found in as many as one of every 300 persons.[58] It is difficult to determine the average age of onset of lentigo maligna from published studies, because histologically verified lesions are heavily biased with lentigo maligna melanoma. The mean age of patients when lesions were first noted, from one large series, was 47.[59] Age is an important consideration in clinical differential diagnosis, because the average age of onset of a lentigo maligna is 2 to 3 decades beyond the age of onset of common acquired nevi.

The tan macule of lentigo maligna is flush to the surface of the skin and has no palpable edge (Fig. 158–17). Macules enlarge slowly over 5 to 10 yr. This phase of intraepithelial growth is referred to as "radial growth." During this phase of melanocytic proliferation, however, the color of macules may darken, fade, or become variegated (Fig. 158–18). Borders that were initially smooth also change, developing irregular notches and indentations.

Histologically, lentigo maligna is characterized by a predominantly non-nesting basal proliferation of atypical melanocytes (Fig. 158–19). Individually disposed cells display mild to moderate pleomorphism. In highly proliferative areas, cells tend to cluster forming ill-

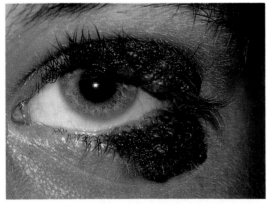

Figure 158–16. Small congenital nevus of upper and lower eyelids (so-called "kissing nevus"). This pigmented verrucous tumor, although large for a typical acquired nevus, is less than 2 cm at its greatest diameter and is thus considered "small" for a congenital nevus.

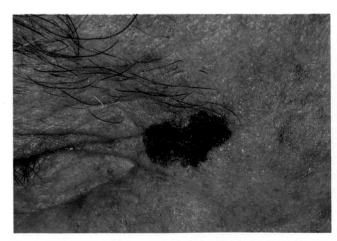

Figure 158–17. Lentigo maligna of the outer canthal skin. The dark brown lesion is flat. (Courtesy of Frank Flowers, M.D.)

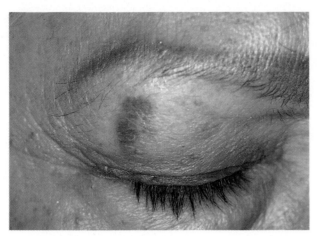

Figure 158–18. Lentigo maligna of the right upper eyelid. The macule has a patchy light tan color.

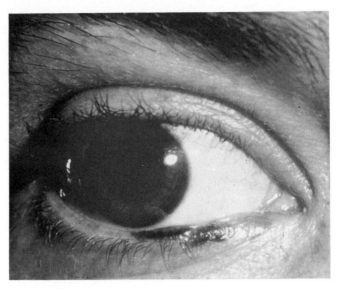

Figure 158–20. Lentigo maligna melanoma of the lower eyelid that had been present for more than 10 yr in a 43-year-old woman. The lesion is deeply pigmented and slightly elevated. (AFIP Accession No. 1240623.)

defined nests, making the distinction with a junctional nevus difficult. Nuclei are hyperchromatic and have irregular shapes, often angulated or spindled. Multinucleated cells may be found. Atypical cells can extend into hair follicles. Fixation artifact makes atypical melanocytes look as if they have retracted from adjacent cells. The dermis usually contains chronic inflammatory cells, mainly lymphocytes and pigmented macrophages.

The natural history of lentigo maligna is not well documented. Most lesions expand slowly over years, but some may undergo rapid radial growth. Most melanomas that arise in lentigo maligna do so 10 to 15 yr after a macule is first noted.[59, 60] The most critical and unfortunately most poorly understood aspect of the behavior of lentigo maligna deals with malignant transformation. The risk of malignant transformation is increased for lesions greater than 4 cm in diameter and for darkly pigmented lesions.[58] Lentigo maligna melanoma has been associated with relative or absolute inability to tan with natural sunlight.[60] Based on epidemiologic data, the lifetime risk of malignant melanoma arising in lentigo maligna is less than 5 percent.[61]

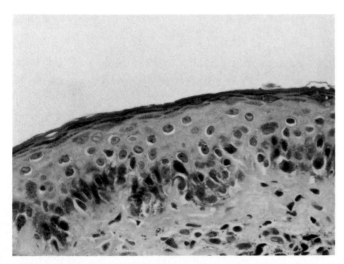

Figure 158–19. Histopathologic features of lentigo maligna showing a proliferation of atypical basal melanocytes.

The first clinical signs of malignant transformation are heralded by surface elevation or frank nodule formation (Fig. 158–20). Subtle distortions of the surface of a lentigo maligna may indicate early dermal invasion. These changes are seen best with oblique lighting or with a hand-held magnifying lens. Unfortunately, some clinically flat macules can demonstrate invasive melanoma when biopsied.

Lentigo maligna must be distinguished from solar lentigo and lentigo simplex. Lentigo maligna is always found on sun-damaged skin and is larger than either a solar lentigo or a lentigo simplex. Because lentigo maligna can be confused with a variety of other pigmented lesions found around the eye, a biopsy should be taken of any suspicious pigmented macule.[62–65]

Surgical removal of lentigo maligna is the most reliable means of extirpation. But the size and location on the eyelids may preclude surgical excision because of cosmetic or functional problems. Alternate therapies including cryotherapy, topical 5-fluorouracil, dermabrasion, and electrodesiccation and curettage are also difficult to apply to the eyelids but may deserve consideration in certain cases. In patients who are chronically ill with stable lesions, or in patients with limited life expectancy, clinical observation is another alternative.

The management of lentigo maligna melanoma is discussed in the section on malignant melanoma.

MALIGNANT MELANOMA

Cutaneous malignant melanoma is the leading cause of death due to primary skin tumors. For reasons that are not fully understood, the incidence of cutaneous malignant melanoma has risen steadily during the last several decades.[66] The clinical and pathologic features of malignant melanoma of the eyelids generally parallel those of cutaneous melanoma elsewhere. Fortunately, cutaneous melanomas rarely occur on the eyelids with 32 cases in the two largest series reported in the literature.[67, 67a] The term malignant melanoma is a redundant expression since "benign melanomas" do not exist.

Cutaneous melanomas usually affect persons between 20 and 60 yr of age, except for lentigo maligna melanoma, which occurs predominantly in the elderly. Cutaneous melanoma has no sexual predilection but is uncommon in blacks and children.[53, 68] The incidence in blacks is approximately one seventh that of whites; orientals are at intermediate risk.

Cutaneous melanomas are divided into four groups according to clinical and histopathologic criteria.[69] Lesions from three of these groups occur on the eyelids: nodular melanoma, superficial spreading melanoma, and lentigo maligna melanoma. The fourth type, acral lentiginous melanoma, involves the distal extremities and is not discussed. The prognosis for each type of cutaneous melanoma depends on many factors. The single most important factor related to survival for localized disease is the anatomic level of invasion within the skin.[69]

Clinically, a superficially spreading melanoma displays a combination of colors, including tan, black, and gray. Dull pink or rose may be the dominant color of some lesions. Unlike lentigo maligna, lesions of superficial spreading melanoma are elevated above the surface of the skin. A definite, although subtle edge is almost always palpable (Fig. 158–21). The elevation of superficial spreading melanomas corresponds to the proliferation of cells within the papillary dermis that occurs early in the course of the disease. Lesions, however, have a prolonged radial growth phase characterized by centrifugual enlargement. Borders are typically irregular and notched. The biologic behavior of superficial spreading melanomas changes with the development of deeper dermal invasion. Nodule formation within a superficial spreading melanoma heralds dermal invasion and thus transformation into the so-called vertical growth phase.

Histologically, the atypical melanocytes of superficial

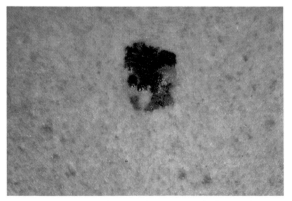

Figure 158–21. Superficial spreading melanoma. The elevated, multinodular lesion is characterized by its variegated colors. Patches of pink and flesh are admixed with dark brown. (Courtesy of Frank Flowers, M.D.)

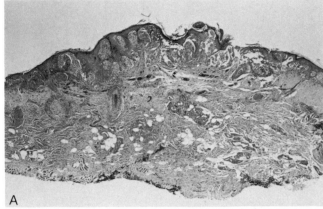

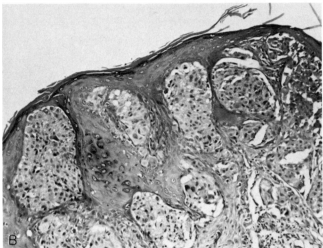

Figure 158–22. *A,* Histologically, a superficial spreading melanoma displays clusters of atypical melanocytes in the epidermis and papillary dermis. *B,* Atypical melanocytes within the epidermis form nests.

spreading melanoma have a tendency to spread into the epidermis, either individually (e.g., pagetoid invasion) or in nests (Fig. 158–22). This pattern of intraepithelial invasion contrasts with the findings in lentigo maligna and lentigo maligna melanoma in which atypical melanocytes are confined to basal layers.

Nodular melanoma evolves much more rapidly than either lentigo maligna or superficial spreading melanoma. They usually have a uniform blue-black color and a spherical, or blueberry-like nodularity. The color may vary, however, from rose-gray to black. Nodular melanomas can be polypoid or irregularly lumpy. Plaque-like lesions of nodular melanoma can be distinguished clinically from typical superficial spreading melanoma by having a more uniform color.

Histologically, two methods are used to express the depth of invasion. Clark and associates,[70] and McGovern[71] developed criteria to ascertain a prognosis by dividing depth of invasion into five anatomic levels (Table 158–2). In situ lesions (Clark level 1) are confined to the epidermis. Level 2 tumors penetrate but do not fill the papillary dermis. Level 3 tumors fill the papillary dermis. Level 4 tumors extend into the reticular dermis, whereas level 5 tumors penetrate subcutaneous tissue.

Table 158–2. CUTANEOUS MALIGNANT MELANOMA

Levels of Invasion*

Level I:	Confined to the epidermis
Level II:	Invasion into the papillary dermis
Level III:	Tumor fills the papillary dermis
Level IV:	Invasion of the reticular dermis
Level V:	Invasion of the subcutaneous fat

*From Clark WH Jr: A classification of malignant melanoma in man correlated with histogenesis and biologic behavior. *In* Montagna W, Hu F (eds): Advances in Biology of Skin. VIII: The Pigmentary System. Oxford, Pergamon Press, 1967, pp 621–647.

Table 158–3. CUTANEOUS MELANOMA: GENERAL STAGING CRITERIA

Stage	Clinical	Histopathology
I	Localized disease; no clinically palpable regional nodes	Absence of tumor in the regional nodes
II	Palpable regional nodes	Tumor present in the regional nodes
III	Evidence of a distant metastasis	Documentation of a distant metastasis

Breslow[72] developed a quantitative method that measures the depth of invasion in millimeters. Measurements are made from the granular cell layer to the deepest tumor cell, using a calibrated micrometer within the microscope. For ulcerated tumors, measurements are taken from the base of the ulcer. The combination of level plus thickness of tumor appears to correlate better with survival than anatomic level of invasion.[73] Patients with tumors less than 0.75 mm thick have nearly a 100 percent survival rate. Tumors thicker than 3 mm have a poor prognosis. The relationship between tumor thickness and survival for tumors between 0.75 and 3 mm is not perfectly linear, however. Tumor thickness is negatively correlated with duration of survival. Thicker tumors have earlier recurrences and shorter duration of survival.[74]

No single prognostic factor can accurately predict the outcome for localized (stage 1) disease.[73] Other clinical and histopathologic features of melanoma also influence the prognosis, although to a lesser degree than tumor thickness. Multivariant analysis has revealed that anatomic location, presence or absence of surface ulceration, and degree of lymphocyte response are independent variables related to outcome.[73–75]

The staging of cutaneous melanoma is based on the presence or absence of region and distant metastasis (Table 158–3). Patients with stages 2 and 3 of the disease have a poor prognosis.[73]

Skin lesions suspected to be melanoma should be photographed for gross morphologic evaluation before biopsy is taken, because photographs permit precise topographical analysis.[76] Photographic assessment of the largest nodule diameter may be a more important prognostic factor than the greatest lesion diameter.[76]

There is a complex interaction between cutaneous melanoma and the host's immune system. Cutaneous melanoma has one of the highest rates of total spontaneous regression of any tumor, estimated to be nearly 15 percent.[77] Partial spontaneous regression is also well documented. Historically, the observation of halos around normal nevi in patients with spontaneously regressed melanomas was the first vivid clinical indication of a host-mediated response to the melanin system.[78] The systemic depigmentation syndromes associated with cutaneous melanoma are considered to be paraneoplastic syndromes. Laboratory studies indicate that the immune response is both cell-mediated and humoral.[79]

The differential diagnosis of cutaneous melanoma of the eyelid is broad and includes a variety of benign and malignant skin lesions (Table 158–4).[62–65] In general, the two most difficult lesions to distinguish from cutaneous melanoma are secondarily pigmented basal cell and squamous carcinomas. Any lesion that is suspicious for melanoma should be photographed, and then a biopsy should be taken and sent for permanent histologic sections.

The optimal form of therapy for localized stage 1 melanoma is not known. The thickness of the primary melanoma is the dominant prognostic factor for clinical stage 1 disease, although survival rates vary according to the specific location of the tumor.[73, 80] The traditional therapy for melanomas involving the papillary dermis is wide surgical excision, usually taking as much as 5 cm of uninvolved skin. The rationale for such large surgical margins has been based on a variety of anecdotal information. Numerous studies addressing the importance of large surgical margins provide conflicting results.[81] Interpretation of the data is difficult because of many compounding and uncontrolled variables. The World Health Organization showed no correlation between the magnitude of surgical margins and mortality rates when corrections were made for anticipated higher mortality rates for thicker tumors.[82] Several other studies, however, do show a trend toward an increasing number of recurrences with narrower margins.[81] Most authorities agree that narrow surgical margins are reasonable if they help to preserve vital structures such as the eyelids, given the lack of correlation between survival and magnitude of margins.[81] There appears to be no advantage to the use of micrographically controlled excision (Mohs' surgery) for eyelid melanomas compared with conventional methods of excision. Survival rates following micrographically controlled excision are similar to those using less time-consuming and costly methods of extirpation.[83, 84]

The role of radical neck dissection in stage 2 melanoma of the head and neck is unclear. Limited data

Table 158–4. LESIONS THAT SIMULATE CUTANEOUS MALIGNANT MELANOMA

Pigmented squamous cell carcinoma
Pigmented basal cell carcinoma
Pigmented seborrheic keratosis
Pigmented actinic keratosis
Pigmented Bowen's disease
Apocrine cystadenoma (blue dome cyst)
Angiokeratoma
Capillary aneurysm (venous lake)

suggest that localized recurrences are reduced when regional lymph nodes are removed, but overall survival may not be improved.[85]

CLINICAL APPROACH: AN OVERVIEW

There is no simple approach to the clinical evaluation of such a broad spectrum of disorders, referred to collectively as "pigmented lesions" of the eyelid. Several principles of clinical evaluation are offered. First and foremost, the greatest patient good is served by being able to diagnose premalignant and malignant lesions at their earliest stage. Thus, clinicians must be familiar with the general symptoms and signs of cutaneous melanoma and its precursor lesions. Because cutaneous melanomas are relatively rare on the eyelids, an ophthalmologist may be uncomfortable in evaluating and diagnosing these lesions. A biopsy must be taken of suspicious lesions, or the patient referred to a dermatologist.

The assessment of pigmented lesions of the skin is usually based on several important features. Pigmented lesions are either congenital or acquired. Lesions present at birth, for all practical purposes, are divided into "congenital nevi" and nevus of Ota. Although the nevus of Ota is, in fact, a type of congenital melanocytic nevus, it has no real propensity for cutaneous malignant transformation. Since all forms of congenital melanocytic nevi, other than the nevus of Ota, are associated with some risk of future malignancy, patients and their families should be referred to a professional experienced in dealing with these skin lesions. Management must be individualized based on the perceived risk of malignant transformation and on the difficulty of surgical excision.

Most pigmented lesions acquired throughout life are benign. Any newly acquired skin lesion after the age of 40 should be viewed suspiciously.

Small flat macules (freckles, solar lentigines, and lentigines simplex) are benign and have no risk of malignant transformation. Tan macules greater than 1.5 cm in diameter that develop in persons over the age of 45 are usually confluent solar lentigines or lentigo maligna. If the clinical distinction is not clear, a biopsy should be taken of the lesion.

There is no real substitute for experience when it comes to evaluating pigmented skin nodules. Included in this group of lesions are malignant melanoma, melanocytic nevi, and a dozen or more lesions that can simulate malignant melanoma (see Table 158–4).

Recent enlargement, darkening, or ulceration of a mole are signs that suggest a malignant change. Unfortunately, these features are usually correlated with tumors that are already deeply invasive and have a poor prognosis. The early detection of primary cutaneous melanoma can be made best by an assessment of the color, borders, and surface features.[86]

Color change is a frequent finding in malignant melanoma, particularly haphazard shades of red, white, or blue. Nodular-type melanomas evolve rapidly and tend to have uniform color (usually bluish-black or bluish-

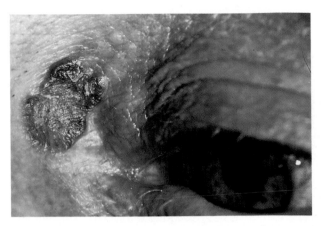

Figure 158–23. Pigmented basal cell carcinoma of the medial canthal skin. This ulcerated, infiltrated tumor cannot be clinically distinguished from a malignant melanoma. (From Resnick RI, Sadun A, Albert DM: Basal cell epithelioma: An unusual case. Ophthalmology 88:1182, 1981.)

red), whereas superficial spreading melanomas are often variegated.

A notch or indentation in the border of an acquired pigmented lesion suggests melanoma, especially the superficial, spreading type.

Irregular surface features are characteristic of melanoma. Irregular topography may be palpable or visible with direct or side illumination.

Many of the features of cutaneous melanoma are seen in pigmented basal cell carcinoma (Fig. 158–23), seborrheic keratosis (Fig. 158–24), and other melanocytic nevi, especially dysplastic nevi. A biopsy must be taken of suspicious lesions, and this should be sent for permanent sections.

Pigmented dermal lesions (e.g., nevus of Ota, blue nevus, cellular blue nevus) are present from birth or are acquired during childhood or adolescence. Any changes in the color, configuration, or topography of these lesions need to be assessed histologically, but keep in

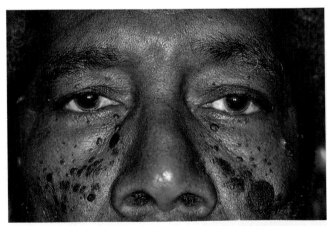

Figure 158–24. Multiple pigmented seborrheic keratoses in a black patient with a pulmonary plasmacytoma. The development of numerous seborrheic keratoses has been associated with visceral malignancies.

mind that malignant transformation is rare in this setting.

SUMMARY

Melanocytes of the eyelids manifest a wide variety of abnormalities owing to developmental and acquired disease. The importance of being familiar with the clinical features of cutaneous melanoma is obvious, because it is a potentially lethal eyelid tumor. Although the basis of neoplastic transformation of melanocytes is not fully understood, the recognition and treatment of precursor lesions reduce the risk of future malignancy. The diagnosis and treatment of cutaneous melanoma in its early stages will minimize morbidity and reduce mortality.

REFERENCES

1. Prota G: Recent advances in the chemistry of melanogenesis in mammals. J Invest Dermatol 75:122, 1980.
2. Fitzpatrick TB, Szabo G: The melanocyte: Cytology and cytochemistry. J Invest Dermatol 32:197, 1959.
3. Szabo G, Gerald AB, Fitzpatrick TB: Racial differences in human pigmentation on the ultrastructural level. J Cell Biol 39:132a, 1968.
4. Szabo G, Gerald AB, Pathak MA, et al: Racial differences in the fate of melanosomes in human epidermis. Nature 222:1081, 1969.
5. Braverman IM: Skin Signs of Systemic Diseases. Philadelphia, WB Saunders, 1979.
6. Poskanzer DC: Heavy metals. In Petersdorf RG, Adams RD, Braunwald E, et al: Harrison's Principles of Internal Medicine, 10th ed. New York, McGraw-Hill, 1983.
7. Sanchez NP, Pathak MA, Sato S, et al: Melasma: A clinical, light microscopic, ultrastructural, and immunofluorescence study. J Am Acad Dermatol 4:698, 1981.
8. Gorlin RJ, Anderson RC, Blaw M: Multiple lentigines syndrome. Am J Dis Child 117:652, 1969
9. Rhodes AR, Silverman RA, Harrist TJ, Perez-Atayde AR: Mucocutaneous lentigines, cardiomucocutaneous myxomas, and multiple blue nevi: The "LAMB" syndrome. J Am Acad Dermatol 10:72, 1984.
10. Traboulsi EI, Maumenee IH: Periocular pigmentation in the Peutz-Jeghers syndrome. Am J Ophthalmol 102:126, 1986.
11. Montagna W, Hu F, Carlisle K: A reinvestigation of solar lentigines. Arch Dermatol 116:1151, 1980.
12. Becker SW: Diagnosis and treatment of pigmented nevi. Arch Dermatol Syphilol 60:44, 1949.
13. Bently-Phillips CB, Marks R: The epidermal component of melanocytic nevi. J Cutan Pathol 3:190, 1976.
14. Mishima Y: Macromolecular changes in pigmentary disorders. Arch Dermatol 91:519, 1965.
15. Pack GT, Lenson N, Berber DM: Regional distribution of moles and melanomas. Arch Surg 65:862, 1952.
16. Allen AC, Spitz S: Histogenesis and clinicopathologic correlation of nevi and malignant melanomas. Arch Dermatol Syphilol 69:150, 1954.
17. Wayte DM, Helwig EB: Halo nevi. Cancer 22:69, 1968.
18. Epstein WL, Sagebiel R, Spitler K, et al: Halo nevi and melanoma. JAMA 225:373, 1973.
19. Weedon D, Little JH: Spindle and epithelioid cell nevi in children and adults: A review of 211 cases of the Spitz nevus. Cancer 40:217, 1977.
20. Sagebiel RW, Chinn EK, Egbert BM: Pigmented spindle cell nevus: Clinical and histologic review of 90 cases. Am J Surg Pathol 8:645, 1984.
21. Hidano A: Persistent mongolian spot in the adult. Arch Dermatol 103:680, 1971.
22. Kopf AW, Weidman AI: Nevus of Ota. Arch Dermatol 85:195, 1962.
23. Hidano A, Kajima H, Ikeda S, et al: Natural history of nevus of Ota. Arch Dermatol 95:187, 1967.
24. Haim T, Meyer E, Kerner H, Zonis S: Oculodermal melanocytosis (nevus of Ota) and orbital malignant melanoma. Ann Ophthalmol 14:1132, 1982.
25. Sang DN, Albert DM, Sober AJ, McMeekin TO: Nevus of Ota with contralateral cerebral melanoma. Arch Ophthalmol 95:1820, 1977.
26. Dorsey CS, Montgomery H: Blue nevus and its distinction from mongolian spot and the nevus of Ota. J Invest Dermatol 22:225, 1954.
27. Kopf AW, Bart RS: Malignant blue (Ota's) nevus. J Dermatol Surg Oncol 8:442, 1982.
28. Roy PE, Schaeffer EM: Nevus of Ota and choroidal melanoma. Surv Ophthalmol 12:130, 1967.
29. Albert DM, Scheie HG: Nevus of Ota with malignant melanoma of the choroid. Arch Ophthalmol 69:774, 1963.
30. Blodi FC: Ocular melanocytosis and melanoma. Am J Ophthalmol 80:389, 1975.
31. Rodriguez HA, Ackerman LV: Cellular blue nevus: Clinical pathologic study of 45 cases. Cancer 21:393, 1968.
32. Hernandez FJ: Malignant blue nevus: A light and electron microscopic study. Arch Dermatol 107:741, 1973.
33. Consensus Conference: Precursors to malignant melanoma. JAMA 251:1864, 1984.
34. Greene MH, Clark WH Jr, Tucker MA, et al: Acquired precursors of cutaneous malignant melanoma: The familial dysplastic nevus syndrome. N Engl J Med 312:91, 1985.
35. Lynch HT, Fusaro RM, Danes BS, et al: A review of hereditary malignant melanoma including biomarkers in familial atypical multiple mole melanoma syndrome. Cancer Genet Cytogenet 8:325, 1983.
36. Lynch HT, Fusaro RM, Pester J, et al: Tumour spectrum in the FAMM syndrome. Br J Cancer 44:553, 1981.
37. Clark WH Jr, Reimer RR, Greene M, et al: Origin of familial malignant melanomas from heritable melanocytic lesions. The B-K mole syndrome. Arch Dermatol 114:732, 1978.
38. Lever WF, Schaumburg-Lever G: Histopathology of the Skin, 7th ed. Philadelphia, JB Lippincott, 1990, p 770.
39. Piepkorn M, Meyer LJ, Goldgar D, et al: The dysplastic nevus: A highly prevalent trait correlating poorly with clinical phenotype. J Cutan Pathol 15:337, 1988.
40. Lynch HT, Fusaro RM: National Institutes of Health consensus report on precursors to malignant melanoma: A difference in opinion. JAMA 252:2872, 1984.
41. Greene MH, Clark WH Jr, Tucker MA, et al: High risk of malignant melanoma in melanoma-prone families with dysplastic nevi. Ann Intern Med 102:458, 1985.
42. Taylor MR, Guerry D 4th, Bondi EE, et al: Lack of association between intraocular melanoma and cutaneous dysplastic nevi. Am J Ophthalmol 98:478, 1984.
43. Margo CE, Rabinowicz IM, Habal MB: Periocular congenital melanocytic nevi. J Pediatr Ophthalmol Strabismus 23:222, 1986.
44. Alper J, Holmes LB, Mihm MC Jr: Birthmarks with serious medical significance: Nevocellular nevi, sebaceous nevi, and multiple café-au-lait spots. J Pediatr 95:696, 1979.
45. Castilla EE, Graca Dutra MD, Orioli-Parreiras IM: Epidemiology of congenital pigmented naevi. I: Incidence rates and relative frequencies. Br J Dermatol 104:307, 1981.
46. Rhodes AR: Neoplasms: Benign neoplasias, hyperplasias, and dysplasias of melanocytes. In Fitzpatrick TB, Eisen AZ, Wolff K, et al (eds): Dermatology in General Medicine, 3rd ed. New York, McGraw-Hill, 1987.
47. Mark GJ, Mihm MC, Liteplo MG, et al: Congenital melanocytic nevi of the small and garment type: Clinical, histologic, and ultrastructural studies. Hum Pathol 4:395, 1973.
48. Lorentzen M, Pers M, Bretteville-Jensen G: The incidence of malignant transformation in giant pigmented nevi. Scand J Plast Reconstr Surg 11:163, 1977.
49. Margo CE, Habal MB: Large congenital melanocytic nevus: Light and electron microscopic findings. Ophthalmology 94:960, 1987.
50. Reed WB, Becker SW, Becker SW Jr: Giant pigmented nevi, melanoma, and leptomeningeal melanocytosis: A clinical and histopathological study. Arch Dermatol 91:100, 1965.
51. Rhodes AR, Silverman RA, Harrist TJ, et al: A histologic

comparison of congenital and acquired nevomelanocytic nevi. Arch Dermatol 121:1266, 1985.

52. Hendrickson MR, Ross JC: Neoplasms arising in congenital giant nevi: Morphologic study of seven cases and a review of the literature. Am J Surg Pathol 5:109, 1981.
53. Trozak DJ, Rowland WD, Hu F: Metastatic malignant melanoma in prepubertal children. Pediatrics 55:191, 1975.
54. Rhodes AR, Sober AJ, Day CL, et al: The malignant potential of small congenital nevocellular nevi: An estimate of association based on a histologic study of 234 primary cutaneous melanomas. J Am Acad Dermatol 6:230, 1982.
55. Elder DE: The blind men and the elephant: Different views of small congenital nevi. Arch Dermatol 121:1263, 1985.
56. Wayte DM, Helwig EB: Melanotic freckle of Hutchinson. Cancer 21:893, 1968.
57. Cramer SF, Kiehn CL: Sequential histologic study of evolving lentigo maligna melanoma. Arch Pathol Lab Med 106:121, 1982.
58. Silvers DN: Focus on melanoma: The therapeutic dilemma of lentigo maligna (Hutchinson's freckle). J Dermatol Surg 2:301, 1976.
59. Clark WH Jr, Mihm MC Jr: Lentigo maligna and lentigo maligna melanoma. Am J Pathol 55:39, 1969.
60. Holman J, Armstrong BK: Pigmentary traits, ethnic origin, benign nevi, and family history as risk factors for cutaneous malignant melanoma. J Natl Cancer Inst 72:257, 1984.
61. Rhodes AR: Neoplasms: Benign neoplasms, hyperplasias, and dysplasias of melanocytes. In Fitzpatrick TB, Eisen AZ, Wolff K, et al (eds): Dermatology in General Medicine, 7th ed. New York, McGraw-Hill, 1987, p 934.
62. Rodrigues-Sains RS, Jakobiec FA, Iwamoto T: Lentigo maligna of the lateral canthal skin. Ophthalmology 88:1186, 1981.
63. Blodi FC, Widner RR: The melanic freckle (Hutchinson) of the eyelid. Surv Ophthalmol 13:23, 1968.
64. Davis J, Pack GT, Higgins GK: Melanotic freckle of Hutchinson. Am J Surg 113:457, 1967.
65. Resnick KI, Sadun A, Albert DM: Basal cell epithelioma: An unusual case. Ophthalmology 88:1182, 1981.
66. Lee JAH: Melanoma. In Schottenfeld D, Fraumeni JF Jr (eds): Cancer Epidemiology and Prevention. Philadelphia, WB Saunders, 1982, pp 984–985.
67. Naidoff MA, Bernadino VB, Clark WH Jr: Melanocytic lesions of the eyelid skin. Am J Ophthalmol 82:371, 1976.
67a. Garner A, Koornneef L, Levene A, Collin JRD: Malignant melanoma of the eyelid skin: Histopathology and behavior. Br J Ophthalmol 69:180, 1985.
68. Reintgen DS, McCarty KM Jr, Cox E, Seigler HF: Malignant melanoma in black American and white American populations. JAMA 248:1856, 1982.
69. Mihm MC Jr, Clark WH Jr, From L: The clinical diagnosis, classification and histogenetic concepts of the early stages of cutaneous malignant melanomas. N Engl J Med 284:1078, 1971.
70. Clark WH Jr, From L, Bernardino EA, et al: The histogenesis and biologic behavior of primary human malignant melanoma of the skin. Cancer Res 29:705, 1969.
71. McGovern VJ: The classification of melanoma and its relationship with prognosis. Pathology 2:85, 1970.
72. Breslow A: Thickness, cross-sectional areas and depth of invasion in the prognosis of cutaneous melanoma. Ann Surg 172:902, 1970.
73. Mastrangelo MJ, Bellet RE, Berd D: Prognostic factors. In Clark WH Jr, Goldman LI, Mastrangelo MJ (eds): Human Malignant Melanoma. New York, Grune & Stratton, 1979.
74. Day CL Jr, Mihm MC Jr, Sober AJ, et al: Predictors of late deaths among patients with clinical stage I melanoma who have not had bony or visceral metastases within the first 5 years after diagnosis. J Am Acad Dermatol 8:864, 1983.
75. Balch CM, Soong SJ, Murad TM, et al: A multifactorial analysis of melanoma. II: Prognostic factors in patients with stage I (localized) melanoma. Surgery 86:343, 1979.
76. Day CL Jr, Mihm MC Jr, Sober AJ, et al: Skin lesions suspected to be melanoma should be photographed: Gross morphological features of primary melanoma associated with metastases. JAMA 248:1077, 1982.
77. Nathanson L: Spontaneous regression of malignant melanoma: A review of the literature of incidence, clinical features and possible mechanisms. Natl Cancer Instit Monograph 44:67, 1976.
78. Pellegrini JR, Wagner RF, Nathanson L: Halo nevi and melanoma. Am Fam Physician 30:157, 1984.
79. Sober AJ: Immunology and cutaneous malignant melanoma. Int J Dermatol 15:1, 1976.
80. Day CL Jr, Mihm MC Jr, Lew RA, et al: Cutaneous malignant melanoma: Prognostic guidelines for physicians and patients. CA 32:113, 1982.
81. Day CL Jr, Mihm MC Jr, Sober AJ, et al: Narrower margins for clinical stage I malignant melanoma. N Engl J Med 306:479, 1982.
82. Cascinelli N, van der Esch EP, Breslow A, et al: Stage I melanoma of the skin: The problem of resection margin. Eur J Cancer 6:1079, 1980.
83. Mohs FE: Chemosurgery for skin cancer: Fixed tissue and fresh tissue technique. Arch Dermatol 112:211, 1976.
84. Mohs FE: Microscopically controlled surgery for periorbital melanoma: Fixed-tissue and fresh-tissue techniques. J Dermatol Surg Oncol 11:284, 1985.
85. Turkule LD, Woods JE: Limited or selective nodal dissection for malignant melanoma of the head and neck. Am J Surg 148:446, 1984.
86. Mihm MC Jr, Fitzpatrick TB, Brown MML, et al: Early detection of primary cutaneous malignant melanoma: A color atlas. N Engl J Med 289:989, 1973.

Chapter 159

■

Unusual Eyelid Tumors

JOSEPH W. SASSANI, AHMED A. HIDAYAT, and FREDERICK A. JAKOBIEC

This chapter features six eyelid lesions: angiosarcoma, Kaposi's sarcoma, nodular fasciitis, Merkel cell tumor, metastatic tumors, and the phakomatous choristoma. These diverse lesions are considered collectively because they are uncommon, and their confusion with similar appearing masses can have serious consequences. Angiosarcoma, Kaposi's sarcoma, and Merkel cell tumor are primary malignancies. Confusing them with benign-appearing "look-alikes" results in delay in diagnosis, during which time tumor metastasis may occur. Conversely, nodular fasciitis is a benign, but locally invasive, reactive lesion, which if confused with malignancy may result in unnecessary disfiguring surgery. Finally, although metastatic lesions are malignant, they are usually best treated with local excision, radiation therapy, or in conjunction with systemic chemotherapy. Confusing metastatic lesions with primary malignancies may also lead to unnecessary disfiguring surgery that poses no hope of cure for the patient.

Malignant soft tissue tumors of the head and neck are distinctly uncommon. Makino found only 23 malignant lesions among 651 soft tissue tumors originating in the head and neck.[1] Viewed from another perspective, soft tissue sarcomas of the head and neck represent less than 5 percent of such tumors in adults.[2–6] In their review of 176 head and neck sarcomas at the Memorial Sloan-Kettering Cancer Center between 1950 and 1985, Farhood and associates found 6 percent and 3 percent involving the cheek and orbit, respectively.[6] Only 10 percent of all the head and neck sarcomas in their study were angiosarcomas; however, they noted that 37 percent of malignant vascular neoplasms (hemangiosarcoma and hemangiopericytoma) arose on the face.

Angiosarcoma, hemangiopericytoma, and Kaposi's sarcoma are the most common malignant vasoformative lesions of the head and neck.[7] The differential diagnosis of these lesions is presented with the discussion of Kaposi's sarcoma.

ANGIOSARCOMA

Holden and colleagues analyzed 72 cases of angiosarcoma involving the face and scalp.[8] Enzinger and Weiss have also offered a comprehensive review of this subject.[8a] The upper face and scalp were the most common tumor locations in their study, representing 65 percent of lesions in men and 82 percent of those in women. The midface was much more frequently involved in men (33 percent) than in women (11 percent); the eyelids are rarely involved (Fig. 159–1A–E). Although others have emphasized a varied clinical presentation for the tumor,[8] Hodgkinson and associates recognized three clinical types: superficial spreading, nodular, and ulcerating.[9] The tumor appears to be more common in males[10, 11] and has a poor prognosis; it may be multiple

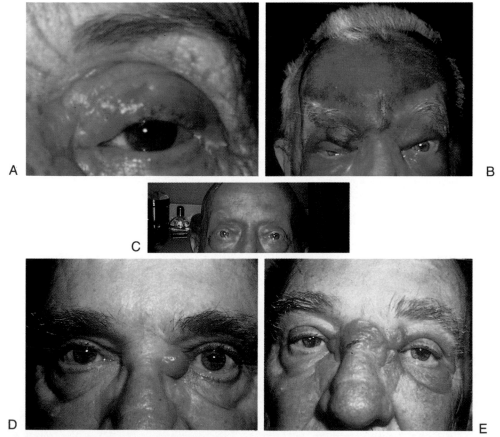

Figure 159–1. Angiosarcoma. A, There is a nodular thickening of the left upper eyelid extending from the medial canthus and the nose to the lateral aspect of the lid. There is also slight ptosis and periorbital edema. B, Multicentric tumor of the forehead and eyelids with an ecchymotic appearance. C, The same patient shown in Figure 159–1B after receiving a course of definitive external beam radiation therapy of 4600 rads. There is considerable regression of the tumor, but dermatochalasis of the eyelids persist. D, A 76-year-old man had a 1-yr history of a left medial canthal lesion arising in the region of the lacrimal sac. There was patent irrigation through the nasolacrimal drainage apparatus. A wide local excision was performed. E, The tumor recurred and has spread across the bridge of the nose to the contralateral medial canthal region. The tumor was poorly responsive to radiotherapy, and the patient eventually succumbed from intracranial extension. (A, Courtesy of C. I. Hood, M.D.; B and C, Courtesy of J. Caya, M.D.; D and E, Courtesy of S. Searl, M.D., and R. Kennedy, M.D.)

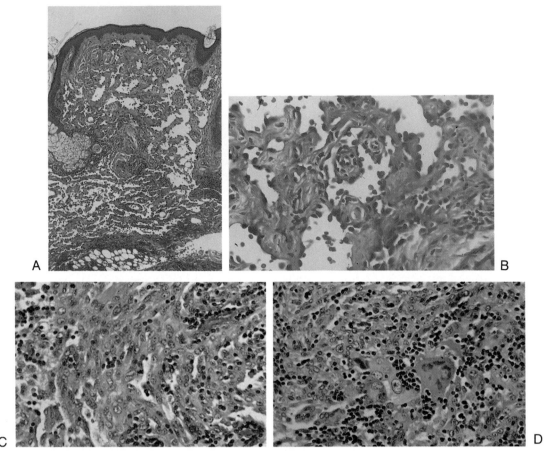

Figure 159–2. Histopathologic features of angiosarcoma. *A,* The dermis is infiltrated by a tumor composed of irregular and interanastomosing vascular channels that create a network of sinusoids. *B,* The vascular channels are lined by malignant endothelial cells with large and hyperchromatic nuclei. In some areas, the malignant cells have piled up along the lumens creating papillations that are typical of angiosarcoma. *C,* Hyperchromatic tumor cells forming solid masses as well as slitlike vascular spaces have an eosinophilic cytoplasm, sometimes leading to the designation of epithelioid-histiocytoid hemangioendothelioma. Note the background infiltration of lymphocytes. *D,* More pleomorphic region of the tumor with less obvious lumen formation and pleomorphic giant cell formation. In some instances, angiosarcomas can be high-grade tumors that are difficult to distinguish from carcinomas or pleomorphic fibrosarcomas. The demonstration of ulex or factor VIII positivity can help to make the correct diagnosis. (*C* and *D,* Courtesy of S. Searl, M.D.)

in 50% of cases.[8a] Holden and colleagues noted an 88 percent overall tumor mortality at 5 yr, and 50 percent of patients were dead within 15 mo of presentation.[8]

Histologically, angiosarcoma is characterized by atypical endothelial cells lining freely anastomosing vascular channels admixed with spindle cell areas and areas lacking differentiation.[12] Other areas show a pile-up of cells creating papillae (Fig. 159–2*A–D*). On the basis of electron microscopic features of numerous pinocytotic vesicles, well-developed cellular junctions, and tubulated bodies, Rosai and associates believed that the tumor was of endothelial cell origin.[12] The tumor cells may be factor VIII and ulex positive.

It has been difficult for authors to make specific recommendations regarding the treatment of angiosarcoma, because of its high mortality rate regardless of therapy. Maddox and Evans suggested that accessibility of the tumor to complete surgical excision was the main factor determining survival rate in their patients.[13] Similarly, Panje and colleagues emphasized the poorly circumscribed nature of the tumor and recommended total surgical excision using frozen section control.[11] Cervical lymph node dissection has been suggested by Hodgkin-

son and colleagues for lateralized lesions or for patients with palpable lymphadenopathy, because of the frequency of spread to cervical lymph nodes.[9] Holden and associates cite the utility of radical radiotherapy, involving wide-field electron beam therapy, in achieving apparent local tumor eradication and prolonged patient survival.[8] In general, radical surgery has been endorsed for solitary lesions and radiotherapy for multiple ones.[8a]

KAPOSI'S SARCOMA

Until recently, Kaposi's sarcoma in the United States was an indolent disease most often affecting males of Ashkenazic Jewish and Mediterranean descent.[14–16] Most patients were middle-aged or older. Typically, focal reddening or purpura of the skin progressed to a darker, more elevated lesion. The lesions usually began at the periphery of a lower extremity, progressed centrally, and eventually erupted in multiple locations before the disease evolved to visceral involvement.[13, 14] In their study of 50 patients, Cox and Helwig found lower extremity involvement in 41 patients and upper extremity lesions in 16 patients. Multiple cutaneous lesions were found in 39 patients. Only seven patients developed head and neck lesions, and only one patient had conjunctival involvement. In 1984 Gnepp and associates found only nine cases of Kaposi's sarcoma of the head and neck in the files of the Armed Forces Institute of Pathology and an additional 74 cases in the literature.[17]

In the past, death caused by Kaposi's sarcoma often resulted from intercurrent disease rather than visceral involvement or other complications of Kaposi's sarcoma. In their study of 70 patients seen at the Mayo Clinic over a 38-yr period, Reynolds and colleagues reported that 29 patients had died. Kaposi's sarcoma was directly related to the cause of death in only eight of these patients.[15] The average duration of disease in the 29 patients who had died was 10 yr.

The demographics and natural history of Kaposi's sarcoma have changed dramatically since the initial reports of opportunistic infections in homosexual men heralded the acquired immunodeficiency syndrome (AIDS) epidemic.[18-20] Kalinske and Leone were able to identify fewer than 30 cases of ocular involvement with Kaposi's sarcoma in the world literature prior to 1982. Yet, in 1989, Jabs and colleagues reported on 200 patients with AIDS who had been examined for ophthalmic manifestations of the disease from 1983 to 1988.[21] Kaposi's sarcoma was present in 13.5 percent of the total patient population, of whom three patients had eyelid involvement and two patients had conjunctival lesions. In a prospective study of 100 homosexuals with AIDS-related Kaposi's sarcoma, Shuler and associates found 20 patients with ophthalmic lesions, of which the eyelid lesion was the presenting evidence of Kaposi's sarcoma (Fig. 159–3A–C).[22] These findings are comparable with other studies regarding the incidence of eyelid and conjunctival involvement in AIDS-related Kaposi's sarcoma.[23-25, 25a]

Patients with AIDS-related Kaposi's sarcoma are much younger than patients with traditional Kaposi's sarcoma (mean age of 38 yr versus 63 yr), are less likely to present with a lower extremity lesion (21 percent versus 76 percent of patients), and survive for a much shorter time after the diagnosis of Kaposi's sarcoma (26 percent mortality within 2 yr versus an average survival of 8 to 13 yr).[17]

Kaposi's sarcoma involving the eyelids is most likely to be encountered in the patient with AIDS. Therapy should be guided by the overall clinical setting. Shuler and associates recommend systemic therapy for multifocal disease.[22] In such cases the periocular lesion may be followed as an indicator of the overall success of the systemic treatment. Focal radiation therapy is recommended if systemic therapy fails, if the disease is limited to ocular structures, or if immediate regression is required.

Kaposi's sarcoma is believed to be a tumor of vasoformative mesenchymal tissue with pericyte and endothelial cell components (Fig. 159–4A–F).[26, 27] Rosai and associates have presented a differential diagnosis of angiosarcoma, Kaposi's sarcoma, and histologically similar-appearing skin lesions.[12] Included in the differential diagnosis are squamous spindle cell carcinoma, metastatic lesions (particularly renal cell carcinoma and choriocarcinoma), multifocal pyogenic granuloma, and angiolymphoid hyperplasia with eosinophilia.[12, 28] Other lesions that should be considered are hemangiopericytoma[29] and intravascular papillary endothelial hyperplasia.[30, 31]

NODULAR FASCIITIS

The first published report of nodular fasciitis (initially called pseudosarcomatous fibromatosis [fasciitis]) was made by Konwaler and associates in 1955.[32] Those authors, however, credit the pathologists of the Memorial Hospital in New York City for recognizing the lesion at least 5 yr previously. Price and colleagues claim that Shuman used the term "nodular fasciitis" to designate some of these lesions as early as 1951.[33] It is a benign and quasineoplastic proliferation of problems developing over a 1- to 2-wk period, and the most common tumor of the fibroblast. It is usually solitary and often tender and occurs preferentially in the age group between 20 and 35 yr.

Nodular fasciitis is a relatively common lesion. Holds

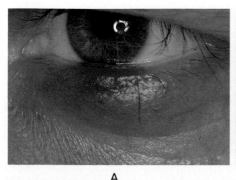 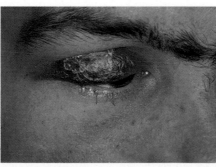 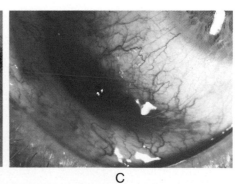

A   B   C

Figure 159–3. Kaposi's sarcoma. *A,* An indurated erythematous lesion of the lower eyelid in a patient with AIDS. *B,* An eschar-like thickening with surface hyperkeratosis and a deep violaceous hue of the upper eyelid in Kaposi's sarcoma. *C,* In the conjunctiva, a typical location for Kaposi's sarcoma in patients with AIDS is seen in the inferior fornix, where a much brighter and beefier red lesion is presented, owing to the transparency of the overlying nonkeratinizing squamous epithelium. (*A* and *B,* Courtesy of H. Perry, M.D.)

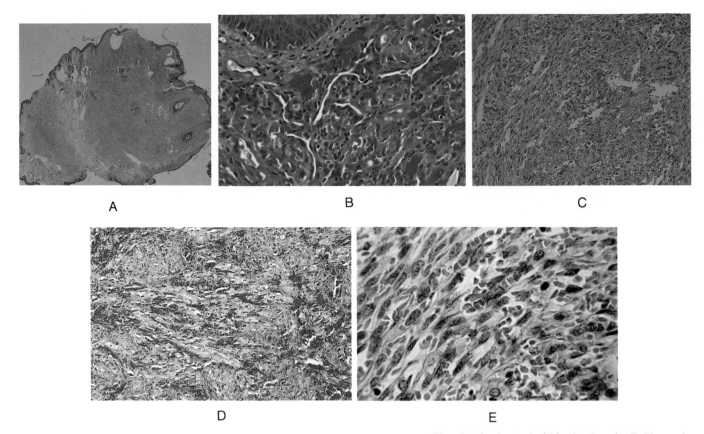

Figure 159–4. Histopathologic features of Kaposi's sarcoma. *A,* A hypercellular proliferation is situated within the dermis. *B,* The early stages of Kaposi's sarcoma may be difficult to distinguish from granulation tissue. Note above that the lesion consists of numerous proliferating capillaries with plump endothelial cells and a wispy proliferation of more immature spindle cells around the newly formed vessels. *C,* This hypercellular tumor consists of a combination of spindled areas blending with angiomatous areas. The spindled areas resemble a well-differentiated fibrosarcoma, except that they contain slitlike vascular spaces containing erythrocytes and merge with attenuated vascular lumina lined by recognizable endothelium. *D,* There is less evidence of lumen formation in this tumor, which consists predominantly of spindle cells. The extensive hemorrhagic foci and occasional clefts within the lesion are useful artifacts pointing toward the probable diagnosis of Kaposi's sarcoma. *E,* Spindle cells without clearcut lumen formation have many percolating erythrocytes between them. Hemosiderin deposits may also form from extravasated erythrocytes. (*B,* Courtesy of H. Perry, M.D.)

and associates, in 1990, found 680 cases reported in two large series and a prior review.[34] It most commonly presents as a rapidly growing, approximately 2 cm, subcutaneous lesion of the upper extremity, except in infants and children in whom the head and neck regions are the most common.[32, 33, 35–37] Its cause is not known and it rarely involves the eyelids, conjunctiva, or orbit (Fig. 159–5A).

Histologically, the lesion is a nonencapsulated nodule that consists of a proliferation of cytologically active-appearing fibroblasts that vary in size and shape (see Fig. 159–5B–D). The cells often grow as if in "tissue culture." Cells may be slender or plump. The more plump cells have abundant cytoplasm, large nuclei, small nucleoli, and lightly staining chromatin. Even the pattern of cell proliferation may vary. A myxoid ground substance is frequently found and is helpful diagnostically. Newly formed capillaries are present in large numbers.[32, 33, 35–37] Dahl and Akerman have suggested that the cytologic appearance is sufficiently characteristic to permit reliable diagnosis by fine needle aspiration.[38]

Based on these histologic characteristics, Bernstein and Lattes identified four histologic variants of nodular fasciitis in their series of 134 cases: (1) reactive type; (2) densely cellular type; (3) lesions with osteoid or cartilaginous metaplasia; and (4) proliferative fasciitis.[36] Shimizu and associates recognize three subtypes: (1) myxoid; (2) cellular; and (3) fibrous.[37] Although such classification systems may be helpful to the individual studying the pathophysiology of the lesion or to the histopathologist confronted with a lesion that has various histologic manifestations, nodular fasciitis uniformly has a favorable prognosis independent of the histologic variant.[37]

Because nodular fasciitis should be cured by local resection, the clinician is advised to question the diagnosis if the lesion recurs. Upon histologic review of 18 such recurrent cases, Bernstein and Lattes found that all 18 had been misdiagnosed as nodular fasciitis, of which 14 could be correctly classified based on review of the original histologic specimens.[36] The appropriate diagnoses were: malignant fibrous histiocytoma (5), fibromatosis (2), and one each: fibrosarcoma, benign fibrous histiocytoma, leiomyoblastoma, neurilemoma, lymphangiosarcoma, neurofibroma, and epithelioid sarcoma.

Nodular fasciitis frequently has been reported to be misdiagnosed as a malignant lesion. In their 1961 review of 65 cases diagnosed as nodular fasciitis from the files of the Armed Forces Institute of Pathology, Price and colleagues noted that 20 patients were misdiagnosed by the pathologist as having malignant lesions. The initial diagnoses in these cases were: fibrosarcoma (14), liposarcoma (2), myxosarcoma (1), and sarcoma not otherwise specified (3).[33] As a result of these misdiagnoses as malignancies, 12 patients received "radical" therapy consisting of wide local excision, excision followed by radiation to the excision site, or by radical reexcision of the area. An even higher frequency of misdiagnosis of malignancy in nodular fasciitis was reported by Soule.[35] Overall, Dahl and Jarlstedt noted a 50 percent misdiagnosis rate of sarcoma in several series of nodular fasciitis cases published until 1972.[39]

Nodular fasciitis seldom involves the head and neck and rarely is found near the eye. In their review of 680 cases in published series, Holds and associates noted 61 (9 percent) involving the head and neck region and only approximately 2 percent located in the ocular region. Font and Zimmerman reported 10 cases of nodular fasciitis of the eye and adnexa, the first and largest such series.[40] They noted that the lesion, when located near the eye, tended to be somewhat smaller in size when excised but otherwise was similar clinically and histologically to that occurring at other anatomic sites. Their series included lesions involving canthus (2); eyelid (2); periorbita (2); canthus and lacrimal sac (1); eyebrow (1); limbus with intraocular extension (1); and scleral insertion of rectus muscle (1). Other authors have reported lesions involving episclera,[34] Tenon's capsule,[41, 42] eyelid,[43] eyebrow,[44] and orbit.[45, 46]

In summary, nodular fasciitis is a benign, often rapidly growing fibroblastic lesion of uncertain cause that rarely recurs and never metastasizes. Failure to recognize its benign nature can result in misdiagnosis as a malignancy, particularly a sarcoma, resulting in unnecessary radical surgery.

MERKEL CELL TUMOR (NEUROENDOCRINE OR TRABECULAR CARCINOMA OF THE SKIN)

In 1875 Merkel described clear, oval, nondendritic, epidermal cells that he believed served as sensory receptors for touch.[47] Histologically, the cell is characterized by clear organelle-rich cytoplasm, and a lobulated nucleus.[48] Electron microscopically, it forms desmosomal attachments to adjacent cells, has poorly developed rough endoplasmic reticulum but many free ribosomes, contains cytoplasmic "spikes" containing filaments, and is usually associated with nerve terminations. A characteristic finding is the presence of membrane-bound cytoplasmic granules that measure 70 to 110 nm in diameter and that are believed to be neurosecretory granules. The presence of these neurosecretory granules has led to analogies between Merkel cells and those

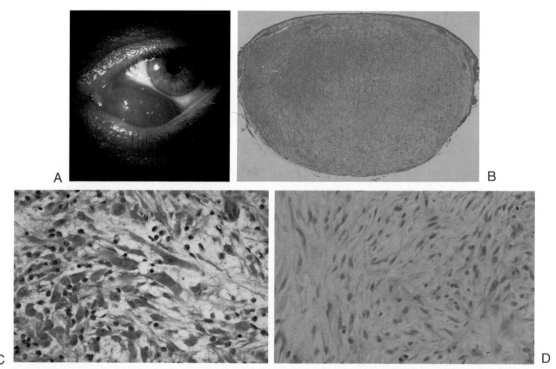

Figure 159–5. Nodular fasciitis. *A,* A rapidly developing violaceous mass situated in the inferior fornix and inferior palpebral conjunctiva. *B,* The excised nodule displays cellular regions alternating with paler myxoid areas. *C,* Somewhat immature and pleomorphic-looking cells are proliferating and extend cytoplasmic processes in a loose matrix, which is often alcian blue positive because of the presence of hyaluronic acid. Note the infiltrating lymphocytes. *D,* A looser proliferation of fibroblasts without a conspicuous inflammatory infiltrate. A mitotic figure is shown toward the bottom of the field. (*A* to *C,* Courtesy of A. Ferry, M.D.)

comprising the *amine precursor uptake decarboxylation* (APUD) system.[49]

In 1972, Toker described trabecular carcinoma of the skin, which is an undifferentiated lesion exhibiting frequent mitoses and composed of anastomosing trabeculas and nests of cells in the dermis.[50] Subsequently, Tang and Toker reported the ultrastructural findings in three of these lesions and demonstrated the presence of neurosecretory granules suggesting a neurocrest origin for the tumor, probably from the Merkel cell.[51] Warner and associates produced further evidence for the Merkel cell origin of trabecular carcinoma by noting the presence of filament-rich straight cytoplasmic "spikes" in the cytoplasm of trabecular carcinoma.[52] Such spikes are a normal finding in Merkel cells.

Some tumors consistent with Merkel cell lesions have exhibited squamous differentiation, as well as other morphologic and immunohistochemical features suggesting similarities to poorly differentiated small cell squamous cell carcinoma, oat cell carcinoma of the lung, or adnexal carcinoma.[53, 54]

The histopathologic differential diagnosis includes malignant lymphoma of skin, myelogenous leukemia, Ewing's sarcoma, embryonal rhabdomyosarcoma, small cell malignant melanoma, neuroblastoma, oat cell carcinoma, metastatic carcinoid, sweat gland carcinoma, and sebaceous carcinoma.[52, 54] Transmission electron microscopy and immunohistochemistry may be necessary in differentiating these lesions. Particularly helpful in diagnosing Merkel cell tumors are the presence of low molecular weight cytokeratin in a paranuclear, dotlike distribution; and positive staining for neuron-specific enolase.[55–60]

Clinically, a Merkel cell tumor often presents as a solitary rapidly growing, red-blue to purple skin nodule on sun-exposed skin. The nodule occasionally ulcerates (Fig. 159–6A–F). In their 1984 literature review of 78 previously reported cases, Searl and associates noted

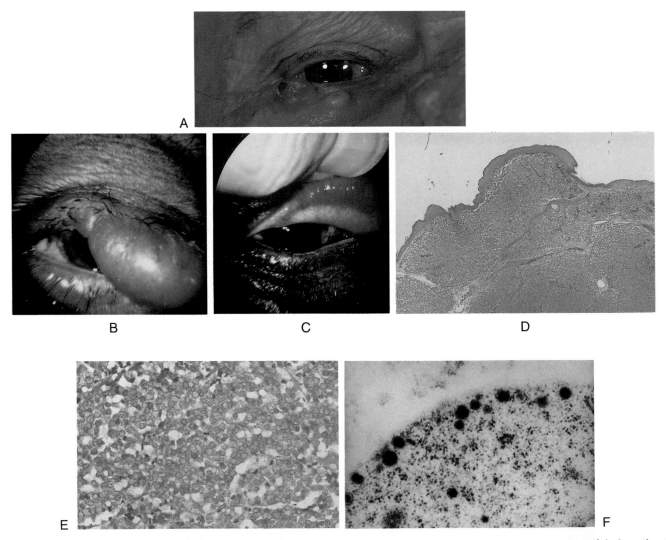

Figure 159–6. Merkel cell tumors. *A,* The red color of this tumor in an older patient is a common feature, but the partial ulceration is atypical. Adnexal carcinomas, such as mucinous adenocarcinoma, should be considered in the clinical differential diagnosis. *B,* The surface of this bulky lesion is smooth and shiny without ulceration, and there are telangiectatic vessels scattered throughout. In contrast to sebaceous carcinoma, the cilia are preserved. *C,* On eversion of the eyelid of the patient shown in *B,* a more obvious reddish discoloration of the base of the lesion is observed. *D,* The dermis is infiltrated by sheets of small round cells. *E,* The tumor consists of uniformly round cells with pale vesicular nuclei, sparse cytoplasm, and many mitotic figures. Both large round cell lymphoma and amelanotic melanoma are frequently offered as mistaken diagnoses. *F,* An electron micrograph displaying several membrane-bound neurosecretory granules along the cytoplasmic border of a tumor cell. (*A,* Courtesy of G. Klintworth, M.D.)

that 43 percent of lesions for which a site was identified were located in the head and neck regions.[61] Lesions varied in size from 0.6 to 4.5 cm. Nine percent (six tumors) were located on the eyelids, and 48 percent were located elsewhere on the body. The average patient age was 66.8 yr (range of 24 to 84 yr). All reported patients for whom race was known were white. The number of published cases involving the eyelid had increased to eight by 1989, and one tumor that involved the eyebrow had also been reported.[62] Subsequently, Whyte and colleagues reported a Merkel cell tumor masquerading as a chalazion.[63] Finally, Kivela and Tarkkanen[63a] have provided a review of periocular cases: 31 in the eyelid, 4 in the inner and outer canthi, 1 in the supraorbital and 5 in the infraorbital regions, with an average age of 77 yr (range of 54 to 95). When located on the eyelid, squamous cell carcinoma, basal cell carcinoma, lymphoma, amelanocytic melanoma, sebaceous gland carcinoma, and metastatic lesions should be among the lesions considered in the differential diagnosis of Merkel cell tumor.

Merkel cell tumor has a relatively poor prognosis because of local recurrence and extensive early lymph node metastases. Optimal management has not definitely been established, although surgical excision with frozen section control has been recommended.[61] Shaw and Rumball reviewed 30 reports of the lesion and described five more cases.[64] They noted that after excision alone of the primary tumor, 39 percent recurred locally and 46 percent recurred regionally. Treatment by excision plus adjuvant node dissection or radiation therapy resulted in a local recurrence rate of 26 percent and a regional recurrence of 22 percent. "Locoregional" recurrence was associated with a 67 percent tumor-related mortality. It is interesting to note that a 44 percent survival for a mean of 40 mo was achieved with node dissection, with or without supplemental radiation therapy for individuals who either presented with regional disease or who later developed regional disease. Other authors also have supported the value of wide local resection, lymph node removal, and supplemental radiation therapy.[65, 66] Some authors recommend a wider role for radiation therapy in the treatment of Merkel cell tumors.[67-70] Similarly, chemotherapy has not been widely recommended; however, some authors have reported favorable results.[71, 72]

METASTATIC TUMORS

Metastatic lesions to the eyelid are very uncommon. In their review of 892 eyelid lesions, Aurora and Blodi noted that 24 percent were malignant, of which only four metastatic tumors were found.[73] They represented 1.4 percent of malignant lesions and 0.3 percent of all lesions. Similarly, Weiner and associates found three metastatic tumors among 2023 eyelid lesions examined over a 14-yr period.[74] Only 15 such lesions were found in the literature until 1970.[75]

Because lesions metastatic to the eyelid are so uncommon, few large series of such cases have been reported. Mansour and Hidayat conducted a clinicopathologic study of 31 patients with metastatic eyelid lesions (Fig. 159–7A–E).[76] Females outnumbered males 4:1. Although most patients were elderly (mean age of 69 yr), one child of 3 yr of age was included in the study. The breast was the most frequently encountered primary site (35 percent); followed by the skin (16 percent); and gastrointestinal and genitourinary sites (10 percent each). In 45 percent of cases, the eyelid lesion was the presenting lesion.

Mansour and Hidayat also summarized the 88 previously reported cases of tumors metastatic to the eyelid.[76] They noted the following primary sites: breast (41), gastrointestinal system (12), respiratory system (9), skin (6), and genitourinary system (4). They stated that referral bias might, in part, explain the relatively low incidence of metastatic breast disease and the high incidence of metastatic disease presenting as an eyelid lesion in their series.[76]

Ferry and Font reported 227 cases of carcinoma metastatic to the eye or orbit.[77] The most frequently encountered primary sites were the breast (40 percent) and the lung (29 percent). There appears to be a much higher frequency of metastasis of lung tumors to the eye and orbit than to the eyelid.

Three general categories of presentation of metastatic eyelid lesions were described initially by Riley.[75] Arnold and associates utilized this system in classifying the clinical presentation of previously reported lesions: (1) most commonly (62 percent) as a solitary, painless nodule that might be confused with a chalazion or primary skin tumor; (2) as a diffuse nontender induration (30 percent); and (3) as an ulcerating lesion of the eyelid skin or conjunctiva (8 percent).[78]

In summary, metastatic tumors to the eyelid can have extremely varied presentations. They should be suspected in any patient with an eyelid mass and a history of previous malignant tumor even if the malignancy is somewhat remotely separated in time from the more recent eyelid mass. All atypical eyelid lesions should be biopsied to ascertain their origin.

Extensive and disfiguring surgery seldom is justified for metastatic lesions. Their therapy is usually by local excision or radiation therapy, or appropriate systemic therapy for other metastatic foci once the primary lesion has been identified. Such therapy is usually best supervised by an oncologist.

PHAKOMATOUS CHORISTOMA
(Fig. 159–8)

In 1979, Zimmerman[79] described three unusual infantile or childhood eyelid lesions that consisted of tissue that had an appearance similar to disorganized lens cells. He called the condition a phakomatous choristoma and believed that it had a malformational basis. Since then, approximately nine other cases have been reported in the literature[80-86] or else have been presented to ophthalmic pathology societies, including the case most recently presented by Eagle to the 1992 Verhoeff Society meeting in San Diego.

All of these lesions share two common features: (1)

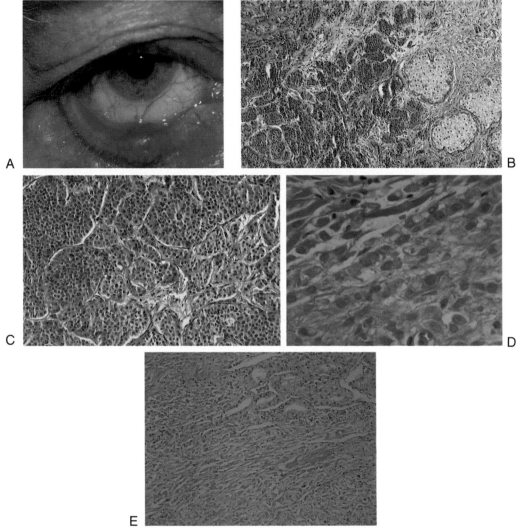

Figure 159–7. Metastatic carcinoma to the eyelids. *A,* The lesion closely resembles a chalazion and was caused by a carcinoid deposit. *B,* A lobular pattern of infiltrating metastatic carcinoid is present on the left and is invading the tarsal plate on the right with its meibomian glands. *C,* Metastatic carcinoid tumor cells are arranged in lobules and have indistinct cytoplasmic borders. A typical feature of carcinoid cells is stippling of their nuclear chromatin. *D,* In this metastatic breast carcinoma, the tumor cells have a tendency to be arranged in short cords (Indian file pattern). The cytoplasm of some of the tumor cells contains a vacuole, which frequently has an alcian-blue or mucicarmine-positive content. Under low power, such tumors frequently look histiocytoid or inflammatory in character, but histiocytes do not possess mucinous inclusions in their cytoplasm. *E,* In this metastatic renal cell carcinoma, there is a glandular pattern in some areas. The tumor cells are pale to vacuolated cytoplasm, which is due in part to the presence of either glycogen or lipid inclusions. (*A,* Courtesy of W. Stafford, M.D.)

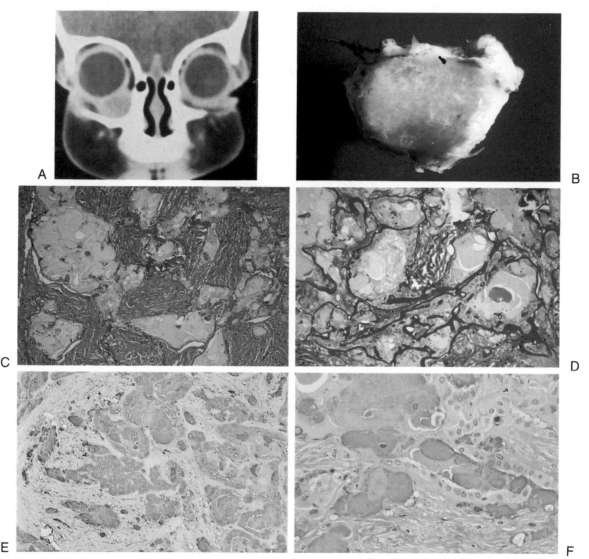

Figure 159–8. Phakomatous choristoma. *A,* Computed coronal tomogram of a lesion that was palpable through the inferomedial eyelid and extends to the equator of the globe. It measured approximately 1.5 cm in greatest diameter. *B,* The excised specimen is unencapsulated but has good circumscription. Note the trabeculation throughout the cut surface, indicating the alternation of collagen with collections of tumor cells. *C,* Large swollen bladder cells (like cataractous Wedl cells) are present in the central portions of the lobules of the tumor cells and are surrounded on their outer perimeter by a low cuboidal epithelium. Note the fibrotic stroma. *D,* The PAS stain outlines a thickened basement membrane, very much simulating the capsule of the lens. *E,* Positive staining of most of the lobular cellular masses with an antibody to cytoplasmic α lens protein (crystallin). *F,* Positive staining for β-protein (crystallin) tends to spare the outer cuboidal cells. (*A, B, E,* and *F;* Courtesy of R. Eagle, M.D., and Gerry Shields, M.D.)

location in the inferomedial lid in the subcutaneous tissues, and (2) frequent extension as disclosed in computed tomographic studies into the anterior inferior orbit. The lesions are firm and present a circumscribed but nonencapsulated margin. Clinical differential diagnoses include, in the neonatal period, capillary hemangioma, rhabdomyosarcoma, juvenile xanthogranuloma, fibrous tumors, peripheral nerve sheath tumors, and leukemic deposits, including granulocytic sarcoma.

Histopathologically the tumors consist of islands of eosinophilic cells with an outer cuboidal rimming layer surrounded by a variably thickened PAS-positive basement membrane. The central cells become bloated and occasionally degenerated and tend to resemble bladder or Wedl cells encountered in human cataracts. The stroma is densely fibrotic, and there may be scattered calcific deposits reminiscent of psammoma bodies.

From the initial report by Zimmerman,[79] and reinforced by subsequent reports, the impression has been gained that these cells are not of epithelial adnexal origin in the skin but rather represent dystopias or persistences of embryonic lens epithelium. If so, then the lens vesicle forms from presumptive inferomedial eyelid embryonic epidermis. The thickened PAS-positive basement membrane is held to be analogous to the lens capsule, and ultrastructural studies[82, 85] have disclosed many cytoplasmic filaments and cellular imbrications that are consistent with lens fiber cells.

Immunohistochemical studies have shown positivity for vimentin but erratic or negative results on staining for cytokeratins, neuron-specific enolase, glial fibrillary acidic protein, and epithelial membrane antigen. At Eagle's Verhoeff presentation, he reported clear-cut positive results of staining for anti–α-crystallin, which reacted centrally both with the outer cuboidal cells and smaller Wedl cells. Beta-crystallin reactivity was generally restricted to the central contents of the epithelial islands, with sparing of the outer cuboidal and occasionally columnar cells.

The therapy for the tumor is wide local excision. It can recur if it is not completely excised, but it is not known to undergo malignant transformation.

REFERENCES

1. Makino Y: A clinicopathological study on soft tissue tumors of the head and neck. Acta Pathol Jpn 29:389, 1979.
2. Goepfert H, Lindberg RD, Sinkovics JG, et al: Soft tissue sarcoma of the head and neck after puberty. Arch Otolaryngol 103:365, 1977.
3. Greager JA, Patel MK, Briele HA, et al: Soft tissue sarcomas of the adult head and neck. Cancer 56:820, 1985.
4. Weber RS, Benjamin RS, Peters LJ, et al: Soft tissue sarcomas of the head and neck in adolescents and adults. Am J Surg Pathol 152:386, 1986.
5. Freeman AM, Reiman HM, Woods JE: Soft-tissue sarcomas of the head and neck. Am J Surg 158:367, 1989.
6. Farhood AI, Hajdu SI, Shiu MH, et al: Soft tissue sarcomas of the head and neck in adults. Am J Surg 160:365, 1990.
7. Batsakis JG, Rice DH: The pathology of head and neck tumors. Part 9B: Vasoformative tumors. Head Neck Surg 3:326, 1981.
8. Holden CA, Spittle MF, Jones EW: Angiosarcoma of the face and scalp, prognosis and treatment. Cancer 59:1046, 1987.
8a. Enzinger FM, Weiss SW: Soft Tissue Tumors. Washington, DC, CV Mosby, 1988, pp 545–561.
9. Hodgkinson DJ, Soule EH, Woods JE: Cutaneous angiosarcoma of the head and neck. Cancer 44:1106, 1979.
10. Bardwill JM, Mocega EE, Butler JJ, et al: Angiosarcoma of the head and neck region. Am J Surg 116:548, 1968.
11. Panje WR, Moran WJ, Bostwick DG, et al: Angiosarcoma of the head and neck: Review of 11 cases. Laryngoscope 96:1381, 1986.
12. Rosai J, Sumner HW, Kostianovsky MCM, et al: Angiosarcoma of the skin: A clinicopathologic and fine structural study. Hum Pathol 7:83, 1976.
13. Maddox JC, Evans HL: Angiosarcoma of the skin and soft tissue: A study of fourty-four cases. Cancer 48:1907, 1981.
14. Cox FH, Helwig EB: Kaposi's sarcoma. Cancer 12:289, 1959.
15. Reynolds WA, Winkelmann RK, Soule EH: Kaposi's sarcoma: A clinicopathologic study with particular reference to its relationship to the reticuloendothelial system. Medicine 44:419, 1965.
16. Mitsuyasu RT, Groopman JE: Biology and therapy of Kaposi's sarcoma. Semin Oncol 11:53, 1984.
17. Gnepp DR, Chandler W, Hyams V: Primary Kaposi's sarcoma of the head and neck. Ann Intern Med 100:107, 1984.
18. Centers for Disease Control: *Pneumocystis* pneumonia—Los Angeles. MMWR 30:250, 1981.
19. Gottlieb MS, Schroff R, Schanker HM, et al: *Pneumocystis carinii* pneumonia and mucosal candidiasis in previously healthy homosexual men: Evidence of a new acquired cellular immunodeficiency. N Engl J Med 305:1425, 1981.
20. Masur H, Michelis MA, Greene JB, et al: An outbreak of community-acquired *Pneumocystis carinii* pneumonia. Initial manifestation of cellular immune dysfunction. N Engl J Med 305:1431, 1981.
21. Jabs DA, Green WR, Fox R, et al: Ocular manifestations of acquired immune deficiency syndrome. Ophthalmology 96:1092, 1989.
22. Shuler JD, Holland GN, Miles SA, et al: Kaposi sarcoma of the conjunctiva and eyelids associated with the acquired immunodeficiency syndrome. Arch Ophthalmol 107:858, 1989.
23. Holland GN, Pepose JS, Pettit TH, et al: Acquired immune deficiency syndrome: Ocular manifestations. Ophthalmology 90:859, 1983.
24. Palestine AG, Rodrigues MM, Macher AM, et al: Ophthalmic involvement in acquired immunodeficiency syndrome. Ophthalmology 91:1092, 1984.
25. Centers for Disease Control: Update: Acquired immunodeficiency syndrome—United States. MMWR 35:17, 1986.
25a. Dugel PU, Gill PS, Frangieh GT, Rao N: Treatment of ocular adnexal Kaposi's sarcoma in the acquired immunodeficiency syndrome. Ophthalmology 99:1127–1132, 1992.
26. Hashimoto K, Lever WF: Kaposi's sarcoma: Histochemical and electron microscopic studies. J Invest Dermatol 43:539, 1964.
27. Weiter JJ, Jakobiec FA, Iwamoto T: The clinical and morphologic characteristics of Kaposi's sarcoma of the conjunctiva. Am J Ophthalmol 89:546, 1980.
28. Hidayat AA, Cameron JD, Font RL, et al: Angiolymphoid hyperplasia with eosinophilia (Kimura's disease) of the orbit and adnexa. Am J Ophthalmol 96:176, 1983.
29. McMaster MJ, Soule EH, Ivins JC: Hemangiopericytoma: A clinicopathologic study and long-term follow-up of 60 patients. Cancer 36:2232, 1975.
30. Sorenson RL, Spencer WH, Stewart WB, et al: Intravascular papillary endothelial hyperplasia of the eyelid. Arch Ophthalmol 101:1728, 1983.
31. Font RL, Wheeler TM, Boniuk M: Intravascular papillary endothelial hyperplasia of the orbit and ocular adnexa: A report of five cases. Arch Ophthalmol 101:1731, 1983.
32. Konwaler BE, Keasbey L, Kaplan L: Subcutaneous pseudosarcomatous fibromatosis (fasciitis): Report of 8 cases. Am J Clin Pathol 25:241; 1955.
33. Price EB, Silliphant WH, Shuman R: Nodular fasciitis: A clinicopathologic analysis of 65 cases. Am J Clin Pathol 35:122, 1961.
34. Holds JB, Mamalis N, Anderson RL: Nodular fasciitis presenting as a rapidly enlarging episcleral mass in a 3-year-old. J Pediatr Ophthalmol Strabismus 27:157, 1990.
35. Soule EH: Proliferative (nodular) fasciitis. Arch Pathol 73:17, 1962.
36. Bernstein KE, Lattes R: Nodular (pseudosarcomatous) fasciitis, a nonrecurrent lesion: Clinicopathologic study of 134 cases. Cancer 49:1668, 1982.

37. Shimizu S, Hashimoto H, Enjoji M: Nodular fasciitis: An analysis of 250 patients. Pathology 16:161, 1984.
38. Dahl I, Akerman M: Nodular fasciitis. A correlative cytologic and histologic study of 13 cases. Acta Cytologica 25:215, 1981.
39. Dahl I, Jarlstedt J: Nodular fasciitis in the head and neck: A clinicopathological study of 18 cases. Acta Otolaryngol 90:152, 1980.
40. Font RL, Zimmerman LE: Nodular fasciitis of the eye and adnexa: A report of ten cases. Arch Ophthalmol 75:475, 1966.
41. Tolls RE, Mohr S, Spencer WH: Benign nodular fasciitis originating in Tenon's capsule. Arch Ophthalmol 75:482, 1966.
42. Ferry AP, Sherman SE: Nodular fasciitis of the conjunctiva apparently originating in the fascia bulbi (Tenon's capsule). Am J Ophthalmol 78:514, 1974.
43. Vestal KP, Bauer TW, Berlin AJ: Nodular fasciitis presenting as an eyelid mass. Ophthalmic Plast Reconstr Surg 6:130, 1990.
44. Meacham CT: Pseudosarcomatous fasciitis. Am J Ophthalmol 77:747, 1974.
45. Levitt JM, deVeer JA, Oguzhan MC: Orbital nodular fasciitis. Arch Ophthalmol 81:235, 1969.
46. Perry RH, Ramani PS, McAllister V, et al: Nodular fasciitis causing unilateral proptosis. Br J Ophthalmol 59:404, 1975.
47. Merkel F: Tastzellen un Tastkorperchen bei den Hausthieren und beim Menschen. Arch fur Mikroskopische Anatomie (Bonn) 11:636, 1875.
48. Winkelmann RK, Breathnach AS: The Merkel cell. J Invest Dermatol 60:2, 1973.
49. Winkelmann RK: The Merkel cell system and a comparison between it and the neurosecretory or APUD cell system. J Invest Dermatol 69:41, 1977.
50. Toker C. Trabecular carcinoma of the skin. Arch Dermatol 105:107, 1972.
51. Tang C-K, Toker C: Trabecular carcinoma of the skin: An ultrastructural study. Cancer 42:2311, 1978.
52. Warner TFCS, Uno H, Hafez GR, et al: Merkel cells and Merkel cell tumors: Ultrastructure, immunocytochemistry, and review of the literature. Cancer 52:238, 1983.
53. Heenen PJ, Cole JM, Spagnolo DV: Primary cutaneous neuroendocrine carcinoma (Merkel cell tumor): An adnexal epithelial neoplasm. Am J Dermatopathol 12:7, 1990.
54. Jones EW: Some special skin tumours in the elderly. Br J Dermatol 122 (Suppl 35):71, 1990.
55. Sibley RK, Dahl D: Primary neuroendocrine (Merkel cell?) carcinoma of the skin. II: An immunocytochemical study of 21 cases. Am J Surg Pathol 9:109, 1985.
56. Layfield L, Ulich T, Liao S, et al: Neuroendocrine carcinoma of the skin: An immunohistochemical study of tumor markers and neuroendocrine products. J Cutan Pathol 13:268, 1986.
57. Moll R, Osborn M, Hartschuh W, et al: Variability of expression and arrangement of cytokeratin and neurofilaments in cutaneous neuroendocrine carcinomas (Merkel cell tumors): Immunocytochemical and biochemical analysis of twelve cases. Ultrastruct Pathol 10:473, 1986.
58. Pettinato G, De Chiara A, Insabato L, et al: Neuroendocrine (Merkel cell) tumor of the skin: Fine-needle aspiration cytology, histology, electron microscopy, and immunohistochemistry of 12 cases. Appl Pathol 6:17, 1988.
59. Balaton AJ, Capron F, Baviera EE, et al: Neuroendocrine carcinoma (Merkel cell tumor?) presenting as a subcutaneous tumor: An ultrastructural and immunohistochemical study of three cases. Pathol Res Pract 184:211, 1989.
60. Skoog L, Schmitt FC, Tani E: Neuroendocrine (Merkel cell) carcinoma of the skin: Immunocytochemical and cytomorphologic analysis of fine-needle aspirates. Diagn Cytopathol 6:53, 1990.
61. Searl SS, Boynton JR, Markowitch W, et al: Malignant Merkel cell neoplasm of the eyelid. Arch Ophthalmol 102:907, 1984.
62. Mamalis N, Medlock RD, Holds JB, et al: Merkel cell tumor of the eyelid: A review and report of an unusual case. Ophthalmic Surg 20:410, 1989.
63. Whyte IF, Orrell JM, Roxburgh ST: Merkel cell tumour of the eyelid masquerading as a chalazion. J R Coll Surg Edinb 36:129, 1991.
63a. Kivela T, Tarkkanen A: The Merkel cell and associated neoplasms in the eyelids and periocular regions. Surv Ophthalmol 35:171, 1990.
64. Shaw JH, Rumball E: Merkel cell tumor: Clinical behavior and treatment. Br J Surg 78:138, 1991.
65. Meland NB, Jackson IT: Merkel cell tumor: Diagnosis, prognosis, and management. Plast Reconstr Surg 77:632, 1986.
66. Bourne RG, O'Rourke MG: Management of Merkel cell tumour. Aust N Z J Surg 58:971, 1988.
67. Pople IK: Merkel cell tumour of the face successfully treated with radical radiotherapy. Eur J Surg Oncol 14:79, 1988.
68. Knox SJ, Kapp DS: Hyperthermia and radiation therapy in the treatment of recurrent Merkel cell tumors. Cancer 62:1479, 1988.
69. Hasle H: Merkel cell carcinoma: The role of primary treatment with radiotherapy. Clin Oncol (R Coll Radiol) 3:114, 1991.
70. Brierley JD, Stockdale AD, Rostom AY: Merkel cell (trabecular) carcinoma of the skin treated by radiotherapy. Clin Oncol (R Coll Radiol) 3:117, 1991.
71. Grosh WW, Giannone L, Hande KR, et al: Disseminated Merkel cell tumor: Treatment with systemic chemotherapy. Am J Clin Oncol 10:227, 1987.
72. Wynne CJ, Kearsley JH: Merkel cell tumor: A chemosensitive skin cancer. Cancer 62:28, 1988.
73. Aurora AL, Blodi FC: Lesions of the eyelids: A clinicopathological study. Surv Ophthalmol 15:94, 1970.
74. Weiner JM, Henderson PN, Roche J: Metastatic eyelid carcinoma. Am J Ophthalmol 101:252, 1986.
75. Riley FC: Metastatic tumors of the eyelids. Am J Ophthalmol 69:259, 1970.
76. Mansour AM, Hidayat AA: Metastatic eyelid disease. Ophthalmology 94:667, 1987.
77. Ferry AP, Font RL: Carcinoma metastatic to the eye and orbit. I: A clinicopathologic study of 227 cases. Arch Ophthalmol 92:276, 1974.
78. Arnold AC, Bullock JD, Foos RY: Metastatic eyelid carcinoma. Ophthalmology 92:114, 1985.
79. Zimmerman LE: Phakomatous choristoma of the eyelid: A tumor of lenticular anlage. Am J Ophthalmol 71:169–177, 1971.
80. Filipic M, Silva M: Phakomatous choristoma of the eyelid. Arch Ophthalmol 88:172–175, 1972.
81. Greer CH: Phakomatous choristoma of the eyelid. Aust J Ophthalmol 94:1778–1781, 1976.
82. McMahon RT, Font RL, McLean IW: Phakomatous choristoma of the eyelid. Arch Ophthalmol 94:1778–1781, 1976.
83. Baggesen LH, Jensen OA: Phakomatous choristoma of the lower eyelid. Ophthalmologica 175:231–235, 1977.
84. Tripathi RC, Tripathi BJ, Ringus J: Phakomatous choristoma of the lower eyelid with psammoma body formation. Ophthalmology 88:1198–1206, 1981.
85. Sinclair-Smith CC, Emms M, Morris HB: Phakomatous choristoma of the lower eyelid: A light and ultrastructural study. Arch Pathol Lab Med 113:1175–1177, 1989.
86. Eustis HS, Karcioglu ZA, Dharma S, Hoda S: Phakomatous choristoma: Clinical, histopathologic and ultrastructural findings in a 4-month-old boy. J Pediatr Ophthalmol Strabismus 27:208–211, 1990.

Chapter 160

■

Upper Eyelid Malpositions: Acquired Ptosis

DAVID B. LYON and RICHARD K. DORTZBACH

Acquired ptosis is the most common form of upper eyelid malposition and accounts for a large percentage of ptosis cases. Although aponeurogenic ptosis is the most prevalent form, there are many other diverse, yet less common, causes that must be properly identified to ensure proper management.

True acquired ptosis is caused by some disturbance of the upper lid retractors, the levator and/or Müller's muscle, and is best classified according to its primary etiology, which includes: (1) mechanical, (2) myogenic, (3) neurogenic, and (4) aponeurogenic.[1–3] Some patients have ptosis with contributions from more than one of these categories. Traumatic ptosis and pseudoptosis deserve special mention. Ptosis resulting from trauma, despite its many and variable forms, should be classified in one of the four aforementioned categories. Pseudoptosis, which is not a form of true acquired ptosis, is due to abnormalities other than those found in the lid elevators. Dermatochalasis (Fig. 160–1), hypotropia, and eye or orbital volume disturbances (microphthalmos, enophthalmos, phthisis bulbi, anophthalmos) commonly cause pseudoptosis.

MECHANICAL ACQUIRED PTOSIS

Mechanical ptosis may be caused by lid tumors, cicatrix, or blepharochalasis. Both benign and malignant tumors of the upper eyelid and orbit may cause ptosis as a result of increased weight in the lid. The contour of the lid usually reflects the tumor position with greater ptosis in the area of the mass. Treatment is directed toward the tumor primarily, with correction of any residual ptosis following tumor therapy considered secondarily or concurrently.

Cicatricial ptosis is caused by disease involving the conjunctiva of the tarsus and superior fornix. Surgical and nonsurgical trauma and conjunctival shrinkage syndromes (e.g., Stevens-Johnson or ocular cicatricial pemphigoid) account for most of these cases. If correction is deemed wise, the general approach usually starts with scar revision or excision combined with conjunctival or other mucous membrane grafts.

Blepharochalasis is a rare condition that affects young people and is of unknown etiology. It is usually hereditary and is manifest by repeated transient attacks of eyelid edema and erythema, which often start around puberty. During attacks, the lid edema may cause ptosis. After repeated attacks, permanent changes in the lids develop, including thinning, wrinkling, and discoloration

of the skin, prolapse of orbital fat and the lacrimal gland into the lid, and attenuation or dehiscence of the levator aponeurosis and canthal ligaments.[4] Management may include blepharoplasty, aponeurotic ptosis repair, resuspension of the lacrimal gland, and canthal reconstruction. Further attacks may cause a recurrent ptosis necessitating reoperation.

MYOGENIC ACQUIRED PTOSIS

Ptosis is a common manifestation of myopathic conditions involving the levator muscle or myoneural junction. Chronic progressive external ophthalmoplegia (CPEO), myasthenia gravis and myasthenic syndromes, myotonic dystrophy, and oculopharyngeal dystrophy account for most cases of myogenic ptosis. Further discussion of the diagnosis and management of these disorders is found in the Neuro-ophthalmology section.

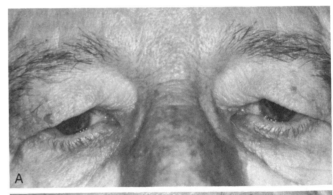

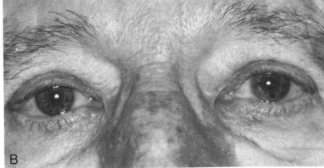

Figure 160–1. A, Pseudoptosis resulting from dermatochalasis. Excess upper eyelid skin and orbicularis muscle hang over upper lid margin of both eyes. B, After correction of dermatochalasis with a bilateral upper eyelid blepharoplasty.

NEUROGENIC ACQUIRED PTOSIS

Dysfunction of the third cranial nerve, which supplies the levator, or the sympathetic innervation to Müller's muscle may cause neurogenic ptosis. Additionally, ptosis may develop on a synkinetic basis caused by aberrant regeneration after third-nerve palsies. Neurogenic ptosis is discussed more fully in Chapter 215.

APONEUROGENIC ACQUIRED PTOSIS

As mentioned earlier, this is the most common form of acquired ptosis and most often affects the elderly. Aponeurotic defects can occur in younger patients as the result of trauma, orbital or eyelid swelling, pregnancy, blepharochalasis, prior ocular surgery, or chronic ocular inflammation. They have also been reported in congenital ptosis.[5]

Jones, Quickert, and Wobig[6] were the first to report that aponeurotic pathology was responsible for this form of acquired ptosis. A dehiscence in the central part of the aponeurosis, with a horizontal dividing line separating the upper and lower parts of the aponeurosis, was described. Disinsertion of the aponeurosis from the tarsus may produce a similar "white line." Thinning and stretching, termed attenuation or rarification, of the aponeurosis, without a true dehiscence or disinsertion produces a similar clinical appearance.[6, 7] Histopathologic work by Dortzbach and Sutula has confirmed the surgical findings of disinsertion and attenuation.[8]

This spectrum of aponeurotic defects and the many terms used to describe them has caused confusion and disagreement among ptosis surgeons. At surgery, the white edge of the dehisced or disinserted aponeurosis is often, but not always, identified. However, a thin sheet of aponeurotic tissue posterior to the white edge may remain attached to the anterior tarsal surface. Carroll,[9] reporting on 250 consecutive lids with involutional ptosis, found a true dehiscence or disinsertion of the aponeurosis in less than 5 percent of cases. The aponeurosis was often very attenuated, but nevertheless, it was intact. Carroll believes that the high incidence of aponeurotic dehiscence and disinsertion reported in the literature is iatrogenic from the surgical technique, likely from scissors or cotton-tipped applicator dissection.

Remembering the upper lid anatomy helps one to understand some of these conflicting ideas. The levator aponeurosis extends inferiorly from the muscular levator below Whitnall's ligament and fans out to its eyelid attachments. It consists of collagenous sheets, or lamellae, that separate to attach to the posterior orbicular fascia and septa between pretarsal orbicularis muscle bundles anteriorly, forming the lid crease, and to the anterior tarsal surface posteriorly. Controversy exists as to which of these insertion sites is more important.[7, 10] Nevertheless, if we think of the aponeurosis as a group of tendinous sheets, and not as a single layer, a mixture of attenuation, dehiscence, and disinsertion within the same eyelid can easily be appreciated. An accumulation of a variety of small aponeurotic defects within the lamellae is probably necessary to create ptosis.

There are certain clinical features that distinguish aponeurogenic acquired ptosis (Fig. 160–2). Historically, the ptosis is acquired, usually after age 55, and precipitating factors, such as orbital and lid edema from trauma, ocular surgery, or blepharochalasis, may exist. The upper lid crease is elevated or absent due to weakened aponeurotic attachments to the tarsus and/or orbicularis when the levator contracts. Similarly, the superior sulcus may be deepened from superior migration of the orbital septum and preaponeurotic fat pad. Upper lid excursion, or levator function, is good and usually measures 12 mm or more. Occasionally, the supratarsal portion of the upper lid is thinned, allowing the color of the iris to be seen through the lid or the superior tarsal border to be discretely palpable. Müller's superior tarsal muscle function is intact.

Although aponeurogenic acquired ptosis may develop or worsen following almost any type of ocular surgery, its occurrence following cataract surgery has received

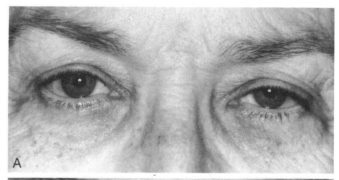

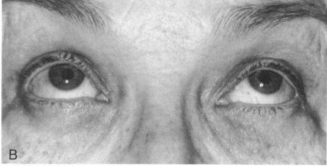

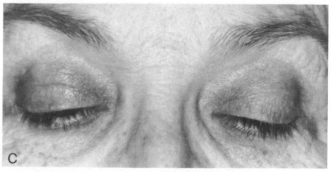

Figure 160–2. Asymmetric bilateral aponeurogenic ptosis. A, Primary gaze. B, Upgaze. C, Downgaze. Note the good upper lid excursion (levator function) and asymmetry of the upper lid creases (left upper lid crease higher than right).

the most study. Paris and Quickert[11] were the first to describe this, and others have analyzed the causative factors.[12–14] Regardless of the surgical technique, significant ptosis can develop in susceptible patients after cataract surgery, and this should be remembered when obtaining informed consent.

Involutional ptosis is a term generally used synonymously with acquired aponeurogenic ptosis. However, degenerative processes other than pure aponeurotic defects have also been identified in subgroups of patients with involutional ptosis. Dehiscence of the medial limb of Whitnall's ligament, lateral shift of the upper lid tarsal plate, and fatty degeneration of the levator muscle were identified at surgery by Shore and McCord in a group of patients with classic findings of involutional ptosis.[15] Historically, these patients had no predisposing factors for aponeurotic defects, such as prior ocular surgery, trauma, or orbital swelling. Fatty infiltration of both Müller's muscle and the levator muscle also has been well described.[16] Such patients had fair to good levator function (mean of 8.9 mm), no lid crease elevation, poor response to topical 10 percent phenylephrine, and intact, but often thinned, levator aponeuroses.

We have noted these myopathic changes at the time of aponeurotic ptosis repair in conjunction with a variety of aponeurotic defects. These cases with multiple causes often require adjustments in surgical technique to achieve the best results.

At the present time, the most widely accepted approach in treating aponeurotic ptosis is correction of the underlying anatomic defect: reattachment of the aponeurosis to the tarsus if it is disinserted, or tucking or small resection if the aponeurosis is dehisced or attenuated.

Clinical Evaluation

As with all medical encounters, the patient's history is taken first to help determine the onset, duration, variability, and severity of the ptosis. Specific inquiry should be made regarding past ocular or lid disease or surgery, trauma, family history of ptosis, and anesthetic history (including malignant hyperthermia). Review of old photographs helps to confirm the duration and severity of the ptosis.

A comprehensive ophthalmic examination should be done on all patients with ptosis with particular emphasis on certain lid measurements and ocular protective mechanisms. Head posture and eyebrow position should be noted first. Patients with severe ptosis instinctively assume a chin-up head position to overcome their visual obstruction and may use their frontalis muscle to help lift the upper lid by anterior lamellar traction.[17] Brow ptosis may increase dermatochalasis of the upper lids, adding a mechanical component to the ptosis.

Lid measurements should be done with the face held in the frontal plane and with the frontalis muscle relaxed. If any frontalis muscle contraction is evident in an effort to partially overcome ptosis or dermatochalasis obstructing vision, it should be neutralized by the examiner by holding the brows in their relaxed position. If there is dermatochalasis obscuring the lid margins, the examiner can lift the brows to observe the lid levels for measurements, again making sure that the patient does not use the frontalis muscle, which may introduce confusing variables. Severe eyebrow ptosis requires some form of browplasty to give a good foundation for supporting the upper lids prior to ptosis repair. A patient with unilateral ptosis may use compensatory unilateral brow elevation, especially if the ptosis is on the side of the dominant eye; this habit should cease after successful ptosis repair.

Lid measurements should include the margin reflex distance (MRD), vertical palpebral fissure (PF), upper lid excursion, and the upper lid crease distance from the lid margin. MRD is the distance in millimeters between the central corneal light reflex and the upper lid margin with the eyes in primary gaze. The amount of ptosis is more accurately determined using the MRD than the PF, because errors from lower lid malpositions are eliminated. A normal MRD is approximately +4 to +5 mm, corresponding to an upper lid level 1 to 2 mm below the superior corneal limbus.

Upper lid excursion is a measure of levator function and records the vertical movement of the upper lid margin from extreme downgaze to extreme upgaze with the frontalis muscle nullified by the examiner's thumb or finger. Classically, levator function is categorized as poor (0 to 5 mm), fair (6 to 11 mm), or good (> 12 mm). In the patient with presumed aponeurogenic ptosis, an upper lid excursion of less than 11 to 12 mm should arouse suspicion as to the cause of the ptosis or should suggest combined mechanisms.

The upper lid crease is measured in the central part of the lid from the cilia while the patient looks down. The crease may be absent, elevated, depressed, or multiple. Normal measurements are 7 to 8 mm in males and 9 to 10 mm in females, although there is considerable variability. An elevated or absent lid crease suggests an underlying aponeurotic attenuation and is often associated with a deepening of the superior sulcus.

Specific notation should also be made regarding the amount of upper lid dermatochalasis and orbital fat prolapse, the upper lid position on downgaze, and the status of the tarsus and superior fornix. A reconstructive blepharoplasty is often needed in elderly patients in conjunction with the ptosis repair to avoid increased pseudoptosis postoperatively. In unilateral acquired ptosis, the ptotic lid is at the same or lower level than the contralateral normal lid on downgaze. Retraction or lag of the ptotic lid on downgaze is due to levator muscle fibrosis, suggesting congenital ptosis. Eversion of the upper lid allows masses or cicatrix in the superior fornix to be ruled out. Symblepharon or vertical shortening of the tarsus may be seen if a previous ptosis repair has been performed by a posterior approach (Fig. 160–3).

Preoperative evaluation should also assess the status of ocular protective mechanisms. Orbicularis muscle function, Bell's phenomenon, and corneal sensation should be intact. Tear film adequacy is confirmed using the tear breakup time and basic secretion tests.

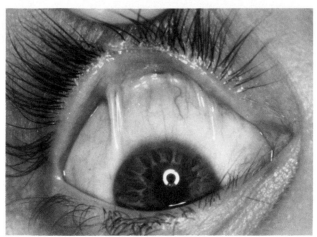

Figure 160–3. Superior fornix symblepharon and vertical shortening of the upper lid tarsus following posterior approach ptosis repair.

If one desires to document visual obstruction caused by ptosis, visual field testing is done. It is important to have the patient relax the frontalis muscle to accurately document the field. Some insurance carriers require repeating the fields with the upper lids taped or held at a normal anatomic level to show the extent of visual field improvement that can be expected following ptosis repair. This also confirms that the field loss is due to the upper lid position. Preoperative photographs with the eyes in the primary position, upgaze, and downgaze are routinely taken to document the findings and are also often required by insurance company review boards.

Ancillary pharmacologic testing for Horner's syndrome (cocaine, hydroxyamphetamine) or myasthenia gravis (tensilon) is indicated if the history or examination suggest these conditions instead of aponeurogenic ptosis. These tests are discussed fully in the Neuro-ophthalmology section.

We routinely perform the manual elevation and phenylephrine tests in unilateral or asymmetric (≥ 2-mm difference in MRD) bilateral cases of acquired ptosis. Manual elevation of the ptotic, or the more ptotic, lid to a normal anatomic position is done while observing the contralateral lid height and recording any change in it. Two drops of phenylephrine 2.5 percent are then instilled in the ptotic eye. After 10 min, both lid heights (MRD) are recorded. If the ptotic lid is raised to a desired level by this stimulation of Müller's superior tarsal muscle, a partial resection of this muscle could be considered to correct the ptosis. If the contralateral lid drops in the manual elevation or phenylephrine test, the patient should be advised of this possibility after correction of the ptotic lid. Also, the surgeon may use this information when doing the ptosis repair to adjust for the expected contralateral lid drop when trying to achieve symmetry.

Bodian has reported a measurable drop in the contralateral lid height (average 2.1 mm) in almost 10 percent of a series of 115 unilateral ptosis repairs.[18] This series included ptosis of all etiologies and surgical correction using a variety of procedures. This phenomenon has been explained by the suggestion that the levator muscles obey Hering's law of equal innervation for paired yoke muscles.[18, 19] The levator subnucleus of the oculomotor complex is known to be a midline structure with bilateral projections, and if there is ptosis in nuclear third-nerve palsies, it is bilateral. If ptosis results in increased innervation to the levators to clear the visual axis, both lids elevate, which may even cause contralateral lid retraction.[20, 21] After ptosis repair, the innervational input is diminished, again bilaterally, and a contralateral lid drop may occur. The stimulus that leads to the initial increased innervation in this subgroup of patients with ptosis is uncertain, but eye dominance may play a role.[20]

To help predict which patients with unilateral ptosis may be predisposed to a contralateral lid fall, we have been studying the possible influence of eye dominance. We posed the following questions: does the nonptotic lid position change more after phenylephrine is instilled in the ptotic eye if the ptotic eye is dominant? Patients with unilateral or asymmetric bilateral ptosis (≥ 2-mm difference in MRD) are candidates for the study. Early results of this ongoing study in 33 patients certainly suggest that the chance for a contralateral lid fall is greater if ptosis affects the dominant eye. This would be anticipated if the level of levator innervation is set by the dominant eye. The stimulus for the dominant eye to increase levator input is unknown but might include clearing of the visual axis for central acuity, retinal illumination level, or peripheral field loss.

Management

Correction of acquired ptosis usually is surgical. The ophthalmologist must first be confident with the classification of a patient's ptosis and must then ascertain the needs and goals of the patient before determining the most appropriate surgical procedure. There are many useful ptosis procedures, some of which are indicated only for specific causes. For aponeurogenic ptosis, we prefer to use the anterior approach to levator surgery almost exclusively.

Preoperative Consent. When discussing ptosis repair with the patient and family, we review the nature of the problem, outline the surgical technique, and present the potential benefits, risks, and complications. More specifically, complications such as hemorrhage, which can threaten vision, infection, and over- or undercorrection, are mentioned. Patients are told that many variables, some controllable and some not, influence their result and that the outcome is sometimes unpredictable. For this reason, possible early revision of the lid height or contour in the office 3 or 4 days postoperatively is presented as a technique for "fine tuning" or "touch up" to maximize favorable results.

Anesthesia. Aponeurotic ptosis repair is done using subcutaneous infiltration of 1 percent xylocaine with epinephrine 1:100,000 for local anesthesia and intravenous sedation with monitored anesthesia care. Limited anesthetic, usually about 1 ml, is used to minimize the protractor paralysis and prevent the spread of anesthetic into the muscular portion of the levator. The patient is sedated just enough so that he or she can relax during the anesthetic injection, but oversedation is avoided. Epinephrine is included in the anesthetic mixture to aid hemostasis, although it may also stimulate Müller's superior tarsal muscle.

Operative Technique (Fig. 160–4). The patient is placed in the supine position, and the whole face is prepared and draped so that there is no tension from the drapes on the brows or lids. The upper lid crease incisions are marked with a fine-tipped skin marking pen at the desired level, length, and contour. If a blepharoplasty is being done in addition, as is often needed in these typically elderly patients, additional markings are made to outline the myocutaneous tissue to be excised. Local anesthetic is injected under the lid crease and in the central pretarsal area followed by gentle massage for a minimum of 5 min.

An optional central lid margin suture of 4–0 silk may be placed to hold the lid on downward traction. Skin incisions are made with a scalpel. A monopolar electro-

cautery with a needle tip is used for both hemostasis and dissection, using the coagulating and cutting current, respectively. Dissection is carried through the orbicularis muscle, and myocutaneous tissue is excised if previously marked. The plane of excision is at the level of the posterior orbicular fascia. The orbital septum is now identified, with the underlying preaponeurotic fat pad and levator aponeurosis often visible through it. After widely opening the septum high in the lid, the preapo-neurotic fat pad is gently dissected away from the underlying levator aponeurosis up to Whitnall's liga-ment. The attachments between the levator and the fat pad are usually avascular and filmy. Care should be taken to identify any fibrous sheets of tissue along the undersurface of the fat, which may be anterior lamellae of the aponeurosis that have separated from the rest of the aponeurosis. Failure to include these layers in the aponeurotic repair may make it impossible to achieve the desired correction. Blunt dissection with cotton-tipped applicators is avoided.

If the aponeurosis is dehisced or disinserted, its distal edge usually appears as a white line inferior to the level at which the septum fuses with the aponeurosis. How-ever, the aponeurosis may appear normal, thinned, or

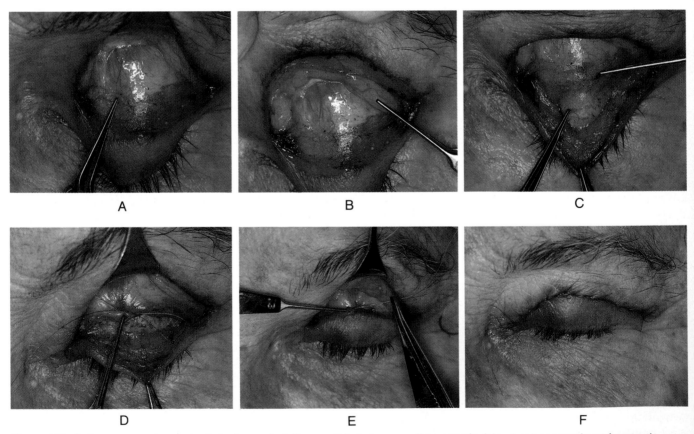

Figure 160–4. Aponeurogenic acquired ptosis repair, left upper lid. *A,* An upper lid crease incision has been made and myocutaneous tissue excised for a blepharoplasty. The orbital septum has been opened, and the preaponeurotic fat pad is retracted superiorly. Forceps point to the levator aponeurosis. *B,* Forceps point to the preaponeurotic fat pad. The "whiter" medial upper lid fat pad can also be seen at the medial (left) corner of the incision. *C,* Pretarsal skin and orbicularis muscle dissected and retracted to expose the tarsal plate (lower forcep). The upper forcep points to the distal end of the levator aponeurosis. *D,* Levator aponeurosis reattached to the tarsus with a central cardinal 6–0 blue prolene suture. The suture is tied with a temporary knot. *E,* Supratarsal fixation suture placed between the pretarsal orbicularis and anterior surface of the levator aponeurosis at the desired height. *F,* Skin closed with a running 6–0 blue prolene suture.

infiltrated with fat or may not be visible at first if it has retracted under the fat pad. If there is uncertainty in identifying the aponeurosis, the patient is asked to look upward, the contraction of the levator muscle thus confirming the location of the aponeurosis. The pretarsal orbicularis is then dissected off the superior half of the tarsal plate. If disinserted, no attachment of the aponeurosis to the tarsus is discernible. Often, however, there is at least some portion of the aponeurosis still attached to the tarsus, and these remnants are carefully preserved. Care should be taken to avoid damaging the peripheral arterial arcade that runs anterior to Müller's muscle along the superior tarsal border. Occasionally, the aponeurosis needs to be carefully dissected away from the underlying Müller's muscle for a few millimeters to allow its free border to be advanced downward.

With the dissection now complete, the aponeurosis is repaired by reattachment to the tarsus, regardless of whether the aponeurosis was dehisced, disinserted, or attenuated. This may require a small resection of the central aponeurosis in cases of attenuation. We no longer simply tuck the aponeurosis, because this creates no raw surface for strong adhesions and thus increases the likelihood of recurrent ptosis.

Three or more horizontal mattress sutures of 6–0 blue prolene are placed to attach the levator to the tarsus. We believe that only a nonabsorbable suture should be used in levator surgery.[22] The central cardinal suture is placed first, being passed vertically through the aponeurosis 3 to 4 mm up from its free edge in an anterior to posterior direction, then horizontally in a partial-thickness bite through the tarsus about 3 mm below its superior border, and finally vertically back through the aponeurosis from posterior to anterior to exit 2 to 3 mm lateral to the first aponeurotic pass. The suture is tied with a temporary knot, and the lid height and contour are examined with the eyes in the primary position and then in upgaze. The lid levels may be evaluated with the patient supine and then sitting up on the operating room table to allow for the effects of gravity, dermatochalasis, and brow ptosis. It is important to remove the operating lights from the field when checking lid position so that the patient does not squint. Oversedation may diminish the patient's effort and cooperation.

There are general guidelines for determining the appropriate lid margin level. In bilateral surgery, the upper lid margins are placed at or 1 mm below the superior limbus in the primary position and upgaze; in unilateral surgery, the margin of the ptotic lid is placed 1 to 2 mm above that of the contralateral lid in primary position and upgaze. This allows for an expected 1- to 2-mm drop in the lid level upon return of function of the anesthetized, paralyzed orbicularis muscles. If the central suture fails to give the appropriate lid height, it is removed and replaced higher or lower through the aponeurosis or tarsus to achieve the desired lid level. In most cases, proper placement of the central suture also gives the desired lid contour. If the suture passes too low on the tarsus, an ectropion may be induced. Once a satisfactory lid level has been obtained, the central suture is tied permanently, and supporting sutures are placed in a similar fashion both medial and lateral to the central cardinal suture. Once again, these are tied temporarily at first and made permanent only after rechecking the lid height and contour. Irregularities of the lid contour are usually best discerned with the eyes in an upgaze position.

With the critical judgment portion of the procedure now complete, additional anesthetic can be injected as needed for fat resection or repair of a prolapsed orbital lobe of the lacrimal gland. If the aponeurosis is significantly advanced, excess aponeurotic tissue below the tarsal sutures is trimmed. Supratarsal fixation of the lid crease is then performed with three buried interrupted sutures of an absorbable 6–0 material. These sutures attach the pretarsal orbicularis muscle edge to the desired level on the anterior surface of the levator aponeurosis to establish the location of the upper lid crease and tip the eyelashes up into proper position. A running suture of 6–0 prolene is used for skin closure. Antibiotic or antibiotic/steroid ointment is applied to the suture line and in the operated eye, and iced gauze compresses are placed before the patient is moved to the recovery area.

Postoperative Orders. Continuous iced gauze compresses are used for the first 24 to 48 hr after surgery, and the head is kept elevated on a minimum of two pillows. Ointment is applied to the suture line three to four times a day, and analgesics are supplied as needed. Patients are instructed to call immediately if there is severe pain, visual loss, or a sudden change in bleeding or bruising. All patients are examined in the office on the third or fourth postoperative day.

Early Postoperative Revision. On the first postoperative visit, the MRD, lid contour, upper lid excursion, lid edema and ecchymosis, lid closure, and corneal status are noted. If the lid height or contour are unacceptable, provided marked edema or hemorrhage are absent, an office revision may be performed quite easily without anesthetic (before closure). Local anesthetic significantly affects lid function and makes judgment of lid levels and contours more difficult. Cutaneous sutures are removed; the wound is spread apart gently; and levator aponeurosis sutures are revised without discomfort in the absence of local anesthesia. Thus, lid evaluation during the office revision under these circumstances is more accurate. The lid margin is placed at the final desired level. After all lid level and contour determinations have been completed, local anesthetic may be injected as needed prior to wound closure. A detailed account of this technique and its excellent results has been presented.[23]

We believe that key principles in the primary repair, such as monopolar cautery dissection (reducing operative and postoperative edema) and use of blue prolene sutures (more easily seen during a revision), make office revision at this early time accurate and relatively quick. Patient acceptance has been very good, at least in part due to the fact that patients are informed preoperatively of this possibility. This technique is recommended primarily for aponeurotic ptosis surgery, because dissection and postoperative edema are less. However, this method

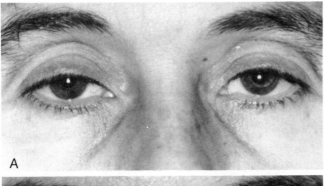

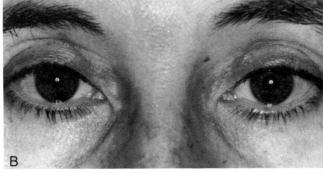

Figure 160–5. *A,* Bilateral aponeurogenic acquired ptosis. *B,* After repair of levator dehiscence in both upper eyelids using the anterior approach.

has also been used successfully in a limited number of patients who have had levator resections. If an early revision is contraindicated, unsuccessful, or deemed unnecessary and an unacceptably low lid height or contour is identified later, we wait at least 6 wk before considering a secondary procedure. If there is an overcorrection causing significant exposure keratopathy that responds poorly to lubricants at any time after surgery, an upper lid recession is indicated.

SUMMARY

The aponeurotic approach to repair of ptosis has greatly enhanced surgical results and decreased the need for reoperation (Fig. 160–5). Nevertheless, any surgeon who performs ptosis repair realizes that results are not always consistent or predictable. The variables involved in ptosis repair have been well described, and several authors have compared operative and postoperative lid levels and developed methods of "early" postoperative adjustment.[24–27] Our revision procedure is unique in its early (3- to 4-day) undertaking and in its lack of anesthetic injection. Continued scientific studies of the pathophysiology and treatment of acquired ptosis hopefully will continue to improve our primary surgical results.

REFERENCES

1. Dortzbach RK, Levine MR, Angrist RC: Approach to acquired ptosis. *In* Smith BC (ed): Ophthalmic Plastic and Reconstructive Surgery. St. Louis, CV Mosby, 1987.
2. Dortzbach RK, McGetrick JJ: Diagnosis and Treatment of Acquired Ptosis. Module 10, Focal Points 1984, American Academy of Ophthalmology, 1984.
3. Frueh BR: The mechanistic classification of ptosis. Ophthalmology 87:1019, 1980.
4. Custer PL, Tenzel RR, Kowalczyk AP: Blepharochalasis syndrome. Am J Ophthalmol 99:424, 1985.
5. Anderson RL, Gordy DD: Aponeurotic defects in congenital ptosis. Ophthalmology 86:1493, 1979.
6. Jones LT, Quickert MH, Wobig JL: The cure of ptosis by aponeurotic repair. Arch Ophthalmol 93:629, 1975.
7. Anderson RL, Beard C: The levator aponeurosis attachments and their clinical significance. Arch Ophthalmol 95:1437, 1977.
8. Dortzbach RK, Sutula FC: Involutional blepharoptosis: A histopathological study. Arch Ophthalmol 98:2045, 1980.
9. Carroll RP: Cautery dissection in levator surgery. Ophthalmic Plast Reconstr Surg 4:243, 1988.
10. Kuwabara T, Cogan DG, Johnson CC: Structure of the muscles of the upper eyelid. Arch Ophthalmol 93:1189, 1975.
11. Paris GL, Quickert MH: Disinsertion of the aponeurosis of the levator palpebrae superioris muscle after cataract extraction. Am J Ophthalmol 81:337, 1976.
12. Kaplan LJ, Jaffe NS, Clayman HM: Ptosis and cataract surgery: A multivariant computer analysis of a prospective study. Ophthalmology 92:237, 1985.
13. Lemke BN, Stasior OG, Rosenberg PN: The surgical relations of the levator palpebrae superioris muscle. Ophthalmic Plast Reconstr Surg 4:25, 1988.
14. Lemke BN: Blepharoptosis Following Cataract Surgery: Retrobulbar versus Peribulbar Block. Oral presentation at the ASOPRS 20th Annual Scientific Symposium, New Orleans, 1989.
15. Shore JW, McCord CD: Anatomic changes in involutional blepharoptosis. Am J Ophthalmol 98:21, 1984.
16. Cahill KV, Buerger GF, Johnson BL: Ptosis associated with fatty infiltration of Müller's muscle and levator muscle. Ophthalmic Plast Reconstr Surg 2:213, 1986.
17. Lemke BN, Stasior OG: Eyebrow considerations in blepharoptosis. Adv Ophthalmic Plast Reconstr Surg 1:55, 1982.
18. Bodian M: Lid droop following contralateral ptosis repair. Arch Ophthalmol 100:1122, 1982.
19. Gay AJ, Salman ML, Windsor CE: Hering's law, the levators, and their relationship in disease states. Arch Ophthalmol 77:157, 1967.
20. Schechter RJ: Ptosis with contralateral lid retraction due to excessive innervation of the levator palpebrae superioris. Ann Ophthalmol 10:1324, 1978.
21. Gonnering RS: Pseudoretraction of the eyelid in thyroid-associated orbitopathy. Arch Ophthalmol 106:1078, 1988.
22. Lemke BN, Dortzbach RK: Study of Long-Acting, Absorbable, Polydioxanone Suture in Levator Palpebrae Superioris Surgery. Oral presentation at the ASOPRS 19th Annual Scientific Symposium, Las Vegas, 1988.
23. Dortzbach RK, Kronish JW: Early Revision in the Office for Adults Having Levator Ptosis Surgery. Oral presentation at the ASOPRS 21st Annual Scientific Symposium, Atlanta, 1990.
24. Berris CE: Adjustable sutures for the correction of adult-acquired ptosis. Ophthalmic Plast Reconst Surg 4:171, 1988.
25. Linberg JV, Vasquez RJ, Chao GM: Aponeurotic ptosis repair under local anesthesia: Prediction of results from operative lid height. Ophthalmology 95:1046, 1988.
26. Jordan DR, Anderson RL: A simple procedure for adjusting eyelid position after aponeurotic ptosis surgery. Arch Ophthalmol 105:1288, 1987.
27. Shore JW, Bergin DJ, Garrett SN: Results of blepharoptosis surgery with early postoperative adjustment. Ophthalmology 97:1502, 1990.

Chapter 161

■

Upper Eyelid Malpositions: Retraction

JEMSHED A. KHAN

EYELID RETRACTION

Upper eyelid retraction exists when, in the presence of a globe of normal size and position, the upper lid margin rests at such a height that white sclera is visible above the iris while the gaze is directed, without staring, in the primary position.[1] The appearance mimics that usually associated with anger, staring, or intense surprise.

Etiology and Pathogenesis

CONGENITAL

Essential Infantile Eyelid Retraction

Although the newborn eyelid fissure is narrow at birth, within a few weeks it widens remarkably,[2] and the upper eyelid margin reportedly lies well above the cornea.[1] Lid retraction, then, may be a normal finding during infancy. The infant palpebral fissure also seems larger than the adult fissure owing to a lesser horizontal width and greater rounding.[2] Stimulation of Müller's muscle may have helped to foster the belief that lid retraction is normal during infancy, in that infants may be easily startled by the approach of an unfamiliar examiner obtaining fissure measurements. The upper eyelid descends during youth, eventually settling 1 to 3 mm below the superior limbus. There is little subsequent alteration in the vertical height of the palpebral fissure.[2-4]

Unilateral Congenital Eyelid Retraction

The primary feature of unilateral congenital eyelid retraction is fixed and persistent retraction of an upper or lower eyelid that is present at birth.[5] Despite lagophthalmos in downgaze, only 20 percent of patients have symptoms of corneal exposure.[5] Other causes of lid retraction should be excluded, and treatment is usually deferred until the patient is at least 4 yr of age, when such patients can cooperate with postoperative manipulation of final lid height via massage. Treatment usually consists of a levator lengthening procedure.[5] The cause of unilateral congenital eyelid retraction is unknown, and the levator muscle appears to be normal during a routine histologic examination.[5]

Cyclic Oculomotor Paralysis and Spasm

Cyclic upper eyelid retraction may be a prominent feature of cyclic oculomotor spasm and paralysis—a rare disorder in which all of the intraocular structures and some of the extraocular structures innervated by the third cranial nerve alternate between spastic and paralytic phases.[6] Almost always, this condition is first noted either at birth or before 2 yr of age and is unilateral.[7] During the paralytic phase, which usually lasts from 1 to 3 min, the pupil dilates and the ciliary body relaxes.[8] The lid usually droops, and the eye is exotropic. Within a few minutes, the upper eyelid begins to twitch, heralding the onset of the spastic phase. During the spastic phase, which usually lasts for 30 to 100 sec, the upper eyelid may retract, the pupil always constricts, and, in about one fourth of cases, the medial rectus constricts.[8] As the spastic phase ends, the upper eyelid once again twitches, signalling a return to the paralytic phase. This condition is benign and lifelong and persists during sleep.[8]

Congenital Hyperthyroidism

Although quite rare, congenital hyperthyroidism occurs occasionally in the newborn offspring of mothers who have a history of hyperthyroidism.[9, 10] Characteristic features of the affected infant include eyelid retraction, goiter, tachycardia, restlessness, diarrhea, ravenous appetite, and failure to gain weight.[9] The disorder has been postulated to result from the transplacental transfer of maternal long-acting thyroid stimulator (LATS) substances or other humoral factors.[11] This disorder is usually self-limiting and lasts from 3 to 6 mo.[12]

A second and more serious form of congenital Graves' disease occurs, in which there is often a family history of thyroid disorder but the mother may or may not be affected.[12] This form is not self-limited and may persist, resulting in premature fusion of cranial sutures, microcephaly, short stature, and emotional and mental retardation.[10, 12]

Miscellaneous

Synkinetic eyelid retraction may accompany Duane's syndrome and Marcus-Gunn jaw-winking.[10]

ACQUIRED LID RETRACTION

Neurogenic

Pretectal Syndrome. Neurogenic lid retraction is most often encountered with damage to the supranuclear posterior commissure, which results in the *pretectal syndrome*.[13] Other features of the pretectal syndrome

1831

may include upward gaze palsy, pupillary light-near dissociation, convergence-retraction nystagmus, skew deviation, and upbeat nystagmus.[13] Although the eponym *Parinaud's syndrome* is often attached to the aforementioned findings,[14, 15] Keane prefers the term *pretectal syndrome*. Keane argues that Parinaud's descriptions of the syndrome were not the first, were general and vague, did not define the syndrome, and incorrectly localized the site of neuroanatomic dysfunction.[13]

Supranuclear lid retraction occurs bilaterally and symmetrically, and its severity parallels the degree of upward gaze palsy. The clinical appearance of bilateral symmetric lid retraction has been termed *Collier's sign*[16] and *posterior fossa stare* (Fig. 161–1).[17] The lid retraction results from the patient's normal levator-superior rectus synkinesis. In an attempt to overcome the upward gaze palsy and maintain the globe in the primary position, excessive innervation must flow to the superior rectus, and thus, also flows to the levator palpebrae superioris, resulting in disproportionate eyelid elevation. Therefore, the supranuclear origin of lid retraction is confirmed by documenting an invariably present upward gaze palsy and noting an often-present disappearance of lid retraction on downgaze.[13] Keane reported lid retraction in 40.3 percent of 206 patients with the pretectal syndrome.[13]

Diagnostic considerations should center about the posterior commissure and include stroke, tumor (Fig. 161–2), encephalitis, infection (often cysticercosis, but also secondary central nervous system [CNS] infections in patients with acquired immunodeficiency syndrome [AIDS]), bulbar poliomyelitis, hydrocephalus, multiple sclerosis, kernicterus, Wernicke's syndrome, Bassen-Kornzweig syndrome, and closed head injury (Table 161–1).[13]

Seventh-Nerve Paralysis. Loss of orbicularis oculi muscle tone in congenital or acquired seventh-nerve palsy may result in eyelid retraction on the basis of unopposed levator muscle and Müller muscle activity. When the seventh-nerve palsy occurs prior to early childhood, the cornea may occasionally tolerate complete exposure without any discomfort or evidence of

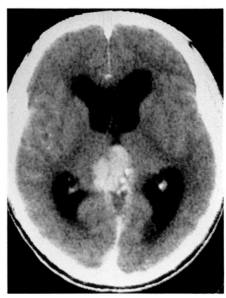
Figure 161–2. A pineal tumor is demonstrated in a CT scan of a patient with pretectal syndrome. (Courtesy of J.R. Keane, M.D.)

exposure keratitis. In older patients, the degree of lid retraction may be obscured by an associated brow ptosis.

The goal of management should be to maintain an adequate corneal epithelial surface. When corneal epithelial breakdown results from an inadequate blink, then temporary or permanent improvement in corneal coverage should be pursued. Medical management[18] may include taping, artificial tears, lubricating ointment,

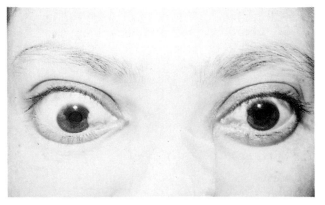
Figure 161–1. Eyelid retraction due to pretectal syndrome in a patient with cysticercal hydrocephalus. (Courtesy of J.R. Keane, M.D.)

Table 161–1. CAUSE OF PRETECTAL SYNDROME

Cause		No. of Patients
Hydrocephalus		80
Hydrocephalus—untreated	54	
Shunt obstruction	26	
(Hydrocephalus and obstruction due to cysticercosis)	(47)	
Stroke		53
Thalamic hemorrhage	32	
Primary pretectal hemorrhage	2	
Infarction	19	
Tumor		45
Pineal	18	
Thalamic	16	
Midbrain/third ventricle	11	
(Metastases)	(3)	
Infection		7
Encephalitis	2	
Ventriculitis	1	
Abscess	4	
(1 bacterial, 1 tuberculous, 2 toxoplasmosis—AIDS)		
Tentorial herniation		9
Trauma		3
Arteriovenous malformation—demonstrated		2
Congenital (?kernicterus)		2
Wernicke's syndrome		1
Bassen-Kornzweig syndrome		1
Unknown		3

Reprinted with permission from Keane JR: The pretectal syndrome: 206 patients. Neurology 40:684–690, 1990.

patching, wrap-around eyeglasses, moisture chamber, therapeutic contact lenses, and humidification of the environment.

More aggressive measures[18-22] include botulinum toxin form A, 1.25 to 2.5 units, injection to induce a protective ptosis,[23] punctal occlusion, modified palpebral spring,[24] upper eyelid loading with a gold weight,[25] tarsorrhaphy, temporalis muscle transposition,[25] nerve transfer,[25] facial reanimation,[25] Gunderson flap,[26] dermal graft,[27] and so forth. The choice of procedure should be based on the probability of spontaneous recovery of seventh-nerve function,[24] corneal stability and sensitivity, tear production, and the patient's wishes. When this form of lid retraction results in only a cosmetic defect, then it is often amenable to correction via a müllerectomy and a small lateral marginal tarsorrhaphy.

Aberrant Regeneration CN III. Upper eyelid retraction may be a prominent feature of aberrant regeneration of the oculomotor nerve. Aberrant regeneration results from misdirection of sprouting axons during the reparative phase following third-nerve injury due to trauma, aneurysm, or tumor. Misdirected axons may result in lid elevation during attempted adduction or infraduction. Aberrant regeneration without an antecedent third-nerve palsy is diagnostic of intracavernous aneurysm or meningioma.[28, 29]

Other Neurogenic Forms of Eyelid Retraction

Fisher's Syndrome. Bilateral external ophthalmoplegia, ataxia, and areflexia compose Fisher's syndrome.[30] Bilateral and symmetric upper eyelid retraction may accompany the external ophthalmoplegia, which is characterized by fixation of gaze in the primary position. Fisher's syndrome is believed to represent either a variant of Guillain-Barré[31] syndrome or a form of parainfectious brain stem encephalitis characterized by both supranuclear and oculomotor nerve disturbances.[32, 33]

Smith and Walsh[34] describe several typical features: (1) adult male preponderance; (2) antecedent respiratory infection; (3) total external ophthalmoplegia, although downward gaze is sometimes spared; (4) normal pupillary light responses; (5) diplopia; (6) cerebellar ataxia; (7) generalized areflexia; (8) absence of motor weakness of the extremeties; (9) absence of mental changes; (10) minimal or no sensory impairment; and (11) spontaneous recovery within 7 to 12 wk.

Variable features include facial palsy, migratory parasthesias, often of the trunk and upper extremities, and cerebrospinal fluid albuminocytologic dissociation. CNS abnormalities are sometimes found on computed tomography (CT) scanning or on magnetic resonance imaging.[31]

Contralateral Ptosis and Pseudolid Retraction. When there is ptosis of the dominant eye, the nondominant upper eyelid often retracts, and the ptotic eye appears normal. This situation of pseudoretraction arises because Hering's law dictates simultaneous and equal innervation of both levator muscles; thus, when an increased levator tone is necessary to raise the ptotic lid to a normal height, this innervation also flows to the normal eyelid, causing it to retract (Fig. 161-3).

This condition of masked ptosis presenting as contra-

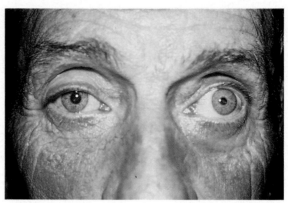

Figure 161-3. Pseudoretraction of the left upper eyelid in a patient with third-nerve palsy of the dominant and fixating right eye.

lateral eyelid retraction may be diagnosed by (1) visually occluding the nonretracted eye, sometimes for a prolonged period, and observing the return of the retracted eyelid to a normal position,[35, 36] or by (2) instilling 2.5 percent topical phenylephrine hydrochloride in the nonretracted eye and observing the return of the retracted eyelid to a normal height,[37] or (3) manually elevating the ptotic lid.[38] If myasthenic ptosis is suspected, edrophonium chloride may be administered as a diagnostic maneuver.[39]

Causes are the same as those considered in any unilateral ptosis. This condition has been diagnosed in patients with dysthyroid unilateral ptosis[37, 40] and myasthenic ptosis.[39, 41]

Proper treatment requires recognizing that the retracted eyelid is in fact normal. Further efforts are directed toward raising the ptotic lid.

Miscellaneous. Periodic lid retraction due to clonic spasm of the levator palpebrae superioris muscles may occur with chorea, impending tentorial herniation, epileptic discharges including petit mal and myoclonic seizures, and oculogyric crises.[17]

Phasic lid opening is observed occasionally in comatose patients. The eyes of these patients are wide open, yet the patient is unresponsive—so-called coma vigil.[17]

Cicatricial

Posttraumatic. Posttraumatic upper eyelid retraction results from contracture of scar tissue or tethering of eyelid structures by scar tissue. If the wound was superficial, then only cutaneous cicatricial tissues may be responsible for eyelid retraction. With deeper injuries, adhesions may involve the tarsus, levator, septum, and so forth.

Postsurgical. Postsurgical upper eyelid retraction may occur following upper eyelid skin excision (i.e., blepharoplasty), levator resection or advancement (i.e., ptosis overcorrection), and müllerectomy or Müller muscle advancement (i.e., tarsoconjunctival flap repair of lower eyelid defects), or as a result of recession of the superior rectus muscle.

Postchemical/Thermal Burn. Eyelid burns are found

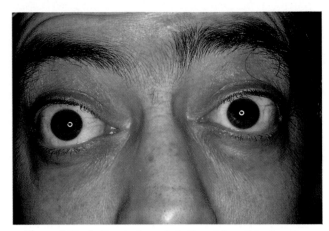

Figure 161–4. Proptosis and dysthyroid eyelid retraction.

in two thirds of patients with thermal facial burns.[42] Half of such burns are superficial partial-thickness injuries that usually heal spontaneously within 1 wk.[42] Among more severe burns, however, ectropion is the most common complication.[43, 44] Visual loss from direct burns of the globe and cornea is rare compared with visual loss caused by corneal infection and exposure secondary to ectropion.[43, 44] Direct globe injury is more common with chemical burns.

The late management of eyelid deformities in burn patients is directed toward functional and esthetic rehabilitation of the eyelids. See Management.

Dysthyroid

Eyelid retraction (Dalrymple's sign) is the most frequent eye finding in patients with Graves' disease[45] and is seen in one third to two thirds of such patients (Fig. 161–4). Among patients with dysthyroid orbitopathy, over 90 percent demonstrate eyelid retraction.[46] When the lid retraction is caused by contracture or fibrosis of the levator tissues, failure of the upper lid to smoothly follow the globe on downgaze (lid lag, i.e., von Graefe's sign) often occurs (Fig. 161–5A, B). Dysthyroid retraction of the upper eyelid is characteristically greatest at the outer one third of the eyelid (see Fig. 161–4). When eyelid retraction accompanies exophthalmos, luxation of the globe can occur (Fig. 161–6A, B). Eyelid retraction may result from proptosis alone, without any eyelid abnormality.

Etiology

Several factors putatively contribute to eyelid retraction with Graves' disease (Table 161–2).

Many of the clinical features of Graves' disease are believed to represent the sequelae of a poorly understood underlying autoimmune reaction against the extraocular muscles.[47] An early feature of this autoimmune attack is the stimulation of endomysial fibroblasts, resulting in mucopolysaccharide deposition restricted to the extraocular muscles.[48] Later on, these fibroblasts produce excess collagen, which strangulates the muscle cells and causes fibrosis and enlargement of the muscle bellies (Figs. 161–7 to 161–10). Engorgement of the muscle bellies, inflammatory processes, increased orbital pressure, and venous congestion favor the development of interstitial edema that manifests as eyelid swelling, herniation of eyelid fat pads, chemosis, and lacrimal gland enlargement.[47]

Pathophysiology. Three anatomic sites of dysfunction have been identified in dysthyroid eyelid retraction: the skeletal muscle fibers of the levator palpebrae superioris,[49] Müller's muscle,[50–52] and the levator muscle and aponeurosis along with adjacent eyelid tissue planes.[51, 52] Each site is considered separately in the following discussion.

Levator Muscle. Skeletal muscle changes in the levator palpebrae superioris appear histologically distinct from those reported in the oculorotary muscles. For example, there is little inflammation or fibrosis of the levator muscle.[49, 51, 52] The primary findings reported are enlargement of individual muscle fibers and expansion of the extracellular space,[49] as well as areas of fatty infiltration and degeneration of striated muscle fibers.[51, 52]

Rundle and Pochin, in their 1944 autopsy study, established a correlation between lid retraction and levator muscle volume.[53] More recently, however, CT imaging in 76 patients in one study and 16 patients in another study showed no correlation between the degree

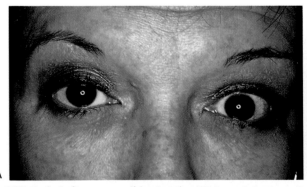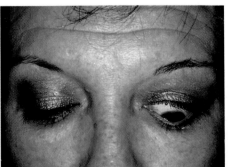

Figure 161–5. A, Left upper eyelid retraction (Dalrymple's sign). B, On downgaze, lid lag is evident (von Graefe's sign).

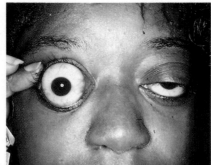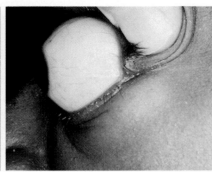

Figure 161–6. *A,* This patient with exophthalmos and eyelid retraction can induce luxation of the globe by increasing eyelid retraction via lateral canthal traction. *B,* Same patient, lateral view.

of lid retraction and volume of the levator-superior rectus complex.[54, 55]

Müller's Muscle. Müller's muscle has also been implicated in the development of dysthyroid lid retraction. Overstimulation of Müller's muscle in the hyperthyroid state causes lid retraction that resolves in the euthyroid state. More permanent structural alterations of Müller's muscle may accompany the eyelid inflammation of Graves' disease and persist in the euthyroid state. In Müller's muscle specimens from patients with dysthyroid lid retraction, Kagoshima and coworkers found electron microscopic evidence of smooth muscle cell contractile and degenerative changes.[50] They believed that these changes were analogous to the degenerative smooth muscle changes described in the arterioles of hypertensive rats.

In contrast, Grove reported that by light microscopy, except for some fatty infiltration, Müller's muscle is relatively uninvolved in dysthyroid lid retraction.[51, 52] Rootman and coworkers studied 66 Müller's muscle specimens from patients with dysthyroid lid retraction and reported an increased mast cell population, occasional lymphocytic cell infiltration, and rare fibrosis.[54] Both Grove and Rootman commented on the paucity of Müller's muscle abnormalities in the specimens that they reviewed.

Levator and Eyelid Tissues. The clinical abnormalities most commonly encountered during surgical correction of dysthyroid lid retraction involve adhesions between the levator and adjacent tissue planes, such as the orbital septum and orbicularis oculi.[51, 52] These adhesions are found in 50 percent of dysthyroid eyelids and may contribute greatly to upper eyelid retraction, lid lag, and lagophthalmos.[51, 52] Specifically, scarring between the levator and septum is thought to tether the eyelid in a

retracted position and limit normal eyelid closure during sleep or blinking.[51, 52] Such adhesions may be appreciated clinically by directing the patient's gaze inferiorly, grasping the lashes of the upper eyelid, and gauging the resistance of the eyelid tissues when tugging inferiorly (Grove's sign).

Eyelid crease malpositions also occur in Graves' disease. Frueh and coworkers reported a higher upper eyelid crease (mean of 1.6 mm) that correlated with the degree of exophthalmos in patients with thyroid eye disease.[4] They concluded that the higher upper eyelid crease indicated that compensatory levator aponeurosis defects occurred in patients with thyroid eye disease. Although aponeurotic ptosis occurs in dysthyroid eye disease, such cases are the exception to the rule. Furthermore, aponeurotic defects have not been routinely identified during the surgical repair of dysthyroid lid retraction.[51, 52, 56–58]

I would offer an alternate explanation for their results: the elevated lid crease represents fibrotic contracture of the anterior insertion of the levator aponeurosis into the upper eyelid skin fold. Because the tarsus is relatively inelastic and opposed in its upward movement by the orbicularis oculi, it does not stretch in response to the chronic upward stress of levator fibrosis and contracture. The eyelid skin, on the other hand, is thin and elastic and expands in its vertical dimension in response to contracture of its levator insertion, thus producing the

Table 161–2. FACTORS PUTATIVELY CONTRIBUTING TO DYSTHYROID EYELID RETRACTION

Hyperthyroidism
Enhanced sensitivity of Müller's muscle to adrenergic stimulation
Proptosis
Secondary levator muscle and superior rectus overactivity in order to overcome inferior rectus restriction
Levator muscle contracture and fibrosis
Adnexal fibrosis

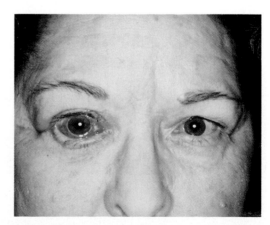

Figure 161–7. Right-sided exophthalmos and lid retraction due to unilateral dysthyroid orbitopathy.

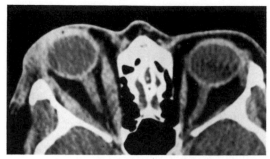

Figure 161–8. Axial CT scan shows fusiform enlargement of horizontal rectus muscle bellies in the dysthyroid right orbit versus normal-sized muscles of the left orbit (same patient as in Figure 161–7).

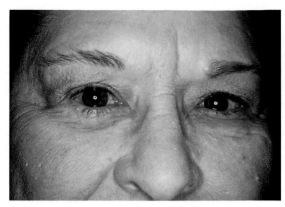

Figure 161–10. Same patient as in previous figures following right orbital decompression and irradiation. Note that the lid retraction has diminished greatly as a result of diminished proptosis. No eyelid surgery was performed.

higher upper eyelid fold characteristic of Graves' disease.

Sisler, Jakobiec, and Trokel postulate that the fibrosis found between the eyelid tissue planes results from the percolation of interstitial fluids and inflammatory cells from the orbit into the eyelid tissues.[48] Interestingly, the posterior orbital fat in dysthyroid orbitopathy is relatively spared from the ravages of inflammation. This suggests that, since the remainder of the orbit is devoid of lymphatics, there is an *efferent* role of the eyelid lymphatics in the development of the eyelid changes of Graves' disease.

Examination of the patient should elucidate the cause of eyelid retraction, quantify the degree of dysthyroid eyelid retraction, and help to determine the urgency or necessity of surgical or medical repositioning of the eyelids.

Hepatic Cirrhosis

Paul, in 1865, first reported an association between what he presumed to be a clinical appearance of thyrotoxicosis and liver disease.[59] Summerskill and Molnar, in 1962, studied 110 cirrhotic patients and found lid lag and lid retraction in 12 percent of patients.[60] They believed that eyelid retraction could occur on the basis of liver disease alone. Bartley and Gorman reviewed some of Summerskill and Molnar's cases and found evidence of thyroid dysfunction.[61] Bartley and Gorman concluded that Summerskill and Molnar's cases probably represented dysthyroid eyelid retraction, which was not easily diagnosed with the tests of 30 yr ago.

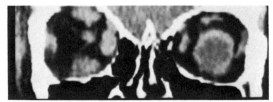

Figure 161–9. Coronal CT scan shows enlarged extraocular muscles in the dysthyroid right orbit compared with the normal-sized muscles of the left orbit. Note that the right levator/superior rectus complex is enlarged. The posterior left globe is seen, but the right globe is displaced anteriorly due to proptosis (same patient as in Figure 161–8).

Drug-Induced and Metabolic

A number of drugs including sympathomimetics—topical neosynephrine,[37] thyroid replacement therapy, and apraclonidine[62]—can induce a temporary eyelid retraction by stimulating Müller's muscle. Corticosteroids, edrophonium chloride, prostigmine, and succinylcholine have also been associated with eyelid retraction, as have the metabolic derangements of hyperkalemic periodic paralysis.[10]

Management

The proper management of upper eyelid retraction requires finding the cause and then effecting an appropriate cure. In neurologic causes, metabolic causes, and pseudoeyelid retraction, treatment should be directed toward the underlying disorder.

When there is marked synkinetic upper eyelid retraction, the levator may have to be completely disinserted and tarsofrontalis suspension provided. Eyelid retraction of 2 mm or less, which is due to seventh-nerve palsy, may be treated by Müller muscle excision and a cosmetic lateral tarsorrhaphy. Greater degrees of eyelid retraction may require lid loading with a gold weight, palpebral spring, temporalis muscle transfer, or levator recession.

Upper eyelid retraction due to cutaneous cicatricial changes or following burns should be treated by excision and release of all scarred tissues accompanied by correction of the skin defect (e.g., Z-plasty, free skin graft, skin flap). Eyelid retraction due to deeper trauma requires excision and release of scarred tissues.

When dysthyroid lid retraction occurs in the milieu of hyperthyroidism, return of the patient to the euthyroid state sometimes resolves the lid retraction. Surgical intervention should, if possible, be deferred until the patient is euthyroid, and the lid retraction is stable rather than progressive.

Dysthyroid eyelid retraction of 3 mm or less without marked adhesion of the levator to the orbital septum may be treated by a posterior approach Müller muscle

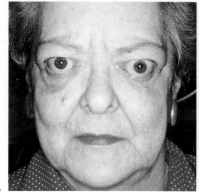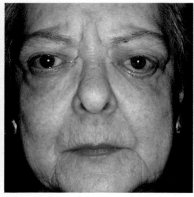

Figure 161–11. *A,* Dysthyroid eyelid retraction resulting in symptomatic corneal exposure keratitis. *B,* Same patient, following anterior approach levator recession, division of septum-levator adhesions, and Müller muscle excision of both upper eyelids.

A   B

excision, possible levator tenotomy, and small lateral tarsorrhaphy.

Greater degrees of dysthyroid upper eyelid retraction or eyelid retraction with septal-levator adhesions require an anterior approach levator recession, division of adhesions, and müllerectomy (Fig. 161–11*A, B*). Success depends on an aggressive and complete dissection, preservation of the lacrimal gland ductules, and early (within 1 wk) readjustment of an unsatisfactory eyelid height. In the author's experience as well as that of others,[51, 52, 58] spacer materials are unnecessary in the upper eyelid (Fig. 161–12). Because one cannot predict the degree to which tissues will spontaneously reapproximate themselves during healing that proceeds from the apex or narrowest aspect of an incision to its widest aspect, levator tenotomy or myotomy incisions, in my hands, lack predictability and adjustability (Fig. 161–13*A, B*).

I favor complete levator disinsertion and recession; specifically, Char's modification of the approach of Harvey and Anderson, with the exception that the sutures extend from the recessed levator edge to the tarsal plate (see Fig. 161–11*A, B*).[63] This approach allows ready readjustment during the early perioperative period—an important consideration since unpredictability is the surgeon's bane when dealing with dysthyroid eye disease. An adjunctive small lateral tarsorrhaphy is

often also used in order to diminish lateral "flare" and elevate the lower eyelid. In order to appreciate the many nuances and avoid the myriad pitfalls of dysthyroid eyelid retraction surgery, the reader is strongly encouraged to review the primary references before attempting surgery.[51, 52, 56–58, 64]

Because stimulation of Müller's muscle contributes to dysthyroid eyelid retraction, pharmacologic disruption of the adrenergic action of norepinephrine on Müller's muscle can diminish eyelid retraction. Topical agents include phentolamine,[65] thymoxamine hydrochloride,[66] guanethidine sulfate,[67, 68] propranolol,[67] and bethanidine.[69]

Topical guanethidine has been most widely used and studied.[68, 70–73] Although effective after several days and well tolerated in 86 percent of patients (i.e., guanethidine monosulfate, 2 or 5 percent solution, 1 gtt b.i.d. to q.i.d.), unwanted local effects, including miosis (100 percent), burning sensation upon instillation (17 percent), visible conjunctival hyperemia (74 percent), discomfort (5 percent), punctate keratitis (4 percent), and marked conjunctival hyperemia due to sensitization (4 percent),[71] have dampened enthusiasm for its routine use in dysthyroid eyelid retraction.[73]

An alternative pharmacologic approach to eyelid retraction targets the skeletal muscle of the levator palpebrae superioris. Botulinum toxin-A interferes with acetylcholine release from the motor nerve terminal,[74] effectively creating a flaccid paralysis that lasts several weeks. Complete ptosis of the upper eyelid can be induced by injecting botulinum toxin-A (Oculinum), 1.2 to 2.5 units, into the tissues lying 25 mm posterior to the midportion of the superior orbital rim and between the belly of the levator palpebrae superioris muscle and the orbital roof.[75] In dysthyroid upper eyelid retraction, botulinum toxin-A injection has met with limited success owing to a marked prolonged ptosis, failure to reverse lid retraction associated with tethering of the levator to the septum, vertical diplopia due to toxin diffusion into the superior rectus, and an impermanent effect.[76]

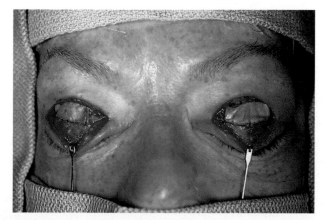

Figure 161–12. Scleral spacer grafts interposed between the superior borders of the tarsal plates and the inferior edge of the recessed levator aponeurosis.

ENTROPION

Entropion is an inward rotation of the eyelid margin such that the cilia brush against the globe. The constant abrasion of the cilia against the cornea risks keratitis or

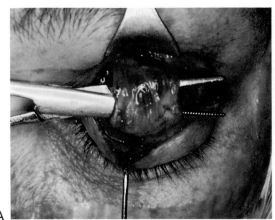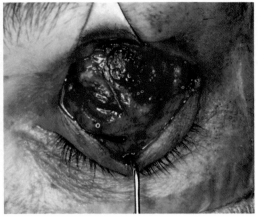

Figure 161–13. *A,* Levator muscle and aponeurosis isolated from the dysthyroid upper eyelid. *B,* Same eyelid as in *A.* Appearance of the levator muscle immediately after levator lengthening by two relaxing myotomy incisions.

ulceration. Even if the cilia are destroyed, keratinized eyelid skin may still irritate the cornea.

Except for unusual cases (i.e., rare involutional cases),[77, 78] congenitally absent skin fold,[79] and tarsal kink syndrome[80, 81] (Figs. 161–14 to 161–17), upper eyelid entropion results from a relative vertical shortage of posterior lamellae tissues (i.e., tarsus, conjunctiva, and eyelid retractors).[82]

Etiology

The usual causes of acquired upper eyelid entropion seen in an international eyelid practice are listed in Table 161–3.[82] Trachoma, often seen in immigrants and older Americans, is the most common cause.

An extensive discussion of the subtleties of all of the various causes of upper eyelid entropion is beyond the scope of this chapter, and the reader is referred elsewhere in the text for a more detailed discussion of individual entities.

Nonetheless, a thorough history, clinical examination, and if necessary, conjunctival biopsy, should establish the cause in most cases. With trachoma, for example, there is often a history of youthful days spent in an endemic area. On examination, Arlt's lines, superficial fibrovascular pannus, and Herbert's pits are often evident. Herpes zoster ophthalmicus is usually evident because of the typical prodrome, unilateral dermatome pattern of vesicular eruption, seasonal occurrence, and occasional characteristic keratitis and uveitis.

Chronic blepharoconjunctivitis often has typical slit-lamp findings, such as lid margin telangiectasia, scurf, collarettes, sebum, meibomian foam, punctate keratitis, papillary conjunctivitis, and marginal corneal infiltrates.

Erythema multiforme major (Stevens-Johnson syndrome), often triggered by a bacteria, virus, or antibiotic, is characterized as cutaneous and mucosal bullous lesions that may heal with significant scarring, dry eye, and symblepharon.

Ocular cicatricial pemphigoid, characterized by bilateral progressive subepithelial conjunctival scarring, is best diagnosed by fresh conjunctival biopsy findings of linear deposition of antibasement membrane antibodies.

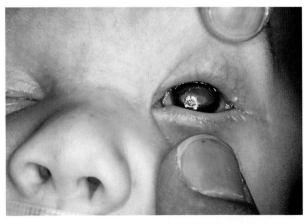

Figure 161–14. Right eyelids and opacified cornea of a 6-week-old infant who was treated since birth for unilateral right-sided conjunctivitis. The right upper eyelid margin is completely inverted due to tarsal kink syndrome.

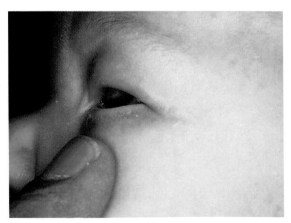

Figure 161–15. The same patient is shown. A lateral view shows complete inversion of the distal upper eyelid.

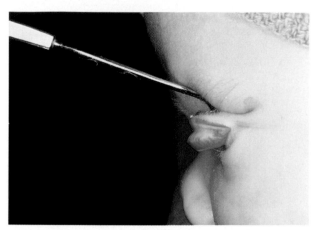

Figure 161–16. The same patient is shown. Eversion of the eyelid over a Desmarres retractor demonstrates the horizontally oriented kink that plicates the eyelid.

Cicatricial vernal conjunctivitis encompasses the usual findings of vernal conjunctivitis, that is, seasonal recurrent giant papillary conjunctivitis in a child or young adult, in addition to cicatricial changes. Dysthyroid, posttraumatic, and alkali-induced entropion can be diagnosed from the history and presentation.

Classification

Classification of the degree of structural distortion of eyelid tissues is an essential ingredient when formulating the surgical plan.[82] "Minimal" entropion is characterized by apparent migration of meibomian glands, conjunctivalisation of the eyelid margin, and lash/globe contact on upgaze. "Moderate" entropion includes the addi-

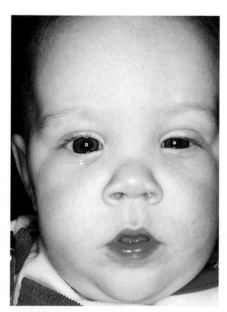

Figure 161–17. The same patient is shown. Corneal opacity and entropion corrected following a posterior approach horizontal wedge resection and eyelid rotation. The residual ptosis is characteristic of tarsal kink syndrome. In anticipation of future ptosis repair, a posterior approach was used in order to leave the levator undisturbed.

Table 161–3. CAUSES OF UPPER EYELID ENTROPION IN AN INTERNATIONAL PRACTICE

Infectious (65% of total)	
1. Trachoma	(40%)
2. Chronic blepharoconjunctivitis	(22%)
3. Herpes zoster ophthalmicus	(3%)
Trauma (19% of total)	
1. Chemical injury/radiant	(7%)
2. Iatrogenic	(5%)
3. Mechanical	(4%)
4. Anophthalmic socket	(3%)
Immunologic (17% of total)	
1. Erythema multiforme	(8%)
2. Ocular cicatricial pemphigoid	(4%)
3. Cicatricial vernal conjunctivitis	(3%)
4. Dysthyroid	(2%)

Modified from Kemp EG, Collin JRO: Surgical management of upper lid entropion. Br J Ophthalmol 70:575–579, 1986.
Totals add to 101% because of decimal place rounding.

tional findings of lash/globe contact in primary position, thickening of the tarsal plate, and lid retraction. In "severe" entropion, one finds gross distortion of the eyelid margin, metaplastic lashes (i.e., distichiasis), keratin plaques, and lagophthalmos (Table 161–4).

Management

MILD ENTROPION

Minimal entropion requires little more than surgical repositioning of the anterior lamellae in order to effect

Table 161–4. CLASSIFICATION AND MANAGEMENT SCHEME DEVISED BY KEMP AND COLLIN FOR UPPER EYELID ENTROPION

Degree of Entropion	Clinical Signs	Operation Procedure
Minimal	Apparent migration of meibomian glands Conjunctivalisation of lid margin Lash/globe contact on upgaze	Anterior lamellar ± lid split at gray line
Moderate	Apparent migration of meibomian glands	Anterior lamellar reposition + lid split + tarsal wedge resection
	Conjunctivalisation of lid margin Lash/globe contact in primary position	or
	Thickening of tarsal plate Lid retraction	Lamellar division
Severe	Gross lid distortion Metaplastic lashes	Rotation of terminal tarsoconjunctiva and posterior lamella advance
	Presence of keratin plaques	or
	Lid retraction causing incomplete closure	Rotation of terminal tarsoconjunctiva and posterior lamellar graft

From Kemp EG, Collin JRO: Surgical management of upper lid entropion. Br J Ophthalmol 70:575–579, 1986.

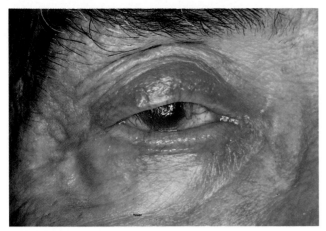

Figure 161–18. Moderate upper eyelid entropion secondary to trachoma. Eyelashes abrade the cornea, and there is a loss of corneal luster.

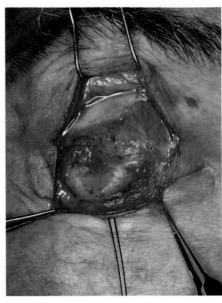

Figure 161–20. The same eyelid is shown. At the time of surgery, the tarsal plate is exposed before a horizontal wedge resection and rotation. Note that the tarsus is curled up like a corn chip. The following are also visible—fatpad, underlying edge of the dehisced levator aponeurosis, and expanse of Müller's muscle visible between the levator edge and upper border of the tarsus.

an upward rotation of the eyelashes.[82] The surgeon enters the eyelid through a lid crease incision and divides the anterior lamellae from the levator and tarsus. Dissection proceeds inferiorly in this plane. In order to avoid damage to the lash follicles, the surgical plane is terminated before approaching within 2 mm of the lid margin. Everting sutures extending into the upper aspect of tarsal plate are placed, and excess skin is excised prior to wound closure. When further eyelid margin rotation is necessary, the eyelid margin may be split at the gray line to a depth of 2 mm.[82]

MODERATE ENTROPION

Because of lash/globe contact in primary gaze and (often) thickening and curling of the tarsal plate, moderate ectropion requires recession of the anterior lamella, with or without a tarsal wedge resection and rotation (Figs. 161–18 to 161–20).[82] During the lid-splitting portion of this surgery, the surgeon should consider cryosurgical application to the distal posterior lamella in order to eradicate metaplastic lashes.[83]

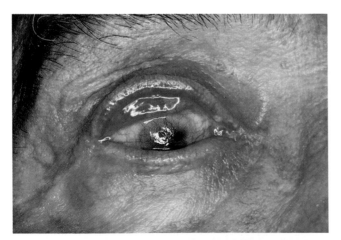

Figure 161–19. The same eyelid is shown. Eversion of the upper eyelid reveals a thickened eyelid and a curled tarsal plate.

SEVERE ENTROPION

Severe entropion is characterized by total disorganization of the lid margin, metaplastic lashes or trichiasis, lid retraction, and occasional keratin plaque formation involving the conjunctiva.[82] Treatment often involves transverse tarsotomy incision of the posterior lamella, outward rotation of the distal tarsoconjunctiva (up to 180 degrees), and correction of tarsal shortening via posterior lamellae grafting.[82] The treatment of keratinized areas is described later.

CONJUNCTIVAL LEUKOPLAKIA AND MARGINAL EPIDERMALIZATION

Scarring and metaplasia of the eyelid margin can produce a roughened surface that abrades the cornea and produces an uncomfortable punctate keratopathy in the absence of trichiasis or distichiasis.[84, 85] This disorder can be treated successfully by dermabrasion of the involved lid margin, excision of scar tissue and metaplastic epithelium, and overgrafting with full-thickness buccal mucous membrane grafts.[84, 86]

Frank keratinization of the tarsal conjunctiva is characterized by moist white keratin patches called leukoplakia (Fig. 161–21). Keratinization may be treated by excision and overgrafting,[86] curette and cryotherapy,[83, 85, 87] and topical retinoic acid.[88]

DESTRUCTION OF LASH FOLLICLES

When the primary problem consists of either lash misdirection (trichiasis) or distichiasis, rather than eyelid margin rotation, surgery can be limited to destruction or repositioning of the offending lashes. Mere epilation,

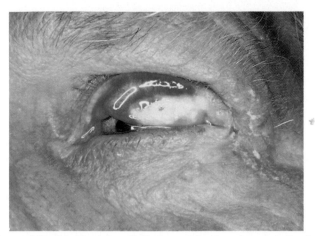

Figure 161–21. Frank keratinization of the tarsal conjunctiva by moist white keratin plaques called leukoplakia.

which has undoubtedly been practiced since time immemorial, provides up to 6 wk of relief before the indomitable lash reemerges to joust with the cornea. This observation has resulted in numerous treatments directed toward the ideal of selective destruction of the lash follicle.

The hardy lash follicle is difficult to eradicate without inducing injury to adjacent normal eyelid structures. The inadequacy of current therapies is best illustrated by noting how the champions of each particular follicle-destructive therapy enthusiastically catalog, in the opening paragraphs of their reports, the shortcomings of all other therapies.

Methods of selective lash follicle destruction include cryotherapy, electrolysis, microscopic "cold steel" excision, laser thermal ablation, and x-ray ablation.[83, 87, 89–97]

Successful cryoablation of lashes demands proper technique. Cryosurgery should be applied to the involved lashes twice, as a rapid freeze monitored by thermocouple to −20° to −25°C degrees followed by a slow thaw to room temperature (Table 161–5).[83, 89, 90, 98] Nitrous oxide–cooled retinal probes and carbon dioxide probes do not reliably cool eyelid tissues to such temperatures.[89, 90] Liquid nitrogen spray or nitrous oxide–cooled probes with rapid flow rates and freezing surface area greater than 0.8 sq cm routinely chill eyelid tissues to −20°C.[89] Tissue temperature monitoring via a thermocouple needle, vasoconstrictive anesthesia, and two-cycle rapid freeze/slow thaw technique should result in a 90 percent success rate.[88, 89]

Unfortunately, cryotherapy of the eyelid is not without significant risks. Blinding acceleration of pemphigoid symblepharon and painful reactivation of trigeminal herpes zoster[87] owing to cryotherapy may occur. Other complications are reported in Wood and Anderson's series of 70 patients, including induction of trichiasis in the eyelid adjacent to the treatment site (9 percent), visual loss, lid notching, corneal ulcer, acceleration of symblepharon, xerosis, cellulitis, skin depigmentation, and marked tissue reaction.[87] Complications are most frequent (68 percent) and severe in patients with conjunctival shrinkage, leading McCord and associates to suggest treatment to only −10°C, if at all, in patients with pemphigoid.[84]

Electrolysis performed under the microscope, although generally satisfactory,[99] carries a 30 to 50 percent recurrence rate[89, 100] and is sometimes associated with eyelid and tarsal scarring.

Laser thermal ablation,[95] popularized by Ewan,[94] is the most selective method of lash follicle destruction. Recurrence rates of up to 50 percent have been reported with current techniques,[97] and ideal treatment settings have yet to be determined. Nonetheless, laser ablation is ideally suited for patients in whom only a few lashes need to be treated and in whom retreatment is feasible. X-ray epilation lost favor because of frequent and serious complications.[101] However, x-ray epilation is still used with relative success in western Australia and the United States. Apparently, fewer side effects have resulted using contemporary fractionated doses with total treatments of 2800 to 3200 rad.[96] Complications, despite proper dosage and shielding, include persistent lashes and conjunctival leukoplakia.

Techniques of surgical exposure of lash follicles followed by microscopically controlled lash follicle ablation are beginning to gain favor as surgeons gravitate toward selective follicle destruction for distichiasis.[91–93]

ECTROPION

Etiology and Pathogenesis

CICATRICIAL ECTROPION

Ectropion of the upper eyelid occurs less frequently than its lower eyelid counterpart, probably because gravity, eyelid squeezing, Müller's muscle, and greater tarsal height all maintain eyelid stability. The everted upper eyelid may distract the upper punctum from the tear film, promote conjunctival epithelialization or exuberant granulation-like masses, and fail to protect the cornea from exposure.[77] Upper eyelid ectropion usually occurs either in instances of severe cicatricial skin changes following cutaneous injury (e.g., zoster ophthalmicus [Figs. 161–22 and 23], trauma, burns) or in instances of tremendous eyelid laxity, (e.g., floppy eyelid syndrome).

Table 161–5. TEMPERATURE-DEPENDENT EFFECTS OF CRYOTHERAPY

Temperature	Effect	Comment
−10° C	Minimal lash destruction	Useful in pemphigoid[86]
−15 to −20° C	Dermal melanocyte depigmentation	In dark-skinned patients, consider lid splitting[83]
−20° C	Lash follicle destroyed	Requires rapid freeze followed by slow thaw, applied twice[89]
−40 to −70° C	Tarsus and lacrimal outflow damage[86]	Not recommended

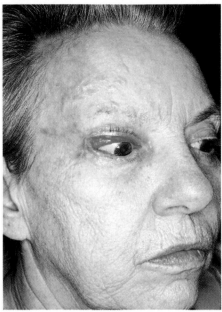

Figure 161–22. Upper eyelid ectropion, cutaneous scarring, and partial loss of an eyebrow in a patient with severe neuralgia following an attack of zoster ophthalmicus.

FLOPPY EYELID SYNDROME

Floppy eyelid syndrome,[102] which usually afflicts obese men, is characterized by a loose "rubbery" tarsus, spontaneous eyelid eversion or loss of lid-to-globe contact at night, chronic papillary conjunctivitis, meibomian gland dysfunction, and loose and easily everted upper eyelids (Fig. 161–24).[102–104] Associations have been noted with sleep apnea,[105] hyperglycinemia,[106] and blepharochalasis.[107] The conjunctivitis can be managed by patching at night, by full-thickness wedge resection of the

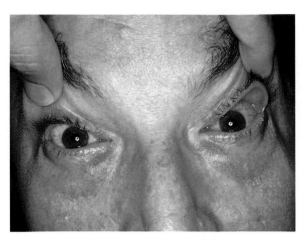

Figure 161–24. A patient with unilateral left chronic papillary conjunctivitis due to floppy eyelid syndrome. Superior traction on the eyelids reveals increased laxity of the floppy eyelid that is loose, rubbery, and everts easily.

upper eyelid,[107] or by any other upper eyelid "tightening" procedure that prevents the upper eyelid from everting or falling away from the globe during sleep (Fig. 161–25).[108]

Management

Trauma that eventually results in ectropion is usually severe enough, in the acute phase, that the eyelids are swollen shut and the cornea is temporarily protected.[44] Even with corneal exposure, conservative management with ointment, goggles, taping, or bandage lenses often suffices. In the case of eyelid burns, it is important to grade the depth of burn, because this guides subsequent management.[42] When the cornea is at risk, early release of scar tissue, combined with skin grafting, is preferable

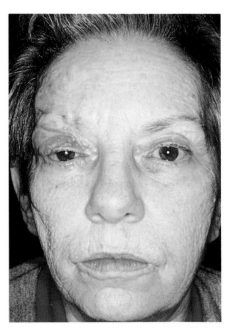

Figure 161–23. The same patient after the release of cicatrix and the placement of a free skin graft. Return of eyelid to a normal position resulted in complete cessation of neuralgia.

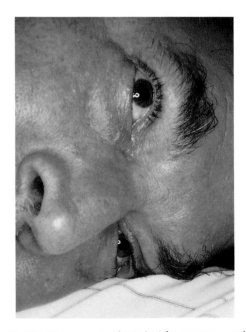

Figure 161–25. The same patient, but in repose; gravity allows the loose eyelid to fall away from the globe.

to relying on a tarsorrhaphy, which often tears and deforms the lid margin, thus complicating subsequent reconstruction.[42]

If the cornea is not in jeopardy, it may be possible to delay reconstructive surgery for several months or longer until inflammation has subsided and the scar tissue has matured. During this waiting period, one may consider massage of tissues and steroid injection in order to enhance remodeling of scar tissues. The "waiting period" ends once the hypertrophic scars pale, soften, and begin diminishing in size. At this point, there is often mobility of the scar, which is indicative of a subcicatricial plane of loose connective tissue. Dissection within this relatively bloodless plane facilitates controlled excision of scar and reconstructive skin grafting.[109]

Cicatricial ectropion is managed by excision of scar, release of skin, free skin grafting (see Figs. 161–22 and 161–23) or skin flaps, Z-plasty, and a variety of other techniques.[44]

REFERENCES

1. Duke-Elder S, MacFaul PA: Disorders of motility. *In* Duke-Elder S, MacFaul PA (eds): System of Ophthalmology. Vol XIII, Part 1: Diseases of the Eyelids. St. Louis, CV Mosby, 1974, pp 568–573.
2. Fox SA: The palpebral fissure. Am J Ophthalmol 62:73–78, 1966.
3. Hill JC: An analysis of senile changes in the palpebral fissure. Can J Ophthalmol 10:32–35, 1975.
4. Frueh BR, Musch DM, Garber FW: Lid retraction and levator aponeurosis defects in Graves' eye disease. Ophthalmic Surg 17:216–220, 1986.
5. Collin JRO, Allen L, Castronuovo S: Congenital eyelid retraction. Br J Ophthalmol 74:542–544, 1990.
6. Rampoldi R: Singolarissimo caso di squilibrio motorio oculopalpebrale. Ann Ottal 13:463–469, 1884.
7. Hicks AM, Hosford GN: Cyclic paralysis of the oculomotor paralysis. Arch Ophthalmol 17:213–222, 1937.
8. Susac JO, Smith JL: Cyclic oculomotor paralysis. Neurology 24:24–27, 1974.
9. Lewis IC, Macgregor AG: Congenital hyperthyroidism. Lancet 1:14–16, 1957.
10. Shields CL, Nelson LB, Carpenter GC, Sheilds JA: Neonatal Graves' disease. Br J Ophthalmol 72:424–427, 1988.
11. Waller RR, Samples JR, Yeatts RP: Eyelid malpositions in Graves' ophthalmopathy. *In* Gorman CA, Waller RR, Dyer JA (eds): The Eye and Orbit in Thyroid Disease. New York, Raven Press, 1984.
12. Hollingsworth DR, Mabry CC, Eckerd JM: Hereditary aspects of Graves' disease in infancy and childhood. J Pediatr 81:446–459, 1972.
13. Keane JR: The pretectal syndrome: 206 patients. Neurology 40:684–690, 1990.
14. Parinaud H: Paralysis des mouvements associés des yeux. Arch Neurologie 4:145–172, 1883.
15. Parinaud H: Paralysis of the movement of convergence of the eyes. Brain 9:330–341, 1886.
16. Collier J: Nuclear ophthalmoplegia with especial reference to retraction of the lids and ptosis and to lesions of the posterior commissure. Brain 50:488–498, 1927.
17. Walsh FB, Hoyt WF: The ocular motor system. *In* Walsh FB, Hoyt WF (eds): Clinical Neuro-Ophthalmology, 3rd ed, Vol 1. Baltimore, Williams & Wilkins, 1969, pp 304–307.
18. Wesley RE, Jackson CG: Facial palsy. *In* Hornblass A (ed): Oculoplastic, Orbital and Reconstructive Surgery, Vol 1. Baltimore, Williams & Wilkins, 1988, pp 325–340.
19. Conley J: Perspectives in facial reanimation. *In* May M (ed): The Facial Nerve. New York, Thieme, 1986, pp 645–664.
20. Levine RE: Eyelid reanimation surgery. *In* May M (ed): The Facial Nerve. New York, Thieme, 1986, pp 681–694.
21. Jelks GW, Smith BC, Bosniak S: The evaluation and management of the eye in facial palsy. Clin Plast Surg 6:397–419, 1979.
22. Lisman RD, Smith BC, Baker D, Arthurs B: Efficacy of the surgical treatment for paralytic ectropion. Ophthalmology 94:671–681, 1987.
23. Kirkness CM, Adams GGW, Dilly PN, Lee JP: Botulinum toxin A-induced protective ptosis in corneal disease. Ophthalmology 95:473–480, 1988.
24. Levine RE: Management of lagophthalmos with the palpebral spring and Silastic elastic prosthesis. *In* Hornblass A (ed): Oculoplastic, Orbital and Reconstructive Surgery, Vol 1. Baltimore, Williams & Wilkins, 1988, pp 384–392.
25. May M: Surgical rehabilitation of facial palsy: Total approach. *In* May M (ed): The Facial Nerve. New York, Thieme, 1986.
26. Gunderson T: Conjunctival flaps in the treatment of corneal disease with reference to a new technique of application. Arch Ophthalmol 60:880–887, 1958.
27. Khan JA: Dermal graft: Alternative to Gunderson flap allows fitting scleral shell over sensitive cornea. Ophthalmic Plast Reconstr Surg 6:260–264, 1990.
28. Cox TA, Wurster JB, Godfrey WA: Primary aberrant oculomotor regeneration due to intracranial aneurysm. Arch Neurol 36:570–571, 1979.
29. Schatz NJ, Savino PJ, Corbet JJ: Primary aberrant oculomotor regeneration: A sign of intracavernous meningioma. Arch Neurol 34:29–32, 1977.
30. Fisher M: An unusual variant of acute idiopathic polyneuritis. N Engl J Med 255:56–65, 1956.
31. Zasorin NL, Yee RD, Baloh RW: Eye-movement abnormalities in ophthalmoplegia, ataxia, and areflexia (Fisher's syndrome). Arch Ophthalmol 103:55–58, 1985.
32. Pessin MS, Logigian EL, Brown MT, et al: CNS dysfunction on Fisher's syndrome. Neurology 39:998–999, 1989.
33. Al-Din AM, Amderson M, Bickerstaff ER, et al: Brain stem encephalitis and the syndrome of Miller Fisher. Brain 105:481–495, 1982.
34. Smith JL, Walsh FB: Syndrome of external ophthalmoplegia, ataxia and areflexia (Fisher). Arch Ophthalmol 58:109–114, 1957.
35. Jain IS: Lid retraction in the non-paretic eye in acquired ophthalmoplegia. Br J Ophthalmol 47:757–759, 1963.
36. Lewallen WM: Lid retraction syndrome. Am J Ophthalmol 45:565–567, 1958.
37. Gonnering RS: Pseudoretraction of the eyelid in thyroid-associated orbitopathy. Arch Ophthalmol 106:1078–1080, 1988.
38. Schechter RJ: Ptosis with contralateral lid retraction due to excessive innervation of the levator palpebrae superioris. Ann Ophthalmol 10:1324–1328, 1978.
39. Gay AJ, Salmon ML, Windsor CE: Herring's law, the levators, and their relationship in disease states. Arch Ophthalmol 77:157–160, 1967.
40. Lohman LL, Burns JA, Penland WR, Cahill KV: Unilateral eyelid retraction secondary to contralateral ptosis in dysthyroid ophthalmopathy. J Clin Neuro-ophthalmol 4:163–166, 1984.
41. Kansu T, Subutay N: Lid retraction in myasthenia gravis. J Clin Neuro-ophthalmol 7:145–148, 1987.
42. Frank DH, Wachtel T, Frank HA: The early treatment and reconstruction of eyelid burns. J Trauma 23:874–877, 1983.
43. Smith DJ, Robson MC, Heggers JP: Reconstruction of head, face, and neck. *In* Boswick J (ed): The Art and Science of Burn Care. Rockville, MD, Aspen Pub Co, 1987.
44. Smith DJ, Robson MC: Eyelid burns. *In* Spoor TC, Nesi FA (eds): Management of Ocular, Orbital, and Adnexal Trauma. New York, Raven Press, 1988, pp 427–435.
45. Char DH: Eye signs and diagnosis. *In* Char DH: Thyroid Eye Disease. Baltimore, Williams & Wilkins, 1985.
46. Day RM: Ocular manifestations of thyroid disease: Current concepts. Trans Am Ophthalmol Soc 57:572–601, 1959.
47. McCord CD, Tanenbaum M: Graves' ophthalmopathy. *In* McCord CD, Tanenbaum M (eds): Oculoplastic Surgery, 2nd ed. New York, Raven Press, 1987, pp 169–196.
48. Sisler HA, Jakobiec FA, Trokel SL: Ocular abnormalities and orbital changes of Graves' disease. *In* Duane TD (ed): Clinical Ophthalmology, Vol 2. Philadelphia, Harper & Row, 1987.
49. Small RG: Enlargement of levator palpebral superioris muscle fibers in Graves' ophthalmopathy. Ophthalmology 96:424–430, 1989.

50. Kagoshimi T, Hori S, Inoue Y: Qualitative and quantitative analyses of Müller's muscle in dysthyroid ophthalmopathy. Jpn J Ophthalmol 31:646–654, 1987.
51. Grove AS: Levator lengthening by marginal myotomy. Arch Ophthalmol 98:1433–1438, 1980.
52. Grove AS: Upper eyelid retraction and Graves' disease. Ophthalmology 88:499–506, 1981.
53. Rundle FF, Pochin EE: The orbital tissues in thyrotoxicosis: Quantitative analysis relating to exophthalmos. Clin Sci 5:51–74, 1944.
54. Rootman J, Patel S, Berry K, Nugent R: Pathological and clinical study of Müller's muscle in Graves' ophthalmopathy. Can J Ophthalmol 22:32–36, 1986.
55. Feldon SE, Levin L: Graves' ophthalmopathy. V: Aetiology of upper eyelid retraction on Graves' ophthalmopathy. Br J Ophthalmol 74:484–485, 1990.
56. Putterman A: Surgical treatment of thyroid-related upper eyelid retraction. Ophthalmology 88:507–512, 1981.
57. Doxanas MT, Dryden RM: The use of sclera in the treatment of dysthyroid eyelid retraction. Ophthalmology 88:887–894, 1981.
58. Harvey JT, Anderson RA: The aponeurotic approach to eyelid retraction. Ophthalmology 88:513–524, 1981.
59. Paul W: Zur Basedow'schen Krankheit. Ber klin Wchnschr 2:277–280, 1965.
60. Summerskill WH, Molnar GD: Eye signs in hepatic cirrhosis. N Engl J Med 266:1244–1248, 1962.
61. Bartley GB, Gorman CA: Hepatic cirrhosis as a doubtful cause of eyelid retraction. Am J Ophthalmol 111:109–110, 1991.
62. Robin AL: Short-term effects of unilateral 1% apraclonidine therapy. Arch Ophthalmol 106:1069–1073, 1988.
63. Char, DH: Surgical management of eyelid retraction. In Char DH: Thyroid Eye Disease. Baltimore, Williams & Wilkins, 1985.
64. Hurwitz JJ, Rodgers KJ: Prevention and management of postoperative lateral upper-lid retraction in Graves' disease. Can J Ophthalmol 18:329–332, 1983.
65. Lee WY, Morimoto PK, Bronsky D, Waldstein LL: Studies of thyroid and sympathetic nervous system interrelationships. I: The blepharoptosis of myxedema. J Clin Endocrinol Metab 21:1402–1412, 1961.
66. Dixon RS, Anderson RA, Hatt MU: The use of thymoxamine in eyelid retraction. Arch Ophthalmol 97:2147–2150, 1979.
67. Sneddon JM, Turner P: Adrenergic blockade and eye signs of thyrotoxicosis. Lancet 2:525–527, 1966.
68. Gay AJ, Wolkstein MA: Topical guanethidine therapy for endocrine lid retraction. Arch Ophthalmol 76:364–367, 1966.
69. Gay AJ, Salmon ML, Wolkstein MA: Topical sympatholytic therapy for pathologic lid retraction. Arch Ophthalmol 77:341–345, 1967.
70. Crombie AL, Lawson AA: Long-term trial of local guanethidine in treatment of eye signs of thyroid dysfunction and idiopathic lid retraction. Br Med J 4:592–595, 1967.
71. Cant JS, Lewis DR: Unwanted pharmacological effects of local guanethidine in the treatment of dysthyroid upper lid retraction. Br J Ophthalmol 53:239–245, 1969.
72. Haddad HM: Lid retraction therapy with a guanethidine solution. [Letter] Arch Ophthalmol 107:169, 1989.
73. Gonnering RS: Lid retraction therapy with a guanethidine solution. [Reply] Arch Ophthalmol 107:169, 1989.
74. Kao I, Drachman DB, Price DL: Botulinum toxin: Mechanism of presynaptic blockade. Science 193:1256–1258, 1976.
75. Kirkness CM, Adams GW, Dilly PN, Lee JP: Botulinum toxin A-induced protective ptosis in corneal disease. Ophthalmology 95:473–480, 1988.
76. Scott AB: Injection treatment of endocrine orbital myopathy. Doc Ophthalmol 58:141–145, 1984.
77. Duke-Elder S, MacFaul PA: Abnormalities of the palpebral aperture. In Duke-Elder S, MacFaul PA (eds): System of Ophthalmology. Vol XIII, Part 1: Diseases of the Eyelids. St. Louis, CV Mosby, 1974, pp 573–586.
78. Miller DG, Hesse RJ: Involutional entropion of the upper lid. Ophthalmic Plast Reconstr Surg 6:16–20, 1990.
79. Hollsten A, Glover AT: An unusual form of upper lid entropion. [Abstract] Ophthalmic Plast Reconstr Surg 6:285, 1990.
80. Kettesy A: Entropion in infancy caused by folding of the tarsus. Arch Ophthalmol 39:640–642, 1948.
81. Bosniak SL: Tarsal kink syndrome. In Hornblass A (ed): Oculoplastic, Orbital and Reconstructive Surgery. Baltimore, Williams & Wilkins, 1988, pp 151–155.
82. Kemp EG, Collin JRO: Surgical management of upper lid entropion. Br J Ophthalmol 70:575–579, 1986.
83. Anderson RT, Harvey JT: Lid splitting and posterior lamella cryosurgery for congenital and acquired distichiasis. Arch Ophthalmol 99:631–634, 1981.
84. McCord CD, Tanenbaum M, Dryden RM, Doxanas MT: Eyelid malpositions. In McCord CD, Tanenbaum M (eds): Oculoplastic Surgery, 2nd ed. New York, Raven Press, 1987, pp 279–324.
85. Maumenee AE: Keratinization of the conjunctiva. Trans Am Ophthalmic Soc 77:133, 1979.
86. McCord CD, Chen WP: Tarsal polishing and mucous membrane grafting for cicatricial entropion, trichiasis and epidermalization. Ophthalmic Surg 14:1021–1025, 1983.
87. Wood JR, Anderson RL: Complications of cryosurgery. Arch Ophthalmol 99:460–463, 1981.
88. Nelson ME: Topical retinoic acid treatment for conjunctival squamous metaplasia. [Photoessay] Arch Ophthalmol 106:1723, 1988.
89. Sullivan JH: The use of cryotherapy for trichiasis. Trans Am Acad Ophthal Otol 83:708–712, 1977.
90. Sullivan JH, Beard C, Bullock JD: Cryosurgery for treatment of trichiasis. Am J Ophthalmol 82:117–121, 1976.
91. Dortzbach RK, Butera RT: Excision of distichiasis eyelashes through a tarsoconjunctival trapdoor. Arch Ophthalmol 96:111–112, 1978.
92. Call MB, Gardner B: Distichiasis revisited. [Abstract] Ophthalmic Plast Reconstr Surg 6:285, 1990.
93. Gossman MD: CO_2 laser combined with conventional microsurgery in the treatment of congenital distichiasis. [Abstract] Ophthalmic Plast Reconstr Surg 6:285–286, 1990.
94. Ewan KJ: Argon laser treatment of trichiasis. Ophthalmic Surg 17:658–660, 1986.
95. Berry J: Recurrent trichiasis: Treatment with laser photocoagulation. Ophthalmic Surg 1979;10:36–38, 1979.
96. Hartzler J, Neldner KH, Forstot SL: X-ray epilation for the treatment of trichiasis. Arch Dermatol 120:620–624, 1985.
97. Bartley G, Bullock JD, Olsen TG, Lutz PD: An experimental study to compare methods of eyelash ablation. Ophthalmology 94:1286–1289, 1987.
98. Gill W, Fraser J, Carter DC: Repeated freeze-thaw cycles in cryosurgery. Nature 219:410–413, 1968.
99. Scheie HG, Albert DM: Distichiasis and trichiasis: Origin and management. Am J Ophthalmol 61:718–720, 1966.
100. Hecht SD: Cryotherapy of trichiasis with use of the retinal cryoprobe. Ann Ophthalmol 90:1501–1503, 1977.
101. McDonald JE, Wilson FM: Ocular therapy with beta particles. Trans Am Acad Ophthalmol Otolaryngol 63:468–485, 1959.
102. Culbertson WW, Ostler HB: The floppy eyelid syndrome. Am J Ophthalmol 92:568–571, 1981.
103. Parunovic A: Floppy eyelid syndrome. Br J Ophthalmol 67:264–266, 1983.
104. Gonnering RS, Sonneland PR: Meibomian gland dysfunction on floppy eyelid syndrome. Ophthalmic Plast Reconstr Surg 3:99–103, 1987.
105. Woog JJ: Obstructive sleep apnea and the floppy eyelid syndrome. Am J Ophthalmol 110:314–315, 1990.
106. Gerner EW, Hughes SM: Floppy eyelid syndrome with hyperglycinemia. Am J Ophthalmol 98:614–616, 1984.
107. Goldberg R, Seiff S, McFarland J, et al: Floppy eyelid syndrome and blepharochalasis. Am J Ophthalmol 102:376–381, 1986.
108. Moore MB, Harrington J, McCulley JP: Floppy eyelid syndrome, management including surgery. Ophthalmology 103:184–188, 1986.
109. Converse JM, McCarthy JG, Dobrkovsky M, Larson DL: Facial burns. In Converse JM (ed): Reconstructive Plastic Surgery, Vol 3. Philadelphia, WB Saunders, 1977, pp 1595–1642.

Chapter 162

Lower Eyelid Malpositions*

WILLIAM L. WHITE and JOHN J. WOOG

ENTROPION

Entropion is characterized by a turning inward of the eyelid margin. It may be either unilateral or bilateral and may involve the upper or lower eyelid (although it is much more frequent in the lower lid). Associated ocular inflammation and tearing may result from trichiasis (inturning of the cilia with lashes in direct contact with the cornea) or from contact of keratinized epithelium of the eyelid margin with the ocular surface. In order to successfully care for the patient with entropion, the specific cause of the entropion must be appreciated. In this regard, it is useful to classify entropion into congenital, spastic, cicatricial, and involutional categories. In this chapter we discuss common clinical features and selected treatment options for several of the frequently encountered forms of entropion.

Congenital

Congenital entropion is a developmental abnormality that usually involves the lower eyelids, although upper eyelid involvement has been reported.[1] Two general types of congenital turning inward of the eyelids are most often recognized. Epiblepharon is characterized by redundancy of pretarsal skin and pretarsal orbicularis muscle, which results in inward rotation of the eyelid margin. Epiblepharon is more common in individuals of Asian descent and is most frequently appreciated in childhood. It may demonstrate spontaneous resolution with growth in facial structures. Epiblepharon can be relatively subtle and in some cases may only be appreciated in downgaze (Fig. 162–1).[2] Surgical management of this condition, when necessary, generally includes excision of an ellipse of skin and pretarsal orbicularis muscle.

The tarsal kink syndrome is a more severe form of congenital entropion in which the inferior portion of tarsus of the upper eyelid is bent inward toward the cornea. Diagnosis of this condition is often difficult, and corneal complications are not unusual. Surgical correction may entail placement of full-thickness eyelid eversion sutures or a transverse blepharotomy with marginal rotation. The latter may be performed either with or without excision and reversal of the tarsal kink, posterior lamella grafting, or both.[3]

Congenital entropion affecting the lower eyelids may occasionally occur solely on the basis of lower eyelid

retractor disinsertion.[4, 5] Management can include placement of eyelid margin rotation sutures either with or without tarsoconjunctival incision.[6]

One other condition, congenital distichiasis, may simulate congenital entropion. In this disorder, an extra row of lashes is noted to emanate from the meibomian gland orifices.[4] It may be associated with a number of developmental anomalies, including lymphedema.[7] Individuals with congenital distichiasis may be completely asymptomatic. This condition is discussed further in Chapter 163.

Spastic

Spastic entropion is caused by increased orbicularis muscle tone leading to inturning of the eyelid margin. It can be associated with ocular inflammation or prolonged patching, and may be antedated by cataract surgery, retinal detachment repair, or other ocular procedures.[4]

The treatment of spastic entropion generally involves placement of absorbable full-thickness eyelid sutures

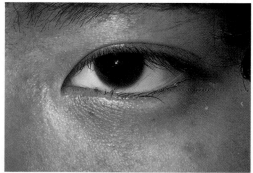

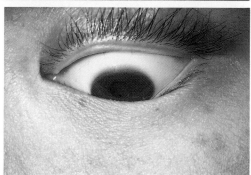

Figure 162–1. In this patient with epiblepharon, note the tendency toward entropion in the primary position of gaze (*A*), with frank entropion in downgaze (*B*).

*The opinions of assertions contained herein are the private views of the authors and are not to be construed as reflecting the views of the Department of the Army or the Department of Defense.

that evert the lid margin,[8] and the underlying disease process is appropriately addressed. Spastic entropion can be a harbinger of early involutional entropion in predisposed individuals.

Cicatricial

The cicatricial type of entropion is characterized by tarsoconjunctival scarring and contraction, which rotates the eyelid margin inward. Cicatricial entropion frequently occurs with trichiasis (misdirected lashes originating in the anterior lamella) and distichiasis (abnormal lashes originating in the posterior lamella). Other associated findings include symblepharon (scar formation between adjacent tarsal and bulbar conjunctival surfaces), ankyloblepharon (cicatrization between the conjunctiva and eyelid margins), and epidermalization (keratinization of the eyelid margin). Etiologic conditions include anophthalmia, previous eyelid surgery, Stevens-Johnson syndrome, ocular pemphigoid, trachoma, bacterial infection, chemical burns, herpes zoster, trauma, radiation, Sjögren's syndrome, and phospholine iodide use.[4] Digital pressure on the skin of the eyelid will evert most entropic lids but will not produce lid eversion if established cicatricial entropion is present. This simple test may confirm a diagnosis of cicatricial entropion initiated on the basis of a suspicious history and slit-lamp examination.[9]

Usual approaches to the treatment of cicatricial entropion include lid splitting with tarsal advancement, internal lamella lengthening with or without free grafts, and lid margin rotation with partial or full-thickness blepharotomy.[10, 11] Surgical repair for cicatricial entropion secondary to ocular pemphigoid may be associated with a higher recurrence rate than other types of cicatricial entropion.[11] In our experience, it has been helpful in the setting of cicatricial pemphigoid to delay corrective surgery pending the institution of appropriate systemic treatment for the underlying disease.

Cryotherapy for trichiasis may also be useful in this group of patients, with good results being achieved with double freeze-thaw applications to $-20°$ to $-25°C$.[4, 11, 12]

Involutional

Pathophysiologic factors underlying the development of involutional entropion include (1) horizontal eyelid laxity, (2) lower eyelid retractor disinsertion, and (3) preseptal orbicularis muscle overriding a portion of the pretarsal orbicularis muscle. In addition, relative enophthalmos secondary to atrophy of orbital fat may be an important factor in some cases.[13–15] These abnormalities will be discussed in detail further on.

Laxity in the lower eyelid is a common finding in involutional entropion. The lateral canthal tendon has been observed to be the primary anatomic site of abnormality in many cases, although medial canthal tendon laxity and, less commonly, horizontal elongation of the tarsal plate itself may be present as well. Lateral canthal

tendon abnormalities may range from simple elongation or thinning of the tissues to complete disruption of the tendon insertion.[16, 17]

A medially displaced lateral canthal angle can be an indication that the lateral palpebral tendon is lax. The normal angle is usually less than 5 mm from the lateral orbital rim. Similarly, lateral traction on the lid should not move the punctum more than 3 mm with a normal medial canthal tendon insertion.[17] The lower eyelid tension can be assessed by pulling the lid away from the globe and observing the subsequent return of the eyelid to its resting position. Eyelids with normal tone should quickly "snap back" into apposition with the globe.[18] Similarly, in a patient with normal lower eyelid tone, the lid can be distracted no more than 6 mm from the globe.[19] In most instances, a qualitative assessment of the horizontal laxity will suffice in determining if it is a component underlying an eyelid malposition.[20, 21]

Detachment, attenuation, or dehiscence of the capsulopalpebral fascia has also been shown to lead to involutional entropion and has been observed to be present in up to 50 percent of cases.[15, 16, 22, 23] When disinserted, the lower lid retractors may be visible through the conjunctiva as a gray area several millimeters below the inferior tarsal border.[15, 24] Diminished lower eyelid excursion in downgaze, attenuation of the lower eyelid crease, or both, may be noted in association with lower eyelid retractor disinsertion as well. Orbicularis muscle hypertrophy has been noted histopathologically in patients with involutional entropion.[25] Anatomically, this may correspond to overriding of the preseptal portion over the pretarsal portion of the orbicularis muscle.

Numerous surgical procedures have been devised for the correction of involutional entropion and yield acceptable results. One general category consists of lower lid tightening procedures, which may involve either tucking the lateral canthal tendon or full-thickness resection of lower eyelid tissue. The latter is usually performed at the lateral canthus. Reattachment of the disinserted lower lid retractors is another type of repair that may also be done either alone or in combination with lower lid tightening. This procedure has also been

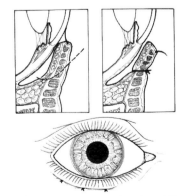

Figure 162–2. Quickert sutures create a band that repproximates the lower eyelid retractors to the inferior tarsal border and prevents overriding of the preseptal over the pretarsal orbicularis.

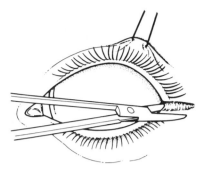

Figure 162–3. A lateral canthotomy is performed.

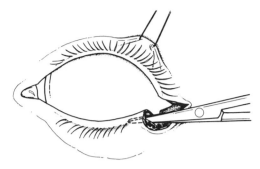

Figure 162–5. Skin and orbicularis muscle are dissected from the anterior surface of the tarsal plate.

performed in conjunction with excision of a strip of skin and a band of preseptal orbicularis muscle.[16, 21, 26–29]

Management

QUICKERT SUTURES

Full-thickness eversion sutures for the lower eyelid, commonly referred to as Quickert sutures (Fig. 162–2),[8] are customarily placed with the patient under local anesthesia. The procedure may in fact be conveniently performed at the bedside when necessary. Following subconjunctival and subcutaneous injection of anesthetic, the periorbital region is prepared in the usual sterile fashion. A scleral shell is placed to protect the globe, and the upper eyelid is retracted. Double-armed 4–0 chromic sutures on a large needle are then placed in a full-thickness fashion. Each arm of each double-armed suture is passed through the conjunctiva of the inferior fornix and engages the lower eyelid retractors prior to passing anterosuperiorly through the eyelid to exit approximately 3 mm inferior to the cilia. Each arm of each double-armed suture is separated by a distance of approximately 3 mm, and two or three such sutures may be placed in each eyelid. The sutures are tied carefully to allow for a slight operative overcorrection. The scleral shell is removed and antibiotic ointment is applied along the suture line. The ointment is continued for 7 to 10 days postoperatively. The slightly everted eyelid usually returns to a normal position during this period. If mild overcorrection persists, the chromic sutures may be removed 1 wk following the surgical

procedure, and gentle eyelid massage can be used to return the lid to a more anatomically correct location.

TARSAL STRIP PROCEDURE

The tarsal strip procedure (Figs. 162–3 to 162–13) was originally described for treating involutional or paralytic eyelid laxity and has been enthusiastically received.[14, 30] It has since been found to be useful for eyelid laxity associated with anophthalmos and entropion.[31]

The procedure is typically initiated with subcutaneous and subconjunctival infiltration anesthesia in the lower eyelid and lateral canthal region. A scleral shell is placed to protect the globe and a lateral canthotomy is performed. This is followed by cantholysis of the inferior crus of the lateral canthal tendon. Meticulous hemostasis is maintained with cautery throughout the procedure. The lateral aspect of the lower eyelid is freed from all attachments to the lateral orbital rim and is subsequently overlapped laterally at the site of the new lateral canthal angle. The amount of lax lateral lower eyelid is noted at the eyelid margin. Following this, the skin and orbicularis muscle are carefully separated from the anterior surface of the tarsus to the area previously demarcated. The lid margin epithelium is then carefully excised from the superior portion of the tarsal strip and the conjunctival epithelium is scraped from its posterior aspect. The tarsal strip is then trimmed to a vertical height of approximately 3 mm. A tunnel is then created beneath the superior crus of the lateral canthal tendon with scissors, and the tarsal tongue is drawn through this

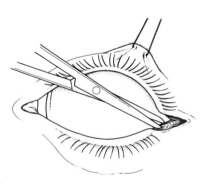

Figure 162–4. Canthotomy is followed by division of the inferior crus of the lateral canthal tendon.

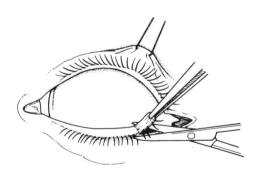

Figure 162–6. The lid margin epithelium is removed including the eyelashes.

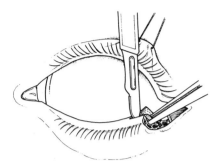

Figure 162–7. The conjunctival epithelium is removed from the posterior surface of the tarsus.

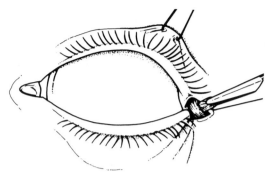

Figure 162–9. The tarsal strip is withdrawn through the tunnel beneath the superior crus of the lateral canthal tendon.

tunnel. The tarsal strip is secured to the periosteum of the lateral orbital rim in the vicinity of the lateral orbital tubercle with a horizontal mattress suture of nonabsorbable material such as 4–0 Teflon impregnated braided polyester fiber (Polydek). Additional absorbable sutures may be placed to re-form the lateral canthal angle and to close the orbicularis muscle. The skin edges are then closed with a suitable suture such as 6–0 nylon.

ECTROPION

Ectropion is a turning out of the eyelid margin away from the globe. Successful treatment of ectropion depends on recognition of the underlying pathophysiology. Types of ectropion to consider include mechanical, cicatricial, paralytic, and involutional.

Mechanical

Mechanical ectropion may be caused by eyelid tumors, herniated orbital fat, or extravasation of fluid into the eyelid. It may also be caused by traction on the anterior lamella by eyeglasses. Treatment of mechanical ectropion is dependent upon elimination of the specific underlying cause and cannot be generalized.[9]

Cicatricial

Foreshortening or loss of tissue in the anterior lamella of the eyelid is common to all cases of cicatricial ectropion. Etiologic factors leading to cicatricial ectropion include thermal or chemical injury, skin disease (e.g., ichthyosis), contracture secondary to chronic (involutional or mechanical) ectropion, excessive skin removal from previous lid surgery (usually lower lid blepharoplasty), and tumors.[4] Proper preoperative assessment of lower eyelid laxity, as well as horizontal shortening of those lids that are lax (at the time of blepharoplasty), should eliminate many cases of ectropion following blepharoplasty.[32–34]

Treating patients with mild cicatricial ectropion by a lower eyelid tightening procedure that does not sacrifice lid tissue can yield acceptable results.[14, 17] More severe cases of cicatricial ectropion will require lengthening of the anterior lamella of the lower lid, usually by skin grafting or local flaps.[4] Infrapunctal excision of an ellipse of conjunctiva and subconjunctival tissue with closure of the resultant defect may be helpful in repairing varying degrees of medial eyelid ectropion with good results.[35] Likewise, a procedure has been developed to lengthen the anterior lamella with a flap while tightening the eyelid via a wedge resection lateral to the punctum, thus inverting the punctum without the use of a skin graft.[36]

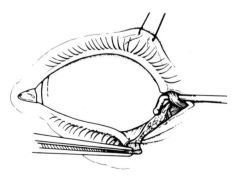

Figure 162–8. A tunnel is created beneath the superior crus of the lateral canthal tendon.

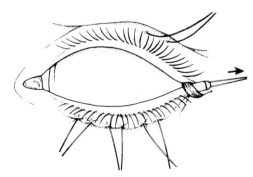

Figure 162–10. A horizontal mattress suture of a nonabsorbable material is passed through the tarsal strip. In this patient, three Quickert sutures have been placed as well.

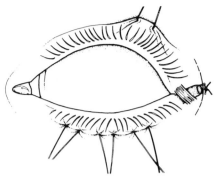

Figure 162–11. The tarsal strip is secured to the periorbita at the lateral orbital tubercle.

Paralytic

Paralytic ectropion occurs when orbicularis muscle and facial nerve function are disrupted and may occur secondary to a variety of causes, including Bell's palsy and after acoustic neuroma resection. Many devices have been developed to treat this problem, some of which include weights, magnets, springs, and encircling devices. A lateral canthal tightening procedure alone or in combination with a medial or lateral canthoplasty will often suffice as a primary procedure,[4] whereas the techniques using implanted devices are best left for unresponsive cases.

Involutional

Etiologic factors underlying involutional ectropion can be similar to those of involutional entropion, with the primary abnormality being laxity of the lateral canthal tendon. Punctal malposition, vertical skin tightness, medial canthal laxity, orbicularis paresis, and disinsertion or laxity of the lower lid retractors also contribute variably.[37, 38] Medial eyelid ectropion with resultant punctal malposition may be a part of a generalized involutional ectropion (Fig. 162–14) but can occur independently.[35]

Earlier procedures used to correct involutional ectropion shortened the eyelid and usually removed a full-thickness midtarsal portion, which is seldom the anatomically abnormal area. Possible complications associated with such procedures included recurrence of laxity,

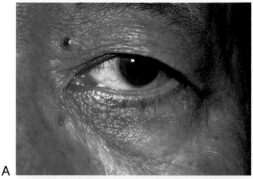
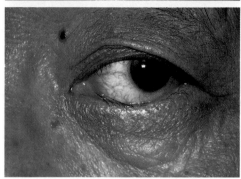

Figure 162–13. Right lower eyelid entropion before (A) and after (B) repair with the combined tarsal strip and Quickert sutures.

eyelid notching, and rounded canthal angles.[14] Approaches currently favored include lower lid shortening at the lateral canthus[37] and a medial spindle excision that causes punctal inversion.[38] Reattachment of the lower lid retractors to the tarsal plate by a conjunctival approach may be indicated when ectropion exists and retractor detachment is apparent clinically.[24]

Management

Correction of punctal eversion via excision of conjunctiva and subconjunctival tissue (Fig. 162–15) is best performed using local anesthesia. It is often used in conjunction with a horizontal eyelid shortening procedure. A scleral shell is placed to protect the globe. Subcutaneous and subconjunctival infiltration of anes-

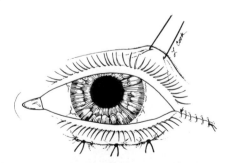

Figure 162–12. The orbicularis muscle and skin layers have been closed, and the Quickert sutures have been tied.

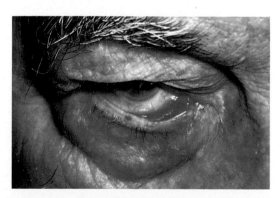

Figure 162–14. Increased horizontal eyelid laxity is noted, with medial ectropion and punctal eversion.

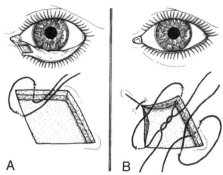

Figure 162–15. A diamond-shaped piece of conjunctiva and subconjunctival tissue is excised inferior to the everted punctum (A). The defect is closed with buried sutures, resulting in punctal inversion (B).

thetic is carried out in the medial portion of the lower eyelid. A spindle is outlined measuring approximately 5 × 2.5 mm on the conjunctiva below the punctum. The highest point of the ellipse is located directly posterior and inferior to the punctum and is separated from the punctum by at least 4 mm. The ellipse of conjunctiva and subcutaneous tissue is then excised, and hemostasis is achieved with cautery. The defect is then closed with multiple 6–0 buried polyglycolic acid sutures. An antibiotic ointment is used for 5 to 7 days postoperatively.

REFERENCES

1. Firat T, Ozkan S: Bilateral congenital entropion of the upper eyelids. Br J Ophthalmol 57:753, 1973.
2. Johnson CC: Epiblepharon. Am J Ophthalmol 66:1172–1175, 1968.
3. Bosniak S, Hornblass A, Smith B: Re-examining the tarsal kink syndrome: Considerations of its etiology and treatment. Ophthalmic Surg 16:437–440, 1985.
4. Nowinski T, Anderson RL: Advances in eyelid malpositions. Ophthalmic Plast Reconstr Surg 1:145–148, 1985.
5. Tse DT, Anderson RL, Fratkin JD: Aponeurosis disinsertion in congenital entropion. Arch Ophthalmol 101:436–440, 1983.
6. Quickert MH, Wilkes DI, Dryden RM: Nonincisional correction of epiblepharon and congenital entropion. Arch Ophthalmol 101:778–781, 1983.
7. Kolin T, Johns KJ, Wadlington WB, et al: Hereditary lymphedema and distichiasis. Arch Ophthalmol 109:980–981, 1991.
8. Quickert MH, Rathbun E: Suture repair of entropion. Arch Ophthalmol 85:304–305, 1971.
9. American Academy of Ophthalmology: Basic and Clinical Science Course. Sect. 9. Orbit, Eyelids and Lacrimal System. San Francisco, 1987, pp 165–175.
10. McCord CD, Chen WP: Tarsal polishing and mucous membrane grafting for cicatricial entropion, trichiasis and epidermalization. Ophthalmic Surg 14:1021–1025, 1983.
11. Millman AL, Katzen LB, Putterman AM: Cicatricial entropion: An analysis of its treatment with transverse blepharotomy and marginal rotation. Ophthalmic Surg 20:575–579, 1989.
12. Sullivan JH, Beard C, Bullock JD: Cryosurgery for treatment of trichiasis. Am J Ophthalmol 82:117–121, 1976.
13. Schaefer AJ: Variation in the pathophysiology of involutional entropion and its treatment. Ophthalmic Surg 14:653–655, 1983.
14. Lordan DR, Anderson RL: The lateral tarsal strip revisited. Arch Ophthalmol 107:604–606, 1989.
15. Dortzbach RK, McGetrick JJ: Involutional entropion of the lower eyelid. In Bosniac SL, Smith BC (eds): Advances in Ophthalmic Plastic and Reconstructive Surgery, vol. 2. New York, Pergamon Press, 1983, pp 257–267.
16. Hsu WM, Liu D: A new approach to the correction of involutional entropion by pretarsal orbicularis oculi muscle fixation. Am J Ophthalmol 100:802–805, 1985.
17. Dryden RM, Edelstein JP: Lateral palpebral tendon repair for lower eyelid ectropion. Ophthalmic Plast Reconstr Surg 4:115–118, 1988.
18. Hill JC: Treatment of epiphora owing to flaccid eyelids. Arch Ophthalmol 97:323–324, 1979.
19. Liu D, Staslor OG: Lower eyelid laxity and ocular symptoms. Am J Ophthalmol 95:545–551, 1983.
20. Hurwitz JJ: Senile entropion: The importance of eyelid laxity. Can J Ophthalmol 18:235–237, 1983.
21. Schaefer AJ: Lateral canthal tendon tuck. Trans Ophthalmol Otolaryngol 86:1879–1882, 1979.
22. Jones LT, Quickert MH, Tsujimura JK: Senile entropion. Am J Ophthalmol 55:463, 1963.
23. Schaefer AJ: Variation in the pathophysiology of involutional entropion and its treatment. Ophthalmic Surg 14:653–655, 1983.
24. Wesley R: Tarsal ectropion from detachment of the lower eyelid retractors. Am J Ophthalmol 93:491–495, 1982.
25. Sisler HA, Labay GR, Finlay JR: Senile ectropion and entropion: A comparative histopathological study. Ann Ophthalmol 8:319–322, 1976.
26. Dryden RM, Leibson J, Wobig J: Senile entropion. Arch Ophthalmol 96:1883–1885, 1978.
27. Wesly RE, Collins JW: Combined procedure for senile entropion. Ophthalmic Surg 14:401–405, 1983.
28. Jackson ST: Surgery for involutional entropion. Ophthalmic Surg 14:322–326, 1983.
29. Markovits AS: Variations of the theme of involutional entropion and the Quickert repair. Ann Ophthalmol 12:1028–1040, 1980.
30. Anderson RL, Gordy DD: The tarsal strip procedure. Arch Ophthalmol 97:2192–2196, 1979.
31. Anderson RL: Tarsal strip procedure for correction of eyelid laxity and canthal malposition in the anophthalmic socket. Ophthalmol 88:895–903, 1981.
32. Rees T: Prevention of ectropion by horizontal shortening of the lower lid during blepharoplasty. Ann Plast Surg 11:17–23, 1983.
33. Dortzbach R: Lower blepharoplasty by the anterior approach—Prevention of complications. Ophthalmology 90:223–229, 1983.
34. McCord C, Shore JW: Avoidance of complications in blepharoplasty. Ophthalmology 90:1039–1046, 1983.
35. Kristan RW, Staslor OG: Infracanalicular full-thickness transverse blepharotomy for medial ectropion. Ophthalmic Plast Reconstr Surg 3:127–129, 1987.
36. Meltzer MA: Medial ectropion repair. Ophthalmic Plast Reconstr Surg 5:182–185, 1989.
37. Frueh BR, Shoengarth LD: Evaluation and treatment of the patient with ectropion. Ophthalmology 89:1049–1054, 1982.
38. Putterman AM: Ectropion of the lower eyelid secondary to Müller's muscle—capsulopalpebral fascia detachment. Am J Ophthalmol 85:814–817, 1978.
39. Tse DT: Surgical correction of punctal malposition. Am J Ophthalmol 100:339–341, 1985.

Chapter 163

Disorders of the Eyelashes and Eyebrows

PETER A.D. RUBIN

The cilia or eyelashes arise from hair follicles just anterior to the tarsus, approximately 2 mm from the eyelid margin, and emerge through the skin at the level of the anterior eyelid margin (Fig. 163–1). The cilia are distributed in two or three irregularly placed rows. In the upper lid, the cilia are more numerous (100 to 150) and longer (8 to 12 mm). Fewer (50 to 75) and shorter (6 to 8 mm) cilia are found in the lower eyelid. The cilia are typically darker than the hair of the scalp and are more resistant to graying with age. The rate of growth is very slow, and they are renewed about every 3 to 5 mo.

The eyebrow region possesses large well-vascularized follicles. In addition to the scalp, the brow and cilia are among the first follicles in the body to elaborate terminal hairs; however, in adulthood, approximately half of the follicles in the brow produce only vellus hairs. In adulthood, the eyebrow cilia typically arise below the level of the upper orbital margin medially and cross above the orbital rim laterally. The wide-ranging appearance of the brows is due to the direction of growth, the distribution, and the position of the eyebrow hairs. Although minimally functional, the eyebrows greatly influence facial expression and aesthetics. Most variations of eyebrow appearance are of no clinical significance, but some are associated with developmental defects or are components of well-recognized syndromes.

Disturbances of the eyebrows and eyelashes can be grouped as disorders of abundance, deficiency, misdirection, pigmentation, or texture.

ABUNDANT GROWTH

Excessive growth of hair at any site on the body, when it is longer, denser, or coarser than is commonly found for a given age, sex, and race, is termed *hypertrichosis*. Although *hirsutism* and *hypertrichosis* are often incorrectly used interchangeably, hirsutism is a more specific disorder of children or adult women in which coarse terminal hairs grow in the adult male distribution pattern.

In congenital hypertrichosis (hypertrichosis lanugosa), the fine fetal lanugo hairs are not replaced by vellus ("peach fuzz") and terminal hairs but persist throughout life. This condition is extremely rare and is marked by the presence of excessively long and silky hairs distributed abundantly on the forehead, eyebrows, eyelids, and eyelashes. It appears to be inherited in an autosomal dominant pattern with variable penetrance and is frequently associated with hypodontia or adontia.[1] When acquired in adulthood, this rare condition of excessive growth of lanugo-type hair is frequently associated with an internal malignancy of the gastrointestinal tract or lung. Although the diagnosis of an internal malignancy typically predates the altered hair growth, the clinical appearance of hypertrichosis lanuginosa may be the initial manifestation of systemic disease. In milder forms, this condition may initially present with the new growth of fine silky hairs confined to the eyelids, nose, and glabella, which all are normally hairless. These hairs may grow very rapidly, as much as 2.5 cm per week, and achieve lengths of more than 10 cm.[2]

Hypertrichosis localized to the periorbital area may be seen with melanocytic nevi. In these cases, the associated hairs are often thicker and darker than the surrounding vellus and terminal hairs.

Other causes of localized hypertrichosis include chronic mechanical or chemical (i.e., corticosteroid) irritation.

Abundant Eyebrows

Prominent and thick eyebrows may be present as a dominantly inherited familial characteristic. Hypertrophy of the eyebrow resulting in fusion of the eyebrows

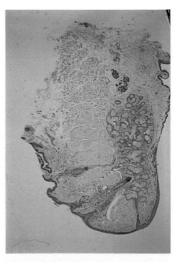

Figure 163–1. Histopathologic cross section of an eyelid demonstrates the follicular origin of the cilia within the midlamella of the eyelid, just anterior to the tarsus.

across the midline is termed *synophrys* (Greek for "with meeting eyebrows"). This condition may occur as an isolated finding or may be part of a more generalized hypertrichosis. Hypertrichosis of the brow and forehead is found in hereditary disorders of Hurler's syndrome, Cornelia de Lange's syndrome (pathologic dwarfism) (Fig. 163–2), porphyria, Waardenburg's syndrome, and autosomal recessive cone-rod dystrophy.[3]

Duplication supercilia, characterized by two separate parallel rows of eyebrows, have also been observed.[4]

Systemic Disorders

Malnutrition, either primary or secondary to malabsorptive states, anorexia nervosa, and dermatomyositis, has been associated with hypertrichosis.

Isolated Abundant Eyelashes

Congenital hypertrichosis of the cilia may be characterized by an increased length of cilia (trichomegaly) (Fig. 163–3), extra rows of cilia (polytrichia), or an ectopic location. Ectopic cilia may emerge anteriorly through the eyelid skin away from the margin, posteriorly through the meibomian orifices (distichiasis), or through the conjunctiva.

Pharmacologic Factors

Several pharmacologic agents have been noted to induce growth of hairs that are between vellus and terminal hairs in quality. The abnormal hair growth typically reverts to a normal pattern within 6 mo to 1 yr after a cessation of the medication. This type of hypertrichosis should be differentiated from drug-induced hirsutism, which results in increased terminal hairs in the male secondary sexual distribution, sparing the periorbital region. This type of hair growth typically is not reversible. Phenytoin, diazoxide, streptomycin, cortisone, penicillamine, minoxidil, and cyclosporin A[5] have been found to contribute to acquired hypertrichosis.

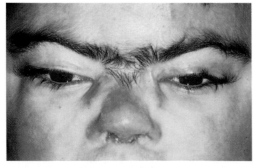

Figure 163–2. Synophrys, or fusion of the brows, may be an inherited familial finding or may be associated with specific congenital defects, as in this case of Cornelia de Lange's syndrome. (Courtesy of John Woog, M.D.)

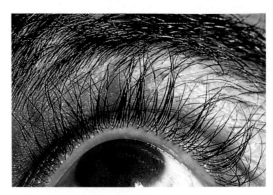

Figure 163–3. Trichomegaly: abnormally long and luxuriant eyelashes.

Treatment

Initial management of hypertrichosis should include a search for any reversible underlying cause of this condition. Typically, none is found, and patients should be counseled to pursue one of several therapeutic options. Bleaching the hairs can camouflage the hypertrichosis, but bleaching agents should be avoided in the periocular area. Mechanical epilation, depilatories, shaving, and epilating waxes all are useful but may cause folliculitis when chronically used. Electrolysis is the only commonly used technique that offers permanent hair removal. If electrolysis is performed in the periorbital region, great caution should be exercised because aggressive treatment can result in puncture scarring of the thin eyelid skin. Because hypertrichosis of the periorbital area is typically one manifestation of a generalized condition, it is best managed by a skilled dermatologist and an endocrinologist, especially if systemic therapy is pursued.

DEFICIENCY OF EYEBROWS AND EYELASHES

Congenital absence of eyelashes and eyebrows as an isolated anomaly is extremely rare. It may be part of a generalized absence of hair (alopecia adnata) or may be associated with hereditary ectodermal dysplasia, progeria, or cryptophthalmos.[6] Unilateral or partial absence of eyelashes may occur with congenital hemifacial atrophy or colobomas of the lids.

Alopecia Syndromes

Alopecia is the absence of hair in regions where hair is usually located. The term typically refers to loss of terminal hairs on the scalp, but involvement of the cilia and eyebrows is common in the alopecia syndromes. The alopecias are generally classified into cicatricial and noncicatricial varieties. In the noncicatricial types, the hair follicles are retained and the potential for regrowth of the hairs remains, whereas in the cicatricial alopecias the hair follicle is destroyed and the hair loss is perma-

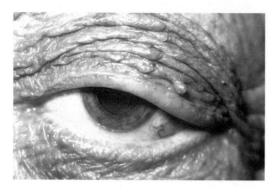

Figure 163–4. Alopecia areata, with complete loss of the eyelashes.

nent. With time, noncicatricial alopecia may evolve to cicatricial alopecia.

Alopecia areata initially occurs episodically, most commonly in patients between the ages of 5 and 40 yr. It is characterized by loss of hair in a slowly enlarging area without evidence of scaling or local infection. Any region of the body may be affected. The most common sites of involvement include the scalp, eyebrows, eyelashes, and beard (Fig. 163–4). Most cases are limited to one or a few small patches of alopecia, which repopulate with normal hair growth within 6 to 12 mo without any specific treatment. In 5 to 10 per cent of cases, hair loss eventually afflicts the entire scalp, brows, and lashes and is termed *alopecia totalis*. In these cases, especially in the pediatric population, the prognosis for return of hair is extremely unfavorable. When coupled with the loss of all body hair, this condition is referred to as *alopecia universalis*. No specific cause has been found for these conditions, although infection, autoimmunity, atopy, and psychologic and genetic factors have been suggested. Multiple therapeutic regimens including systemic and intralesional steroids, ultraviolet radiation, topical minoxidil, and chemical sensitization have been used with only limited, if any, success.[7] Psychiatric counseling, especially for children, is useful in adjusting to the cosmetic deformity.

Hair loss present in, but not limited to, the eyelashes and brows due to a destructive process is termed *madarosis* (Greek for "bald"). Whenever loss of the cilia and lashes occurs, it is important to search for an underlying local or systemic cause. The spectrum of potential causes of hair loss, in addition to the alopecia syndromes previously mentioned, includes infections, chemicals and drugs, endocrinopathies, nutritional and metabolic disorders, systemic diseases, neurotic behavior, and local trauma.

INFECTIONS

General systemic infections may result in localized cilia and brow loss. Secondary and tertiary syphilis have classically been described as causing loss of the temporal aspect of the brow. Similarly, leprosy, tuberculosis, and typhoid may be accompanied by madarosis. Localized pyogenic infections of the skin including carbuncles and furuncles or chronic blepharitis may result in a localized hair loss attributed to a direct toxic effect of staphylococcal toxins.[8]

Superficial bacterial infections such as impetigo usually do not cause hair loss. Fungal dermatophytes including the genera *Microsporum* (ringworm infections), *Trichophyton*, and *Epidermophyton* can contribute to local hair loss. Among the viruses, herpes zoster, with its associated obliterative dermal vasculitis, can cause profound cicatricial alopecia.

ENDOCRINE CAUSES

Endocrine disorders, especially hypothyroidism, have been known to cause brow alopecia, notably within the temporal brow. Interestingly, hyperthyroid, hypopituitary, and hyperparathyroid states may also cause alopecia.

SYSTEMIC DISEASES

Noninfectious dermatoses, including psoriasis, seborrheic dermatitis, exfoliative dermatitis, and follicular dermatitis, as well as dermatomycetes and systemic lupus erythematosus, may also contribute to hair loss (Fig. 163–5).

CHEMICALS AND DRUGS

Numerous drugs and chemical agents have been associated with alopecia via systemic or topical exposure. These include thallium, nitrogen mustard, cancer chemotherapeutic agents (e.g., methotrexate, cyclophosphamide, and vinca alkaloids), excessive vitamin A, thyroid antagonists, anticoagulants, and boric acid. Chronic malnutrition and mineral deficiencies of iron and zinc can also contribute to hair loss.

LOCAL FACTORS

Local factors such as chronic blepharitis or neoplasms that invade the dermis and disrupt the hair follicles, such as basal, squamous, and sebaceous cell carcinomas, can lead to loss of lashes. Focal loss of eyelashes attributable to "inflammation" should always be sus-

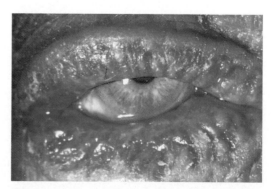

Figure 163–5. Chronic dermatitis with severe eczematous thickening of the eyelid margins accounts for the extensive madarosis.

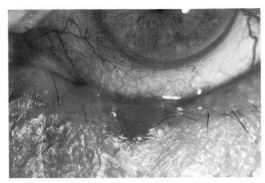

Figure 163–6. Neoplastic loss of cilia may occur from invasion and destruction of the follicles situated at the anterior face of the tarsus.

pected of heralding an undiagnosed underlying malignancy. In this setting, a full-thickness biopsy of the eyelid with fresh tissue stained for fat is particularly useful to rule out the possibility of a sebaceous gland carcinoma or other neoplasm (Fig. 163–6).

TRAUMA

Traumatic causes of alopecia include lacerations and thermal burns. The iatrogenic factors include excessive undermining of the anterior lamella to within 2 mm of the eyelid margin and follicular radiation exposure of greater than 1200 rad. Segmental alopecias are a common side effect of proton beam radiation for uveal melanoma (Fig. 163–7).

NEUROSIS

In rare cases, patients, typically children, pull out the hairs of the scalp and brow, as well as the cilia. This behavior, if suspected, can be confirmed by close observation of patients. Patients with this condition, termed *trichotillomania*, may not be aware of their habit of autoepilation. Therefore, ophthalmologists should counsel these patients and in severe cases recommend psychiatric consultation.

Hair Loss Treatment

The loss of brows or lashes, even when complete, such as in alopecia totalis, typically does not result in a significant functional deficit. Some patients may complain of perspiration getting into their eyes owing to the lack of a "sweat band" effect from the brows. Others may report a frequent foreign body sensation in their eyes because they do not have cilia to serve as a physical barrier to screen out small airborne particles in the region of the eyes. The aesthetic deficit should not be minimized, and it is imperative that a physician work closely with patients to determine the cause of hair loss, its potential reversibility, and a range of treatment options. Hair loss can often be reversed if the underlying infectious, endocrine, nutritional, or pharmacologic factors are directly treated. Unfortunately, the treatment

of alopecia areata and its related disorders has been very disappointing.

If the cilia or brow loss is due to a local inflammatory or infectious process, aggressive topical treatment with eyelid hygiene or topical systemic antibiotics may be curative. In regions of the eyelids where the cilia are sparse but not absent, eyeliner or blepharopigmentation (tattooing) may produce the desired appearance of more luxuriant growth. In cases of permanent or prolonged hair loss, the judicious use of eyeliner, brow pencils, or false eyelashes may yield acceptable cosmetic results.

SURGICAL TREATMENT

Loss of Eyelashes

Surgical options offer a more permanent result. Regions of the eyelids where the cilia are sparse but not absent may be adequately camouflaged with permanent blepharopigmentation (tattooing), giving the appearance of more abundant growth.

In cases of segmental lash loss, such as in congenital colobomas, as a result of trauma, or as a sequela to proton beam irradiation of choroidal melanomas, the defect can be corrected by full-thickness resection of the involved portion of the eyelid.

Transplantation of hairs to areas devoid of lashes is an alternative technique. Brow hairs and their follicles, which are matched for length and direction of growth, may be transplanted into the pretarsal region of the eyelid.[9, 10] Four rows of cilia are typically grafted to allow for the anticipated atrophy of the outer rows. Alternatively, temporal eyelashes, which are less cosmetically apparent, may be transplanted to cover a defect of cilia in the central portion of the eyelid. These techniques are tedious and often do not yield the desired results; therefore, alternative techniques for correction of deficient cilia should be pursued before choosing this option. After successful grafting, misdirected cilia, which commonly appear, can be obliterated by electrolysis.

Loss of Eyebrow

When possible, local transposition of eyebrows is preferable because it can most closely match the nu-

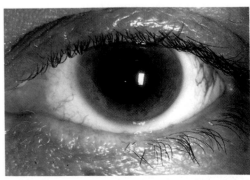

Figure 163–7. Radiation madarosis and focal depigmentation in the medial portion of the lower eyelid occurred after proton beam irradiation for a uveal melanoma.

merous properties of these hairs; including color, texture, shortness, slow growth, acute angle between skin and hair shaft, and direction of growth. Hair direction in the brow is complicated and must be accurately matched to achieve the optimal cosmetic result. In the medial portion of the brow, the hairs are directed superolaterally, but more superiorly and laterally, the orientation changes from lateral to inferolateral. Segmental loss of the eyebrows following trauma or excision of brow lesions is optimally reconstructed with a subcutaneous pedicle flap from the ipsilateral brow.[11]

Larger defects can be covered by composite free grafting from the nape of the neck or postauricular area.[12] Alternatively, in cases of total bilateral eyebrow loss, a bipedicled scalp flap has also been described.[13] These techniques are complicated by variable viability of the hair follicles, especially in free grafts, and failure to match the subtle eyebrow features of direction and length.

MISDIRECTION

Although the eyelashes are among the shortest and finest hairs on the body, they potentially pose the most hazards, for in cases of chronic misdirection of cilia, the resulting ocular surface disease can lead to blindness. The cilia normally arise from follicles located just anterior to the tarsus, emerge through the anterior lamella, and are directed away from the globe. In several distinct conditions, the cilia are misdirected toward the globe. These include congenital distichiasis, epiblepharon, acquired distichiasis, and entropion. It is important to identify the cause of misdirected cilia so that appropriate specific intervention can be administered (Table 163–1).

Distichiasis

Distichiasis is a rare congenital anomaly in which fully formed or smaller and less pigmented eyelashes emerge from the openings of the meibomian glands (Fig. 163–8). This defect may result when a primary epithelial

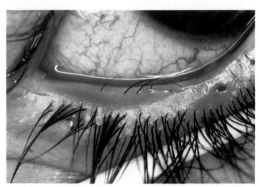

Figure 163–8. Congenital distichiasis. Normally formed cilia are emerging from meibomian gland orifices.

germ cell destined to differentiate into a specialized meibomian sebaceous gland of the tarsus develops into a complete pilosebaceous unit. Distichiasis is frequently inherited in an autosomal dominant pattern with high penetrance and variable expressivity. Although usually occurring as an isolated disorder, this condition has also been reported in association with mandibulofacial dysostosis,[14] ptosis, strabismus, congenital heart defects,[15] and trisomy 18.[16] During infancy, these fine misdirected cilia are usually well tolerated despite their apposition to the globe. Clinical presentation may be delayed until 5 yr of age, when patients may complain of chronic ocular irritation. Treatment can be deferred until symptoms develop.

ACQUIRED DISTICHIASIS

The concept of acquired distichiasis has not achieved widespread acceptance, but its presence, if distichiasis is defined as aberrant cilia emerging through the meibomian orifices, is well established.[17] Acquired distichiasis occurs most prominently in the setting of chronic inflammation, especially in cases of ocular cicatricial pemphigoid and Stevens-Johnson syndrome and after chemical injuries of the eyelid. Unlike congenital distichiasis, the cilia of acquired distichiasis tend to be nonpigmented and stunted and are more likely to cause symptomatic ocular surface irritation. It is theorized that under certain stimuli, possibly immunologic, chemical, or physical, the sebaceous meibomian gland undergoes metaplastic transformation into a pilosebaceous gland, producing hairs. This condition should be differentiated from trichiasis, in which the misdirected lashes have their origin in the anterior lamellae. This distinction is important because specific therapies, such as posterior lamella cryotherapy, can be directly used to eliminate acquired distichiatic cilia.[18]

Trichiasis

Trichiasis (Greek for "hair condition") is an acquired aberrant growth of the cilia that emanate from the anterior lamella and are misdirected toward the ocular surface (Fig. 163–9). It is distinguished from other

Table 163–1. DIFFERENTIAL DIAGNOSIS OF EYELASHES DIRECTED AGAINST THE GLOBE

Term	Features
Distichiasis	Eyelashes emerging from meibomian gland orifices
Congenital	Fine pigmented cilia
Acquired	Cilia often nonpigmented, stunted
	Associated conditions: Stevens-Johnson syndrome, ocular cicatricial pemphigoid
Epiblepharon	Congenital fold of pretarsal skin applies cilia of normal origin against globe
Trichiasis	Cilia emerge from normal anterior lamella location
	Commonly associated with trachoma
Entropion	Abnormal rotation of entire eyelid margin toward globe
	Etiologies: congenital, spastic, involutional, cicatricial

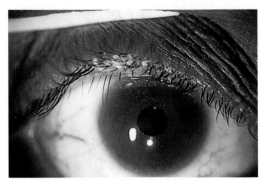

Figure 163–9. Trichiasis. Cilia emerging from a normal anterior lamellar location are misdirected toward the globe. Trichiasis in this case was due to underlying trachoma.

causes of lash misdirection because the lid margin is in a normal position. Prolonged inflammation, as noted with acquired distichiasis, usually contributes to this condition. Traditionally, chronic infections, most notably trachoma, may result in trichiasis. Along with tear deficiency and cicatricial entropion, trichiasis can contribute toward blinding complications in the advanced stages of this disease.

Epiblepharon

Epiblepharon[19] is characterized by congenital redundancy of the pretarsal skin and orbicularis muscle, which may override the eyelid margin and apply the cilia against the globe (Fig. 163–10). An additional cause of this condition may be the absence of insertion of the eyelid retractors into the anterior lamella, preventing marginal migration of the skin and orbicularis. Epiblepharon often does not require treatment, because it may resolve spontaneously with growth of the face. Symptomatic cases can be treated with lid crease–forming sutures[20, 21] or with a small elliptical excision of skin and orbicularis near the eyelid margin combined with a tarsal fixation closure.

Entropion

Entropion is distinguished from the other disorders that result in lashes misdirected toward the globe by abnormal rotation of the eyelid margin toward the ocular surface (Fig. 163–11). Thus, despite normal origins and growth patterns of the lashes, the rotation of the eyelid margin results in misdirection of the cilia toward the globe. The underlying cause of the marginal malposition can typically be attributed to congenital, spastic, involutional, or cicatricial factors. Involutional entropion is the most common cause of this type of eyelid malposition. In involutional cases, lower eyelid involvement is overwhelmingly more frequent, primarily because the greater height of tarsus in the upper eyelid provides more stability and resistance to the tendency of eyelid rotation. It is interesting to note that in some cases of significant laxity of the upper eyelid, such as in the floppy eyelid syndrome, upper eyelid lash ptosis (without contacting the ocular surface) in the absence of an apparent eyelid malposition may be a sign of eyelid instability (Fig. 163–12). The cicatricial entropions encountered with chronic inflammation (i.e., cicatricial ocular pemphigoid and Stevens-Johnson syndrome) and characterized by posterior lamella foreshortening also commonly feature trichiasis and acquired distichiasis (Fig. 163–13).

Management of Misdirected Cilia

Naturally, if misdirection of the cilia is not primary, the underlying cause (i.e., entropion or epiblepharon) should be initially addressed. If there are no symptoms or signs of ocular irritation due to misdirected cilia, treatment can be deferred. In individuals awaiting treatment, aggressive lubrication with ointments or use of a therapeutic contact lens may provide temporary relief. Removal of offending cilia can be categorized into modalities of epilation—surgery, electrolysis, cryosurgery, and surgical extirpation.

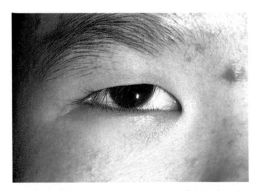

Figure 163–10. Epiblepharon. A redundant fold of pretarsal skin and underlying orbicularis muscle overrides the eyelid margin and applies the cilia of the lower eyelid against the globe. (Courtesy of J. Woog, M.D.)

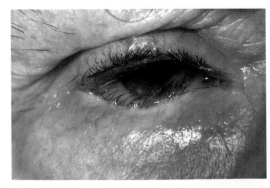

Figure 163–11. Involutionary entropion. Rotation of the entire lower eyelid margin against the globe. Thickening of the lower eyelid margin and narrowing of the horizontal palpebral aperture are reflective of an overriding preseptal orbicularis muscle and a lateral canthal dehiscence, respectively.

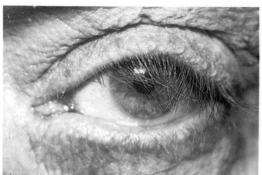 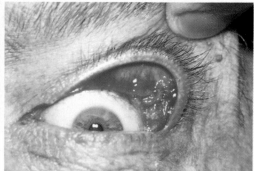

Figure 163–12. *A*, Eyelash ptosis. The upper eyelid cilia are in a vertical configuration yet are not contacting the ocular surface. *B*, The upper eyelid's marked laxity, contributing to the eyelash malposition, is apparent in this case of floppy eyelid syndrome.

EPILATION

Epilation, especially in cases of limited involvement, provides temporarily relief but is rarely curative. In cases of chronic and recurrent misdirection of cilia, patients and their families can often be taught to recognize and epilate offending cilia to provide temporary relief if ophthalmic care is not immediately accessible.

ELECTROLYSIS

In cases of limited aberrant cilia, electrolysis may effectively eliminate the lashes. After local anesthesia, a fine needle (approximately 30 gauge) is introduced into the offending follicle and low current is applied to cause follicular destruction (Fig. 163–14). With effective application of this method, the cilia are easily epilated. Aggressive treatment should be avoided because it may lead to eyelid notching or destruction of adjacent follicles and resultant focal madarosis.

CRYOTHERAPY

Although not as selective as electrolysis, cryotherapy seems to be the most effective method of destroying aberrant cilia, especially when extensive obliteration is needed. This technique ideally uses a large bevel-tipped cryoprobe positioned at the lid margin, combined with a nitrous oxide or carbon dioxide cryogen source. Follicular freezing to a temperature of $-20°$ C is usually sufficient for permanent destruction of the follicles. A thermocouple probe can confirm the intensity of freezing; however, a double application of a 30- to 45-sec freeze and slow thaw has been shown empirically to be an effective cryosurgical treatment.[22]

Complications of this procedure may include lid depigmentation (especially notable in more darkly pigmented patients), lid notching, symblepharon, lid edema, and intense postoperative pain. When the aberrant cilia are located within the posterior lamella (distichiasis), lid splitting and direct cryoprobe applications to the posterior lamella can serve to selectively destroy the posteriorly routed aberrant cilia, preserve the normally positioned cilia emerging from the anterior lamella, and minimize the risk of lid depigmentation.[18]

SURGICAL EXTIRPATION

If trichiatic cilia are only present segmentally, a limited full-thickness resection of the aberrant area can be curative. This situation is commonly encountered in focal lid notching following traumatic laceration, prior full-thickness lid repair, and localized conjunctival scarring. In these cases, full-thickness repair also yields a significant cosmetic improvement because the lid contour can be restored.

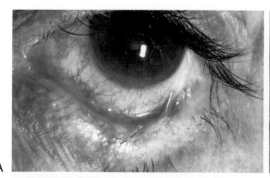 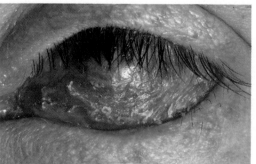

Figure 163–13. *A*, Trichiasis and acquired distichiasis are present along with a dense inferior symblepharon in this case of ocular cicatricial pemphigoid. *B*, Severe trichiasis, cicatricial entropion, and diffuse ocular surface keratinization are found in this advanced case of Stevens-Johnson syndrome.

Direct surgical excision of aberrant follicles by an external approach has been advocated; however, this technique usually requires microscopic control.[23] Others have described correction of distichiasis through excision of eyelashes using a transconjunctival approach.[24] Both of these techniques are tedious and complicated by a high rate of recurrence.

DISORDERS OF PIGMENTATION

Unlike hair on other parts of the body, the cilia and eyebrows are resistant to graying until late age. Ultrastructurally, graying, termed *canities*, reflects minimal saturation of apparently normal melanosomes with melanin. In white hair, melanocytes are scarce or absent.

Poliosis

Poliosis is distinguished from physiologic canities by its focal nature and the total absence of melanin in a group of neighboring follicles (Fig. 163–15). Clinically, this is reflected in localized depigmentation of hairs and a resultant patch of white hairs. Numerous causes of acquired poliosis are known, including vitiligo, localized irradiation, severe dermatitis, tuberous sclerosis, neurofibromatosis and the uveitis syndrome of Vogt-Koyanagi-Harada, and sympathetic ophthalmia.[25] When present in the periocular region, poliosis is usually associated with patches of vitiligo.

Piebaldism

Congenital poliosis limited to the anterior scalp margin is referred to as *piebaldism*. It is typically inherited as an autosomal dominant trait and is of no medical significance. However, in Waardenburg's syndrome,[26] it

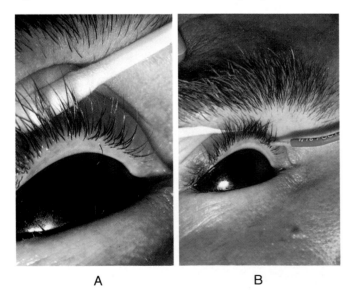

Figure 163–14. *A,* Focal trichiasis in the upper eyelid. *B,* Electroepilation of a trichiatic cilium. A corneal/scleral shell is placed to protect the globe.

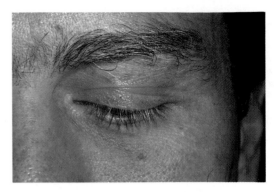

Figure 163–15. Poliosis. Segmental depigmentation of the eyelash and brow cilia.

is associated with congenital deafness and hypertelorism. This syndrome is transmitted in an autosomal dominant pattern with the variable penetrance of its associated anomalies. It accounts for approximately 1 to 2 percent of congenital deafness. Among the associated ophthalmic abnormalities are synophrys and iris heterochromia.[27]

DISORDERS OF TEXTURE

A structural defect in the hair shaft that causes the hair to twist on its own axis is referred to as *pili torti*. The hairs, including the cilia, emerge at oblique angles and are fragile, short, and sparse. Cases may be inherited in an autosomal dominant pattern or may be sporadic. In Menke's syndrome, also referred to as *kinky hair disease*,[28] the basic abnormality appears to be related to copper storage and is inherited through an X-linked recessive gene.

REFERENCES

1. Beighton P: Congenital hypertrichosis lanuginosa. Arch Dermatol 101:669, 1970.
2. Hedgedus SI, Schorr WF: Acquired hypertrichosis lanuginosa and malignancy. Arch Dermatol 106:84, 1970.
3. Jalili IK: Cone-rod congenital amaurosis associated with congenital hypertrichosis: An autosomal dominant condition. J Med Genet 26:504, 1989.
4. Cascio G: Sur la "duplicato supercilii." Ophthalmologica 130:231, 1955.
5. Weaver DT, Bartley GB: Cyclosporine-induced trichomegaly. Am J Ophthalmol 109:239, 1990.
6. Ebling FJG, Dawber R, Rook A: The hair. *In* Rook A, Wilkinson DS, Ebling FJG, et al (eds): Textbook of Dermatology, 4th ed, vol. 3. Oxford, Blackwell Scientific Publications, 1986, pp 1973–2000.
7. Orentrich N: Treatment of alopecia areata. JAMA 238:347, 1977.
8. Butterworth T, Fowler JC: Postfuruncular alopecia. AMA Arch Dermatol 80:570, 1959.
9. Mutou Y, Boo-Chai K: Transplantation of hair for eyelash replacement. Plast Reconstr Surg 29:573, 1962.
10. Santos JG, Matus RR, Vera AS: Correction of alopecia of eyebrows in leprous patients. Plast Reconstr Surg 27:316, 1961.
11. Kasai K, Ogawa Y: Partial eyebrow reconstruction using subcutaneous pedicle flaps to perserve the natural hair direction. Ann Plast Surg 24:117, 1990.
12. System of ophthalmology, *In* Duke-Elder S (ed): The Ocular Adnexa, vol. XIII. St. Louis, CV Mosby, 1974, pp 381–382.

13. Brent B: Reconstruction of ear, eyebrow, and sideburn in the burned patient. Plast Reconstr Surg 55:312, 1975.
14. Bartley GB, Jackson IT: Distichiasis and cleft palate. Plast Reconstr Surg 84:129, 1989.
15. Goldstein S, Qazi QH, Fitzgerald J, et al: Distichiasis, congenital heart defects, and mixed peripheral vascular anomalies. Am J Genet 20:283, 1985.
16. Mehta L, Shannon RS, Duckett DP, Young ID: Trisomy in a 13-year-old girl. J Med Genet 23:256, 1986.
17. Scheie HG, Albert DM: Distichiasis and trichiasis: Origin and management. Am J Ophthalmol 61:718, 1966.
18. Anderson RL, Harvey JT: Lid splitting and posterior lamella cryo-surgery for congenital and acquired distichiasis. Arch Ophthalmol 99:631, 1981.
19. Levitt JM: Epiblepharon and congenital entropion. Am J Ophthalmol 44:112, 1957.
20. Quickert MH, Wilkes DI, Dryden RM: Non-incisional correction of epiblepharon and congenital entropion. Arch Ophthalmol 101:778, 1983.
21. Hayasaka S, Noda S, Setogawa T: Epiblepharon with inverted eyelashes in Japanese children. II: Surgical repairs. Br J Ophthalmol 73:128, 1989.
22. Sullivan JH, Beard C, Bullock JD: Cryosurgery for the treatment of trichiasis. Am J Ophthalmol 82:117, 1976.
23. Wolfley D: Excision of individual follicles for management of congenital distichiasis and localized trichiasis. J Pediatr Ophthalmol Strabismus 24:22, 1987.
24. Dortzbach RK, Butera RT: Excision of distichiasis eyelashes through a transconjunctival trapdoor. Arch Ophthalmol 96:111, 1978.
25. Albert DM, Nordland JJ, Lerner AB. Ocular abnormalities occurring with vitiligo. Ophthalmology 86:1145, 1979.
26. Waardenburg PJ: A new syndrome combining developmental anomalies of the eyelids, eyebrows, and nose root with pigmentary defects of the iris and ear hair and with congenital deafness. Am J Hum Genet 3:195, 1951.
27. Cant JS, Martin AJ. Waardenberg's syndrome: Report of a family. Br J Ophthalmol 51:755, 1967.
28. Danks DM, Campbell J, Walker-Smith BJ, et al: Menkes' kinky hair syndrome. Lancet 1:1100, 1972.

Chapter 164

■

Eyelid Manifestations of Systemic Disease

JANEY L. WIGGS and FREDERICK A. JAKOBIEC

Many systemic disorders can cause abnormalities of the eyelids (Table 164–1). Often, such lesions may be the first indication of an underlying disease. Familiarity with these lesions allows the ophthalmologist to detect potentially severe systemic illness. This chapter reviews eyelid lesions associated with some systemic disorders including hyperlipidemia, vasculitis and connective tissue disease, amyloidosis, sarcoidosis, and eyelid lesions associated with systemic malignancy.

XANTHOMATOUS LESIONS

Xanthelasmas

Patients affected by essential hyperlipidemia and secondary hyperlipidemia resulting from diabetes or biliary cirrhosis can develop xanthomas. When xanthomas occur on the eyelid, they are referred to as xanthelasmas. Eyelid xanthelasmas typically appear in middle-aged or elderly patients as bilateral flat, yellowish soft plaques on the inner canthi (Fig. 164–1). These lesions consist of foamy histocytes with a surrounding localized inflammatory reaction.[1] Eyelid xanthelasmas are frequently seen in patients with type II hyperlipidemia and are less typically seen in patients with the type IV phenotype.[2] Normolipemic patients can also develop these lesions, and many of these patients have lipoprotein abnormalities that may result in an enhanced atherogenic potential.[3,4] In a study

of 41 normolipemic patients with eyelid xanthelasmas, significantly decreased levels of high-density lipoprotein cholesterol (HDL-C) were found. This population of patients had three to four times the risk of cardiac

Table 164–1. EYELID FINDINGS ASSOCIATED WITH SYSTEMIC DISEASE

Xanthelasmas	Hyperlipidemias
Multiple nodules of the eyelids	Lipoid proteinosis
Ptosis, purpura of the eyelid skin	Amyloidosis
Edema, ptosis, and retraction of the lower lid	Wegener's granulomatosis
Pseudorheumatoid nodules of the eyelids	Granuloma annulare
Rapidly enlarging nodule of the eyelid	Nodular fasciitis
Focal infarction of the eyelid skin	Polyarteritis nodosa
Lax-appearing but firm and immobile eyelids	Scleroderma
Heliotrope discoloration of the upper eyelid skin	Dermatopolymyositis
Fine telangiectases of the upper eyelid	Systemic lupus erythematosus eyelid
"Millet seed" nodules of the eyelids	Sarcoidosis
Keratoacanthomas; sebaceous tumors	Muir-Torre syndrome (colon carcinoma)
Trichilemmomas	Cowden's syndrome (breast, thyroid, gastrointestinal carcinomas)
Multiple basal cell carcinomas	Basal nevoid syndrome (medulloblastoma)

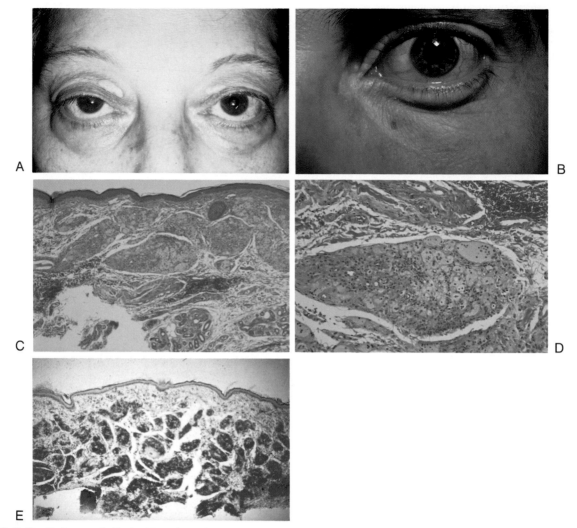

Figure 164–1. Xanthelasma. *A,* Typical location of yellow plaques in the superomedial aspects of the eyelids, seen best on the right. *B,* Extensive xanthelasmatous deposits of the upper and lower eyelids, extending onto the upper cheek. The eyelids have been thickened, and there is corrugation of the eyelid margin in the inner aspect of the upper eyelid. *C,* A biopsy specimen of xanthelasma discloses lobules of pale-staining histiocytic cells. *D,* Each lobule is composed of mononucleated and multinucleated histiocytic cells, many of which have been totally bloated by myriad cytoplasmic vacuoles and are therefore referred to as *foam cells.* A gigantic multinucleated foam cell is shown at the outer periphery on upper right. *E,* Oil red O stain of fresh frozen tissue demonstrates that the cytoplasmic vacuoles contain lipid. Most of the lobules are arranged around a central capillary.

disease compared with a control group of normolipemic patients without xanthelasmas.[5] These studies demonstrate the high probability of lipid abnormalities and increased cardiovascular risk in patients with xanthelasmas.

Surgical excision of eyelid xanthelasmas results in definitive treatment in approximately 50 percent of cases. A recurrence is likely if the patient is affected by an underlying hyperlipidemia syndrome.[6]

Xanthoma Tuberosum

Tuberous xanthoma is another lesion that frequently occurs in patients with types II and III hyperlipidemias. This lesion can also be found in association with an IgG dysproteinemia in which a low serum complement level, elevated cryoglobulinemia, and leukopenia as well as hyperlipemia are also sometimes seen.[7, 8]

Tuberous xanthomas, or necrobiotic xanthogranuloma, appear as plaque-like nodules on the eyelids as well as on the buttocks, elbows, knees, and fingers. Histopathologically, these lesions are found in deeper layers of the skin than xanthelasma. Tuberous xanthomas consist of foamy histiocytes, Touton giant cells, extracellular cholesterol deposits, and fibrous inflammatory cells. Studies have suggested that the accumulation of lipid in these lesions is a direct result of the elevated levels of lipid in the blood of these patients.[9]

Erdheim-Chester Disease

Erdheim-Chester disease, or lipoid granulomatosis, is a disorder characterized by elevated blood lipid levels and lipogranuloma formation with reactive inflammatory involvement of the long bones, lungs, heart, and kidneys. The ophthalmic manifestations of the disease include bilateral xanthelasma, exophthalmos, ophthalmoplegia, edema and atrophy of the optic nerve, and retinal striae.[10] The histopathologic lesion that characterizes Erdheim-Chester disease is a fibrosing xanthogranulomatous process composed of xanthomatous histiocytes, numerous Touton giant cells, and areas of fibrosis.[11]

DEPOSITIONS

Lipoid Proteinosis

Lipoid proteinosis, also referred to as Urbach-Wiethe syndrome, is a disorder characterized by the formation of numerous papules and nodules on the skin of the face, knees, elbows, and the mucous membranes of the lips, pharynx, and larynx. Similar lesions have also been described involving the gastrointestinal tract, pancreas, and testes.[12] The radiographic finding of bilateral sickle-shaped calcifications of the skull is characteristic of the disease.[13] The ophthalmic manifestations of this disorder are primarily the formation of many small nodules lining the margins of all four eyelids. These nodules can become confluent and typically have a waxy or semi-translucent appearance (Fig. 164–2). Histopathologic analysis of these lesions shows thickened capillary walls with basement membrane deposition of a hyaline material.[14, 15] This condition may be inherited as an autosomal recessive trait.[16]

Amyloidosis

Primary systemic amyloidosis may have many clinical manifestations including alopecia, macroglossia, pallor of the skin, and abnormalities of the nails. The ophthalmic manifestations of the disease include ptosis and complete external ophthalmoplegia secondary to amyloid deposits in the extraocular muscles and purpura of the eyelids, which may occur spontaneously or following minor trauma.[17, 18] The purpuric lesions are caused by blood vessels that easily rupture because of deposited amyloid. The skin of the eyelids is also a common site for the characteristic eruption of primary systemic amyloidosis.[19] These lesions are symmetric, bilateral confluent papules with a waxy appearance (Fig. 164–3). The finding of hemorrhagic papules involving the skin of the eyelids strongly suggests the diagnosis of primary systemic amyloidosis.[20, 21] Rarely intraorbital amyloidosis has been described with associated levator muscle involvement and proptosis.[22] Treatment of local involvement of the eyelids and conjunctiva by amyloidosis is controversial. In a small study, local radiation treatment was found to result in some shrinkage of these lesions.[23]

VASCULITIS AND CONNECTIVE TISSUE DISORDERS

Wegener's Granulomatosis

Wegener's granulomatosis is a systemic arteritis in which the lungs, kidneys, upper respiratory system, and sinuses can be affected by a necrotizing vasculitis. Orbital and ocular lesions are also associated with lesions of the head and neck. Ophthalmic involvement can be quite varied in this disease and includes orbital inflammation, scleritis and episcleritis, corneal ulceration and inflammation, and conjunctival hemorrhage.[24] Eyelid involvement is seen in approximately 20 percent of patients with Wegener's granulomatosis and consists of edema, ptosis, and retraction of the lower lid (Fig. 164–4).[25] Treatment with corticosteroids and immunosuppressive agents has dramatically improved the prognosis of affected patients, although substantial mortality and ocular morbidity are still associated with this disease.

Granuloma Annulare

Granuloma annulare, or pseudorheumatoid nodules, are subcutaneous lesions that can be found in the head and neck region of otherwise healthy children or young adults. These nodules can be found in the eyelid and

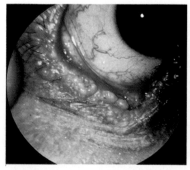 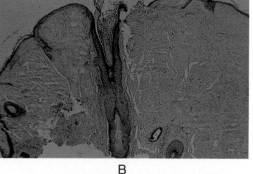

A   B

Figure 164–2. Lipoid proteinosis. *A,* All four eyelids are characteristically involved in this process. The eyelid margins are beset with confluent pearly nodules. *B,* A biopsy specimen reveals replacement of the upper and lower dermis of the eyelid by a hyaline/amorphous material that has destroyed most of the adnexal structures, with a single eyelash being preserved. This hyaline material is a PAS-positive glycoprotein that is diastase-resistant and may be the result of dermal fibroblasts synthesizing noncollagenous proteins at the expense of collagens. The material may also contain lipidic material and is weakly positive on Congo red staining.

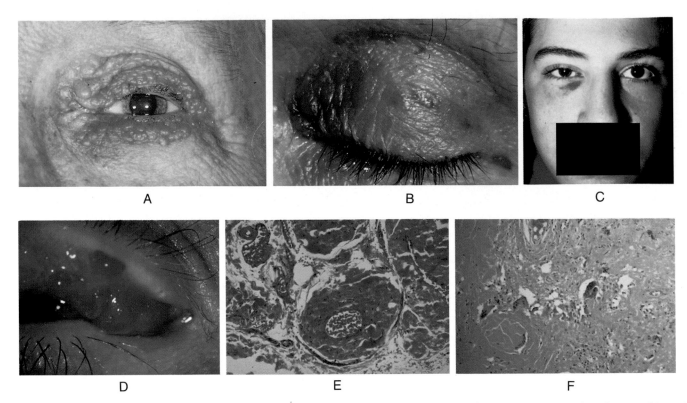

Figure 164–3. Cutaneous involvement with amyloidosis. *A,* An elderly patient presented with yellow nodules of all four eyelids and was not known to have a systemic ailment. Systemic amyloidosis was ultimately diagnosed. (Courtesy of Dr. Alan Proia.) *B,* Hemorrhagic papules of the eyelid skin in a patient with amyloidosis. *C,* This teenaged patient presented with a hemorrhage of the lower eyelid and a reddish mass in the caruncular region. *D,* On everting the eyelids, hemorrhagic and yellowish deposits are identified in the conjunctiva of the same patient shown in *C.* In contradistinction to cutaneous eyelid involvement, conjunctival amyloid deposits are generally not associated with systemic disease, which was not discovered in this patient. *E,* Characteristic Congophilic perivascular deposits of amyloid material. *F,* A multinucleated foreign body giant cell response has been mounted to amorphous deposits of amyloid material.

periorbital region, often showing a predilection for the lateral upper eyelid and outer canthus.[26] Granuloma annulare have a cystic consistency and histopathologically consist of multiple, confluent, necrobiotic granulomata. A zonal pattern showing three distinct areas can be found in some nodules, with the innermost area showing necrobiosis of collagen, the middle portion composed of fibroblasts and histiocytes, and the outer area containing sclerotic blood vessels. The surrounding stroma usually shows an infiltrate of chronic inflammatory cells and eosinophils. These lesions are similar clinically and histopathologically to the subcutaneous nodules of rheumatoid arthritis; however, these patients do not develop the other systemic symptoms of this disease.[27] Generally, granuloma annulare follow a benign clinical course and local excision, usually performed for diagnostic purposes, is the only treatment indicated.

Nodular Fasciitis

Nodular fasciitis is a benign reactive proliferation of fibroblasts and vascular elements involving the subcutaneous tissue. Clinically, the lesions appear as rapidly growing nodules associated with slight tenderness. These lesions usually occur in young adults and typically affect the upper extremities, chest, and back. Nodular fasciitis of the head and neck is more common in infants and children. In these patients it can affect the ocular adnexa, and approximately 50 percent of these cases involve the eyelid.[28] Histopathologically, the lesions consist of fibroblasts surrounding large cystoid spaces containing an intercellular myxoid ground substance. Treatment is by local excision, and the syndrome rarely recurs.[29]

Polyarteritis Nodosa

Polyarteritis nodosa is a multisystem disorder characterized by necrotizing arteritis of medium and small muscular arteries. The ocular manifestations of this disease depend on which ophthalmic vessels are involved. Optic nerve and retinal ischemia, scleritis, episcleritis, corneoscleral ulcers, and orbital inflammation have all been observed.[24] Lid involvement is usually in the form of focal infarction of the skin of the eyelids.

Scleroderma

Scleroderma is a progressive systemic disorder that results in inflammatory, fibrotic, and degenerative

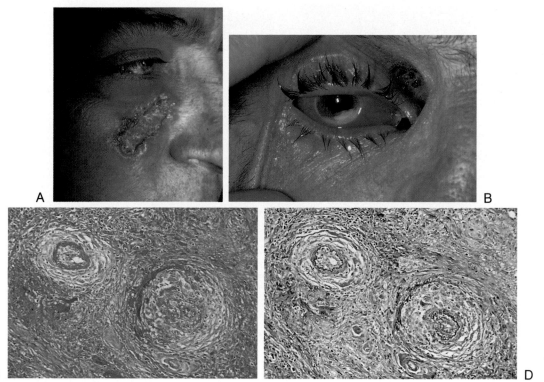

Figure 164–4. Wegener's granulomatosis. *A,* A cutaneous infarct from underlying vasculitis with ulcer formation and erythema of the eyelids. *B,* There is active scleritis with a peripheral ulcerative keratitis in this patient with retraction of the eyelids toward a fistula in the caruncular area that opens into the ethmoid sinus. This patient had extensive sinus and orbital destructive vasculitis. *C,* Two blood vessels in an orbital biopsy with granulomatous vasculitis, as well as granulomatous elements present in the interstitium. *D,* An elastic stain identifies surviving remnants of the internal elastica. (*C* and *D,* Courtesy of Dr. Ralph Eagle.)

changes of connective tissue, skin, synovium, gastrointestinal organs, lungs, and kidneys. The cause of this disease is unknown but is considered to be related to an abnormal cell-mediated immune reaction to collagen.[30] The skin of the face and eyelids may be affected by the sclerodermatous process, resulting in lax-appearing lids that are actually firm and immobile (see Chapter 238). Despite the decreased excursion of the eyelids in advanced cases, lagophthalmos and exposure keratitis do not develop.[31] Involvement of blood vessels in the skin of the eyelids may also lead to the development of telangiectases.[32]

Dermatomyositis

Polymyositis is an inflammatory disease of muscle characterized by progressive symmetric muscle weakness, dysphagia, and arthralgias. When typical skin lesions of macular erythema and telangiectases affecting the face, neck, and upper trunk accompany the muscle disease, the disorder is called dermatomyositis. When seen in patients older than 40 yr of age, dermatomyositis is associated with malignancy in a high percentage of cases.[33] Involvement of the eyelids is frequent in patients affected by dermatomyositis. Typical findings are "heliotrope" discoloration of the upper eyelid skin along with eyelid and periorbital edema (Fig. 164–5).[34] Diagnosis of this syndrome is made by serum analysis for elevated muscle enzymes and the demonstration of

characteristic pathology in a muscle biopsy. The appropriate treatment involves corticosteroid therapy after a search for occult systemic malignancy has been made.[33]

Systemic Lupus Erythematosus

Systemic lupus erythematosus is an autoimmune disorder that can affect many different organ systems. Ocular involvement may also be widespread and can include the cornea, sclera, retina, optic nerve, and visual pathways within the brain as well as the eyelids. The most characteristic findings of the lid skin are telangiectases of the superficial cutaneous vessels of the vascular marginal arcade of the upper eyelid. These fine erythematous lines form a horizontal band just above the lashes of the upper lids (Fig. 164–6). The lid skin may be part of the general cutaneous reaction seen in these patients, including the typical "butterfly rash."[35] Edema of the eyelids may be an early finding in individuals affected with lupus erythematosus.[36] Blepharospasm, which worsens with exacerbations of the disease and improves with immunosuppressive therapy, may also be an unusual finding in affected patients.[37, 38]

SARCOIDOSIS

Sarcoidosis is a disease of unknown cause characterized by noncaseating epithelioid tubercles, which occur

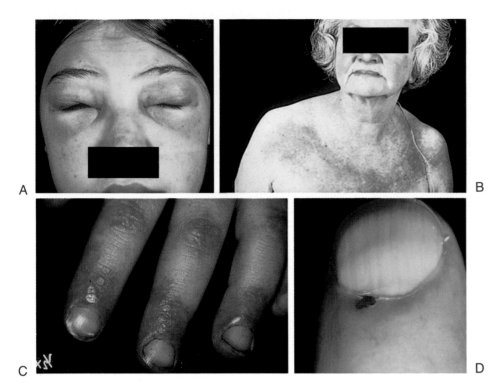

Figure 164–5. Dermatomyositis. *A,* Eyelid erythema (heliotrope) with a distinctive violaceous hue, and profound edema. *B,* Erythema of the chest skin associated with underlying atrophy of the muscles. *C,* Distinctive periungual erythema with erythematous nodules of the knuckles (Gottron's papules). *D,* In contradistinction to dermatomyositis, other systemic autoimmune diseases may present with focal cutaneous and periungual ulcers from an underlying vasculitis, as in this patient with systemic rheumatoid arthritis.

in many organs and tissues and by immunologic abnormalities that can also have systemic manifestations. Sarcoidosis can affect virtually all ocular structures.[39, 40] Inspection of the eyelid skin may demonstrate the characteristic "millet seed" cutaneous nodules (Fig. 164–7).[41] The lacrimal sac and nasolacrimal duct may become infiltrated by sarcoid granulomas, producing epiphora

and dacryocystocutaneous fistulas.[42] Symblepharon may develop as a consequence of severe conjunctival inflammation.[43] Eyelid swelling may be an early manifestation of ocular sarcoidosis,[44] and nodular lesions of the eyelids representing noncaseating granulomas may be the only ocular evidence of the disease.[45, 46] Immunohistochemical staining for the angiotensin-converting enzyme may be

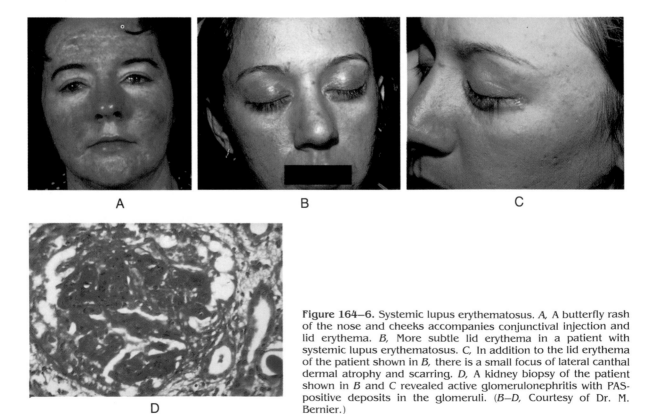

Figure 164–6. Systemic lupus erythematosus. *A,* A butterfly rash of the nose and cheeks accompanies conjunctival injection and lid erythema. *B,* More subtle lid erythema in a patient with systemic lupus erythematosus. *C,* In addition to the lid erythema of the patient shown in *B,* there is a small focus of lateral canthal dermal atrophy and scarring. *D,* A kidney biopsy of the patient shown in *B* and *C* revealed active glomerulonephritis with PAS-positive deposits in the glomeruli. (*B–D,* Courtesy of Dr. M. Bernier.)

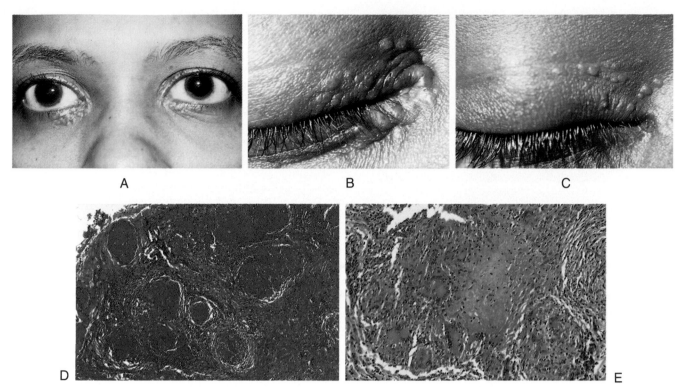

Figure 164–7. Sarcoidosis. *A,* Multiple small, confluent dermal papules of all four eyelids. *B,* The papules are located in the superficial lid dermis beneath the epidermis and can cause release of pigment from the epidermis (incontinentia pigmenti). (*A* and *B,* Courtesy of Dr. D. Morris.) *C,* Small nonconfluent papules of the dermis can invite the mistaken diagnosis of milia. *D,* The granulomas in sarcoidosis elicit a prominent fibroblastic response. In this modified trichrome stain, the granulomas stain intensely red, owing to the presence in the cytoplasm of filaments (vimentin) and numerous cytoplasmic organelles. *E,* Multinucleated giant cells are not infrequently associated with the sarcoid nodules. In general, there is a light lymphocytic and plasmacytic infiltrate associated with the nodules ("naked granulomas").

helpful in differentiating sarcoid granulomas of the lid and conjunctiva from granulomatous tissue caused by a chalazion.[47] Cosmetically disfiguring sarcoid dermatitis may be treated with intradermal triamcinolone if systemic prednisone therapy is not warranted.[48]

EYELID DISORDERS ASSOCIATED WITH SYSTEMIC MALIGNANCY

Muir-Torre Syndrome

Muir and coworkers' originally observed the association of cutaneous keratoacanthomas with visceral carcinoma, particularly of the colon.[49] Torre noted the association of multiple cutaneous sebaceous tumors and internal malignancy.[50] Muir-Torre syndrome has subsequently been recognized as the occurrence of sebaceous hyperplasia, adenoma and carcinoma, basal cell carcinoma with sebaceous differentiation, or keratoacanthoma in association with visceral cancer.[51]

Patients affected with this syndrome have involvement of the skin of the lids with sebaceous tumors (50 percent) or keratoacanthomas (50 percent) (Fig. 164–8).[52] Jakobiec has also reported a sebaceous adenoma of the meibomian glands in a patient with a history of colonic

carcinoma.[53] Benign sebaceous tumors of the ocular adnexa are extremely rare under usual circumstances, and when seen they ought to raise the possibility of associated internal carcinoma. In 50 percent of patients with the syndrome, there will be only one cutaneous sebaceous tumor.[53]

Patients with Muir-Torre syndrome have a high incidence of carcinoma of the colon. In addition, carcinomas of the endometrium, ovary, bladder, stomach, prostate, breast, and uterine cervix have also been described. Fifty percent of the associated cancers are located in the colon. Men are affected more frequently than women by a ratio of 2:1.[54, 55] In a large study by Finan and Connolly, 25 of 59 patients with sebaceous adenoma, sebaceous epithelioma, or sebaceous carcinoma developed visceral cancer, most commonly colonic cancer, and 72 percent of these patients had a history of visceral cancer in family members. It has been observed that these patients have a prolonged survival time compared with patients with similar tumors (but without the other manifestations of the syndrome), suggesting a low degree of malignancy in Muir-Torre syndrome. Interestingly, these patients have a tendency toward benign adenomatous and fibrous proliferations such as thyroid adenomas, adenofibromatous hyperplasia of the prostate, fibrocystic disease of the breast, uterine fibroids, Peyronie's disease, Dupuytren's contracture, carpal tunnel syndrome, and fibromyxoid jaw tumor.[56]

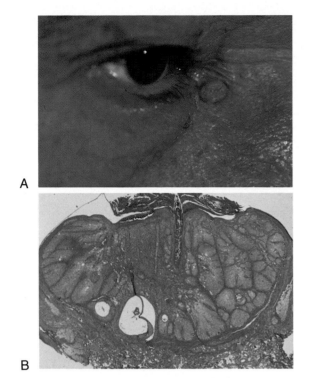

Figure 164–8. *A*, Keratoacanthoma of the lower lid in a patient with Muir-Torre syndrome. *B*, Photomicrograph of a keratoacanthoma from a patient with Muir-Torre syndrome.

As noted earlier, many patients affected with Muir-Torre syndrome have family members who are similarly affected, suggesting an inheritable genetic predisposition to tumor formation in these individuals. Most reports describing families with this syndrome suggest an autosomal dominant mode of transmission with high penetrance.[57] The observation that patients affected with Muir-Torre syndrome have multiple tumors of several tissue types suggests that such patients carry a germline, or constitutional mutation in a specific gene, that leads to the occurrence of tumors in those tissues. The localization and characterization of this putative gene would be an important step toward understanding the pathogenesis of human neoplasia.

Cowden's Disease

Cowden's disease is inherited as an autosomal dominant trait and is characterized by the development of multiple benign and malignant tumors. The disease has also been called the "multiple hamartoma syndrome" because of the presence of multiple hamartomatous anomalies of various organs. The disorder represents a complex mixture of ectodermal, mesodermal, and endodermal hamartomatous lesions of which mucocutaneous, breast, thyroid, and gastrointestinal tumors are most often encountered.[58]

Multiple trichilemmomas, benign tumors of the hair follicle, found in the skin around the eyelids are believed to be diagnostic of Cowden's disease (Fig. 164–9).[59, 60] In a review of 14 cases of Cowden's disease, all the patients examined had multiple trichilemmomas in the skin surrounding the eyelids. No patient with a solitary trichilemmoma has been reported to have Cowden's disease. Only one patient with more than one trichilemmoma has been reported *not* to have Cowden's disease, and this patient had only two lesions. No differences have been observed between the histologic pattern of the multiple trichilemmomas of Cowden's disease and that of solitary trichilemmomas. Recognition of multiple trichilemmomas as a component of Cowden's disease may facilitate the early diagnosis of cancer in patients with this syndrome.[61] Other ocular abnormalities have rarely been reported in association with Cowden's disease, and these include angioid streaks (in two patients) and a retinal glioma (in one patient).[62–64]

Patients affected with Cowden's disease have many systemic findings including goiter, hypothyroidism, thyroid adenoma, ovarian cysts, uterine leiomyomas, gastrointestinal polyps, and breast disease. Thyroid abnormalities were noted in 67 percent of patients with Cowden's disease, and men and women were equally affected. Of female patients with the disorder, 76 percent had breast lesions. Gastrointestinal tract lesions were noted in 41 percent of patients, whereas genitourinary system abnormalities were noted in 55 percent of patients. Skin changes, which are characterized by progressive verrucous, papular, and lichenoid lesions involving mucosal and cutaneous surfaces, have been frequently described in this disorder.[65]

In families affected with Cowden's disease, the inher-

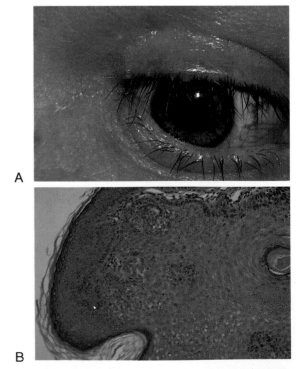

Figure 164–9. *A*, Multiple trichilemmomas of the upper lid in a patient with Cowden's disease. *B*, Photomicrograph of a trichilemmoma excised from a patient with Cowden's disease. (*A*, From Bardenstein D, McLean I, Nerney J, Boatwright R: Cowden's disease. Published courtesy of Ophthalmology 95:1038, 1988.)

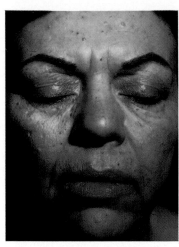

Figure 164–10. Multiple basal cell carcinomas in a patient with the basal nevoid syndrome. (Courtesy of Dr. L. Shapiro.)

itance of the tumor-predisposing trait suggests autosomal dominant transmission.[66] It is likely that a specific genetic defect results in this disease, but the location of such a gene has yet to be determined.

Basal Cell Nevus Syndrome and Medulloblastoma

This disease is characterized by the early onset of multiple basal cell carcinomas that may be present in childhood. Individuals with this syndrome have an increased chance of developing ovarian tumors, including fibromas, ovarian fibrosarcomas, fibrosarcoma of the jaws, and medulloblastoma. The significant ocular findings in this syndrome are multiple basal cell carcinomas located around the eyes in the skin of the lids and forehead (Fig. 164–10). In patients affected with this syndrome, basal cell carcinomas are more likely to develop in regions of the skin that have been irradiated. Systemically, patients with this syndrome have a higher incidence of medulloblastoma, ovarian tumors, jaw cysts, ectopic calcification, cutaneous pits of the hands and feet, and developmental skeletal defects. Men are affected more frequently than women. These patients generally develop medulloblastoma at a younger age than do patients with medulloblastoma without the associated syndrome. Like Muir-Torre syndrome, long survival is a common feature of these patients. This syndrome is inherited as an autosomal dominant trait with reported penetrance to be as high as 97 percent.[67, 68] A specific genetic defect has yet to be located.

REFERENCES

1. Segal P, Insull W Jr, Chambless LE, et al: The association of dyslipoproteinemia with corneal arcus and xanthelasma. Circulation 73:1108–1118, 1986.
2. Depot MJ, Jakobiec FA, Dodick JM, Iwamoto T: Bilateral and extensive xanthelasma palpebrum in a young man. Ophthalmology 91:522–527, 1984.
3. Fredrickson DS, Levy RI, Lees RS: Fat transport in lipoproteins: An integrated approach to mechanisms and disorders. N Engl J Med 276:34–44, 1967.
4. Couste-Blaxy P, Marcel YL, Cohen L, et al: Increased frequency of Apo E-ND phenotype and hyperbeta-lipoproteinemia in normolipidemic subjects with xanthelasmas of the eyelids. Ann Intern Med 96:164–169, 1982.
5. Bates MC, Warren SG: Xanthelasma: Clinical indicator of decreased levels of high-density lipoprotein cholesterol. South Med J 82:570–574, 1989.
6. Mendelson BC, Masson JK: Xanthelasma: Follow-up on results after surgical excision. Plast Reconstr Surg 58:535–538, 1976.
7. Codere F, Lee RD, Anderson RL: Necrobiotic xanthogranuloma of the eyelid. Arch Ophthalmol 101:60–63, 1983.
8. Bullock JD, Bartley GB, Campbell RJ, et al: Necrobiotic xanthogranuloma with paraproteinemia: Case report and a pathogenetic theory. Trans Am Ophthalmol Soc 84:342–354, 1986.
9. Parker F, Odland GF: Experimental xanthoma: A correlative biochemical, histologic, histochemical and electron microscopic study. Am J Pathol 53:537–566, 1968.
10. Simpson FG, Robinson PJ, Hardy GJ, Losowsky MS: Erdheim-Chester disease associated with retroperitoneal xanthogranuloma. Br J Radiol 52:232–235, 1979.
11. Jaffe HL: Lipid (cholesterol) granulomatosis. In Jaffe HL: Metabolic, Degenerative and Inflammatory Diseases of Bones and Joints. Philadelphia, Lea & Febiger, 1972, pp 535–541.
12. Francois J, Bacskulin J, Follmann P: Manifestations oculaires du syndrome d'Urbach-Wiethe hyalinosis cutis et mucosae. Ophthalmologica 155:433–448, 1968.
13. Hofer PA, Larsson PA, Goller H, et al: A clinical and histopathological study of twenty-seven cases of Urbach-Wiethe disease: Dermatologic, gastroenterologic, neurophysiologic, ophthalmologic and roentgendiagnostic aspects, as well as the results of some clinico-chemical and histochemical examinations. Acta Pathol Microbiol Scand 245:1–87, 1974.
14. Charlin C, Fernandez FL: Le syndrome d'Urbach-Wiethe. Arch Ophthalmol (Paris) 35:521–526, 1975.
15. Feiler-Ofry V, Lewy A, Regenbogen L, et al: Lipoid proteinosis (Urbach-Wiethe syndrome). Br J Opthalmol 63:694–698, 1979.
16. Jensen AD, Khodadoust AA, Emery JM: Lipoid proteinosis: Report of a case with electron microscopic findings. Arch Ophthalmol 88:273–277, 1972.
17. Raflo GT, Farrell TA, Sioussat RS: Complete ophthalmoplegia secondary to amyloidosis associated with multiple myeloma. Am J Ophthalmol 92:221–224, 1981.
18. Milutinovich J, Wu W, Savory J: Periorbital purpura after renal biopsy in primary amyloidosis. JAMA 242:2555, 1979.
19. Fett DR, Putteerman AM: Primary localized amyloidosis presenting as an eyelid margin tumor. Arch Ophthalmol 104:584–585, 1986.
20. Brownstein MH, Elliott R, Helwig EB: Ophthalmologic aspects of amyloidosis. Am J Ophthalmol 69:423–430, 1970.
21. Brownstein MH, Helwig EB: The cutaneous amyloidoses. I: Localized forms; II: Systemic forms. Arch Dermatol 102:8–19, 1970.
22. Liesegang TJ: Amyloid infiltration of the levator palpebrae superioris muscle: Case report. Ann Ophthalmol 15:610–613, 1983.
23. Pecora JL, Sambursky JS, Vargha Z: Radiation therapy in amyloidosis of the eyelid and conjunctiva: A case report. Ann Ophthalmol 14:194–196, 1982.
24. Watson PG, Hayreh SS: Scleritis and episcleritis. Br J Ophthalmol 60:163, 1976.
25. Bullen CA, Liesegang TJ, McDonald TJ, De Remee RA: Ocular complications of Wegener's granulomatosis. Ophthalmology 90:279–290, 1983.
26. Rao NA, Font RL: Pseudorheumatoid nodules of the ocular adnexa. Am J Ophthalmol 79:471–478, 1975.
27. Ross MJ, Cohen KL, Peiffer RL, Grimson BS: Episcleral and orbital pseudorheumatoid nodules. Arch Ophthalmol 101:418–421, 1983.
28. Font RL, Zimmerman LE: Nodular fasciitis of the eye and adnexa. Arch Ophthalmol 75:475–481, 1966.
29. Enzinger FM, Weiss SW: Benign tumors and tumor-like lesions of blood vessels. In Enzinger FM, Weiss SW (eds): Soft Tissue Tumors. St. Louis, CV Mosby, 1983.
30. Stuart JM, Postlethwaite AE, Kang AH: Evidence of cell-mediated immunity to collagen in progressive systemic sclerosis. J Lab Clin Med 88:601, 1976.

31. Horan EC: Ophthalmic manifestations of progressive systemic sclerosis. Br J Ophthalmol 53:388, 1969.

32. West RH, Barnett AJ: Ocular involvement in scleroderma. Br J Ophthalmol 63:845–847, 1979.

33. Bohan A, Peter JB: Polymyositis and dermatomyositis. N Engl J Med 292:344, 403, 1975.

34. Susac JO, Garcia-Mullin R, Glaser JS: Ophthalmoplegia in dermatomyositis. Neurology 23:305, 1973.

35. Grossman J, Callerame ML, Condemi JJ: Skin immunofluorescence studies on lupus erythematosus and other antinuclear-antibody-positive diseases. Ann Intern Med 80:496, 1974.

36. Nowinski T, Bernardino V, Naidoff M, Parrish R: Ocular involvement in lupus erythematosus profundus (panniculitis). Ophthalmology 89:1149–1154, 1982.

37. Jankovic J, Patten BM: Blepharospasm and autoimmune diseases. Mov Disord 2:159–163, 1987.

38. Rajagopalan N, Humphrey PR, Bucknall RC: Torticollis and blepharospasm in systemic lupus erythematosus. Mov Disord 4:345–348, 1989.

39. Obernauf CD, Shaw HE, Sydnor CF, Kinktworth GK: Sarcoidosis and its ophthalmic manifestations. Am J Ophthalmol 86:648–655, 1978.

40. Hertzberg R: Sarcoidosis. Aust J Ophthalmol 11:58–59, 1983.

41. Ryan SJ, Maumenee AE: Ocular sarcoidosis. In Ryan SJ, Smith RE (eds): Selected Topics on the Eye in Systemic Disease. New York, Grune and Stratton, 1974, pp 235–249.

42. Neault RW, Riley FC: Report of a case of dacryocystitis secondary to Boeck's sarcoid. Am J Ophthalmol 70:1011, 1975.

43. Flach A: Symblepharon in sarcoidosis. Am J Ophthalmol 85:210–214, 1978.

44. Diestelmeier MR, Sausker WF, Pierson DL, Rodman DG: Sarcoidosis manifesting as eyelid swelling. Arch Dermatol 118:356–357, 1982.

45. Brownstein S, Liszauer AD, Carey WD, Nicolle DA: Sarcoidosis of the eyelid skin. Can J Ophthalmol 25:256–259, 1990.

46. Imes RK, Reifschneider JS, O'Connor LE: Systemic sarcoidosis presenting initially with bilateral orbital and upper lid masses. Ann Ophthalmol 20:466–467, 469, 1988.

47. Immonen I, Friberg K, Gronhagen-Riska C, et al: Angiotensin-converting enzyme in sarcoid and chalazion granulomas of the conjunctiva. Acta Ophthalmol (Copenh) 64:519–521, 1986.

48. Bersaani TA, Nichols CW: Intralesional triamcinolone for cutaneous palpebral sarcoidosis. Am J Ophthalmol 99:561–562, 1985.

49. Muir EG, Bell AJY, Barlow KA: Multiple primary carcinomata of the colon, duodenum, and larynx associated with keratoacanthomata of the face. Br J Surg 54:191, 1967.

50. Torre D: Multiple sebaceous tumors. Arch Dermatol 98:549, 1968.

51. Graham R, et al: Torre-Muir syndrome—An association with isolated sebaceous carcinoma. Cancer 55:2868, 1985.

52. Fahmy A, Burgdorf WHC, Schosser RH, Pitha J: Muir-Torre syndrome: Report of a case and reevaluation of the dermatopathologic features. Cancer 49:1898, 1982.

53. Jakobiec FA, et al: Unusual eyelid tumors with sebaceous differentiation in the Muir-Torre syndrome. Ophthalmology 95:1543, 1988.

54. Anderson DE: An inherited form of large bowel cancer in Muir's syndrome. Cancer 45:1103, 1980.

55. Grignon DJ, Shum DT, Bruchschwaiger O: Transitional cell carcinoma in the Muir-Torre syndrome. J Urol 138:406, 1987.

56. Finan MC, Connolly SM: Sebaceous gland tumors and systemic disease: A clinicopathologic analysis. Medicine 63:232, 1984.

57. Lynch T, et al: Muir-Torre syndrome in several members of a family with a variant of the cancer family syndrome. Br J Dermatol 113:295, 1985.

58. Weary PE, Gorlin RJ, Gentry WC, et al: Multiple hamartoma syndrome (Cowden's disease). Arch Dermatol 106:682, 1972.

59. Bardenstein DS, McLean IW, Nerney J, Boatwright RS: Cowden's disease. Ophthalmology 95:1038, 1988.

60. Reifler DM, Ballitch HA, Kessler DL, et al: Trichilemmoma of the eyelid. Ophthalmology 94:1272, 1987.

61. Brownstein MH, Wolf M, Bikowski JB: Cowden's disease—A cutaneous marker of breast cancer. Cancer 41:2393, 1978.

62. Aram H, Zidenbaum M: Multiple hamartoma syndrome (Cowden's disease). J Am Acad Dermatol 9:774, 1983.

63. Allen BS, Fitch MH, Smith JG Jr: Multiple hamartoma syndrome: A report of a new case with associated carcinoma of the uterine cervix and angioid streaks of the eyes. J Am Acad Dermatol 2:303, 1980.

64. Nuss DD, Aeling JL, Clemons DE, Weber WN: Multiple hamartoma syndrome (Cowden's disease). Arch Dermatol 114:743, 1978.

65. Thyresson HN, Doyle HA: Cowden's disease (multiple hamartoma syndrome). Mayo Clin Proc 56:179, 1981.

66. Gentry WC, Eskritt NR, Gorlin RJ: Multiple hamartoma syndrome (Cowden's disease). Arch Dermatol 109:521, 1974.

67. Howell JB: Nevoid basal cell carcinoma syndrome: Profile of genetic and environmental factors in oncogenesis. J Am Acad Dermatol 11:98, 1984.

68. Naguib MG, Sung JH, Erickson DL, et al: Central nervous system involvement in the nevoid basal cell syndrome: Case report and review of the literature. Neurosurgery 11:52, 1982.

SECTION IX

Orbit

Edited by
DANIEL J. TOWNSEND and FREDERICK A. JAKOBIEC

Chapter 165

Basic Anatomy of the Orbit

MARLON MAUS

Traditionally, orbital anatomy is taught in terms of the various systems that compose the human body. First, the bony skeleton is described and then layers are added almost independent of one another. Thus, we find diagrams of "the arteries" floating in a vacuum or "the nerves" with no other features except the fact that one can recognize them because they are yellow. Although this approach is acceptable for the memorization needed to pass examinations, it does little to help the clinician analyze a patient's complaint. As radiologists have discovered, the orbit lends itself remarkably well to division into "compartments." The most obvious being the "intraconal" and "extraconal" spaces, referring to the area within and without the extraocular muscle "cone."

This chapter divides the orbit into compartments that have some clinical or pathologic significance. This is not, however, a true anatomic division. The supratemporal area of the orbit, e.g., is often the site of tumors that present with signs that are directly related to the presence of certain structures. Dermoid cysts (found at bony sutures), lacrimal gland tumors, and lymphoproliferative processes are just some examples of what may be termed the *supratemporal orbital mass syndrome*. Another example is the intraconal tumor, which produces noticeable axial proptosis even when relatively small. There is also a definite tendency for inflammatory pseudotumors, tumors, and cysts of the orbit to occur predominantly in the upper compartment.

Proposed compartments of the orbit include (1) the globe, (2) the superior extraconal orbit, (3) the inferior extraconal orbit, and (4) the intraconal orbit (Fig. 165–1).

GLOBE

The globe is the raison d'etre for the orbit. All structures of the orbit must be thought of in the context in which they contribute to the activities of the globe and its main function—vision.

In the adult, the globe measures about 24 mm in the anteroposterior diameter and 23 mm in the vertical diameter. The horizontal diameter is slightly longer—about 23.5 mm. The volume of the globe is 7 cu cm and that of the orbit is about 30 cu cm.

The position of the globe in the orbit is determined by the need to allow the visual axis to attain its physiologic angle. Although the angle between the lateral walls of both orbits is 90 degrees, that of the medial and lateral wall of a single orbit is 45 degrees. This means

that the visual axis and the orbital axis are 23 degrees apart. In addition, the visual axis is not the same as the optic axis because of the temporal location of the fovea centralis (Fig. 165–2).

There is a fascial sheath, or Tenon's capsule, that surrounds the globe and separates it from the orbital fat. It is connected to the sclera by thin bands and creates the potential episcleral space. The firmest attachments in the anterior portion are 1.5 mm posterior to the limbus, and posteriorly, they are located at the point that it fuses to the optic nerve sheath. The extraocular muscles, nerves, and blood vessels must first pierce the fascial sheath before ultimately reaching the globe. All the muscles are encased in a sleeve of fascia. In addition, the ones around the lateral and medial rectus muscles send projections to the zygomatic and the lacrimal bones called the *check ligaments*. The inferior fascia is considerably thickened and is called the suspensory ligament of Lockwood. It joins the check ligaments to serve as a cradle for the globe (Fig. 165–3).

Superiorly, the sheath is condensed around the superior rectus muscle and the levator palpebrae superioris, forming the upper lid retractor complex. Inferiorly, the lower lid retractor is formed by the projection of fascia from the inferior rectus muscle to the lower border of tarsus.

The globe lies only partially within the orbit. The reason for this is that the vertical distance between the orbital rims is 35 mm and lies at the level of the cornea. However, the width is 40 mm, yet the lateral orbital rim

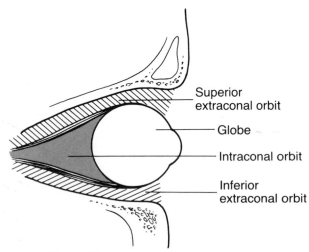

Figure 165–1. Compartments of the orbit.

- Superior extraconal orbit
- Globe
- Intraconal orbit
- Inferior extraconal orbit

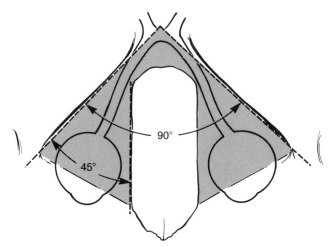

Figure 165–2. Angular relationships of the orbit.

covers only two thirds of the globe, making this the area most exposed to trauma.

SUPERIOR EXTRACONAL ORBIT

There are seven bones that form the orbital walls: the frontal, sphenoid, maxillary, palatine, zygomatic, ethmoid, and lacrimal. The sphenoid bone is present in three of the walls and contributes some of the most important structures. It is also involved in neurofibromatosis, in which it may be partially lacking. The volume of the orbit is 25 to 30 cu ml (Fig. 165–4).

The roof of the orbit is a triangle formed by the lesser wing of the sphenoid and the frontal bone (Fig. 165–5). It gently slopes down medially and laterally into the walls of the orbit. The lateral wall is composed of the greater wing of the sphenoid and the zygomatic bone. The theoretical border with the roof is the zygomaticofrontal suture anteriorly and the superior orbital fissure

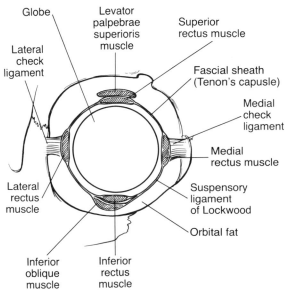

Figure 165–3. Fascial architecture of the orbit.

posteriorly. The medial wall consists of the ethmoid bone, the lacrimal bone, a small part of the lesser wing of the sphenoid, and the tip of the maxilla. Its limit superiorly is the frontoethmoidal suture. As the roof slopes posteriorly, it incorporates the optic canal, which is contained by the lesser wing of the sphenoid. This is the apex of the orbit, which Whitnall called the "stalk" of the pear-shaped orbit. It is here that the four rectus muscles take their origin at the annulus of Zinn, which is further described in the section on the Intraconal Compartment.

There are several important landmarks contained in the bony skeleton of the superior extraconal compartment. The orbital roof is 3 mm thick anteriorly and thins significantly posteriorly at the point that it separates the orbit from the anterior cranial fossa. The anterior and posterior ethmoidal canals are located within the frontoethmoidal suture. The anterior canal is 20 mm behind the anterior orbital margin, and the posterior canal is 12 mm behind this (see Fig. 165–5). They are the passages for the anterior and posterior ethmoidal arteries and the anterior ethmoidal nerve. The arteries are branches of the ophthalmic artery. The posterior ethmoidal artery supplies the posterior ethmoidal air cells, the dura of the anterior cranial fossa, and the upper part of the nasal mucosa. The anterior ethmoidal artery enters the anterior cranial fossa and then, through the cribiform plate, reaches the nose.

The anterior ethmoidal nerve is a sensory branch of the nasociliary nerve, supplying the anterior ethmoidal air cells, the mucous membrane of the upper part of the nose, and finally the dorsum and tip of the nose. It is responsible for involvement of the tip of the nose in herpes zoster ophthalmicus (Hutchinson's sign) (Fig. 165–6).

The trochlear fossa (fovea) is the depression in which the trochlea of the superior oblique tendon is found. It is a cartilaginous structure located supramedially about 4 to 5 mm from the rim. The fossa of the lacrimal gland is located in the frontal bone, supratemporally (see Fig. 165–5). The zygomaticofrontal suture shows the most inferior and lateral limits.

The medial wall is the thinnest one in the orbit. The lamina papyracea provides very little protection from extension of infection from the ethmoidal sinus air cells. Extensions of the sphenoid and maxillary sinuses often can also be found behind the medial walls (Fig. 165–7; see also Fig. 165–5).

The lateral wall is, in contrast, the strongest one. The zygomatic bone is very thick at the orbital rim; however, it becomes thinner by the time it articulates with the greater wing of the sphenoid. Externally, this thin plate is part of the temporalis fossa. The greater wing of the sphenoid is strongest in its most lateral part but becomes thinner posteriorly when it separates the orbit from the middle cranial fossa.

The lateral orbital tubercle or Whitnall's tubercle, is found in the most anterior part of the wall, 11 mm below the frontozygomatic suture (see Fig. 165–3). It serves as the site of attachment for the check ligament of the lateral rectus muscle, the suspensory ligament of the globe (Lockwood's ligament), the lateral palpebral

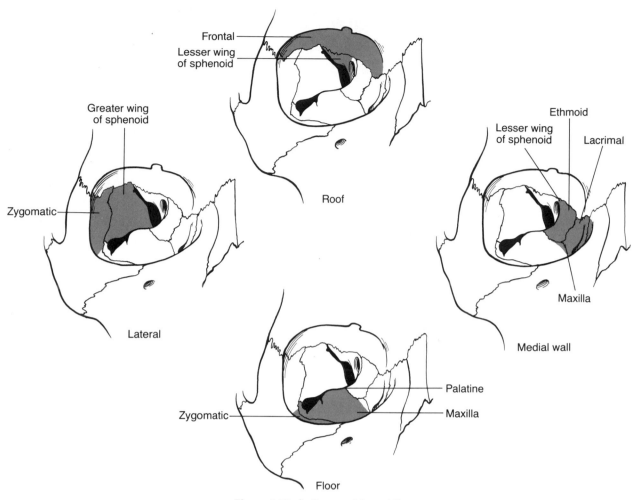

Figure 165—4. Bones of the orbit.

ligament, and the levator muscle aponeurosis. A short distance behind the tubercle the zygomatic canal is found. This structure transmits the zygomatic nerve and branches of the infraorbital artery. The zygomatic nerve is a branch of the maxillary nerve, arising in the ptery-

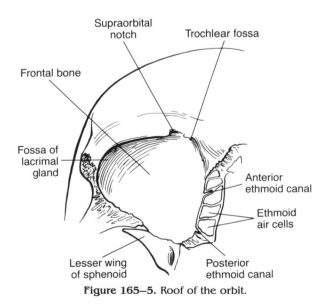

Figure 165—5. Roof of the orbit.

gopalatine fossa. It divides into the zygomaticotemporal and the zygomaticofacial nerves within the orbit before supplying the skin on the forehead and cheek. It also sends a branch to the lacrimal nerve containing postganglionic parasympathetic fibers from the pterygopalatine ganglion (Figs. 165–8 and 165–9).

The last foramen of the bones of the superior compartment is the anteriorly located supraorbital foramen or notch. It transmits the supraorbital nerve which is the terminal branch of the frontal nerve, a part of the ophthalmic division of cranial nerve V. It supplies the skin and conjunctiva of the upper lid and the skin of the forehead and scalp. It also sends a twig to the frontal sinus through the frontal bone (Fig. 165–10).

The four foramina found in this compartment are thus the anterior ethmoidal foramen, the posterior ethmoidal foramen, the zygomatic foramen, and the supraorbital foramen.

The extraconal part of the superior orbital fissure is included in this compartment because it is formed by the greater and lesser wings of the sphenoid bone and transmits nerves supplying superior structures, including the lacrimal nerve, the frontal nerve, and the trochlear nerve (Fig. 165–11).

The lacrimal nerve is the smallest of the three branches of the ophthalmic division of the trigeminal

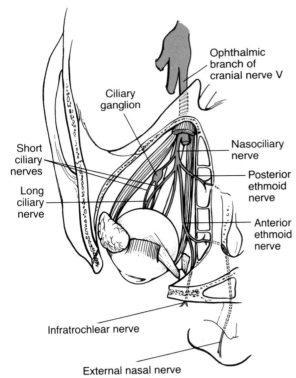

Figure 165–6. The ophthalmic division of cranial nerve V, which is the origin of the nasociliary nerve.

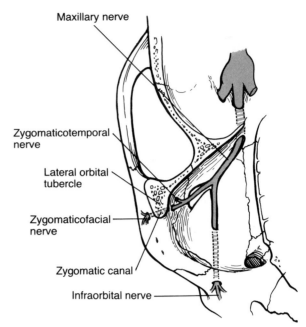

Figure 165–8. Maxillary division of cranial nerve V.

nerve (cranial nerve V). It courses along the superior border of the lateral rectus muscle accompanied by the lacrimal artery. It receives the branch, previously described, from the zygomaticofacial nerve. These parasympathetic fibers are the secretory fibers for the lacrimal gland (see Fig. 165–9).

The frontal nerve is the largest branch of the ophthalmic division of cranial nerve V. It lies on the superior surface of the levator palpebrae superioris. It gives off a small supratrochlear branch halfway into the orbit. This branch travels over the trochlea and supplies

the skin of the upper lid and the forehead, as well as the conjunctiva (Fig. 165–12).

The trochlear nerve (cranial nerve IV) is the only cranial nerve that lies outside the annulus supplying an extraocular muscle. It enters the muscle as a series of branches quite posteriorly in the orbit (see Fig. 165–12).

Most of the structures in the orbit have a vascular supply from the ophthalmic artery. After it originates from the internal carotid artery, it enters the orbit through the optic canal below and lateral to the optic

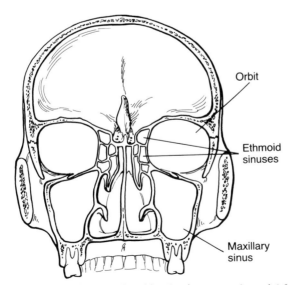

Figure 165–7. Orbital relationships to sinuses and cranial fossa.

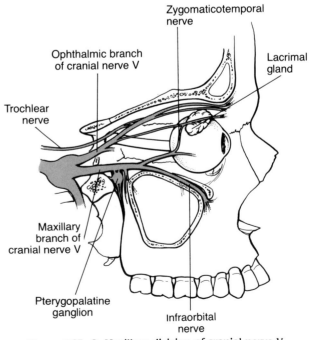

Figure 165–9. Maxillary division of cranial nerve V.

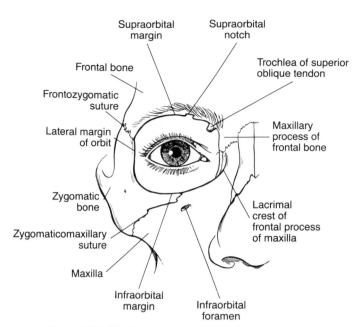

Figure 165–10. External landmarks of the bony orbit.

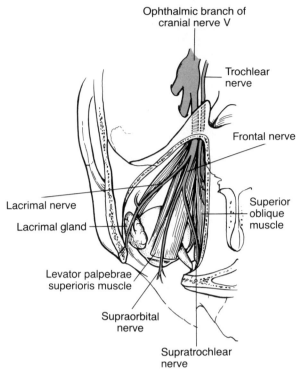

Figure 165–12. Superior branches of the ophthalmic division of cranial nerve V and the trochlear nerve (cranial nerve IV).

nerve. Within the orbit, it first lies between the lateral rectus muscle and the optic nerve; it then crosses over the nerve and lies below the superior rectus muscle. As it reaches the medial wall of the orbit, it is accompanied by the nasociliary nerve. In its most anterior part, it divides into its terminal branches—the supratrochlear and dorsal nasal arteries. There is great variation in the branches of the ophthalmic artery (and their locations), but the most usual are as follows (Fig. 165–13): (1) central retinal artery, (2) lacrimal artery, (3) muscular branches, (4) ciliary arteries, (5) supraorbital artery, (6) posterior ethmoidal artery, (7) anterior ethmoidal ar-

tery, (8) meningeal branch, (9) medial palpebral artery, (10) supratrochlear artery, and (11) dorsal nasal artery.

There is a rich anastomotic plexus between the internal carotid and the external carotid arteries on the face and scalp. An occlusion of the internal carotid will thus rarely result in sudden blindness.

The venous drainage of the orbit is also divided into

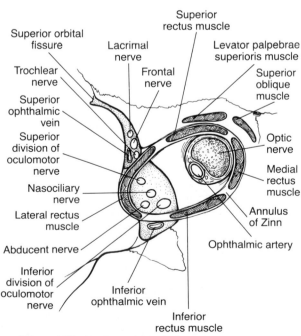

Figure 165–11. Posterior orbit: the annulus of Zinn.

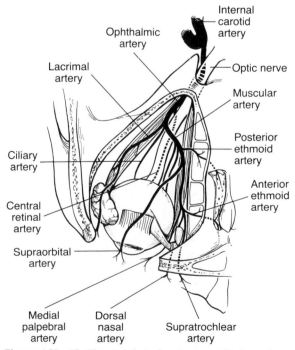

Figure 165–13. The ophthalmic artery and its branches.

two compartments. The superior compartment is drained by the larger superior ophthalmic vein. It arises anteriorly from the supraorbital vein and part of the facial vein. As it moves posteriorly, it receives branches accompanying the ophthalmic artery, and finally it usually receives the inferior ophthalmic vein before exiting through the upper portion of the superior orbital fissure. It empties into the cavernous sinus. Other veins that communicate with the sinus are the inferior cerebral, superficial middle cerebral, and middle meningeal veins.

Within the cavernous sinus, several structures lead to the orbit. The internal carotid syphon gives off the ophthalmic artery just after it emerges from the cavernous sinus. Its lateral wall contains the oculomotor, trochlear, abducens, and ophthalmic and maxillary divisions of the trigeminal nerve (Fig. 165–14).

The superior compartment contains the lacrimal gland. According to Whitnall, it measures 20 mm × 12 mm × 5 mm. It is divided into a large orbital part and a smaller palpebral part by the lateral horn of the aponeurosis of the levator palpebrae. The orbital part is encased superiorly by the bone of the lacrimal fossa and inferiorly by the aponeurosis of the levator and the lateral rectus muscle. Laterally and anteriorly it borders the orbital septum, at which point it is easily reached surgically (Fig. 165–15).

The palpebral part of the lacrimal gland lies under the aponeurosis of the levator and over the conjunctiva of the superior fornix. It is here, 4 to 5 mm from the superior tarsal border, that the 12 ducts from the orbital lobe empty through the palpebral lobe. The ducts from the palpebral lobe empty separately into the fornix. The entire gland has a pseudocapsule derived from the periorbita. Whitnall's ligament and the levator aponeurosis provide additional support for the gland. Whitnall's ligament attaches high on the lateral orbital wall, at which point it must be protected during surgery to prevent the gland from prolapsing. The gland has a pinkish gray appearance and can be distinguished from orbital fat both by color and consistency (see Fig. 165–15).

The lacrimal artery, and sometimes the infraorbital artery, supply the lacrimal gland (see Fig. 165–13). The

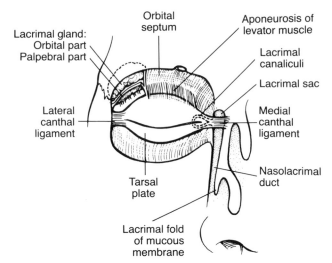

Figure 165–15. Gland and drainage anatomy of the lacrimal system.

venous drainage is into the superior ophthalmic vein. Lymphatic drainage is into the superficial parotid lymph nodes through the conjunctival plexus. There are small collections of lymphoid tissue within the gland. There are normally no other lymphatics within the orbit.

The nerve supply to the lacrimal gland has two components. The autonomic system is responsible for both baseline and reflex lacrimation. The lacrimal gland is thought to provide mostly reflex secretion. The parasympathetic nerve originates from the lacrimatory nucleus of the facial nerve, and it reaches the nerve of the pterygoid canal through the great petrossal branch of the facial nerve. It then synapses at the pterygopalatine ganglion before sending postganglionic fibers into the maxillary nerve, the zygomaticotemporal nerve, and finally the lacrimal nerve. The sympathetic postganglionic fibers arise from the superior cervical ganglion; they join the deep petrosal nerve, after which they parallel the parasympathetic fibers (Fig. 165–16).

Sensory branches from the ophthalmic division of the trigeminal nerve are also found in the lacrimal nerve (see Fig. 165–9).

Histologically, this serous gland consists of lobules separated by loose connective tissue. The acini have central lumina surrounded by columnar cells. The intralobular ducts are cuboidal cells surrounded by myoepithelial cells, and they drain into interlobular ducts that have a two-layered epithelial lining.

Although the concept of compartments is useful to the clinician analyzing a problem, the anatomist finds a connective tissue framework spanning the entire orbit. Koornneef, using extremely meticulous studies and building upon the work of previous anatomists, described this framework in detail. The first part is Tenon's capsule, which surrounds the globe and extraocular muscles in the anterior orbit. This was described in the section on the Globe. It must be noted that posterior to the globe, the intermuscular septa are very thin or lacking, and thus a true muscle cone is not present (Fig. 165–17).

The anterior orbital connective tissue connects Ten-

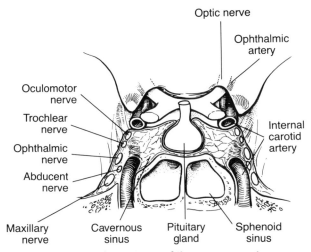

Figure 165–14. Anatomy of the cavernous sinus.

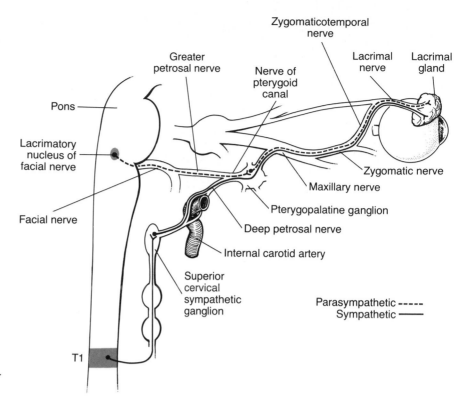

Figure 165–16. Autonomic supply to the lacrimal gland.

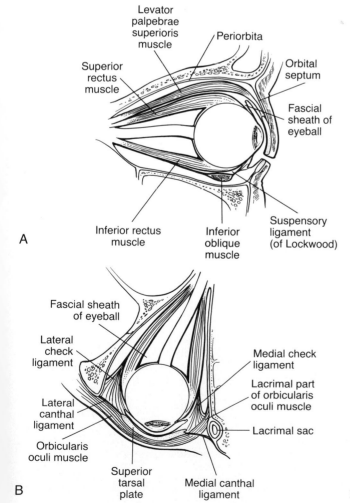

Figure 165–17. *A* and *B,* Fascia and ligaments of the orbit.

on's capsule to the periorbita near the anterior orbital margin. These are connective tissue septa that are present 360 degrees around the globe, condensing into the suspensory ligaments (i.e., of Lockwood) and other stabilizing structures (see Fig. 165–17).

The third part is the extraocular muscle connective tissue system, which anteriorly forms the check ligaments of the medial and lateral rectus muscles and the intermuscular fibrous septum. This system is extremely complex as it progresses from the apex to the anterior orbit. There are attachments between muscles and the orbital walls, between muscles, and between the globe and the muscle sheaths.

The orbital septum is the anatomic boundary of the anterior orbit. It originates at the orbital rim from the thick periorbita called the arcus marginalis. It also attaches to both the anterior and posterior lacrimal crests. Superiorly, it fuses with the levator aponeurosis; inferiorly, it fuses with the capsulopalpebral fascia before attaching to the lower border of tarsus.

The orbital fat is separated by the septa previously described and is held in a posterior position by the orbital septum. The fat pad overlying the levator aponeurosis, or preaponeurotic fat pad, is limited medially by fascia originating from the trochlear region. Laterally, the lacrimal gland can be confused with the temporal aspect of the preaponeurotic fat pad during blepharoplasty or ptosis surgery. There are three lower lid fat pads, the nasal one being the largest. It is crossed by fascial attachments from the inferior oblique muscle.

Various relations are found to the bony orbit. Superiorly, the frontal bone contains the frontal sinuses, and occasionally even some ethmoidal air cells are present. The frontal lobe of the brain lies above the roof of the orbit. Medially, the orbit is next to the nasal cavity, ethmoidal sinuses, and sphenoidal sinus. Laterally, the orbital wall abuts the temporal fossa with the temporal muscle and the middle cranial fossa containing the temporal lobe. Under the orbital floor is the maxillary sinus (see Fig. 165–7).

INFERIOR EXTRACONAL ORBIT

The floor of the orbit is made up of the maxillary, zygomatic, and palatine bones. It does not extend all the way to the apex of the orbit. The most important landmark is the infraorbital canal, which is the continuation of the infraorbital groove. The latter starts 2.5 to 3 cm from the orbital rim. The canal starts 1.5 cm from the rim and opens into the face as the infraorbital foramen. The floor is very thin, particularly medial to the infraorbital canal, and consists mostly of the orbital plate of the maxilla. It overlies the maxillary sinus and is 0.5 to 1 mm thick (Fig. 165–18).

The sides of the floor gently slope onto the medial and lateral orbital walls. Medially, it joins the lacrimal bone, ethmoid bone, and lesser wing of the sphenoid bone. A projection of the maxillary bone, the frontal process, also forms part of the medial wall. It is here that the fossa for the lacrimal sac is found. The lacrimal bone is divided into two portions by the posterior

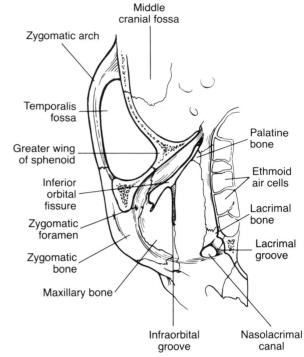

Figure 165–18. Floor of the orbit.

lacrimal crest. The posterior portion articulates with the ethmoid bone, the anterior portion forms the floor of the lacrimal sac fossa, which is extremely thin and easily broken during surgery (Fig. 165–19).

The opening of the nasolacrimal canal from the nasolacrimal fossa is defined by the hamular process of the posterior lacrimal crest and the lacrimal notch of the maxilla. The canal is 18 mm long and is directed 15

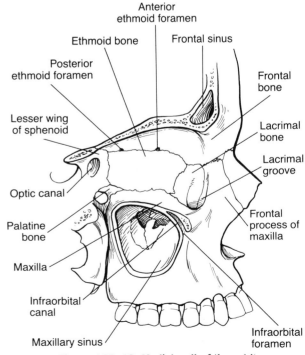

Figure 165–19. Medial wall of the orbit.

degrees backward, downward, and laterally. It empties into the nose at the level of the inferior meatus, at which point it is guarded by a mucous membrane, the plica lacrimalis or valve of Hasner. The anterior lacrimal crest becomes continuous with the inferior orbital margin, whereas the posterior crest is continuous with the medial margin.

The lacrimal sac, which is 13 to 15 mm long, has the opening for the lacrimal canaliculi on its lateral aspect. It is enclosed by a fascial sheath that attaches to the anterior and posterior lacrimal crests (see Fig. 165–10). It is surrounded by a venous plexus. Anterior to the fascia is the medial palpebral ligament (or canthal ligament), and posterior to it is the lacrimal part of the orbicularis oculi, a posterior limb of the pretarsal muscle. The fundus of the sac is 3 to 5 mm above the indistinct upper border of the palpebral tendon. The angular vein, which becomes the facial vein, crosses anterior to the medial palpebral ligament. The lacrimal sac is composed of a double layer of columnar epithelium with goblet cells. As it continues into the nasolacrimal duct, it becomes a double-layered epithelium with cilia (see Fig. 165–15).

The lacrimal portion of the pretarsal orbicular muscle of the eye is responsible for much of the pumping mechanism during blinking. It pulls the lid medially and the sac laterally while also positioning the puncta into the tear lake. The complete pumping mechanism has several components: a portion of preseptal orbicularis muscle is anterior to the sac (Jones muscle), the superficial and deep heads of the lacrimal part of the pretarsal orbicularis muscle (the deep one is Horner's muscle), and the periorbita around the sac called the *lacrimal diaphragm*.

The fossa of the origin of the inferior oblique muscle is located just behind the orbital margin and lateral to the nasolacrimal canal. Laterally, the floor joins the sphenoid and zygomatic bones, which form the lateral orbital wall. On the margin of the zygomatic bone, 10 mm below the zygomaticofrontal suture, is the lateral orbital tubercle (of Whitnall). This is the attachment site for the lateral horn of the levator aponeurosis, the lateral canthal ligament, the check ligament of the lateral rectus muscle, and the orbital suspensory ligament of Lockwood.

Posteriorly, the inferior orbital fissure, which measures 20 mm, transmits nerves and vessels into the pterygopalatine and infratemporal fossae. The fissure originates at the orbital apex and extends anteriorly within 15 to 20 mm from the inferior orbital rim (see Fig. 165–18). The inferior orbital vein arises anteriorly from the anterior orbital cavity and has connections with the facial vein. Posteriorly, it empties either into the superior ophthalmic vein or directly into the cavernous sinus. It also has connections via the inferior orbital fissure with the pterygoid venous plexus.

The maxillary division of the trigeminal nerve leaves the cavernous sinus via the foramen rotundum and into the pterygopalatine fossa. Here it sends two branches to the pterygopalatine ganglion and other branches to the teeth and the zygomatic nerve before continuing to the orbit via the inferior orbital fissure. It becomes the infraorbital nerve, which enters the infraorbital groove and canal to supply the lower lid skin and conjunctiva, nasal ala, cheek, and upper lip. Other branches are the middle superior alveolar and the anterior superior alveolar branches (see Figs. 165–9 and 165–10).

The maxillary nerve also carries postganglionic parasympathetic fibers from the pterygopalatine ganglion to the lacrimal nerve, first via the zygomatic nerve and then via the zygomaticotemporal nerve (see Fig. 165–16). Sympathetic fibers innervating the smooth orbital muscle of Horner at the apex also enter the orbit via the inferior orbital fissure.

INTRACONAL ORBIT

The orbital apex is the most posterior part of this compartment, and it contains the most important structures. The rectus muscles originate from the common tendinous ring or annulus of Zinn. The annulus is actually formed by two tendons, an upper and a lower one (of Lockwood and of Zinn, respectively). They attach to the lesser wing of the sphenoid, below the optic foramen, at which point they are continuous with the dura mater of the middle cranial fossa. This is the origin of the inferior rectus and the inferior part of the medial and lateral rectus muscles (see Fig. 165–11).

As the annulus is followed laterally, it bridges the superior and inferior orbital fissures, attaching laterally onto the greater wing of the sphenoid. There is a small spine at the lower edge of the superior orbital fissure at the point that the lateral rectus muscle attaches. The annulus then bridges the medial end of the superior orbital fissure. It then continues toward the optic canal at which point it is continuous with the optic nerve sheath. The superior rectus and medial rectus muscles attach in this portion of the annulus. The levator palpebrae originates above the superior rectus muscle, and although it is not part of the annulus, the muscles form a functional unit as they proceed anteriorly (see Fig. 165–11).

The various structures that enter the muscle cone at the apex include the optic nerve with its meningeal cover and subarachnoid space, the ophthalmic artery, and a surrounding sympathetic plexus through the optic canal. The upper and lower divisions of the oculomotor nerve, the nasociliary nerve, and the abducent nerve enter through the superior orbital fissure within the cone. As mentioned previously, the superior orbital fissure outside the cone transmits the trochlear nerve, the frontal nerve, and the lacrimal nerve (see Fig. 165–11).

The optic canal connects the middle cranial fossa to the orbit. The direction of the canal is parallel to the lateral orbital wall. The canal is formed by the two roots of the lesser wing of the sphenoid. The roof of the canal is below the frontal lobe and the olfactory tract. Medially, the sphenoid and ethmoid sinuses abut the canal. The infralateral aspect of the canal is made by the optic strut, which is the bone joining the lesser wing to the body of the sphenoid. The length of the canal is from 5 to 11 mm. The medial wall is thinnest, making it most approachable surgically this way. The optic nerve is extremely well anchored to the canal by the optic nerve sheath that attaches to the nerve and bone.

The optic nerve is 4.5 to 5 cm long and about 4 mm in diameter. It has four portions: the intraocular segment, which measures 1 mm; the intraorbital part, which is 30 mm; the intracanalicular portion, which is 5 to 6 mm; and the intracranial segment, which is 10 mm. The redundancy of the nerve results in an S-shaped course within the orbit. The central retinal artery enters the nerve inferomedially 10 mm behind the globe. The blood supply to the nerve is variable, but anteriorly it is from the posterior ciliary arteries, of which there are 15 to 20, and the central retinal artery. More posteriorly, the central retinal artery and collateral branches supplying the pia mater also supply the nerve (see Fig. 165–13).

The rectus muscles are approximately 40 mm in length. They have varying lengths of tendon, which attach firmly onto the sclera. The insertions form the spiral of Tillaux, with the medial rectus having the shortest distance to the limbus and the superior rectus the longest. The nerve serving each muscle enters the internal surface of the muscle at its posterior third. The inferior rectus and oblique muscles are served by the inferior division of the oculomotor nerve. The lateral rectus muscle is innervated by the abducens, and the superior rectus and the medial rectus muscles are innervated by the superior division of the oculomotor nerve. The superior oblique muscle is innervated by the trochlear nerve, which lies outside the cone.

The muscular branches of the ophthalmic artery, of which there are two, provide the vascular supply to the muscles in the form of their terminal branches—the anterior ciliary arteries. There are two of these arteries/muscle, except for the lateral rectus muscle, which has only one.

The inferior oblique muscle courses posteriorly and laterally from its origin in the fossa, which was previously described in the discussion of the anteromedial orbital floor. It shares a fascial cover with the inferior rectus as it courses posteriorly on its way to its posterior attachment. This fascia forms an important element of Lockwood's ligament.

The nasociliary nerve, the third branch of the ophthalmic nerve from cranial nerve V, enters the orbit through the annulus of Zinn. It crosses over the optic nerve at which point it sends branches to the medial orbital wall. It then sends a sensory branch to the ciliary ganglion, whose fibers then enter the globe via the short posterior ciliary nerves. More anteriorly, the nasociliary nerve has two or three branches, the long ciliary nerves, which supply anterior globe structures. They also carry sympathetic nervous fibers to those structures. The nerve then exits the cone to supply anteromedial orbital structures.

The ciliary ganglion, which lies between the lateral aspect of the optic nerve and the lateral rectus muscle in the posterior orbit, is mainly a parasympathetic ganglion (Fig. 165–20). Only the preganglionic parasympathetic fibers arising from the Edinger-Westphal nucleus of the oculomotor nerve synapse in the ciliary ganglion. They reach the ganglion via the oculomotor branch to the inferior oblique muscle. The postganglionic fibers supply the iris sphincter muscle and ciliary body by way of the short posterior ciliary nerves, of which there are 8 to 20. As described previously, the sensory fibers pass

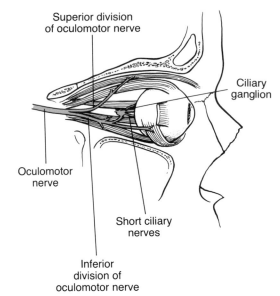

Figure 165–20. The oculomotor nerve (cranial nerve III).

through the ciliary ganglion but do not synapse there. The sympathetic postganglionic fibers, which originate from the superior cervical ganglion and reach the orbit via the internal carotid and ophthalmic arteries, also pass through the ciliary ganglion on their way to the globe.

CONCLUSIONS

This chapter has tried to present a slightly different approach to orbital anatomy. The separation of the orbit into compartments is a useful, but limited, tool for the clinician. It is useful because when analyzing a pathologic process in a specific area of the orbit, it will be possible to find all structures involved in a single section of this chapter. It is limited because, much to our chagrin, no pathologic process respects our arbitrary borders. Finally, the unifying force in all anatomic descriptions must be the diagrams that accompany the text. It is truly the case of a picture being worth a thousand words.

BIBLIOGRAPHY

American Academy of Ophthalmology: Basic and Clinical Science Course, vol. 1. San Francisco, CA, 1992.

Doxanas MT, Anderson RL: Clinical Orbital Anatomy. Baltimore, Williams & Wilkins, 1984.

Duke-Elder S, Wybar KC: The anatomy of the visual system. *In* Duke-Elder S (ed): System of Ophthalmology. St. Louis, CV Mosby, 1961.

Jones IS, Jakobiec FA, Nolan BT: Patient examination and introduction to orbital disease. *In* Duane TD (ed): Clinical Ophthalmology. Hagerstown, Harper & Row, 1976, pp 1–14.

Koornneef L: Orbital septa: Anatomy and function. Ophthalmology 86:876–880, 1979.

Rootman J: Basic anatomic considerations. *In* Rootman J (ed): Diseases of the Orbit. Philadelphia, JB Lippincott, 1988, pp 3–18.

Snell RS, Lemp MA: Clinical Anatomy of the Eye. Cambridge, Blackwell Scientific, 1989.

Zide BM, Jelks GW: Surgical Anatomy of the Orbit. New York, Raven Press, 1985.

Chapter 166

∎

Approach to Orbital Disorders and Frequency of Disease Occurrence

RICHARD L. DALLOW
and STEVEN G. PRATT

The anatomic bony orbital space contains a large variety of tissues that have potential for development of a wide spectrum of diseases. In addition to the globe, with its neural and uveal components, the anterior orbit is composed of the lid and adnexa with epithelial and secretory elements, conjunctiva, lacrimal gland, and lacrimal sac and duct. Posterior orbit components include the cushioning fat and supportive fibrous tissue, the optic nerve and other sensory and motor cranial nerves, the extraocular muscles and lid muscles, and arteries and veins related to the carotid, dural, and facial systems. The paranasal sinuses surround much of the orbit circumference, and cranial structures surround the rest, with the cavernous sinus, carotid artery, and pituitary gland being especially noteworthy. Nearly all of these tissue elements and structures can be the origin of or participants in structural deformities, benign or malignant neoplasms, arteriovenous malformations, or inflammatory and congestive processes. They also may be damaged by trauma.

A concept of orbital disorders in broad categories is helpful in analyzing the significance of clinical symptoms and signs and in directing appropriate laboratory and imaging investigations. The major questions for consideration in orbital disorders are as follows: (1) Have orbital tissues or bones suffered *traumatic* alteration (fracture, displacement, or hemorrhage)? (2) Is an *infection* (cellulitis or abscess) present? (3) Is a *neoplasm* present (benign versus malignant; local versus invasive versus disseminated)? (4) Can an *inflammatory* or *congestive* process (Graves' disease, pseudotumor, arteriovenous shunts) be identified?

ORBITAL SYMPTOMS AND HISTORY

History and physical examination can supply many clues for distinguishing among the important general categories of orbit diseases. Proptosis of a globe is the most dramatic orbital symptom, especially if it occurs abruptly. Often, however, proptosis may be subtle or so slowly developing that a patient is unaware of it. Acquaintances may comment on it, and comparison with old photographs is instructive. A patient's age has a very definite influence on diagnostic considerations.

Children from birth to 20 yr old have a different statistical distribution of orbital disorders compared with older adults, as documented later in this chapter.

Symptoms of special importance for orbital disorders are globe proptosis, pain, and vision changes. One should try to establish the approximate duration of exophthalmos and its progression or stability to distinguish whether the responsible process is acute or chronic. Pain should be assessed for its location, character, and severity. Surface discomfort due to corneal exposure often causes more severe and deeper pain than might be expected. Significant pain accompanies most inflammatory orbital processes. Many tumors cause little orbital discomfort unless they invade the orbital periosteum. Vision changes should be analyzed for alterations in visual acuity, visual fields, and color discrimination, as well as for diplopia.

Previous medical history can be quite instructive, because many orbital disorders relate to systemic diseases. Head or orbit trauma, even remote in time, can cause secondary effects of bony defects, extraocular muscle imbalances, and arteriovenous malformations. Febrile illnesses may herald orbit infections. Pertinent systemic review includes thyroid disorders or symptoms, diabetes mellitus, other tumors, inflammatory or autoimmune disorders, and other adenopathy or skin lesions. Smoking habits are important not only when considering lung tumors but also Graves' disease. Family history of thyroid abnormality is very significant, because up to 30 percent of Graves' disease is familial.

PHYSICAL EXAMINATION OF ORBITS

On physical examination of the orbits, as with other eye problems, vision parameters are essential. Visual acuity, color discrimination, visual fields, and pupillary reactions may be altered by compromise of the optic nerve or by compression of the globe peripherally or posteriorly. Exophthalmos must be documented in a reproducible manner for later comparisons. Hertel's type of exophthalmometer provides accurate quantitation of corneal apex measurements relative to the bony lateral orbital rim (Fig. 166–1). Absolute measurements less than 20 mm are generally normal for whites, but

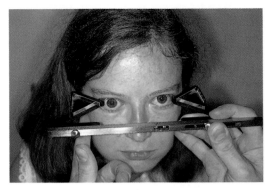

Figure 166–1. Measurement of exophthalmos with Hertel's instrument incorporating 45-degree angled mirrors to visualize the eyes laterally on a millimeter scale against a horizontal base distance scale.

higher levels are common for blacks, Asians, and other races with shallow bony orbits. Higher readings imply orbit disorders. Asymmetry greater than 1.5 mm between the two orbits is considered abnormal also, regardless of the absolute value.

General inspection of an orbit may reveal a visible bulge of tumor or inflammation that is focal or generalized. Palpation around the globe and orbit rim is useful for detecting anteriorly located masses and helps to clarify characteristics of the lesion such as its size and contour, whether it is circumscribed or infiltrative,

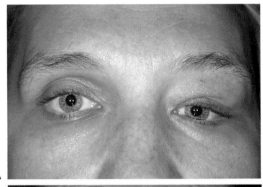

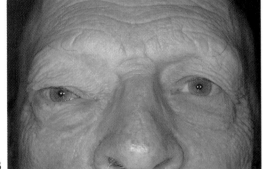

Figure 166–2. Benign anterior orbit tumors. *A*, Bulging mass in upper temporal quadrant of left orbit that is chronic, asymmetric, firm, circumscribed, and movable, indicating a benign tumor of the lacrimal gland (pleomorphic adenoma). *B*, Upper medial quadrant mass of right orbit that is chronic, soft, and compressible but immobile and causing globe displacement, consistent with a frontoethmoidal sinus mucocele.

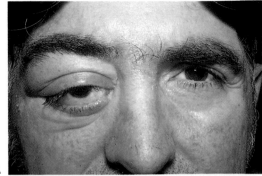

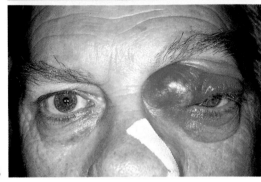

Figure 166–3. Malignant anterior orbit tumors. *A*, Lacrimal gland mass of recent onset and rapid growth with pain and vision and motility compromise, representing an adenoid cystic carcinoma. *B*, Sinus mass extending into the orbit (squamous cell carcinoma), causing secondary mucopyocele.

whether it is fixed to adjacent tissues or freely mobile, and whether it is tender. Posteriorly located masses are less likely to be palpable. Increased orbital resistance on retropulsion of the globe is a nonspecific finding of almost any kind of posterior orbital abnormality. The orbit quadrant in which findings are most prominent provides definite clues about the tissue involved (i.e., upper temporal quadrant—lacrimal gland, dermoid; upper medial quadrant—sinus mucocele; lower medial quadrant—lacrimal sac) (Figs. 166–2 and 166–3). The position of a displaced globe also suggests the location of an orbit abnormality and implicates certain tissues. Globe position may be dramatically influenced by either restriction or paralysis of extraocular muscles. Head deformities such as temporal fossa protuberance supply clues about intracranial involvement by tumors.

Generalized orbit congestion or inflammation accompanies cellulitis, pseudotumor, Graves' disease, and arteriovenous malformations. Fever, palpable warmth, and erythema characterize infections. Passive congestion without these signs is more suggestive of the other processes. Conjunctival chemosis and vascular injection of the globe, particularly over the extraocular muscles, are nonspecific inflammatory-congestive signs (Figs. 166–4 to 166–6). Rhythmic pulsation of the globe implies an arteriovenous fistula or a cranial bone defect. Subtle pulsations are more readily detectable with applanation tonometry. Intraocular pressures may be elevated with any orbital process, particularly with generalized congestion. An audible bruit over the orbit or temporal fossa of the head is evidence of a high-flow fistula.

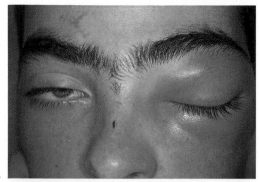

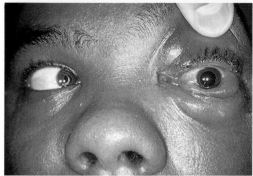

Figure 166–4. Acute inflammatory orbit disorders. A, Cellulitis secondary to sinusitis with fever, diffuse erythema, and swelling, requiring intense systemic antibiotics, decongestants, and surgical drainage of the sinus. B, Pseudotumor (idiopathic orbit inflammation) producing congested lids and conjunctiva and ocular motility compromise, all promptly reversible with systemic corticosteroids.

IMAGING STUDIES

The fundamental essential tests for orbital disorders are soft tissue imaging studies. These are preceded, however, by the physical examination and medical laboratory evaluation, including, as appropriate, thyroid function tests (free T_4, thyroid-stimulating hormone), autoimmune disease tests, and investigation for disseminated tumors, in addition to routine blood count. Not all patients with orbit symptoms require imaging studies—for example, those with identifiable Graves' disease and stable clinical findings.

Imaging study options have evolved over the decades from radiography (1890s), to B-scan ultrasonography (1960s), to computed tomography (CT) scan (1970s) and magnetic resonance imaging (MRI) (1980s). In general, CT scan is the most useful imaging study for the orbit because it depicts bony structure as well as soft tissue masses and inflammatory signs (Figs. 166–7 and 166–8). It is essential to evaluate both axial and coronal section planes to fully explore the orbital roof and floor. MRI is helpful for orbital apex lesions and intracranial lesions and to further define tumor vascularity (Fig. 166–9). Ultrasonography is a readily accessible initial imaging test to detect tumors, characterized as circumscribed or invasive, and to define inflammatory signs of muscle or fat involvement. Radiography has a very limited role now, being largely supplanted by CT for bone evaluation. Special imaging studies for vascular lesions are Doppler ultrasonography and contrast injection techniques of venography and arteriography. Radioisotopes

Alterations of eyelid position are instructive, with lid ptosis implying either mechanical involvement of levator muscle or palsy and lid retraction suggesting a disorder of the thyroid or central nervous system. A diagram annotating measurements of eyelid excursions is useful. Lid edema, inflammation, fat prolapse, or a focal lesion should be observed.

Ocular motility impairment may be caused by cranial nerve paresis in the orbit intracranially or by restriction of extraocular muscles due to inflammation, fibrosis, or tumor infiltration. Distinguishing paretic from restrictive causes is aided by forced duction testing of extraocular muscles with forceps using topical anesthesia or by observing intraocular pressure alterations in different fields of gaze. Specific extraocular muscle limitations may be documented on a relative scale or with careful prism measurements of horizontal, vertical, and cyclorotary components. Trigeminal nerve sensation should also be tested.

Ocular fundus findings with orbit disorders are caused by compression or ischemia of the globe or optic nerve or by periocular inflammation. Globe compression produces choroid folds in the posterior pole and may result from swelling of orbital fat as well as from tumor masses. Optic nerve head elevation can result from generalized orbit congestion or inflammation, from tumor intrinsic to the optic nerve, or from tumor surrounding it. Shunt vessels may be encountered with orbital meningiomas. Retinal vascular congestion is nonspecific.

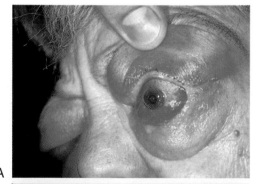

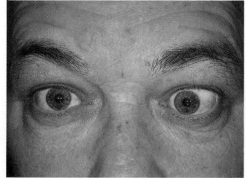

Figure 166–5. Thyroid-related exophthalmos (Graves' disease). A, Severe acute phase with active inflammation and congestion of orbits, lids, conjunctiva. B, Chronic phase with exophthalmos, lid retraction, and strabismus (left eso- and hypodeviations from muscle restrictions).

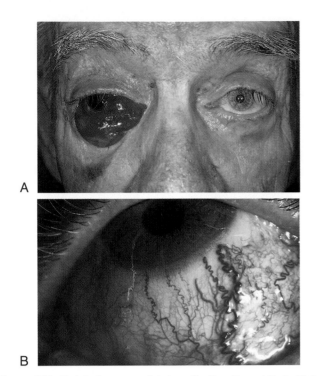

Figure 166–6. Arteriovenous fistulas affecting the orbit. *A,* High-flow carotid-cavernous fistula with acute congestion and cranial nerve palsies. *B,* Low-flow dural shunt with congestion of conjunctival vessels in characteristic radial pattern and corkscrew configuration but minimal orbital signs except mild exophthalmos.

ocular proptosis. One must realize that the conclusions reached by any orbital survey vary according to source of the material and the age group studied, the percentage of biopsy-proven entities, the geographic area encompassed, the speciality and type of practice of the researchers, and the scope of diagnostic modalities used to evaluate the patients enrolled in the series. As a result, it is easy to understand the differences encountered when reviewing and comparing such material. Most of the material and all of the tables in this chapter come from our series analyzing 2000 consecutive patients evaluated for suspected orbital disease. These patients were referred by more than 300 physicians in the New England area, and all were examined by the same clinician (RLD) during an 8-yr period (1972–1980). The referral sources represent multiple medical institutions and specialities. Two diagnostic modalities have revolutionized the scope and accuracy of orbital evaluation—ultrasonography and CT. Our series began during their inception and paralleled their rapid sophistication. Although the unequivocal diagnosis of orbital disease can be made only by histopathologic examination, current noninvasive procedures can provide a correct general diagnosis in most cases.

Table 166–3 lists our findings on the incidence of orbital disease by decade of life. The age distribution in our series ranges from birth to 92 yr, with a median age of 47 yr. It is informative to correlate our data in Table 166–1 with Henderson's orbital tumor series from the Mayo Clinic and with Rootman's series from British

are useful for detecting some disseminated tumors. Dacryocystography of the lacrimal sac defines patency and tumors of the nasolacrimal system.

Although imaging studies graphically illustrate tissue definition, pathology can be assessed definitively only by obtaining tissue specimens surgically. This can be accomplished by open biopsy, tumor excision, or fine-needle aspiration. The decision about whether to perform needle aspiration or an incisional biopsy versus complete tumor excision with an intact capsule is very important, because some tumors might be disseminated by an inappropriate surgical approach, leading to unnecessary tumor recurrence. Imaging studies together with clinical assessment provide guidelines for surgical approaches (Table 166–1). Tumors that appear circumscribed and chronic are best excised intact if practical. It is often advisable to obtain a biopsy sample of tumors that appear infiltrative or acute and are therefore likely to be either inflammatory or malignant (Table 166–2). Definitive treatment is then determined after the pathology has been fully evaluated. Surgical techniques and treatment options are addressed elsewhere in this text in chapters about specific orbital diseases.

FREQUENCY OF ORBITAL DISORDERS

Through the years, many comprehensive studies have investigated the incidence of orbital tumors or causes of

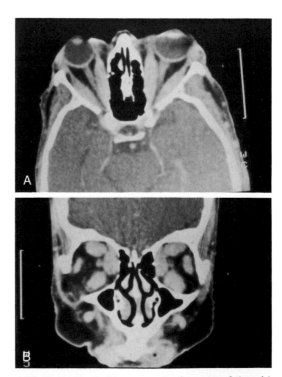

Figure 166–7. Computed tomography images of thyroid-related exophthalmos (Graves' disease). Axial section *(A)* and coronal section *(B)* planes depict asymmetric enlargement of extraocular muscles with crowding of the optic nerve at the orbit apex. Both scan planes are essential for defining orbit pathology.

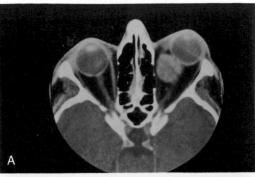

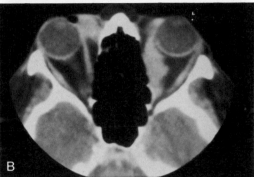

Figure 166–8. Computed tomography images of orbit tumors. A, Circumscribed mass posterior to the globe and displacing normal structures, characteristic of a benign tumor (hemangioma). B, Irregular mass extending deeply into the orbit, indicating an infiltrative neoplasm (lymphoma).

Table 166–1. GUIDELINES FOR ORBITAL TUMOR DIAGNOSIS

	Benign Tumors	Malignant Tumors
Duration of symptoms	Long (years)	Short (months)
Pain	None	Present
Vision impairment	Little	Present
Motility impairment	Little	Present
Degree of exophthalmos	Minor	Marked
Imaging findings	Circumscribed mass Bone intact	Infiltrative mass Bone eroded

orbital tumor survey, whereas Henderson's review of 764 tumors lists a female:male ratio of 12:13.

Seventy percent of the orbital disease in our overall series is benign, although one must use the term with caution. For instance, benign mixed tumor of the lacrimal gland and sclerosing pseudotumor are benign histologically, but their clinical behavior can be quite destructive. Silva found 58 percent of the tumors in his series to be benign histologically, although his review includes only biopsy-proven cases and thus excludes a large number of inflammatory disorders.

A broad overview of our series is shown in Table 166–4. Inflammatory orbital disease represents 51 percent of our entire series, with orbital mass lesions accounting for 32 percent of our survey. The vascular subdivision in Table 166–2 comprises such entities as dural and carotid-cavernous sinus fistulas, as well as aneurysms. Traumatic orbital hemorrhages make up most of our trauma category. In 6 percent of our series, pseudoproptosis is the diagnosis arrived at by investigation. Seven percent of the subjects in our study had an undetermined cause of their orbital findings after ruling out all identifiable causes and with a minimum follow-up period of 5 yr. A more comprehensive discussion of the previously mentioned topics is undertaken in the following paragraphs of this chapter.

The most common orbital disorders found in our series are listed in Table 166–5. Graves' ophthalmopathy ranks first, followed in decreasing frequency by idiopathic inflammatory pseudotumor, pseudoproptosis, vascular anomalies, orbital cellulitis, meningiomas, non-Hodgkin's lymphoma, metastatic lesions, dermoid-epidermoids, sinus mucopyoceles, and traumatic mass lesions. In his study of unilateral exophthalmos, Palmer combined eight previous series and found the five most common causes to be vascular, inflammatory, lymphomas and other blood tumors, metabolic, and

Columbia. In these studies, the second decade of life shows the lowest incidence of orbital disorders and the incidence of orbital disease steadily increases from the third through sixth decade. Fifty-three percent of all tumors in Henderson's series occur between 40 and 70 yr of age, whereas 52 percent of all patients in our series are in a similar age range. In Hou and Garg's review of 193 orbital tumors from the University of Iowa, 48 percent of the patients were between 40 and 70 yr of age. Sixty-six percent of the patients in our series are female. After excluding all patients with Graves' disease, an entity with a 4:1 female prevalence, we still found 57 percent of the patients to be female. Female patients account for 57 percent of the subjects in Silva's

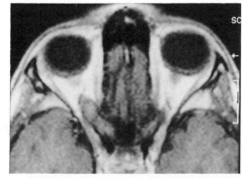

Figure 166–9. Magnetic resonance imaging scan of an orbital apex tumor extending through the optic canal and into the optic chiasm intracranially (glioma).

Table 166–2. SURGICAL DECISIONS FOR ORBIT TUMORS

Biopsy Specimen	Complete Excision Intact
Malignancy suspected	Benignity suspected
Infiltrative appearance	Encapsulated appearance
Solid consistency	Cystic or solid mass
Complex surgical approach	Accessible surgical approach

Table 166–3. DISTRIBUTION OF ORBITAL DISEASE BY DECADE

Age (Years)	%
0–10	8
11–20	7
21–30	10
31–40	11
41–50	16
51–60	19
61–70	18
71–80	9
>80	2

meningiomas. In a histopathologic series of 504 expanding lesions of the orbit, Reese lists the most common cause as granuloma, followed by hemangioma, lymphoma, lymphangioma, and rhabdomyosarcoma. Wright's series from Moorfields Eye Hospital in London lists dysthyroid eye disease as the most frequent cause of orbital disease, followed in decreasing order by vascular causes, pseudotumors, inflammatory causes, and fractures and trauma. A series by Moss, which contains a combination of clinical, radiographic, and pathologic diagnoses, reports thyroid ophthalmopathy as the most frequent cause of expanding lesions of the orbit, followed by hemangioma, lymphosarcoma (lymphoreticular), pseudotumor, and lacrimal gland epithelial tumors. Among Rootman's 1409 cases, thyroid-related orbitopathy accounts for 47.1 percent, followed by neoplasia at 22.3 percent, structural abnormalities 13.8 percent, inflammatory disorders 10.2 percent, vascular lesions 2.8 percent, and degenerative changes 1.7 percent.

Vascular mass lesions make up approximately two thirds of the vascular subdivision noted in Table 166–5. Vascular disorders not associated with a discrete orbital mass can also lead to orbital disease. Such entities as dural-cavernous sinus fistula, aneurysm, intracranial arteriovenous malformations, cavernous sinus syndrome, and carotid-cavernous sinus fistula all have been attended by pathologic orbital findings.

Three of the five orbital disorders in Table 166–3 are inflammatory in nature (i.e., Graves' ophthalmopathy, idiopathic inflammatory pseudotumor, and orbital cellulitis). Table 166–6 is a summary of the inflammatory orbital disease in our series. By including inflammatory mass lesions in this category, inflammatory orbital disease accounts for 54 percent of our entire orbital survey.

Table 166–4. INCIDENCE OF ORBITAL DISORDERS

	Cases	%
Mass lesions	549	32
Inflammatory	869	51
Vascular	33	2
Trauma	33	2
Pseudoproptosis	107	6
Undetermined cause	117	7
	1707	100
Negative findings	292	
Total series	2000	

Table 166–5. COMMON ORBITAL DISORDERS

	Cases	%
Graves' disease	590	32
Pseudotumors	107	6
Pseudoproptosis	107	6
Vascular	101	6
Orbital cellulitis	91	5
Undetermined	117	6
Meningioma (primary-secondary)	52	3
Non-Hodgkin's lymphoma	50	3
Metastatic	50	3
Dermoid-epidermoid	42	2
Sinus mucocele-pyocele	33	2
Traumatic mass lesions	33	2
All others	452	24
Total	1825	100

Jakobiec and Jones lend support to our findings by stating, "Non-organismal inflammations and infections collectively cause well over 50 percent of cases of orbital disease and proptosis."

As noted in Table 166–7, pseudoproptosis is not an uncommon cause for referral to an orbital specialist. One must be alert for the wide variety of common entities that may be overlooked while searching for a nonexisting orbital disease. We found globe asymmetry, cranial nerve paralysis, and congenital facial asymmetry to be the three most common causes of pseudoproptosis. Unilateral or asymmetric bilateral myopia accounts for most cases of globe asymmetry. Congenital craniostenosis, essential facial hemiatrophy (Parry-Romberg's syndrome), and previous orbital-facial fractures can be responsible for facial asymmetry. Unilateral ptosis may suggest contralateral proptosis, and lid retraction can give a false impression of globe prominence.

Some researchers subdivide orbital tumors into primary, secondary, metastatic, and generalized (part of a multifocal process). We believe a more useful clinical

Table 166–6. INFLAMMATORY ORBITAL DISORDERS

		Cases	%
Graves' disease		590	64
Pseudotumor		107	12
Diffuse without mass	52		
Acute	30		
Chronic	22		
Dacryoadenitis	18		
Mass—resolved on steroids	19		
Myositis	11		
Fibrosing	7		
Orbital cellulitis		91	10
Scleritis-uveitis		15	1
Miscellaneous		126	13
Optic nerve	11		
Sjögren's syndrome	5		
Abscess	5		
Sarcoidosis	3		
Wegener's syndrome	2		
Vasculitis	2		
Dacryocystitis	1		
Others	97		
Total		929	100

Table 166–7. CAUSES OF PSEUDOPROPTOSIS

		Cases	%
Globe asymmetry		78	72
Nerve paralysis		17	17
Third	12		
Sixth	5		
Congenital facial asymmetry		6	5
Orbital fracture		3	3
Lid retractions		1	1
Poststrabismus surgery		1	1
Myasthenia gravis		1	1
Total		107	100

approach is to combine the last three previously mentioned subdivisions into a "secondary" category. Using this classification, 58 percent of the orbital mass lesions in our series are primary and 42 percent are secondary. By comparison, primary orbital tumors account for 68 percent of Illif's reviews and 48 percent of Hou and Garg's series. Orbital mass lesions are an important subdivision of orbital disease. Our experience in this area is summarized in Table 166–8. The six most common categories in our series are neurogenic, cystic, vascular, lymphoreticular, inflammatory, and metastatic. By comparison, analysis of a series by Reese and Henderson show vascular lesions to be the most common category, followed by neurogenic and then cystic masses. In Silva's study in Mexico City, cystic lesions are the most common subdivision, followed by inflammatory and neurogenic etiologies.

In our neurogenic category, meningiomas are the most frequent entity, followed by optic nerve lesions and then neurofibroma. Henderson lists a similar distribution among the neurogenic masses in his orbital tumor series. Reese lists neurofibroma as the most common neurogenic tumor, followed by meningioma and then glioma. An orbital tumor survey from the Neurological Institute of Columbia-Presbyterian Medical Center lists optic nerve glioma as the most common orbital tumor, followed in order of frequency by meningioma, neurofibroma, carcinoma, carotid-cavernous fistula, and encephalocele. This neurosurgical series by Housepian and Trokel includes patients of all ages and is not limited to cases approached surgically.

Table 166–8. ORBITAL MASS LESIONS (549 CONSECUTIVE CASES)

	Cases	%
Neurogenic	97	18
Cysts	95	17
Vascular	68	12
Lymphoreticular	66	12
Inflammatory	60	11
Metastatic	50	9
Secondary epithelial	28	5
Lacrimal-intrinsic neoplasms	16	3
Osseous-cartilage	10	2
Miscellaneous	24	4
Undetermined	35	7
Total	549	100

In our series, the most common cystic mass lesions are dermoid-epidermoid cysts, followed by sinus mucocele-pyocele and then lipodermoid. The most prevalent cystic mass in Henderson's series is mucocele, followed by dermoid-epidermoid cyst and hematic cysts. Mucoceles account for 8.5 percent of all lesions in Henderson's tumor series and 6 percent of all lesions in our series of 549 orbital masses. Although patients with mucoceles often receive their primary care from an otolaryngologist, ophthalmologists should remain alert for this frequent secondary orbital mass.

In decreasing order of frequency, cavernous hemangioma, lymphangioma, and capillary hemangioma are the three most frequent vascular mass lesions in our series. Cavernous hemangiomas are the most prevalent hemangiomas in adults, whereas capillary hemangioma is the most common childhood hemangioma.

In decreasing order of frequency, our lymphoreticular category is composed of non-Hodgkin's lymphoma, lymphoid hyperplasia, plasmacytoma, and granulocytic sarcoma. Non-Hodgkin's lymphoma represents 9 percent of our orbital tumor series and 7.5 percent of Henderson's orbital tumor survey. Lymphoid hyperplasia is a relatively recent subdivision of lymphoreticular disease. *Granulocytic sarcoma* is a newer term for the older and more widely used clinical term *chloroma*.

As shown in Table 166–8, inflammatory lesions account for 11 percent of our orbital tumor series. Idiopathic inflammatory pseudotumors make up 73 percent of all inflammatory masses in our study, and they represent 8 percent of our 549 orbital mass lesions. By comparison, inflammatory mass lesions account for 8 percent of Henderson's orbital tumor series, whereas orbital pseudotumors represent 5 percent of his entire tumor survey.

A brief discussion of metastatic orbital disease is appropriate, because this entity represents a significant subdivision of orbital mass lesions. Metastatic tumors are responsible for 9 percent of the orbital tumors in our study and for approximately 7.5 percent of the orbital masses in Henderson's series at the Mayo Clinic. Metastatic tumors account for 12 percent of the orbital masses in Hou and Garg's pathologic review. The most common tumor to metastasize to the orbit in adults is breast carcinoma, followed in frequency by carcinoma of the lung. Neuroblastoma is the most common childhood entity to metastasize to the orbit.

In decreasing order of frequency, our secondary epithelial tumor category includes neoplasm from the paranasal sinuses, periorbital skin–conjunctiva, nasopharynx, and nasal cavity. In our series, paranasal sinus neoplasms account for 54 percent of the previously mentioned subdivision. Paranasal sinus neoplasms represent 41 percent of Henderson's secondary epithelial neoplasms. Secondary epithelial neoplasms account for 5 percent of our total orbital masses while representing 14 percent of the total orbital tumors in Henderson's survey.

Our lacrimal-intrinsic neoplasm category includes only those tumors whose origin is traced to functional components of the lacrimal gland. It accounts for 3 percent

Table 166–9. FREQUENCY OF SPECIFIC MASS LESIONS (549 CONSECUTIVE CASES)

		Cases	%
Meningioma (primary-secondary)		52	9
Metastatic		50	9
Non-Hodgkin's lymphoma		50	9
Pseudotumor		44	8
Hemangioma		43	8
Cavernous	33		
Capillary	10		
Dermoid-epidermoid		42	8
Sinus mucocele-pyocele		33	6
Lacrimal-intrinsic neoplasms		16	3
Optic nerve glioma		16	3
Inflammatory—others		16	3
Sjögren's syndrome	5		
Abscess	5		
Sarcoidosis	3		
Wegener's syndrome	2		
Dacryocystitis	1		
Paranasal sinus neoplasms		15	3
All others		172	31
Total		549	100

Table 166–11. BILATERAL ORBITAL MASS LESIONS

Glioma	Amyloidosis
Meningioma	Leukemia
Lymphoreticular	Wegener's syndrome
Pseudotumor	Sjögren's syndrome
Cysts	Neuroblastoma
Metastatic	Fibrosis
Sarcoidosis	Vasculitis

of the orbital masses in our series. By comparison, such neoplasms account for 5 percent of the orbital tumors in Henderson's survey. These neoplasms are an infrequent cause of orbital mass lesions.

Osseous and cartilaginous causes of orbital masses are uncommon, fibrous dysplasia being the most frequent in our series. In Henderson's study, orbital osteoma is the most common lesion within this subdivision.

A further breakdown of orbital mass lesions is presented in Table 166–9. Meningiomas are the most common tumor in our series. Other common masses are non-Hodgkin's lymphoma, pseudotumor, hemangioma, dermoid-epidermoid, and paranasal sinus mucopyocele. Henderson also lists meningioma as the most common orbital tumor, followed by mucocele, secondary squamous cell carcinoma, lymphoma, hemangioma, metastatic lesions, pseudotumor, and arteriovenous fistula.

Evidence of bilateral orbital disease involvement is a valuable clinical finding that implies a somewhat different emphasis that is reflected in Table 166–10 from our series. Inflammatory-congestive processes account for most bilateral orbital disorders. This category is dominated in adults by Graves' disease and inflammatory pseudotumor. Simultaneous bilateral orbital involvement with pseudotumor-like manifestations carries a potential for eventual diagnosis of systemic disorders such as polyarteritis nodosa, Graves' disease or endocrine exophthalmos, Wegener's granulomatosis, sarcoi-

dosis, amyloidosis, dysproteinemia, and systemic lupus erythematosus. Several entities might account for bilateral orbital mass lesions (Table 166–11). The majority of bilateral orbit disorders not associated with a mass are benign. On the other hand, bilateral orbital mass lesions often signify a neoplastic process or serious systemic disease that is likely to be malignant.

Childhood orbital disorders show a distinct distribution that differs from adulthood. Table 166–12 lists the most common categories for the age group from birth to 20 yr in our series. Inflammatory (37 percent) and mass lesions (37 percent) categories are the most common, followed by trauma 6 percent, vascular 2 percent, bony developmental 2 percent, general diseases 1 percent, and pseudoproptosis 8 percent. By comparison, inflammatory disease accounts for 44 percent of Crawford's review of childhood orbital diseases, followed by neoplastic 20 percent, bony developmental 9 percent, trauma 9 percent, general diseases 7 percent, and vascular causes 7 percent. Crawford's childhood orbital disease survey from the Toronto Hospital for Sick Children resembles our series because it discusses this topic as it relates to proptosis, thus including entities other than biopsy-proven disorders.

In our series, orbital cellulitis is the most common childhood inflammatory disorder, followed in frequency by idiopathic inflammatory pseudotumor and Graves' ophthalmopathy. In Crawford's study, orbital cellulitis is also the most prevalent inflammatory entity, followed by Graves' disease. Although Crawford's series does not include any cases of idiopathic inflammatory pseudotumor, this is the second most common inflammatory disease in our childhood survey. Pseudotumor is not uncommon in childhood; 6 to 16 percent of the patients in the series dealing with orbital pseudotumor have been 20 yr of age or younger.

Table 166–10. BILATERAL ORBITAL DISORDERS

Inflammatory
    Graves' disease
    Pseudotumor
Mass lesions
Vascular shunts
Congenital
Pseudoproptosis

Table 166–12. CHILDHOOD ORBITAL DISORDERS (257 CONSECUTIVE CASES)

	Cases	%
Inflammatory	95	37
Mass lesions	95	37
Trauma	15	6
Vascular	6	2
Bone development	5	2
General diseases	2	1
Pseudoproptosis	21	8
Unknown	18	7
Total	257	100

Table 166–13. CHILDHOOD ORBITAL DISORDERS: MASS LESIONS (95 CONSECUTIVE CASES)

		Cases	%
Dermoid-epidermoid cysts		35	37
Neurogenic		22	24
Glioma	15		
Neurofibroma	4		
Schwannoma	3		
Vascular		20	21
Hemangioma	14		
Lymphangioma	6		
Rhabdomyosarcoma		5	5
Lymphoreticular		4	4
Mucocele		4	4
Others		5	5
Total		95	100

A further analysis of childhood orbital mass lesions appears in Table 166–13. In both our series and Iliff and Green's summary of four reviews of childhood orbital tumors, the three most common categories of childhood orbital masses are cystic, neurogenic, and vascular. Cystic lesions are the most prevalent subdivision and represent more than one third of both series. In each study, neurogenic tumors are more prevalent than vascular mass lesions. Rootman's series of childhood orbit mass lesions lists inflammatory 12.9 percent, dermoid-epidermoid 11.2 percent, thyroid 10 percent, capillary hemangioma 9.5 percent, and malignant tumors 7.1 percent. We found dermoid-epidermoid cysts to be the most common mass, followed by optic nerve glioma, capillary hemangioma, lymphangioma, and rhabdomysarcoma. In decreasing order of frequency, Iliff and Green list dermoid, hemangioma, rhabdomyosarcoma, optic nerve glioma, neurofibroma, neuroblastoma, and lymphangioma. The most common malignant orbital tumors in childhood are rhabdomyosarcoma, lymphoreticular lesions, and metastatic neuroblastoma. Metastatic neuroblastoma, although uncommon, is reported to spread to the orbit in 11 to 38 percent of cases, with a possible ratio of bilateral to unilateral metastases of 4:3.

Table 166–14 demonstrates the distribution of childhood tumors in relationship to benign versus malignant and primary versus secondary. A similar analysis of Crawford's series reveals 30 percent of the masses to be primary orbital and 60 percent to be secondary. An equal incidence of benign and malignant tumors is reported in Crawford's study. In both subdivisions, the principal reason for such a large disparity between series is the paucity of dermoid-epidermoid in Crawford's study.

Table 166–14. ORBITAL MASS LESIONS IN CHILDHOOD (95 CONSECUTIVE CASES)

Primary versus secondary	
87%	14%

Benign versus malignant	
86%	14%

Orbital hemorrhage accounts for a majority of traumatic orbital problems in childhood. Such entities as arteriovenous malformation, aneurysms, Sturge-Weber syndrome, and hemorrhage associated with systemic disease cause most childhood vascular orbit disorders that are not associated with a discrete orbital mass. Congenital structural anomalies such as craniostenosis, meningocele, cephalocele, and Crouzon's disease account for most cases of bony developmental childhood orbital diseases. Under the general disease category are such entities as Hand-Schüller-Christian disease, eosinophilic granuloma, and Letterer-Siwe disease. Finally, pseudoproptosis is a fairly common finding in childhood cases being evaluated for potential orbital disorders.

In summary, orbital disease offers clinicians a challenging field in which to pursue diagnostic, medical, and surgical modalities. Inflammatory orbital disease accounts for a significant percentage of both childhood and adult orbital disorders. Among adults, Graves' disease is the leading cause of either unilateral or bilateral exophthalmos. In children, orbital cellulitis is the most common entity causing orbital disease. Cystic, neurogenic, and vascular mass lesions are the common tumor subdivisions in both adults and children. Fortunately, orbital mass lesions are benign in the majority of cases.

BIBLIOGRAPHY

Anderson SR, Seedorff HH, Halberg P: Thyroiditis with myxedema and orbital pseudotumor. Acta Ophthalmol 41:120, 1963.

Blodi FC, Gass JDM: Inflammatory pseudotumor of the orbit. Br J Ophthalmol 52:79, 1968.

Brenner EH, Shock JP: Proptosis secondary to systemic lupus erythematosus. Arch Ophthalmol 91:81, 1974.

Bullen CI, Liesegant TJ, McDonald TJ: Ocular complications of Wegener's granulomatosis. Ophthalmology 90:279, 1983.

Chavis RM, Garner A, Wright JE: Inflammatory orbital pseudotumor. Arch Ophthalmol 96:1817, 1978.

Crawford JS: Disease of the orbit. In Toronto Hospital for Sick Children, Department of Ophthalmology: The Eye in Childhood. Chicago, Year Book Medical Publishers, 1967, pp 331–364.

Dallow RL: Reliability of orbital diagnostic tests: Ultrasonography, computerized tomography, and radiography. Ophthalmology 85:1218, 1978.

Dallow RL, Momose KJ, Weber AL, Wray SH: Comparison of ultrasonography, computerized tomography (EMI scan), and radiographic techniques in evaluation of exophthalmos. Trans Am Acad Ophthalmol Otolaryngol 81:305, 1976.

Duke-Elder S: System of Ophthalmology, vol XIII, Part II. Lacrimal, Orbital, and Para-Orbital Diseases. Chapter XI. St. Louis, CV Mosby, 1974, pp 774–810.

Ferry AP, Font RL: Carcinoma metastatic to the eye and orbit. I: A clinicopathologic study of 227 cases. Arch Ophthalmol 92:276, 1974.

Henderson JW, Farrow GM: Orbital Tumors, 2nd ed. New York, Thieme-Stratton, 1980, p 1–690.

Houspian EM, Trokel S: Tumors of the orbit. In Youmans JR (ed): Neurological Surgery. Philadelphia, WB Saunders, 1973, pp 1275–1296.

Hou PK, Garg MP: Tumors of the orbit: A report of 193 consecutive cases. In Blodie FC (ed): Current Concepts in Ophthalmology. St. Louis, CV Mosby, 1972, pp 176–185.

Iliff WJ, Green WR: Orbital tumors in children. In Jakobeic FA (ed): Ocular and Adnexal Tumors. Birmingham, Aesculapius, 1978, pp 669–684.

Iliff CE, Ossofsky HJ: Tumors of the orbit. Trans Am Ophthalmol Soc 55:505, 1957.

Jakobiec FA, Jones IS: Orbital inflammations. In Duane TD (ed):

Clinical Ophthalmology, 2nd ed. New York, Harper & Row, 1980, pp 1–75.

Kassman T, Sundmark E: Orbital pseudotumors with amyloid. Acta Ophthalmol 45:220, 1967.

Little JM: Waldenstroms macroglobinemia in the lacrimal gland. Trans Am Acad Ophthalmol Otolaryngol 71:875, 1967.

Lloyd GAS: CT scanning in the diagnosis of orbital disease. Comput Tomogr 3:227, 1979.

Melmonk L, Goldberg JS: Sarcoidosis with bilateral exophthalmos as the initial symptom. Am J Med 33:158, 1962.

Morrow-Lippa L, Jakobiec FA, Smith M: Idiopathic inflammatory orbital pseudotumor in childhood. II: Results of diagnostic tests and biopsies. Ophthalmology 88:565, 1981.

Mottow LS, Jakobiec FA: Idiopathic inflammatory orbital pseudotumor in childhood. I: Clinical characteristics. Arch Ophthalmol 96:1410, 1978.

Moss HM: Expanding lesions of the orbit: A clinical study of 230 consecutive cases. Am J Ophthalmol 54:761, 1962.

Palmer BW: Unilateral exophthalmos. Arch Ophthalmol 82:415, 1965.

Reese AB: Expanding lesions of the orbit (Bowman lecture). Trans Ophthalmol Soc UK 91:85, 1971.

Rootman J: Diseases of the Orbit. Philadelphia, JB Lippincott, 1988, pp 1–612.

Shields JA, Bakewell B, Augsburger JJ, et al: Space occupying orbital masses in children: A review of 250 consecutive biopsies. Ophthalmology 93:379, 1986.

Silva D: Orbital tumors. Am J Ophthalmol 65:318, 1968.

Susal AL: Vascular studies of the orbital cavity. Ophthalmology 88:548, 1981.

Trokel SL, Jakobiec FA: Correlation of CT scanning and pathologic features of ophthalmic Graves' disease. Ophthalmology 88:553, 1981.

Van Wien S, Merz EH: Exophthalmos secondary to periarteritis nodosa. Am J Ophthalmol 56:204, 1963.

Weiter J, Farkas T: Pseudotumor of the orbit as the presenting sign in Wegener's granulomatosis. Surv Ophthalmol 17:106, 1972.

Wright JE: The role of ultrasound in the investigation and management of orbital disease. In Thijssen JM, Verbeek AM (eds): Documenta Ophthalmologica Proceedings Series. Dordrecht, Dr. W Junk Publishers, 1981, pp 273–276.

Chapter 167

■

Orbital Surgical Techniques

DANIEL J. TOWNSEND

Appropriate orbital surgery depends on a fundamental understanding of ocular, adnexal, and orbital anatomy combined with a familiarity with the differential diagnosis and relative incidence of orbital disease processes. This knowledge, combined with radiologic and laboratory information, can allow the patient the least traumatizing method of diagnosis and treatment.

Improved instrumentation and anesthesia techniques, higher quality operating microscopes and fiberoptic illumination, and more accurate preoperative noninvasive imaging techniques have significantly advanced the armamentarium of the orbital surgeon in the past few decades.

ORBITAL SURGICAL TECHNIQUES

Orbital surgery in the modern era consists of two basic types of surgical approaches to the orbit: anterior orbitotomy and lateral orbitotomy. Neurosurgical or transfrontal approaches to the orbital apex are not discussed here. These topics are covered in neurosurgery textbooks. Reese,[1] in 1971, reported that more than 90 percent of all expanding processes of the orbit can be adequately evaluated with one or both of these surgical approaches.

There are believed to be four surgical spaces within the orbit: two real spaces and two potential spaces.[2] The first potential space of the orbit is the episcleral or Tenon space, which is the area between Tenon's capsule and the sclera, which lies beneath it. The second is the subperiosteal space; this lies between the orbital bones and the overlying periosteum. Both the potential spaces of the orbit, in general, do not play a large role in orbital surgery.

The real spaces of the orbit include the area outside the muscle cone of the orbit, involving the space between the intramuscular septa of the extraocular muscles and the periosteum of the periorbital bones, and the central space, which includes the muscle cone and the space within it. These two real spaces are important in orbital surgery because most orbital pathologic processes can be found within them.

ANESTHESIA

General anesthesia is preferred in most orbital surgical cases, although local blocks can be used in easily accessible anterior pathologic processes. Hypotensive techniques are recommended to improve hemostasis as well.

ANTERIOR ORBITOTOMY

Anterior orbital surgery can be approached in two main surgical techniques: either a transconjunctival anterior approach or an anterior transcutaneous approach through the lids along the orbital rim (Fig. 167–1). Bone removal can be obtained with either method. The decision to use one technique over the other usually depends

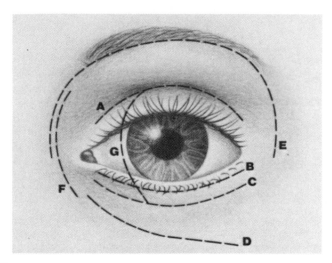

Figure 167–1. Surgical approaches for anterior orbitotomy. *A,* Upper eyelid crease incision; *B,* subciliary incision; *C,* lower eyelid crease incision; *D,* lower orbital rim incision; *E,* orbital rim incision; *F,* medial incision; *G,* transconjunctival incision. (From Kohn R: Textbook of Ophthalmic Plastic and Reconstructive Surgery. Philadelphia, Lea & Febiger, 1988, p 300. Reprinted with permission.)

on the actual location of the orbital lesion, whether it can be easily palpable through the skin or through conjunctiva, and whether partial excision or biopsy versus complete total excision of the tumor mass is anticipated.

The transconjunctival approach can be used to enter the orbit between the globe and the orbital rim, and it allows access to pathology located along the globe itself, especially in cases involving problems such as orbital lymphoma and perimuscular tumors such as schwannomas and other neurogenic tumors. It can also provide exposure of lesions along the muscle cone. Usually a lateral canthotomy is required, with dissection through conjunctiva, orbicularis muscle, and orbital septum. Prolapsed orbital fat and damage to the oblique muscles are potential surgical problems.

Orbital rim or anterior orbital skin incisions can be made either superiorly along the eyebrow itself, just beneath the eyebrow cilia, or inferiorly through an orbital rim or infraciliary approach, in which a large skin flap can be constructed before entering the orbital rim inferiorly. With superior incisions along the eyebrow itself, attention must be given to the important anatomic attachments superiorly, including the supraorbital vascular bundle and the trochlea, which lies 4 mm behind the orbital rim superonasally.

Once dissection is carried out to the level of the periosteum, the periosteum can be elevated with a periosteal elevator, entering the potential space between bone and the periosteum, with care being taken in the supranasal region; damage to the trochlea and superior oblique muscle can result in binocular torsional diplopia. It is important to close the periosteum with absorbable sutures superiorly to maintain normal suspension of upper eyelid structures.

Inferior orbital rim incisions can be made directly at the level of the orbital rim or can be performed using the infraciliary approach; again care must be taken to avoid damage to the infraorbital nerve and vessels. Although the inferior approach does not, in general, allow good access to posteriorly displaced structures within the orbit or with lacrimal gland and other lateral tumors, it is an excellent approach to excise an anteriorly displaced tumor such as an orbital dermoid, to treat orbital fractures, and to obtain biopsy specimens of infiltrative tumors of the orbit (i.e., potential metastatic orbital processes).

LATERAL ORBITOTOMY

Lateral orbitotomy and variations of it have been used in ophthalmology for more than 100 yr. Although Kronlein[3] is generally thought to have been the first to develop a technique of lateral orbitotomy, history reveals that other surgeons in Germany (Wagner) and France (Passavant) also contributed to the development of methods allowing access to the retrobulbar space by removing the lateral bone rim and orbital wall.[4]

Kronlein[3] first described a surgical technique for the removal of orbital dermoid cysts in 1888; he reported that a crescentic incision in the lateral orbit provided access to the retrobulbar space. Over the years, several modifications of this basic technique have been developed, with the most important modification offered by Burke and Reese[4] in the 1950s.

The current technique for lateral orbitotomy, in general, involves a combination of a lazy S-shaped or curvilinear incision in a vertical plane along the lateral orbital rim, with extension of this incision in a horizontal manner from the level of the lateral canthus toward the ear (Fig. 167–2A). Sometimes lateral canthotomies with isolation and retraction of the lateral canthal tendon may be necessary for improved orbital exposure.

The lateral orbitotomy skin incision can be made in a curvilinear manner in the lateral two thirds of the eyebrow at the level of the bone orbital rim. The incision should be continued below the insertion in the lateral canthal tendon and carried posteriorly for 4 to 4.5 cm (Fig. 167–2A–C). Dissection can be then be performed through the various subcutaneous layers, including the orbicularis muscle, to the level of the periosteum along the frontal-zygomatic suture line.

At this point, traction sutures or a self-retaining retractor may be used to retract the skin muscle flap at the level of the temporalis muscle. The periosteum can then be incised parallel to the orbital margin. Careful elevation of the periosteum both anteriorly and posteriorly along the orbital rim will allow exposure of the orbital cavity. The key bony anatomic structure exposed is the suture line, which is composed of the lateral aspect of the frontal bone and the frontal process of the zygoma (see Fig. 167–2C). The temporalis muscle must also be elevated and reflected posteriorly after the muscle is partially disinserted by incising the periosteum.

At this time, a 25- to 30-mm segment of orbital bone containing the frontal-zygomatic suture line can be removed (see Fig. 167–2D and E). Malleable retractors

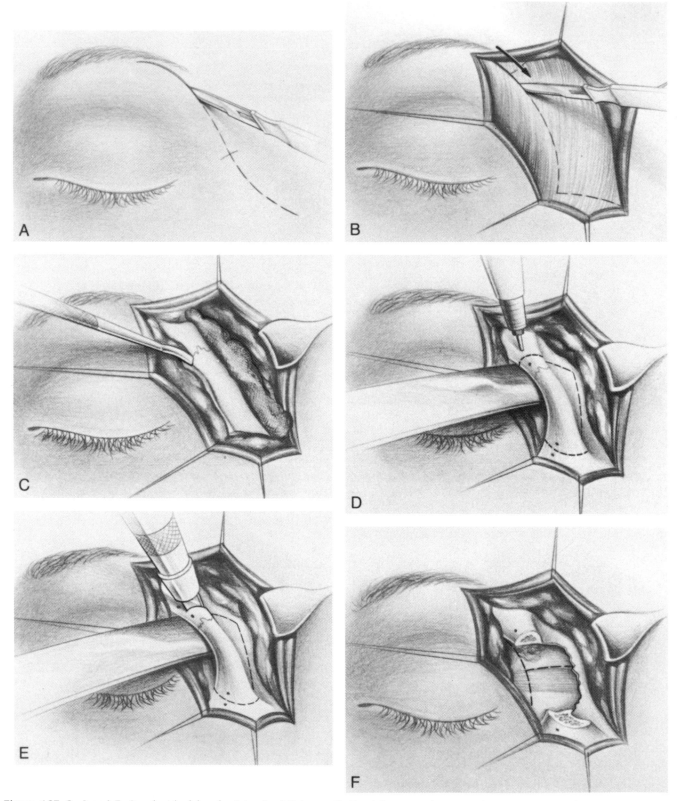

Figure 167–2. *A* and *B,* Surgical incision for lateral orbitotomy. *C,* Frontal-zygomatic suture line. *D* and *E,* Orbital bone removal. *F,* Incision of periorbita.

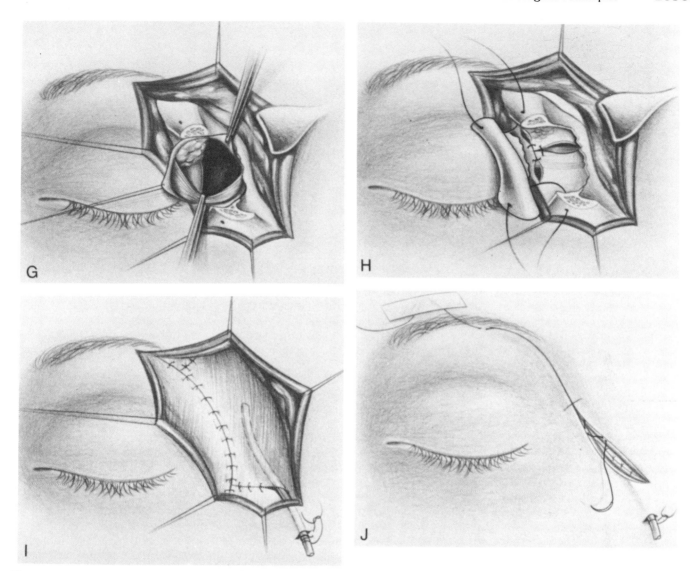

Figure 167–2 *Continued. G,* Incision of periorbita. *H* and *I,* Replacement of lateral bone wall fragment. *J,* Insertion of surgical drain.

can be used to protect the orbital contents posteriorly. The rotary or circular saw can be used to make horizontal cuts in the superior and inferior bony margins. A bone rongeur can then be used to rock the bony segment back and forth to break the hinge. If more posterior bone resection to the level of the sphenoid is necessary, further bites can be obtained with the bone ronguer. Up to 50 percent more exposure can be achieved using this method. Care must be taken at this point to avoid excessive orbital bleeding either from the subperiosteal space or as a result of temporalis muscle trauma.

The periorbita can now be seen. To enter the orbital contents, the periorbita can be incised by making a T-shaped incision with the T on its side (see Fig. 167–2F and G). The lateral rectus muscle may be tagged at this point to provide better orientation of orbital structures. The orbital contents must be very carefully dissected because the lateral rectus muscle and multiple intramarginal adhesions between the fat and other neurosensory

structures may be found here, with potential damage to adjacent ocular structures. This portion of surgery should be completed by closure of the periorbita using absorbable sutures, with some allowance being made for the escape of blood or serous fluid.

The lateral wall bone fragment can be replaced, if necessary, by drilling burr holes in the adjacent stable facial bone and passing 26- or 28-gauge orthodontic steel wire through in an effort to reposition the lateral bony orbital rim (see Fig. 167–2A–I). The Synthes Corporation (Paoli, PA) has produced a titanium mesh implant to provide similar bony stabilization laterally. In cases such as orbital decompression associated with thyroid disease or malignant proptosis, it is best not to replace the bone because this will detract from the decompressive effects. Usually minimal cosmetic blemish is noted postoperatively despite the loss of bone.

The periosteum should be closed, if possible, with absorbable sutures. Placement of a rubber catheter or

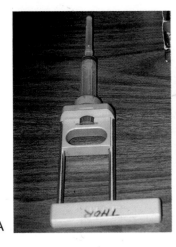
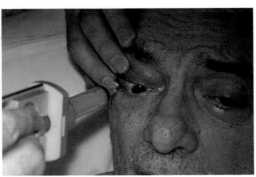

Figure 167–3. *A* and *B,* Fine-needle aspiration device.

Penrose drain for blood drainage should also be considered (see Fig. 167–2 *J*). The subcutaneous tissue is closed at this time and a light dressing is applied as well; one must monitor visual acuity and check for the presence of intraorbital hemorrhage and hematomas frequently within the first 24 to 48 hr. Orbital drains can be removed at that time.

MEDIAL ORBITOTOMY

In certain situations, excellent exposure can be obtained with a transconjunctival medial approach, removing the insertion of the medial rectus muscle after tagging it with a traction suture. This allows the surgeon to gain significantly more exposure posteromedially and along the muscle cone itself to search for any processes that could involve medial tumors or trauma to the medial aspect of the orbit. In addition, optic nerve sheath fenestrations (discussed in Section 11) can be performed using this approach.

Other approaches for accessing the medial orbital space, including the ethmoid or Lynch transcutaneous incision or the transantral Caldwell-Luc operation, can also be considered. Descriptions of these techniques are found in otolaryngology textbooks. Combined medial and lateral approaches can also be used, especially for the diagnosis of apical tumors and in cases of optic nerve decompression.

NEWER VARIATIONS IN ORBITAL SURGERY

Fine-Needle Aspiration Biopsy of the Orbit

Over the past decade, fine-needle aspiration has evolved as an alternative method of biopsy of orbital masses, especially in cases of lymphoid, metastatic, and inflammatory processes or in blind eyes caused by optic nerve lesions.[5–7]

A 22-gauge, 3.75-cm needle is attached to a 20-ml syringe in a pistol-grip aspiration device, and the needle tip is guided, via direct palpation or radiologic scanning, to the area of pathology (Fig. 167–3*A* and *B*).

Suction is obtained, and the needle tip is gently rocked back and forth to aspirate as much tissue as possible. The biopsy specimen can then be fixed onto a glass slide and undergo pathologic evaluation.

Accurate diagnosis of orbital tumors is reported in up to 80 percent of cases[6]; the combined team approach of a competent cytologist, ophthalmic pathologist, and experienced orbital surgeon will maximize these results.[6] Fibrous tumors (e.g., metastatic scirrhous breast carcinoma) and other orbital processes may not allow sufficient aspiration material for diagnosis.[7]

Fine-needle aspiration biopsy of the orbit is not indicated for lesions anterior to the orbital septum or for benign encapsulated masses of the orbit.[9] Another theoretical contraindication is benign mixed lacrimal gland tumor, which may undergo local metastasis with needle biopsy "tracking."[9]

Potential complications of this technique include orbital hemorrhage, ptosis, motility disturbances, seeding of tumor along the needle tract, and globe penetration (Fig. 167–4).[8, 9]

The current needle length, 3.75 cm, will, it is hoped, avoid the vital structures of the superior orbital fissure (and posterior to it) in adults. It appears that fine-needle

Complications of FNA			
Ophthalmologists*		Non-Ophthalmologists^c	
complications	cases#	complications	cases
orbital hemorrhage	7	orbital hemorrhage	3-1NLP
ptosis	1	perforated globe	2
motility disturbance	1	ptosis	1
prominent scar	1	motility disturbance	2
		blindness	3
		death	3
*138 patients (Liu, 1985)			
^cunknown number of patients			
#no sequellae			

Figure 167–4. Potential complications of fine-needle aspiration. (NLP, no light perception.)

aspiration may be most helpful in identifying or guiding therapy of malignant unresectable orbital neoplasms.[7]

Orbital Endoscopy

Rigid and fiberoptic endoscopy of the sinuses and nasal passages has been effectively used by otolaryngologists for the past decade. This procedure has been used in orbital and lacrimal evaluations, especially as the diameter of the endoscope has decreased, and has generated wider applicability.[10]

REFERENCES

1. Reese AB: Expanding lesions of the orbit. Trans Ophthalmol Soc UK 91:85, 1971.
2. Couper WL, Harris GJ: Clinical ophthalmology (Duane series). *In* Orbital Surgery 1981. pp 1–23.
3. Kronlein RV: Zur pathologic und operativen Behandung der dermoid Cysten der Orbita. Beitr Klin Chir 4:149, 1888.
4. Henderson JW: Orbital Tumors. Philadelphia, WB Saunders, 1973.
5. Kennerdell JS, Dekker A, Johnson BL, Dubois PJ: Fine needle aspiration biopsy: Its use in orbital tumors. Arch Ophthalmol 97:1315, 1979.
6. Kennerdell J, Slamouits T, Dekker A, Johnson BL: Orbital fine needle aspiration biopsy. Am J Ophthalmol 99:547, 1985.
7. Kopelman JE, Shorr N: A case of prostatic carcinoma metastatic to the orbit diagnosed by fine needle aspiration and immunoperoxidase staining for prostatic specific antigen. Ophthalmol Surg 18:599, 1987.
8. Krohel G, Tobin D, Chavis R: Inaccuracy of fine needle aspiration biopsy. Ophthalmology 92:666, 1985.
9. Liu D: Complications of fine needle aspiration of the orbit. Ophthalmology 92:1768, 1985.
10. Norris J, Stewart W: Bimanual endoscopic orbital biopsy: An emerging technique. Ophthalmology 92:34, 1985.

BIBLIOGRAPHY

1. Wright JE, Chavis RM, Krohel GB, Stewart WB: Practical Approach to Diseases of the Orbit. AAO Instruction Course 1981.
2. Rootman J: The Orbit. JB Lippincott, Philadelphia, 1988.
3. Kohn R: Textbook of Ophthalmologic Plastic and Reconstructive Surgery. Lea & Febiger, Philadelphia, 1988.
4. Berke RN: A modified Kronlein operation. Trans Am Ophthalmol Soc 51:193, 1953.
5. Grove AS: Orbital disease: Examination and diagnostic evaluation. Ophthalmology 86:854, 1979.
6. AAO Instruction Booklet 1989, Orbital Anatomy & Physiology, pp 15–27. Eyelids & Orbit.
7. Grove AS: Orbital disorders. *In* Pavan-Langston D (ed): Manual of Ocular Diagnosis and Treatment. Boston, Little, Brown and Company, 1980.

Chapter 168

■

Cystic Lesions of the Orbit

GARY E. BORODIC

DUCTAL CYST OF THE LACRIMAL GLAND (Fig. 168–1)

The ductal cysts of the lacrimal gland are probably the most common cystic lesions occurring in the orbit. These lesions typically occur in the palpebral portion of

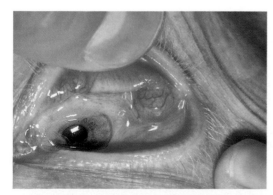

Figure 168–1. Ductal cyst of the lacrimal gland. Example of a typical lacrimal ductal cyst. With the lid everted, the cyst can usually be directly viewed as it extends into the superior fornix and is easily seen. Occasionally, the cyst extends into the orbital portion of the lacrimal gland.

the gland and protrude into the superior fornix, which allows a direct method for both inspection and aspiration of the lesion. The lesions are often bilateral.

Occasionally, if a secondary reason for orbital inflammation occurs such as an infection or a pseudotumor, these lesions can cause confusion with abscess formation or other forms of tumor.

MICROPHTHALMOS WITH A CYST[1]

Microphthalmos with a cyst is thought to arise from incomplete closure of the fetal cleft, which results in a cyst attached to the sclerae. The cyst is lined internally by gliotic retina and externally by a fibrous envelope. The eyes are usually microphthalmic and often demonstrate colobomas of the lens and retinas. A reverse polarity of the layers of neuroretinas can be recognized occasionally within the cyst. Useful vision is highly unlikely secondary to multiple globe deformities. Occasionally, the globe can be of normal size or larger. The cysts are located usually in the inferior orbit and cause the lower lid to bulge.

Therapy for this condition may include removal of

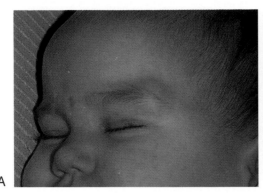 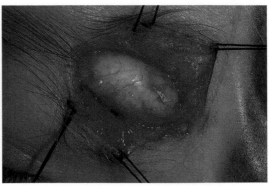

A   B

Figure 168–2. Typical orbital rim epidermoid tumor. *A,* Epidermoid and anterior orbital dermoid tumors typically occur in the superior temporal quadrant of the rim. The lesions are smooth when palpated and can often be moved. These lesions often present during childhood. *B,* The surgical plane is easily established around these well-circumscribed lesions, and efforts should be made to totally remove the lesions to ensure that they do not recur from a residual portion of the tumor.

the cyst and deformed globe, with socket reconstruction when appropriate.

EPIDERMOID AND DERMOID TUMORS (Fig. 168–2*A* and *B*)

Epidermoid and dermoid tumors are the most common cystic tumors occurring in the orbital and periorbital region and are the most common orbital neoplasms in the pediatric age group. These tumors are choristomas—that is, congenital tumors arising from embryonic tissues displaced from usual anatomic locations. The distinction between an epidermoid tumor and a dermoid tumor is based on tissue types found in association with the cyst. The gross architecture of both an epidermoid tumor and a dermoid tumor involves a large single or multiloculated cystic cavity containing keratin and inwardly directed lining of stratified squamous cell epithelium. In developmental terms, epidermoid and dermoid cysts may be the result of sequestration of surface ectoderm pinched off at bone suture lines or along the lines of embryonic closure.[2]

The epidermoid contains only stratified squamous cell epithelium forming the wall of the cyst, whereas the dermoid contains epidermal appendages including hair follicles, sweat glands, and sebaceous glands. A teratoma is a closely related congenital tumor that may have cystic elements but contains histologic elements derived from the three primary germ layers (ectoderm, mesoderm, or endoderm), such as intestinal mucosa, central nervous system tissue, and thyroid tissue.

The lesions often connect to bone sutures by way of fibrous attachments. The frontal/zygomatic suture is the most common attachment for the periorbital dermoid and is consistent with the upper outer periorbital quadrant being the most common location for these lesions. Lesions of the upper outer periorbital quadrants may have deeper projections into the orbit through the temporal fossa. The "dumbbell dermoid" may project anteriorly as a palpable cystic mass, yet the lesion can erode the lateral orbital wall and straddle the orbital and temporal fossa spaces (Fig. 168–3).[3] These lesions may be more susceptible to incomplete surgical removal.

Dermoids are slowly growing lesions that usually occur not only with bone attachments but are also likely to exert a mottling effect on the orbital walls or rim. Fossa formation within the anterior lateral wall of the orbit represents probably the most common bone change, although more extensive bone erosion or even extension into the intracranial space is possible.[4]

The clinical presentation of an epidermoid tumor or a dermoid tumor can occur at any time but is clearly more common in childhood. The constellation of signs and symptoms is dependent on the location of the tumor (periorbital or orbital). The pattern of growth of these tumors is usually very slow. The periorbital lesions are recognized as a discrete, well-circumscribed, freely movable mass. Although the upper outer quadrant is the most characteristic location, these lesions may occur in any periorbital location. Deeper lesions within the orbit may present as an orbital mass with diplopia and proptosis.[5] In such situations, the clinical presentation demands a diagnostic evaluation to characterize the nature of the tumor and any degree of posterior orbital involvement. Another presentation of these tumors is orbital inflammation following blunt trauma. In this situation, trauma results in the rupture of the cyst with the release of its contents into soft tissues. Inflammatory foreign body reaction ensues. Because of the presence of orbital inflammation, infections are suspected; however, radiologic evaluation that reveals a cystic tumor is helpful in suspecting this diagnosis. Tissue evaluation may reveal a foreign body granuloma from keratin debris released from the cyst, as well as chronic inflammatory infiltrates including cholesterol deposition appearing as transparent clefts surrounding this inflammatory reaction.[6] Calcification may also be seen within the lining of the cyst. The latter histologic changes can be noted even in situations without a history of blunt trauma or rupture, indicating a possible subclinical release of cystic contents over an extended period. Similar histologic findings also may be present upon evaluation of a specimen for a patient who had previous surgical procedures in which there was subtotal removal of the lesion.[7] Occasionally, fistulization is seen after incomplete removal of orbital dermoid tumors.

Radiographic Analysis

Typically, the computed tomography (CT) scan appearance of a dermoid is that of a cystic lesion occurring in close approximation to bone. These lesions are extraconal when they occur in the deep orbit. As mentioned earlier, bone changes are frequently present and are helpful in the differential diagnosis. These changes include: (1) fossa formation with bone attenuation, (2) bone erosion, and (3) bone sclerosis.

Fossa formation or orbital wall attenuation suggests chronicity and results from a pressure effect from the slowly growing tumor. The extreme example of this process is erosion into the intracranial space or into the temporal fossa (dumbbell dermoid). Such extreme erosion, however, is uncommon. When erosion is present, the lesion must be differentiated from the malignant process as well as from other cystic lesions associated with large bone wall abnormalities, such as encephalocele or mucocele.

Magnetic resonance imaging (MRI) can be helpful in further characterizing epidermoid and dermoid tumors.

Although bone changes are better resolved with CT scanning, MRI offers a higher degree of resolution in the soft tissue density contrast that may be helpful particularly in evaluating deeper orbital lesions. In general, periorbital dermoids are usually not a difficult diagnostic problem. The surgical approaches are more straightforward. MRI is often not obtained in dermoids occurring in this location. However, when the lesion extends more posteriorly into the orbit, the surgeon must assess the degree of posterior involvement. In this respect, the imaging studies are critical.

The keratin core of these lesions appears on MRI with a single intensity that is variable with each tumor. Some dermoids emit a T_1, T_2 signal similar to that of vitreous, increasing signal hyperintensity on T_2. These lesions can also be hyperintense on the T_1 signal.[8] MRI is particularly useful in defining the cystic nature of the lesion when the lesion presents as an inflammatory orbitopathy with surrounding tissue reaction. Occasionally MRI or CT scan can demonstrate a fluid level within the cyst.[8]

Treatment

Periorbital dermoids are typical and do not represent diagnostic problems, which may be encountered with

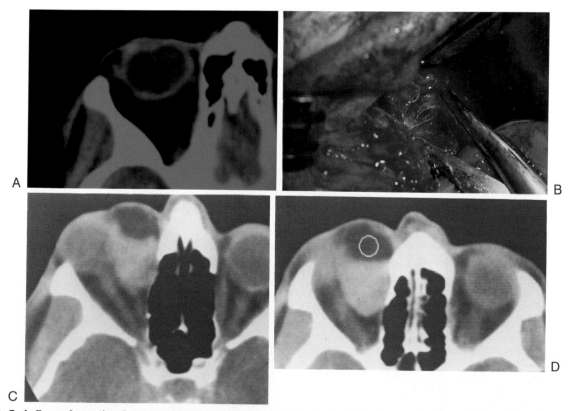

Figure 168–3. *A*, Fossa formation from the anterior-located dermoid (*arrow*). Orbital dermoids frequently cause fossa formation. This phenomenon can be helpful for diagnostic purposes. Occasionally, this attenuation of the lateral wall is so great as to allow penetration of a portion of the epidermoid or dermoid into the temporal fossa (dumbbell dermoid). *B*, During surgical exploration of dermoid tumors, hair can occasionally be seen emerging from the lesion as found in this surgical field. This finding strongly suggests that the lesion is a dermoid tumor. *C* and *D*, Computed tomography (CT) scan of a posterior orbital dermoid tumor. Epidermoid and dermoid tumors arising in the posterior portion of the orbit present with diplopia, proptosis, and globe displacement. At CT, these lesions have sharply defined margins with central low density. Fossa formation and attenuation of adjacent bone can also be characteristic. A fat-fluid level can sometimes be seen on a CT scan, as demonstrated here (*circle*). Varying tissue densities at the core of these lesions constitute a common attribute on CT scans.

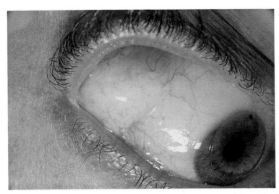

Figure 168–4. Appearance of a typical lipodermoid. This lesion usually occurs on the superior temporal epibulbar region and is often covered by fatty globules under conjunctiva. These lesions can occur occasionally in other positions on the globe and are sometimes associated with Goldenhar's syndrome. Because of the infiltrating nature and poor clinical response to surgical excision, these lesions should not be excised. Unlike epidermoid and dermoid tumors, lipodermoids are not cystic.

deeper lesions. Generally, the removal of periorbital dermoids is useful to confirm the diagnosis. Other reasons for removing these lesions are to relieve symptoms created by a mass in the periorbital region, to eliminate the likelihood of an inflammatory reaction after blunt trauma secondary to cyst rupture, and to improve cosmetics. These lesions are very well circumscribed and can be easily dissected around the circumference, leaving the lesion intact upon excision (see Fig. 168–2B). This lesion is usually attached to a bone or bone suture within the orbital rim. Occasionally, hair can be seen emerging from these lesions during surgical excision, suggesting the lesion's histologic character (see Fig. 168–3B). Complete removal of these lesions on the first surgical attempt is desirable. If the lesion is only partially removed, it can recur. This situation most usually occurs after a portion of the dermoid is left within a bone. Because dermoid tumors can occasionally extend within

bone, the surgeon should be certain that all the walls of the cyst are removed completely from the fossa or its extension within bone. In this situation, it may be necessary to remove a portion of the lateral orbital bone rim to ensure complete tumor excision (see Fig. 168–3A).

Deeper orbital lesions must be removed to confirm the diagnosis, relieve pressure effects on deeper orbital structures, prevent continued bone erosion (possibly into the intracranial space), and relieve possible interference with ocular motility. These lesions can be removed by using lateral orbitotomy. When erosion into the intracranial space or the sinus is present, the orbitotomy can be integrated with a neurosurgical or otolaryngologic procedure to ensure thorough excision. Marsupialization has been advocated as an alternative to complete excision and involves subtotal removal of the tumor with exteriorization of an evacuated cyst.[9] Complete excision of the tumor clearly remains the preferred surgical management technique.

LIPODERMOID (Fig. 168–4)

The lipodermoid is a common choristoma that occurs in the superotemporal epibulbar region and occasionally causes intermittent ocular irritation (see Fig. 168–4). These lesions are often noncystic, however, and contain tissues derived from multiple germ layers (e.g., epidermal appendages, fat, and smooth muscle). Occasionally, epibulbar dermoids are seen in association with Goldenhar's syndrome (consists of preauricular skin tags, lid coloboma, epibulbar dermoids, and skeletal defects).

These lesions infiltrate into the peribulbar region, lid, and surrounding orbital tissues. They should not be surgically excised because they create extensive cicatricial reactions postoperatively.[10] An extensive postoperative cicatricial reaction can lead to globe restriction and lid malformations. Figure 168–5 demonstrates a lid fistula that was created by a surgical attempt to repair a

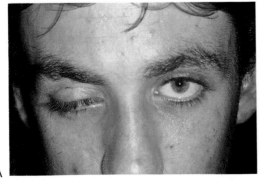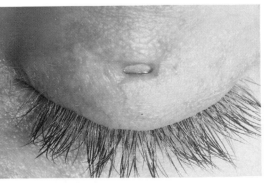

Figure 168–5. *A* and *B,* Excision of lipodermoids has been associated with adverse consequences. The lesions are exceedingly infiltrating for benign tumors and are associated with substantial postoperative scarring. The patient shown here underwent a surgical excision for a superior epibulbar dermoid during childhood. Postoperatively, intense epibulbar scarring led to severe ptosis. After multiple attempts to correct ptosis with levator resections, this young man was left with a full-thickness fistula of the upper lid. Several attempts to close the fistula were unsuccessful. The clinical course of this patient exemplifies the reason why a conservative nonoperative approach is still the preferred method for management of these lesions.

postoperative ptosis, which was created by an attempt at epibulbar lipodermoid excision. When present, these lesions should not be surgically excised.

ENCEPHALOCELE (Fig. 168–6A and B)

Encephalocele is a congenital orbital tumor formed by herniation of the intracranial contents through bone dehiscence at the skull base. When the herniation involves meninges and cerebrospinal fluid, this congenital tumor is called a "meningocele." When a tumor contains brain parenchymal tissue with meninges, the tumor is appropriately called a "meningoencephalocele." These lesions are usually diagnosed during infancy and childhood as a protruding mass within the supramedial portion of the orbit. During straining, bending, or lifting, the mass may protrude significantly as increased intracranial pressure forces more cerebrospinal fluid and tissue through the bone dehiscence. The lesions often pulsate or can create pulsating exophthalmos as the intracranial pulse is transmitted to the orbit through the bone dehiscences. Encephalocele can be categorized as

(1) frontoethmoidal and (2) associated with sphenoid bone dysplasia.

Because the skull-based deformity is a prerequisite for the presence of encephalocele, these patients often have other clinical signs of cranial and facial bone malformation. Hypertelorism, broad nasal bridge, and malar and orbital floor depressions are common coexisting findings (see Fig. 168–6A and B). Many patients with orbital encephalocele are eventually diagnosed with neurofibromatosis. Patients with encephalocele should be inspected carefully for stigmata of neurofibromatosis, such as "café-au-lait" spots, Lisch nodules on the iris, cutaneous fibromas, and periorbital plexiform fibromas of the lid (see Fig. 168–6B). The globe may be ptotic because of an absence of the significant portion of the orbital floor. The globe is often pushed into an inferior lateral position because the encephalocele usually protrudes into the orbit through a superior and medial bone defect. Occasionally, the meningeal herniation is minimal and the orbital contents decompress through the bone defect, resulting in a pulsating enophthalmos. Occasionally, fat atrophy may be associated with this latter condition. Because of pressure communication

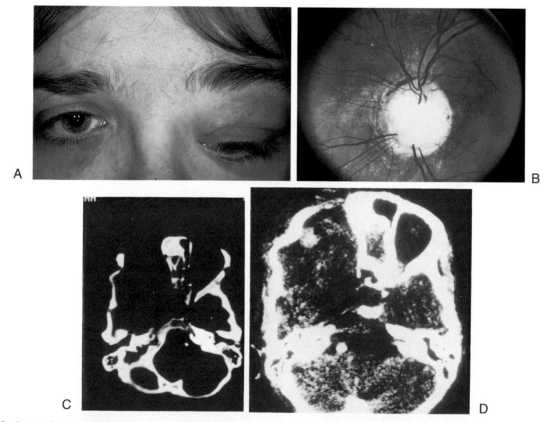

Figure 168–6. *A* and *B*, Encephalocele and meningocele are congenital orbital tumors resulting from herniation of brain contents through a bone defect at the skull base. Encephaloceles may extend into the orbit or oropharynx, and occasionally there are associated colobomas of the optic nerve (*B*). The sphenoorbital encephaloceles are almost exclusively associated with neurofibromatosis. Other signs of neurofibromatosis, such as plexiform neurofibroma of the lid or café-au-lait spots, may be recognized.
The typical physical findings suggestive of sphenoorbital encephalocele include pulsating proptosis, hypertelorism, and telecanthus on the side of the lesion (*A*). Proptosis may increase when the head is in a position of dependency or during the Valsalva maneuver. The globe is depressed inferolaterally by the lesion. *C* and *D*, There is always a defect within the lesser wing of the sphenoid bone, which is seen on the CT scan (*C*). Herniation of the intracranial contents is imaged through the bone defect (*D*). On plain radiographs, the superior orbital fissure and other bone landmarks of the posterior orbit are completely missing.

from the intracranial space into the orbit, the patient experiences intermittent proptosis during the Valsalva maneuver or when the head is in a dependent position.

Encephalocele may occur with other ocular and orbital malformations, such as optic atrophy, optic nerve colobomas, microphthalmos, and optic nerve gliomas (particularly when associated with neurofibromatosis). A specific form of abnormality characterized as an excavated, funnel-shaped, distorted optic disc has been associated with basal encephalocele. This association has been identified as "morning glory syndrome."[11]

This deformity can place the patient at greater risk for intracranial injury as a result of midfacial contusions.[12] The patient shown in Figure 168–7 received a blunt injury during active duty as a police officer. Figure 168–7 demonstrates the extreme amount of proptosis resulting from the orbital edema and hemorrhage that followed. She was aphasic for approximately 48 hr after the injury. A CT scan demonstrated an extensive intracerebral hemorrhage following the periocular contusion.

Radiologic Findings (see Fig. 168–6C, D)

A defect within the anterior cranial fossa may be demonstrated on the CT scan. These frontal sinus encephaloceles are best viewed in conjunction with three-dimensional reconstructions and coronal views. The frontal encephalocele protrudes through the bone defect into the ethmoidal sinus and occasionally into the orbit. This encephalocele may protrude into the nasopharynx and appear as a smooth mass on posterior nasal examination. Frontal ethmoidal encephalocele has been specifically associated with the "morning glory syndrome."

When associated with sphenoid bone dysplasia, there is enlargement of the superior orbital fissure that gives the appearance of the "bare orbit" on plain films. A CT scan examination reveals an enlarged middle cranial fossa. The temporal lobe of the brain may herniate

through the hole of the posterior lateral orbit, forming in effect an intraorbital mass. Enlargement of the pituitary fossa and optic canal has been associated with this bone deformity.[13]

Treatment

Generally, orbital encephaloceles are not removed unless there is extensive involvement within the orbit. When a surgical approach is planned, dural obliteration is needed to close the defect within the sphenoid bone. Frontal encephaloceles are more accessible from a neurosurgical point of view and can be closed with a dural patch.

Globe ptosis can be corrected with the insertion of bone or cartilage grafts in the inferior orbit to help support the globe and produce a superior displacement. Autogenous fascia lata slings have been tried if ptosis remains with poor levator function.

Patients should be warned of the potential damage resulting from blunt trauma to the eye and orbits; protective eyewear should be recommended.

MUCOCELE (Fig. 168–8A–E)

Mucoceles are cystic lesions originating from the paraorbital sinus that slowly enlarges, causing bone deformity with possible erosion into the orbit. Although the size of these lesions can be considerable, a prior history of sinus disease may not necessarily be present. The cause of these cystic growths is probably related to an obstruction of the sinus ostia with internal cystic expansion of the sinus epithelium. The expanded epithelium appears to secrete its mucus into the cystic expansion, causing an increase in the mass of these lesions. With further expansion, the bone walls of the sinus become attenuated and eventually destroyed. These cystic masses may expand into the intracranial

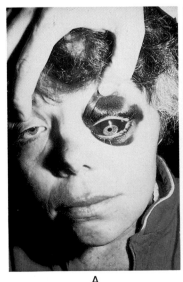
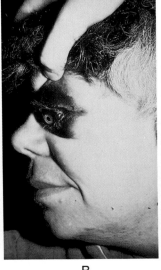
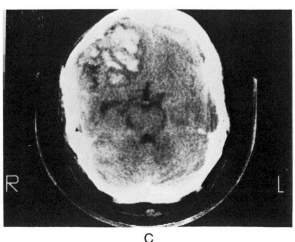

A B C

Figure 168–7. A to C, After blunt contusion to the periorbital region, this patient had a substantial intracranial hemorrhage with neurologic deficits. This patient is also shown in Figure 168–6A. Patients with sphenoorbital encephalocele can sustain considerable intracranial injury with moderate periorbital trauma.

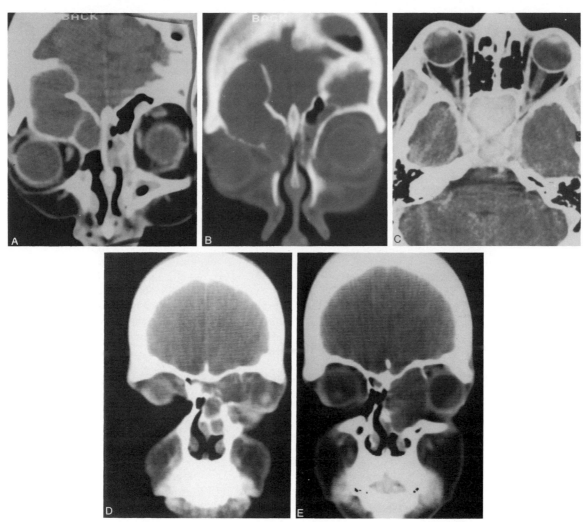

Figure 168–8. *A* and *B,* Frontal sinus mucocele is the most common location for these lesions. The frontal mucocele demonstrated here presented as diplopia associated with proptosis. Other presentations include upper lid discharging fistula from secondary infection (mucopyocele) and meningitis. These lesions often attenuate bone and may extend into the anterior cranial fossa and displace the brain. In the lesion shown here, only a thin membrane separating intracranial contents from the mucocele was noted in the operating room. The mucocele not only displaced the globe but also extended into the neurocranium to displace the frontal lobes. *C,* Sphenoid sinus mucoceles are considerably less common than frontal sinus lesions. As frontal sinus mucoceles, these lesions attenuate surrounding bone and may extend into the orbital apex, compressing neural structures. Compressive optic neuropathy and compressive oculomotor palsies may be the presenting ophthalmic syndromes produced by these lesions. *D* and *E,* Ethmoid sinus mucoceles can displace the eye laterally, causing diplopia and disfigurement. Erosion through the medial orbital wall and into the nasal cavity is a common finding.

space or into the orbit. The core of these lesions contains a yellow mucoid material, and occasionally the lesions can precipitate a purulent infection (mucopyocele). When infected, orbital cellulitis or meningitis may ensue. Intrinsic abnormalities in the microanatomy of the respiratory epithelium may play some role because the condition has been associated with cystic fibrosis, which can produce mucoceles during infancy and early childhood.[14] Although trauma with fractures, infection with scarring, polyps, and other lesions of the nasal cavity can occasionally be associated with mucocele formation, most often there is no clear past history suggesting a cause.

Mucoceles most commonly arise from the frontal and ethmoid sinuses anteriorly. The frontal sinus mucocele, which is probably the most common mucocele, erodes the orbital roof and displaces the globe inferiorly, often causing diplopia. When infected, frontal sinus mucopyoceles have a tendency to form draining fistulas within the upper eyelid. The presenting complaint of a frontal mucocele may be a discharging lesion of the upper lid. This type of presentation should alert the clinician to obtain appropriate radiologic examination. The frontal mucocele may also extend toward the intracranial space, displacing the brain (see Fig. 168–8*A, B*). An anterior ethmoidal mucocele can present as a mass within the medial canthal region, and the appearance of telecanthus (see Fig. 168–8*D, E*). Medial displacement of the globe may be present, and this may result in diplopia. Mucoceles can arise from the sphenoid and posterior ethmoid sinus much less commonly.

The differential diagnosis for cystic medial orbital lesions must also include an encephalocele with a skull base deformity. Direct decompression of an encephalocele would be obviously contraindicated, whereas drainage or obliteration of a mucocele would be an indicated form of therapy. Meningocele and encephalocele are always associated with a congenital skull base deformity, which is best demonstrated on CT scanning with coronal views through the orbits. The proptosis created is often intermittent, worsened when the head is in a dependent position, and occasionally associated with globe and periorbital pulsations.

Unlike lesions arising in the anterior orbit, a posterior location causes a different constellation of symptoms. Compression of the optic nerve with loss of vision and associated visual field abnormalities or other cranial neuropathies with associated diplopia can be seen. Pain can be an associated symptom but is clearly not always present.

Spontaneous, nontraumatic enophthalmos is an important and unique presenting syndrome that can be caused by maxillary sinus mucoceles.[15] Unlike mucoceles presenting in other sinuses, a discrete cystic lesion is often not observed on a CT evaluation, but rather the orbital floor appears to have become eroded and collapsed into the maxillary sinus with mucosal thickening and opacification of the sinus (Fig. 168–9A, B). The radiologic picture may even suggest an eroding neoplasm. As with mucoceles occurring in other locations,

nasal symptoms or past history of sinusitis may not be present. Globe ptosis with deepened superior sulcus is another finding on examination (see Fig. 168–9B to D). Spontaneous diplopia may be the presenting complaint.

The CT appearance of a typical mucocele includes bowing of a sinus wall into the orbit, with attenuation or even erosion of bone associated with a cystic cavity (see Fig. 168–8). With more advanced cases, the erosion into the orbit may be complete and the central mucoid contents of the lesion may resemble a tumor from the paranasal sinus invading the orbit. As mentioned earlier, the syndrome of spontaneous enophthalmos with maxillary sinus mucocele usually fails to demonstrate the typical cystic lesion within the sinus. MRI demonstrates highly variable signal intensities. Some have a low-intensity T_1-weighted image that becomes hyperintense on T_2-weighted sequences. Others are hyperintense on T_1- and T_2-weighted images, whereas others are hypointense on T_1- weighted images and very hypointense on T_2-weighted images. The various magnetic resonance patterns have been discussed in the literature and may relate to sequential changes in chemical composition of the mucus or the presence of fungal concretions within the cyst.[16, 17]

Management of mucoceles requires the reestablishment of normal drainage, removal of the lining of the

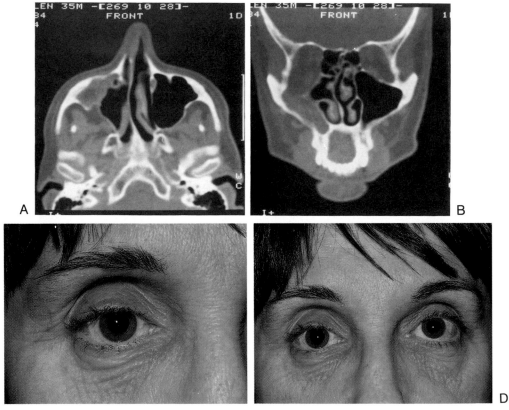

Figure 168–9. A and B, Typical appearance of maxillary sinus mucocele enophthalmos syndrome (Montgomery). Unlike a mucocele that occurs in other sinuses, the maxillary sinus mucocele does not usually have a cystic component and tends to cause an attenuation and collapse of the maxillary sinus (A) and floor of the orbit with attendant globe ptosis and enophthalmos (B). C, Maxillary sinus mucocele often presents as spontaneous enophthalmos with globe ptosis and deepening of the superior sulcus. Diplopia may occur. Management can involve inferior wall reconstruction using autogenous material such as nasal cartilage or bone grafts. The surgeon will find a bowed-down floor on inferior orbitotomy. Resupporting the floor with a bone or cartilage graft will close the floor defect and elevate the globe. When an orbitotomy is performed, drainage of the maxillary sinus with a nasoantral window should be accomplished.

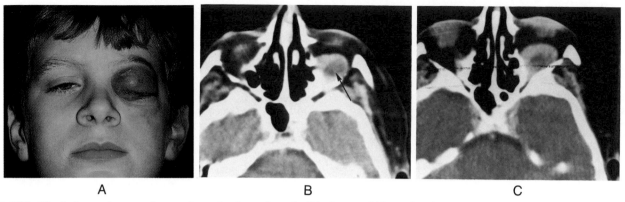

Figure 168–10. *A,* A spontaneous hemorrhage is shown here in this 8-year-old boy. Surgical exploration of the orbit revealed large fluid-filled cystic lesions. The histologic diagnosis was lymphangioma of the orbit. *B* and *C,* Lymphangiomas occur in children and usually present as an orbital mass. The lesions, which usually tend to appear solid on a CT evaluation in most cases, can however occasionally have a somewhat cystic appearance on a CT scan, as demonstrated here. (The *arrow* points to the area of low attentuation in the central portion of the lesion.)

cyst, and preferably obliteration if the frontal sinus is involved.[18] The frontal sinus mucocele can be approached by an osteoplastic flap with a sinus exposure, removal of the entire lining of the cyst, and obliteration of the sinus cavity with abdominal fat. With ethmoidal mucoceles, decompression can be performed into the nasal cavity with complete removal of the cyst lining via ethmoidectomy. Sphenoid sinus mucoceles require posterior ethmoidectomy with ethmoidal drainage into the nasal cavity and sphenoidotomy with complete removal of the cyst wall. Decompression of the lesion may provide benefit from pressure effects on vital neural structures in the region of the orbital apex. In the case of spontaneous enophthalmos associated with a maxillary sinus mucocele, a maxillary sinus decompression may be accomplished with the Caldwell-Luc approach and a nasoantral window for drainage. The orbital floor may be reconstructed with autogenous grafts of nasal cartilage taken from a submucosal nasal septal resection and bone fragment from the Caldwell-Luc procedure,

or a partial thickness calvarial bone graft. Alternatively, alloplastic materials such as titanium plate fixated anteriorly to the orbital rim may be used to elevate the globe and thus restore a normal globe position.

VASCULAR AND LYMPHATIC LESIONS OF THE ORBIT WITH CYSTIC CHARACTERISTICS
(Fig. 168–10*A* to *C*)

Occasionally, a vascular or lymphatic lesion of the orbit may present as a cystic tumor. In a child, the most notable lesion would be a lymphangioma with a cystic component. Such a lesion presents during early childhood with proptosis, with lid disfigurement and globe displacement in the coronal plane. Spontaneous hemorrhage within this lesion can be the presenting clinical picture. Neuroradiographic analysis demonstrates an infiltrating lesion with a cystic component (see Fig. 168–

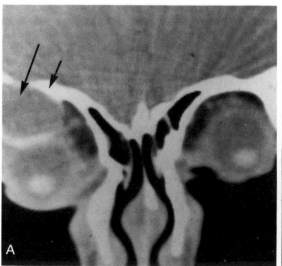
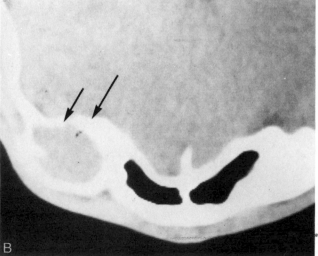

Figure 168–11. *A* and *B,* The appearance of a cholesterol granuloma of the orbit is shown here on a computed tomography (CT) scan. An erosive and destructive cystic lesion is seen at the orbital rim on a CT scan, with a soft tissue mass extending into the the orbit. The superior orbital rim is the most common location.

10B, C). Surgical exploration reveals an infiltrating tumor with cystic components filled with fluid.

In addition to lymphangiomas, orbital varix and arteriovenous malformation may appear cystic on CT scanning. These lesions tend to produce intermittent proptosis and dependent proptosis. Occasionally, intermittent compression of the optic nerve can lead to transient loss of vision associated with an afferent pupillary sign. Occasionally, these lesions present with acute proptosis with a spontaneous orbital hemorrhage (see Fig. 168–10A).

Hematic Cyst (Fig. 168–11A, B)

Hematic cysts (e.g., cholesterol granuloma, reactive xanthomatous lesion, cholesteatoma) are intraosseous lesions that occur at the superior orbital rim within the frontal bone and may expand within the subperiosteal space and displace soft tissues within the orbit (Fig. 168–11). These lesions have also been described in the temporal bone. The lesion is thought to arise from an intradiploic focus that is thought to erode and expand through the inner and outer tables of the frontal bone. Surgical exploration reveals oily brown fluid with crystals and yellow tissues. The pathologic examination demonstrates granulomatous inflammation with giant cells and needle-like cholesterol clefts.

Cholesterol granuloma appears as a cystic lesion on CT scans or on MRI, although associated bone erosion and destruction often cause a malignant neoplasm to be considered in the differential diagnosis. On MRI, the T_1- and T_2-weighted signal hyperintensity was consistent with blood products within the cyst.[8]

Therapy involves surgical exploration with a brow incision approach to gain access to the lesion in order to establish the pathologic diagnosis and curet and excise the lesion.

When the lesion extends into the anterior cranial fossa, an combined orbitomy with a craniotomy may be needed.

Aneurysmal Bone Cyst[19]

Aneurysmal bone cysts are lytic and expansile mass lesions that usually occur in the roof of the orbit in adolescent patients. These lesions are known to occur in long bones, but occasionally they occur in the skull region. Although the pathogenesis remains unknown, several theories on the pathogenesis have included alterations in hemodynamics, bleeding into preexisting bone lesions, and abnormal bone formation. These lesions can occasionally be associated with a rapid mass effect on the eye, which is usually considered secondary to intralesional hemorrhage. Proptosis, diplopia, and compressive syndromes on cranial nerves may lead the patient to seek medical attention. Because bone destruction is often seen on neuroradiologic evaluation, these lesions should often be distinguished from a malignant process, particularly a invasive lacrimal gland tumor.

The CT scan appearance of these lesions includes bone lysis and a soft tissue mass, often with sharply defined borders. Because of the high degree of vascularity, these lesions may contrast enhance.

Echinococcosis (Hydatid Cyst)

Echinococcosis is the most common orbital parasitic infestation worldwide. This condition occurs most commonly in temperate climates and in the Middle East. The lesions present with a mass effect or less commonly as an acute inflammatory orbital response from a ruptured cyst after an injury. Efforts should be made to establish a systemic diagnosis in a patient originating from an endemic area with a cystic orbital mass.

Malignant Tumors with Cystic Components

From a surgical perspective, malignant neoplasms arising from a number of tissue types can assume a cystic growth pattern. Although these tumors may not present as typical cystic orbital lesions, multiloculated cystic cavities may appear in the surgical field. I have observed this pattern in squamous cell carcinoma, rhabdomyosarcoma, and metastatic adenocarcimona.

REFERENCES

1. Mann I: Developmental Abnormalities of the Eye, 2nd ed. Philadelphia, JB Lippincott, 1957.
2. Yanoff M, Fine BS: Ocular Pathology, 3rd ed. Philadelphia, Harper & Row, 1988, p 520.
3. Cullen JF: Orbital diploe dermoids. Br J Ophthalmol 58:105–106, 1974.
4. Pfeiffer RL, Nicholl RJ: Dermoid and epidermoid tumors of the orbit. Arch Ophthalmol 46:39, 1948.
5. Grove AS: Giant dermoid cyst of the orbit. Ophthalmology 86:1513–1520, 1979.
6. Rootman J: Diseases of the Orbit. Philadelphia, JB Lippincott, 1988, p 489.
7. Sherman RP, Rootman J, LaPoint JS: Dermoids: Clinical presentation and management. Br J Ophthalmol 68:642–652, 1984.
8. Newton TH, Bilaniuck LT: Radiology of the Eye and Orbit. New York, Raven Press, 1990.
9. Kennedy RE: Marsupialization of inoperable orbital dermoids. Am Ophthalmol Soc 68:146, 1970.
10. Sullivan G: Caveat Chirurgicus. Trans Am Ophthalmol Soc 70:328–336, 1972.
11. Goldhammer Y, Smith JL: Optic nerve anomalies and basal encephalocele. Arch Ophthalmol 93:115–118, 1975.
12. Bienfang DC, Borodic GE: Pulsating exophthalmos after closed head injury. N Engl J Med 311(8):520–527, 1983.
13. Binet EF, Kiefer SA, Martin SH, Peterson HO: Orbital dysplasia in neurofibromatosis. Radiology 93:829–833, 1969.
14. Stoll S, Kertesz E, Sibinga M, et al: Exophthalmos due to pyocele of the sinus in children with cystic fibrosis. Trans Am Acad Ophthalmol Otolaryngol 70:811, 1966.
15. Montgomery WW: Mucocele of the maxillary sinus causing enophthalmos. Eye Ear Nose Throat Monthly 43:41–44, 1964.
16. Van Tassel P, Lee Y, Jing B, DePena CA: Mucoceles of the paranasal sinuses: MR imaging with CT correlation. AJNR 10:607–612, 1989.
17. Zinreich SJ, Kennedy DW, Malat J, et al: Fungal sinusitis: Diagnosis with CT and MR imaging. Radiology 169:439–444. 1988.
18. Montgomery WW: Osteoplastic frontal sinus operation: Coronal incision. Ann Otol Rhinol Larygol 74:821–831, 1965.
19. Klepach GL, Ho REM, Kelly JK: Aneurysmal bone cyst of the orbit. J Clin Neuro Ophthalmol 4:49–52, 1984.

Chapter 169

■

Management of Thyroid Ophthalmopathy (Graves' Disease)

RICHARD L. DALLOW and PETER A. NETLAND

GENERAL CONSIDERATIONS

Orbitopathy related to thyroid disorders, known widely by the eponym of Graves' disease, is an autoimmune process that is progressive but self-limited, with a variable course extending over 1 to 3 yr generally and having possible vision-threatening complications. The earliest descriptions of hyperthyroid patients with congestive exophthalmos and infiltrative dermopathy were published by Parry (1825 posthumously) and by Graves (1835) in the English literature and by von Basedow (1840) in the German literature. Thyroid ophthalmopathy is the most common orbital disorder, accounting for greater than 85 percent of bilateral exophthalmos and up to 50 percent of unilateral exophthalmos as documented in several large series of patients. Many patients who appear to have unilateral involvement clinically actually show evidence of bilateral orbit involvement when studied by current soft tissue imaging techniques of ultrasonography, computed tomography, or magnetic resonance. This orbit disorder typically affects young or middle-aged women within 1 yr of development of hyperthyroidism. The age range extends, however, from the teens to 80 yr of age, and the female to male ratio is 4:1. Some factors influencing its development include heredity, stress, smoking, and environmental stimuli. Full descriptions of Graves' disease physiology, pathology, clinical signs, disease course, and differential diagnosis are covered elsewhere (see Chap. 248). This chapter deals with therapeutic approaches including local measures, medical therapy, radiation, and surgical options.

It is important to distinguish treatment of the thyroid gland abnormality from treatment of the orbital disorder. Although these two aspects of Graves' disease may be related as an autoimmune process, perhaps based on similar antigens or proximity of genes, the clinical course of orbital involvement may seem to proceed independently of thyroid gland dysfunction and treatment. Multiple clinical studies have shown that reversal or exacerbation of hyperthyroidism may have little effect on progress of the ophthalmopathy. There is little convincing evidence of any consistent effect of any one type of thyroid treatment on the development, progression, or improvement of ophthalmopathy. Thyroid gland treatment affects only one of the end organs of this disease process and does not alter the fundamental autoimmune process causing orbitopathy. The clinical impression of worsening ophthalmopathy after thyroid gland ablation by radioiodine or surgery may represent simply the natural course of the orbit disease regardless of thyroid treatment. Some reports suggest, however, that thyroid gland destruction by radioiodine may stimulate increased antigen-antibody responses that aggravate the autoimmune disease activity. Profound changes in thyroid functional status, particularly hypothyroidism, may, indeed, activate eye problems. Frequently, in managing these patients, treatment of the thyroid gland must be simultaneous but independent of treatment for ophthalmopathy. Achievement of euthyroid status under management by an endocrinologist is generally desirable before performing definitive eye care but is not absolutely essential.

Clinical signs of Graves' ophthalmopathy are summarized by Werner's classification, adopted by the American Thyroid Association in 1977, which provides a useful format of increasing severity (Table 169–1): class 0 represents subclinical disease without signs or symptoms; class 1 includes signs of eyelid retraction and stare; class 2 includes soft tissue edema and inflammation; class 3 includes exophthalmos; class 4 includes ocular motility imbalance and diplopia from restrictive myopathy; class 5 covers exposure keratopathy; and class 6 represents optic neuropathy with potential blindness. This classification is often referred to by the mnemonic NOSPECS, based on the first letter of each item in Werner's original table. In reality, clinical signs do not always progress in this sequence. The disease process may be quite asymmetric between the two orbits and may undergo spontaneous exacerbations and remissions. The major clinical problems of this disorder are optic neuropathy, diplopia, corneal exposure, and cosmesis. The first three of these problems are vision-

Table 169–1. GRAVES' DISEASE OPHTHALMOPATHY: WERNER'S CLASSIFICATION

Class*	Description
0	No signs or symptoms
1	Only signs (eyelid retraction)
2	Soft tissue periorbital swelling
3	Proptosis of eyes
4	Extraocular muscle involvement, diplopia
5	Corneal involvement, exposure
6	Sight loss by optic nerve compromise

*Classes 0 and 1 are noninfiltrative disease. Classes 2–6 are infiltrative disease.

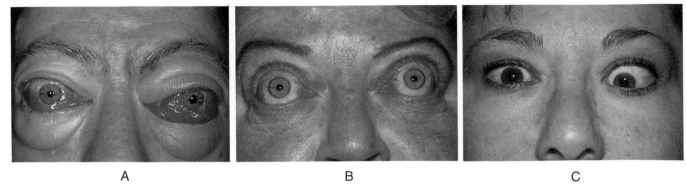

A   B   C

Figure 169–1. Clinical appearances of orbitopathy of Graves' disease. *A,* Acute inflammatory and congestive phase with marked bilateral eyelid retraction, conjunctival chemosis, exophthalmos, and optic nerve compromise. *B,* Chronic stable phase with eyelid retraction and edema and firm exophthalmos. *C,* Chronic phase with marked strabismus from restrictive myopathy, resulting in hypotropia and esotropia deviations and corresponding diplopia.

threatening. The cosmetic aspect is certainly not trivial, however, because it has a significant impact on a patient's self-image and confidence and causes chronic irritation with some functional impairment.

Orbitopathy of Graves' disease has two broad phases. Initially, there is an acute, active inflammatory and congestive phase lasting 6 to 18 mo but continuing up to 3 yr in a small group of patients (Fig. 169–1). This phase is mediated predominantly by lymphocytes and fibroblasts and is partially responsive to treatment with corticosteroids, immunosuppression, and local radiation therapies. The acute phase is followed by a chronic, stable phase with hypertrophy and fibrosis of extraocular muscles, lacrimal glands, and orbital fat, together with subcutaneous eyelid changes. These later phase changes are permanent and will not regress or progress spontaneously, and they are unresponsive to any suppressive treatment. Surgical repair is necessary to improve this second phase.

Because thyroid eye disease tends to fluctuate in severity, an evaluation of uncontrolled clinical studies is difficult to make. Eyelid retraction as a result of sympathomimetic stimulation may improve in up to 50 percent of patients, whereas exophthalmos from orbital soft tissue changes usually remains stable after reaching its maximum degree. Corneal exposure is often controllable with topical lubricants and other measures. Ocular motility imbalance may show marked fluctuations with edema, inflammation, and fibrosis involving each of the extraocular muscles variably. In general, patients should be observed for periods of 6 mo or more before any definitive therapeutic intervention, although suppression of inflammation with systemic corticosteroids may be considered in the interim. Three exceptions that require prompt early therapy are optic neuropathy, severe exposure keratopathy, and "malignant" exophthalmos, the latter being rapid, severe orbital inflammation and congestion. The threat of possible permanent visual loss from these latter problems and the unlikely possibility of their spontaneous improvement mandate urgent medical, radiation, or surgical therapy.

All therapies for Graves' orbitopathy have some potential undesirable side effects systemically or locally, and none have been established to suppress the course of orbitopathy other than temporarily. Because the fundamental disease course cannot be altered significantly, caution must be observed in considering the use of major systemic therapy or local tissue-altering therapy for orbit involvement. Local measures are directed initially at protecting the eyes from exposure and minimizing discomfort while awaiting spontaneous stabilization of the disease process. Antiinflammatory and immunosuppressive medications and orbital irradiation may be used for palliative effects or for prompt, albeit temporary, disease suppression. Later treatment of the end products of the disease process for visual or cosmetic improvement may involve multiple surgical procedures. Approximately 33 percent of these patients benefit ultimately from some surgery for eye problems.

LOCAL TREATMENT MEASURES

Local measures can be useful for mild ophthalmopathy or for temporizing effects before definitive therapy. Ocular discomfort is due largely to corneal and conjunctival exposure and often responds to topical lubrication. Methylcellulose artificial teardrops may be used during the day, and ointment may be used at night. Taping eyelids closed at night or using goggles to provide a humidified chamber is helpful, if manageable. Photophobia may be relieved by darkened glasses with side protection. Corneal exposure can be controlled frequently with minor measures. When there is evidence of corneal epithelial breakdown, close observation with prompt and effective treatment is indicated, including topical antibiotic ointment and even partial eyelid closure with surgical tarsorrhaphy. In severe situations, surgical levator and Müller's muscle recessions and lower eyelid retractor muscle recessions or orbital decompression may be required.

Periorbital soft tissue edema is often most marked in the morning after a period of recumbency with accumulation of some dependent edema. Head elevation at night by using extra pillows or elevating the head of the bed 5 to 10 degrees may be helpful for reducing edema. Patients who sleep prone may notice some improvement with a supine sleeping position. Diuretics can provide some nonspecific fluid elimination for patients with mild swelling, but they are generally minimally effective in this disease.

Mild eyelid retraction may be alleviated transiently by use of topical adrenergic blocking agents. These agents are helpful because, before fibrosis later in the course of the disease, increased α-adrenergic stimulus to Müller's muscle may contribute to eyelid retraction. Guanethidine sulfate eye drops can produce a lid ptosis of approximately 1.5 mm. This effect is transient and reversible, so therapy ranging from one drop every other day to three drops per day must be continued to maintain the desired ptosis. Side effects include local toxicity leading to superficial punctate keratitis, miosis, and dilation of conjunctival vessels. These side effects are minimized if lower concentrations (2 or 5 percent) are used. Although not as widely used as guanethidine, other adrenergic agents including bethanidine sulfate and thymoxamine may have an effect on eyelid retraction. Topical guanethidine is useful in acute or subacute management of mild eyelid retraction, but surgical correction is usually required for chronic, stable eyelid retraction.

Diplopia from extraocular muscle restrictive imbalances is most troublesome in the primary straightforward gaze position and in downgaze, the most functional gaze positions. The most commonly affected muscles are inferior and medial rectus restrictions producing tethering effects and causing hypo- and esodeviations that are noncomitant. Less often, superior rectus or lateral rectus involvement causes hyper- and exodeviations. Oblique muscle deviations are seldom of major importance in this disease. Monocular occlusion or intentionally fogging one eye with glasses will eliminate diplopia but reduces useful vision. Prisms can be incorporated into glasses to correct diplopia in one gaze position only, which may be adequate for small degrees of diplopia. Prism measurements should be made using a Maddox rod in both vertical and horizontal directions for primary gaze and for downgaze, providing maximal measurements in the most functional gaze positions. There is some clinical art, subjectivity, and flexibility in prescribing prisms for this problem. Differences will be apparent for separate distance and reading prescriptions. Prisms may be divided between the two sides in any practical combinations, because only the net result is important. Up to 8 prism diopters total correction in each direction may be ground into glasses satisfactorily. Higher prisms, often up to 30 prism diopters, require Fresnel stick-on prisms. Frequent changes in prisms may be necessary as the disease evolves. Medical therapy and radiation have minimal effects on the ocular motility disturbances. Strabismus surgery for larger deviations of restrictive myopathy can be considered after the deviation has been documented as unchanged over 6 mo to 1 yr.

MEDICAL MANAGEMENT

Corticosteroids

Corticosteroids are the mainstay of pharmacologic therapy for Graves' ophthalmopathy and may be used alone or in combination with other immunosuppression, radiation, or surgery. Steroid suppression of lymphocytes and fibroblasts that mediate the autoimmune response presumably reduces local orbital inflammation and edema. Soft tissue changes may improve rapidly with corticosteroids, although high doses are required initially to obtain significant clinical effects. In a typical regimen, prednisone, 60 to 100 mg orally, is given in three to four divided doses daily for several days and then tapered over several weeks (Fig. 169–2). Steroid administration once daily or on alternate days is not sufficiently effective in suppressing this disease process. In some clinical studies, megadose intravenous prednisolone has been effective for acute, severe "malignant" exophthalmos. The effect of corticosteroids is only temporary and is effective only while the drug is being given. The disease process rebounds promptly with cessation of therapy unless therapy is extended over many months or years with very gradual tapering. Such extended therapy is usually impractical because of side effects.

Steroid therapy is particularly useful for patients with acute inflammatory eye symptoms or signs and optic neuropathy, as well as patients with continued disease progression despite radiation or surgical therapy. Although optic neuropathy usually improves with corticosteroid therapy, this problem will likely rebound as the dose is tapered below 40 mg of prednisone daily; however, this dose threshold varies with different individuals. Several repeat steroid treatment courses are usually preferable to extended therapy. Radiation or surgical treatment should be considered as a more permanent remedy. Although corticosteroids have little effect on exophthalmos or on strabismus, perioperative corticosteroids are frequently useful in patients undergoing orbital decompression to limit the inflammatory response to surgical trauma. Not all patients respond well to corticosteroids, especially those with chronic orbit changes that are no longer inflammatory in nature. It may be difficult to wean successfully treated patients off corticosteroids without subsequent use of radiation therapy or immunosuppressive therapy. In general, ophthalmopathy continues to recur unless corticosteroid monotherapy is given continuously for the 1- to 3-yr period over which the disease may stabilize spontaneously.

Corticosteroid therapy, although effective in Graves' ophthalmopathy, has many contraindications and complications to be considered (Table 169–2). Long-term steroid therapy is impractical in most patients. Patients become Cushingoid on even low doses, and these effects are slow to resolve. Other common problems include gastrointestinal ulceration and hemorrhage, aggravation of diabetes and hypertension, generalized myopathy, weight gain, sleeplessness, psychosis or euphoria, and drug interactions. Less frequent problems of tuberculosis activation, vertebral spine collapse, and aseptic necrosis of the hips must be considered also. All patients receiving high-dose steroids require careful monitoring and consideration of alternative therapies. Starting corticosteroid treatment represents a commitment that should not be undertaken casually. Weaning patients

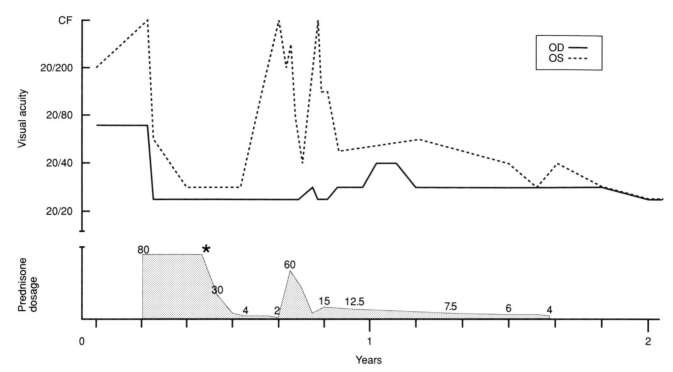

Figure 169–2. Response of visual acuity to systemic corticosteroids in a patient with Graves' disease and with bilateral optic nerve compromise. Horizontal axis is a time scale over 2 yr. Lower vertical axis plots daily prednisone dosage. Upper vertical axis plots visual acuity of each eye separately. A prompt dramatic improvement of visual acuity occurred with high-dose steroids. Dosage was tapered when duodenal ulcer developed (*asterisk*). Vision deteriorated at lower steroid dose and responded again to elevated dose. Steroid dose was successfully tapered, with stabilization of vision over 2 yr. No other therapy was used for the ophthalmopathy. (OD, right eye; OS, left eye; CF, counting fingers acuity.)

off steroids presents problems also because the symptoms of Graves' disease may return.

There have been attempts to reduce the systemic effects of corticosteroids using local administration by retrobulbar injection. Although soft tissue signs may improve, the response rate with local injection is much lower in comparison with systemic administration of corticosteroids. Suppression of the systemic autoimmune process causing orbitopathy is less likely to occur with local steroids. Furthermore, injection risks are increased significantly with the tight, congestive, and inflexible orbital tissues found in Graves' disease. A clinical situation in which local injection of corticosteroids may be helpful is when systemic therapy is contraindicated and other therapies are not immediately effective.

Other Immunosuppressive Therapy

Immunosuppression of Graves' orbitopathy may be partially achieved with other agents, most notably cyclosporine. Reports using cyclosporine have shown variable results. A randomized clinical trial demonstrated a 61 percent response to corticosteroid therapy compared with a 22 percent response using cyclosporine alone. Because corticosteroids are more effective, monotherapy with cyclosporine may be indicated only when other therapies are impractical. Lower doses of cyclosporine may be useful in combination with corticosteroids for longer-term maintenance therapy or to reduce disease relapse after steroid taper and cessation. Side effects of nephrotoxicity and hypertension must be considered with cyclosporine therapy. Cyclophosphamide, methotrexate, and azathioprine have been used with equivocal results. Serious complications of these agents, including bone marrow suppression and sterility, limit their usefulness. In general, immunomodulation may reduce orbital inflammation modestly but have little effect on exophthalmos.

Table 169–2. SYSTEMIC CORTICOSTEROIDS: SIDE EFFECTS AND COMPLICATIONS

Cushingoid appearance
Weight gain, increased appetite, sodium retention
Mental status alterations (sleeplessness, psychosis, depression, euphoria)
Gastrointestinal irritation, ulceration, hemorrhage
Drug interactions, especially anticoagulants
Hypertension
Diabetes mellitus
Infection susceptibility (tuberculosis, fungi, bacteria)
Cataracts
Glaucoma
Vertebral spine collapse
Aseptic necrosis of hips
Adrenal gland suppression (vulnerability to stress, surgery)
Steroid dependence (risk of abrupt discontinuation of medication)
Death
Failure to improve the condition

Bromocriptine, a dopamine receptor binding agent, has a variety of effects, including suppression of prolactin levels, inhibition of thyroid-stimulating hormones, and anti–T lymphocyte action, that are theoretically beneficial for Graves' disease. Reported results using bromocriptine are modestly encouraging and without any significant side effects.

Plasmapheresis, or plasma exchange therapy, is based on the concept that removal of humoral factors in an autoimmune process may lead to clinical improvement. It can be effective in acute forms of Graves' orbitopathy, but rebound of the disease process is likely if plasma exchange is not followed with immunosuppressive therapy. Although rapid improvement seems evident with this treatment, interpretation of studies is difficult because of concurrent steroid or cytotoxic drug therapy. Recurrence in greater than 35 percent of patients so treated required repeated courses of plasmapheresis, albeit with shorter courses of immunosuppression. Disadvantages of plasmapheresis include expense, hospitalization, and potentially fatal complications.

ORBITAL RADIATION THERAPY

Local radiation therapy for orbit diseases has been used for more than 50 yr. Application in the early 1970s of newer megavoltage delivery systems producing a collimated photon beam permitted more discrete low-dose treatment regimens with fewer undesirable effects. Use of orbital radiation has become increasingly popular for treatment of Graves' orbitopathy as a substitute for or as an adjunct to corticosteroids and surgery. Evaluation of the effect of radiation is frequently complicated, however, by concurrent use of other treatments.

The mechanism of radiation's therapeutic effect in Graves' orbitopathy appears to be suppression of pathogenic orbit lymphocytes that are exquisitely sensitive and possibly suppression of fibroblasts also. Active orbit inflammation and congestion are reduced but with minimal improvement of swollen extraocular muscles and fat. Although similar to the local effects of corticosteroids, radiation effects are often less dramatic but more prolonged than the transient effects of steroids. Dose and delivery systems for low-dose orbital radiation generally follow the protocol of Donaldson and colleagues reported in 1973 (Fig. 169–3). A computed tomographic (CT) scan is used for dosimetric mapping. The radiation field is concentrated in the posterior orbit incorporating an area from the lateral bony rim anteriorly to the border of the sella turcica posteriorly. Right and left treatment fields are individualized to avoid unintended cross-radiation of the opposite orbit, and secondary blocking shields are used to avoid the lens and retina as much as practical. A cobalt-60 unit delivers a well-collimated photon beam with total dose of 2000 cGy (or rads) delivered in 10 fractions over 2 wk.

Interpretation of data on orbital radiation therapy is complicated by several factors. There is a lack of standardized protocol of treatment and no consensus on clinical criteria for judging results. The stage of the disease at the time of treatment has a major influence on effectiveness. Early treatment of active inflammation is very successful, whereas late treatment of chronic orbit changes is almost completely ineffective. Use of adjunctive corticosteroids or other immunosuppression or orbit surgery preceding, concurrent with, or after radiation makes separation of effects of each modality impossible. Because the effectiveness of radiation tends to parallel the results of high-dose systemic corticosteroids, a steroid trial serves as a useful test for consideration of radiation therapy.

Trends of radiation therapy that have emerged consistently are as follows: (1) Active orbit inflammation and congestion are reduced significantly in 75 to 85 percent of cases; (2) optic neuropathy is improved in 65 to 85 percent of cases, with the most severely affected eyes showing the greatest degree of improvement (Figs.

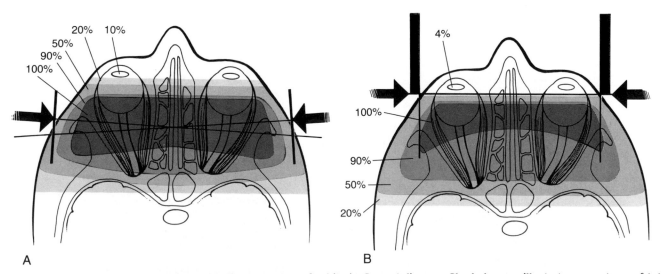

Figure 169–3. Radiation dosimetry mapping for treatment of orbits in Graves' disease. Shaded areas illustrate percentage of total radiation dose that is delivered to different portions of the orbits. *Arrows* indicate radiation beam directions from both sides. Crossover radiation is included in calculations. *A,* Angled collimated external radiation beam concentrates delivery to the posterior orbit. *B,* Lead shields are used to block radiation from anterior globes.

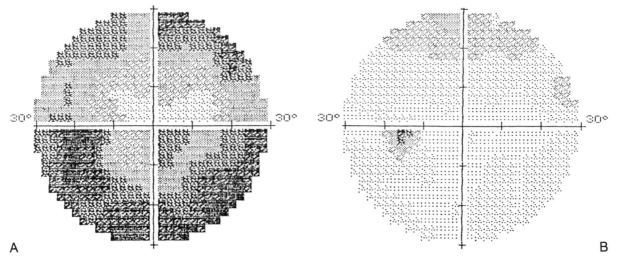

Figure 169–4. Visual field plots of a patient with Graves' disease with optic nerve compromise (left eye). *A*, Pretreatment visual field defects demonstrate generalized depression of sensitivity, peripheral constriction, and an inferior altitudinal hemianopia. Visual acuity was 20/80 with minimal dyschromatopsia and afferent pupillary defect. Opposite right eye had similar findings of lesser degree. *B*, Visual field plot of same eye 6 wk after completion of orbital radiation treatment shows complete resolution of field defects. Visual acuity, color perception, and pupillary response recovered to normal. There was no recurrence of this problem.

169–4 and 169–5); (3) exophthalmos improves very minimally with only 1 to 2 mm of proptosis reduction; (4) strabismus generally shows little change; (5) chronic orbit changes show no improvement. Beneficial effects of radiation occur within 1 to 8 wk of treatment. Changes after that time may be attributable to the fundamental disease course. Repeat radiation treatment is not advisable because of cumulative dose-related complications.

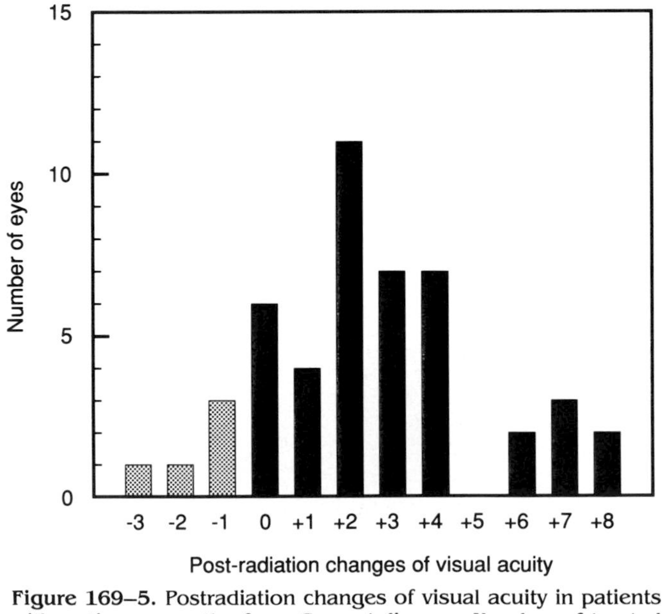

Radiation therapy usually eliminates corticosteroid dependency and permits patients to be tapered off steroids rapidly and completely. Low-dose radiation does not seem to increase orbital fibrosis, as some clinicians had thought, and, in fact, seems to make the effects of subsequent surgery more predictable and more effective by reducing inflammatory reaction first.

Complications of orbital radiation treatment are rare and usually relate to some sensitizing influences that accentuate radiation effects (Table 169–3). Secondary tumors do not occur at these low-dose levels. Cataracts and dry eyes are minimized with anterior orbital blocking techniques. Induced optic neuropathy has not been documented at these low doses. The primary risk is radiation-induced microangiopathy of the retinal vessels, which is manifested by macular hemorrhages, exudates, capillary nonperfusion, and neovascularization (Fig. 169–6). Development of retinopathy is generally delayed an average of 3 yr after exposure, although it has been described as early as 3 wk and as late as 7 yr after the treatment. Radiation retinopathy may occur at doses exceeding 3500 cGy but has been reported without extenuating circumstances only once at a dose level of 2000 cGy. Risk factors for this problem include systemic

Figure 169–5. Postradiation changes of visual acuity in patients with optic neuropathy from Graves' disease. Number of treated eyes are plotted vertically. Changes in Snellen's visual acuity lines are plotted horizontally. Of 47 treated eyes, visual acuity improved in 36, remained stable in 6, and worsened in 5. Eyes with the worst pretreatment vision improved the most. Eyes that worsened had additional problems of hypertensive or diabetic retinopathy. No other retina or optic nerve problems developed over 5 yr of follow-up.

Table 169–3. ORBITAL IRRADIATION: SIDE EFFECTS AND COMPLICATIONS

Skin burns and hair loss
Keratoconjunctivitis sicca
Corneal scarring
Cataracts
Retinal microangiopathy (accentuated by diabetes, chemotherapy)
Optic neuropathy
Pituitary gland dysfunction
Secondary malignant tumors
Growth retardation
Failure to improve the condition

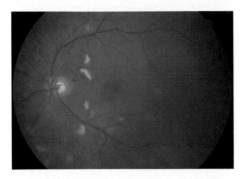

Figure 169–6. Retinopathy developing after orbital radiation therapy for lymphoma. Retina findings developed 2 yr after radiation and are characterized by exudates, hemorrhages, and capillary hypoperfusion indicating microangiopathy.

chemotherapy, which potentiates radiation effects, and microvascular vulnerability associated with diabetes mellitus. Because of potential undesirable radiation effects, caution must be observed in recommending this treatment for a benign and self-limited disease process. Several investigators experimented with lower-dose radiation protocols to reduce risks, but data are insufficient to judge therapeutic effectiveness. Because radiation dose effects are cumulative, repeat treatment should be avoided unless regarded as absolutely essential to preserve vision.

Although complications of low-dose radiation therapy are infrequent, avoidance of problems requires careful attention to technique, dosimetry, and risk factors by an experienced radiation therapist. Radiation is useful as a secondary or even a primary treatment modality for orbitopathy of Graves' disease. By reducing inflammation and congestion, radiation therapy creates an opportunity to wean patients off corticosteroids and also serves a useful preparation for orbit surgery to minimize postoperative inflammation.

SURGICAL MANAGEMENT

Introduction

Surgery can improve several aspects of the orbitopathy of Graves' disease. Unlike medical or radiation therapies that attempt to reduce inflammation and congestion, surgery produces mechanical alterations of distorted tissues in a definitive and permanent manner to relieve orbit pressure and to improve restricted functions. Surgical orbit decompression can relieve exophthalmos, exposure problems, globe prolapse anteriorly, and, most important, optic nerve compression. Strabismus repair can improve the noncomitant diplopia from restrictive myopathy of extraocular muscles. Eyelid adjustments of both upper and lower lids can provide better corneal protection, reduced exposure symptoms, and improved cosmesis. In addition to marked functional improvement and rehabilitation, the psychological benefits of surgery are often profound.

The major clinical problems to be addressed surgically are, in order of clinical importance, (1) optic neuropa-

thy, (2) diplopia, (3) corneal exposure, and (4) cosmesis. Different surgical procedures are required for each of these purposes, and they must be performed sequentially with a coordinated overall plan. If orbit decompression is deemed necessary, then it must be performed first because the decompression may alter the strabismus and lid position, often aggravating the former and improving the latter. After an appropriate interval for orbit soft tissue stabilization, strabismus repair is performed second and may require multiple procedures. Eyelid adjustments are the last procedures to be performed, proceeding from lid lengthening and tarsorrhaphy to blepharoplasty and anterior fat removal.

Applying conservative criteria for surgery in our patient population of Graves' orbitopathy, we found that approximately 33 percent of patients benefited from some surgical correction. Orbit decompression for medical necessity, rather than cosmetic improvement, was required by 10 percent of patients, strabismus repair by 11 percent, and eyelid procedures by 26 percent. Some patients had all three types of surgery and occasional repeat procedures. In most patients, lid procedures alone are quite sufficient to relieve exposure and improve cosmesis.

The timing of surgery is most important. Surgery during the acute phase of orbital inflammation and congestion is seldom advisable because the reactive process may be aggravated by surgery, and the results are likely to be suboptimal and unpredictable. Urgent surgery may be necessary on rare occasions for vision-threatening problems of optic neuropathy or corneal ulceration that have not responded adequately to other forms of therapy, but these situations are certainly exceptional. In general, surgery should await stabilization of the orbital disease process and be used to repair the consequences of the disease. Treatment before surgery with corticosteroids, immunosuppression, or radiation is often helpful in achieving a quiescent status that will permit more useful and predictable surgical results.

Orbit Decompression Surgery

Surgical decompression of the orbit produces mechanical enlargement of the confining space by partial removal of bony walls and periosteum, allowing prolapse of posterior orbital soft tissue into adjacent spaces and relieving pressure on the optic nerve and the globe. By this method, soft tissue pressure is relieved and the globe can be reposited up to 15 mm posteriorly, although generally 5 to 6 mm is achieved. Excessive decompression is undesirable because of significant secondary problems.

The primary indications for orbit decompression by conservative criteria are severe exophthalmos, globe prolapse anterior to the lids, exposure keratopathy, and, most important, optic nerve compression. Decompression for cosmetic purposes also has some advocates, but the procedure does have potential complications to consider. Patients with exophthalmos greater than 24 mm are often candidates for orbit decompression, whereas less proptotic eyes can usually be aided adequately by lid procedures alone. Surgery is most effective with a stabilized orbit that is no longer inflamed or progressive, and it often follows pretreatment medically or with radiation. Conversely, chronic fibrotic orbit tissues achieve less effect from decompression compared with softer, congested tissues, so that optimal timing does influence results.

Anatomic surgical approaches for orbit decompression are multiple. The bony orbit configuration resembles a cone with four definable walls that are surrounded by ethmoid sinus medially, maxillary antrum inferiorly, temporal fossa laterally, and cranial cavity superiorly. Any of the walls are available for partial removal to facilitate orbit soft tissue prolapse into the adjacent spaces (Fig. 169–7). The air-filled spaces of the sinuses offer the best opportunities for greatest volume prolapse, whereas the temporal fossa provides more space than suspected, and the orbit roof provides the least. Each procedure can be referred to by its anatomic location or the eponym of its originator.

The Krönlein orbitotomy for removal of the lateral orbital rim is performed via a 2-cm skin incision extending from the lateral canthus toward the ear (Fig. 169–8A). Temporalis muscle and periosteum are separated from bone on both sides of the rim. An oscillating saw and a heavy rongeur facilitate removal of a 2½ × 3-cm section of bone laterally, which may include the orbital rim. Alternatively, the rim may remain in place or be replaced by wiring. Lateral orbital periosteum is incised widely to allow generous prolapse of orbital fat into the temporal fossa of the skull, which provides a fairly generous space. Closure of this orbitotomy involves only subcutaneous layers and skin, leaving the deeper tissue widely separated.

The orbital floor and medial wall can be approached by several routes. An inferior fornix conjunctival incision or an external lower eyelid skin incision will allow access to the orbital floor, where periosteum is then elevated to expose the entirely bony orbital floor and the lower half of the medial wall (see Fig. 169–8B). Chisels and rongeurs are used to create a large osteotomy. Generally, it is necessary only to remove the medial orbit floor, stopping at the inferoorbital neurovascular bundle, and extending to a depth of 3½ cm posteriorly. The osteotomy may then be extended posterior to the lacrimal sac and medially along the ethmoid sinus, stopping short of the ethmoidal arteries. Maxillary antrum mucosa and ethmoid air cells are removed to create large spaces into which orbital fat is prolapsed by incising periosteum. Only the conjunctiva or skin require closure.

An alternative for even wider and deeper medial orbital wall removal of the optic canal posteriorly is an external ethmoidectomy approach via a medial skin incision with or without removal of the nasal turbinates (see Fig. 169–8C). A Caldwell-Luc procedure popularized by Ogura may be performed by entry into the maxillary antrum through a bone window created over the gums (see Fig. 169–8D). The orbital floor is removed from below, avoiding the infraorbital neurovascular bundle, and the osteotomy is carried up onto the medial orbital wall into the ethmoid sinus. Visualization toward

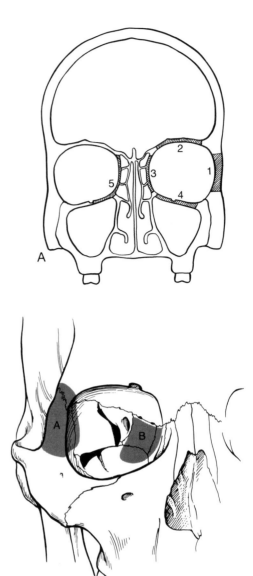

Figure 169–7. Skull diagrams of orbit decompression procedures. *A*, Frontal section of the orbits depicts cross-hatched areas of bone removal with various surgical approaches: (1) lateral orbitotomy (Krönlein's operation); (2) orbit unroofing via craniotomy (Naffziger's operation); (3) medial wall removal and ethmoidectomy; (4) orbit floor removal; (5) combined ethmoidectomy and medial orbit floor (Ogura). *B*, Three-quarter view of skull with shaded areas of bone removal using lateral *(A)*, and medial, with a partial orbit floor combination *(B)* to achieve a 2½ wall decompression.

the orbital apex is somewhat limited through this approach, and only a partial ethmoid decompression may result. Advancing technology of nasal endoscopic surgery makes possible an inferomedial orbital decompression via the nasal mucosa (see Fig. 169–8E). Using video control through the endoscope, small scalpels and rongeurs are used for a complete ethmoidectomy, medial orbital wall removal, and a partial orbital floor removal. Naffziger's procedure for orbital roof removal requires a frontotemporal craniotomy approach. This procedure has higher risks and morbidity and achieves less decompression effect than the other procedures. It is seldom performed as the primary procedure for this

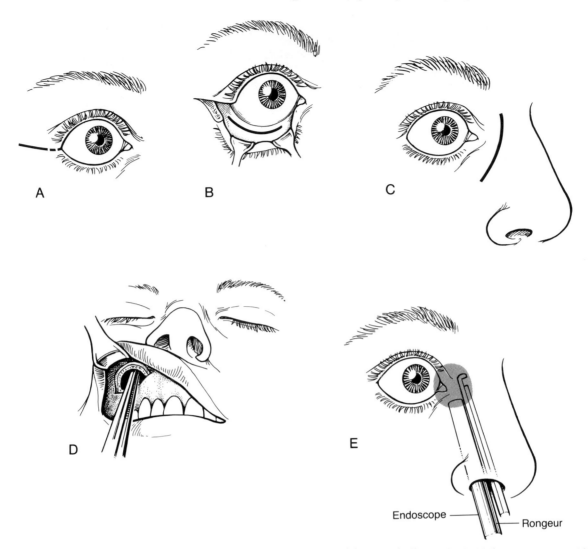

Figure 169–8. Surgical approaches for orbit decompression procedures. Incisions are indicated by bold lines. *A,* Lateral skin incision with or without severing of the canthus for removal of the temporal orbit wall. Bony rim of the orbit may be removed or replaced optionally. *B,* Inferior fornix conjunctival incision with or without lateral canthoplasty for orbit floor removal and partial inferomedial wall removal. Access is insufficient for a complete ethmoidectomy. *C,* Skin incisions for a complete external ethmoidectomy and medial orbit wall removal along with partial orbit floor removal. Orbit apex is accessible by this approach. *D,* Caldwell-Luc approach via superior gums with osteotomy into the maxillary antrum with exposure from below of orbit floor and medial orbit wall to the orbit apex. *E,* Nasal endoscopic approach via nasal mucosa for exposure of entire medial orbit wall and limited medial orbit floor.

purpose but may be used in severe cases to supplement other decompression procedures.

With surgical orbital decompressions, the bone removal area approximates 2 × 3 cm on each wall with most techniques. It is important to leave some bone support for the globe inferiorly to prevent its subluxation. Periosteum incisions and active prolapse of orbital fat with breakup of fibrous septae are essential to achieving good decompression effect. Extraocular muscles prolapse also but do so passively and less dramatically than the fat. Drainage of the surgical areas is usually unnecessary, and packing is contraindicated. Systemic steroids are continued in the perioperative period if the patient has been taking steroids previously. Antibiotics are an option but may not be essential in many patients.

Each surgical approach has its merits and deficiencies. Surgeons commonly combine two or three approaches

to achieve adequate decompression and to distribute the prolapse of tissues into more than one direction for a balanced result (Fig. 169–9). The procedures are tailored to the needs of individual patients, with consideration of the degree of desired decompression, the desirability of reaching the orbital apex (as with optic neuropathy), and the suitability of skin incisions or hidden incisions. Inferomedial and lateral approaches are most popular, whereas the superior orbital roof approach is currently seldom used except occasionally in combination with other walls. Individual surgeons have their own preferences for approaches and techniques.

Complications of orbital decompression surgery are infrequent but can be serious. Postoperative hemorrhage, infection, and exacerbation of the Graves' inflammatory process are usually readily treated problems. Damage to the infraorbital nerve and artery or to the

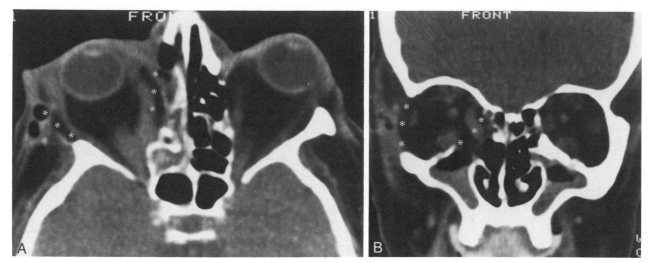

Figure 169–9. Computed tomographic scans after unilateral right-sided orbit decompression illustrating areas of bone removal and soft tissue prolapse. *A,* Axial scan with removal of lateral orbit wall and medial wall combined with ethmoidectomy. *B,* Coronal scan plane with additional depiction of partial orbit floor removal medially. *Asterisks* indicate previous bone locations.

nasolacrimal drainage system are generally avoidable with good visualization during surgery. Contraction scarring or keloid formation may result from skin incisions, and fistulas may develop with mucosal approaches. Excessive displacement of the globe, extraocular muscles, and eyelids can result from large decompression procedures, creating significant difficulties later. Secondary enophthalmos from aggressive decompression is extremely difficult to correct. It is not infrequent, however, for strabismus to be aggravated by any orbit decompression and to require later repair for correction of diplopia. The most severe operative complications result from inadvertent perforation of the cribriform area causing cerebrospinal fluid leak or subarachnoid hemorrhage or from direct damage to the optic nerve at the orbital apex causing loss of vision. Experienced surgical technique in a carefully controlled nonaggressive approach is essential to minimizing these potential surgical complications. Surgery is often facilitated by combined ophthalmology, otolaryngology, and neurosurgery participation.

Strabismus Surgery

Diplopia is one of the most functionally disabling aspects of Graves' disease. Because it is due to asymmetric restriction of the extraocular muscles, the motility imbalance is complex and noncomitant with both vertical and horizontal components. This differs significantly from a paretic muscle problem. It also fluctuates unpredictably because, like the orbitopathy in general, the motility imbalance goes through an acute inflammatory phase that may be prolonged before stabilizing into a chronic fibrotic phase. Similarly, initial therapy of the strabismus must be temporary, perhaps using changeable prisms, and definitive treatment with surgery must await the later stable phase of the disease. Steroids, immunosuppression, and radiation tend to have little impact on the ocular motility imbalance. Muscle surgery is the only definitive treatment. Premature surgical in-

tervention, however, can be counterproductive and very difficult to correct later.

All of the extraocular muscles of both orbits are probably affected to some degree in Graves' disease. For unknown reasons, the inferior rectus and the medial rectus muscles are the most commonly affected, resulting in hypotropia and esotropia deviations. It is probably more than coincidence that these are the most frequently used muscles for normal functioning of downgaze and convergence, and their involvement produces symptomatic diplopia. Occasionally, superior and lateral recti are affected predominantly, causing hyper- and exodeviations. In contrast, involvement of the oblique muscles is rarely significant clinically. Apparent unilaterality or asymmetry of muscle involvement between the two orbits is more relative than real because several muscles are usually involved, but with the resulting imbalance implicating one or two muscles most prominently. CT imaging correlates reasonably well with individual muscle involvement, identifying the more swollen muscles producing the most restriction.

The degrees of muscle imbalance vary tremendously. As little as 2 prism diopters of strabismus can be symptomatic for vertical deviations and esodeviations, sometimes only as the perception of "blurred" vision. Cyclodeviations exceeding 10 degrees are symptomatic also. Dramatic large deviations may exceed 40 prism diopters, with the most affected muscle incapable of any motion. Plotting diplopia fields with a Hess chart or Lancaster red-green testing is helpful in assessing the degree of surgery that may be useful. The muscle imbalance may be aggravated by orbital decompression surgery. Whenever there is extensive removal of an orbital wall, the adjacent rectus muscle prolapses into the enlarged space and becomes functionally shortened, thus increasing the restrictive effect of that muscle. This is particularly notable for medial and inferior recti, producing increased esotropia after ethmoidal decompression or hypotropia after antral decompression (Fig. 169–10).

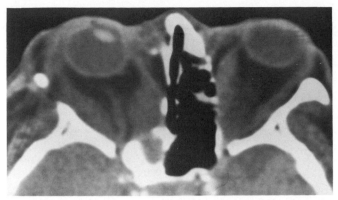

Figure 169–10. Computed tomographic scan after a combined lateral, medial, and inferomedial decompression of right orbit. Markedly enlarged medial rectus muscle has prolapsed toward the nasal septum with relief of optic nerve compression. Muscle prolapse has accentuated esotropia by functionally shortening this restrictive muscle.

The goal of strabismus treatment is to create adequate muscle balance for fusion of images in straightforward and downgaze positions. Because it is seldom possible to relieve diplopia in all gaze positions, there is frequently residual diplopia in upgaze and lateral gaze. A limited area of fusion may be achieved with the use of prisms in glasses, as previously described, for smaller angles of deviation below 8 to 10 prism diopters. This often requires combined horizontal and vertical prisms. Larger deviations generally require strabismus surgery.

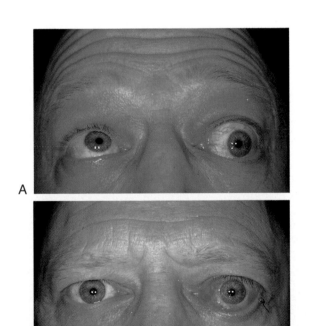

Figure 169–11. Strabismus surgical correction for restrictive myopathy in Graves' disease. A, Preoperative findings demonstrate restriction of left inferior rectus muscle on attempted upgaze. B, Postoperative recession of inferior rectus muscle achieves vertical alignment and fusion of images. Retraction of lower eyelid results from most inferior rectus recessions and may be corrected by minimal lid surgery at the initial procedure or later.

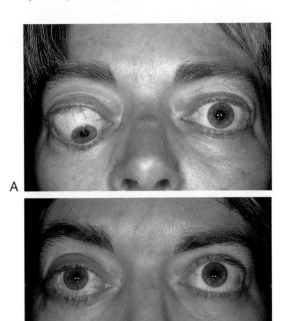

Figure 169–12. Orbitopathy of Graves' disease with asymmetric exophthalmos, eyelid retraction, and strabismus. A, Hypotropia and esotropia deviations of the right eye are characteristic. B, Postoperative right orbit decompression, strabismus repair (recession of inferior and medial recti), and lid correction (levator recession) result in fusion of images in primary and downgaze positions and acceptable general appearance with relief of exposure.

These strabismus deviations should be stable by reproducible prism measurements for 6 mo to 1 yr before considering surgery.

Guidelines for surgical corrections of this strabismus are to seek a slight undercorrection of hypotropia, and, conversely, slight overcorrection of hyperdeviation, whereas esodeviations are best overcorrected slightly and exodeviations undercorrected (Figs. 169–11 and 169–12). These principles relate to the preeminent importance of the primary and downgaze positions and the reserve capabilities of globe depression and convergence. A and V patterns are of less importance than the dominant vertical and horizontal deviations. Muscle recessions are the preferable technique, with marginal myotomies as supplementary procedures. Muscle resections should be avoided if possible, because all the muscles are likely to be partially involved in the fibrotic process.

Criteria for the amount of muscle surgery are (1) preoperative prism measurements that are maximized with use of the Maddox rod and (2) forced-duction testing of individual muscles at the time of surgery, which is best accomplished under general anesthesia or complete muscle block anesthesia. The effect of muscle surgery varies between 2.5 to 4.0 prism diopters per millimeter of muscle relocation. More restrictive muscles tend to yield more effect per millimeter of relocation. An average effect of 3 prism diopters per millimeter can be used in most calculations. Conservative maximal amounts of muscle recession should be used to avoid locating muscles too close to the globe equator, thus altering the mechanical fulcrum of muscle action and reducing its range of motion. Inferior and medial recti can be recessed safely up to 6 to 7 mm; superior and lateral recti can be recessed further, if necessary. Adjustable sutures are an individual surgeon preference that may be helpful, although they may be limited to one muscle in each eye and may be difficult to manage in thyroid patients with increased anxiety (Fig. 169–13). Furthermore, the strabismus status on the first postoperative day is not always representative of the result obtained after several months when the muscle has undergone continued fibrosis or advancement.

Combined horizontal and vertical muscle surgery is often performed simultaneously, taking into account that some of the adducting influence of the inferior rectus will be altered by its recession. Limiting surgery to two rectus muscles for each eye is probably a wise precaution to reduce the risk of anterior segment ischemia, which may be accentuated with these already abnormal extraocular muscles. A series reported by Rootman and colleagues had 63 percent combined vertical and horizontal deviations. The frequency of pro-

cedures on individual muscles was 49 percent for medial rectus, 41 percent for inferior rectus, 8 percent for superior rectus, 1 percent for lateral rectus, and 0 percent for oblique muscles. One muscle was operated in 50 percent of patients, two muscles in 27 percent, and three or more muscles (two eyes) in 23 percent.

Approximately 80 percent of patients achieve adequate correction with one operation if all components of the strabismus are addressed at once. Later changes in strabismus may occur, however, and require reoperation. This may be due to disease progression with more muscles becoming involved, more muscle restriction, or spontaneous advancement of muscle insertions by fibrosis. Secondary strabismus repairs for deviations exceeding 8 to 10 prism diopters may be necessary in about 10 percent of patients but should be delayed 6 mo or more unless a muscle is grossly misaligned. Lower eyelid retraction is an inevitable consequence of large recessions of the inferior rectus. Treatment of this is discussed later in the chapter and may be simultaneous with strabismus surgery.

Botulinum toxin treatment to produce partial temporary denervation of restricted muscles may have a limited role in the early course of Graves' disease. Such denervation has been proposed to reduce development of muscle fibrosis, but this effect is speculative. Results of botulinum injections are difficult to evaluate. There is no adequate series of treated patients, effects tend to be nonspecific and unpredictable for individual muscles, and complications include a spreading effect of the drug and undesired lid effects. Caution is best observed in considering this experimental approach. Ultimately, strabismus surgery is likely to be necessary for most of these patients.

Eyelid Surgery

Eyelid retraction often dominates the clinical appearance of Graves' disease patients, giving them the characteristic "stare." In addition to cosmetic disfigurement, lid retraction causes exposure symptoms of dry eyes and can lead to incomplete lid closure and corneal ulceration or scarring. The components of lid retraction are the smooth Müller's muscle, the striated levator muscle of the upper lid, and the analogous retractor muscle of the lower lid. These muscles are initially subject to the sympathomimetic effects of hyperthyroidism. This phase may improve spontaneously with metabolic stabilization. Guanethidine eye drops may provide temporary relief but are not very satisfactory in most patients.

With development of congestive orbitopathy, the eyelid muscles undergo the same pathologic changes as do the rectus muscles, proceeding from acute inflammation to chronic fibrosis and restriction. The restrictive effect produces typical lid lag on downgaze and may be accentuated by accompanying exophthalmos and by a restrictive inferior rectus muscle. Lid retraction can give the false impression of more globe proptosis than is actually present. Steroids and radiation have minimal effects on lid retraction. Treatment is basically surgical after the lids have stabilized.

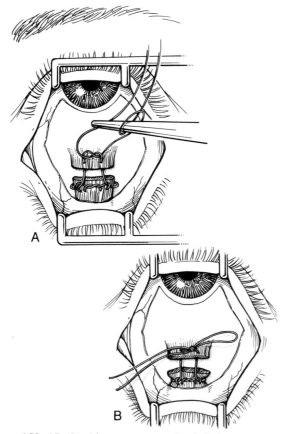

Figure 169–13. Strabismus surgery for inferior rectus muscle recession using an adjustable suture. *A,* The muscle is detached after securing a suture through the muscle tendon near its insertion. Sutures may be reinserted directly into sclera at the predetermined distance posteriorly. *B,* Alternatively, the suture may be placed lax at the original insertion with a slipknot and then adjusted within a few hours using prisms to determine its desired location.

The timing of lid surgery, as with other aspects of Graves' disease, is most important. Surgery too early in the disease course may have to be readjusted or entirely reversed later. Any anticipated orbital decompression or strabismus surgery must be completed before lid surgery. Orbital decompression may improve the component of lid retraction that is due to distortion from the proptotic globe. Strabismus surgery may relieve the compensatory component related to restrictive extraocular muscles, particularly when inferior rectus restriction accentuates upper eyelid retraction by excessive attempts by the patient to elevate the globe. Conversely, large recessions of the inferior rectus muscle nearly always cause more lower lid retraction because of common attachments to the capsulopalpebral fascia.

Several surgical procedures are available to improve eyelid retraction, often in combinations. The options include (1) lateral tarsorrhaphy, (2) Müller's and levator muscle lengthening, (3) lower eyelid elevation, and (4) blepharoplasty with orbital fat excision. Tarsorrhaphy is a simple nondestructive option that is easily reversible and, therefore, may serve as a temporary or permanent lid correction. It consists of fusion of opposing tarsal surfaces of upper and lower lids at the lateral canthus and extending medially a distance of 5 to 8 mm. Variations include shaving or splitting the tarsus and joining the surfaces with a mattressed suture secured on a bolster, preferably preserving the lashes of both lid margins. The net effect of tarsorrhaphy is greater in elevating the lower lid rather than lowering the upper lid, which has stronger opposing forces of the levator muscle. Tarsorrhaphy alone may suffice for minor exposure problems and may be combined with other procedures also. Müllerectomy alone may suffice for smaller degrees of lid retraction, augmented by levator recession for a larger effect.

The elevating muscles of the upper lid, Müller's and levator, are often greatly reinforced in their actions by the restrictive myopathy of Graves' disease. The surgical goal of weakening or lengthening these muscles to relieve eyelid retraction can be achieved in several ways with coarsely graded results. Unfortunately, however, all methods are somewhat arbitrary rather than truly quantitative. The muscles can be detached partially or entirely from their attachments to tarsus and skin. Müller's muscle can be excised in a horizontal strip to weaken it definitively without any reattachment (Fig. 169–14). Levator aponeurosis can be resuspended by sling sutures to the tarsal edge after achieving the desired spacing to relieve lid retraction, or the levator can be lengthened instead by marginal myotomies (Fig. 169–15). Spacer materials using bank sclera or other materials can be placed between the detached muscle and the tarsal border as a lengthening procedure (Fig. 169–16). The lateral aspect of the lid must be lengthened the most, along with cutting of the lateral horn of levator aponeurosis. These procedures alter the skin folds and result unavoidably in elevation of the lid crease.

The choice of operative technique for Müller's and levator muscles is based on the degree of lid retraction. Müllerectomy and modest levator lengthening can be accomplished via a posterior conjunctival approach,

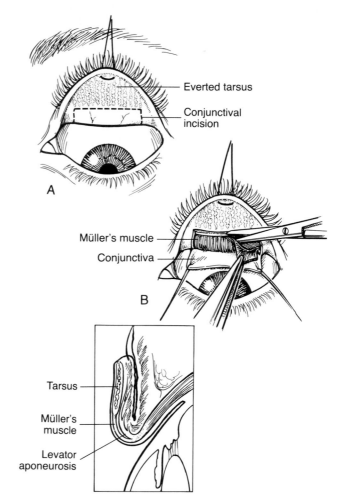

Figure 169–14. Upper eyelid lengthening surgery through a posterior approach. *A,* Eversion of the eyelid on a traction suture exposes the superior tarsal border, along which a conjunctival incision is made extending the entire width of the lid. *B,* Müller's muscle is dissected free of tarsus anteriorly and conjunctiva posteriorly a distance of 1 to 1½ cm, and a horizontal strip of the muscle is excised. Levator aponeurosis is then incised horizontally across its lateral two thirds, combined with a radial cut of the lateral canthal tendon attachment. Preservation of an intact medial portion of levator is desirable. Placing the lid on traction for several days postoperatively accentuates the ptosis effect.

whereas larger corrections require external skin approach for thorough access to the entire levator aponeurosis. The lacrimal gland ductules must be respected and avoided to prevent producing dry-eye problems. Upper lid retraction more than 3 mm above the limbus will likely require an external skin approach, whereas lesser degrees may be done via the posterior conjunctival approach with less elaborate procedures (Fig. 169–17). Lid traction for several days postoperatively is useful to maintain the surgical effect, because the lids have a tendency to repair themselves toward their former preoperative positions, obviating any improvement.

Lower eyelid elevation involves detachment and recession of lower lid retractor muscles and capsulopalpebral fascia across the entire width of the lid. The muscle edge can be reattached to orbicularis muscle 6 to 8 mm posteriorly, or spacer material (sclera or nasal,

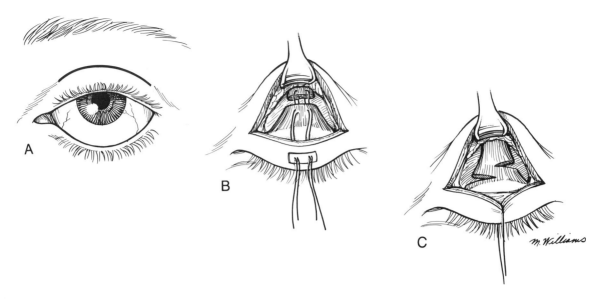

Figure 169–15. Upper eyelid lengthening surgery through an anterior approach. *A,* Skin incision is located in the upper lid crease to expose tarsus and levator aponeurosis posteriorly. *B,* Levator may be detached completely and resuspended to tarsus with sling sutures adjusted to produce adequate lengthening. *C,* Levator may be lengthened by staggered marginal myotomies crossing the midline.

buccal, or ear cartilage) can be inserted, as with the upper lid. Again, lid traction postoperatively helps preserve the surgical effect and prevent contracture of tissues during the early healing phase. The lower lid correction can be augmented with some lateral tarsorrhaphy.

Blepharoplasty has a modified role in Graves' orbitopathy, but must be performed with caution. The goal of blepharoplasty in this setting is to excise prolapsing orbital fat and tighten the lids horizontally but not vertically. The inflammatory disease process causes skin and fat to be more fibrous or less pliable than normal. Fat can be excised generously through lid incisions as

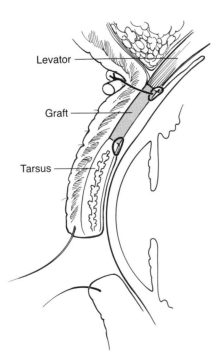

Figure 169–16. Cross-section diagram of upper eyelid anatomy depicts detachment of Müller's muscle and levator with insertion of graft material between levator and tarsus to produce lengthening of the upper lid.

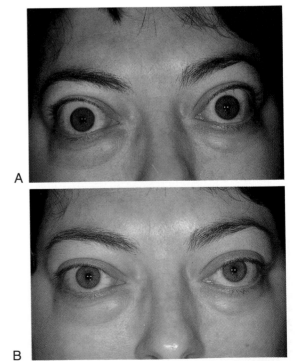

Figure 169–17. Surgical correction of upper eyelid retraction in Graves' disease. *A,* Preoperative bilateral eyelid retraction shows typical lateral accentuation. *B,* Postoperative levator and Müller's recessions via posterior approach produced a more normal eyelid level with adequate closure.

long as orbital structures are not incorporated and hemostasis is maintained. Minimal skin excision is usually best to avoid foreshortening the abnormal lid tissues too much.

Surgical eyelid corrections are the most common procedures performed for Graves' patients and often suffice to provide adequate corneal protection, relief of external exposure symptoms, and cosmetic improvement that masks small degrees of exophthalmos. The most common complication of eyelid surgery for Graves' disease is some asymmetry of lid position on comparison of the two sides. Usually the overall improvement of lid position overshadows minor degrees of asymmetry. Occasionally, significant lid asymmetry requires reoperation several months later. Elevation of the upper eyelid fold is inevitable with many of the lid operations. Other postoperative problems include eyelid thickening or edema, suture granuloma, or wound infection. Extrusion of or reaction to a lid implant may require its removal. More serious problems that can be avoided with careful surgical technique are loss of eyelashes, dry eye from lacrimal ductules transection, and epiphora from canalicular transection. The positive psychologic effects of eyelid improvement can be profound in many patients who lose much of their anxiety over this disease when their eyelids are improved.

SUMMARY

The orbitopathy of Graves' disease spans a spectrum from minor eye signs and symptoms to severe, disabling, vision-threatening problems. Patients with all degrees of this disorder can be helped through a variety of topical measures, medications (corticosteroids, immunosuppressives), local radiation, and surgical procedures. Surgery is very effective in improving the difficult problems of eyelid retraction, exophthalmos, diplopia, corneal exposure, and optic neuropathy.

The Graves' disease process is prolonged, however. The disease course itself, which cannot be altered substantially, extends over 1 to 3 yr, and the sequence of treatments extends for several months. The sequence and timing of treatment are important to obtain optimal results. Although restoration of complete normality may not be entirely practical, essentially all patients with Graves' orbitopathy can be rehabilitated functionally and cosmetically.

BIBLIOGRAPHY

For sections General Considerations, Local Treatment Measures, and Medical Management

Agapitos PJ, Hart IR: Long-term follow-up of ophthalmic Graves' disease. Can Med Assoc J 136:369, 1987.
Apers RC, Oosterhuis JA, Bierlaagh JJM: Indications and results of prednisone treatment in thyroid ophthalmopathy Ophthalmologica 173:163, 1976.
Atkinson S, Holcombe M, Kendall-Taylor P: Ophthalmopathic immunoglobulin in patients with Graves' ophthalmopathy. Lancet 2:374, 1984.
Bahn RS, Garrity JA, Bartley GB, Gorman CA: Diagnostic evaluation of Graves' ophthalmopathy. Endocrinol Metab Clin North Am 17:527, 1988.

Bahn RS, Gorman CA: Choice of therapy and criteria for assessing treatment outcome in thyroid-associated ophthalmopathy. Endocrinol Metab Clin North Am 16:391, 1987.
Bartalena L, Marcocci C, Bogazzi F, et al: Use of corticosteroids to prevent progression of Graves' ophthalmopathy after radioiodine therapy for hyperthyroidism. N Engl J Med 321:1349, 1989
Bartalena L, Marcocci C, Chiovato L, et al: Orbital cobalt irradiation combined with systemic corticosteroids for Graves' ophthalmopathy: Comparison with systemic corticosteroids alone. J Clin Endocrinol Metab 56:1139, 1983.
Bigos ST, Nisula BC, Daniels GH: Cyclophosphamide in the management of advanced Graves' optic neuropathy. Ann Intern Med 90:921, 1979.
Brabant G, Peter H, Becker H, et al: Cyclosporin in infiltrative eye disease [letter]. Lancet 1:515, 1984.
Brown J, Coburn JW, Wigod RA, et al: Adrenal steroid therapy of severe infiltrative ophthalmopathy of Graves' disease. Am J Med 34:786, 1963.
Buffam FV, Rootman J: Lid retraction—Its diagnosis and treatment. Int Ophthalmol Clin 18:75, 1978.
Cant JS, Lewis DR: Unwanted pharmacological effects of local guanethidine in the treatment of dysthyroid upper lid protraction. Br J Ophthalmol 53:239, 1969.
Cant JS, Lewis DR, Harrison MT: Treatment of dysthyroid ophthalmopathy with local guanethidine. Br J Ophthalmol 53:233, 1969.
Carlson RE, Scheribel KW, Hering PJ, et al: Exophthalmos, global luxation, rapid weight gain: Differential diagnosis. Ann Ophthalmol 14:724, 1982.
Cartlidge NE, Crombie A, Anderson J, et al: Critical study of 5 percent guanethidine in ocular manifestations of Graves' disease. Br J Med 4:645, 1969.
Char DH: Thyroid Eye Disease, 2nd ed. New York, Churchill Livingstone, 1990.
Char DH, Norman D: The use of computed tomography and ultrasonography in the evaluation of orbital masses. Surv Ophthalmol 27:49, 1982.
Dallow RL: Evaluation of unilateral exophthalmos with ultrasonography: Analysis of 258 consecutive cases. Laryngoscope 85:1905, 1975.
Dallow RL: Eye Problems Associated With Thyroid Disorders. Boston, Thyroid Foundation of America, 1987.
Dallow RL: Reliability of orbital diagnostic tests: Ultrasonography, computerized tomography, and radiography. Ophthalmology 85:1218, 1978.
Dallow RL, Momose KJ, Weber AL, Wray SH: Comparison of ultrasonography, computerized tomography (EMI scan), and radiographic techniques in evaluation of exophthalmos. Trans Am Acad Ophthalmol Otolaryngol 81:305, 1976.
Dallow RL, Pratt SG: Approach to Orbital Disorders and Frequency of Disease Occurrence. *In* Albert DM, Jakobiec FA (eds): The Principles and Practice of Ophthalmology. Philadelphia, WB Saunders, 1993.
Dandona P, Marshall NJ, Bidey SP, et al: Successful treatment of exophthalmos and pretibial myxoedema with plasmapheresis. Br J Med 1:374, 1979.
Dandona P, Marshall N, Bidey S, et al: Treatment of acute malignant exophthalmos with plasma exchange. *In* Stockigt JR, Nagataki S (eds): Thyroid Research VIII. Canberra, Australian Academy of Science, 1980.
Day RM, Carroll FD: Corticosteroids in the treatment of optic nerve involvement associated with thyroid dysfunction. Trans Am Ophthalmol Soc 65:41, 1976.
Dixon RS, Anderson RL, Hatt MU: The use of thymoxamine in eyelid retraction. Arch Ophthalmol 97:2417, 1979.
Duke-Elder S: System of Ophthalmology, vol. 13. St Louis, CV Mosby, 1972.
Eden KC, Trotter WR: Lid-retraction in toxic diffuse goiter. Lancet 2:385, 1942.
Falconer MA, Alexander WS: Experiences with malignant exophthalmos: Relationship of the condition to thyrotoxicosis and the pituitary thyrotropic hormone. Br J Ophthalmol 35:253, 1951.
Feldon SE, Muramatsu S, Weiner JM: Clinical classification of Graves' ophthalmopathy; identification of risk factors for optic neuropathy. Arch Ophthalmol 102:1469, 1984.
Garber MI: Methylprednisolone in the treatment of exophthalmos. Lancet 1:958, 1966.

Gay AJ, Wolkstein MA: Topical guanethidine therapy for endocrine lid retraction. Arch Ophthalmol 76:364, 1966.

Glinoer D, Etienne-Decerf J, Schrooyen M, et al: Beneficial effects of intensive plasma exchange followed by immunosuppressive therapy in severe Graves' ophthalmopathy. Acta Endocrinol (Copenh) 111:30, 1986.

Glinoer D, Schrooyen M: Plasma exchange therapy for severe Graves' ophthalmopathy. Horm Res 26:184, 1987.

Glinoer D, Schrooyen M, Winand RJ: The role of plasmapheresis in Graves' ophthalmopathy. In Wall JR, How J (eds): Graves' Ophthalmopathy. Boston, Blackwell Scientific, 1990.

Gonnering RS: Pseudoretraction of the eyelid in thyroid-associated orbitopathy. Arch Ophthalmol 106:1078, 1988.

Gorman CA: Temporal relationship between onset of Graves' ophthalmopathy and diagnosis of thyrotoxicosis. Mayo Clin Proc 58:515, 1983.

Gorman CA, Waller RR, Dyer JA: The Eye and Orbit in Thyroid Disease. New York, Raven Press, 1984.

Grove AS: Evaluation of exophthalmos. N Engl J Med 292:1005, 1975.

Hales IB, Rundle FF: Ocular changes in Graves' disease: A long-term follow-up study. Q J Med 29:113, 1960.

Hamilton HE, Schultz RD, DeGowin EL: The endocrine eye lesion in hyperthyroidism. Arch Intern Med 105:675, 1960.

Hamilton RD, Mayberry WE, McConahey WM, et al: Ophthalmopathy of Graves' disease: A comparison between patients treated surgically and patients treated with radioiodine. Mayo Clin Proc 42:812, 1967.

Hay ID: Clinical presentations of Graves' ophthalmopathy. In Gorman CA, Waller RR, Dryer JA (eds): The Eye and Orbit in Thyroid Disease. New York, Raven Press, 1984, pp 129–142.

Henderson JW: Optic neuropathy of exophthalmic goiter (Graves' disease). Arch Ophthalmol 59:471, 1958.

Henderson JW: Orbital Tumors, 2nd ed. New York, Thieme-Stratton, 1980.

Hiromatsu Y, Fukazawa H, Wall JR: Cytotoxic mechanisms in autoimmune thyroid disorders and thyroid-associated ophthalmopathy. Endocrinol Metab Clin North Am 16:269, 1987.

Hiromatsu Y, Wang PW, Wosu L, et al: Mechanisms of immune damage in Graves' ophthalmopathy. Horm Res 26:198, 1987.

Howlett TA, Lawton NF, Fells P: Deterioration of severe Graves' ophthalmopathy during cyclosporin treatment [letter]. Lancet 2:1101, 1984.

Jacobson DH, Gorman CA: Diagnosis and management of endocrine ophthalmopathy. Med Clin North Am 69:973, 1985.

Jakobiec FA, Jones IS: Orbital inflammations. In Duane TD (ed): Clinical Ophthalmology. Hagerstown, MD, Harper & Row, 1980, vol. 2, Chapter 35, pp 1–75.

Jones DIR, Munro PS, Wilson GM: Observations on the course of exophthalmos after ¹³¹I therapy. Proc R Soc Med 62:15, 1969.

Kadlubowski M, Irvine WJ, Rowland AC: The lack of specificity of ophthalmic immunoglobulins in Graves' disease. J Clin Endocrinol Metab 63:990, 1986.

Kahaly G, Lieb W, Müller-Forell W, et al: Ciamexone in endocrine orbitopathy. A randomized double-trial placebo-controlled study. Acta Endocrinol [Copenh] 122:13, 1990.

Kahaly G, Schrezenmeir J, Krause B, et al: Cyclosporine and prednisone. V. Prednisone in treatment of Graves' ophthalmopathy: A controlled, randomized and prospective study. Eur J Invest 16:415, 1986.

Karlsson FA, Dahlberg PA, Jansson R, et al: A study of cyclosporin in endocrine ophthalmopathy. In Schindler R (ed): Cyclosporin in Autoimmune Diseases. Berlin, Springer-Verlag, 1985.

Kelly W, Longson D, Smithard D, et al: An evaluation of plasma exchange for Graves' ophthalmopathy. Clin Endocrinol [Oxf] 18:484, 1983.

Kendall-Taylor P: The pathogenesis of Graves' ophthalmopathy. Clin Endocrinol Metab 14:331, 1985.

Kendall-Taylor P, Crombie AL, Stephenson AM, et al: Intravenous methylprednisolone in the treatment of Graves' ophthalmopathy. Br Med J 297:1574, 1988.

Kodama K, Sikorska H, Bandy-Defoe P, et al: Demonstration of a circulating auto antibody against a soluble eye-muscle antigen in Graves' ophthalmopathy. Lancet 2:1353, 1982.

Kolodziej-Maciejewska H, Reterski Z: Positive effect of bromocrip-

tine treatment in Graves' disease orbitopathy. Exp Clin Endocrinol 86:241, 1985.

Kuzuya N, DeGroot LJ: Effect of plasmapheresis and steroid treatment on thyrotropin binding inhibitory immunoglobulins in a patient with exophthalmos and a patient with pretibial myxedema. J Endocrin Invest 5:373, 1982.

Kvetny J, Frandsen NE, Johnson T, et al: Treatment of Graves' ophthalmopathy with cyclosporin A. Acta Med Scand 220:189, 1986.

Lawton NF: Exclusion of dysthyroid eye disease as a cause of unilateral proptosis. Trans Ophthalmol Soc UK 99:226, 1979.

Lessell S: Current concepts in ophthalmology: Optic neuropathy. N Engl J Med 299:533, 1978.

Levitt MD, Edis AJ, Agnello R, McCormick CC: The effect of subtotal thyroidectomy on Graves' ophthalmopathy. World J Surg 12:593, 1988.

Lewis RA, Slater N, Croft DN: Exophthalmos and pretibial myxedema not responding to plasmapheresis. Br Med J 2:390, 1979.

Lopatynsky MO, Krohel GB: Bromocriptine therapy for thyroid ophthalmopathy. Am J Ophthalmol 107:680, 1989.

McGregor AM, Beck W, Weetman AP: Cyclosporin in the management of Graves' ophthalmopathy. In Schindler R (ed): Cyclosporin in Autoimmune Diseases. Berlin, Springer-Verlag, 1985.

Mulherin JL Jr, Temple TE Jr, Lundey DW: Glucocorticoid treatment of progressive infiltrative ophthalmopathy. South Med J 65:77, 1972.

Netland PA, Dallow RL: Thyroid Ophthalmopathy. In Albert DM, Jakobiec FA (eds): The Principles and Practice of Ophthalmology. Philadelphia, WB Saunders, 1993.

Panzo GJ, Tomsak RL: A retrospective review of 26 cases of dysthyroid optic neuropathy. Am J Ophthalmol 96:190, 1983.

Pequegnat IP, Mayberry WE, McConahey WM, et al: Large doses of radioiodine in Graves' disease: Effect on ophthalmopathy and long-acting thyroid stimulation. Mayo Clin Proc 42:802, 1967.

Perros P, Weightman DR, Crombie AL, et al: Azathioprine in the treatment of thyroid-associated ophthalmopathy. Acta Endocrinol [Copenh] 122:8, 1990.

Peter SA: Euthyroid Graves' disease: Report of a case observed over a 12-year period. Am J Med 80:1197, 1986.

Pope RM, McGregor AM: Medical Management of Graves' Ophthalmopathy. Boston, Blackwell Scientific, 1990.

Prummel MF, Mourits MP, Berghout A, et al: Prednisone and cyclosporine in treatment of severe Graves' ophthalmopathy. N Engl J Med 321:1353, 1989.

Rootman J: Diseases of the Orbit. Philadelphia, JB Lippincott, 1988.

Sawers JS, Irvine WJ, Toft AD, et al: Plasma exchange in conjunction with immunosuppressive drug therapy in the treatment of endocrine exophthalmos. J Clin Lab Immunol 6:245, 1981.

Schrooyen M, Winand R, Glinoer D: Plasma exchange therapy for severe Graves' ophthalmopathy. Orbit 5:105, 1986.

Sergott RC, Glaser JS: Graves' ophthalmopathy: A clinical and immunologic review. Surv Ophthalmol 26:1, 1981.

Shields CL, Nelson LB, Carpenter GC, Shields JA: Neonatal Graves' disease. Br J Ophthalmol 72:424, 1988.

Shine B, Fells P, Edwards OM, Weetman P: Association between Graves' ophthalmopathy and smoking. Lancet 335:1261, 1990.

Shumak KH, Rock GA: Therapeutic plasma exchange. N Engl J Med 310:762, 1984.

Skalka HW: The use of ultrasonography in the diagnosis of endocrine orbitopathy. Neurol Ophthalmol 1:109, 1980.

Skinner SW, Miller JE: Permanent improvement of thyroid-related upper eyelid retraction from bethanidine. Am J Ophthalmol 67:764, 1969.

Spaulding SW, Lippes H: Hyperthyroidism; Causes, clinical features, and diagnosis. Med Clin North Am 69:937, 1985.

Sridama V, DeGroot LJ: Treatment of Graves' disease and the course of ophthalmopathy. Am J Med 87:70, 1989.

Stevens JT: The roentgen rays and radium in toxic goiter and hyperthyroidism. JAMA 97:1689, 1931.

Streeten DHP, Anderson GH Jr, Reed GF, Woo P: Prevalence, natural history and surgical treatment of exophthalmos. Clin Endocrinol 27:125, 1987.

Tallstedt L, Lundell G, Torring O, et al: Occurrence of ophthalmopathy after treatment for Graves' hyperthyroidism. N Engl J Med 326:1733, 1992.

Thomas ID, Hart JK: Retrobulbar repository corticosteroid therapy in thyroid ophthalmopathy. Med J Aust 2:484, 1974.

Trobe JD, Glaser JS, Laflamme P: Dysthyroid optic neuropathy. Clinical profile and rationale for management. Arch Ophthalmol 96:1199, 1978.

Utech C, Wulle KG, Bieler EU, et al: Treatment of severe Graves' ophthalmopathy with cyclosporin A. Acta Endocrinol [Copenh] 110:493, 1985.

Utech C, Wulle KG, Panitz Z, et al: Immunosuppressive treatment of Graves' ophthalmopathy with cyclosporine A. Transplant Proc 20:173, 1988.

Utech C, Wulle KG, Pfannenstiel P, et al: Ciamexon-treatment in endocrine ophthalmopathy. Acta Endocrinol [Suppl] [Copenh] 281:342, 1987.

von Graffenried B, Harrison WB: Cyclosporin in autoimmune diseases—Side-effects (with emphasis on renal dysfunction) and recommendations for use. In Schindler R (ed): Cyclosporin in Autoimmune Diseases. Berlin, Springer-Verlag, 1985.

Wall JR, Henderson J, Strakosch CR, et al: Graves' ophthalmopathy. Can Med Assoc J 124:855, 1981.

Wall JR, How J (eds): Graves' Ophthalmopathy. Current Issues in Endocrinology and Metabolism. Boston, Blackwell Scientific, 1990.

Wall JR, Strakosch CR, Fang SL, et al: Thyroid binding antibodies and other immunological abnormalities in patients with Graves' ophthalmopathy: Effect of treatment with cyclophosphamide. Clin Endocrinol 10:79, 1979.

Weetman AP, Fells P, Shine B: T and B cell reactivity to extraocular and skeletal muscle in Graves' ophthalmopathy. Br J Ophthalmol 73:323, 1989.

Weetman AP, McGregor AM: Autoimmune thyroid disease: Developments in our understanding. Endocr Rev 5:309, 1984.

Weetman AP, McGregor AM, Ludgate M, et al: Cyclosporin improves Graves' ophthalmopathy. Lancet 2:486, 1983.

Weightman D, Kendall-Taylor P: Cross-reaction of eye muscle antibodies with thyroid tissue in thyroid-associated ophthalmopathy. J Endocrinol 122:201, 1989.

Werner SC: The eye changes of Graves' disease. Mayo Clin Proc 47:969, 1972.

Werner SC: Modification of the classification of the eye changes of Graves' disease. Am J Ophthalmol 83:725, 1977.

Werner SC: Modification of the classification of the eye changes of Graves' disease: Recommendations of the Ad Hoc Committee of the American Thyroid Association [Editorial]. J Clin Endocrinol Metab 44:203, 1977.

Werner SC: The Thyroid, 3rd ed. New York, Harper & Row, 1971.

Werner SC, Feind CR, Aida M: Graves' disease and total thyroidectomy: Progression of severe eye changes and decrease in serum long acting thyroid stimulator after operation. N Engl J Med 276:132, 1967.

Wiersinga WM: Novel drugs for treatment of Graves' ophthalmopathy. In Wall JR, How J (eds): Graves' Ophthalmopathy. Boston, Blackwell Scientific, 1990, pp 111–126.

Wiersinga WM, Smit T, van der Gaag R, Koornneef L: Temporal relationship between onset of Graves' ophthalmopathy and onset of thyroidal Graves' disease. J Endocrinol Invest 11:615, 1988.

Wiersinga WM, Smit T, van der Gaag R, et al: Clinical presentation of Graves' ophthalmopathy. Ophthalmic Res 21:73, 1989.

Wright P: Adverse reactions to guanethidine eye drops. Br J Ophthalmol 71:323, 1987.

Yamamoto K, Saito K, Takai T, et al: Diagnosis of exophthalmos using orbital ultrasonography and treatment of malignant exophthalmos with steroid therapy, orbital radiation therapy and plasmapheresis. Prog Clin Biol Res 116:189, 1983.

BIBLIOGRAPHY

For section Orbital Radiation Therapy

Bagan SM, Hollenhorst RW: Radiation retinopathy after irradiation of intracranial lesions. Am J Ophthalmol 88:694, 1979.

Barret L, Glatt HJ, Burde RM: Optic nerve disease in thyroid eye disease: CT. Head Neck Radiol 167:503, 1988.

Bartalena L, Marcocci C, Chiovato L, et al: Orbital cobalt irradiation combined with systemic corticosteroids for Graves' ophthalmopathy: Comparison with systemic corticosteroids alone. J Clin Endocrinol Metab 56:1139, 1983.

Beierwaltes WH: X-ray treatment of malignant exophthalmos: A report on 28 patients. J Clin Endocrinol Metab 13:1090, 1953.

Brennan MW, Leone CR, Janake L: Radiation therapy for Graves' disease. Am J Ophthalmol 96:195, 1983.

Brown GC, Shields JA, Sanborn G, et al: Radiation retinopathy. Ophthalmology 89:1494, 1982.

Chacko DC: Considerations in the diagnosis of radiation injury. JAMA 245:1255, 1981.

Chan RC, Shukovsky LJ: Effects of irradiation on the eye. Radiology 120:673, 1976.

Covington E, Lobes L, Sudarsanam A: Radiation therapy of exophthalmos: Report of seven cases. Radiology 122:797, 1976.

Donaldson SS, Bagshaw MA, Kriss JP: Supervoltage orbital radiopathy for Graves' ophthalmopathy. J Clin Endocrinol Metab 37:276, 1973.

Donaldson SS, Glick JM, Wilbur JR: Adriamycin activating a recall phenomenon after radiation therapy. Ann Intern Med 81:407, 1974.

Gedda P, Lindgren M: Pituitary and orbital roentgen therapy in the hyperophthalmopathic types of Graves' disease. Acta Radiol 42:211, 1954.

Glaser JS: Graves' ophthalmopathy. Arch Ophthalmol 102:1448, 1984.

Hurbli T, Char DH, Harris J, et al: Radiation therapy for thyroid eye diseases. Am J Ophthalmol 99:633, 1985.

Jones A: Orbital x-ray of progressive exophthalmos. Br J Radiol 24:637, 1951.

Kazim M, Trokel S, Moore S: Treatment of acute Graves' orbitopathy. Ophthalmology 98:1443, 1991.

Kinyoun JL, Kalina RE, Brower SA, et al: Radiation retinopathy after orbital irradiation for Graves' ophthalmopathy. Arch Ophthalmol 102:1473, 1984.

Konishi J, Iida Y, Kasagi K, et al: Clinical evaluation of radiotherapy for Graves' ophthalmopathy. Endocrinol Jpn 33:637, 1986.

Kriss JP, McDougall IR, Donaldson SS: Graves' ophthalmopathy. In Krieger DT, Bardin W (eds): Current Therapy in Endocrinology. New York, Decker, 1984, pp 104–109.

Lloyd WC, Leone CR: Supervoltage orbital radiotherapy in 36 cases of Graves' disease. Am J Ophthalmol 113:374, 1992.

Miller ML, Goldberg SH, Bullock JD: Radiation retinopathy after standard radiotherapy for thyroid related ophthalmopathy. Am J Ophthalmol 112:600, 1991.

Nikoskelainen E, Joensuu H: Retinopathy after irradiation for Graves' ophthalmopathy. Lancet 2:690, 1989.

Olivotto IA, Ludgate CM, Allen LH, Rootman J: Supervoltage radiotherapy for Graves' ophthalmopathy: CCABC technique and results. Int J Radiat Oncol Biol Phys 11:2085, 1985.

Palmer D, Greenberg P, Cornell P, Parker RG: A retrospective analysis. Int J Radiat Oncol Biol Phys 13:1815, 1987.

Petersen IA, Kriss JP, McDougall IR, Donaldson SS: Prognostic factors in the radiotherapy of Graves' ophthalmopathy. Int J Radiat Oncol Biol Phys 19:259, 1990.

Pigeon P, Orgiazzi J, Berthezene F, et al: High voltage orbital radiotherapy and surgical orbital decompression in the management of Graves' ophthalmopathy. Horm Res 26:172, 1987.

Pinchera A, Bartalena L, Chiovato L, Marcocci C: Radiotherapy of Graves' ophthalmopathy. In Gorman CA, Waller RR, Dyer JA (eds): The Eye and Orbit in Thyroid Disease. New York, Raven Press, 1984, pp 301–316.

Ravin JG, Sisson JC, Knapp WT: Orbital radiation for the ocular changes of Graves' disease. Am J Ophthalmol 79:285, 1975.

Rinchera A, Bartalena L, Chiovato L, Marcocci C: Radiotherapy of Graves' ophthalmopathy. In Gorman CA, Waller RR, Dyer JA (eds): The Eye and Orbit in Thyroid Disease. New York, Raven Press, 1984, pp 301–316.

Shukovsky LJ, Fletcher GH: Retinal and optic nerve complications in a high dose irradiation technique of ethmoid sinus and nasal cavity. Radiology 104:629, 1972.

Sisson JC: Mechanisms by which retrobular fibroblasts are stimulated by lymphocytes: Role of cyclic nucleotide. Proc Soc Exp Biol Med 154:386, 1977.

Sisson JC, Vanderberg JA: Lymphocyte-retrobulbar fibroblast interaction: Mechanisms by which stimulation occurs and inhibition of stimulation. Invest Ophthalmol 11:15, 1972.

Stevens JT: The roentgen rays and radium in toxic goiter and hyper-thyroidism. JAMA 97:1689, 1931.

Teng CS, Crombe AL, Hall R, Ross WM: An evaluation of super-voltage orbital irradiation for Graves' orbitopathy. Clin Endocrinol 13:545, 1980.

Teoh R, Woo J: Combined irradiation and low-dose cyclophospha-mide in the treatment of Graves' ophthalmopathy. Postgrad Med J 63:777, 1987.

Trobe JD, Glaser JS: Dysthyroid optic neuropathy. Arch Ophthalmol 96:1199, 1978.

van Ouwerkerk BM, Wijngaarde R, Hennemann G, et al: Radiother-apy of severe ophthalmic Graves' disease. J Endocrinol 13:545, 1980.

BIBLIOGRAPHY

For section Surgical Management

Carter KD, Frueh BR, Hessburg TP, Musch DC: Long term efficacy of orbital decompression for compressive optic neuropathy of Graves' eye disease. Ophthalmology 98:1435, 1991.

DeSanto LW, Gorman CA: Selection of patients and choice of operation in Graves' ophthalmopathy. Laryngoscope 83:2051, 1973.

Dyer JA: The oculorotary muscles in Graves' disease. Trans Am Ophthalmol Soc 74:425, 1976.

Dunn WJ, Arnold AC, O'Connor PS: Botulinum toxin for the treatment of dysthyroid ocular myopathy. Ophthalmology 93:470, 1986.

Fells P: Orbital decompression for severe dysthyroid eye disease. Br J Ophthalmol 71:107, 1987.

Flanagan JC: Bank sclera in oculoplastic surgery. Ophthalmic Surg 5:45, 1974.

Garrity J, Gorman CA: Pitfalls associated with orbital decompression for thyroid related orbitopathy. Exp Clin Endocrinol 97:338, 1991.

Garrity JA, Saggau DD, Gorman CA, et al: Torsional diplopia after transantral orbital decompression and extraocular muscle surgery associated with Graves' orbitopathy. Am J Ophthalmol 113:363, 1992.

Grove AS: Levator lengthening by marginal myotomy. Arch Oph-thalmology 98:1433, 1980.

Jampolsky A: Recent advances in strabismus management, strabismus reoperation techniques. Trans Am Acad Ophthalmol Otolaryngol 79:704, 1975.

Kennedy DW, Goodstein ML, Miller NR, Zinreich SJ: Endoscopic transnasal orbital decompression. Arch Otolaryngol Head Neck Surg 116:275, 1990.

Kennerdell JS, Maroon JC: An orbital decompression for severe dysthyroid exophthalmos. Ophthalmology 89:467, 1982.

Kennerdell JS, Maroon JC, Buerger GF: Comprehensive surgical management of proptosis in dysthyroid orbitopathy. Orbit 6:153, 1987.

Kennerdell JS, Rosenbaum AE, Hoshy MH: Apical optic nerve decompression of dysthyroid optic neuropathy on computed tomog-raphy. Arch Ophthalmol 99:807, 1981.

Koorneff L: Eyelid and orbital fascial attachments and their signifi-cance. Eye 2:130, 1988.

Leone CR: The management of ophthalmic Graves' disease. Oph-thalmology 91:770, 1984.

Long JA, Baylis HI: Hypoglobus following orbital decompression for dysthyroid ophthalmopathy. Ophthalmic Plast Reconstr Surg 6:185, 1990.

McCord CD: Current trends in orbital decompression. Ophthalmology 92:21, 1985.

Michel O, Bresgen K, Russmann W, et al: Endoscopic controlled endonasal decompression of the orbit in endocrine ophthalmopathy. Laryngol Rhinol Otol [Stuttg] 70:656, 1991.

Morax S, Hurbli T: Choice of surgical treatment for Graves' disease. J Craniomaxillofac Surg 15:174, 1987.

Ogura J, Wessler S, Avioli V: Surgical approach to the ophthalmop-athy of Graves' disease. JAMA 216:1627, 1971.

Putterman AM: Surgical treatment of thyroid related upper lid retrac-tion. Ophthalmology 88:507, 1981.

Scott AB: Injection treatment of endocrine orbital myopathy. Doc Ophthalmol 58:499, 1981.

Scott WE, Martin-Casals A, Jackson OB: Adjustable sutures in strabismus surgery. J Pediatr Ophthalmol 14:71, 1977.

Scott WE, Thalacker JA: Diagnosis and treatment of thyroid myopa-thy. Ophthalmology 88:493, 1981.

Seiff SR, Shorr N: Nasolacrimal drainage system obstruction after orbit decompression. Am J Ophthalmol 106:204, 1988.

Shorr N, Neuhaus RW, Baylis H: Ocular motility problems after orbital decompression for dysthyroid ophthalmopathy. Ophthal-mology 89:323, 1982.

Skov CMB, Mazov ML: Managing strabismus in endocrine eye dis-ease. Can J Ophthalmol 19:269, 1984.

Stabile JA, Trokel SL: Increase in orbital volume obtained by de-compression in dried skulls. Am J Ophthalmol 95:327, 1983.

Sterk CC, Bierlach JMM, Breukman CJ, deKeizer RJW: Orbital decompression and motility disturbances in endocrine ophthalmop-athy. Doc Ophthalmol 61:229, 1986.

Trokel SL, Cooper WC: Orbital decompression: Effect of motility and globe position. Ophthalmology 86:2064, 1979.

Trokel S, Moore S, Kazim M: Diplopia in Graves' disease. Am Orthoptic J 38:159, 1988.

Waller RR, Anderson RL: Thyroid ophthalmopathy and orbital decompression. In Stewart WB (ed): Ophthalmic Plastic and Re-constructive Surgery. San Francisco, American Academy of Oph-thalmology, 1984.

Walsh TE, Ogura JH: Transantral orbital decompression for malignant exophthalmos. Laryngoscope 67:544, 1957.

Warren JD, Spector JG, Burde R: Long term follow up and recent observations on 305 cases of orbital decompression for dysthyroid ophthalmopathy. Laryngoscope 99:35, 1989.

Young JD: Ocular complications of transantral decompression for thyrotoxic exophthalmos. Proc R Soc Med 64:929, 1971.

Chapter 170

Noninfectious Orbital Inflammations and Vasculitis

NEAL G. SNEBOLD

Patients may present to the clinician with signs and symptoms of orbital inflammation resulting from any one of a number of local or systemic disorders (Table 170–1). Navigating through the differential diagnosis of diseases that can cause or mimic orbital inflammation can seem a daunting task, particularly because many of these conditions may share common clinical characteristics. However, a meticulous history and physical examination in combination with appropriate laboratory, imaging, and histopathologic studies will greatly facilitate the diagnostic process. Once the correct diagnosis has been achieved, a rational treatment plan can be devised.

NONSPECIFIC IDIOPATHIC ORBITAL INFLAMMATION (ORBITAL PSEUDOTUMOR)

General Considerations

Since antiquity, proptosis has been considered prima-facie evidence of orbital neoplasm. However, in the late 1800s, several patients with presumed orbital tumors were observed who demonstrated unexpected improvement. The unusual clinical course of these patients was attributed to homeopathic cures or spontaneous remission. Other patients undergoing orbital exenteration for presumed tumors were found to have benign orbital inflammation in lieu of neoplasia. Panas coined the term *pseudoplasma* to describe these puzzling cases.[1] In 1930, Birch-Hirschfeld published an analysis of 30 such cases and introduced the concept of orbital pseudotumor.[2] Cases were divided into three categories: (1) spontaneous resolution of suspected tumor without pathologic confirmation, (2) no surgically identifiable tumor mass but histopathology showing a diffuse benign cellular infiltrate, and (3) tumor mass identified at surgery with histopathologic findings of inflammation rather than neoplasia. The concept of orbital pseudotumor subsequently became entrenched in the literature but was of limited clinical usefulness because of the heterogeneity of reported cases and overlapping characteristics with other lymphoid, neoplastic, and inflammatory diseases.

Clinical observations and improvements in diagnostic technology resulted in a more precise definition of orbital pseudotumor.[3–6] Orbital pseudotumor may be defined as a nonspecific, idiopathic, benign inflammatory process characterized by a polymorphous lymphoid in-filtrate with varying degrees of fibrosis.[7, 8] This definition excludes specific local and systemic causes of orbital inflammation. The clinical course of the disorder may be acute, subacute, or chronic. Although it can occur in childhood, the peak incidence is during the fourth and fifth decades of life. There is no sex predilection.

Diseases of the orbit with lymphocytic infiltration as a common feature range from benign idiopathic pseudotumor and Graves' orbitopathy to malignant lymphoma. Benign reactive hyperplasia and atypical lymphoid hyperplasia are lymphoproliferative disorders that lie on a continuum between the two extremes. Although atypical lymphoid hyperplasia is considered a lymphoid neoplasm, the categorization of reactive lymphoid hyperplasia in this schema is controversial. Some authorities consider benign reactive lymphoid hyperplasia a variant of idiopathic orbital pseudotumor.[5–7] Others believe that benign reactive lymphoid hyperplasia should be grouped with the lymphoid neoplasms.[9, 10]

Patients with benign reactive lymphoid hyperplasia carry a 6 percent risk of mortality in 5 yr and a 15 to 25 percent chance of eventual systemic involvement. Atypical reactive lymphoid hyperplasia carries a 19 percent risk of mortality and a 40 percent chance of systemic disease in 5 yr.[10] In view of the increased risk of mortality and systemic involvement in so-called benign reactive

Table 170–1. DIFFERENTIAL DIAGNOSIS OF ORBITAL INFLAMMATORY DISEASE

Inflammatory Disorders
  Graves' orbitopathy
  Infection
    Bacterial
    Fungal
    Parasitic
  Idiopathic pseudotumor
  Granulomatous disease
    Sarcoidosis
    Idiopathic noninfectious granulomatous inflammation
    Erdheim-Chester disease
    Necrobiotic xanthogranulomatosis
  Sjögren's syndrome
  Vasculitis
  Miscellaneous
    Foreign-body reaction
    Ruptured dermoid cyst
    Sinus mucocele
Noninflammatory Disorders
  Neoplasia
  Vascular disorders
    Dural-cavernous sinus arteriovenous fistula
    Orbital varix

lymphoid hyperplasia, it appears reasonable to classify it as a lymphoid neoplasm and exclude it from the category of benign idiopathic orbital pseudotumor. This distinction has important diagnostic, prognostic, and therapeutic implications.[11, 12]

Pathology and Pathogenesis

The pathologic findings in the acute, subacute, and chronic forms of idiopathic pseudotumor differ depending on the degree of inflammatory and fibrovascular response. Tissues throughout the orbit may be involved, and clinical manifestations of the disease will vary accordingly. Histologic findings in the acute form of the disease consist of a hypocellular polymorphous infiltrate composed of mature lymphocytes, plasma cells, macrophages, and polymorphonuclear leukocytes. Eosinophils may also be present.[13] Eosinophil degranulation is believed to contribute to tissue fibrosis.[14] Multinucleated foreign-body giant cells secondary to fat necrosis have also been described.[5] The cellular infiltrate of orbital pseudotumor tends to be diffuse and multifocal. In contrast, lymphoid neoplasms are characterized by a hypercellular monomorphous infiltrate with scant stroma. Rarely, a component of true vasculitis limited to the orbit may be seen in idiopathic orbital pseudotumor.[7, 9, 15, 16] Small arteries and arterioles are primarily affected, and the condition is histologically similar to hypersensitivity vasculitis. This condition is termed type I pseudotumor in Henderson's classification and is rarely associated with any systemic disease.[7]

In the subacute and chronic forms of idiopathic pseudotumor, increasing amounts of fibrovascular stroma are present. Normal muscle, fat, and glandular elements are replaced with fibrous tissue. This desmoplastic response may ultimately result in dense fibrosis with entrapment of orbital structures and mass effect. Lymphoid follicles with germinal centers may be observed, particularly in the chronic phase.[10] Stepwise progression from acute inflammation to chronic fibrosis may occur. However, some cases of nonspecific idiopathic orbital inflammation are primarily sclerotic in nature and may present insidiously without passing through a prior acute inflammatory phase.[17] The pathogenesis of orbital pseudotumor remains unknown. Viral, allergic, and immunologic causes have been proposed.[18]

Clinical Manifestations

The clinical manifestations of idiopathic orbital pseudotumor are chiefly determined by the degree of inflammatory response and the particular orbital tissues involved. The acute form of the disease is characterized by the abrupt onset of pain, lid swelling, and redness, which usually bring the patient to medical attention within hours to days. Diplopia and decreased vision may also be present. If the inflammatory process contains a desmoplastic component, the presentation may be subacute or chronic. The greater the fibrovascular response, the more chronic the illness and the less evident are signs of orbital inflammation. Signs and symptoms of insidious onset evolving over weeks to months are largely the result of mass effect and entrapment caused by fibrosis. Patients typically present with slowly progressive visual loss, diplopia, or proptosis. Orbital pseudotumor is usually a monophasic illness, but it can be recurrent, particularly in children. Recurrent disease is uncommon in adults but has been reported up to 10 yr after the initial episode (Figs. 170–1 and 170–2).[5, 19]

In idiopathic orbital inflammation, various "target tissues" within the orbit may come under immunologic attack, resulting in distinctive patterns of disease.[9, 20] Orbital inflammation may be localized or diffuse. Localized forms of idiopathic pseudotumor involve the anterior or posterior orbit, extraocular muscles, and lacrimal gland.

Involvement of the *anterior orbit* is one of the most common localized forms of inflammatory pseudotumor (see Fig. 170–2). This pattern of inflammation has been termed periscleritis, sclerotenonitis, and anterior inflammatory pseudotumor.[20, 21] Tenon's capsule and the periscleral tissues are primarily affected, but scleral involvement may also occur. Clinical findings vary depending on the primary locus of the inflammatory process. When the tissues of the anterior orbit are primarily involved, signs of orbital inflammation are the prominent features on examination. With significant posterior scleral involvement, signs of ocular inflammation may dominate the clinical picture. Because of overlapping signs and symptoms, anterior inflammatory pseudotumor and posterior scleritis can at times be difficult to differentiate clinically. These entities may represent variations of the same disease process.[22, 23]

Common presenting symptoms in acute anterior in-

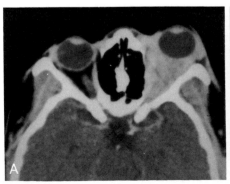
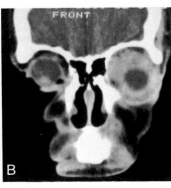

Figure 170–1. A 19-year-old woman experienced the acute onset of pain, redness, and swelling of the left eye with diplopia. *A,* Contrast-enhanced computed tomographic (CT) scan, axial view, demonstrating panorbital infiltrate characteristic of diffuse orbital pseudotumor. Systemic medical evaluation was negative. Signs and symptoms of orbital inflammation completely resolved with oral corticosteroid therapy. *B,* CT scan, coronal view.

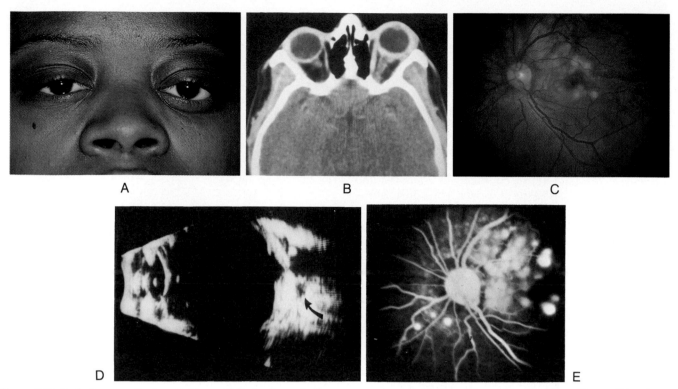

Figure 170–2. *A*, Same patient as in Figure 170–1 returned after an asymptomatic hiatus of 2 yr with painful swelling, mild redness, ophthalmoparesis, and decreased vision of the left eye. Symptoms were less severe than during the previous episode. *B*, Contrast-enhanced axial computed tomographic scan demonstrates ragged periocular infiltrate typical of anterior inflammatory pseudotumor. *C*, Fundus photograph shows fluffy white subretinal infiltrates and serous retinal elevation in the peripapillary and macular regions of the left eye. *D*, B-scan ultrasonogram demonstrates thickening of the uveoscleral coat and effusion in Tenon's space at the neuroocular junction (T sign). *E*, Fluorescein angiogram demonstrates multiple small hyperfluorescent lesions in the peripapillary and macular areas of the left eye. Systemic medical evaluation was again negative, and findings resolved with oral corticosteroid therapy.

flammatory pseudotumor are pain with redness and swelling of the eye and ocular adnexa. The pain, which is sometimes excruciating, is of rapid onset and is referable to the eye and orbit. In posterior scleritis, the pain may radiate more to the temporal region.[13] Less common presenting symptoms include diplopia and visual loss. Patients often complain of generalized malaise but are afebrile and otherwise in good health.

External examination shows edema and erythema of the lids (especially the upper lids) and periorbital region without induration or lymphadenopathy. Ptosis, proptosis, and decreased orbital resilience with pain on ballottement of the globe are common findings. Slit-lamp examination shows conjunctival chemosis and injection. Signs of uveitis may be evident. Iridocyclitis, pars planitis, and posterior uveitis have been reported in both posterior scleritis and anterior idiopathic pseudotumor.[21, 23, 24] Funduscopic findings may include annular or localized choroidal detachment, choroidal striae, retinal elevation simulating a mass lesion, exudative retinal detachment, and cystoid macular edema (see Fig. 170–2C).[23] Choroidal osteomas have also been reported.[25] Extraocular muscle involvement results in myositis with painful ophthalmoparesis. Inflammation surrounding the optic nerve results in perineuritis or papillitis with signs of optic nerve dysfunction.

Glaucoma may occur in association with anterior

inflammatory pseudotumor by several mechanisms. Annular choroidal detachment may rotate the lens-iris diaphragm forward, resulting in angle closure. Secondary open-angle glaucoma can occur as a result of obstruction of the trabecular meshwork by uveitic inflammatory cells. Inflammation involving the trabecular meshwork, Schlemm's canal, or episcleral vessels may produce a relative obstruction of aqueous outflow with increased intraocular pressure.[21, 26, 27]

A contrast-enhanced computed tomographic (CT) scan of the orbits typically shows a ragged infiltrate that involves the soft tissue of the anterior orbit and surrounds the globe (see Fig. 170–2B). Scleral enhancement and thickening may be evident. Optic nerve, extraocular muscles, and lacrimal gland may also be involved.[9, 20] B-scan ultrasonogram may demonstrate choroidal or retinal detachment and thickening of the sclerouveal coat in cases of posterior scleral involvement.[23] Widening of the potential space between the episclera and Tenon's capsule by effusion is seen with sclerotenonitis. Perineural and sub-Tenon's effusion at the neuroocular junction results in the so-called T sign (see Fig. 170–2D).[28] Fluorescein angiography shows patchy choroidal filling in the early phase followed by punctate areas of fluorescein leakage, which gradually collects in the subretinal space in the late phase (see Fig. 170–2E). Macular edema may also be present.[23]

In acute *dacryoadenitis*, the lacrimal gland is the primary focus of inflammation. Patients commonly present with the acute onset of pain localized to the supratemporal region of the orbit accompanied by upper lid swelling and redness. Examination reveals lid edema, warmth, and erythema, but there is no induration to suggest cellulitis. A characteristic S-shaped deformity with ptosis of the upper lid is seen. The lacrimal gland may be palpable and exquisitely sensitive to touch. The enlarged and erythematous palpebral lobe of the lacrimal gland is easily visualized in the supratemporal conjunctival fornix. Lateral conjunctival chemosis and injection are usually present as well. Involvement of the adjacent lateral rectus muscle results in painful ophthalmoparesis and diplopia. Proptosis and decreased visual acuity are usually absent. Lacrimal inflammation may also be subacute or chronic, evolving over weeks to months and presenting with a painless lacrimal fossa mass.

CT shows enhancement and enlargement of the lacrimal gland (Fig. 170–3). The enlarged gland appears elongated and molded to surrounding structures. Infiltration of the surrounding tissues is common with involvement of Tenon's capsule and the lateral rectus muscle. There is no erosion of adjacent bone. B-scan ultrasonography shows lacrimal enlargement with a homogeneous acoustic appearance.[9, 20]

Orbital *myositis* is another common variant of nonspecific idiopathic orbital inflammation. Diplopia and pain exacerbated by eye movement are hallmark presenting complaints in the acute form. Examination reveals restriction of ocular movement in the field of action of the affected muscles. Forced-duction testing may be positive. Proptosis with increased resistance and pain on ballottement of the globe is common. Point tenderness in the supranasal orbit has been reported in a case of superior oblique myositis with peritrochlear

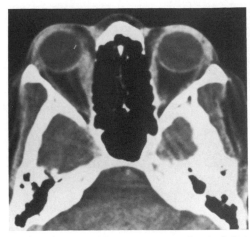

Figure 170–4. A 41-year-old woman complained of diplopia and pain of the right eye exacerbated with eye movement, which lasted for 8 wk. Systemic evaluation was negative. Contrast-enhanced axial computed tomographic scan of the orbits demonstrates enlargement and enhancement of the right medial rectus muscle and tendon characteristic of myositis.

inflammation.[29] Localized conjunctival injection and chemosis may be seen at the tendinous insertion of the involved muscle. Single or multiple muscles may be involved in either one or both orbits, and the illness may be recurrent.[19, 30] Various antecedent conditions such as upper respiratory tract infection, sinusitis, asthma, allergic rhinitis, Crohn's disease, serum sickness, and trauma have been reported in association with orbital myositis.[30–32] In contrast to acute myositis, symptoms may develop slowly over several months in subacute and chronic cases.[33, 34] Rarely, orbital myositis may be complicated by orbital hemorrhage and lid ecchymosis.[35]

CT scanning shows diffuse enlargement of one or more extraocular muscles (Fig. 170–4). There is a pre-

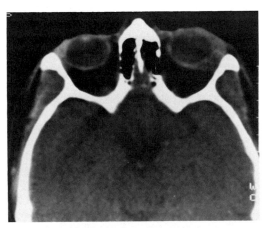

Figure 170–3. Previously healthy 34-year-old woman complained of pain, swelling, and redness of the left upper eyelid for 1 wk. Examination revealed edema and erythema of the left upper eyelid; mildly enlarged lacrimal gland painful to palpation; and injection and chemosis of the lateral bulbar conjunctiva. Axial computed tomographic scan of the orbit shows elongated enlargement of the lacrimal gland consistent with acute dacryoadenitis. Medical evaluation was unremarkable except for mild elevation of sedimentation rate. Findings rapidly resolved with oral corticosteroid therapy.

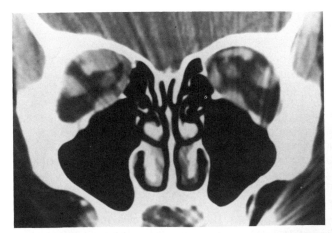

Figure 170–5. A 61-year-old woman with a 1-mo history of intermittent diplopia and pain of the right eye. Examination revealed mild proptosis, chemosis, and restriction of elevation of the right eye. Contrast-enhanced coronal computed tomographic scan of the orbit shows enlargement and enhancement of the levator–superior rectus complex. Extensive medical evaluation was negative, and diagnosis of idiopathic orbital myositis was made. All clinical and radiographic findings completely resolved with corticosteroid therapy.

Figure 170–6. A 55-year-old man with progressive painless proptosis of the left eye and diplopia of 6 months duration. Examination was significant for proptosis, increased resistance to ballottement of the globe, chemosis, and restricted abduction. A, Contrast-enhanced axial computed tomographic (CT) scan of the orbit shows an infiltrating lesion in the posterior orbit of the left eye. B, Coronal CT scan demonstrates an infiltrating lesion of the inferolateral posterior orbit. Biopsy showed nonspecific idiopathic orbital inflammation. Recurring symptoms after discontinuation of corticosteroids necessitated the use of low-dose radiation for control.

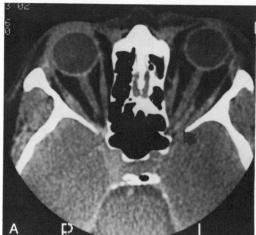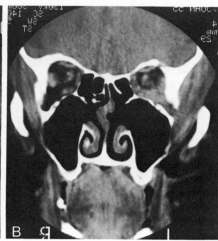

dilection for pseudotumor to involve the medial and superior recti (Fig. 170–5). Classically, the entire muscle is involved, including the belly and tendon. A ragged soft tissue infiltrate may be seen involving tissues adjacent to the muscles.

The *posterior* pattern of acute pseudotumor presents primarily with clinical signs and symptoms of the orbital apex syndrome with optic neuropathy and ophthalmoplegia (Figs. 170–6 and 170–7). Pain, proptosis, and external inflammatory signs are less prominent features than in the anterior form of pseudotumor.[20] Optic nerve dysfunction results from inflammation of the perineural tissues or compression via mass effect. Signs of optic nerve involvement include decreased visual acuity, dyschromatopsia, visual field defects, relative afferent pupillary defect, and disc edema. Efferent pupillary defects secondary to presumed damage to the ciliary ganglion have also been reported.[19] Contrast-enhanced CT scanning shows enlargement and enhancement of the optic nerve sheath with infiltration of perineural orbital fat and connective tissue.[36, 37] The infiltrate may also involve the extraocular muscles in the orbital apex.[38]

The *chronic sclerosing variant* of idiopathic pseudotumor is well-described and may represent the sequela of previous episodes of acute orbital inflammation or may occur in a de novo manner.[7, 17, 39] Histologically, it consists of a polymorphous infiltrate with a dense collagenous stroma. There appears to be a predilection for this sclerotic mass to involve the posterior orbit, although in some cases a firm mass may be palpable anteriorly. The insidious onset of decreasing vision, diplopia, and proptosis is a common presentation. Pain is a variable feature. Entrapment of extraocular muscles and orbital soft tissue by the fibrotic mass results in restrictive myopathy and diplopia. The presence of a mass lesion in the orbital apex produces compressive optic neuropathy, dysfunction of the ocular motor nerves, and proptosis. Orbital venous drainage may be obstructed, resulting in signs of orbital congestion.

The clinical manifestations and response to treatment of the chronic sclerosing form may be considerably different than in acute forms of orbital pseudotumor. Intracranial extension with bony erosion has been reported.[40–44] This has led some authorities to suggest that the chronic sclerosing variant of orbital pseudotumor be considered as a separate clinical entity.[17, 41, 45] The sclerosing variant of pseudotumor has been reported to occur in association with multifocal fibrosclerosis.[8, 45, 46] The latter is a systemic disease that may manifest as retroperitoneal and mediastinal fibrosis, sclerosing cholangitis, Riedel's thyroiditis, and pachymeningitis. Some cases of the sclerosing form of orbital pseudotumor may represent a manifestation of this disorder.[46–48]

The relationship between idiopathic orbital pseudotumor and *paranasal sinus disease* is controversial. Orbital myositis may be preceded by an upper respiratory

Figure 170–7. A 47-year-old man with a history of mild Graves' orbitopathy complained of increasing proptosis of the right eye and worsening diplopia. A, Contrast-enhanced axial computed tomographic (CT) scan of the orbit shows a lesion in the apex. B, Coronal CT scan demonstrates the mass displacing the inferior rectus and optic nerve. Results of biopsy were consistent with nonspecific idiopathic orbital inflammation. The lesion responded poorly to corticosteroids, but radiation therapy was successful.

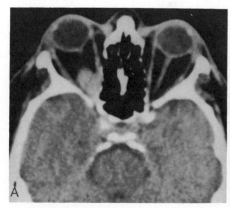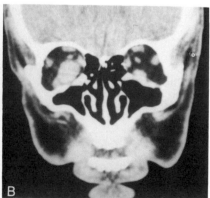

tract infection or sinusitis.[30-32] Orbital pseudotumor following chronic paranasal sinusitis complicated by orbital cellulitis and subperiosteal abcess has been reported.[49] Despite these reports, most cases of idiopathic orbital inflammation lack clinical and radiographic evidence of sinus involvement. A definite causal relationship between sinus disease and idiopathic orbital pseudotumor has yet to be established.[5, 8]

Simultaneous occurrence of idiopathic pseudotumor in the orbit and sinuses is unusual but can occur.[50-52] The orbital inflammatory process is believed to involve the sinuses secondarily via small communicating blood vessels between the orbit and sinuses. Orbital inflammation may mimic primary sinus diseases such as invasive carcinoma or sinusitis.[53] Chronic intranasal cocaine use may result in inflammatory sinus disease that secondarily involves the orbit. Chronic osteolytic sinusitis and optic neuropathy are hallmark features of this disorder.[54, 55]

Pediatric orbital pseudotumor is uncommon but is not a rarity. Approximately 6 to 16 percent of orbital pseudotumors occur during the first and second decades of life.[5, 56] Several distinguishing characteristics are unique to occurrence of orbital pseudotumors in the pediatric population. There is a higher incidence of bilateral orbital involvement without evidence of underlying systemic illness. Anterior uveitis and optic disc edema are more common and are often associated with bilateral orbital inflammation. Patients with bilateral involvement and iritis experience a greater incidence of recurrence and morbidity. Trauma or upper respiratory tract infection may precede the onset of orbital pseudotumor in some cases.[56] Eosinophilia of the peripheral blood is present in approximately one third of cases. Similarly, increased numbers of eosinophils may be found in tissue specimens obtained at orbital biopsy.[14, 57] Uncommonly, spontaneous orbital hemorrhage can occur as a complication of idiopathic orbital pseudotumor.[58]

Differential Diagnosis

A variety of disease entities may result in orbital inflammation or mimic orbital inflammatory disease in clinical presentation. Thus, a number of disorders must be excluded before the diagnosis of nonspecific idiopathic orbital inflammation can be made (see Table 170–1). Such an array of diagnostic possibilities often makes the diagnosis of orbital inflammatory disorders challenging. Consideration of the patients' pattern of orbital involvement, clinical course, and systemic signs and symptoms aids in this process. First, a meticulous history and physical examination are required. These data are supplemented by appropriate laboratory and radiographic testing. Biopsy of orbital lesions may also be necessary.

The *orbitopathy of Graves' disease* is the most commonly encountered cause of orbital inflammation. Distinguishing Graves' orbitopathy from idiopathic pseudotumor is usually not difficult. However, in some instances, differentiating the two may be extremely challenging. For example, Graves' disease may present with prominent signs of orbital inflammation simulating the appearance of acute anterior pseudotumor or with long-standing myopathic changes suggesting chronic orbital myositis. The absence of demonstrable thyroid dysfunction in euthyroid patients and the occasional unilateral occurrence of Graves' orbitopathy may add to the confusion. Clinical features helpful in differentiating these entities are outlined in Table 170–2.

Infection is a common cause of orbital inflammation and may result in serious morbidity and mortality. *Orbital cellulitis* may be complicated by subperiosteal or orbital abcess formation and potentially fatal cavernous sinus thrombosis. It is, therefore, imperative that infectious causes be excluded when pursuing the diagnosis of idiopathic pseudotumor. The most common cause of bacterial orbital cellulitis is paranasal sinusitis. Other causes include contiguous spread of infection from the face, ocular adnexa, and oropharynx; penetrating orbital foreign bodies; and septicemia. The presence of any of these predisposing conditions in a patient with signs of orbital inflammation should suggest the possibility of infection. Findings consistent with orbital infection include marked malaise with a "toxic"-appearing patient, fever, and a complete blood count, with differential showing leukocytosis with a shift to the left.

Immunocompromised and debilitated patients are prone to *fungal infections* of the upper respiratory tract and sinuses. *Rhinoorbital mucormycosis* may occur as a complication of diabetic ketoacidosis and may be life-threatening. This is an aggressive infection characterized by the rapid development of orbital pain and inflammatory signs, culminating in an apex syndrome with ophthalmoplegia and visual loss.[59] Examination of the nasal mucosa or palate may reveal a black eschar representing tissue necrosis. *Aspergillus* may invade the orbit from an infected sinus, resulting in a slowly progressive infiltrating mass lesion. Involvement of the posterior orbit by *Aspergillus* can produce a corticosteroid-responsive apex syndrome similar to the chronic sclerosing variant of idiopathic orbital pseudotumor. Delayed diagnosis of *Aspergillus* infection may result in a fatal outcome.[60, 61] Although uncommon, tuberculous and syphilitic involvement of the orbit in the form of periostitis or infiltration can occur.

A variety of *granulomatous disorders* may result in signs and symptoms of orbital inflammation. These conditions can be differentiated from idiopathic pseudotumor by characteristic ophthalmic, systemic, and histologic features. Sarcoidosis is the most commonly encountered disorder and is discussed in a subsequent section. A form of noninfectious idiopathic granulomatous inflammation without evidence of systemic involvement has been described.[16, 62] Erdheim-Chester disease is a multisystem xanthogranulomatous disorder occurring in adults that may result in orbital infiltration and cicatrization.[63, 64] Biopsy of orbital lesions reveals cholesterol-laden histiocytes, Touton giant cells, lymphocytes, plasma cells, and fibrosis. Infiltration of heart, lung, kidney, and bone can occur. The presence of xanthelasma-like lid lesions and systemic involvement aid in the recognition of this uncommon disorder.[65]

Table 170–2. CLINICAL FEATURES OF ORBITAL PSEUDOTUMOR AND GRAVES' ORBITOPATHY

Variable	Idiopathic Pseudotumor	Graves' Orbitopathy
Sex predilection	None	3:1 female
Mode of onset	Acute, subacute, chronic	Chronic
Pain	Often present, may be severe	Painless, unless with keratitis or marked orbital congestion
Laterality	Usually unilateral	Usually bilateral
Lid signs	Lid edema, erythema, ptosis	Lid and periorbital edema, lid retraction, lid lag, lagophthalmos
Systemic symptoms	Malaise	Generally well; symptoms of thyroid disease
Laboratory findings	Elevated ESR*	Abnormal thyroid function in most cases
Radiographic findings	Infiltrate or mass; uveoscleral enhancement; EOM† enlargement, including tendonous insertion; any muscle, particularly superior and medial recti	Spindle-shaped EOM† enlargement, sparing tendon, especially inferior and medial recti; increased orbital fat volume
Ultrasonography	Uveoscleral thickening; sub-Tenon's effusion	May detect enlarged EOM† before CT‡ scan

*ESR, erythrocyte sedimentation rate
†EOM, extraocular muscle
‡CT, computed tomography

Necrobiotic xanthogranuloma is a disorder occurring in older patients having paraproteinemia associated with monoclonal gammopathy or myeloma. Clinical findings include firm-, waxy-, and injected-appearing subcutaneous nodules of the lids. The conjunctiva and orbit may be involved.[66, 67]

Other specific causes of orbital inflammation such as the *vasculitides* and *connective tissue diseases* may also masquerade as idiopathic pseudotumor. Primary orbital vasculitis limited to the orbit without systemic manifestations can also occur.[7, 15, 16] These entities may be diagnosed by characteristic clinical, histologic, and laboratory findings as discussed later.

A variety of *neoplastic disorders* may present with clinical features resembling orbital inflammation such as pain, lid edema, ptosis, conjunctival injection and chemosis, and proptosis. The clinical course will generally be subacute or chronic. Diagnostic possibilities include lymphoproliferative disorders; metastatic tumors, most commonly breast and lung carcinoma; secondary invasion of the orbit by tumors from adjacent structures; and primary orbital tumors. In children, rhabdomyosarcoma and the chloroma of acute myelogenous leukemia may progress extremely rapidly, mimicking an acute orbital inflammatory process. Orbital lymphoma has a predilection for the retrobulbar and superior orbital regions and exhibits a tendency to spread along the contours of the globe or other orbital structures. It has a characteristic putty-like or molded appearance on CT scan without evidence of bone erosion.[68] In cases of metastatic or invasive carcinoma, CT scanning with bone window technique may reveal bony erosion, which is not a feature of idiopathic pseudotumor.

The most common vascular abnormality to be confused with orbital pseudotumor is the low-flow *dural arteriovenous malformation of the cavernous sinus.* This disorder occurs most commonly in middle-aged women with a history of systemic hypertension and atherosclerotic vascular disease. The mode of onset is usually subacute or chronic. Painful orbital congestion with lid swelling, ptosis, proptosis, and conjunctival chemosis may simulate orbital inflammation. The corkscrew "arterialized" conjunctival vessels, which are pathognomonic for this disorder, are not seen in idiopathic pseudotumor. Although elevated intraocular pressure is sometimes seen in orbital pseudotumor, it commonly occurs with dural venous shunts because of elevated episcleral venous pressure associated with retrograde flow through the superior and inferior orbital veins. Marked pulsation of the mires pattern when performing applanation tonometry may be seen with dural arteriovenous fistulas. This finding is due to elevated pulse pressure, which can also be demonstrated with pneumotonography. Other features suggestive of a dural arteriovenous fistula include ophthalmoplegia resulting from extraocular muscle edema or ocular motor nerve paresis; signs of anterior segment ischemia with aqueous cell and flare, rubeosis, corneal edema, and progressive cataract; and venous stasis retinopathy. CT scans may show enlargement of the superior ophthalmic vein, diffuse extraocular muscle enlargement, and bulging of the cavernous sinus.[69] A sudden and marked exacerbation of orbital pain and swelling may signify thrombosis of the superior ophthalmic vein, which can be visualized with magnetic resonance imaging (MRI) scanning.[70] This event signifies resolution of the shunt, and patients will subsequently enjoy a marked improvement. Rarely, an *orbital varix* may present with acute pain and proptosis and be confused with pseudotumor. Valsalva maneuver may produce distention of the varix that can be observed clinically and demonstrated with CT.

Dacryoadenitis may be due to a variety of inflammatory processes. Bacterial, viral, fungal, tuberculous, and syphilitic infections of the lacrimal gland can occur. Bacterial infection, usually from *Staphylococcus aureus* or *Streptococcus*, may occur as a result of spread from the ocular adnexa, trauma, or bacteremia.[8, 71] The most common viral cause is mumps, although mononucleosis and herpes zoster may also be causative. With infectious causes, fever, lymphadenopathy, and leukocytosis will generally be present as opposed to nonspecific idiopathic lacrimal inflammation in which the only systemic findings are generalized malaise and elevated sedimentation rate. Noninfectious causes of lacrimal inflammation to be excluded in the diagnosis of idiopathic pseudotumor include sarcoidosis, Sjögren's syndrome, and Wegener's granulomatosis. The majority of noninfectious cases, however, are idiopathic in nature.[16] Primary lacrimal neoplasia or lymphoid tumor should be considered in cases of chronic lacrimal gland enlargement. The radiographic appearance of epithelial lacrimal tumors on CT scan is a rounded or globular expansion of the gland. Approximately 80 percent of these tumors will result in erosion of adjacent bone. In contrast, lymphoid tumors and idiopathic pseudotumor produce an oblong or elongated enlargement of the gland with molding to surrounding structures. Lymphoid neoplasms tend to be localized, whereas pseudotumor is often multifocal with accompanying myositis, sclerotenonitis, or optic perineuritis. Bone involvement is rare except in sclerosing pseudotumor.[72] Bilateral lacrimal gland involvement should raise the possibility of Sjögren's syndrome, sarcoidosis, lymphoid tumors, or idiopathic inflammation.

The clinical picture of *orbital myositis* may be due to a host of disorders. Graves' orbitopathy is the most common disorder confused with the myositic variant of idiopathic pseudotumor. Often, characteristic patterns of muscle involvement noted on CT scan will aid in differentiating these two conditions (see Table 170–2). Graves' orbitopathy causes enlargement of the muscle belly and spares the tendon. In Graves' disease, single or multiple muscles may be affected, and involvement of both orbits is common. Classically, idiopathic inflammatory pseudotumor involves both the extraocular muscle and tendon (see Fig. 170–4). Unfortunately, this is not true in all cases. In fact, bilateral orbital involvement with sparing of the muscle tendon probably occurs more commonly in myositis than previously thought, making the radiographic distinction between myositis and Graves' orbitopathy difficult in some cases.[73, 74] Ultimately, one cannot rely solely on imaging data, and integration of clinical and radiographic findings is necessary for accurate diagnosis.

Signs of orbital inflammation, ophthalmoplegia, and extraocular muscle enlargement can also occur with cavernous sinus thrombosis, carotid-cavernous sinus fistulas, orbital cellulitis, and tumors of extraocular muscle.[75] Tumors involving extraocular muscle may be primary (rhabdomyosarcoma), metastatic, or lymphoid.[76–78] Serum sickness, Crohn's disease, vasculitis, herpes zoster, sarcoidosis, Lyme disease, and giant cell polymyositis have been associated with orbital myositis.[30, 33, 79–84] Details of the history, physical examination, and radiographic appearance will facilitate differentiation of these diverse causes.[85] Conditions resulting in extraocular muscle enlargement are listed in Table 170–3.[16, 74, 86–88]

Lesions of the *posterior orbit* usually present with progressive findings of an orbital apex syndrome, which include ophthalmoplegia, optic neuropathy, and proptosis. Diagnostic considerations in the evaluation of a lesion in the orbital apex include orbital neoplasm, either primary or secondary invasion or metastatic; lymphoid tumor; optic nerve glioma or sheath menin-

Table 170–3. CONDITIONS ASSOCIATED WITH EXTRAOCULAR MUSCLE ENLARGEMENT

Inflammatory
  Graves' orbitopathy
  Myositis
  Orbital cellulitis
  Sarcoidosis
  Vasculitides
Neoplastic
  Primary tumor of muscle—rhabdomyosarcoma
  Metastasis
  Lymphoid tumors
Vascular
  Carotid-cavernous sinus fistula
  Dural-cavernous sinus arteriovenous malformation
  Venous obstruction secondary to orbital apex tumor
Miscellaneous
  Acromegaly
  Amyloidosis
  POEMS* syndrome
  Trichinosis
  Lithium therapy

*POEMS, syndrome of peripheral neuropathy, organomegaly, endocrinopathy, monoclonal gammopathy, and skin changes.

gioma; Wegener's granulomatosis; sarcoidosis; and idiopathic pseudotumor, particularly the sclerosing variant.[89] Infectious processes such as aspergillosis may mimic an orbital apex mass, as discussed previously.[61, 62]

Analogous to orbital pseudotumor, nonspecific idiopathic inflammation may occur in the region of the superior orbital fissure and anterior cavernous sinus. Known as the *Tolosa-Hunt syndrome*, this disorder may produce pain and ophthalmoplegia as seen with lesions of the orbital apex. Visual loss, however, rarely occurs, and external signs of orbital inflammation are absent. Proptosis, if present, is usually minimal. This syndrome of painful ophthalmoplegia may be produced by a variety of inflammatory, infectious, neoplastic, and vascular disorders. Thus, the diagnosis of Tolosa-Hunt syndrome is one of exclusion, and a salutary response to a trial of corticosteroid is not necessarily diagnostic.[90–92] MRI has demonstrated abnormal signals in the cavernous sinus in a significant number of patients with clinical features of Tolosa-Hunt syndrome.[93, 94] Thus, MRI may provide helpful diagnostic information in the evaluation of patients with presumed Tolosa-Hunt syndrome.

Bilateral involvement in suspected idiopathic orbital pseudotumor raises the specter of underlying systemic disease. Clearly, children exhibit a high incidence of bilaterality, with up to 45 percent having simultaneous or sequential involvement of both orbits but without evidence of systemic illness.[56, 95] Bilaterality in adults occurs less commonly but is thought by many authorities to have an increased association with systemic disease.[4, 5, 8, 48] Others have found that this is not the case.[6] Disorders to be considered in the differential diagnosis of bilateral orbital inflammation include Graves' disease; sarcoidosis; lymphoid tumor; metastasis; primary orbital or systemic vasculitis; Sjögen's syndrome; Erdheim-Chester disease; syphilis; tuberculosis; and multifocal sclerosis with retroperitoneal fibrosis.

Diagnosis

Idiopathic orbital pseudotumor is a diagnosis of exclusion. Specific local and systemic causes of orbital inflammation as well as conditions mimicking inflammatory disease must be excluded. A meticulous history and physical examination are the first steps in diagnosis. The information thus gained may be used to identify clinical syndromes or specific systemic associations with orbital inflammatory disease. A rational plan for subsequent medical, surgical, laboratory, and radiologic investigations may then be formulated.[85]

Medical evaluation and laboratory testing are tailored to the clinical presentation and differential diagnostic possibilities. Tests that may be helpful but not necessarily indicated in all cases include complete blood count with differential; sedimentation rate; antinuclear antibody; thyroid function tests; serum protein electrophoresis; assessment of renal function with blood urea nitrogen, creatinine, and urinalysis; Veneral Disease Research Laboratory test or FTA-ABS test; and purified protein derivative with control. The supersensitive thyroid-stimulating hormone is an excellent screen for thyroid dysfunction in the ambulatory patient. A chest radiograph may reveal evidence of tuberculosis, sarcoidosis, neoplasia, vasculitis, or Wegener's granulomatosis. In suspected cases of sarcoidosis, serum calcium, angiotensin converting enzyme (ACE), serum lysozyme, and gallium scanning may be useful. The antineutrophil cytoplasm antibody (ANCA) may be positive in a large percentage of patients with Wegener's granulomatosis.

Orbital imaging studies useful in the diagnosis of inflammatory disease are CT and MRI. High-resolution CT scanning remains an excellent modality for evaluating orbital inflammatory disease.[96] CT scanning provides good delineation of orbital anatomy and useful diagnostic information concerning orbital masses and infiltrates. The size and location of abnormal tissue densities, contrast enhancement, and the presence of calcium, bone erosion, or hyperostosis are demonstrated by CT scan. The CT findings in idiopathic orbital pseudotumor have been described previously here.[36–38] For orbital diagnosis, a CT scan with axial and coronal views and contrast enhancement is required. Bone window technique is helpful in demonstrating bony involvement.

Experience with MRI in orbital diagnosis is growing rapidly. The use of high-field-strength magnets, surface coils, contrast agents, and fat-suppression techniques has resulted in superb orbital images. The signal-intensity characteristics of orbital tissues reveal more specific information concerning pathologic alteration than CT scanning.[96] The increased specificity of MRI allows differentiation among hemorrhage, neoplasia, and inflammation.[97] Other advantages of MRI compared with CT scanning include improved image resolution, particularly adjacent to dense cortical bone or in the orbital apex and cavernous sinus regions; less dental artifact; no radiation exposure; and ability to obtain axial, coronal, and sagittal views without repositioning the patient. Disadvantages are long exposure times, higher cost, sensitivity to movement artifact, poor imaging of bone,

and inability of claustrophobic patients to tolerate the procedure. MRI is contraindicated in patients with ferromagnetic aneurysm clips, cardiac pacemakers, or ocular and orbital metallic foreign bodies. Relative contraindications are metallic prosthetic heart valves and pregnancy.[96]

The issue of *orbital biopsy* often arises when evaluating the patient with orbital inflammatory disease. In acute and subacute cases with the typical signs and symptoms of idiopathic orbital inflammation and a negative medical evaluation for specific cause, orbital biopsy is usually not required.[11, 16] A salutary response to corticosteroid therapy may be both therapeutic and diagnostic.[13] Chronic orbital lesions should undergo biopsy to establish a tissue diagnosis of nonspecific inflammatory pseudotumor.[98] This information is useful in determining diagnosis and prognosis and in planning treatment. Other instances in which biopsy should be considered include lesions recurrent or refractory to treatment; presence of a discrete mass on CT or MRI, particularly when accompanied by bone involvement or extraorbital extension; history of carcinoma; and isolated lacrimal enlargement. In view of the relatively high incidence of lacrimal involvement by systemic and neoplastic processes and the low morbidity of the procedure, biopsy is recommended for isolated lacrimal lesions.[20]

The primary goal of the biopsy is to obtain adequate tissue for diagnosis without damage to orbital structures. Thus, an incisional rather than excisional biopsy is performed. An exception to this strategy is if the surgeon unexpectedly encounters a primary epithelial tumor of the lacrimal gland. For example, a benign mixed tumor of the lacrimal gland would require complete excision.[16] Optimally, at least 1 cm^3 volume of tissue should be obtained for pathologic analysis.[99] This may be difficult in some cases. Frozen sections can be helpful in identifying and characterizing abnormal orbital tissue intraoperatively. The majority of biopsies may be performed via an anterior orbitotomy under general or local anesthesia. Lesions in the posterior orbit may necessitate using a Krönlein lateral orbitotomy, an anterior approach through the ethmoid sinus and lamina papyracea or, rarely, unroofing the orbit via craniotomy. Orbital inflammation may be markedly exacerbated by open biopsy. The administration of high-dose corticosteroids in the perioperative period will help in avoiding this potentially sight-threatening complication.[8]

Fine-needle aspiration biopsy has been advocated for the diagnosis of orbital lesions, but its use remains controversial.[12, 98, 100] This technique carries a relatively low risk of complications and may be performed under local anesthesia. The availability of an experienced cytopathologist is essential for proper interpretation of the results. Because of the small volume of tissue obtained, the results may be inconclusive and preclude the use of immunohistopathologic techniques.[12] Additional tissue must then be removed via open biopsy or a second fine-needle aspiration. In general, an open biopsy is preferred, but fine-needle aspiration may be helpful in select cases.

A portion of the tissue obtained at biopsy should be preserved in *formalin* for permanent paraffin sections, because light microscopy remains the method by which the majority of pathologic diagnoses are made. Another specimen should be sent to the laboratory in *saline* for immunohistopathologic analysis. These techniques allow categorization of lymphoid lesions in terms of clonality and cell type based on cell surface markers on T cells and kappa or lambda light chain immunoglobulins in the case of B cells.[18] Monoclonal lesions are malignant, and polyclonal lesions are generally believed to be benign. Immunohistopathologically benign lesions may undergo malignant transformation. Molecular genetic analysis has shown that some of these lesions may harbor small clones of monoclonal B lymphocytes.[101]

Patients found at biopsy to have a lymphoid tumor require further investigation for possible systemic involvement. Oncologic consultation should be requested. Serum immunoelectrophoresis, bone marrow aspiration, and abdominal CT scan should be obtained.[99] Bone scan and liver-spleen scan, intravenous pyelography, and lymphoangiography may also be indicated.[12] The potential for systemic involvement exists in all patients with lymphoproliferative lesions, even so-called benign reactive lymphoid hyperplasia.[101] Continued long-term medical surveillance for potential multisystem disease is, therefore, prudent.[12, 98, 99, 101]

Treatment

The primary goal in the treatment of nonspecific inflammation of the orbit is rapid and effective suppression of the inflammatory process. Corticosteroids are the mainstay of therapy, and adequate doses must be administered to achieve the desired results. Inadequate treatment may result in a higher rate of recurrence and increased visual morbidity from cicatrization of orbital tissues.[13] Once the desired effect has been achieved, the medication is slowly tapered over a period of weeks and is then discontinued. Chronic corticosteroid therapy with its attendant systemic complications is to be avoided. Refractory or recurrent cases may be better managed by other modalities such as as low-dose radiation or chemotherapy.

With the exception of isolated lacrimal involvement, the majority of patients with acute and subacute cases and presenting with the typical historic, physical, laboratory, and radiographic findings of nonspecific idiopathic orbital inflammation may be treated without biopsy. Patients with severe cases may require rapid institution of treatment. Once sufficient data have been obtained to exclude an infectious cause, treatment may be initiated with corticosteroids barring any medical contraindication. An initial dose of oral prednisone, 60 to 100 mg/day in divided doses, should be used in most adults.[13, 98, 102] Alternatively, 1.0 to 1.5 mg/kg/day may also be used to calculate the initial dose of oral prednisone.[9] Doses as low as 40 to 60 mg/day have been found to be effective for myositis and dacryoadenitis.[16] Patients usually have marked symptomatic improvement within 48 to 72 hr of starting treatment. However, high-dose

corticosteroids should be continued for 2 to 3 wk to suppress the inflammation adequately. This may lower the likelihood of recurrence and decrease long-term morbidity. If at this point a salutary effect has been achieved, the corticosteroids may then be slowly tapered over the next few weeks. Generally, reducing the prednisone by 10 mg/wk will prevent rebound, but each case must be approached individually. If the patient experiences a rebound of signs or symptoms, the dose of corticosteroids must be increased and then tapered more gradually. Indomethacin is reportedly effective in mild cases of orbital myositis as a substitute for corticosteroids.[103]

Anterior inflammatory pseudotumor may be complicated by increased intraocular pressure as described previously. As the orbital inflammation responds to corticosteroid therapy, this complication will resolve. Decreasing aqueous formation with a topical β-blocker and oral carbonic anhydrase inhibitor will bring intraocular pressure under control while awaiting the corticosteroid response. A topical cycloplegic should be added if angle closure resulting from choroidal effusions is present.

Cases that are recurrent or refractory to treatment require orbital biopsy to confirm the diagnosis of nonspecific orbital inflammation. Recurrent cases may then be treated appropriately with repeated courses of oral prednisone, but long-term treatment with corticosteroids is to be assiduously avoided. Low-dose orbital radiation is an excellent alternative means of suppressing orbital inflammation in refractory and steroid-dependent cases or in instances in which the use of corticosteroids is medically contraindicated. A poor response to corticosteroids does not necessarily preclude a salutary effect by radiation. Total radiation doses of 1000 to 3000 cGy have been advocated, with many lesions responding to 1500 to 2000 cGy.[9, 13, 20, 98, 102, 104–106] The globe should be shielded, and the total dose should be fractionated and delivered over a 10- to 14-day course to avoid complications. Potential complications of radiation therapy include cataract formation, dry eye, and radiation retinopathy. Patients with a preexisting microangiopathy, such as diabetes mellitus, or a history of treatment with cytotoxic chemotherapeutic agents may be at higher risk of the development of radiation retinopathy.

Cytotoxic agents are of value in select cases of orbital inflammation. Cyclophosphamide has been used to control primary vasculitis of the orbit refractory to corticosteroids and radiotherapy.[15] Low-dose cyclosporine therapy has been shown to be effective in suppressing recurrent or corticosteroid-resistant inflammatory orbital pseudotumor with minimal side effects (mild hypertrichosis).[107, 108] Cyclosporine therapy in diabetic patients not only avoids the hyperglycemia associated with corticosteroids but may result in improved regulation of serum blood sugar.[109]

Chronic cases of idiopathic orbital inflammatory disease require biopsy to determine the correct diagnosis and to plan treatment. If the lesion is nonsclerosing, high-dose corticosteroid treatment as outlined previously may be successful. Radiotherapy is used if the lesion proves recurrent or refractory to corticosteroids.

Sclerosing lesions with their higher potential for morbidity and progression require more aggressive treatment. A generous incisional biopsy followed by combined corticosteroid and radiation therapy is recommended for these lesions.[98] Lesions located in the anterior orbit may be amendable to safe surgical excision. Unfortunately, sclerosing lesions have a predilection for the posterior orbit, and any attempt at extirpation would likely result in loss of vision and ophthalmoplegia. Cytotoxic drugs such as methotrexate and cyclophosphamide may be beneficial in particularly resistant cases.[98] Rarely, radical excision to debulk the tumor mass or orbital exenteration is required to control aggressive lesions.

SARCOIDOSIS

Sarcoidosis is an idiopathic disorder characterized by granulomatous inflammation involving multiple organ systems. The most commonly affected tissues are the lungs, hilar lymph nodes, eyes, and skin. The disease is most commonly seen in young adults 20 to 40 yr of age with a peak incidence at age 30. In the United States, sarcoidosis is at least 10 times more frequent in blacks than in whites. The incidence of ocular involvement is higher in blacks as well. Epidemiologic studies suggest that living in a rural environment may increase the risk of acquiring sarcoidosis.

The pathogenesis of sarcoidosis involves a defect in cell-mediated immunity. An antigen, which is yet to be identified, results in stimulation of T helper cells and inhibition of T suppressor cells. The high incidence of hilar adenopathy and pulmonary involvement in sarcoidosis suggests that this inciting agent may be inhaled. The stimulated T helper cells activate monocytes, which form epithelioid and multinucleated giant cells. These cells, in turn, form the characteristic histopathologic lesion of sarcoidosis, the noncaseating epithelioid cell granuloma. Humoral immunity is also abnormal in sarcoidosis with increased B cell activity resulting in hypergammaglobulinemia.

Clinically, sarcoidosis manifests in acute, subacute, and chronic forms. The acute form consisting of hilar lymphadenopathy with erythema nodosum and polyarthritis is usually benign and self-limited. Patients with chronic sarcoidosis have had the disease for more than 2 yr, tend to be older, and have a higher incidence of extrapulmonary involvement. Pulmonary involvement is the most common systemic manifestation of the disease. Patients may complain of dry cough, dyspnea, wheezing, and constitutional symptoms such as malaise, weight loss, and fever. Radiographic evidence of sarcoidosis is present in approximately 90 percent of cases, but in more than 35 to 40 percent respiratory symptoms may be absent, with the disease being detected on routine chest x-ray film. Although the lung, eyes, and skin are most commonly affected, other organ systems may be involved, including the liver, heart, and central nervous system. Ocular involvement occurs in approximately 25 to 50 percent of patients with sarcoidosis.[16, 110–113] The majority of patients with ocular involvement in sarcoi-

dosis have evidence of uveal tract inflammation in the anterior or posterior segment. The reader is referred to Volume 2, Chapter 86, and Volume 5, Chapter 254, for further details concerning the ocular and systemic manifestations of sarcoidosis.

Orbital involvement in sarcoidosis is uncommon but has been well-documented in the literature.[114–120] Granulomatous infiltration of orbital fat and connective tissue occurs in less than 1 percent of cases. However, up to 25 percent of patients with ophthalmic manifestations of sarcoidosis may have involvement of the orbit and related structures such as lacrimal apparatus, eyelids, extraocular muscle, and optic nerve.[111] Sarcoidosis of the orbit most commonly presents with signs and symptoms of acute or subacute orbital inflammation (Fig. 170–8). The clinical picture may be similar to that seen in idiopathic nonspecific inflammatory disease of the orbit (pseudotumor) with pain, proptosis, ophthalmoparesis, and visual loss. CT scanning may demonstrate involvement of lacrimal gland, extraocular muscle, and orbital soft tissue (see Fig. 170–8B).[118, 120–124] Bone destruction may also be seen.[125] Sarcoidosis occurring in the paranasal sinuses may secondarily involve the orbits.[126]

The lacrimal gland is the most commonly affected orbital tissue, with palpable enlargement of the gland being present in 10 percent of cases. A higher incidence of lacrimal involvement is found if the patient is tested for abnormalities in reflex lacrimation. Lacrimal gland enlargement in sarcoidosis is generally painless and often bilateral (see Fig. 170–8C). Lacrimal sac involvement is rare.[127] The skin is frequently involved in sarcoidosis, and subcutaneous nodules or masses may sometimes be palpated in the eyelids.[120] Infiltration of the extraocular muscles results in ophthalmoparesis because of a restrictive myopathy.[121] Involvement of the levator palpebrae–superior rectus muscle complex can cause blepharoptosis.[122] Optic neuropathy occurs in 5 percent of cases and may be due to infiltration, direct compression by granuloma, or angiitis.[128–134]

Isolated extralacrimal orbital granulomas that are histopathologically indistinguishable from the typical lesions of systemic sarcoidosis can occur. These lesions have been termed "orbital sarcoid" or "sarcoid reaction pattern" and in some cases may represent a separate entity unassociated with systemic sarcoidosis.[7, 8] However, most patients with apparently isolated orbital sarcoid, whether lacrimal or extralacrimal, will eventually be found to have systemic sarcoidosis.[119]

A presumptive diagnosis of sarcoidosis can be made when the patient presents with the typical clinical, laboratory, and radiographic findings of the disease. In 90 percent of patients, the chest radiograph will be abnormal. Although not specific for sarcoidosis, an elevated serum ACE may be found in 50 to 80 percent of patients. Gallium scanning may show abnormal uptake in the lacrimal glands and pulmonary hila.[112, 113] Characteristic gallium uptake in combination with an elevated ACE is more than 90 percent specific for sarcoidosis. Other supportive findings include anergy to cutaneous skin testing, hypercalcemia, hypergammaglobulinemia, elevated serum lysozyme, and abnormal

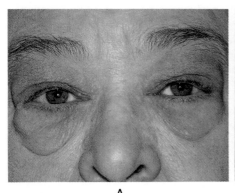
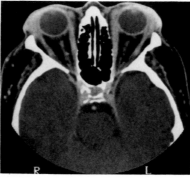
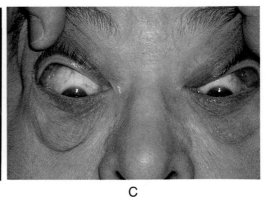

A   B   C

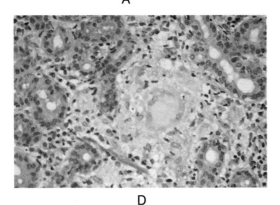

D

Figure 170–8. *A,* A 67-year-old Caucasian woman complained of puffiness of the eyelids and pressure sensation around the eyes which lasted for 6 wk. Examination was significant for visual acuity of 20/50 in both eyes; intraocular pressures of 40 mmHg in both eyes; mild exophthalmos; lacrimal gland enlargement; and conjunctival injection and chemosis. *B,* Contrast-enhanced axial computed tomographic scan demonstrates anterior orbital infiltrate involving the lacrimal glands and the medial rectus muscles bilaterally. *C,* Bilateral enlargement of the palpebral lobe of the lacrimal gland. *D,* Lacrimal gland biopsy specimen with noncaseating granulomas consistent with sarcoidosis. Positive lacrimal biopsy obviated the need for a more invasive procedure for pulmonary lesion biopsy. Oral corticosteroid therapy resulted in rapid resolution of signs and symptoms.

pulmonary function testing. However, histopathologic confirmation via tissue biopsy remains the gold standard in the diagnosis of sarcoidosis.

Depending on the clinical presentation, biopsy specimens may potentially be obtained from several ocular structures including conjunctiva, lacrimal gland, eyelid skin, or orbit. Establishing the diagnosis of sarcoidosis in this manner spares the patient from more invasive procedures such as transbronchial or mediastinal biopsy. If conjunctival nodules are present, biopsy of these lesions may confirm the diagnosis. A random conjunctival biopsy in which no lesions are visible will be positive less than 10 percent of the time.[135] The lacrimal gland may undergo biopsy via an anterior orbitotomy or transconjunctival approach.[136, 137] If the palpebral portion of the gland is enlarged, the latter technique may be used (see Fig. 170–8C and D). Care must be taken not to damage or transect the isthmus of the gland through which the lacrimal ductules course, because this can result in dry eye. Biopsy of eyelid skin nodules and subcutaneous masses may also yield a diagnosis. Biopsy of the minor salivary glands in the oral mucosa of the lower lip may be positive for sarcoidosis in up to 60 percent of cases.[138] Sarcoidosis has also been confirmed by skeletal muscle biopsy.[139]

Orbital involvement by sarcoidosis generally responds well to a course of oral corticosteroid. Prednisone, 30 to 60 mg/day in divided doses, tapered over 8 to 12 wk, is effective in most cases. Injection of orbital or lid lesions with triamcinolone has been advocated.[140] Response to treatment is assessed by the clinical examina-

tion. Serum ACE and lysozyme levels may also be helpful as an index of disease activity.

VASCULITIS

The vasculitides are a diverse group of diseases that share the common feature of inflammation or necrosis involving blood vessels. In these conditions, an angiocentric inflammatory response occurs, resulting in cellular infiltration of blood vessel walls and the perivascular tissues. Arteries and veins of various sizes in any organ system may be involved depending on the clinical syndrome. The vascular infiltrate consists of polymorphonuclear leukocytes in the acute stage, followed by the appearance of lymphocytes, plasma cells, and monocytes as the lesions evolve. Fibrinoid deposition and necrosis of the vessel wall in combination with endothelial damage result in narrowing, obliteration, or thrombosis of the vessel lumen, with subsequent signs and symptoms of ischemia. Giant cells and granuloma formation may also occur in certain syndromes such as giant cell arteritis and Wegener's granulomatosis.

The cause of systemic vasculitis is unknown in most cases, but many of the vasculitis syndromes are thought to be immune complex–mediated. An abnormal immune response to an antigenic stimulus produces immune complex formation and initiates an immunologic cascade culminating in inflammation and destruction of blood vessels. Disorders of cell-mediated immunity may play a role in certain conditions as well.

The vasculitides that most commonly have orbital manifestations are Wegener's granulomatosis, polyarteritis, hypersensitivity vasculitis, and giant cell arteritis. Virtually any of the vasculitic syndromes may produce signs and symptoms of orbital inflammation resembling idiopathic orbital pseudotumor. Because many of these diseases can result in serious morbidity or mortality, it is imperative that they be considered in the differential diagnosis of orbital inflammatory disease. Analysis of clinical, histopathologic, and laboratory findings will aid in timely and accurate diagnosis. The orbital manifestations of each disease are discussed later. For an in-depth review of the systemic and ocular features of of these disorders, the interested reader is referred to Volume 5, Section 237, The Eye and Systemic Disease, and reviews in the literature.[141-145]

WEGENER'S GRANULOMATOSIS

Wegener's granulomatosis is a disorder characterized by necrotizing granulomatous inflammation and vasculitis primarily affecting the entire respiratory tract and kidneys. Although the cause is unknown, it is thought to be an immune complex–mediated hypersensitivity disease. Cytotoxic effects of neutrophils and eosinophils may contribute to the vascular insult.[146] The peak incidence is in the fifth decade of life, and men are twice as likely as women to acquire the disease.

The classic triad of disseminated Wegener's granulomatosis consists of necrotizing granulomatous inflammation of the upper and lower respiratory tracts and glomerulonephritis. Clinical manifestations include sinusitis, bone destruction with saddle nose deformity, epistaxis, otitis media, respiratory mucosal ulcerations, and pneumonitis. Renal failure is a common cause of mortality. A focal small-vessel vasculitis affecting other organ systems is also usually present.[147] Eyes, joints, skin, heart, and peripheral nerves are the most frequently affected extrapulmonary sites.

Wegener's granulomatosis also occurs in a limited form, which is more common in females with a less severe clinical course than the disseminated form. There is primarily upper and lower respiratory tract involvement; renal and other extrapulmonary manifestations are less common. However, the incidence of ocular involvement is equal to that of disseminated Wegener's granulomatosis and its recognition can be important in making the diagnosis.[148]

Ocular involvement in Wegener's granulomatosis is common, occurring in approximately 50 percent of patients.[144, 149] Ocular manifestations, which are often bilateral, include conjunctivitis, marginal ulcerative keratitis, episcleritis, scleritis, uveitis, retinal vasculitis, and optic neuropathy.[149-151]

Orbital signs and symptoms occur in approximately 50 percent of patients with ocular manifestations of Wegener's granulomatosis.[151] Contiguous spread of inflammation to the orbit from the paranasal sinuses or nasopharynx is the most common mechanism of orbital involvement. Less commonly, Wegener's granulomatosis can occur in the orbit as an isolated phenomenon and *may be the initial sign of the disease.*[150-155]

Common signs and symptoms of orbital involvement in Wegener's granulomatosis include proptosis, pain, redness, orbital congestion, and ophthalmoparesis. Bilateral orbital involvement is common. Wegener's granulomatosis may also be manifest in the orbit as a chronically progressive orbital apex syndrome presenting with pain, ophthalmoparesis, and decreased vision (Fig. 170–9).[16, 156] Extraocular muscle dysfunction may be due to direct vasculitic involvement of the muscles or to cranial neuropathy.[157-159] Eyelid granulomas, dacryoadenitis, and nasolacrimal duct obstruction may be seen with involvement of the ocular adnexa.[150]

The diagnosis of Wegener's granulomatosis may be

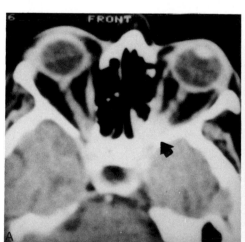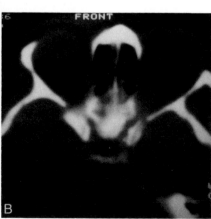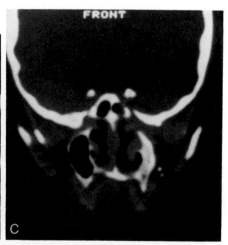

Figure 170–9. A 69-year-old woman complained of malaise, left-sided facial pain, and decreased vision of the left eye, which lasted for 6 mo. *A*, Contrast-enhanced axial computed tomographic (CT) scan of the orbits demonstrates an infiltrative lesion involving the left orbital apex and adjacent paranasal sinuses. *B*, Axial CT, bone window technique. *C*, Coronal CT, bone window technique, demonstrates bony erosion in the wall of the sphenoid sinus. Ethmoidal biopsy revealed necrotizing granulomatous inflammation and vasculitis consistent with the diagnosis of Wegener's granulomatosis.

suspected in a patient presenting with the constellation of findings outlined previously. Unfortunately, the classic features of disseminated Wegener's granulomatosis may not be present, particularly in the limited form of the disease. Therefore, the clinician must maintain a high index of suspicion when evaluating patients presenting with signs and symptoms of orbital inflammatory disease. The presence of concomitant sinus disease (>90 percent of cases) and bilaterality should alert one to consider the diagnosis of Wegener's granulomatosis. Wegener's granulomatosis may present with orbital findings similar to idiopathic orbital pseudotumor. Thus, a case of presumed pseudotumor that responds inadequately or only transiently to corticosteroid therapy should raise the possibility of Wegener's granulomatosis.

Nonspecific laboratory findings in Wegener's granulomatosis include anemia, leukocytosis, thrombocytosis, elevated sedimentation rate, and C-reactive protein. Microscopic hematuria may also be present. The antineutrophil cytoplasmic antibody (ANCA) is a very useful serologic test with a high sensitivity and specificity for Wegener's granulomatosis. Approximately 60 to 90 percent of patients with the disease will have a positive ANCA result.[160–163] Histopathologic confirmation of the diagnosis is necessary in cases in which serologic testing is inconclusive. Common biopsy sites are the nasal mucosa, sinus mucosa, and orbit. A spectrum of histopathologic findings other than the classic Wegener's triad of vasculitis, granulomatous inflammation, and tissue necrosis may be found on biopsy of orbital lesions. Correlation of orbital histopathology with the clinical presentation, ANCA result, and extraorbital biopsy results is important.[164]

Serious manifestations of Wegener's granulomatosis have been found to respond well to a combination cyclophosphamide and corticosteroid regimen. ANCA titers are useful in monitoring disease activity.[165] Sight-threatening proptosis sometimes encountered with aggressive orbital involvement may require urgent surgical orbital decompression.[150, 166] Nasolacrimal duct obstruction may be relieved via dacryocystorhinostomy if the disease is quiescent.[167]

POLYARTERITIS (PERIARTERITIS NODOSA)

Polyarteritis is an immune complex–mediated systemic necrotizing vasculitis that affects predominantly middle-aged men. The disease is characterized by panmural inflammation and fibrinoid necrosis affecting small and medium-sized arteries. Vascular involvement is segmental, with a propensity to involve the bifurcations. Endothelial proliferation and fibrosis occur as the lesions heal, resulting in occlusion of the lumen. Aneurysm formation results from partial involvement of the arterial wall in 10 to 15 percent of cases; hence, the term *nodosa* was used to describe these lesions.

Multiple organ systems may be involved, often resulting in protean signs and symptoms. The most frequently affected organ is the kidney (70 percent), followed by the musculoskeletal system (64 percent), peripheral nerve (51 percent), gastrointestinal tract (44 percent), skin (43 percent), heart (36 percent), and central nervous system (23 percent).[145] Presenting symptoms are usually constitutional: weight loss, fever, anorexia, malaise, abdominal pain, myalgias, and arthralgias. Signs of renal dysfunction are common and include proteinuria, hematuria, renal vascular hypertension, and perirenal or retroperitoneal hemorrhage. Myocardial infarction, congestive heart failure, and pericarditis may occur as manifestations of cardiac involvement. Damage to the vasa nervorum results in peripheral neuropathy, which may occur as a mononeuritis multiplex. Cutaneous manifestations include palpable purpura, livedo reticularis, ulcerations, and subcutaneous nodules. Signs of central nervous system involvement occur late in the course of the disease.

Ocular involvement occurs in approximately 10 to 20 percent of cases of polyarteritis.[144] Signs of retinal and choroidal ischemia secondary to systemic vascular hypertension or local vasculitis are common findings.[168, 169] Necrotizing scleritis, uveitis, and peripheral corneal ulceration can also be seen.[170, 171]

Orbital vasculitis secondary to polyarteritis may have a variety of manifestations. Presenting signs and symptoms such as orbital congestion, proptosis, and ophthalmoparesis may be identical to those seen with nonspecific idiopathic orbital inflammation. This may confound the diagnosis, particularly if systemic manifestations are not yet apparent.[172] Pain is a variable feature. Visual loss can occur secondary to optic nerve ischemia or inflammation.[173] Anterior and posterior forms of ischemic optic neuropathy have been reported.[170, 174–176] An orbital apex syndrome with painful proptosis, ophthalmoparesis, and visual loss has been described in a patient with polyarteritis.[177] Orbital vasculitis can also cause intermittent reductions of blood supply to the optic nerve, retina, or choroid resulting in amaurosis fugax.[178]

The diagnosis of polyarteritis may be suspected in patients presenting with constitutional symptoms and signs of multisystem dysfunction as outlined previously. Features particularly suggestive of systemic vasculitis are skin lesions, peripheral neuropathy, jaw claudication, and renal sediment abnormalities.[142] Leukocytosis with neutrophilia, anemia, thrombocytosis, and elevated sedimentation rate are common laboratory abnormalities. Angiographic evidence of segmental arterial narrowing and aneurysm formation may be supportive of the diagnosis of polyarteritis, but these findings are nonspecific. Short of histopathologic confirmation, there is no specific laboratory test for polyarteritis.

Clinically involved tissues such as skin, peripheral nerve, testes, or muscle may undergo biopsy to establish the diagnosis definitively. Temporal artery biopsy has been of value in rare instances.[179, 180] Because of the segmental nature of the disease, multiple tissue sections must be examined so as not to overlook involved areas.

The prognosis in untreated polyarteritis is poor, with only 13 percent survival at 5 yr. In cases with limited or nonprogressive disease, moderate doses of corticosteroid may be sufficient. In more severe cases, combined regimens of corticosteroid and cytotoxic agents such as cyclophosphamide have greatly reduced morbidity and increased 5-yr survival rates to 80 percent.

GIANT CELL ARTERITIS

Giant cell arteritis is a systemic vasculitis characterized by focal nonnecrotizing granulomatous inflammation of small to medium-sized arteries, particularly the cranial arteries arising from the aortic arch. The vessels are involved in a segmental manner. The inflammatory response is thought to be a cell-mediated reaction to an antigen associated with the arterial wall. Histopathologic findings include granulomatous lesions with epithelioid and giant cells, a nonspecific inflammatory infiltrate, intimal fibrosis, and fragmentation of the internal elastic lamina. These pathologic changes in the arterial wall lead to obliteration or thrombosis of the vessel lumen.

Giant cell arteritis is a disease affecting older patients at an average age of 70 yr and rarely occurs before the age of 50. It is also rare in blacks and Asians. Systemic symptoms include headache with scalp tenderness, jaw claudication or tongue pain, malaise, anorexia, weight loss, fever, myalgias, and depression.[181] Neurologic manifestations of giant cell arteritis occur in approximately 30 percent of patients and consist of stroke, transient ischemic attacks, and peripheral neuropathy.[182] Cardiac involvement is probably more common than previously believed and can result in angina pectoris, congestive heart failure, or myocardial infarction.[183, 184] Patients admitted to the hospital for visual loss may continue to deteriorate with successive stroke and fatal myocardial infarction even while receiving intravenous methylprednisolone therapy.

Ophthalmologic manifestations in giant cell arteritis are common; visual loss is the most frequently encountered. Anterior ischemic optic neuropathy is by far the most common cause of visual loss in giant cell arteritis, accounting for 80 to 90 percent of cases. This is the result of involvement of the ophthalmic artery or its branches, particularly the posterior ciliary arteries. Less frequent causes are central and branch retinal artery occlusion and chiasmal and retrochiasmal field deficits.[185] Approximately 15 percent of patients experience diplopia resulting from ocular motor nerve, brain stem, or extraocular muscle ischemia.

Orbital involvement in giant cell arteritis is due to vasculitic occlusion of its carotid or ophthalmic arterial blood supply. This results in ocular and orbital ischemia. Ocular signs and symptoms are identical to those seen in the ocular ischemic syndrome associated with atherosclerotic vascular occlusive disease.[186] Signs of anterior segment ischemia include conjunctival injection, corneal edema, aqueous cell and flare, rubeosis iridis, progressive cataract, and hypotony.[187, 188] Venous stasis retinopathy and choroidal ischemia may occur with posterior segment involvement.[189, 190] Generalized orbital ischemia may produce a clinical picture simulating orbital inflammation with pain, chemosis, proptosis, ophthalmoplegia, and visual loss.[191–193] Ophthalmoparesis resulting from extraocular muscle ischemia or necrosis can occur in giant cell arteritis.[194–197] Tonic pupils secondary to ciliary ganglion ischemia have been reported in giant cell arteritis.[198]

The diagnosis and institution of treatment in giant cell arteritis should be as expeditious as possible to avoid visual loss and potentially serious systemic complications. Visual loss secondary to ischemic optic neuropathy in giant cell arteritis is irreversible in most cases. However, the orbital manifestations of giant cell arteritis respond well to corticosteroids. Signs and symptoms of ocular ischemic syndrome, extraocular muscle ischemia, and generalized orbital ischemia may completely resolve with high-dose corticosteroid therapy.[186] A detailed discussion concerning the diagnosis and treatment of giant cell arteritis may be found in Volume 5, Section 236, of this textbook.

HYPERSENSITIVITY VASCULITIS

Hypersensitivity vasculitis, also referred to as small-vessel vasculitis or leukocytoclastic angiitis, is the most common cause of blood vessel inflammation. Hypersensitivity vasculitis is characterized by widespread necrotizing vasculitis involving arterioles, capillaries, and, in particular, venules. The disease process is initiated when antibodies are produced in reaction to a circulating antigen such as a drug, microbe, or tumor antigen, although in many cases a specific antigen cannot be demonstrated. Deposition of circulating immune complexes in the vascular wall results in polymorphonuclear leukocytic infiltration. This inflammatory response produces fibrinoid necrosis of the vessel wall, increased vascular permeability, and extravasation of erythrocytes, resulting in microinfarction and hemorrhagic lesions in affected tissues.

Hypersensitivity vasculitis may produce a number of syndromes with widely varying clinical manifestations depending on the extent of the disease and the target organs involved. Examples of hypersensitivity vasculitis include the vasculitis associated with connective tissue diseases such as systemic lupus erythematosus (SLE) and rheumatoid arthritis; serum sickness and drug reactions; Henoch-Schönlein purpura; the vasculitis associated with subacute bacterial endocarditis and malignancies; and essential mixed cryoglobulinemia. Multiple organs may be affected, but skin involvement is a predominant feature, with palpable purpura being the cardinal manifestation.[141, 143]

SLE is a chronic relapsing and remitting multisystem inflammatory disorder of unknown cause. It is nine times more common in females, occurring most frequently in girls and young women. Increased B cell activity and a defect in T cell suppression produce autoantibody formation and immune complex deposition, resulting in a necrotizing vasculitis affecting small vessels and capillaries. The most common systemic manifestations of SLE involve the musculoskeletal system, skin, and kidneys. Ocular involvement occurs in approximately 20 percent of patients with SLE. Retinopathy is the most common manifestation, with cotton-wool spots being a hallmark feature. Other ocular findings in SLE are choroidopathy, scleritis, episcleritis, and optic neuropathy.[144, 199]

Orbital vasculitis secondary to SLE is uncommon but has been described.[16, 81, 200–203] Patients may present with signs and symptoms of anterior orbital inflammation such as pain, proptosis, chemosis, and ophthalmoparesis. Involvement may be unilateral or bilateral. Extraocular muscle dysfunction as a result of associated myositis may be present.[81, 204] In contrast to this dramatic presentation, painless chemosis and periorbital edema may be the presenting signs of SLE.[205]

The clinical diagnosis of SLE may be made when four or more of the American Rheumatism Association diagnostic criteria are met.[206, 207] Antinuclear antibodies are present in more than 90 percent of SLE cases, but may be present in other connective tissue diseases as well. However, detection of antibodies to double-stranded DNA (present in 75 percent of SLE patients) has a positive predictive value of 95 percent that the patient has the disease. The LE cell test is no longer considered useful.

Therapeutic intervention in SLE is aimed at relief of symptoms and prevention of complications. Mild manifestations of the disease such as myalgias and arthralgias may be controlled with salicylates, nonsteroidal antiinflammatory drugs, or hydroxychloroquine. The latter is also useful in managing dermatologic complications. High-dose corticosteroids are used in severe cases. Various cytotoxic drugs and plasmaphoresis have also been used.

Primary orbital vasculitis may occur in the absence of associated systemic findings. The clinical presentation is similar to that seen in nonspecific anterior orbital pseudotumor with the acute or subacute onset of pain, swelling, and redness of the lids and periorbital tissues, ptosis, conjunctival injection, and chemosis. Proptosis may also be present.[7, 15, 16] Histopathologic findings are suggestive of hypersensitivity vasculitis. Henderson termed this entity type I orbital pseudotumor.[7] Ophthalmoparesis and severe visual loss can also occur in some cases.[15] Primary orbital vasculitis will often respond well to systemic corticosteroid therapy.[16] Low-dose radiation and immunosuppressive agents such as cyclophosphamide may be useful in cases refractory to corticosteroids.[7, 15]

SJÖGREN'S SYNDROME

Sjögren's syndrome is an autoimmune disorder characterized by chronic inflammation of the lacrimal and salivary glands, resulting in keratoconjunctivitis sicca and xerostomia (sicca complex). Sjögren's syndrome was originally described as the triad of dry eye, dry mouth, and rheumatoid arthritis. It is now recognized that the sicca complex can occur in the absence of associated connective tissue disease. This is known as primary Sjögren's syndrome. Secondary Sjögren's syndrome is defined as the sicca complex in association with a connective tissue disease such as rheumatoid arthritis, scleroderma, SLE, polymyositis, or polyarteritis nodosa.[144, 208] The majority of patients affected are middle-aged and elderly women. The cause is unknown, but Epstein-Barr virus and cytomegalovirus infection may play a role.[209]

In Sjögren's syndrome, a lymphoid infiltrate composed of lymphocytes and plasma cells results in loss of the normal tubuloacinar architecture of the lacrimal gland. The immunophenotypic composition of the lymphocytic infiltrate has been demonstrated to be B cells and T helper cells.[209] Destruction of glandular elements results in dysfunction of the lacrimal, salivary, and exocrine glands throughout the body, resulting in an autoimmune exocrinopathy.[210]

Sjögren's syndrome may have a variety of systemic manifestations.[211] Involvement of the salivary glands results in decreased salivation and xerostomia. Complications of xerostomia include difficulties with chewing, swallowing, and phonation; ulceration of the oral mucosa; fissures of the tongue and lips; and frequent dental caries. The dryness may extend to the mucosa of the nasopharynx and the entire tracheobronchial tree, resulting in recurrent bronchitis and pneumonitis. Other systemic manifestations include cutaneous vasculitis, Raynaud's phenomenon, thyroiditis, pancreatitis, hepatitis, nephritis, adult celiac disease, and gastric achlorhydria. Peripheral neuropathy may also be present; involvement of the trigeminal nerve is common.[212, 213] Corneal hypoesthesia resulting from trigeminal neuropathy increases the likelihood of corneal complications associated with dry eye. Patients with Sjögren's syndrome are also at increased risk of acquiring lymphoproliferative disorders including malignant lymphoma.

Laboratory findings in Sjögren's syndrome include positive antinuclear antibodies in approximately 70 percent of patients, with antibodies to Ro (SS-A) and La (SS-B) being highly suggestive of primary Sjögren's syndrome. Assay for rheumatoid factor is positive in 50 percent of patients with primary Sjögren's syndrome and in the majority of patients with associated rheumatoid arthritis. Anemia of chronic disease, hypergammaglobulinemia, and cryoglobulinemia may also be present.

The primary ocular manifestation of Sjögren's syndrome is keratoconjunctivitis sicca resulting from impaired function of the lacrimal gland and the accessory lacrimal glands of the conjunctiva. Decreased tear production results in symptoms of chronic ocular irritation with burning, a sandy or gritty sensation, and redness. Severe discomfort may make it difficult for the patient even to keep the eyes open. Symptoms are exacerbated by wind, low humidity, anticholinergic medications, and activities that decrease the blink rate such as reading, viewing television, and driving. Signs of dry eye include debris in the corneal tear film, decreased tear breakup time, reduced tear meniscus along the margin of the lower lid, conjunctival injection, and filamentary keratopathy. Fluorescein staining may be used to demonstrate punctate keratopathy, and devitalized epithelium can be assessed with rose bengal staining. Conjunctival symblepharon formation and corneal ulceration with perforation can occur in severe cases. Ocular infections are also more frequent in Sjögren's syndrome.

The Schirmer test can be used to demonstrate decreased lacrimation but may be diagnostic in only 50 percent of cases. If performed without anesthesia, the test measures both basal and reflex tearing. A Schirmer's test without anesthesia showing 3 mm or less of wetting in 5 min has proved to be 100 percent specific for keratoconjunctivitis sicca.[214] Measurements of tear osmolarity have proven highly sensitive and specific for keratoconjunctivitis sicca.[215] Biopsy of the labial accessory salivary glands, conjunctiva, or lacrimal gland may be helpful in confirming the diagnosis in uncertain cases.

Clinically detectable enlargement of the lacrimal gland in Sjögren's syndrome is uncommon. However, when it occurs, the presentation may resemble mild dacryoadenitis in combination with findings of the sicca syndrome.[16] In the evaluation of the patient with bilateral lacrimal enlargement, Sjögren's syndrome should be considered along with other diagnostic possibilities such as sarcoidosis, lymphoproliferative disease, nonspecific orbital inflammation, syphilis, and tuberculosis. Details concerning the therapy of dry eye may be found in Volume 1, Section 14 of this textbook.

REFERENCES

1. Duke-Elder S: System of Ophthalmology, vol. XIII. London, Henry Kimpton, 1974.
2. Birch-Hirschfeld A: Zur diagnostic and pathologic der orbital tumoren. Ber Dtch Ophthalmol Ges 32:127, 1905.
3. Coop ME: Pseudotumor of the orbit: A clinical and pathologic study of 47 cases. Br J Ophthalmol 45:513, 1961.
4. Jellinek EH: The orbital pseudotumor syndrome and its differentiation from endocrine exophthalmos. Brain 92:35, 1969.
5. Blodi FC, Gass JD: Inflammatory pseudotumor of the orbit. Trans Am Acad Ophthalmol Otolaryngol 71:303, 1967.
6. Chavis RM, Garner A, Wright JE: Inflammatory orbital pseudotumor: A clinicopathologic study. Arch Ophthalmol 96:1817, 1978.
7. Henderson JW: Orbital Tumors. New York, Thieme-Stratton, 1980.
8. Jakobiec FA, Jones IS: Orbital inflammations. In Duane TD (ed): Clinical Ophthalmology, vol 2. Hagerstown, MD, Harper & Row, 1989, pp 1–75.
9. Kennerdell JS, Dresner SC: The nonspecific orbital inflammatory syndromes. Surv Ophthalmol 29:93, 1984.
10. Jakobiec FA: Lymphoid tumors. In Spencer WH (ed): Ophthalmic Pathology: An Atlas and Textbook, vol 3. Philadelphia, WB Saunders, 1986, pp 2663–2711.
11. Maureillo JA, Flanagan JC: Pseudotumor and lymphoid tumor: Distinct clinicopathologic entities. Surv Ophthalmol 34:142, 1989.
12. Loeffler M, Hornblass A: Lymphoid proliferative disorders of the orbit. Ophthalmol Clin North Am 4:125, 1991.
13. Jakobiec FA: Non-infectious orbital inflammations. In Spencer WH (ed): Ophthalmic Pathology: An Atlas and Textbook, vol 3. Philadelphia, WB Saunders, 1986, pp 2777–2795.
14. Noguchi H, Kephart GM, Campbell J, et al: Tissue eosinophilia and eosinophile degranulation in orbital pseudotumor. Ophthalmology 98:928, 1991.
15. Garrity JA, Kennerdell JS, Johnson BL, et al: Cyclophosphamide in the treatment of orbital vasculitis. Am J Ophthalmol 102:97, 1986.
16. Rootman J: Diseases of the Orbit. Philadelphia, JB Lippincott, 1988.
17. Weissler MC, Miller E, Fortune MA: Sclerosing orbital pseudotumor: A unique clinicopathologic entity. Ann Otol Rhinol Laryngol 98:496, 1989.
18. Jakobiec FA, Lefkowitch J, Knowles DM: B- and T-lymphocytes in ocular disease. Ophthalmology 91:635, 1984.
19. Braig RF, Romanchuk KG:Recurrence of orbital pseudotumor after 10 years. Can J Ophthalmol 23:187, 1988.
20. Rootman J, Nugent R: The classification and management of acute orbital pseudotumors. Ophthalmology 89:1040, 1982.
21. Bertelsen TI, Acute sclerotenonitis and ocular myositis complicated by papillitis, retinal detachment, and glaucoma. Acta Ophthalmol 38:136, 1960.
22. Rush JA, Kennerdell JS, Donin JF: Acute periscleritis—A variant of idiopathic orbital inflammation. Orbit 1:221, 1982.
23. Benson WE: Posterior scleritis. Surv Ophthalmol 32:297, 1988.
24. Allen JC, France TD: Pseudotumor of the orbit and peripheral uveitis. J Pediatr Ophthalmol 14:33, 1977.
25. Katz RS, Gass JD: Multiple choroidal osteomas developing in association with recurrent orbital inflammatory pseudotumor. Arch Ophthalmol 101:1724, 1983.
26. Gass JD: Retinal detachment and narrow-angle glaucoma: Secondary to inflammatory pseudotumor or the uveal tract. Am J Ophthalmol 64:612, 1967.
27. Wilhelmus KR, Grierson I, Watson PG: Histopathologic and clinical associations of scleritis and glaucoma. Am J Ophthalmol 91:697, 1981.
28. Kenny AH, Halfner JN: Ultrasonic evidence of inflammatory thickening and fluid collection within the retrobulbar fascia: The T sign. Ann Ophthalmol 91:1557, 1977.
29. Tychsen L, Tse D, Ossoinig K, et al: Trochleitis with superior oblique myositis. Ophthalmology 91:1075, 1984.
30. Ludwig I, Tomsak RL: Acute recurrent orbital myositis. J. Clin Neuro Ophthalmol 3:41, 1983.
31. Purcel JJ, Taulbee WA: Orbital myositis after upper respiratory tract infection. Arch Ophthalmol 99:437, 1981.
32. Slavin ML, Glaser JS: Idiopathic orbital myositis: Report of six cases. Arch Ophthalmol 100:1261, 1982.
33. Weinstein GS, Dresner SC, Slamovits TL, et al: Acute and subacute orbital myositis. Am J Ophthalmol 96:209, 1983.
34. Bullen CL, Younge BR: Chronic orbital myositis. Arch Ophthalmol 100:1749, 1982.
35. Reifler DM, Leder D, Rexford T: Orbital hemorrhage and eyelid ecchymosis in acute orbital myositis. Am J Ophthalmol 107:111, 1989.
36. Curtin HD: Pseudotumor. Radiol Clin North Am 25:583, 1987.
37. Trokel SL, Hilal SK: Submillimeter resolution CT scanning of orbital diseases. Ophthalmology 87:412, 1980.
38. Nugent RA, Rootman J, Robertson WD, et al: Acute orbital pseudotumors: Classification and CT features. Am J Radiol 137:957, 1981.
39. Cervellini P, Volpin L, Curri D, et al: Sclerosing orbital pseudotumor. Ophthalmologica 193:39, 1986.
40. Edwards MK, Zauel DW, Gilmore RL, et al: Invasive orbital pseudotumor-CT demonstration of extension beyond orbit. Neuroradiology 23:215, 1982.
41. Abramovitz JN, Kasdon DL, Sutula F, et al: Sclerosing orbital pseudotumor. Neurosurgery 12:463, 1983.
42. Kaye AH, Hahn JF, Craciun A, et al: Intracranial extension of inflammatory pseudotumor of the orbit. J Neurosurg 60:625, 1984.
43. Frohman LP, Kupersmith MJ, Lang J, et al: Intracranial extension and bone destruction in orbital pseudotumor. Arch Ophthalmol 104:380, 1986.
44. Noble SC, Chandler WF, Lloyd RV: Intracranial extension of orbital pseudotumor: A case report. Neurosurgery 18:798, 1986.
45. Brazier DJ, Sanders MD: Multifocal fibrosclerosis associated with supracellar and macular lesions. Br J Ophthalmol 67:292, 1983.
46. Berger JR, Snodgrass S, Glaser J, et al: Multifocal fibrosclerosis with hypertrophic intracranial pachymeningitis. Neurology 39:1345, 1989.
47. Coming DE, Shubi KB, van Eyes J, et al: Familial multifocal fibrosclerosis: Findings suggesting that retroperitoneal fibrosis, mediastinal fibrosis, sclerosing cholangitis, Riedel's thyroiditis, and pseudotumor of the orbit may be different manifestations of a single disease. Ann Intern Med 66:884, 1967.
48. Richards AB, Shalka HW, Roberts FJ, et al: Pseudotumor of the orbit and retroperitoneal fibrosis: A form of multifocal fibrosclerosis. Arch Ophthalmol 98:1617, 1980.
49. Reidy JJ, Giltner J, Apple DJ, et al: Paranasal sinusitis, orbital abcess, and inflammatory tumors of the orbit. Ophthalmic Surg 18:363, 1987.

50. Eshaghian J, Anderson RL: Sinus involvement in inflammatory orbital pseudotumor. Arch Ophthalmol 99:627, 1981.
51. Bussone G, LaMantia L, Parati EA, et al: Orbital pseudotumor, chronic sinusitis, and idiopathic paraproteinemia. Orbit 3:115, 1984.
52. Pillai P, Saini JS: Bilateral sino-orbital pseudotumor. Can J Ophthalmol 23:177, 1988.
53. Weisberger EC, Zauel DW, Gilmor RL, et al: Otolaryngologists' role in diagnosis and treatment of orbital pseudotumor. Otolaryngol Head Neck Surg 93:536, 1985.
54. Newman NM, DiLoretto DA, Ho JT, et al: Bilateral optic neuropathy and osteolytic sinusitis: Complications of cocaine abuse. JAMA 259:72, 1988.
55. Goldberg RA, Weisman JS, McFarland JE, et al: Orbital inflammation and optic neuropathies associated with chronic sinusitis of intranasal cocaine abuse. Arch Ophthalmol 107:831, 1989.
56. Mottow LS, Jakobiec FA: Idiopathic inflammatory orbital pseudotumor in childhood. I: Clinical characteristics. Arch Ophthalmol 96:1410, 1978.
57. Mottow-Lippa L, Jakobiec FA, Smith M: Idiopathic inflammatory orbital pseudotumor in childhood. Ophthalmology 88:565, 1981.
58. Linberg JV, Mayle M: Spontaneous orbital hemorrhage associated with idiopathic inflammatory pseudotumor. Am J Ophthalmol 109:103, 1990.
59. Bray WH, Giangiacomo J, Ide CH: Orbital apex syndrome. Surv Ophthalmol 32:136, 1987.
60. Nielson EW, Weisman RA, Savino PJ, et al: Aspergillosis of the sphenoid sinus presenting as orbital pseudotumor. Otolaryngol Head Neck Surg 91:699, 1983.
61. Slavin ML: Primary aspergillosis of the orbital apex. Arch Ophthalmol 109:1502, 1991.
62. Krohel GB, Carr EM, Webb RM: Intralesional corticosteroids for inflammatory lesions of the orbit. Am J Ophthalmol 101:121, 1986.
63. Alper MG, Zimmerman LE, LaPiana FG: Orbital manifestations of Erdheim-Chester disease. Trans Am Ophthalmol Soc 81:64, 1983.
64. Rozenberg I, Wechsler J, Koenig S, et al: Erdheim-Chester disease presenting as malignant exophthalmos. Br J Radiol 59:173, 1986.
65. Shields JA, Karcioglu ZA, Shields CL, et al: Orbital and eyelid involvement with Erdheim-Chester disease: A report of two cases. Arch Ophthalmol 109:850, 1991.
66. Robertson DM, Winkelmann RK: Ophthalmic features of necrobiotic xanthogranuloma with paraproteinemia. Am J Ophthalmol 97:173, 1984.
67. Bullock JD, Bartley GB, Campbell RJ, et al: Necrobiotic xanthogranuloma with paraproteinemia. Ophthalmology 93:123, 1986.
68. Yeo JH, Jakobiec FA, Abbott GF, et al: Combined clinical and computed tomographic diagnosis of orbital lymphoid tumors. Am J Ophthalmol 94:235, 1982.
69. Keltner JL, Satterfield D, Dubin AB, et al: Dural and carotid cavernous sinus fistulas: Diagnosis, management, and complications. Ophthalmology 94:1585, 1987.
70. Sergott RC, Grossman RI, Savino PJ, et al: The syndrome of paradoxical worsening of dural-cavernous sinus arteriovenous malformations. Ophthalmology 94:205, 1987.
71. Harris GJ, Snyder RW: Lacrimal gland abcess. Am J Ophthalmol 104:193, 1987.
72. Jakobiec FA, Yeo JH, Trokel SL, et al: Combined clinical and computed tomographic diagnosis of primary lacrimal fossa lesions. Am J Ophthalmol 94:785, 1982.
73. Dresner SC, Rothfus WE, Slamovits TL, et al: Computed tomography of orbital myositis. AJR 143:671, 1984.
74. Patrinely JR, Osborn AG, Anderson RL, et al: Computed tomographic features of nonthyroid extraocular muscle enlargement. Ophthalmology 96:1038, 1989.
75. Spoor TC, Hartel WC: Orbital myositis. J Clin Neuro Ophthalmol 3:67, 1983.
76. Divine RD, Anderson RL: Metastatic small cell carcinoma masquerading as orbital myositis. Ophthalmic Surg 13:483, 1982.
77. Capone A, Slamovits TL: Discrete metastasis of solid tumors to extraocular muscles. Arch Ophthalmol 108:237, 1990.
78. Hornblass A, Jakobiec FA, Reifler DM, et al: Orbital lymphoid tumors located predominantly within extraocular muscles. Ophthalmology 94:688, 1987.
79. Young RS, Hodes BL, Cruse RP, et al: Orbital pseudotumor and Crohn's disease. J Pediatr 99:250, 1981.
80. Volpe NJ, Shore JW: Orbital myositis associated with herpes zoster. Arch Ophthalmol 109:471, 1991.
81. Grimson BS, Simons KB: Orbital inflammation, myositis, and systemic lupus erythematosus. Arch Ophthalmol 101:736, 1983.
82. Seidenberg KB, Leib ML: Orbital myositis with Lyme disease. Am J Ophthalmol 109:13, 1990.
83. Noel LP, Clarke WN: Orbital myositis with Lyme disease. Am J Ophthalmol 110:98, 1990.
84. Kattah JC, Zimmerman LE, Kolsky MP: Bilateral orbital involvement in fatal giant cell polymyositis. Ophthalmology 97:520, 1990.
85. Mauriello JA, Flanagan JC: Management of orbital inflammatory disease. A protocol. Surv Ophthalmol 29:104, 1984.
86. Trokel SL, Hilal SK: Recognition and differential diagnosis of enlarged extraocular muscles in computed tomography. Am J Ophthalmol 87:503, 1979.
87. Rothfus WE, Curtin HD: Extraocular muscle enlargement: A CT review. Radiology 151:677, 1984.
88. Dick AD, Atta H, Forrester JV: Lithium induced orbitopathy. Arch Ophthalmol 110:452, 1992.
89. Burde RM: Double vision, visual loss, and an enhancing orbital apex. Surv Ophthalmol 33:55, 1988.
90. Kline LB: The Tolosa-Hunt syndrome. Surv Ophthalmol 27:79, 1982.
91. Spector RH, Fiandaca MS: The "sinister" Tolosa-Hunt syndrome. Neurology 36:198, 1986.
92. Campbell RJ, Okazaki H: Painful ophthalmoplegia (Tolosa-Hunt variant): Autopsy findings in a patient with necrotizing intracavernous carotid vasculitis and inflammatory disease of the orbit. Mayo Clin Proc 62:520, 1987.
93. Yousem DM, Atlas SW, Grossman RI, et al: MR imaging of the Tolosa-Hunt syndrome. AJNR 10:1181, 1989.
94. Goto Y, Hosokawa S, Goto I, et al: Abnormality in the cavernous sinus in three patients with Tolosa-Hunt syndrome: MRI and CT findings. J Neurol Neurosurg Psychiatry 53:231, 1990.
95. Grimson BS, Cohen KL, Peiffer RL, et al: Isolated, bilateral orbital mass lesions during childhood. J Pediatr Ophthalmol Strabismus 19:42, 1982.
96. Purdy EP, Bullock JD: Magnetic resonance imaging and computed tomography in orbital diagnosis. Ophthalmol Clin North Am 4:89, 1991.
97. Atlas SW, Grossman RI, Savino PJ, et al: Surface-coil MR of orbital pseudotumor. AJR 148:803, 1987.
98. Kennerdell JS: Management of nonspecific inflammatory and lymphoid orbital lesions. Inter Ophthalmol Clin 31:7, 1991.
99. White V, Rootman J, Quenville N, et al: Orbital lymphoproliferative and inflammatory lesions. Can J Ophthalmol 22:362, 1987.
100. Warren FA, Kennerdell JS: Orbital fine needle aspiration biopsy. In Hornblass A (ed): Oculoplastic, Orbital, and Reconstructive Surgery. Baltimore, Williams & Wilkins, 1990, p 803.
101. Jakobiec FA, Neri A, Knowles DM: Genotypic monoclonality in immunophenotypically polyclonal orbital lymphoid tumors. Ophthalmology 94:980, 1987.
102. Leone CR, Lloyd WC: Treatment protocol for orbital inflammatory disease. Ophthalmology 92:1325, 1985.
103. Noble AG, Tripathi RC, Levine RA: Indomethacin for the treatment of idiopathic orbital myositis. Am J Ophthalmol 108:336, 1989.
104. Sergott RC, Glaser JS, Charyulu K: Radiotherapy for idiopathic inflammatory pseudotumor. Arch Ophthalmol 99:853, 1981.
105. Orcutt JC, Garner A, Henk JM, et al: Treatment of idiopathic inflammatory orbital pseudotumor by radiotherapy. Br J Ophthalmol 67:570, 1983.
106. Lanciano R, Fowble B, Sergott RC, et al: The results of radiotherapy for orbital pseudotumor. Int J Radiat Oncol Biol Phys 18:407, 1990.
107. Diaz-Llopis M, Menezo JL: Idiopathic inflammatory orbital pseudotumor and low-dose cyclosporine. Am J Ophthalmol 107:547, 1989.

108. Bielory L, Frohman LP:Low-dose cyclosporine therapy of granulomatous optic neuropathy and orbitopathy. Ophthalmology 98:1732, 1991.
109. Herold KC, Rubenstein AH: Immunosuppression for insulin-dependent diabetes. N Engl J Med 318:701, 1988.
110. Crick RP, Hoyle C, Smellie H: The eyes in sarcoidosis. Br J Ophthalmol 45:461, 1961.
111. Obenauf CD, Shaw HE, Snydor CF, et al: Sarcoidosis and its ophthalmic manifestations. Am J Ophthalmol 86:648, 1978.
112. Jabs DA, Johns CJ: Ocular involvement in chronic sarcoidosis. Am J Ophthalmol 102:297, 1986.
113. Karma A, Huhti E, Poukkula A: Course and outcome of ocular sarcoidosis. Am J Ophthalmol 106:467, 1988.
114. Melmon K, Goldberg J: Sarcoidosis with bilateral exophthalmos as the presenting symptom. Am J Med 33:158, 1962.
115. Leino M, Tuovinen E, Romppanen T: Orbital sarcoidosis. Acta Ophthalmol 60:809, 1982.
116. Khan JA, Hoover DL, Giangiacomo J, et al: Orbital and childhood sarcoidosis. J Pediatr Ophthalmol Strabismus 23:190, 1983.
117. Wolk RB: Sarcoidosis of the orbit with bone destruction. AJNR 5:204, 1984.
118. Signorini E, Cianciulli E, Ciorba E, et al: Rare multiple orbital localizations of sarcoidosis. Neuroradiology 26:145, 1984.
119. Collison JMT, Miller NR, Green WR: Involvement of orbital tissues by sarcoid. Am J Ophthalmol 102:302, 1986.
120. Imes RK, Reifschneider JS, O'Connor LE: Systemic sarcoidosis presenting initially with bilateral orbital and upper lid masses. Ann Ophthalmol 20:466, 1988.
121. Stannard K, Spalton DJ: Sarcoidosis with infiltration of the external ocular muscles. Br J Ophthalmol 69:562, 1985.
122. Snead JW, Seidenstein L, Knific RJ, et al: Isolated orbital sarcoidosis as a cause of blepharoptosis. Am J Ophthalmol 112:739, 1991.
123. Hammerschlag SB, Hesselink JR, Weber AL: Inflammatory disease. In Computed Tomography of the Eye and Orbit. Norwalk, CT, Appleton-Lange, 1983, pp 159–205.
124. Sacher M, Lanzieri CF, Sobel LL, et al: Computed tomography of bilateral lacrimal gland sarcoidosis. J Comput Assist Tomogr 8:213, 1984.
125. Wolk RB: Sarcoidosis of the orbit with bone destruction. AJNR 5:204, 1984.
126. Bronson LJ, Fisher YL: Sarcoidosis of the paranasal sinuses with orbital extension. Arch Ophthalmol 94:243, 1976.
127. Harris GJ, Williams GA, Clarke GP: Sarcoidosis of the lacrimal sac. Arch Ophthalmol 99:1198, 1981.
128. Gudeman SK, Selhorst JB, Susac JO, et al: Sarcoid optic neuropathy. Neurology 32:597, 1982.
129. Caplan L, Corbett J, Goodwin C, et al: Neuro-ophthalmic signs in the angiitic form of neurosarcoidosis. Neurology 33:1130, 1983.
130. Beardsley TL, Brown SWL, Sydnor CF: Eleven cases of sarcoidosis of the optic nerve. Am J Ophthalmol 97:62, 1984.
131. Graham EM, Ellis CJK, Sanders MD, et al: Optic neuropathy in sarcoidosis. J Neurol Neurosurg Psychiatry 49:756, 1986.
132. Mansour AM: Sarcoid optic disc edema and optocilliary shunts. J Clin Neuro Ophthalmol 6:47, 1986.
133. Galetta S, Schatz NJ, Glaser JS: Acute sarcoid optic neuropathy with spontaneous recovery. J Clin Neuro Ophthalmol 9:27, 1989.
134. Matjucha ICA, Katz B: The optic neuropathy of sarcoidosis. Semin Ophthalmol 7:60, 1992.
135. Weinreb RN, Tessler H: Laboratory diagnosis of ophthalmic sarcoidosis. Surv Ophthalmol 28:653, 1984.
136. Weinreb RN: Diagnosing sarcoidosis by transconjunctival biopsy of the lacrimal gland. Am J Ophthalmol 97:573, 1984.
137. Karma A: Diagnosing sarcoidosis by transconjunctival biopsy of the lacrimal gland [letter]. Am J Ophthalmol 98:640, 1984.
138. Nessan VJ, Jacoway JR: Biopsy of minor salivary glands in the diagnosis of sarcoidosis. N Engl J Med 301:922, 1979.
139. Cheng KH, Brinkman CJJ, Rothova A: An unusual case of neurosarcoidosis confirmed by a muscle biopsy specimen. Am J Ophthalmol 110:574, 1990.
140. Bersani TA, Nichols CW: Intralesional triamcinolone for cutaneous palpebral sarcoidosis. Am J Ophthalmol 99:561, 1985.
141. Haynes BF, Allen NB, Fauci AS: Diagnostic and therapeutic approach to the patient with vasculitis. Med Clin North Am 70:355, 1986.
142. Conn DL: Update on systemic necrotizing vasculitis. Mayo Clin Proc 64:535, 1989.
143. Conn DL, Hunder GG: Vasculitis and related disorders. In Kelley WN, Harris ED Jr, Ruddy S, Sledge CB (eds): Textbook of Rheumatology, 3rd ed. Philadelphia, WB Saunders, 1989, pp 1167–1199.
144. Jabs DA: The rheumatic diseases. In Schachat AP, Murphy RP, Patz A (eds): Retina. St. Louis, CV Mosby, 1989, Vol 2, pp 457–480.
145. Cupps TR, Fauci AS: The vasculitic syndromes. Adv Intern Med 27:315, 1982.
146. Trocme SD, Bartley GB, Campbell RJ, et al: Eosinophil and neutrophil degranulation in ophthalmic lesions of Wegener's granulomatosis. Arch Ophthalmol 109:1585, 1991.
147. Wolff SM, Fauci AS, Horn RG, et al: Wegener's granulomatosis. Ann Intern Med 81:513, 1974.
148. Coutu RE, Klein M, Lessell S, et al: Limited form of Wegener's granulomatosis: Eye involvement as a major sign. JAMA 233:868, 1975.
149. Haynes BF, Fishman ML, Fauci AS, et al: The ocular manifestations of Wegener's granulomatosis: Fifteen years experience and review of the literature. Am J Med 63:131, 1977.
150. Bullen CL, Leisgang TJ, McDonald TJ, et al: Ocular complications of Wegener's granulomatosis. Ophthalmology 90:279, 1983.
151. Robin JB, Schanzlin DJ, Meisler DM, et al: Ocular involvement in the respiratory vasculitides. Surv Ophthalmol 30:127, 1985.
152. Weiter J, Farkas TG: Pseudotumor of the orbit as a presenting sign of Wegener's granulomatosis. Surv Ophthalmol 17:106, 1972.
153. Allen JC, France TD: Pseudotumor as the presenting sign of Wegener's granulomatosis in a child. J Pediatr Ophthalmol 14:158, 1977.
154. Parelhoff ES, Chavis RM, Friendly DS: Wegner's granulomatosis presenting as orbital pseudotumor. J Pediatr Ophthalmol Strabismus 22:100, 1985.
155. Coppeto JR, Yamase H, Monteiro MLR: Chronic ophthalmic Wegener's granulomatosis. J Clin Neuro Ophthalmol 5:17, 1985.
156. Scully RE, Mark EJ, McNeely BU: Case records of the Massachusetts General Hospital. N Engl J Med 305:999, 1981.
157. Pinchoff BS, Spahlinger DA, Bergstrom TJ, et al: Extraocular muscle involvement in Wegener's granulomatosis. J Clin Neuro Ophthalmol 3:163, 1983.
158. Kirker S, Keane M, Hutchinson M: Benign recurrent multiple mononeuropathy in Wegener's granulomatosis. J Neurol Neurosurg Psychiatr 52:918, 1989.
159. Scully RE, Mark EJ, McNeely WF, et al: Case records of the Massachusetts General Hospital. N Engl J Med 318:760, 1988.
160. Cross CE, Lillington GA: Serodiagnosis of Wegener's granulomatosis: Pathobiologic and clinical implications. Mayo Clin Proc 64:119, 1989.
161. Nolle B, Specks U, Ludermann H, et al: Anticytoplasmic autoantibodies: Their immunodiagnostic value in Wegener's granulomatosis. Ann Intern Med 111:28, 1989.
162. Pulido JS, Goeken JA, Nerad JA, et al: Ocular manifestations of patients with circulating antineutrophil cytoplasmic antibodies. Arch Ophthalmol 108:845, 1990.
163. Soukiasian SH, Foster CS, Niles JL, et al: Diagnostic value of antineutrophil cytoplasmic antibodies in scleritis associated with Wegener's granulomatosis. Ophthalmology 99:125, 1992.
164. Kalina PH, Lie JT, Campbell RJ, et al: Diagnostic value and limitations of orbital biopsy in Wegener's granulomatosis. Ophthalmology 99:120, 1992.
165. Cohen Tervaert JW, van der Woude FJ, Fauci AS, et al: Association between active Wegener's granulomatosis and anticytoplasmic antibodies. Arch Intern Med 149:2461, 1989.
166. Thawley SE: Wegener's granulomatosis: Unusual indication for orbital decompression. Laryngoscope 89:145, 1979.
167. Hardwig PW, Bartley GB, Garrity JA: Surgical management of nasolacrimal duct obstruction in patients with Wegener's granulomatosis. Ophthalmology 99:133, 1992.
168. Morgan CM, Foster CS, D'Amico, et al: Retinal vasculitis in polyarteritis nodosa. Retina 6:205, 1986.

169. Kinyoun JL, Kalina RE, Klein ML: Choroidal involvement in systemic necrotizing vasculitis. Arch Ophthalmol 105:939, 1987.
170. Haskjold E, Froland S, Egge K: Ocular polyarteritis nodosa: Report of a case. Acta Ophthalmol 65:749, 1987.
171. Purcell JJ Jr: Polyarteritis nodosa. In Gold DH, Weingeist TA (eds): The Eye in Systemic Disease. Philadelphia, JB Lippincott, 1990, pp 51–53.
172. Van Wien S, Merz EH: Exophthalmos secondary to polyarteritis nodosa. Am J Ophthalmol 56:204, 1963.
173. Miller NR: Walsh and Hoyt's Clinical Neuro-Ophthalmology, 4th ed., vol. 4. Baltimore, Williams & Wilkins, 1991.
174. Goldstein I, Wexler D: Bilateral atrophy of the optic nerves in periarteritis nodosa. Arch Ophthalmol 18:767, 1937.
175. Kimbrell OC Jr, Wheliss JA: Polyarteritis nodosa complicated by bilateral optic neuropathy. JAMA 201:139, 1967.
176. Bagegni A, Lyness RW, Johnston PB, et al: Visual recovery in orbital vasculitis. Br J Ophthalmol 72:737, 1988.
177. Hayasaka S, Uchida M, Setogawa T, et al: Polyarteritis nodosa presenting as orbital apex syndrome. Orbit 9:117, 1990.
178. Newman NM, Hoyt WF, Spencer WH: Macula-sparing monocular blackouts. Clinical and pathological investigations of intermittent choroidal vascular insufficiency in a case of periarteritis nodosa. Arch Ophthalmol 91:367, 1974.
179. Coppeto JR, Miller D: Polyarteritis nodosa diagnosed by temporal artery biopsy. Am J Ophthalmol 102:541, 1986.
180. Sedwick LA, Margo CE: Sixth nerve palsies, temporal artery biopsy, and necrotizing vasculitis. J Clin Neuro Ophthalmol 9:119, 1989.
181. Goodman BW: Temporal arteritis. Am J Med 67:839, 1979.
182. Caselli RJ, Hunder GG, Whisnant JP: Neurologic disease in biopsy-proven giant cell arteritis. Neurology 38:352, 1988.
183. Save-Soderbergh J, Malmvall B-E, Andersson R, et al: Giant cell arteritis as a cause of death. JAMA 255:493, 1986.
184. Hupp SL, Nelson GL, Zimmerman LE: Generalized giant cell arteritis with coronary artery involvement and myocardial infarction. Arch Ophthalmol 108:1385, 1990.
185. Mehler MF, Rabinowich L: The clinical neuro-ophthalmologic spectrum of temporal arteritis. Am J Med 85:839, 1988.
186. Hamed LM, Guy JR, Moster ML, et al: Giant cell arteritis in the ocular ischemic syndrome. Am J Ophthalmol 113:702, 1992.
187. Zion VM, Goodside V: Anterior segment ischemia with anterior ischemic optic neuropathy. Surv Ophthalmol 19:19, 1974.
188. Radda TM, Bardach H, Riss B: Acute ocular hypotony. A rare complication of temporal arteritis. Ophthalmologica 182:148, 1981.
189. Spolaore R, Gaudric A, Coscas G, et al: Acute sectoral choroidal ischemia. Am J Ophthalmol 98:707, 1984.
190. Mack HG, O'Day J, Currie JN: Delayed choroidal perfusion in giant cell arteritis. J Clin Neuro Ophthalmol 11:221, 1991.
191. Stein R, Regenbogen L, Romano A, et al: Orbital apex syndrome due to cranial arteritis. Ann Ophthalmol 12:708, 1980.
192. Clark AE, Victor WH: An unusual presentation of temporal arteritis. Ann Ophthalmol 19:343, 1987.
193. Laidlaw DAH, Smith PEM, Hudgson P: Orbital pseudotumor secondary to giant cell arteritis: An unreported condition. Br Med J 300:784, 1990.
194. Wagener HP, Hollensorst RW: The ocular lesions of temporal arteritis. Am J Ophthalmol 45:617, 1958.
195. Barricks MR, Travisa DB, Glaser JS, et al: Ophthalmoplegia in cranial arteritis. Brain 100:209, 1977.
196. Dimant J, Grob D, Brunner NG: Ophthalmoplegia, ptosis, and miosis in temporal arteritis. Neurology 30:1054, 1980.
197. Goldberg RT: Ocular muscle paresis—An unusual case. Ann Ophthalmol 15:240, 1983.
198. Coppeto JR, Greco T: Mydriasis in giant cell arteritis. J Clin Neuro Ophthalmol 9:267, 1989.
199. Gold DH, Morris DA, Henkind P: Ocular findings in systemic lupus erythematosus. Br J Ophthalmol 56:800, 1972.
200. Burkhalter E: Unique presentation of systemic lupus erythematosus. Arthritis Rheum 16:428, 1973.
201. Brenner EH, Shock JP: Proptosis secondary to systemic lupus erythematosus. Arch Ophthalmol 91:81, 1974.
202. Wilkinson LS, Panush RS: Exophthalmos associated with systemic lupus erythematosus. Arthritis Rheum 18:188, 1975.
203. Bankhurst AD, Carlow TJ, Reidy RW: Exophthalmos in systemic lupus erythematosus. Ann Ophthalmol 16:669, 1984.
204. Evans OB, Lexow SS: Painful ophthalmoplegia in systemic lupus erythematosus. Ann Neurol 4:584, 1978.
205. Leahey AB, Connor TB, Gottsch JD: Chemosis as a presenting sign of systemic lupus erythematosus. Arch Ophthalmol 110:609, 1992.
206. Tan EM, Cohen AS, Fries JF, et al: The 1982 revised criteria for the classification of systemic lupus erythematosus. Arthritis Rheum 25:1271, 1982.
207. Schur PH: Clinical features of SLE. In Kelley WN, Harris ED Jr, Ruddy S, Sledge CB (eds): Textbook of Rheumatology, 3rd ed. Philadelphia, WB Saunders, 1989, pp 1101–1129.
208. Whaley K, Alspaugh MA: Sjögren's syndrome. In Kelley WN, Harris ED Jr, Ruddy S, Sledge CB (eds): Textbook of Rheumatology, 3rd ed. Philadelphia, WB Saunders, 1989, pp 999–1020.
209. Pepose JS, Akata RF, Pflugfelder SC, et al: Mononuclear cell phenotypes and immunoglobulin gene rearrangements in lacrimal gland biopsies from patients with Sjögren's syndrome. Ophthalmology 97:1599, 1990.
210. Strand V, Talal N: Advances in the diagnosis and concept of Sjögren's syndrome (autoimmune exocrinopathy). Bull Rheum Dis 30:1046, 1980.
211. Pokorny G, Nemeth J, Marczinovits I, et al: Primary Sjögren's syndrome from the view-point of an internal physician. Int Ophthalmol 15:401, 1991.
212. Alexander GE, Provost TT, Stevens MB, et al: Sjögren's syndrome: Central nervous system manifestations. Neurology 31:1391, 1981.
213. Alexander EL, Provost TT, Stevens MB, et al: Neurologic complications of primary Sjögren's syndrome. Medicine 61:247, 1982.
214. Farris RN: Sjögren's syndrome. In Gold DH, Weingeist TA (eds): The Eye in Systemic Disease. Philadelphia, JB Lippincott, 1990, pp 70–71.
215. Gilbard JP, Farris RL, Santamaria J: Osmolarity of tear microvolumes in keratoconjunctivitis sicca. Arch Ophthalmol 96:677, 1978.

Chapter 171

■

Infectious Processes of the Orbit

CHRISTOPHER T. WESTFALL, ANN SULLIVAN BAKER,
and JOHN W. SHORE

Infections of the orbit and periorbital tissues are a particularly important subset of orbital inflammatory disease, not only because of the frequency of presentation but also because these potentially life-threatening conditions demand prompt, specific therapeutic management. The orbit may be infected by bacteria, fungi, or parasites. Modes of presentation, inciting factors, and treatment options differ for each of these groups, although diagnostic modalities are largely the same. Each group is addressed separately in this chapter.

BACTERIAL INFECTION

Of the infections that the practicing ophthalmologist can expect to encounter, the most common are those caused by bacteria. There are a host of bacteria that have been reported to lead to orbital and periorbital infection. Clinical circumstances often provide the necessary clues to determine the offending organism and to allow initiation of treatment pending culture results. It is best to categorize bacterial orbital infections by patient age, site of origin, and anatomic location, because these factors serve to indicate the most likely organism, direct antibiotic selection, and determine the prognosis.

The pathophysiology of bacterial infections is directly linked to the anatomy of the midface. The sinuses structurally represent walls of the orbit. The ethmoid sinuses in particular, with their exquisitely thin lamina papyracea, predispose the orbit to extension from sinus infection.[1-4] The second anatomic consideration relates to the absence of venous valves in the midface, which allows direct posterior spread of any infectious process. The valveless inferior and superior ophthalmic veins provide a direct conduit through the orbit.[1-4] Infection reaches the orbit by one of three methods: implantation, local extension, or hematogenous spread.[1] Implantation occurs usually in association with a traumatic break in the skin. Local extension is exemplified by spread from a contiguous sinusitis, and hematogenous spread may occur from a multiplicity of distant sites.

At the outset, it is important to clarify the terms, "site or origin" and "anatomic location" as they are used in this chapter. "Site of origin" refers to the nidus of infection that led to involvement of orbital and periorbital tissues. Common sites of origin for orbital and periorbital infection include sinusitis, skin trauma, and dental infection. In contrast, "anatomic location" refers to the specific periorbital and orbital tissues infected. The anatomic location of infection depends on the natural barrier provided by the orbital septum. The simplest classification scheme categorizes infections by preseptal (periorbital) or postseptal (orbital) location. Further categorization yields five subsets of orbital infection: inflammatory edema, orbital cellulitis, subperiosteal abscess, orbital abscess, and cavernous sinus thrombosis.[1, 4, 5] In this chapter, infections anterior to the orbital septum are referred to as "preseptal" or "periorbital," whereas those that have extended posterior to the septum are termed "postseptal" or "orbital" infections.

Pediatric Bacterial Infections

CLINICAL PRESENTATION

The clinical presentation of a child with an orbital infection is usually that of pain, heat, redness, and swelling of the tissues surrounding the involved orbit (Fig. 171–1). There is typically fever and an elevation of the white blood cell count.[6] History of trauma, lacrimal outflow obstruction, upper respiratory tract infection, or sinusitis should be carefully elicited. *Haemophilus* infection is frequently characterized by a purple hue to the skin. The presence of a demarcation line corresponding to the arcus marginalis suggests an orbital (postseptal) infection. The presence of proptosis, ophthalmoplegia, conjunctival chemosis, or loss of vision are also suggestive of orbital involvement, but postseptal extension may exist in the absence of any of these findings.[7] Orbital apex syndrome or cavernous sinus thrombosis must be considered in more severe cases, particularly if loss of vision occurs. Finally, signs of meningitis such as opisthotonos and lethargy must be sought as complications of an orbital infection with intracranial extension.

ANATOMIC CLASSIFICATION

Preseptal cellulitis tends to occur in children younger than 5 yr of age, with postseptal involvement occurring predominantly in children over 5 yr of age. Orbital infections in older children are commonly associated with sinusitis,[2] and the ethmoid sinuses are most frequently implicated.[1, 8]

BACTERIOLOGY

In the pediatric age group, *Staphylococcus aureus*, *Streptococcus* sp., and *Haemophilus influenzae* are the most commonly encountered bacteria.[6] The successful isolation of an organism from any given infection de-

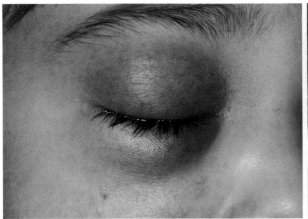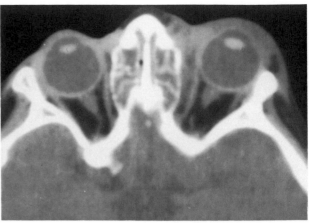

Figure 171–1. A, Presentation of a 3-year-old infant with pain, local heat, redness, and edema of the periorbital tissues is typical of bacterial infection. Decreased ocular motility was suggestive of orbital involvement. Note the sharp demarcation line corresponding to the origin of the orbital septum, the arcus marginalis. This finding is frequently seen in postseptal infection. B, The CT scan demonstrates ethmoid sinusitis with extension of the infectious process through the lamina papyracea into the medial orbit. There is no evidence of abscess formation. The child responded to antibiotics given intravenously.

pends on the tissue cultured—soft tissue aspirate, sinus drainage, or blood. Rates for positive culture seem to relate to both the site of origin and to the location of the infection. In one series,[6] aspirates from preseptal cellulitis yielded S. aureus, Streptoccoccus sp., and H. influenzae, among other organisms, whereas only a single isolate of S. aureus was recovered from patients with postseptal cellulitis. Blood cultures yielded H. influenzae and streptococci. Positive cultures were seen in periorbital cellulitis 18 percent of the time but in only 5 percent of postseptal cases.[6] Other isolates identified in this study included Moraxella, E. coli, E. aerogenes, and anaerobic bacteria, Bacteroides sp., Peptostreptococcus, Fusobacterium, and Propionibacterium acnes. Primary infection with Streptococcus faecalis has also been reported.[9] Anaerobic infections can be particularly devastating; recent mortality in the pediatric age group has been reported.[10]

An unusual infectious process, botryomycosis, or more correctly, pseudomycosis, may involve the orbits of both children and adults. It is thought that this entity is caused by an encapsulated form of Staphylococcus, which is particularly resistant to conventional medical therapy.[11]

Mycobacterium hominis or atypical mycobacteria may infect the orbits in any age group.[12–16] The absence of pulmonary involvement does not rule out granulomatous orbital infection.[14] Proptosis, bone erosion, and cutaneous fistula in particular should arouse suspicion.[16] Purified protein derivative (PPD) skin testing should always be considered in the diagnostic work-up of orbital cellulitis.[15]

DIAGNOSIS

Ancillary diagnostic methods available for evaluating children with orbital and periorbital infections include physical examination (motility, vision, proptosis, fever), white blood cell count with differential, cultures (pus, blood, and sinus drainage), orbital ultrasound and com-

puted tomography (CT) scan. Lumbar puncture is reserved for children who have meningeal signs.[17] As a predictor of whether an infection is orbital or periorbital, fever and white blood cell count are of little help.[6] The CT scan has supplanted plain sinus films as the imaging study of choice. Orbital cellulitis has been demonstrated radiographically in the absence of proptosis, ophthalmoplegia, or decreased visual acuity.[7] It should also be noted that the presence or absence of an abscess in a patient with orbital cellulitis is suggested but by no means defined by a CT scan. Cases in which an abscess was suspected radiographically but not confirmed at surgery have been reported.[18] Air fluid levels are unusual, even in the presence of an abscess.[19]

THERAPY

The therapy of orbital infection in the pediatric age group depends on the severity of the infection, site of origin, and site of involvement, as well as the suspected organism. Therapy is obviously best directed at the underlying cause, if known. Sinusitis should be treated with the appropriate antibiotic and possibly with surgical drainage (Fig. 171–2). Consultation with an otorhinolaryngologist is appropriate. Surface wounds are associated with a high incidence of S. aureus and streptococcal infection. A penicillinase-resistant penicillin such as nafcillin is the drug of choice. Bites demand additional coverage for gram-negative organisms and anaerobes. The risk of H. influenzae and the threat of meningitis for children younger than 5 yr of age requires that chloramphenicol, a second or third-generation cephalosporin, or ampicillin be included as therapy.[6] Resistance to ampicillin must be taken into consideration when selecting therapy for infections caused by H. influenzae. Most abscesses should be drained; several subperiosteal abscesses, defined by CT scan, have been successfully managed medically. In carefully selected cases, this may be an acceptable alternative to surgical drainage.[20]

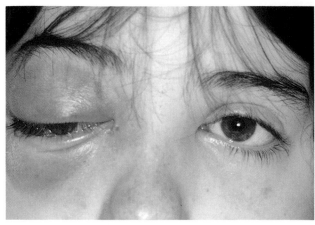 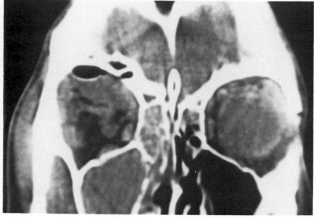

Figure 171–2. *A,* Marked proptosis, ptosis, ophthalmoplegia, and decreased visual acuity were presenting findings in a child with pansinusitis and an abscess in the superior orbit. *B,* CT scan shows maxillary and ethmoid sinus opacification as well as orbital inflammation and abscess. Prompt surgical drainage of the orbital abscess, anterior ethmoidectomy, and maxillary antrostomy followed by a prolonged course of antibiotics were necessary for resolving this life-threatening infection.

Adult Bacterial Infections

ANATOMY

The orbital septum provides convenient demarcation not only in reference to the anatomic location of infection but also with regard to the severity of disease. Orbital (postseptal) infections may be thought of as a continuum of diffuse inflammation, localized inflammatory mass or phlegmon, and finally, abscess—either subperiosteal or extraperiosteal. Orbital apex involvement or extension of the infectious process intracranially as meningitis, abscess, or cavernous sinus thrombosis are particularly severe manifestations of orbital infection. Identification of the anatomic location and the extent of infection define the severity of the disease, the prognosis, and the appropriate course of therapy. Loss of vision or ophthalmoplegia mandates a search for orbital apex or cavernous sinus involvement.[21, 22]

Subperiosteal abscesses are an interesting subset of orbital infection. Antibiotics penetrate poorly into the subperiosteal space, and rapid expansion of the abscess can lead to early visual compromise.[23] As noted elsewhere in this chapter, a CT scan may inaccurately diagnose phlegmon or hematoma as a subperiosteal abscess.[18, 23] Coagulase positive and negative *Staphylococcus, H. influenzae, Streptococcus* sp., *Brahamella catarrhalis, Klebsiella pneumoniae,* and *Eikenella corrodens* have been identified in one study of this subset of orbital infections.[23]

PATHOPHYSIOLOGY

Orbital infection may originate from any number of sites. Most series have reported sinus involvement in 60 to 70 percent,[3, 4, 24] with ethmoid involvement predominating.[3, 25] However, a group from Ann Arbor reported sinus involvement in 29 percent of their cases, differentiating this entity from upper respiratory tract infection, seen in 28 percent of the series.[25] Trauma to the eye or periocular tissues was seen in 24 percent, and otitis was present in 9 percent of infected patients.[25] There have been case reports of orbital cellulitis associated with strabismus surgery,[26] blepharoplasty,[27, 28] dacryocystitis,[29] subacute bacterial endocarditis,[30] panophthalmitis,[31] and phlebitis from a scalp vein needle in an infant.[32] Dental abscess is a well-known precursor to orbital infection.[33] Recent mortality secondary to septic cavernous sinus thrombosis in a patient with gingivitis and parapharyngeal abscess has been reported.[34] Periorbital cellulitis has also been identified secondary to fracture of the medial maxillary wall with outflow obstruction and development of sinusitis.[35] Posterior sphenoethmoiditis may lead to orbital apex syndrome and early visual compromise.[21]

Origination of an orbital cellulitis from an infected sinus must be differentiated from orbital involvement with a sinus mucocele or mucopyocele.[36] A mucocele represents a collection of mucus within an obstructed sinus cavity. The term mucopyocele implies the presence of purulent material. An obstruction may be the result of chronic infection, tumor, or trauma.[36] Chronicity leads to an expansion of the cavity and to thinning of the bony sinus walls. Expansion into the orbit or contiguous inflammation may result in orbital findings. Specifically, sphenoid sinus involvement may compress the optic nerve and cause visual loss or visual field loss.[37] Most commonly involved are the frontal and anterior ethmoid sinuses, resulting in a superonasal mass effect.[36] Appropriate imaging studies for mucoceles and mucopyoceles include both CT scan and magnetic resonance imaging (MRI) scans.[37] Treatment involves surgery.

BACTERIOLOGY

The organisms most commonly isolated in adult bacterial infections include *S. aureus* and streptococcal species.[38] *Bacillus cereus* panophthalmitis and *Clostridium perfringens* infection are devastating processes that may extend to involve orbital tissues.[31, 39] The periorbital cellulitis seen with *Streptococcus* can be particularly virulent and has been reported in association with lid necrosis,[40] specifically when combined with *Staphylococcus* to cause a synergistic gangrene.[41] Lid necrosis has also been reported with *Pseudomonas aeruginosa* and with *Proteus*.[41, 42] Animal bites or other contact with animal secretions may lead to infection with *Pasteurella multocida*.[43]

CLINICAL EVALUATION

The interview of a patient with orbital infection should identify recent trauma, current antibiotics, systemic complaints, and recent infection of any type, but especially upper respiratory tract or sinus infection.

Clinical findings are the key to determining whether an infection is preseptal or postseptal in location. Most bacterial orbital infections present with periorbital pain, swelling, heat, and redness. Both preseptal and postseptal infections share these findings. Fever is commonly present. Postseptal infections tend to be characterized by ophthalmoplegia, proptosis, and chemosis (Fig. 171–3). Loss of vision may indicate an abscess or cavernous sinus thrombosis. A peripheral demarcation line corresponding to the arcus marginalis heralds a postseptal infection. Fluctuance suggests an abscess, but CT scanning is usually required to make this diagnosis.

DIAGNOSTIC STUDIES

Ancillary studies include white blood cell count with differential; cultures of blood, periorbital tissue, pus, and sinus drainage; ultrasound; sinus films; and CT scanning. The use of sinus films has mainly been supplanted by the CT scan. Thin (2.5 mm) axial and coronal cuts with contrast material are appropriate.[3, 19] An abscess that is not visible on a CT scan has been clinically suspected and surgically proven.[44] Conversely, infectious masses or hematomas may be misinterpreted as abscesses. The authors of one article suggest that the diagnosis of an orbital abscess made from a CT scan

should, in some cases, lead to a trial of antibiotic therapy under close clinical observation.[18] Surgical drainage may be reserved for cases that fail to respond in a timely manner.[18]

THERAPY

Treatment of adults with orbital infection parallels that for children. Consultation with the appropriate subspecialist is appropriate if sinus disease, otitis, or oral pathology are present. As a rule, undrained pus must be treated surgically, although it must be reemphasized that the specificity of CT scanning for an abscess is less than 100 percent. Antibiotic selection depends on the clinical setting. Jones and Steinkuller suggest the schema represented in Figure 171–4, and the treatment regimen outlined in Table 171–1.[45] Particularly in animal and human bites, anaerobic organisms and *Pasteurella* must be covered.[46] An adult with mild preseptal cellulitis may be treated on an outpatient basis with oral antibiotics. Orbital (postseptal) cellulitis, particularly if the presence of phlegmon or abscess is suspected, is best treated with intravenous antibiotics. Close clinical follow-up dictates the timing and necessity for surgical drainage.

FUNGAL INFECTIONS

In contrast with bacterial infections, which tend to occur in otherwise healthy individuals, fungal infections have a predilection for the debilitated host. Human orbital infections have been caused by the *Phycomycetes* (*Mucor* and *Rhizopus* sp.), *Ascomycetes* (*Aspergillus* sp.), *Blastomyces*,[47] *Sporothrix* sp.,[48, 49] and *Phaeohyphomycoses* (*Bipolarina* sp.)[50] The greatest clinical significance is attached to those caused by the *Phycomycetes* and *Ascomycetes* classes of fungi.

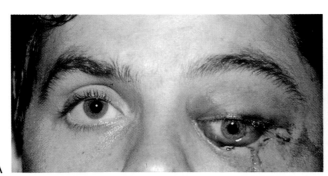
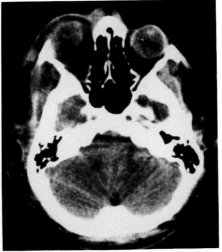

Figure 171–3. *A,* Surgical repair of a zygomatic arch fracture preceded the development of subperiosteal orbital abscess. Note the depression of the globe, secondary to mass effect. *B,* Extension of the infectious process from the temporal fossa is evident on the CT scan. Prompt surgical drainage followed by a prolonged course of antibiotics led to resolution without functional sequelae.

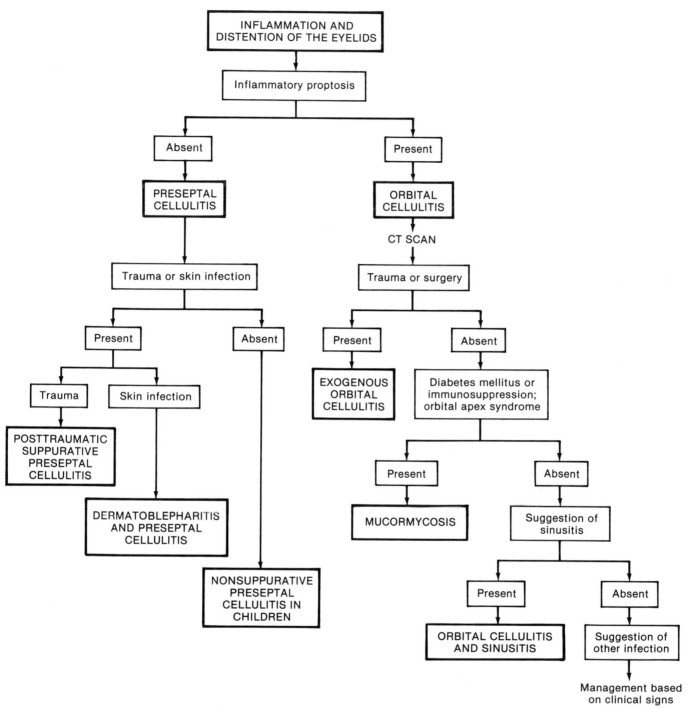

Figure 171–4. Algorithm proposed by Steinkuller and Jones for the evaluation of orbital infection. (From Jones DB, Steinkuller PG: Strategies for the initial management of acute preseptal and orbital cellulitis. Trans Am Ophthalmol Soc 86:94–112, 1988.)

Table 171–1. THERAPEUTIC OPTIONS AS PROPOSED BY STEINKULLER AND JONES

Principal Entities in Preseptal Cellulitis			
Route	*Entity*	*Etiology*	*Initial Therapy*
Exogenous	Posttraumatic	*Staphylococcus aureus*	Nafcillin
	Secondary to dermatoblepharitis	*Staphylococcus pyogenes*	
Endogenous	Nonsuppurative in children	*Haemophilus influenzae*	Cefuroxime or ampicillin and
		Streptococcus pneumoniae	chloramphenicol

Principal Entities in Orbital Cellulitis			
Route	*Entity*	*Etiology*	*Initial Therapy*
Exogenous	Posttraumatic	*Staphylococcus aureus*	Nafcillin and tobramycin
	Postsurgical		
Endogenous	Secondary to sinusitis	*Streptococcus pneumoniae*	Nafcillin and chloramphenicol
		Other streptococci	
		Staphylococcus aureus	
		Haemophilus influenzae	
		Non–spore-forming anaerobes	

From Jones DB, Steinkuller PG: Strategies for the initial management of acute preseptal and orbital cellulitis. Trans Am Ophthalmol Soc 86:94–112, 1988.

Orbital Infection Secondary to the Phycomycetes

MYCOLOGY

Although mucormycosis is the term commonly used to refer to fungal infections of this class, the correct term is phycomycosis. *Mucor* and *Rhizopus* are two genera of the order *Mucorales*, a subset of the class Phycomycetes, which have been implicated in human orbital infection. Phycomycetes are the most common fungi that infect orbital tissues.[51] They are ubiquitous saprophytic fungi that are normally not pathogenic to humans.[52]

PATHOPHYSIOLOGY

The healthy human host commonly inhales the 3- to 6-μ–diameter spores of the Phycomycetes and promptly eliminates them through phagocytosis.[53] In the pathologic state, phycomycete infection may present as pulmonary, disseminated, gastrointestinal, cutaneous, and rhinoorbital-cerebral forms.[53] The rhinoorbital-cerebral progression begins in the nose, spreads to the maxillary sinus, and then to the ethmoids and orbit.[54, 55] The infection gains entrance to the central nervous system not only through the orbital roof and apex but also through the cribriform plate.[54, 56] The organism invades blood vessel walls, causing necrosis, thrombosis, obstruction, and ultimately, infarction of involved tissues.[55, 56] Internal carotid, middle cerebral, ciliary, and retinal arteries as well as the cavernous sinus are all subject to this progression.[54, 55]

CLINICAL PRESENTATION AND DIAGNOSIS

Infection by the Phycomycetes is characterized by a foul-smelling seropurulent discharge. The involved tissues on intranasal examination are necrotic, with a dark discoloration, resembling clotted blood—the direct effect of vascular thrombosis and tissue infarction.[53, 54, 56]

This characteristic black eschar is usually a late finding, and its absence does not rule out fungal infection.[55, 56] Orbital apex involvement results in both internal and external ophthalmoplegia, ptosis, and periorbital numbness secondary to trigeminal nerve injury.[54, 55] Bilateral orbital involvement has been reported.[56]

Individuals predisposed to infection by the Phycomycetes include diabetics in ketoacidosis, leukemics, patients with lymphoma, multiple myeloma, cancer, septicemia, and burns.[53, 54, 55, 57] It has been reported in a dehydrated infant.[58] Ionizing irradiation, antibiotics, and steroids all favor proliferation of the Phycomycetes, *Mucor*, and *Rhizopus*.[52, 54–56] Bacterial infection may tip the balance of control in patients with diabetes, ultimately resulting in fungal infection. In one series, 13 of 16 cases had antecedent bacterial infections.[53]

Presenting complaints include localized pain, fever, headache, lethargy, as well as the ophthalmic findings of decreased visual acuity, afferent pupillary defect, trigeminal insensitivity, ophthalmoplegia, and proptosis.[54, 57] The most common early signs are sinusitis, pharyngitis, or nasal discharge, seen in 11 of 16 patients reported by Ferry and associates.[53] Orbital or periorbital pain was reported in 6 of 16 patients. It should be noted that in this series, only 18 percent showed evidence of the characteristic black eschar found early in their course.[53] Therefore, the absence of this finding should not prevent the clinician from entertaining the diagnosis of phycomycetal infection. Sedimentation rate and white blood cell count are often elevated. Blood cultures seldom have positive results.[53, 56] Biopsied tissue reveals nonseptate branching hyphae that may be seen on potassium hydroxide (KOH) preparation, Gomori methamine silver (GMS) stain, and hematoxylin and eosin stains. Sabouraud's agar without inhibitors is appropriate for culture.[56, 59] A CT scan is almost indispensable for defining the extent of fungal infection.

THERAPY

Treatment must be promptly instituted. Success demands a combined surgical and medical approach.[60]

Thorough débridement of necrotic tissues in conjunction with the application of antifungal agents is the mainstay of therapy. Recall that the organisms are saprophytic and thrive in hypoxic environments. Although complete excision of necrotic tissues is necessary, exenteration is not mandated. Limited mucormycosis has been successfully managed without exenteration.[55]

Amphotericin is central to medical therapy,[56, 57] but other agents, such as ketoconazole alone or in combination with other drugs, are used.[52] Selection and administration of these toxic agents demands involvement of an appropriately trained internist. Hyperbaric oxygen may have a therapeutic role.[53, 61]

The general management plan for patients with Phycomycetes infections should include: (1) early recognition of clinical signs: (2) correction of acidosis and systemic abnormalities, to include underlying bacterial infection; (3) débridement of necrotic tissues; (4) examination of biopsied material immediately on KOH preparation and GMS stain; (5) culture on appropriate media; (6) establishment of sinus/orbital drainage; and (7) an intravenous antifungal agent.[53, 55] Finally, the aggressive débridement demanded by the disease often requires reconstructive efforts by plastic surgeons: ear, nose, and throat (ENT) plastic surgeons, and ophthalmic plastic surgeons.

PROGNOSIS

The prognosis of the infection depends on the rapidity of diagnosis and the institution of proper treatment. Mortality rates, although less than they were 30 yr ago, are still high. In 1961, mortality was approximately 90 percent, but recent series range from 15 to 35 percent.[56] Even in a series with reportedly successful outcomes, the time from presentation of symptoms to establishment of diagnosis averaged 4 days.[55] The presentation of a diabetic or immunocompromised patient with sinusitis, rhinitis, or facial pain should alert the clinician.[56] Similarly, the obtunded diabetic who does not awaken in response to adequate metabolic control demands that fungal infection be considered.[53, 54, 56, 59] It must be remembered that the poor survival rates associated with this disease are not only due to the aggressive nature of *Mucor* and *Rhizopus* but also to delayed diagnosis.[54, 55]

Orbital Infection Due to *Aspergillus*

MYCOLOGY AND PATHOPHYSIOLOGY

Aspergillus is also a saprophytic, ubiquitous fungus that is normally not pathogenic in humans.[61] When it does appear as a source of infection, the rhinoorbital-cerebral route of entry seems to parallel that of the Phycomycetes. A nasal entry with spread to the anaerobic environment of the maxillary, ethmoid, and sphenoid sinuses precedes orbital extension.[61] An isolated sphenoid sinusitis can lead to involvement of the optic nerve in the optic canal.[65] Attendant arteritis may lead to thrombosis, occlusion, and aneurysm formation.[61]

The organism has a predilection for the compromised host but may also be seen occasionally in otherwise healthy individuals.[60] Cancer patients are at specific risk—72 percent of patients infected with *Aspergillus* have leukemia and 20 percent have lymphoma.[62]

CLINICAL PRESENTATION AND DIAGNOSIS

In contrast to the fulminant infection associated with *Mucor* or *Rhizopus*, *Aspergillus* infections tend to be more indolent, with symptoms lasting from months to years.[60] This slower course belies the severity of the infection that can often lead to blindness and death (Fig. 171–5). The infection has recently been reported as a steroid-responsive optic neuropathy, with fatal outcome.[63] *Aspergillus* infection of the orbit following dental infection similarly led to diagnostic dilemma and death.[64] These cases should serve to alert the clinician to the insidious nature of *Aspergillus* infections, and the disorder should be added to differential diagnosis lists that include pseudotumor[65] and optic neuritis.[63]

Presenting symptoms include a gradually progressive exophthalmos associated with a chronic fibrosing granulomatous inflammation of the sinuses.[66] Visual loss may be the presenting complaint. Correct diagnosis depends on a high index of suspicion and a biopsy demonstrating dichotomously branching septated hyphae.[61] An appropriate laboratory examination includes 10 to 20 percent KOH preparation, GMS stain, and hematoxylin and eosin stain. Calcofluor white has been suggested as an effective fungal stain.[67] Sabouraud's agar without inhibitors such as cyclohexamide is an appropriate fungal culture medium.

THERAPY

The treatment for *Aspergillus* is the same as for Phycomycetes—wide surgical débridement in conjunction with systemic antifungal therapy. Amphotericin B, alone or in combination with 5-fluorocytosine or rifampin, is the option available to the clinician.[60–62] Irrigation of the débrided tissues and reversal of immunosuppression should be accomplished if possible.[62] The mortality associated with the diagnosis is high. Prompt, aggressive management is necessary for therapeutic success.

PARASITES

Parasitic orbital infections are relatively rare in the United States but are endemic in other parts of the world, including South America, Africa, and the Middle East.

Echinococcus

Echinococcosis results from the larval form of the tapeworm, genus *Echinococcus*.[68] The worm lives in the intestine of the dog, shedding its eggs in the dog's feces. Following ingestion by an intermediate host, such as a

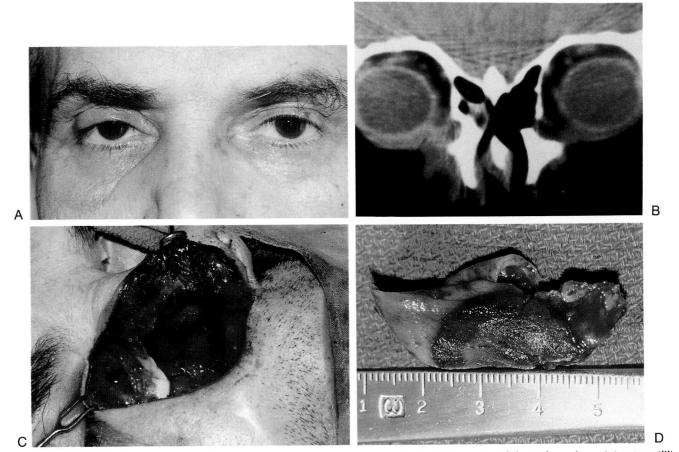

Figure 171–5. *A,* Localized swelling in the nasolabial and infraorbital regions associated with mild ptosis and a minimal motility disturbance was caused by aspergillosis in a 68-year-old patient with leukemia. *B,* A coronal CT scan demonstrates soft tissue inflammation and mucosal thickening. *C,* Wide surgical débridement required resection of the nasal septum. *D,* The resected specimen. Note the area of necrosis.

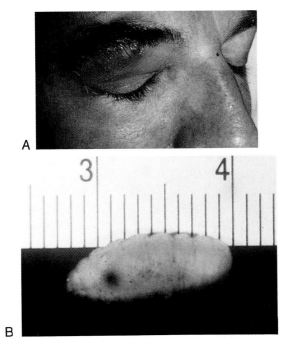

Figure 171–6. *A,* Multiple pruritic papular skin lesions in a middle-aged man 2 wk after a visit to West Africa. Each lesion represented the larval stage of the Tumbu fly. Topical application of petroleum jelly forces the larva to surface, enabling mechanical extraction. *B,* Extracted larva. (*A* and *B,* Courtesy of Monte Mills, M.D.)

cow or sheep, the eggs hatch in the animal's gut. The hydatid cysts undergo hematogenous dissemination to a wide variety of tissues. Subsequent ingestion of these tissues by the definitive host, humans, leads to the final larval stage. Infected human tissues include liver and lungs, but hydatid cysts appear in the orbit in 1 percent of cases of echinococcosis.[68]

Clinical presentation tends to occur in patients under 20 yr of age[68, 69] as a slowly progressive proptosis with or without ophthalmoplegia. Visual acuities range from 20/20 to no light perception.[68, 69] Ultrasound shows a circumscribed cystic structure. A CT scan reveals a cyst of water or cerebrospinal fluid (CSF) density.[68, 69] As long as the parasite remains encysted, serologic results may be negative. Therefore, the absence of positive titers does not rule out infection.[68]

Management is surgical excision.

Cysticercosis

Cysticercus cellulosae eggs from the intermediate host, pigs, are ingested by the human in the form of raw pork. The cysticerci are preferentially disseminated to the eye and brain, with orbital involvement (primarily) of the rectus muscles having been reported.[48, 70] Laboratory work-up may be nondiagnostic.[70] Surgical removal of the cysts or medical therapy with praziquantel and steroids is appropriate to diminish the inflammatory response.[71, 72]

Microfilaria

Diorofilaria rarely infects humans. An insect vector, usually the mosquito, transmits the parasite to the definitive host. The worm has been reported to be a cause of proptosis and chemosis. Treatment is surgical excision.[73]

Myiasis

Myiasis, infection with fly larvae, has been reported in the United States[74] but is more commonly found in other parts of the world.[75] The larvae enter directly through the conjunctiva or the skin and may cause significant tissue destruction (Fig. 171–6).[75]

REFERENCES

1. Hornblass A, Herschorn BJ, Stern K, Grimes C: Orbital abscess. Surv Ophthalmol 29:169–178, 1984.
2. Gamble RC: Acute inflammations of the orbit in children. Arch Ophthalmol 10:483–497, 1933.
3. Clary R, Weber AL, Eavey R, Oot RF: Orbital cellulitis with abscess formation caused by sinusitis. Ann Otol Rhinol Laryngol 97:211–212, 1988.
4. Smith AT, Spencer JT: Orbital complications resulting from lesions of the sinuses. Ann Otol Rhinol Laryngol 57:5–27, 1948.
5. Chandler JR, Langenbrunner DJ, Stevens ER: The pathogenesis of orbital complications in acute sinusitis. Laryngoscope 80:1414–1423, 1970.
6. Weiss A, Friendly D, Eglin K, et al: Bacterial periorbital and orbital cellulitis in childhood. Ophthalmology 90:195–203, 1983.
7. Rubin SE, Slavin ML, Rubin LG: Eyelid swelling and erythema as the only signs of subperiosteal abscess. Br J Ophthalmol 73:576–578, 1989.
8. Weizman Z, Mussaffi H: Ethmoiditis-associated periorbital cellulitis. Int J Pediatr Otorhinolaryngol 11:147–151, 1986.
9. Biedner BZ, Marmur U, Yassur Y: *Streptococcus faecalis* orbital cellulitis. Ann Ophthalmol 18:194–195, 1986.
10. Partamian LG, Jay WM, Fritz KJ: Anaerobic orbital cellulitis. Ann Ophthalmol 15:123–126, 1983.
11. Kallet HA, McKenzie KS, Johnson FD: Bacterial pseudomycosis of the orbit. Am J Ophthalmol 68:504–507, 1969.
12. Levine RA: Infection of the orbit by an atypical *Mycobacterium*. Arch Ophthalmol 82:608–610, 1969.
13. Sen DK: Tuberculosis of the orbita and lacrimal gland: A clinical study of 14 cases. J Pediatr Ophthalmol Strabismus 17:232–238, 1980.
14. Khali M, Lindley S, Matouk E: Tuberculosis of the orbit. Ophthalmology 92:1624–1627, 1985.
15. Oakhill A, Shah KJ, Thompson AG, et al: Orbital tuberculosis in childhood. Br J Ophthalmol 66:396–397, 1982.
16. Spoor TC, Harding SA: Orbital tuberculosis. Am J Ophthalmol 91:644–647, 1981.
17. Antoine GA, Grundfast KM: Periorbital cellulitis. Int J Pediatr Otorhinolaryngol 13:273–278, 1987.
18. Gold SC, Arrigg PG, Hedges TR: Computerized tomography in the management of acute orbital cellulitis. Ophthalmic Surg 18:753–756, 1987.
19. Weber AL, Mikulis DK: Inflammatory disorders of the periorbital sinuses and their complications. Radiol Clin North Am 25:615–630, 1987.
20. Rubin SE, Rubin LG, Zito J, et al: Medical management of orbital subperiosteal abscess in children. J Pediatr Ophthalmol Strabismus 26:21–26, 1989.
21. Slavin ML, Glaser JS: Acute severe irreversible visual loss with sphenoethmoiditis-"posterior" orbital cellulitis. Arch Ophthalmol 105:345–348, 1987.
22. Geggel HS, Isenberg SJ: Cavernous sinus thrombosis as a cause of unilateral blindness. Ann Ophthalmol 14:569–574, 1982.
23. Harris GJ: Subperiosteal inflammation of the orbit: A bacteriological analysis of 17 cases. Arch Ophthalmol 106:947–952, 1988.
24. Bergin DJ, Wright J: Orbital cellulitis. Br J Ophthalmol 70:174–178, 1986.
25. Jackson K, Baker SR: Periorbital cellulitis. Head Neck Surg 9:227–234, 1987.
26. Wilson M, Paul TO: Orbital cellulitis following strabismus surgery. Ophthalmic Surg 18:92–94, 1987.
27. Allen MV, Cohen KL, Grimson BS: Periorbital cellulitis secondary to dacryocystitis following blepharoplasty. Ann Ophthalmol 17:498–499, 1985.
28. Rees TD, Craig SM, Fisher Y: Orbital abscess following blepharoplasty. Plast Reconstr Surg 73:126–127, 1983.
29. Ahrens-Palumbo MJ, Ballen PH: Primary dacryocystitis causing orbital cellulitis. Ann Ophthalmol 14:600–601, 1982.
30. Hornblass A, To K, Coden DJ, Ahn-Lee S: Endogenous orbital cellulitis and endogenous endophthalmitis in subacute bacterial endocarditis. Am J Ophthalmol 108:196–197, 1989.
31. Ullman S, Pflugfelder SC, Hughes RS, Forster RK: *Bacillus cereus* panophthalmitis manifesting as an orbital cellulitis. Am J Ophthalmol 103:105–106, 1987.
32. Harris GJ: Subperiosteal abscess of the orbit. Arch Ophthalmol 101:751–757, 1983.
33. Bullock JD, Fleishman JA: Orbital cellulitis following dental extraction. Trans Am Ophthalmol Soc 87:111–133, 1984.
34. Harbour RC, Trobe JD, Ballinger WE: Septic cavernous sinus thrombosis associated with gingivitis and parapharyngeal abscess. Arch Ophthalmol 102:94–97, 1984.
35. Gatot A, Tovi F, Moshiashvili A: Periorbital cellulitis: Presenting feature of undiagnosed old maxillary fracture. Int J Pediatr Otorhinolaryngol 11:129–134, 1986.
36. Kaufman SJ: Orbital mucopyoceles: Two cases and a review. Surv Ophthalmol 25:253–262, 1981.
37. Stankiewicz JA: Sphenoid sinus mucocele. Arch Otolaryngol Head Neck Surg 115:735–740, 1989.

38. Trono D, Durand M, Baker AS: Unpublished data from the Massachusetts Eye and Ear Infirmary, Boston, MA.

39. Crock GW, Heriot WJ, Janakiraman P, Weiner JM: Gas gangrene infection of the eyes and orbits. Br J Ophthalmol 69:143–148, 1985.

40. Scott PM, Bloome MA: Lid necrosis secondary to streptococcal periorbital cellulitis. Ann Ophthalmol 13:461–465, 1981.

41. Ross J, Kohlhepp PA: Gangrene of the eyelids. Ann Ophthalmol 5:84–88, 1983.

42. Prendiville KJ, Bath PE: Lateral cantholysis and eyelid necrosis secondary to *Pseudomonas aeruginosa.* Ann Ophthalmol 20:193–195, 1988.

43. Weber DJ, Wolfson JS, Swarts MU, et al: *Pasteurella multocida* infections. Report of 34 cases and review of the literature. Medicine 63:133–154, 1984.

44. Hodges E, Tabbara KF: Orbital cellulitis: Review of 23 cases from Saudi Arabia. Br J Ophthalmol 73:205–208, 1989.

45. Jones DB, Steinkuller PG: Strategies for the initial management of acute preseptal and orbital cellulitis. Trans Am Ophthalmol Soc 86:94–112, 1988.

46. McNamara MP, Richie M, Kirmani N: Ocular infections secondary to *Pasteurella multocida.* Am J Ophthalmol 106:361–362, 1988.

47. Vida L, Moel SA: Systemic North American blastomycosis with orbital involvement. Am J Ophthalmol 77:240–242, 1974.

48. Jakobiec FA, Jones IS: Orbital inflammations. *In* Duane TD (ed): Clinical Ophthalmology. Philadelphia, JB Lippincott, 1988.

49. Streeten BW, Rabuzzi DD, Jones DB: Sporotrichosis of the orbital margin. Am J Ophthalmol 77:750–755, 1974.

50. Maskin SL, Fetchick RJ, Leone CR Jr, et al: *Bipolaris hawaiiensis*-caused phaeohyphomycotic orbitopathy. Ophthalmology 96:175–179, 1989.

51. Diaz AG, Hernanz AP, Larregla S, et al: Orbital phycomycosis. Ophthalmologica 182:165–170, 1981.

52. O'Keefe M, Haining WM, Young JDH, Guthrie W: Orbital mucormycosis with survival. Br J Ophthalmol 70:634–636, 1986.

53. Ferry AP, Abedi S: Diagnosis and management of rhino-orbito-cerebral mucormycosis (phycomycosis). Ophthalmology 90:1096–1104, 1983.

54. Schwartze GM, Kilgo GR, Ford CS: Internal ophthalmoplegia resulting from acute orbital phycomycosis. J Clin Neuro-ophthalmol 4:105–108, 1984.

55. Kohn R, Hepler R: Management of limited rhino-orbital mucormycosis without exenteration. Ophthalmology 92:1440–1444, 1985.

56. Bray WH, Giangiacomo J, Ide CH: Orbital apex syndrome. Surv Ophthalmol 32:136–140, 1987.

57. Zak SM, Katz B: Successfully treated spheno-orbital mucormycosis in an otherwise healthy adult. Ann Ophthalmol 17:344–348, 1985.

58. Miller RD, Steinkuller PG, Naegele D: Nonfatal maxillocerebral mucormycosis. Ann Ophthalmol 12:1065–1068, 1980.

59. Lazzaro EC, Sloan B: Mucormycosis: Case presentation and discussion. Ann Ophthalmol 14:660–662, 1982.

60. Dortzbach R, Segrest DR: Orbital aspergillosis. Ophthalmic Surg 14:240–244, 1983.

61. Yumoto E, Kitani S, Okomura H, Yanagihara N, et al: Sino-orbital aspergillosis associated with total ophthalmoplegia. Laryngoscope 95:190–192, 1985.

62. Harris G, Will B: Orbital aspergillosis, conservative debridement and local amphotericin irrigation. Ophthalmic Plast Reconstr Surg 5:207–211, 1989.

63. Spoor TC, Hartel WC, Harding S, et al: Aspergillosis presenting as a corticosteroid-responsive optic neuropathy. J Clin Neuro-ophthalmol 2:103–107, 1982.

64. Case 38–1982, Case records of the Massachusetts General Hospital: A 66-year-old diabetic woman with sinusitis and cranial nerve abnormalities. N Engl J Med 307:806–814, 1982.

65. Nielsen EW, et al: Aspergillosis of the sphenoid sinus presenting as orbital pseudotumor. Otolaryngol Head Neck Surg 91:699–703, 1983.

66. Green WR, Font RL, Zimmerman LE: Aspergillosis of the orbit. Arch Ophthalmol 82:302–313, 1969.

67. Marines HM, Osato MS, Font RL: The value of calcofluor white in the diagnosis of mycotic and acanthamoeba infections of the eye and ocular adnexa. Ophthalmology 94:23–26, 1987.

68. Morales AG, Croxatto JO, Crovetto L, et al: Hydatid cysts of the orbit: A review of 35 cases. Ophthalmology 95:1027–1032, 1988.

69. Kars Z, Kansu T, Ozcan OE, et al: Orbital echinococcosis: Report of two cases studied by computerized tomography. J Clin Neuro-Ophthalmol 2:197–199, 1982.

70. Hamed HH: Orbital affection with cysticercus cellulosae. Bull Ophta Soc Egypt 61:253–255, 1968.

71. Jones TC: Cestodes (tapeworm). *In* Mandell GL, Douglas RG, Bennett J: Principles and Practice of Infectious Diseases, 3rd ed. New York, Churchill Livingstone, 1990, p 2154.

72. Sotelo J, Escobedo F, Rodriguez-Carbajal J, et al: Therapy of parenchymal brain cysticercosis with praziquantel. N Engl J Med 310:1001–1007, 1984.

73. Thomas D, Older JJ, Kanjawalla NM, et al: The dirofilaria parasite in the orbit. Am J Ophthalmol 82:931–933, 1976.

74. Eifrig DE: Ocular myiasis. Arch Ophthalmol 82:137, 1969.

75. Mathur SP, Makhija JM: Invasion of the orbit by maggots. Br J Ophthalmol 51:46, 1967.

Chapter 172

■

Tumors of the Lacrimal Gland and Sac

FRANCIS C. SUTULA

LACRIMAL GLAND TUMORS

Lacrimal gland tumors characteristically present with upper eyelid fullness, alteration of the upper eyelid contour, and downward and nasal displacement of the globe. Because approximately half of all lacrimal fossa masses are inflammatory, the other half are neo-plastic,[1-3] and differentiating between these two groups is imperative.

Symptoms

The two groups usually present quite differently. Erythema, chemosis, pain with extraocular movement,

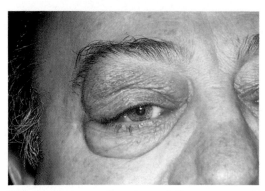

Figure 172–1. The normal contour of the upper eyelid is deformed into an S shape with enlargement of a mass in the lacrimal gland fossa.

and tenderness on palpation usually signify inflammatory disease.[4, 5] The pain associated with perineural invasion in adenocystic carcinoma usually occurs after a mass is noticed or proptosis commences.[6–8] The globe is also relatively free of injection compared with the amount of discomfort present. Eye movement does not significantly modify this complaint. Rarely symptomatic is the diminution in lacrimal gland secretions due to any of these processes.

Signs

Lacrimal fossa lesions are suspected when there is fullness of the upper eyelid, asymmetry of the superior sulci, and alteration of the eyelid contour. An S-shaped contour is quite characteristic (Fig. 172–1). Expansion of the lesion beyond the confines of the lacrimal fossa displaces the globe downward and inward. Spread of the lesion posteriorly produces proptosis.

Palpation of the lateral portion of the upper lid confirms the presence of a mass. Whether the mass is freely mobile, fixed to the orbital rim, smooth and rubbery, or nodular and tender helps differentiate its nature for the clinician.

Other ocular findings are unusual, but globe deformation with resultant refractive error and choroidal folds can develop with masses of significant dimension.

Evaluation

The current standard of care is to evaluate patients with a lacrimal gland mass using computed tomography (CT). CT scans not only define the density and relative homogeneity of the lesion but can also illustrate whether one or both lobes of the gland are involved or if extension beyond the gland has occurred. CT scans can be superior to magnetic resonance imaging (MRI) in identifying changes in bone. Therefore, lacrimal fossa and orbital rim changes are more easily recognizable with CT scanning. Specifically, benign enlargement of the fossa of the pleomorphic adenoma is distinguishable from osteolytic lesions of adenocystic carcinoma.[9]

Inflammation

Although infections of the lacrimal gland are quite rare, they have been recognized as a clinical entity for centuries.[10] Even with this recognition, the mechanism of dacryoadenitis is not altogether understood. Although ascension from the conjunctiva through the lacrimal ductules into the gland is theoretically possible, most cases are associated with systemic infection.[10] Because systemic manifestations are usually minor, the inflamed lacrimal gland is the most significant sign and, therefore, considered to be primary.

Clinically, patients present with fullness and tenderness in the superior aspect of the upper eyelid. Mechanical ptosis and the typical S-shaped curve of the upper eyelid are usually present. Edema may spread into the temporal fossa, and preauricular nodes may be enlarged and tender. Palpation of the lacrimal fossa usually discloses a tender, nut-shaped swelling that is continuous with neither the orbital rim nor the tarsus or ciliary margin. The latter sign distinguishes acute dacryoadenitis from lid abscesses due to involvement of the meibomian, Zeiss's, or Moll's glands. Localization of the erythema and chemosis to the upper and outer quadrant of the lid and protuberance of the easily herniated lacrimal gland confirm the diagnosis. These specific findings attest to the fact that the palpebral lobe is more frequently involved than the orbital lobe.[10]

The normal course of infectious dacryoadenitis is for gradual resolution to take place over several weeks, but several months may pass before the inflammation completely subsides. Although complications are rare, reports have described external cutaneous fistulas in suppurative infections. A fatal case of meningitis was reported after bacterial dacryoadenitis tracked to the cavernous sinus during the preantibiotic era.[10] Consecutive atrophy of the lacrimal acini leading to keratitis sicca has also been described. Lacrimal ductal cysts can form after infections or traumatic insults. I recently observed bilateral dacryops in a patient who, while on sabbatical in Africa 4 mo previously, had had bilateral dacryoadenitis (Fig. 172–2).

The two most common infectious causes of dacryoadenitis are gonorrhea and mumps. Dacryoadenitis due to gonorrhea appears more often in men in their third

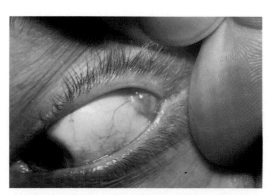

Figure 172–2. Dacryops following dacryoadenitis.

decade of life. Dacryoadenitis due to mumps more often afflicts children, accompanying bilateral parotid swelling. With both agents, the involvement is acute and often bilateral and resolves spontaneously without sequelae. Histoplasmosis, trachoma, mononucleosis, and zoster are among a list of other infectious diseases known to cause dacryoadenitis. Actinomycetic infection must be considered with lacrimal calculus formation.

Noninfectious systemic granulomatous disease can also be associated with enlargement of lacrimal glands. Involvement may be unilateral or bilateral and is usually characterized by painless, slowly progressive growth. The nodules feel firm and the glands freely mobile under the skin. Sarcoidosis[1, 10] is the principal cause of systemic granulomatous disease involving the lacrimal gland but usually affects the gland only after other organs are involved. When the dacryoadenitis is associated with parotitis and uveitis, Heerfordt's syndrome is diagnosed. In contrast, Mikulicz's syndrome has more general distribution.[10] It is marked by chronic bilateral enlargement of both the lacrimal glands and the salivary glands. The cause is obscure. The differential diagnosis includes sardoidosis, tuberculosis, syphilis, lymphoma, mumps, Hodgkin's disease, and Waldenström's macroglobulinemia.

Two nongranulomatous systemic diseases that can enlarge the lacrimal glands are Sjögren's syndrome[11] and thyroid-associated ophthalmopathy. These entities are discussed thoroughly in other sections of this text, but suffice it to say the Sjögren's syndrome may eventually lead to atrophy of the gland substance. Association with lymphoepithelial hyperplasia and even lymphoma is well documented. Thyroid-associated ophthalmopathy may involve the entire orbit bilaterally, albeit asymmetrically.

IDIOPATHIC INFLAMMATORY PSEUDOTUMOR

Idiopathic inflammatory pseudotumor (IIP) is a common cause of lacrimal gland enlargement.[1, 2, 12, 13] In fact, IIP is most likely not one disease but a group that will be reduced in numbers as causes are defined. The merit in this conjecture is based on the fact that early clinicians such as Birsh-Hirshfield and Mikulicz included granulomatous diseases such as sarcoid and tuberculosis and

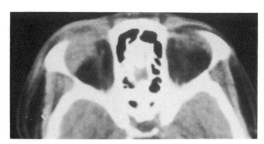

Figure 172–4. Computed tomography scan of the patient in Figure 172–3 showing inflammation confined to the lacrimal gland.

even frank malignancies in their classification. Because of the uncertainty of the cause of the entity and the myriad of clinical and histologic findings, a most inexact term for this condition remains. The word *idiopathic* is temporary, because when the cause is discerned, it will rightfully assume a place in the name of the disease. *Inflammatory* is a word that histologically could not be more broad. *Pseudotumor* itself is an oxymoron. *Tumor* means "firm swelling," and there is nothing false about the firm swelling in idiopathic inflammatory pseudotumor. Jakobiec and Jones[14] astutely suggested that a more accurate designation would be *pseudoneoplasm*, because the real concern is to differentiate a benign inflammatory lesion from a potentially lethal neoplasm. However, because of its wide current use, *pseudotumor* will probably remain popular for some time to come.

IIP of the lacrimal gland tends to present as an erythematous, edematous, and painful upper eyelid. It may be associated with extraocular muscle palsy and subsequent diplopia and ptosis (Figs. 172–3 to 172–5). It can also present with minimal redness or pain. That the orbital lobe is more often affected than the palpebral lobe and that the onset of the symptoms encompasses months rather than days or weeks helps differentiate it from dacryoadenitis.

The histologic features of IIP are diverse. These include the presence of plasma cells, eosinophils, and lymphocytes arranged in sheets or even germinal centers. Capillary proliferation, vasculitis, or dense fibrous tissue can be the predominant finding.[14] All of these are associated with a reactive response rather than neoplas-

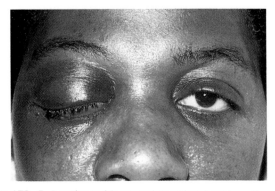

Figure 172–3. A patient with several months' duration of a painful and swollen eyelid. Systemic antibiotic therapy was of no avail.

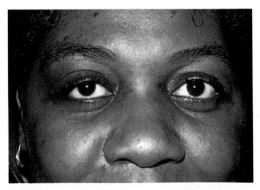

Figure 172–5. The same patient in Figure 172–3 following a short course of systemic corticosteroid therapy for her pseudotumor.

tic growth. These protean forms create difficulty in determining the true incidence of the disorder. For example, if arterial inflammation predominates, the tissue sample may be classified as vasculitis.

Studies for cell surface markers to determine whether or not the lymphocytes involved are monoclonal or polyclonal[15] now represent the standard of care. However, a polyclonal picture does not ensure that the lesion will continue to be benign. A substantial number will evolve into malignancies.[16] Genetic marker investigations[17] have been better able to delineate the parentage of lymphocytic populations.

Satisfactory resolution of the symptoms and signs with a therapeutic trial of high-dose systemic steroids confirms, with some qualifications, the diagnosis of IIP. If response is poor, a biopsy must be performed to rule out neoplasm. Radiotherapy in doses less than for lymphoma can also be used; a favorable response with either regimen does not preclude careful follow-up for many years. Too often a frank neoplasm develops in an area in which a benign histologic picture was seen.

NEOPLASMS OF THE LACRIMAL GLAND

Almost half of all tumors of the lacrimal gland are epithelial in origin.[1, 2, 3, 10, 11] The other tumors are mostly lymphoproliferative and are divided between idiopathic inflammatory pseudotumor and lymphoma. Half of all epithelial tumors are pleomorphic adenomas (mixed cell tumor); the other half are malignant.[13, 14, 18, 19]

Pleomorphic Adenoma

The term *mixed cell tumor* was first used to describe lacrimal gland lesions as early as 1874.[10] The term at first encompassed both malignant and benign lesions but gradually evolved to refer specifically to pleomorphic adenoma. The reason that this lesion was originally called *mixed cell* is that it consists of two distinct elements. One element is the epithelial lining of the ducts, and the other element has an apparently mesenchymal appearance. However, the stroma is actually formed by the outer layer of epithelium that lines the ducts. It is this metaplasia of the epithelium that forms myxoid, fibrous, and even cartilaginous stroma. Many references are made to the "capsule" surrounding mixed cell tumors. This structure is, in reality, a pseudocapsule formed by compression of tissues surrounding the tumor.[2, 13, 14] Infiltration by the tumor through this pseudocapsule is commonly observed microscopically.

The typical age of presentation of patients with mixed cell tumor is 35 years. Fullness of the upper eyelid and gradual downward displacement of the globe will have been noticed for at least 1 yr. Diplopia is caused by mechanical limitation only when gaze is directed toward the lesion. Rarely is any pain associated with this mass. Radiographic findings often demonstrate enlargement of the lacrimal fossa without any bone destruction.

The crucial aspect of management of all lacrimal fossa tumors is to suspect pleomorphic adenoma. Although this tumor is histologically benign, incomplete excision will likely result in relentless recurrences leading to increased orbital dysfunction and even malignant transformation.[2, 10, 14, 20] Therefore, when pleomorphic adenoma is suspected, a lateral orbitotomy is mandatory. The entire tumor with its pseudocapsule, surrounding levator aponeurosis, conjunctiva, and periorbita must be excised en bloc[2, 21, 22] to avoid recurrences and long-term misery for patients.

Other benign epithelial neoplasms of the lacrimal gland are quite rare and are of the types often associated with the other salivary glands. These other tumors are represented by isolated case reports of Warthin's tumor[10] (papillary cystadenoma lymphomatosum) and oncocytoma[23] (oxyphilic adenoma).

As already mentioned, 25 per cent of tumors involving the lacrimal gland are cancerous. These do not show any sex predilection. The age of onset of these lesions can precede or parallel the onset of mixed cell tumors. The majority (60 per cent) of malignant tumors of the lacrimal gland are adenoid cystic carcinoma.[2, 10, 14, 18, 20] Half of the remaining neoplasms are malignant mixed cell tumors, and the remaining 20 per cent are split among adenocarcinoma, undifferentiated carcinoma, squamous cell carcinoma, and mucoepidermoid carcinoma.[24]

Adenoid Cystic Carcinoma

The clinical features of adenoid cystic carcinoma are the associated pain and the short duration of the signs and symptoms from onset to presentation. The reason for the associated pain is early perineural infiltration by the tumor.[1, 2, 10, 14, 18] Radiographic appearance of the lacrimal fossa may show no changes or destructive lesions of the bone.

The name *adenoid cystic carcinoma* and the older term, *cylindroma*, accurately describe the microscopic picture. Closely packed small, densely stained cells aggregate around large ovoid spaces.[7, 4] The spaces contain hyalin or mucin. The separation of these two elements is striking and, even at low power, has been likened to the appearance of Swiss cheese.

Five histologic patterns characterize adenoid cystic carcinoma: cribriform, sclerosing, basaloid, comedocarcinoma, and tubular. The basaloid pattern is associated with the worst prognosis. The more differentiated patterns augur longer survival. Gamel and Font[25] reported that patients whose tumors had a basaloid component had a 5-yr survival rate of only 21 percent. Patients whose tumors contained no basaloid components had a 5-yr survival rate of 71 percent. The overall 5-yr survival rate of all adenoid cystic carcinomas was 47 percent. This number plummets to 22 percent after 15 yr.

The major cause of death due to adenoid cystic carcinoma is intracranial spread, which is hastened by perineural invasion. Metastasis to the lung occurs 5 to 10 yr after the initial diagnosis has been made. Treatment consists of exenteration with or without postoperative radiotherapy. Both the Mayo Clinic series[2] and the series of Font and Gamel[7] show no increase in the survival of patients who have had radiotherapy. Other types of carcinoma of the lacrimal gland include squamous cell and mucoepidermoid carcinoma. Interestingly, these are quite rare in the lacrimal gland but occur much more frequently in the salivary glands.

Malignant Mixed Cell Tumors

Malignant mixed cell tumors account for less than 10 percent of all epithelial tumors of the lacrimal gland. These tumors most often arise within or adjacent to benign pleomorphic adenoma[26] and are more frequently associated with recurrent benign mixed tumors displaying rapid growth.[2, 10] Widespread, uniform malignant aggregations are not seen, giving credence to the belief that malignant transformation occurs within benign tumors rather than de novo. The epithelial carcinomatous change is most often that of adenocarcinoma. Squamous cell carcinoma and sarcomatous changes occur much less frequently.

Lymphoma and Other Reticuloendothelial Tumors

Lymphoma of the lacrimal gland presents as a painless mass involving the lacrimal fossa (Figs. 172–6 to 172–8). The characteristic salmon-colored mass can sometimes be seen in the superior lateral cul-de-sac, but more often, the palpable mass is fixed to the orbital rim and is rubbery in consistency.[1, 2, 10, 11, 12] Radiographic appearance of the bone is usually normal. CT scans usually show a homogeneous consistency with indistinct borders characteristic of the infiltrative nature of this lesion.[27] The tumor often shows a tendency to mold into the contour of the lacrimal fossa and the surrounding bony contour.

The age incidence of lymphoma of the lacrimal gland appears bimodal, with peaks in both the third decade and the sixth. Both unilateral and bilateral presentations are possible. Care must be taken to rule out any extraorbital site of lymphoma. Full-body scanning and bone marrow biopsies are standard early investigative techniques. When an extraorbital site is found, orbital radiotherapy may be curative. Some oncologists argue that lymphoma is a systemic disease that may initially present in the orbit and, therefore, prescribe systemic chemotherapy. The fact that half of all patients with orbital

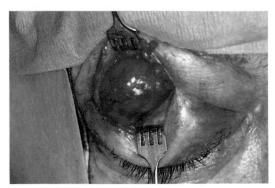

Figure 172–7. Intraoperative photograph of the patient in Figure 172–6 showing the enlarged lacrimal gland.

lymphoma will demonstrate an extraorbital site of involvement within 5 yr lends some credence to this point of view. In any case, these patients must be monitored by both the ophthalmologist and oncologist with examinations and scans for several years before reasonable assurance of cure can be assumed.

The occurrence of Hodgkin's disease in the lacrimal gland is rare. Other lymphoproliferative diseases involving the lacrimal fossa include lymphosarcoma and Burkitt's lymphoma. Interestingly, Burkitt's lymphoma[10] is the most common cause of bilateral lacrimal gland enlargement in Uganda.

Secondary Tumors

Secondary tumors of the lacrimal gland are rare. Sinus tumors rarely invade the gland because of the distance from even the most lateral portion of the frontal sinus. However, basal cell carcinoma at the lateral canthus, squamous cell carcinoma from the conjunctiva, or even sebaceous cell carcinoma from the lid may present with the bulk of its mass in the lacrimal fossa. Biopsy and ensuing surgery should demonstrate the source of the lesion.

In summary, the characteristic presentation of lacrimal fossa masses should enable clinicians to diagnose these tumors. Inflammatory and neoplastic characteristics are helpful in directing the course of action. CT is invaluable in assessing the nature of the lesion, the lobe involved, and any associated osseous changes. Suspicion

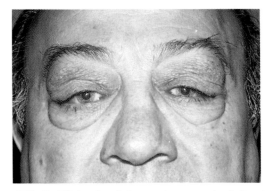

Figure 172–6. Bilateral painless enlargement of the lacrimal glands led to this referral for treatment of mechanical ptosis.

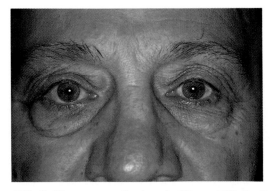

Figure 172–8. The same patient as in Figure 172–6 after chemotherapy for systemic lymphoma.

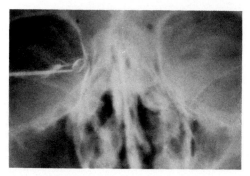

Figure 172–9. A dacryocystogram demonstrating a clear space within the sac. Anteroposterior view.

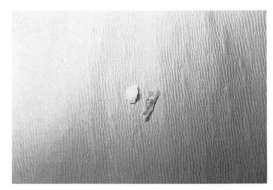

Figure 172–11. The dacryolith in the previous dacryocystograms.

of pleomorphic adenoma will appropriately guide clinicians in their surgical management.

LACRIMAL SAC TUMORS

Lacrimal sac tumors present differently from nasolacrimal duct obstruction in that tumors more often result in intermittent episodes of epiphora and dacryocystitis. A palpable mass within the lacrimal sac cannot be reduced when the mass is a tumor. A dacryocystocele, on the other hand, is reducible (see Figs. 172–16 to 172–21). Patency, as demonstrated by irrigation to the nasopharynx, in the presence of observed epiphora is another suspicious indicator. This sign demonstrates that no duct abnormality is present and may suggest a "ball valve" type of lesion in the sac. Spontaneous bleeding[28, 29] from the punctum must always be regarded with a high index of suspicion.

Dacryocystography

Whenever a mass within or extrinsic to the sac is suspected, dacryocystography is warranted. Bilateral exposures with posteroanterior and lateral views enable comparisons to be made. A late film (30 min) should be taken to help assess the emptying time of the two sides. A low-viscosity contrast medium (Ethiodol or Pantopaque) is superior to aqueous or highly viscous materials[30–34] for this application.

Filling defects may be due to intrinsic masses such as dacryoliths[35] or neoplasia. Lacrimal stones are radiolucent and therefore are demonstrated by a clear space within the sac (Figs. 172–9 to 172–11), referred to as *reduplication of the lacrimal sac shadow.* A tumor within the sac changes the normal concave appearance of the wall to a scalloped border. A lacy filling defect pattern may be seen with polypoid proliferation within the sac (Fig. 172–12). Extrinsic masses compress the sac wall and convert the normal concave outline to one with a convex component.

Histology of the Lacrimal Sac

Review of the histologic features of the lacrimal sac is pertinent before discussing the tumors that involve the structure. The lining of the lacrimal sac is pseudostratified columnar epithelium. The more superficial layer is columnar; the deeper is flattened. The wall of the sac resembles adenoid tissue and contains elastic fibers. It has a rich venous plexus. Additionally, the sac contains scattered goblet cells, mucus secretors, and serous glands. Some intrinsic masses are due to anatomic variations in the sac. Whitnall (Fig. 172–13)[36] and Busse and colleagues[37] reported on the high degree of variation in the configuration of the sac and the duct. The exact incidence of diverticula is uncertain, but their presence has been repeatedly noted during anatomic dissections and surgery. The clinical manifestation of a diverticulum (Fig. 172–14) may be apparent only when a concurrent

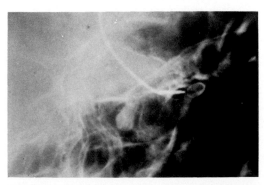

Figure 172–10. Lateral view of the dacryocystogram in Figure 172–9.

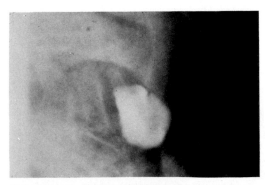

Figure 172–12. Lacy pattern within the sac denoting a papillomatous lesion within the sac.

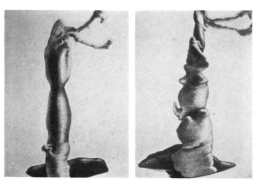

Figure 172–13. Plaster casts with lacrimal systems (after Whitnall) showing the variation in diverticulum.

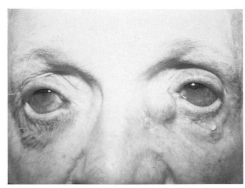

Figure 172–15. A dacryocele associated with idiopathic nasolacrimal duct obstruction.

event causes its inflammation. Diverticulitis of the lacrimal sac has been observed during the latter part of pregnancy. It usually resolves in the postpartum period. Recurrences may be observed during subsequent pregnancies.

The most common cystlike lesion is the mucocele,[28] associated with concurrent nasolacrimal duct obstruction. The secretions of the sac and the tears distend the sac to incredible proportions (Fig. 172–15). When the lumen of the sac becomes infected and purulent secretions fill the sac, the mass is referred to as a *pyocele*.

Other extrinsic cystic lesions may also cause dacryoceles or resemble them. A mucocele arising from the ethmoidal sinus may obstruct the outflow from the lacrimal sac (Figs. 172–16 to 172–21) to the nasolacrimal duct, giving rise to a mucocele of the lacrimal sac. An ethmoidal mucocele may also extend anteriorly without lacrimal sac involvement. When this does occur, the cystic structure can usually be identified superior to the medial canthal tendon. Another external cystic lesion that may impinge on the lacrimal sac is a dermoid cyst.[38] The second most frequent orbital site is at the junction of the frontal bone and the frontal process of the maxillary bone. Rare reported causes of cystic masses

within the lacrimal sac are trauma and congenital malformation. This latter etiology is unique in that the cyst within the sac has a complete and separate wall.

Dacryoliths

Foreign bodies[39] in the sac can be surrounded by epithelial debris and inflammatory tissue to produce a dacryolith of soft, putty-like consistency. The nidus of the dacryolith often is a cilium.[40] Rarer causes of stone formation include brush bristles and argyrosis[41] decompensation products. After chronic application of topical epinephrine,[42] melanin-laden casts have formed within the sac. *Actinomyces*,[43] although more frequently involving the canaliculus (Figs. 172–22 to 172–24), may contribute to stone formation in the sac. *Candida*[44] and *Aspergillus*[45] have also been reported.

GRANULOMAS

Granulomatous disease can, on occasion, produce a mass within the lacrimal sac.[46] Causes include extraorbital manifestations of idiopathic inflammatory pseudotumor and systemic granulomatous diseases. Sarcoidosis[47, 48] has been demonstrated within the lacrimal sac in patients with respiratory manifestations of this

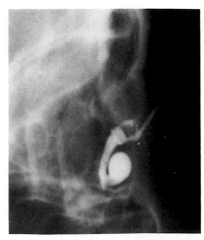

Figure 172–14. Diverticulum in a pregnant patient. The inflammatory aspect resolved in the postpartum period.

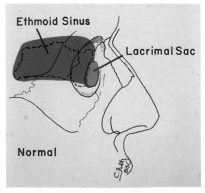

Figure 172–16. The ethmoidal sinus usually terminates posterior to the lacrimal sac.

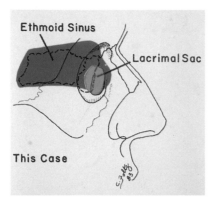

Figure 172–17. Anterior extension of the ethmoidal sinus can extend anteriorly to the lacrimal sac.

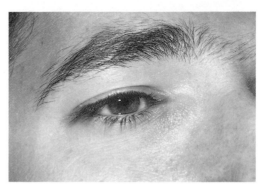

Figure 172–20. Close-up of blue cyst.

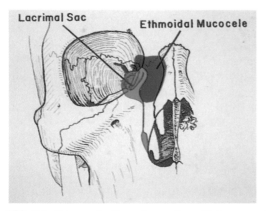

Figure 172–18. Demonstration of an ethmoidal mucocele obstructing the flow from the lacrimal sac to its duct.

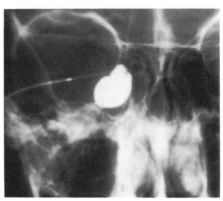

Figure 172–21. Dacryocystogram of the patient in Figure 172–19.

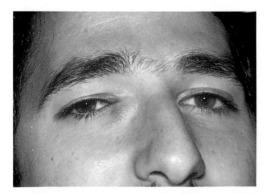

Figure 172–19. A patient with recurrent "blue cyst" in a corner of his right eye. The patient could massage the cyst to reduce it. When he performed this maneuver, he sensed a foul taste in his throat.

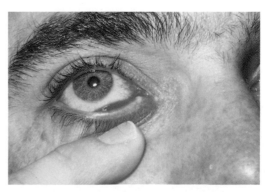

Figure 172–22. A patient with the "pouting" punctum of *Actinomyces*.

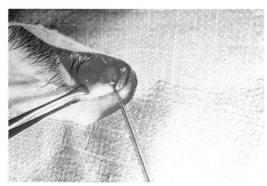

Figure 172–23. Marsupialization of the canaliculus, exposing the stone within.

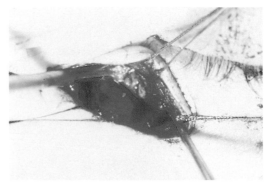

Figure 172–25. A lacrimal sac opened showing the nodularity associated with sarcoidosis.

noncaseating granuloma. Lacrimal sac involvement may present long after respiratory symptoms have resolved (Fig. 172–25). On rare occasions, biopsy of an involved lacrimal sac (Fig. 172–26) may provide the initial sign that a patient harbors this entity.

Patients with Wegener's granulomatosis[49] may also have involvement of the nasolacrimal duct and lacrimal sac (Figs. 172–27 and 172–28). Before successful chemotherapy of this disease, few patients lived long enough to present with epiphora. With longer survival times, involvement of the lacrimal sac (Fig. 172–29) should be suspected in these patients. Successful therapeutic intervention can be offered.

EPITHELIAL TUMORS

Epithelial tumors are the most common neoplasms of the lacrimal sac.[28–29, 50–54] Malignant tumors outnumber benign tumors three to one. The most common benign epithelial tumor is the papilloma.[55] A true papilloma exhibits epithelial papillomatosis and acanthosis. An inflammatory papilloma exhibits granulomatous tissue. Although one third of all epithelial papillomas are indeed benign, recurrent lesions[56] mandate thorough investigation. Patients often have a history of papillomas at the punctum (Fig. 172–30), only to have relentless recurrences.

Inverted papillomas are also called *transitional cell*

carcinoma and *schneiderian papilloma*.[55–56] These can arise de novo in the lacrimal sac but are more commonly associated with extension from the lateral aspect of the nose or maxillary sinus. Although this lesion is not malignant in itself, the recurrence rate is great and mutilation (Figs. 172–31 to 172–34) results if successful therapy is not forthcoming. Additionally, metaplastic transformation to squamous cell carcinoma occurs in 10 to 15 per cent of these cases. Squamous cell[50–53] carcinoma (Figs. 172–35 to 172–44) can also arise within the lacrimal sac without antecedent papillomas.

Other forms of epithelial carcinomas are far less common in the lacrimal sac. These include adenocarcinoma and epidermoid carcinoma. Mucoepidermoid carcinoma (Figs. 172–45 to 172–47)[66] is a rare form of epithelial carcinoma with a grave prognosis. In fact, it appears that except for our reported case,[67] most patients have succumbed to the tumor within 5 yr. The difference between those and ours is that ours was diagnosed by routine biopsy of the lacrimal sac. The other cases already had masses at presentation. This observation illustrates that even though the yield of significant pathology on routine lacrimal sac biopsy is small, it can nevertheless have a profound effect on the life of a patient.

Other reported epithelial tumors include adenoma, pleomorphic adenoma, and oncocytoma.[28–29, 50–53]

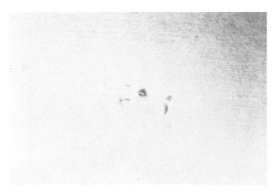

Figure 172–24. Stones from the canaliculi of the patient in Figure 172–23.

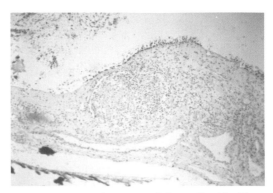

Figure 172–26. The lacrimal sac of the patient in Figure 172–25, demonstrating the noncaseating granuloma of sarcoidosis.

Text continued on page 1965

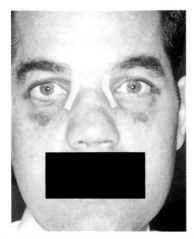

Figure 172–27. Patient with Wegener's granulomatosis in remission shortly after dacryocystorhinostomy for epiphora.

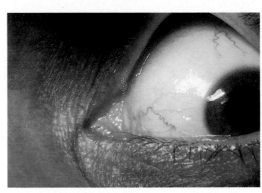

Figure 172–30. The appearance of a papilloma extending from the punctum. This patient has had multiple excisions of papilloma at this site, with rapid recurrences.

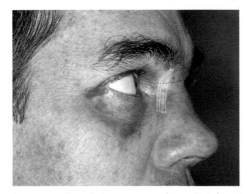

Figure 172–28. Profile of the same patient showing the saddle deformity of Wegener's granulomatosis.

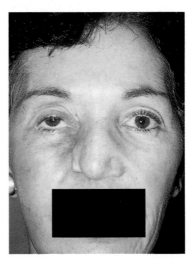

Figure 172–31. A patient with multiple recurrences of inverted papillomatosis showing deformity of her right medial canthal and lateral nasal area.

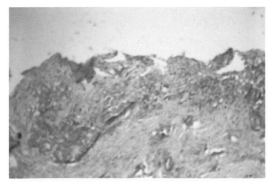

Figure 172–29. The lacrimal sac of the previous patient, showing necrosis, generalized inflammation, and vasculitis.

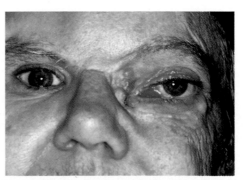

Figure 172–32. A patient with multiple recurrences and incomplete excisions of an inverted papilloma secondarily involving the left nasolacrimal sac.

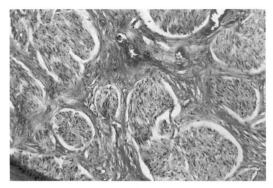

Figure 172–33. The pathology of inverted papillomatosis, exhibiting the inward growth of the papilloma.

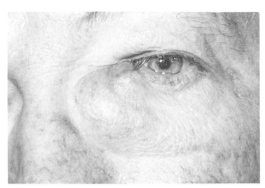

Figure 172–36. A close-up view of the left medial canthal mass.

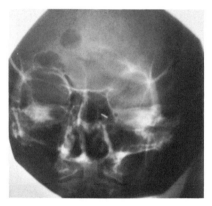

Figure 172–34. A plain radiograph demonstrating clouding of the involved sinuses in the patient pictured in Figure 172–32.

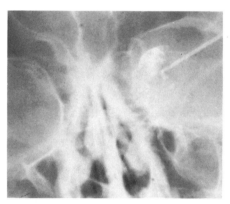

Figure 172–37. A dacryocystogram performed in this patient showed the lacy, scalloping pattern of a papillomatous internal filling defect.

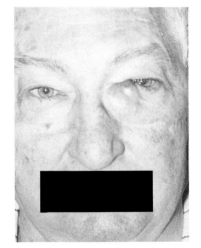

Figure 172–35. A patient with a 20-year history of recurrent papillomas excised at the puncta.

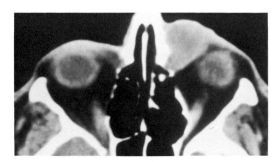

Figure 172–38. An axial computed tomography scan showing the extent of the lesion in the fossa of the lacrimal sac.

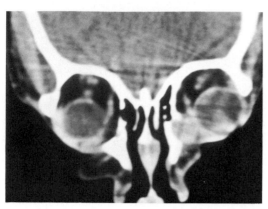

Figure 172–39. A coronal computed tomography scan demonstrating confinement of the mass in the lacrimal fossa area.

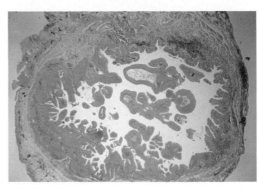

Figure 172–42. The nasolacrimal sac demonstrating the inverted papillomatosis (low power).

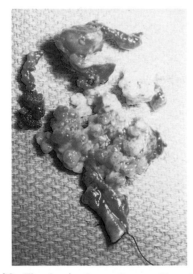

Figure 172–40. The lacrimal sac "opened" and the terminal portion of the nasolacrimal duct after its excision.

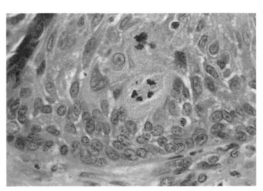

Figure 172–43. Area within lacrimal sac demonstrating squamous metaplasia (high power).

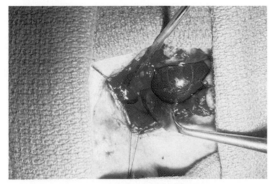

Figure 172–41. Intraoperative photograph demonstrating excision of the canaliculi and the denuded nasolacrimal duct.

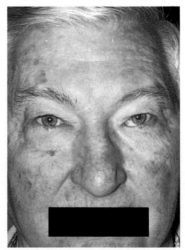

Figure 172–44. Postoperative appearance of the patient shown in Figure 172–35.

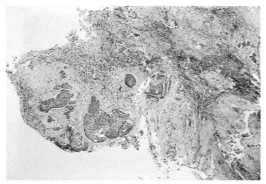

Figure 172–45. Mucoepidermoid carcinoma of the lacrimal sac after routine biopsy during a dacryocystorhinostomy.

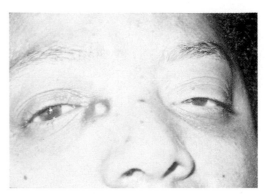

Figure 172–48. A patient with acute dacryocystitis.

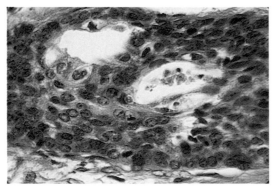

Figure 172–46. Mucoepidermoid carcinoma of a maxillary sinus.

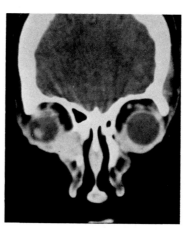

Figure 172–49. Computed tomography scan of the patient pictured in Figure 172–48 revealed a mass in the vicinity of the nasolacrimal duct.

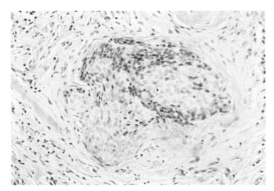

Figure 172–47. Mucoepidermoid carcinoma with a mucicarmine stain. The mucus-secreting cells stain light pink.

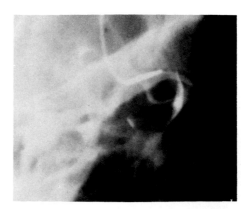

Figure 172–50. A dacryocystogram shows an external indentation on the nasolacrimal sac–duct junction.

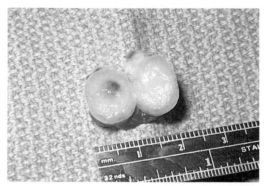

Figure 172–51. An intraoperative photograph showing the bisected schwannoma.

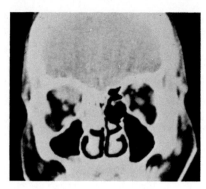

Figure 172–53. An osteoma arising from the ethmoidal sinus, causing secondary nasolacrimal duct obstruction.

LYMPHOPROLIFERATIVE DISORDERS

Lymphoproliferative lesions are the second most common type of tumor causing lacrimal sac–nasolacrimal duct obstruction.[28–29, 58–59] Once again, the discovery of these lesions is often made only after the lacrimal sac is exposed and a tissue diagnosis is made. Lymphoma predominates over benign IIP. Effort should be made to ascertain that the lymphoma is limited to the involved lacrimal system, excluding involvement of additional adjacent or distant sites. If the lesion is localized to the lacrimal sac and duct area, radiotherapy can be administered. With systemic manifestations, chemotherapy is the prescribed treatment.

Lymphomas of the lacrimal sac are sometimes associated with leukemia. Lymphosarcomas, including the reticulum cell variety, have been reported. Although extremely uncommon, Hodgkin's disease has occurred in the sac.[28, 29]

MESENCHYMAL TUMORS

Both benign and malignant tumors of mesenchymal elements have been reported in the lacrimal sac. Capillary and cavernous hemangiomas and even hemangiopericytomas[60] have been represented in the literature. Melanomas,[61–63] neurilemmoma (Figs. 172–48 to 172–54), plexiform neuroma (see Fig. 172–52), and osteoma have involved the sac both intrinsically and extrinsically.

The rare occurrences of fibromas,[65] Kaposi's sarcoma, and other sarcomas are mentioned for completeness.

SECONDARY INVOLVEMENT

Case reports of benign lesions extrinsically causing lacrimal sac masses are numerous. One cause is orbital lymphangioma with anterior extension. An osteoma from the ethmoidal sinus (see Fig. 172–53) can form a mass in the lacrimal sac area.

Deep recurrences of basal cell carcinoma (see Fig. 172–54) and cutaneous squamous cell carcinoma in the canthal area may present as nasolacrimal duct obstruction, especially after incomplete excision and reconstructive efforts have camouflaged the recurrence.

Metastatic tumors to the lacrimal sac are extremely rare. However, obscure neoplasia, including choroidal melanoma,[64] has been observed.

SUMMARY

In summary, intermittent epiphora, sanguineous discharge, or an irreducible mass must lead clinicians to suspect lacrimal sac tumor. CT and MRI scans sometimes help elucidate the diagnosis. Even though the frequency of these lesions is extremely low, pathologic

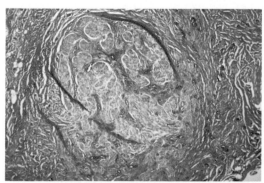

Figure 172–52. A plexiform neuroma discovered incidentally at surgery for nasolacrimal duct obstruction.

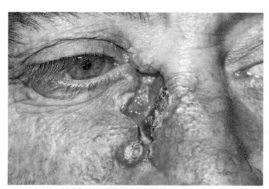

Figure 172–54. Invasion of the nasolacrimal duct and sac area can occur secondary to the spread of cutaneous tumors such as this recurrent basal cell carcinoma.

examination of the lacrimal sac, its duct, and surrounding tissue may have dramatic consequences for patients.

REFERENCES

1. Krohel G, Stewart W, Chavis R: Orbital Disease: A Practical Approach. New York, Grune & Stratton, 1981.
2. Henderson J: Orbital Tumors. Philadelphia, WB Saunders, 1973, pp 409–442.
3. Forrest A: Lacrimal gland tumors. In Duane TD (ed): Clinical Ophthalmology. Hagerstown, Harper & Row, 1976, pp 1, 16, 40.
4. Wright JE, Stewart WB, Krohel GB: Clinical presentation and management of lacrimal gland tumors. Br J Ophthalmol 63:600, 1979.
5. Stewart WB, Krohel GB, Wright JE: Lacrimal gland and fossa lesions: An approach to diagnosis and management. Ophthalmology 86:886, 1979.
6. Font RL, Gamel JW: Epithelial tumors of the lacrimal gland: An analysis of 256 cases. In Jakobiec FA (ed): Ocular and Adnexal Tumors. Birmingham, AL, Aesculapius, 1978, pp 787–805.
7. Font RL, Gamel JW: Adenoid cystic carcinoma of the lacrimal gland: A clinicopathologic study of 79 cases. In Nicholson DH (ed): Ocular Pathology Update. New York, Masson, 1980, pp 277–283.
8. Henderson JW: Intrinsic neoplasms of the lacrimal gland. In Orbital Tumors. New York, Decker/Thieme-Stratton, 1980, pp 394–424.
9. Jakobiec FA, et al: Combined clinical and computed tomographic diagnosis of lacrimal gland lesions. Am J Ophthalmol 94:785, 1982.
10. Duke-Elder S, MacFaul P: The ocular adnexa. In System of Ophthalmology. St. Louis, CV Mosby, 1974, pp 638–672.
11. Milder B: Diseases of the lacrimal gland. In Milder B, Weil B (eds): The Lacrimal System. Norwalk, CT, Appleton-Century-Crofts. 1983, pp 105–110.
12. Harris GJ, Dixon TA, Haughton VM: Expansion of the lacrimal gland fossa by a lymphoid tumor. Am J Ophthalmol 96:546, 1983.
13. Jakobiec FA, Font RL: Lacrimal gland tumors. In Spencer WG (ed): Ophthalmic Pathology: An Atlas and Textbook, vol. 3. Philadelphia, WB Saunders, 1986, p 2496.
14. Jones IS, Jakobiec FA: Diseases of the Orbit. Hagerstown, Harper & Row, 1979.
15. Knowles DM II, Jakobiec FA, Halper JP: Immunologic characterization of ocular adnexal lymphoid neoplasms. Am J Ophthalmol 87:603, 1979.
16. Rootman J: Lymphoproliferative and leukemic lesions. In Rootman J (ed): Diseases of the Orbit. Philadelphia, JB Lippincott, 1988, pp 205–240.
17. White W: Application of genotypic analysis in orbital lymphoid disease. Presented at Symposium on Advances in Genetic Eye Diseases, Boston, January 25, 1992.
18. Zimmerman LE, Sanders TE, Ackerman LV: Epithelial tumors of the lacrimal gland: Prognostic and therapeutic significance of histologic types. Int Ophthalmol Clin 2:337, 1962.
19. Forrest AW: Pathologic criteria for effective management of epithelial lacrimal gland tumors. Am J Ophthalmol 71:178, 1971.
20. Milder B, Smith M: Tumors of the lacrimal gland. In Milder B, Weil B (eds): The Lacrimal System. Norwalk, CT, Appleton-Century-Crofts, 1983, pp 111–116.
21. Jones IS: Surgical considerations in the management of lacrimal gland tumors. Clin Plast Surg 5:561, 1978.
22. Wright JE: Surgical exploration of the orbit. In Stewart WB (ed): Ophthalmic Plastic and Reconstructive Surgery. San Francisco, American Academy of Ophthalmology, 1984.
23. Beskid M, Zarzycka M: A case of onkocytoma of the lacrimal gland. Klin Oczna 29:311, 1959.
24. Thorvaldsson SE, Beahrs OH, Woolner LB, et al: Mucoepidermoid tumors of the major salivary glands. Am J Surg 120:432, 1970.
25. Gamel JW, Font RL: Adenoid cystic carcinoma of the lacrimal gland: The clinical significance of a basaloid histologic pattern. Hum Pathol 13:219, 1982.
26. Forrest AW: Epithelial lacrimal gland tumors: Pathology as a guide to prognosis. Trans Am Acad Ophthalmol Otolaryngol 58:848, 1954.
27. Jakobiec FA, Yeo JH, Trokel SL, et al: Combined clinical and computed tomographic diagnosis of primary lacrimal fossa lesions. Am J Ophthalmol 94:785, 1982.
28. Duke-Elder S, MacFaul P: The ocular adnexa. In System of Ophthalmology. St. Louis, CV Mosby, 1974, pp 724–759.
29. Linberg JV: Disorders of the lower excretory system. In Milder B, Weil B (ed): The Lacrimal System. Norwalk, CT, Appleton-Century-Crofts, 1983, pp 133–143.
30. Milder B, Demorest BH: Dacryocystography. I: The normal lacrimal apparatus. Arch Ophthalmol 51:180, 1954.
31. Demorest BH, Milder B: Dacryocystography. II: The pathologic lacrimal apparatus. Arch Ophthalmol 54:410, 1955.
32. Lloyd GA, et al: Subtraction macrodacryocystography. Br Radiol 47:379, 1974.
33. Rossomojdo RM, Carlton WJ, Trueblood JH, Thomas RP: A new method of evaluating lacrimal drainage. Arch Ophthalmol 88:523, 1972.
34. Milder B: Dacryocystography. In Milder B, Weil B (eds): The Lacrimal System. Norwalk, CT, Appleton-Century-Crofts, 1983, pp 79–91.
35. Berlin AJ, Rath R, Rich L: Lacrimal system dacryoliths. Ophthalmic Surg 11:435, 1980.
36. Whitnall ES: The Anatomy of the Human Orbit. London, Oxford University Press, 1932.
37. Busse H, Muller KM, Kroll P: Radiological and histological findings of the lacrimal passages of newborns. Arch Ophthalmol 98:528, 1980.
38. Hornblass A, Gabry JB: Diagnosis and treatment of lacrimal sac cysts. Ophthalmology 86:1655, 1980.
39. Jones LT: Tear sac foreign bodies. Am J Ophthalmol 60:111, 1965.
40. Jay JL, Lee WR: Dacryolith formation around an eyelash retained in the lacrimal sac. Br J Ophthalmol 60:722, 1976.
41. Gronvall H: On argyrosis and concretion in the lacrimal sac. Acta Ophthalmol (Kbh) 221:247, 1944.
42. Spaeth GL: Nasolacrimal duct obstruction caused by topical epinephrine. Arch Ophthalmol 77:355, 1967.
43. Blanksma LJ, Slijper J: Actinomycotic dacryocystitis. Ophthalmologica 176:145, 1978.
44. Fine M, Waring WS: Mycotic obstruction of the nasolacrimal duct (candida). Arch Ophthalmol 38:39, 1974.
45. Rosenvold LK: Dacryocystitis and blepharitis due to infection by Aspergillus niger. Am J Ophthalmol 25:588, 1942.
46. Nolan J: Granuloma of lacrimal sac: Simulating a neoplasm. Am J Ophthalmol 62:756, 1966.
47. Harris GJ, Williams GA, Clarke GP: Sarcoidosis of the lacrimal sac. Arch Ophthalmol 99:1198, 1981.
48. Neault RW, Riley FC: Report of a case of dacryocystitis secondary to Boeck's sarcoid. Am J Ophthalmol 70:1011, 1970.
49. Spalton DJ, O'Donnell PJ, Graham EM: Lethal midline lymphoma causing acute dacryocystitis. Br J Ophthalmol 65:503, 1981.
50. Flanagan JC, Stokes DP: Lacrimal sac tumors. Trans Am Acad Ophthalmol Otolaryngol 85:1282, 1978.
51. Ryan SJ, Font FL: Primary epithelial neoplasms of the lacrimal sac. Am J Ophthalmol 76:73, 1973.
52. Hornblass A, Jakobiec FA, Bosniak S, et al: The diagnosis and management of epithelial tumors of the lacrimal sac. Ophthalmology 87:476, 1980.
53. Spaeth EB: Carcinomas and tumors of the lacrimal sac. Arch Ophthalmol 57:689, 1952.
54. Ryan SJ, Font RL: Primary epithelial neoplasms of the lacrimal sac. Am J Ophthalmol 76:73, 1973.
55. Karcioglu ZA, Caldwell DR, Reed HT: Papillomas of lacrimal drainage system: A clinicopathologic study. Ophthalmic Surg 15:670, 1984.
56. Verner FL, et al: Epithelial papillomas of the nasal cavities and sinuses. Ann Otolaryngol 70:574, 1959.
57. Harry J, Ashton N: The pathology of tumors of the lacrimal sac. Trans Ophthalmol Soc UK 88:19, 1969.
58. Benger RS, Frue BR: Lacrimal drainage obstruction from lacrimal sac infiltration by lymphocytic neoplasia. Am J Ophthalmol 101:242, 1986.

59. Knowles DM, Jakobiec FA: Orbital lymphoid neoplasms: A clinicopathologic study of 60 patients. Cancer 46:576, 1980.
60. Gurney N, Chalkley T, O'Grady R: Lacrimal sac hemangiopericytoma. Am J Ophthalmol 71:757, 1971.
61. Duguid IM: Malignant melanoma of the lacrimal sac. Br J Ophthalmol 48:394, 1964.
62. Farkas TG, Lamberson RE: Malignant melanoma of the lacrimal sac. Am J Ophthalmol 66:45, 1968.
63. Eitrem E: Innocent, pigmented nevus-cell tumor (melanoma) of the lacrimal sac. Acta Ophthalmol 31:283, 1953.
64. Economides NG, Page RC: Metastatic melanoma of the lacrimal sac. Ann Plast Surg 15:244, 1985.
65. Howcroft MJ, Hurwitz JJ: Lacrimal sac fibroma. Can J Ophthalmol 15:1967, 1980.
66. Ni C, Wagoner MD, Wang WJ, et al: Mucoepidermoid carcinomas of the lacrimal sac. Arch Ophthalmol 101:1572, 1983.
67. Khan JA, Sutula FC, Pilch BZ, Joseph MP: Mucoepidermoid carcinoma involving the lacrimal sac. Ophthalmol Plast Reconstr Surg 4:153, 1988.

Chapter 173

■

Vascular Lesions of the Orbit

I. RAND RODGERS and ARTHUR S. GROVE, Jr.

Vascular lesions comprise 10 to 15 percent of all orbital tumors. Their color, which ranges from striking red to deep blue, and their morphology, which varies from a well-defined mass to infiltrative tumor sheets, attest to their clinical and behavorial heterogeneity. Histologically, vascular tumors run the gamut from the exceedingly benign to locally aggressive to highly anaplastic and malignant.

The history of vascular orbital tumors is likewise rich in diversity. The first incontestable vascular orbital lesion was described by Walton in 1853.[1] Seven years later, Von Graefe extensively reviewed cavernous hemangiomas as an entity.[2] In 1864, Hodges, a Boston surgeon, successfully removed a vascular tumor without sacrificing vision; his incision extended from the lateral canthus to the lateral orbital rim.[3] With Krönlein's[4] 1888 description of a lateral orbitotomy, the orbit and its vascular lesions were more easily accessible. As our sophistication increased, myriad lesions were recognized as arising from vascular anlagen. With advances in imaging, surgical techniques, and immunohistochemical and electron microscopic studies, vascular tumors have been defined and categorized.

CAPILLARY HEMANGIOMA

Capillary hemangiomas are benign orbital hamartomas occurring almost exclusively in children. Infantile or hemangioblastic hemangioma, juvenile hemangioma, strawberry hemangioma, and benign hemangioendothelioma have been used interchangeably in describing this entity. The preferred terminology is capillary hemangioma because it more accurately describes this tumor's ultrastructural findings: a proliferation of true capillary units consisting of endothelial cells surrounded by pericytes.[5]

Capillary hemangiomas occur more commonly in females than in males and may be located in either the eyelid or orbit. The majority of capillary hemangiomas appear at birth or shortly thereafter and enlarge in size

for a variable period before stabilizing. Eventually, most involute, with approximately 30 percent having completely regressed within 3 yr, 60 percent within 4 yr, and 70 percent within 7 yr.[6] Capillary hemangiomas are estimated to occur in 1 to 2 percent of infants, with a higher incidence in low birth weight children. Involvement of the superficial dermis of the lids results in a raised, dimpled intensely red lesion called a strawberry mark (Fig. 173–1). Involvement of the deep dermis and anterior orbit creates a blue-appearing tumor with a spongy texture (Fig. 173–2A). The mass deepens in color and becomes more prominent when the child cries, strains, or is held by the feet with the head down.

Capillary hemangiomas of the eyelid and orbit generally occur in otherwise healthy children. Multiple hemangiomas arising on the skin of the head and neck or within viscera may occur, and a family history of capillary hemangiomas may be elicited.[7] Although there are usually no systemic manifestations of hemangiomatosis in infants, extensive visceral hemangiomas may result in thrombocytopenia and severe hemorrhage as a result of entrapment of platelets within the tumor (Kasabach-Merritt syndrome).[8] Cardiac failure has been reported as the sequela of high-velocity shunting. There

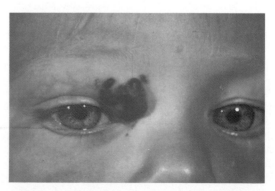

Figure 173–1. A 1-year-old with the classic strawberry nevus, which is confined to the dermis.

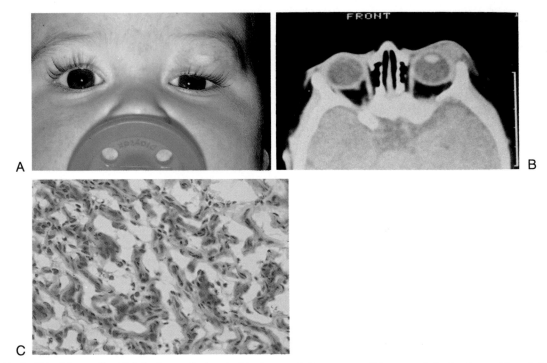

Figure 173–2. *A,* This 10-month-old infant was first noted to have a left upper eyelid mass at 4 wk of age. The violaceous-colored lesion rapidly enlarged over a 20-wk period. Retinoscopy disclosed 4 diopters of astigmatism. *B,* Axial computed tomography demonstrates a smooth-contoured upper eyelid/anterior orbit mass. *C,* The lesion did not involute with intralesional steroids. Because of the high astigmatism, the tumor was excised. Fine endothelially lined vascular channels are apparent on tissue stained with H&E.

is also predilection for orbital hemangiomas to be associated with subglottic hemangiomas, a cause of respiratory tract obstruction.[9]

The capillary hemangioma of the orbits and eyelids is generally unilateral. When confined to the deep orbital tissues, the child may present with proptosis and globe displacement but no other stigmas. Although the extraocular muscles may rarely be involved, diplopia and ocular motility disturbances are not evident. Asymmetric refractive errors are often found. Robb noted a relatively high incidence of myopia, which he attributed to lengthening of the eye resulting from equatorial meridional pressure of the anterior orbital tumor on the glove.[10] Stigmar and colleagues described a high percentage of hyperopia on the involved side.[11] The hyperopia was encountered among patients with large retrobulbar tumors compressing the eye and shortening its anteroposterior length and correlated with keratometric measurements of corneal astigmatism. If a plus cylinder convention is used, the axis of the cylinder points toward the tumor mass. The refractive errors tend to persist even after regression of the hemangioma unless early treatment occurs.

Capillary hemangiomas of the eyelid and anterior orbit can usually be diagnosed on the basis of clinical examination. The differential diagnosis includes nevus flammeus (port-wine stain), congenital hydrops, and rhabdomyosarcoma. Nevus flammeus is associated with the Sturge-Weber syndrome and is flat and noncompressible. Congenital hydrops of the nasolacrimal sac is frequently blue in color and is thus confused with capillary hemangiomas. Congenital hydrops is present at birth, is firm to palpation, and has associated signs and symptoms of nasolacrimal duct obstruction. Deep capillary hemangiomas may be difficult to differentiate from rhabdomyosarcoma, thus necessitating biopsy.

Ultrasonograms and computed tomography may be helpful in defining the extent of the tumor. Ultrasonograms demonstrate an irregular mass with high internal reflectivity. Blood flow is rapid. With pressure exerted by the ultrasonogram probe on the tumor, the mass compresses. Computed tomography reveals an irregular, poorly circumscribed mass, which generally shows marked enhancement (see Fig. 173–2*B*). Angiography, which is no longer necessary, conclusively proves that the lesion is fed by anomalous branches of the internal or external carotid artery. The feeding vessels are frequently enlarged, and early draining veins are seen.

On gross examination, the capillary hemangioma is a circumscribed, soft red mass with a multinodular surface. Large feeding vessels are typically seen and may be the source of extensive bleeding. Microscopically, dense lobules of tumor cells separated by connective tissue septae are found. There is an abundance of well-differentiated endothelial cells and pericytes (see Fig. 173–2*C*). Vascular channels may be occluded because of tumor cell growth. Reticulin stain discloses a limited reticulin sheath around the endothelial cells. Calcification may rarely be seen in long-standing cases. Electron microscopy, seldom necessary for the pathologic diagnosis, reveals proliferating endothelial cells and pericytes.

The management of capillary hemangiomas with orbital involvement is dependent on associated ocular complications if any. Amblyopia and strabismus have been reported to occur at rates between 41 and 80 percent in several large series.[7, 10, 11] Indications for treatment include (1) occlusion of the visual axis secondary to tumor growth, (2) inducement of strabismus, (3) the presence of anisometropia sufficient to cause amblyopia, and (4) a rapidly growing tumor with the potential to occlude the pupillary axis, induce strabismus, or cause anisometropic amblyopia.

In recent years, corticosteroids have become increasingly popular in the treatment of capillary hemangiomas. The value of steroids was recognized by a fortuitous observation. Systemic steroids administered to control bleeding diatheses in patients with Kasabach-Merritt syndrome produced rapid regression of the associated hemangiomas. Zarem and Edgerton[12] in 1967 reported a series of infants treated successfully with systemic prednisone and two patients treated with intralesional steroids. Kushner[13] in 1982 reported large series of capillary hemangiomas treated with intralesional steroids. The recommended dose is 40 mg of triamcinolone and a 6-mg preparation of equal parts of betamethasone sodium phosphate and bethamethasone acetate injected directly into the lesion. Care must be taken to draw back on the syringe before injecting to prevent steroid solution from entering the intravascular space. An attempt should be made to distribute the steroid evenly throughout the tumor through either one or multiple percutaneous punctures with a tuberculin syringe. Most of the involution will occur within 2 wk, but additional regression can occur within 5 to 6 wk.[14] If regression is incomplete or clinically inadequate, an additional injection is then recommended. Corticosteroids are believed to shrink hemangiomas because of their vasoconstricting abilities. Steroids increase vascular bed sensitivity to circulating vasoconstrictor agents. Studies in humans and animals have shown that cortisone produces arteriolar constriction. Steroid injections are, however, contraindicated for retrobulbar hemangiomas. Such steroid injections have been reported to cause central retinal artery occlusion after retrobulbar hemangiomas. Central retinal artery occlusion may occur after steroid embolism to optic nerve vasculature.[15] It is recommended that children receiving systemic or intralesional corticosteroids avoid routine pediatric immunizations with live, attenuated virus for 2 wk before and after steroid administration.

Other treatment modalities include surgery and yttrium aluminum garnet (YAG) laser photocoagulation. Cryotherapy, injection of sclerosing agents, arterial embolization, and radiotherapy are no longer used (Table 173–1).

LYMPHANGIOMAS

Lymphangiomas are thin-walled vascular channels hemodynamically isolated from the arterial and venous orbital circulation. They arouse curiosity because the orbit is normally devoid of lymphatic channels as well as lymphoid follicles. Wright[16] suggested that lymphangiomas are variants of venous malformations, but clinical, hemodynamic, and histopathologic studies strongly suggest that lymphangiomas are distinct orbital hemartomas.[17]

Lymphangiomas are benign tumors that may be found in the conjunctiva, the eyelids, the orbit, or elsewhere in the head and neck region.[18] They most often present during childhood. In the largest reported series by Jones[19] involving 29 cases, 10 patients presented at birth, 11 patients presented between 1 and 5 yr, 5 patients presented between 6 and 15 yr, and 3 patients presented in adulthood (at ages 27, 38, and 44). There is no preference for race, sex, or laterality. Deep lymphangiomatous lesions classically present with acute onset of a fulminant proptosis resulting from spontaneous hemorrhage within the orbit. Proptosis may occur in the presence of an upper respiratory tract infection, reflecting the proliferating lymphoid elements in the connective tissue trabeculas of the tumor.[20]

The infiltrative tumor mass may compress the globe or optic nerve, causing refractive errors, secondary glaucoma, congestion of the optic nerve, and visual field deficits. So-called chocolate cysts may form; these cysts are circumscribed, brown lesions and are the sequelae of hemorrhage.[21] Chocolate cysts have been reported to cause optic nerve compression and visual impairment, necessitating emergency surgery.

Orbital x-ray films are usually normal, although enlargement of the orbit may be evident. Calcifications are occasionally found in long-standing lesions. Ultrasonography demonstrates acoustic hollowness, good

Table 173–1. VASCULAR LESIONS

Capillary Hemangioma
  Benign lid and orbital hamartoma
    1–2% incidence
    Generally unilateral with onset soon after birth
    Kasabach-Merritt syndrome
  Radiologic studies
    Ultrasonogram: high internal reflectivity
    CT* scan: irregular, poorly circumscribed mass
  Treatment modalities
    Observation
    Intralesional steroids/systemic steroids
    Laser/radiation/sclerosing agents
  Pathology
    Microscopic: dense lobules of endothelial cells and
              pericytes
    Electron microscopic: proliferating true capillary units
Lymphangioma
  Benign lid and orbital tumor
    Involve head and neck
    Occur predominantly in children and teenagers
    Chocolate cysts
  Radiologic studies
    Ultrasonogram: cystic pattern
    CT* scan: infiltrative, multilobulated lesion
  Treatment modalities
    Observation
    Steroids
    Surgery

*CT, computed tomography.

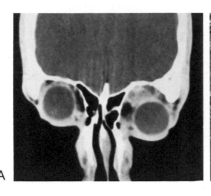 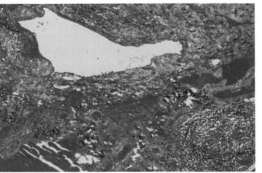

Figure 173–3. *A,* A multilobulated lymphangioma of the superonasal orbit has resulted in globe displacement. Note the differing tissue densities within the tumor. *B,* Lymphatic channels of varying sizes typify the histopathology. In this section, clear lymphatic fluid is present in the largest channel, whereas erythrocytes fill the smaller channels. A lymphatic aggregate is present. H&E, ×80.

sound transmission, and a diffuse or cystic pattern. On computed tomography, an infiltrative, multilobulated cystic tumor with irregular outlines is apparent (Fig. 173–3A). No connections to the arterial or venous circulations are found, and phleboliths may be present.[22]

The management of lymphangiomas is challenging.[23] Systemic steroids have been used in the hope of reducing the size of lymphoid nodules and the onset of inflammation. The overall effect is limited. Radiotherapy has no role in treating these lesions. Complete surgical excision is often difficult if not impossible; because of the infiltrative nature of the tumor, it is virtually impossible to create a cleavage plane allowing total tumor removal without damaging vital orbital structures. Limited success has been achieved with the carbon dioxide laser, which cauterizes while the tumor is being excised.[24] Complications of surgery include optic nerve dysfunction secondary to hemorrhage, orbital fibrosis, and recurrences.

On gross examination, lymphangiomas are unencapsulated tumors composed of cystic spaces filled with blood or clear fluid. On histologic examination, lymphangiomas consist of channels ranging in size from capillary to cavernous; lymphatic fluid is usually found within the tumors, but admixed erythrocytes may be present. The loose connective tissue septa between the vascular channels may contain foci of lymphoid cells. Fine blood vessels are also seen within the septa. Spontaneous rupture of these unsupported vessels leads to the accumulation of chocolate blood cysts (see Fig. 173–3B). Ultrastructurally, there is an absence of pericytes and smooth muscle cells. Characteristic of lymphatic channels, lymphangiomas contain interrupted basement membrane material.[18]

CAVERNOUS HEMANGIOMA

Cavernous hemangiomas are the most common benign orbital tumors of adults.[25, 26] They are generally considered developmental hamartomas. Although a rudimentary lesion may be present at birth, cavernous hemangiomas do not usually become symptomatic until the third to fifth decade of life. The tumor is characteristically unilateral and solitary, although rare reports of multifocal lesions within an orbit exist. There is no predilection for race or ethnicity. In the largest survey reported involving 66 subjects, females were more commonly affected than males.[27]

Cavernous hemangiomas are well-encapsulated and well-tolerated lesions. The typical history is of slowly developing proptosis over a 3- to 5-yr period. Rapid growth may occur during pregnancy.[28] Some degree of blurred vision is generally noted, but patients rarely complain of diplopia or pain.[29] Cavernous hemangiomas are typically located within the retrobulbar space, and thus the proptosis is a purely axial one and averages 5 mm (Fig. 173–4A). The normal to slightly decreased visual acuity on clinical examination results from hyperopia induced by the retrobulbar tumor's compression of the posterior sclera and retina. Visual acuity may be reduced 1 to 2 lines, and visual-field testing may reveal field abnormalities corresponding to those optic nerve axons compressed by the tumor. Ocular motility may be slightly restricted in extreme fields of gaze. The anterior segment examination is unremarkable; even with high grades of proptosis, the cornea is protected by lids that have been stretched over the protracted course of tumor growth. Funduscopic examination may reveal optic nerve swelling and chorioretinal striae (see Fig. 173–4B).

Although the tumor is usually found within the muscle cone, it can occur in the extraconal space. Presenting signs will differ, with axial proptosis replaced by another form of displacement.[30]

Radiologic imaging techniques useful in the evaluation of a suspected cavernous hemangioma include ultrasonography, computed tomography, and magnetic resonance imaging. Ultrasonography documents a round to ovoid tumor with well-defined borders and moderate sound transmission. There are multiple high internal echos on A-scan. Computed tomography generally reveals a discrete lesion with smooth surfaces. Bone displacement may occur in those cases of extraconal cavernous hemangiomas. Because blood flow through the lesion is stagnant and independent from the orbital vascular system, cavernous hemangiomas do not fill with contrast within the first 1 to 2 min;[31] it takes approximately 20 min after contrast injection for the tumor to accumulate dye. On magnetic resonance imaging, the tumor is distinct from the soft tissues, being hypointense to fat on T_1-weighted images (see Fig. 173–4C) and hyperintense to fat and isointense to vitreous on T_2-weighted images (see Fig. 173–4D).[32]

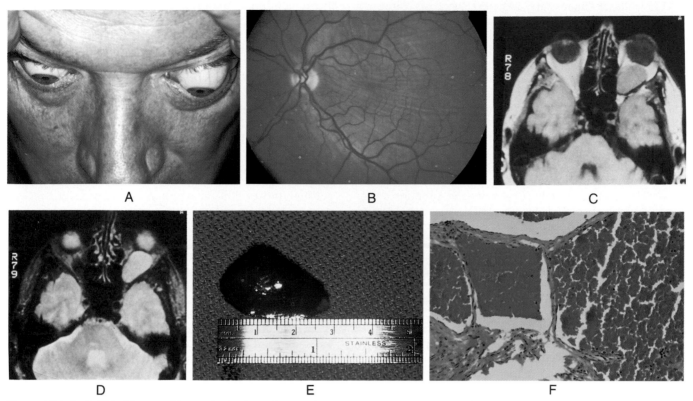

Figure 173–4. *A,* This 42-year-old man had a 5-yr history of gradually increasing axial proptosis. Neither the eyelids nor the globe is inflamed. *B,* The tumor's indentation on the globe produced hyperopia and choroidal striae. *C,* Magnetic resonance imaging depicts an ovoid, intraconal mass. On T_1-weighted images (TR = 800, TE = 20), the tumor is hypointense to fat. *D,* On T_2-weighted images (TR = 2000, TE = 80), the hemangioma is hyperintense to fat and relatively isointense to vitreous. *E,* The tumor was excised via a lateral orbitotomy. Its violaceous hue results from the stagnant and poorly oxygenated blood within it. *F,* Large vascular spaces 500 μ to 1 mm in size are lined by a flattened monolayer of endothelial cells. H&E, ×140.

Surgical treatment is recommended for optic nerve compression as evidenced by visual-field defects, optic nerve swelling, or pallor. Additional indications include diplopia and bothersome cosmesis. The surgical approach is most often a lateral orbitotomy because of the tumor's usual position within the muscle cone. Complete resection of cavernous hemangiomas is generally accomplished because the tumor is so well-encapsulated and relatively few feeding vessels exist. Hemangiomas that lie in the less accessible medial orbit may need to be cut into pieces before being removed. On rare occasions, hemangiomas have involuted spontaneously.

On gross examination cavernous hemangiomas are spongy, well-encapsulated ovoid masses (see Fig. 173–4E). Their violaceous hue results from the stagnation of poorly oxygenated blood within the tumor. The cut surface discloses the surrounding capsule and large vascular channels. On histologic sectioning, large, closely packed, congested vascular spaces are separated by fibrous connective tissue septae. The vascular channels, measuring 500 μ to 1 mm in diameter, are lined by thin, flattened endothelial cells. Intravascular thrombosis may be seen (see Fig. 173–4F). On electron microscopy, endothelial cells ensheathed by one to five layers of muscle cells and containing cytoplasmic filaments are apparent.[33]

The pathogenesis of cavernous hemangiomas is uncertain. One theory espouses that immature sprouts of capillary endothelial cells grow into loose myxoid interstitium. Subsequently, these capillary-sized channels become ectatic and acquire smooth muscle. Others believe that cavernous hemangiomas result from a preexisting vascular malformation, the vessels of which become patent over years as a result of thrombosis, infarction, or inflammation.[34]

Hemangiopericytomas

Hemangiopericytomas were first described by Stout and Murray in 1942.[35] They are exceedingly rare tumors; the orbit is an uncommon site of involvement. Hemangiopericytomas arise from an abnormal and idiopathic proliferation of the pericytes surrounding blood vessels. These tumors may be benign or malignant or share characteristics of both. They are capable of metastasizing to distant organs including lung, bone, and liver and may be fatal.[36]

There are several reports of hemangiopericytomas arising in the orbits of infants, but generally the tumor affects adults.[37] In the largest series of patients (30), reported from the Armed Forces Institute of Pathology

(AFIP) files,[38] males are affected twice as often as females. There is no predilection for race. Patients are symptomatic for a shorter period of time than patients with cavernous hemangiomas. Presenting signs and symptoms include progressive, unilateral proptosis generally associated with downward displacement of the globe. Associated decreased visual acuity, diplopia, and pain may occur. In striking contrast to cavernous hemangiomas, hemangiopericytomas may cause puffiness of the eyelids with a bluish or reddish discoloration of the ocular adnexa; the congestion is not nearly as active as seen in pseudotumor, however.

Orbital computed tomography documents a round to oval orbital mass usually located in the superior orbit. The well-encapsulated lesion, with its large arterial feeding vessels, exhibits dramatic enhancement on injection of contrast material. Hemangiopericytomas may, in rare instances, extend through the orbital bones into the temporal fossa or brain.[39] Calcification may be seen in long-standing cases.[40] On magnetic resonance imaging, these well-delineated tumors are hypointense to fat on T_1-weighted images and hyperintense to fat and isointense to vitreous on T_2-weighted images.

Surgery is indicated for those lesions impairing optic nerve function or mobility. Some investigators recommend surgery whenever a hemangiopericytoma is suggested on clinical examination and imaging.[41] At surgery, hemangiopericytomas are solid and dark blue to violaceous. They may bleed extensively and be exceedingly friable. Complete excision may not be technically possible.

Histologically, hemangiopericytomas may assume one of three configurations: a prominent vascular pattern of sinusoidal spaces, an ostensibly solid pattern in which the vasculature may not be seen, or a combination of the two. The tightly packed cells around the thin-walled blood vessels are lined by flattened endothelial cells (Fig. 173–5). The histologic differential diagnosis includes fibrous histiocytoma, malignant hemangioendothelioma, and angioblastic meningioma. Hemangiopericytomas and fibrous histiocytomas may be confused because they may share storiform patterns. Hemangiopericytomas contain PAS- and reticulin-staining basement membrane material, which surrounds the proliferating pericytes. Fibrous histiocytomas do not contain such basement membrane material. The malignant hemangioendothelioma consists of proliferating endothelial cells that stain profusely with Factor VIII. Angioblastic meningiomas, a neural tumor, will stain with S100 protein.

Hemangiopericytomas can histologically be benign or malignant. Diagnostic criteria include the number of mitotic figures per high-power field, the degree of cellularity, and the degree of nuclear atypia. In the AFIP series,[38] 16 of 30 hemangiopericytomas were histologically benign, containing four or fewer mitotic figures per high-power field; five patients had borderline lesions with evidence of cellular atypia and an increased number of mitotic figures; nine lesions were clearly malignant, displaying an average of 35 to 40 mitotic figures per high-power field, cellular atypia, and nuclear pleomorphism. Although the histologic appearance does not necessarily reflect biologic behavior, the more malignant-appearing tumors have a greater tendency to undergo local recurrence or distant metastasis.

Incomplete excision of hemangiopericytomas occurs and reflects the tumor's infiltrative pattern and propensity to bleed. The management of such cases is controversial and is dependent on the histopathology and the patient's clinical signs and symptoms. If visual function is severely compromised, consideration should be given to exenterating the orbit. If visual function is not impaired, careful observation of the patient may be justified. Incompletely excised tumors have a high frequency of local recurrence. In addition, they are capable of invading the brain. In the AFIP series, patients died of widespread metastases 6 to 32 yr after the onset of symptoms (Table 173–2).

Malignant Hemangioendothelioma

Hemangioendotheliomas comprise less than 1 percent of all soft tissue sarcomas and are among the rarest of orbital neoplasms.[42] This tumor is both locally aggressive and capable of metastatic spread.[43] Children and young adults are preferentially affected.[44] Clinical signs and symptoms include rapidly developing proptosis, globe displacement, and ophthalmoplegia.[45] Messmer and colleagues[46] reported a patient who presented with painful ophthalmoplegia, suggestive of the Tolosa-Hunt syndrome.

Computed tomography reveals a circumscribed or infiltrative mass that enhances with contrast. Histologically, pleomorphic, hyperchromatic endothelial cells form vascular channels that infiltrate the orbital soft tissues. In some cases, the trabeculae of malignant cells may project into the bloodless vascular spaces. Dense fibrous connective tissue divides the mass of tumor cells. Immunohistochemical staining for FVIIIRA (a component of factor VIII) and VEAI (a lectin with a marked affinity for endothelial cell membranes) is helpful in making the diagnosis.[47] The optimal treatment is un-

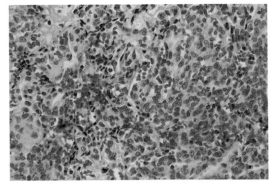

Figure 173–5. This hemangiopericytoma demonstrates an admixture of sinusoidal spaces between which are solid areas of ovoid- to spindle-shaped cells. No mitotic figures or bizarre pleomorphic cells are seen. H&E, × 140.

Table 173–2. VASCULAR LESIONS

Cavernous Hemangioma
  Benign orbital tumor
    Most common orbital lesion in adults
    Well-encapsulated, well-tolerated
  Radiologic studies
    Ultrasonogram: well-defined round tumor with high internal echos
    CT* scan: late enhancement with contrast
    MRI†: hypointense to fat on T_1, hyperintense on T_2
  Treatment
    Observation
    Surgery
  Pathology
    Gross appearance: encapsulated, violaceous lesion
    Microscopic: large, congested vascular spaces
    EM‡: endothelial cells encased by muscle cells
Hemangiopericytoma
  Uncommon tumors
    Orbit is rarely affected
    Metastatic potential
    Inflammatory signs and symptoms
  Radiologic studies
    CT scan: well-defined lesions with dramatic contrast enhancement
    MRI: hypointense to fat on T_1, hyperintense on T_2
  Pathology
    Microscopic: three histologic patterns
    EM: proliferating endothelial cells
Malignant Hemangioendothelioma
  Exceedingly rare orbital tumor
    Locally aggressive and capable of metastatic spread
    Children and young adults preferentially affected
  Radiologic studies
    CT scan: circumscribed or infiltrative mass
  Pathology
    Microscopic: hyperchromatic endothelial cells stain positively for FVIIIRA
Kimura's Disease
  Preferentially afflicts Asian males
    Inflammatory infiltrate
    Skin variant associated with elevated immunoglobulin E levels
  Proliferating capillary units and germinal centers

*CT, computed tomography; †MRI, magnetic resonance imaging; ‡EM, electron microscopy.

known because of a lack of long-term follow-up of the few reported cases. Jakobiec and Font[48] recommend exenteration. Shields[41] recommends wide surgical excision with supplemental radiotherapy if there is a question of residual tumor. Children have a poorer prognosis than adults.

ANGIOLYMPHOID HYPERPLASIA WITH EOSINOPHILIA

This rare tumor, also known as Kimura's disease, is characterized by endothelial cell prolificacy associated with an inflammatory infiltrate. Asian males are preferentially affected and are generally symptomatic from months to years.[49] Orbital signs and symptoms include proptosis typically with globe displacement inferiorly and a palpable mass.[50] This entity also affects the skin of the head and neck, producing subcutaneous nodules. The skin variant, but not the orbital variant, is associated

with bronchial asthma, eosinophilia, and increased serum immunoglobulin E levels.[51] At surgery, the lesions are red in color and tend to bleed extensively. A salmon-colored mass representing lymphoid tissue may be found on the tumor's surface. Histologically, angiolymphoid hyperplasia with eosinophilia is characterized by proliferating capillary units with plump endothelial cells lining lumens of various size. The inflammatory cell aggregate consists of eosinophils and lymphocytes, which may form germinal centers. No necrosis is seen (Fig. 173–6). Electron microscopic studies disclose plump endothelial cells containing numerous mitochondria and prominent villose processes. Some capillaries contain prominent multilaminar basement membrane material.[52] Immunohistochemically, the tumor stains for Factor VIII–related antigen. The histologic differential includes Churg-Strauss syndrome, angiosarcoma, and Wegener's granulomatosis. Treatment includes wide local excision. Radiotherapy and steroids may play a role in treating lesions inaccessible to complete resection. This lesion is considered benign, and there is no evidence of recurrence in completely excised lesions.

ARTERIOVENOUS COMMUNICATIONS: ARTERIOVENOUS MALFORMATIONS, CAROTID-CAVERNOUS FISTULAS, AND DURAL SHUNTS

In arteriovenous (AV) communications, blood flows from the arterial circulation directly into the venous circulation without passage through intervening capillaries. High-flow states are characterized by orbital swelling and chemosis, increased episcleral and intraocular pressure, and pulsatile exophthalmos. Low-flow states display similar signs and symptoms but to a lesser degree.[53] AV communications may be classified as either AV malformations (AVMs), carotid-cavernous sinus fistulas, or dural shunts. Communications located entirely within the orbit are exceedingly rare and are congenital AVMs; such lesions may be found in Wyburn-Mason syndrome and Osler-Weber-Rendu disease. The vast majority of

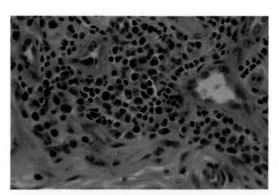

Figure 173–6. Kimura's disease is characterized by proliferating capillary units with plump endothelial cells. Mononuclear inflammatory cells and occasionally eosinophils are present. H&E, ×140.

Table 173–3. ARTERIOVENOUS COMMUNICATIONS

Arteriovenous Malformations
   Direct blood flow from artery to vein
      Occur spontaneously or after trauma
      Pulsatile mass; vascular congestion
   Pathology
      Mature arteries and veins
Carotid-Cavernous Fistulas
   Direct communications between internal carotid and
      cavernous sinus
      Arise spontaneously or as a trauma sequela
      Increased blood flow and pressure
   Treatment
      Balloon
      Embolization
      Surgery
Dural Shunts
   Indirect communications between meningeal branches of
      internal or external carotid artery and cavernous sinus
      Usually arise spontaneously
      Postmenopausal women affected
   Radiologic studies
      Ultrasonogram and CT* scan: enlarged muscles and
        superior ophthalmic vein
   Treatment
      Observation
      Angiography
      Embolization
      Surgery

*CT, computed tomography.

AV communications occur outside the orbit and secondarily affect the orbital veins (Table 173–3).

Arteriovenous Malformations

AVMs are usually supplied by branches of both the internal and external carotid artery. They may occur spontaneously or result from trauma. The venous drainage in these malformations is antegrade and usually results in a high-flow state. An AVM frequently presents as a pulsatile mass within the orbit or eyelids. If the tumor is situated anteriorly in the orbit, it may be visible as a blue pulsating subcutaneous mass. Epibulbar vascular congestion and a bruit may be present. Histologically, the tumor is composed of mature arteries and veins. The vessels are hypertrophied and stain for muscles and elastic fibers. AVMs are often enlarged and are difficult to excise completely because they may recur after apparent obliteration of the feeding vessels.

Carotid-Cavernous Fistulas

Carotid-cavernous fistulas are direct communications between the internal carotid artery and the cavernous sinus. These shunts may arise spontaneously or may be the sequelae of severe head trauma. In either case, a rent is created in the intracavernous portion of the internal carotid artery, allowing blood to flow directly into the cavernous sinus and its encased plexus of veins. The increased blood flow and elevated pressure are transmitted through the sinus to its tributory veins including the ophthalmic vein. Clinical signs and symptoms include chemosis, orbital swelling, episcleral venous congestion, elevated intraocular pressure, and retinal hemorrhages and ischemia. Third- and sixth-nerve palsies may be associated. A thorough evaluation requires the use of contrast angiography with selective injection of the internal and external carotid arteries. Treatment is indicated when vision is threatened. The optimal treatment is the detachable balloon technique through an endoarterial route. The balloon enters the fistula and is inflated until the fistula is closed. Using this technique, more than 90 percent of direct carotid-cavernous fistulas can be successfully closed with virtually no mortality and with morbidity limited to transient motor paresis in one third of patients.[54] Other treatment modalities include embolization, electrothrombosis of the fistula,[55] and direct surgery.

Dural Shunts

Dural shunts are indirect communications between meningeal branches of the internal or external carotid arteries and the cavernous sinus.[56] They usually occur spontaneously and may be characterized hemodynamically as high or low flow, with elevated venous pressure transmitted to the eye via the superior ophthalmic vein. Postmenopausal women are most commonly affected. The clinical features of dural shunts include mild exophthalmos, moderate elevation of intraocular pressure, and episcleral vascular dilatation.[57] Bruits are infrequent; consequently, the condition may be misdiagnosed as pseudotumor. Ocular ischemia and optic disc neovascularization have been reported.[58] Ultrasonogram and computed tomography usually reveal enlargement of the superior ophthalmic vein and extraocular muscles in the involved orbit (Fig. 173–7). The diagnosis is definitively made with selective angiography, although some authors believe that angiographic evaluation may be unwarranted given that most symptoms resolve with time. Others note the resolution of dural shunts after arteriography, although the precise mechanism is unknown.[59] For those patients who acquire progressive proptosis, increased intraocular pressure nonresponsive to antiglaucoma medications, or debilitating diplopia in primary gaze, surgical intervention may be necessary. Balloon occlusion is not possible in such patients because the involved branches of the internal and external carotid are small and numerous. For external carotid feeder vessels, embolization is possible with detachable balloons, isobutylcyanoacrylate, or polyvinyl alcohol particles.[60] Embolization of the internal carotid is not recommended because of the high success rate of embolization of external carotid artery feeders and the borderline patency of the circle of Willis in older patients. Other techniques include electrothrombosis of the fistula and direct surgery[61]; there is, however, a higher rate of failure and morbidity with these techniques. Hanneken and colleagues[62] recommend a transvenous approach with a detachable balloon catheter to the cavernous sinus through the ipsilateral superior ophthalmic vein.

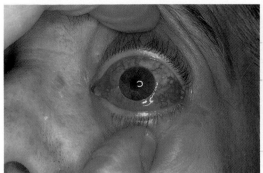
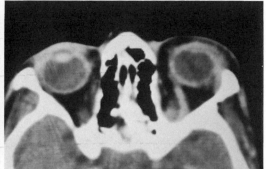

Figure 173–7. *A*, Epibulbar vascular congestion, conjunctival chemosis, and a prominent globe may be mistaken for orbital inflammatory disease, but these signs typify arteriovenous communications. *B*, The right superior ophthalmic vein is dilated in this patient with a dural shunt.

They report limited morbidity and no mortality, but to date their population size is small.

ORBITAL VARIX

Variable proptosis dependent on a change in head position is strongly suggestive of an orbital varix.[63] These anomalies consist of either a single segmental dilatation of a vein or a tangle of ectatic vascular channels. Varices may be primary congenital lesions or secondary acquired lesions, the sequelae of intracranial or orbital AVMs. Lesions with prominent connections to the systemic venous system are distensible and respond to changes in the venous circulation. They present with the classical findings of proptosis and pain, which increase with Valsalva's maneuver.[64] Other varices are nondistensible and lack significant connection to the venous bed. These lesions are characterized by a stagnant circulation and thrombus formation.

Patients with primary varices are typically in their second to third decade of life when they become symptomatic. At rest, patients with distensible varices may be enophthalmic, the result of enlarged orbits and fat atrophy. During periods of extreme engorgement, pain may be apparent. Rarely, there may be a family history of orbital varices, and varices may be present in the neck and shoulder region. Patients with nondistensible varices may present with hemorrhage after rupture of the variceal wall or thrombosis within the lesion, resulting in sudden proptosis and pain. There may be restriction of ocular motility and lid chemosis if the lesion is anteriorly located.

Plain x-ray films may demonstrate orbital enlargement and small, round areas of calcification, the result of organized thrombi. Venography, no longer frequently used, reveals a massively enlarged vein or a mass of tortuous vessels.[65] Computed tomography with contrast will demonstrate the enlarged vessels. Proptosis can be demonstrated by asking the patient to perform Valsalva's maneuver during the imaging procedure.[64]

The management of varices is conservative.[66] Surgery should be performed only when vision is threatened or when the deformity is severe. If the varix is secondary, the deformity may resolve if the cause of the venous dilatation is treated. The carbon dioxide and YAG lasers may facilitate removal of superficial and subcutaneous varices (Table 173–4).

CHOLESTEROL GRANULOMA

Cholesterol granuloma is an idiopathic condition primarily affecting the orbital frontal bone.[67] A variety of terms have been used to describe this entity including hematoma and chronic hematic cyst, but we prefer the term cholesterol granuloma because it most aptly describes the histopathology. The pathogenesis of cholesterol granuloma and its predilection for the frontal bone are enigmatic. Trauma has been cited as the initiating event but probably is unrelated.[68] Whatever the inciting cause, focal hemorrhage into the diploë of bone occurs. Prostaglandins released by platelets initiate resorption of bone and expose additional diplopic blood vessels. These vessels are a continuing source of blood breakdown products causing expansion of the mass.[69]

Cholesterol granulomas preferentially affect males. In the largest series published, by McNab and Wright,[70] cholesterol granuloma occurred in patients ranging in age from 25 to 68 yr, with a mean age of 44 yr (Fig. 173–8*A*). The most common symptom was proptosis

Table 173–4. ADDITIONAL VASCULAR LESIONS

Orbital Varix
  Ectatic vascular channels
    Proptosis associated with change in head position
    Young adults affected
    Exophthalmos or enophthalmos
  Radiologic studies
    Ultrasonogram: calcification
    CT* scan: enlarged vessels
  Conservative treatment
Cholesterol Granuloma
  Idiopathic condition
    Males commonly affected
    Proptosis, diplopia, palpable mass
  Radiologic studies
    CT* scan: superotemporal orbital mass
    Magnetic resonance imaging: high signal intensity of T_1 and T_2 images

*CT, computed tomography.

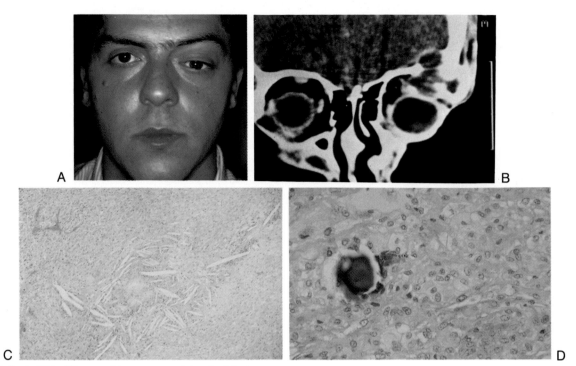

Figure 173–8. A, This 32-year-old man complained of facial asymmetry. Visual acuity was 20/20 OS, but the globe was displaced inferiorly. A fullness was appreciated in the superior orbit. B, Axial computed tomography reveals a cystic-appearing superior orbital mass with erosion of the orbital roof. C, The classical cholesterol clefts, inflammatory cell infiltrate, and erythrocytes of cholesterol granulomas. H&E, ×40. D, High-power magnification using H&E reveals calcium deposits and mononuclear cell infiltrate.

followed by blurred vision and eyebrow ache. On ocular examination, visual acuity was generally unaffected, but decreased acuity secondary to an acquired astigmatism or choroidal folds may occur. The mean amount of proptosis was 4 mm with the globe displaced downward and inward. Mobility was often restricted in upgaze and abduction. In two thirds of the patients, a mass was palpable; it varied in texture from soft and fluctuant to firm.

Plain films disclose a characteristically well-defined osteolytic defect with rounded edges. Computed tomography reveals a mass in the supratemporal orbit. The mass generally appears homogeneous with erosion and expansion of bone. There is either partial or complete loss of the outer table, allowing the mass to expand extraperiosteally into the orbit. If the inner table is eroded, dura may be exposed (see Fig. 173–8B). On magnetic resonance imaging, the lesion emits a high signal intensity on both T_1- and T_2-weighted images. These signal intensities reflect the peripheral accumulation of paramagnetic free methemoglobin.[71]

At surgery, the underlying bone is thinned and the tumor possesses a yellow-red coloration. Fluid often leaks from the lesion. On histologic examination, cholesterol clefts surrounded by mononuclear cells and multinucleated giant cells are found. Hemosiderin and hematodin granules are scattered throughout the lesion and stain with Prussian blue. No evidence of a cystic lining occurs, a factor distinguishing this lesion from an epidermoid cyst (see Fig. 173–8C). Postoperatively, patients do well with no evidence of tumor recurrence.

REFERENCES

1. Duke-Elder S, MacFaul PA: System of Ophthalmology: Vol. 13. The Ocular Adnexa Part II. St. Louis, CV Mosby, 1974.
2. Hodges RM: Cases of tumors. Boston Med J 71:417, 1864.
3. Von Graefe A: Zur Casuistik der Geschwulste. Arch Ophthalmol (Berlin) 7(pt. 2):11, 1860.
4. Krönlein RU: Zur Patholojie Und operativen Behandlung der Dermoidcysten der orbita. Beitr Klin Chir 4:149, 1888.
5. Iwamoto T, Jakobiec FA: A comparative ultrastructural study of the normal lacrimal gland and its epithelial tumors. Hum Pathol 13:236, 1982.
6. Margileth A, Museles M: Cutaneous hemangiomas in children: Diagnosis and conservative management. JAMA 194:523, 1965.
7. Haik GR, Jakobiec FA, Ellsworth RM, Jones IS: Capillary hemangioma of the lids and orbit: An analysis of the clinical features and therapeutic results in 101 cases. Ophthalmology 86:760, 1979.
8. Kasabach HH, Merritt KK: Capillary hemangioma with extensive purpura: Report of a case. Am J Dis Child 59:1063, 1940.
9. Yee RD, Hepler RS: Congenital hemangioma of the skin with orbital and subglottic hemangiomas. Am J Ophthalmol 75:876, 1973.
10. Robb RM: Refractive errors associated with hemangiomas of the eyelids and orbit in infancy. Am J Ophthalmol 83:52, 1977.
11. Stigmar G, Crawford JS, Ward CM, Thomson HG: Ophthalmic sequelae of infantile hemangiomas of the eyelids and orbit. Am J Ophthalmol 85:806, 1978.
12. Zarem HA, Edgerton MT: Induced resolution of cavernous hemangiomas following prednisolone therapy. Plast Reconstr Surg 39:76, 1967.
13. Kushner BJ: Intralesional corticosteroid injection for infantile adnexal hemangioma. Am J Ophthalmol 93:496, 1982.
14. Kushner BJ: Infantile adnexal hemangioma: Eyelid and orbital. In Smith BC, Della Rocca RC, Nes FA, Lisman RD (eds): Ophthalmic Plastic and Reconstructive Surgery. St. Louis, CV Mosby, 1987, pp 846–852.

15. Ellis PP: Occlusion of the central retinal artery after retrobulbar corticosteroid injection. Am J Ophthalmol 85:352, 1978.

16. Wright JE: Orbital vascular anomalies. Trans Am Acad Ophthalmol Otolaryngol 78:606, 1974.

17. Rootman J, Hay E, Grace D, et al: Orbital adnexal lymphangiomas: A spectrum of hemodynamically isolated vascular hamartoma. Ophthalmology 93:1558, 1986.

18. Jakobiec FA, Jones IS: Vascular tumors, malformations, and degenerations. In Jones IS, Jakobiec FA (eds): Diseases of the Orbit. Hagerstown, MD, Harper & Row, 1979, pp 269–308.

19. Jones IS: Lymphangioma of the ocular adnexa: An analysis of 62 cases. Trans Am Ophthalmol Soc 57:602, 1959.

20. Iliff WJ, Green WR: Orbital lymphangiomas. Ophthalmology 86:914, 1979.

21. Reese AD, Howard GM: Unusual manifestations of ocular lymphangioma and lymphangiectasis. Surv Ophthalmol 18:226, 1973.

22. Davis KR, Hesselink JR, Dallow RL, Grove AS: CT and ultrasound in the diagnosis of cavernous hemangioma and lymphangioma of the orbit. J Comput Tomogr 4:98, 1980.

23. Jones IS, Desjardins L: Management of orbital neurofibromas and lymphangiomas. In Jakobiec FA (ed): Ocular and Adnexal Tumors. Birmingham, AL, Aesculapius, 1978, pp 735–740.

24. Kennerdell JS, Maroon JC, Garrity JA, et al: Surgical management of orbital lymphangioma with the carbon dioxide laser. Am J Ophthalmol 102:308, 1986.

25. Forrest AW: Intraorbital tumors. Arch Ophthalmol 41:198, 1949.

26. Shields JA, Bakewell B, Augsburger JJ, et al: Classification and incidence of space occupying lesions of the orbit: A survey of 645 cases. Arch Ophthalmol 102:1606, 1984.

27. Harris GJ, Jakobiec FA: Cavernous hemangioma of the orbit: A clinicopathologic analysis of 66 cases. In Jakobiec FA (ed): Ocular and Adnexal Tumors. Birmingham, AL, Aesculapius, 1978, pp 741–781.

28. Zauberman H, Feinsod M: Orbital hemangioma growth during pregnancy. Acta Ophthalmol 48:928, 1970.

29. Ruchman MC, Flanagan JC: Cavernous hemangioma of the orbit. Ophthalmology 90:1328, 1983.

30. Harris GJ, Jakobiec FA: Cavernous hemangioma of the orbit: An analysis of 66 cases. J Neurosurg 51:219, 1979.

31. Davis KR, Hesselink JR, Dallow RL, Grove AB: CT and ultrasound in the diagnosis of cavernous hemangioma and lymphangioma of the orbit. J Comput Tomogr 4:98, 1980.

32. Gingold MP, Hornblass A, Rodgers IR, Deck M: MRI in the evaluation of orbital tumors. Presented at the annual meeting of The American Society of Ophthalmic Plastic and Reconstructive Surgeons, Las Vegas, NV, 1988.

33. Iwamoto T, Jakobiec FA: Ultrastructural comparison of capillary and cavernous hemangioma of the orbit. Arch Ophthalmol 97:1144, 1979.

34. Hood CI: Cavernous hemangioma of the orbit. A consideration of pathogenesis with an illustrative case. Arch Ophthalmol 83:49, 1970.

35. Stout AD, Murray MR: Hemangiopericytoma: A vascular tumor featuring Zimmerman's pericytes. Ann Surg 116:26, 1942.

36. Henderson JW, Farrow GM: Primary orbital hemangiopericytoma: An aggressive and potentially malignant neoplasm. Arch Ophthalmol 96:666, 1978.

37. Kapoor S, Kapoor MS, Aurora AL, et al: Orbital hemangiopericytoma: A report of a 3 year old child. J Pediatr Ophthalmol Strabismus 15:40, 1978.

38. Croxatto JO, Font RL: Hemangiopericytoma of the orbit: A clinicopathologic study of 30 cases. Hum Pathol 13:210, 1982.

39. Jakobiec FA, Howard G, Jones IS, Wolff M: Hemangiopericytoma of the orbit. Am J Ophthalmol 78:816, 1974.

40. Garrity JA, Kennerdell JS: Orbital calcification associated with hemangiopericytoma. Am J Ophthalmol 102:126, 1986.

41. Shields JA: Vasculogenic tumors and malformations. In Shields JA (ed): Diagnosis and Management of Orbital Tumors. Philadelphia, WB Saunders, 1989, pp 132–134.

42. Enzinger FM, Weiss SW: Soft Tissue Tumors. St. Louis, CV Mosby, 1983.

43. Mortada A: Rare primary orbital sarcomas. Am J Ophthalmol 68:619, 1969.

44. Tsuda N, Takaku I: A case report of malignant vascular tumor of the orbit in a newborn. Folia Ophthalmol Jpn 21:728, 1970.

45. Diallo J, Moliva G: A propos d'une observation de sarcome angioblastique primitif de l'orbite avec metastases chez en enfant de deux ans. Bull Soc Med Afr Noire Lang Fr 15:635, 1970.

46. Messmer EP, Font RL, McCrary JA, et al: Epithelioid angiosarcoma of the orbit presenting as Tolosa-Hunt syndrome. Ophthalmology 90:1414, 1983.

47. Hufnagel T, Ma L, Kuo TT: Orbital angiosarcoma with subconjunctival presentation: Report of a case and literature review. Ophthalmology 94:72, 1987.

48. Jakobiec FA, Font RL: Orbit. In Spenser WH (ed): Ophthalmic Pathology: An Atlas and Textbook. Philadelphia, WB Saunders, 1986, pp 2552–2553.

49. Kimura T, Yoshimura S, Ishikawa E: Unusual granulation combined with hyperplastic change of lymphatic tissue. Trans Soc Pathol Jpn 37:179, 1978.

50. Bostad L, Pettersen W: Angiolymphoid hyperplasia with eosinophilia involving the orbit: A case report. Acta Ophthalmol 60:419, 1982.

51. Moesner J, Pallesen R, Sorensen B: Angiolymphoid hyperplasia with eosinophilia (Kimura's disease). Arch Dermatol 117:650, 1981.

52. Hidayat AA, Cameron DJ, Font RL, et al: Angiolymphoid hyperplasia with eosinophilia (Kimura's disease) of the orbit and ocular adnexa. Am J Ophthalmol 96:176, 1983.

53. Kupersmith MJ, Berenstein A, Flamm E, et al: Neuro-ophthalmologic abnormalities and intravascular therapy of traumatic carotid-cavernous fistulas. Ophthalmology 93:906, 1986.

54. Debron GM, Vinuela AJ, Fox AJ, et al: Indications of treatment from classification of 152 carotid-cavernous fistulae. Neurosurgery 22:285, 1988.

55. Hosobuchi Y: Electrothrombosis of carotid-cavernous fistula. J Neurosurg 42:76, 1975.

56. Newton TH, Hoyt WF: Dural arteriovenous shunts in the region of the cavernous sinus. Neuroradiology 1:71, 1970.

57. Slusher MM, Lennington RB, Weaver RG, Davis CH: Ophthalmic findings in dural arteriovenous shunts. Ophthalmology 86:720, 1979.

58. Harris MJ, Fine SJ, Miller NR: Photocoagulation treatment of proliferative retinopathy secondary to carotid-cavernous fistulas. Am J Ophthalmol 90:515, 1980.

59. Grove AS: The dural shunt syndrome: Pathology and clinical course. Ophthalmology 91:31, 1984.

60. Kuppersmith MJ, Berenstein A, Choi IS, et al: Management of non-traumatic vascular shunts involving the cavernous sinus. Ophthalmology 95:121, 1988.

61. Parkinson D: A surgical approach to the cavernous portion of the carotid artery: Anatomic studies and case report. J Neurosurg 23:474, 1965.

62. Hanneken, AM, Miller NR, Debrun GM, et al: Treatment of carotid-cavernous fistulas using a detachable balloon catheter through the superior ophthalmic vein. Arch Ophthalmol 107:87, 1989.

63. Krohel GB, Wright JS: Orbital hemorrhage. Am J Ophthalmol 88:254, 1979.

64. Winter J, Centeno RS, Bentson JR: Maneuver to aid diagnosis of orbital varix by computerized tomography. AJNR 3:30, 1982.

65. Vignard J, Clay C, Bilaniak LT: Venography of the orbit: An analytic report of 43 cases. Radiology 110:373, 1974.

66. Rootman J, Graeb DA: Vascular lesions. In Rootman J (ed): Diseases of the Orbit. Philadelphia, JB Lippincott, 1988, pp 553–557.

67. Milne HL III, Leone CR, Kincard MC, Brennan MW. Chronic hematic cyst of the orbit. Ophthalmology 94:271, 1987.

68. Shapiro A, Tso MOM, Putterman AM, et al: A clinicopathologic study of hematic cysts of the orbit. Am J Ophthalmol 102:237, 1986.

69. Eugenidis N, Gessaga E, Chrzanowski R: Bone scan and angiography for orbitofrontal cholesterol granuloma. Neuroradiology 19:93, 1980.

70. McNab AA, Wright JE: Orbitofrontal cholesterol granuloma. Ophthalmology 97:28, 1990.

71. Kersten RC, Kersten JL, Bloom HR, et al: Chronic hematic cyst of the orbit: Role of magnetic resonance imaging in diagnosis. Ophthalmology 95:1549, 1988.

Chapter 174

■

Peripheral Nerve Sheath Tumors of the Orbit

LEONARD A. LEVIN and FREDERICK A. JAKOBIEC

Within the orbit, there are cellular elements of both the central and peripheral nervous systems. The optic nerve is a tract of the central nervous system, while the orbital soft tissues are endowed with a luxuriant system of peripheral nerves, including sensory branches (the trigeminal), oculomotor nerves (the third, fourth, and sixth cranial nerves supplying the extraocular muscles), and sympathetic and parasympathetic fibers. Curiously, most benign and malignant orbital peripheral nerve sheath tumors appear to originate from divisions of the trigeminal, because pain is a frequent accompaniment at the time of presentation, and more important, because after their successful removal deficits in the function of the other nerves are not identified, unless there has been collateral intraoperative damage.

The major anatomic and cellular differences between the optic nerve and the orbital peripheral nerves are worth emphasizing. The outermost portion of the optic nerve is constituted by the fibrous dura, which rarely (if ever) is responsible for a primary noninflammatory mass. The innermost layers, between which percolates the cerebrospinal fluid, are the arachnoid and pia. The meningeal tissues are responsible for primary optic nerve meningiomas through the proliferation of meningothelial cells. The intraaxial parenchymal portion of the optic nerve consists of the axons of the retinal ganglion cells, which are enveloped in myelin produced by the oligodendroglial cells, each of which ensheaths several axons. It is an intriguing anomaly that optic nerve tumors of pure oligodendrocytes are virtually unknown. Finally, there are astrocytes that, when transformed, are responsible for optic nerve gliomas. Astrocytes contain cytoplasmic intermediate filaments that immunostain for glial fibrillary acidic protein; they are sometimes called fibrous astrocytes because of these filaments and not because they synthesize collagen. Among other functions, astrocytes intermediate between the axons and the blood vessels and invaginating pial septa. This is discussed further in Chapter 22.

All other orbital nerves, including the sympathetic, oculomotor, and sensory nerves and the nervi vasorum, as well as the ciliary ganglion, are peripheral. Analogous to the optic nerve, peripheral nerves have an outer fibrous sheath called the epineurium, which in all likelihood is not responsible for orbital tumors. Each peripheral nerve is subdivided into bundles by repeating ensheathing perineural circlets. Perineural cells possess both contractile and insulating properties. Within the perineural compartments are Schwann cells, a single cell type that serves in place of both the astrocyte and the oligodendrocyte. Unlike the central nervous system oligodendrocyte, each Schwann cell myelinates only one peripheral axon. Instead of meningeal-type fibroblasts, which line the optic nerve, and fibroblastic pial septae, which intercalate within it, orbital peripheral nerves, like other nerves in the body, contain epineural, perineural, and endoneural fibroblasts, the last of which elaborate a delicate myxoid and fibrillar matrix within the endoneural compartment. The ciliary ganglion is a way-station for intermixing trigeminal fibers, sympathetic fibers, and parasympathetic fibers (only the last of which synapse within the ganglion) on their way to the globe via the short and long posterior ciliary nerves. A bona fide ganglionic tumor of the ciliary ganglion has never been convincingly described, although utterly rare neuroid and paraganglionic tumors have putatively been ascribed as an origin in the ciliary ganglion.

In analyzing cellular typologies and embryologic cellular origins, peripheral nerve tumors outside of the head and neck region have been attributed to neural crest progeny, which include Schwann cells, melanocytes, and peripheral ganglion cells. In the head and neck region, however, there are no paraxial mesodermal somites, so that the neural crest must take up the task of providing many of the connective tissue phenotypes of the head and neck region, including with respect to the eye and ocular adnexa, the corneal stromal keratocytes, the uveal tissues, the sclera, most of the orbital soft tissues with the exception of the striated extraocular muscles, and even the trochlear cartilage and many of the bones of the orbit. The collectivity of the neural crest contributions to these traditionally mesodermally derived elements has been referred to as the ectomesenchyme or mesectoderm.

With respect to tumors of presumptive neural crest offspring, there are two concepts that should be understood. A neurocristopathy is a systemic syndrome with multifocal proliferations of neural crest cells: melanocytes, ganglion cells, and Schwann cells. Some of the most dramatic manifestations of neurocristopathies are neurofibromatosis type 1 (von Recklinghausen's neurofibromatosis, a syndrome with multiple ocular and skin findings localized to chromosome 17; see later) and neurofibromatosis type 2 (a syndrome typically of bilateral acoustic neuromas but without significant ocular findings, localized to chromosome 22). The multiple endocrine neoplasia (MEN) syndromes (especially MEN syndrome type IIb—also called MEN syndrome type III) are other examples with significant ophthalmic manifestations, including thickening of the corneal nerves (in retrospect, not a characteristic of neurofibromatosis type 1). Another aspect of tumors of the neural crest progeny is the APUD system (*a*mine *p*recursor *u*ptake and *d*ecarboxylation); tumors of this system are referred to as apudomas. Besides neural crest lineage, they all share morphologic and biochemical demonstration of cytoplasmic dense-core polypeptide secretory products: pheochromocytomas and chemosensory tumors (paragangliomas) synthesize catecholamine products, whereas medullary carcinoma of the thyroid produces calcitonin. Both medullary carcinoma of the thyroid and pheochromocytoma are features of the MEN syndrome type IIb (see later).

There is also sometimes a tendency to confuse the neural crest and its tumors with neuroectoderm and its neoplasms. The neural crest is a paired mass of cells that delaminate from the embryonic ectoderm on either side of the invaginating neural tube (neuroectoderm). The latter is responsible for the formation of the neuraxis and, with respect to the eye, only for the retina and pigmented and nonpigmented epithelium. Rare tumors and dysontogenetic masses of the orbital and other ocular adnexal soft tissues and bones may occasionally arise from ectopias of true neuroectoderm, such as the rare pigmented retinal choristoma (formerly called the retinal anlage tumor) that has the peculiarity of arising in the maxillary bone but can secondarily invade the orbit.

There are two fundamental types of presentation of benign peripheral nerve sheath tumors: quiet insidious proptosis, in which visual function and extraocular motility are often well preserved and there is very little ocular irritation in the form of lid edema or conjunctival chemosis; and massive overgrowths and hypertrophies of the involved lids and orbit, such as seen in plexiform neurofibromas and diffuse neurofibromas of neurofibromatosis type 1. Peripheral nerve tumors may clinically mimic other ophthalmic pathologies. A schwannoma has been reported in a patient with a slowly enlarging solid medial eyelid margin mass, where the clinical diagnosis was initially chalazion.[1] Ciliary body schwannoma may simulate melanoma,[2] and a schwannoma has presented within the sclera itself.[3] Initial diagnoses of papilloma, basal cell carcinoma, epithelial inclusion cyst, and chronic dacryocystitis were entertained in several cases of superficially situated peripheral nerve tumors of the ocular adnexa.[4] Two lacrimal gland tumors eventually were diagnosed as neurofibromas.[5]

It is worth placing the clinical presentations of peripheral nerve sheath tumors in the context of other simulating orbital neoplasms before taking up a more detailed discussion of the nerve tumors themselves. Both isolated neurofibromas and schwannomas tend to be well-tolerated, rounded, or circumscribed masses. The radiographic differential diagnosis of such rounded lesions includes cavernous hemangioma, fibrous histiocytoma, and hemangiopericytoma. Only the cavernous hemangioma among these closely mimics the presentation of benign peripheral nerve sheath tumors. For example, even when these lesions have been neglected and reach sizable proportions, because of their slow growth the orbital tissues and lid tissues tend to accommodate to them. Thus, corneal exposure will only be

seen very late with the large peripheral nerve sheath tumors and cavernous hemangiomas, because the lid tends to slowly stretch upon the eyeball, and there is very little evidence of congestion of the eyelids and the conjunctiva.

By contrast, equally sized hemangiopericytomas and fibrous histiocytomas create much more evidence of lid and conjunctival congestion and, for a comparable size, more evidence of optic nerve and extraocular dysfunction. In high grades of proptosis the lids will be retracted, leading to corneal and epibulbar exposure. Sometimes malignancies in the orbit can produce a surprisingly circumscribed appearance on imaging studies, such as in primary orbital melanomas and some metastatic carcinomas, but there is invariably more symptomatology produced by these lesions in terms of pain, motility disturbance, and visual decline. Furthermore, the patients will have much shorter symptomatic periods in comparison with patients harboring benign peripheral nerve sheath tumors and cavernous hemangiomas.

With the advent of multiplanar computed tomography (CT) and magnetic resonance imaging (MRI), the distinction between a juxtaoptic nerve tumor and a primary tumor of the optic nerve has been enormously facilitated. Nonetheless, there are situations of clinical or surgical confusion in which a glioma or meningioma of the optic nerve might be confused with a peripheral nerve tumor of the orbit. For example, a surgeon could conceivably incise an optic nerve tumor, thinking he or she had encountered an encapsulated orbital tumor. One clue to the presence of an optic nerve tumor, other than the radiologic appearance, is the disproportion between usually advanced visual loss and low degrees of proptosis (2 to 4 mm).

The other major class of orbital tumor that may well be the most common in adults consists of the lymphoid tumors.[6] In contrast to benign peripheral nerve sheath tumors and cavernous hemangiomas, these benign and malignant conditions tend to arise in the sixth and seventh decades. They produce an insidious proptosis that develops over 4 to 6 mo, unless they are high-grade malignancies. Imaging studies can be particularly helpful in segregating these lesions apart from the previously mentioned ones. Lymphoid tumors have a propensity to arise in the superior orbit and retrobulbar tissues; however, rather than create rounded masses, they tend to replace the orbital fat in an irregular fashion, producing arclike contours and straight lines where they abut fascial planes, bone, and the sclera of the globe. Bone destruction is rare in this class of neoplasm, unless it has arisen from a sinus or from within the bone itself.

TUMOR TYPES

Schwannoma (Neurilemoma)

CLINICAL FEATURES

The schwannoma, or neurilemoma, is a pure proliferation of Schwann cells. These tumors comprise approximately 1 percent of all orbital tumors (Table 174–1) and are found in 1.5 percent of patients with

Table 174–1. PREVALENCE OF PERIPHERAL
NERVE SHEATH TUMORS OF THE ORBIT

Series	n	Schwannomas (%)	Neurofibromas (%)	Other* (%)
Henderson[73]	764	8 (1.0)	18 (2.4)	2 (0.3)
Rootman[74]	1409	14 (1.0)	7 (0.5)	4 (0.3)
Shields[62]	645	5 (0.8)	5 (0.8)	4 (0.6)
Kennedy[75]	820	4 (0.5)	25 (3.0)	0 (0.0)

*Amputation neuroma, granular cell tumor, and malignant schwannoma.

neurofibromatosis type 1.[7] However, they may also present in patients without stigmata of neurofibromatosis type 1,[8] or formes frustes of neurofibromatosis type 1, such as in patients with nondiagnostic numbers of (less than 6) café-au-lait spots.[9] The tumors tend to become clinically symptomatic after the first two decades of life and are therefore usually seen in young to middle-aged adults as a cause of slowly progressive proptosis, sometimes evolving over years (Fig. 174–1). Unless neglected (Fig. 174–2), they cause low-grade exophthalmos of 2 to 4 mm. Uncommonly, they present in childhood.[10] Ocular complaints depend on the location of the tumor and its size. For example, a tumor at the orbital apex or in an intimate juxtaoptic nerve locus (the short posterior ciliary nerves on each side of the optic nerve are a frequent site of spawning for these tumors) can lead to an earlier visual deficit from compressive optic neuropathy (Fig. 174–3) than can tumors located more laterally or superiorly in the orbit.

There may be induced hyperopia with retinal striae (see Fig. 174–1B), but because of their elegant circumscription, extraocular motility is generally not affected until they become bulky. Rarely, a schwannoma may invade an extraocular muscle.[10] In contrast to lesions such as hemangiopericytoma and fibrous histiocytoma, there is less evidence of congestion of the conjunctiva and the eyelids with the benign peripheral nerve sheath tumors. Because they are often located in the superior orbit, they are often associated with hypophthalmos. Rarely, they may present as intraocular tumors, presumably arising from a peripheral nerve, such as the long posterior ciliary nerve.[11] Even more rarely, they may

present in the orbit as an extension from an intracranial tumor, such as a trigeminal ganglion schwannoma.[12] As discussed more comprehensively below, on CT scanning and magnetic resonance imaging, they can appear as circumscribed, partially cystic, round to ovoid lesions, but sometimes as remarkably elongated masses, located behind the globe or in another of the orbital quadrants (Figs. 174–4 to 174–6).

PATHOLOGY

Schwannomas are extremely well encapsulated, owing to the fact that the capsule is formed by the perineural cells of the nerve radicle of origin (Fig. 174–7). At the time of surgery and on examination of fresh tissue in the laboratory, the tumors display a smooth surface, are fluctuant and friable on palpation, and have a translucent fish-flesh to tan coloration; on cut surface, there may be foci of hemorrhage, yellow discoloration, and outright cavity formation (Fig. 174–8). Microscopically, both solid areas (Antoni A) and more myxoid areas (Antoni B) alternate with each other in varying proportions (Fig. 174–9). The more solid areas feature a spindle cell population oriented in fascicles with a delicate background fibrillary character, due predominantly to the interweaving of myriad cell processes, conferring the appearance of a neuropil (Fig. 174–10). The nuclei of the tumor cells are ovoid and may have a fine stippling of the chromatin and a small nucleolus. Lateral palisading of the nuclei is frequently observed (Fig. 174–11A); if this becomes highly regimented, structures called Verocay bodies are produced (see Fig. 174–11B), in which the bipolar interdigitating cell processes become highly organized in a refractile manner, while the nuclei are laterally disposed in ribbons (an almost identical cellular organization can be seen in some uveal melanomas referred to as "fascicular"). In the looser myxoid areas, ovoid, bipolar, and multipolar cells are suspended in a watery matrix. Some of these cells may undergo secondary lipidization, accounting for the yellow hue focally observed on the cut sections of the gross specimens.

Mitoses are absent, and nuclear atypism is unusual except in the cellular schwannoma, a tumor typically of

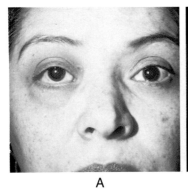
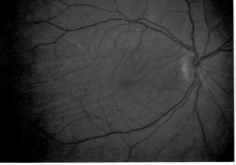
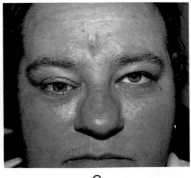

A   B   C

Figure 174–1. Orbital schwannomas (neurilemoma). A, A 42-year-old woman presented with a quiet right proptosis measuring only 2 mm, which is intimated by virtue of the baring of the inferior sclera. Motility was undisturbed and there was no eyelid or conjunctival congestion. B, There was induced hyperopia and accompanying retinal striae. C, A right superior orbital schwannoma of larger dimensions with a 4-yr history and 6 mm of proptosis and marked hypotropia.

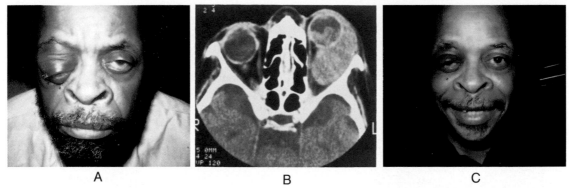

A   B   C

Figure 174–2. Long-standing orbital schwannoma. *A,* A slowly progressive right proptosis developed over a decade and ultimately measured 12 mm. Despite the high-grade proptosis, note that the upper eyelid has commensurately stretched to continue to cover the eyeball. *B,* Axial computed tomography (CT) scan shows a massive ovoid tumor in the lateral and retrobulbar orbital compartments. Note the associated retinal detachment. *C,* After complete removal of the tumor, there is residual upper eyelid ptosis, which the patient refused to have corrected. (*A–C,* Courtesy of Tom Moazed, M.D.)

the paravertebral region, which is more cellular than a normal schwannoma, does not possess Verocay bodies, but has the same benign course.[13, 14] The deposition of collagen in schwannomas is usually less conspicuous than in neurofibromas, and this is responsible for their friability at the time of surgical delivery. The PAS and reticulin stains demonstrate a bounteous investiture of individual cells with strand-like material, which at the ultrastructural level corresponds to the production of basement membrane material. More abundant collagen deposition along with a surprising amount of nuclear pleomorphism can be seen in some older hypocellular lesions, in the absence of mitotic activity; such changes have led to the term "ancient schwannoma." The Mas-

son trichrome stain may show radiating and cruciate depositions of keloidal collagen in these ancient lesions. The alcian blue stain for hyaluronic acid is weakly to nonpositive in the myxoid areas of schwannoma, in comparison with the more vivid positivity of neurofibroma.

The xanthoma-type cells that may be focally detected in schwannoma in all likelihood reflect imbibition by the tumor cells of lipid that leaks out of fenestrated capillaries, rather than the infiltration of true histiocytic xanthoma cells. The capillaries in schwannoma often manifest a thickened PAS-positive sheath, constituted by both redundant basement membrane formation and the accumulation of leaked moieties from the vessels (see Fig. 174–11*C*). These thickened walls are not found in most neurofibromas. The vascular changes can also lead to foci of hemorrhagic degeneration, the collection of hemosiderin-laden macrophages, and massive cystic degeneration in the core of a schwannoma.

Electron microscopy reveals electron-lucent cells with many long delicate cellular processes, which are invested by continuous basement membranes. This basement membrane may contain long-spacing collagen (Luse

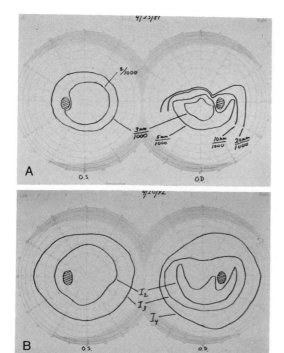

Figure 174–3. Compressive optic neuropathy from an orbital schwannoma *(A),* which improved postoperatively upon the removal of the lesion *(B).*

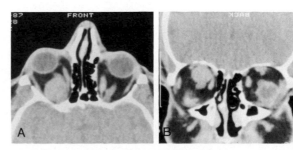

Figure 174–4. Orbital schwannoma. *A,* Axial CT scan displaying an exquisitely rounded tumor at the orbital apex. There is a suggestion of deflection of the optic nerve nasally just behind the globe. *B,* Coronal CT section demonstrates that the optic nerve is separate from the rounded mass; the former structure can be seen adherent on the latter's inferior aspect.

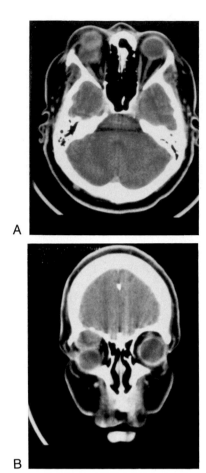

Figure 174–5. Orbital schwannoma. *A,* Axial CT scan depicting a round mass in contact with the posterior aspect of the globe. Note the suggestion of central radiolucency. *B,* A coronal CT section also confirms the radiolucent central region of the lesion, as well as some thinning of the orbital roof. The lesion had been present for many years. The radiolucency suggests the existence of either secondary xanthomatization or cystification within the mass.

bodies) (Fig. 174–12). Myelin figures may be present, befitting this tumor's origin from a myelinating cell. The schwannoma is an almost pure proliferation of Schwann cells, as opposed to the heavy contribution of endo-

neural fibroblasts without basement membranes in neurofibroma; thus, schwannomas are reliably S100 positive, unless there are problems with fixation of the tissue. The tumor cell cytoplasm contains a sparsity of organelles, consisting of short strands of rough surfaced endoplasmic reticulum, scattered cytoplasmic filaments and neurotubules, and a modest number of Golgi complexes and mitochrondia. Lysosomes can be observed, probably subserving a phagocytic capability that becomes fully expressed during wallerian degeneration and in the production of tumoral xanthoma cells. The vimentin stain is positive in schwannoma, but this is not helpful in distinguishing a schwannoma from a neurofibroma or a fibrous histiocytoma, because these other tumors also contain this mesoderm-associated cytoplasmic intermediate filament.

The major differential diagnoses of a schwannoma under the microscope are a fibrous histiocytoma and a leiomyoma, both of which are negative for S100. The fibrous histiocytoma exhibits a twisted, cartwheel, or spiral nebular pattern of tumor cells, which is sometimes referred to as storiform. Fibrous histiocytomas, however, may be focally or even spectacularly myxoid in character, but the cells will not be as wavy as those seen in a neurofibroma; extensive and diffuse myxoid foci are much rarer in schwannoma. Furthermore, nuclear palisading is not typically encountered in a fibrous histiocytoma. Leiomyoma is much more likely to be confused under the microscope with schwannoma, because the thin actin filaments of the leiomyoma cells may simulate the delicate neurophil background of a schwannoma. Both tumors are also capable of exhibiting nuclear palisading; the nuclei of a leiomyoma, however, are ovoid or cigar-shaped, as opposed to pointed (e.g., in fibroblastic and neurofibromatous proliferations), whereas delicate stippling of the chromatin is more marked in a schwannoma. In a leiomyoma, the trichrome stain reveals a much more intense cytoplasmic fuchsinophilia and the smooth muscle intermediate filament desmin can be demonstrated, whereas these features are absent in a schwannoma. In a leiomyoma, if the cellular fascicles are cut in cross-section, one often observes perinuclear halos, due to the shrinkage and

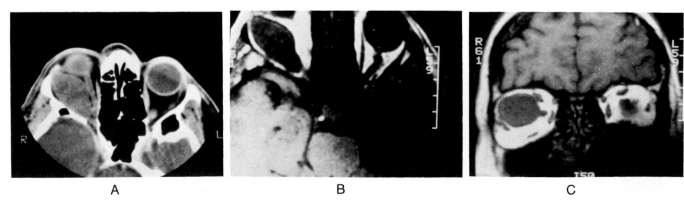

Figure 174–6. Orbital schwannoma. *A,* An elongated and extremely well encapsulated lesion is located in the lateral orbit but extends toward the orbital apex. There is nasal displacement of the optic nerve, which is clearly differentiable from the mass lesion. In addition to a rounded appearance, orbital schwannomas can offer this elongated fusiform shape. *B,* Magnetic resonance imaging (MRI) displays hypointense signals in T₁-weighted images. This lesion was bright in T₂-weighted images, as are most orbital tumors. *C,* MRI in the coronal plane highlights the optic nerve in the orbital fat on the nasal aspect of the lesion, thereby helping to distinguish the tumor from a primary optic nerve glioma (astrocytoma).

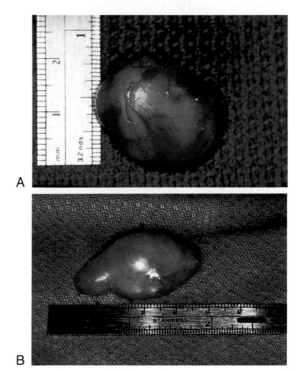

Figure 174–7. Fresh gross appearances of completely excised orbital schwannomas. *A*, A round lesion with a shiny capsule manifesting a fish-flesh appearance. The lesion was fluctuant to palpation. (Courtesy of Peter Rubin, M.D.) *B*, An elongated and well-encapsulated orbital schwannoma. The small proboscoid component on the left extended through the superior orbital fissure. (Courtesy of Richard Lisman, M.D.)

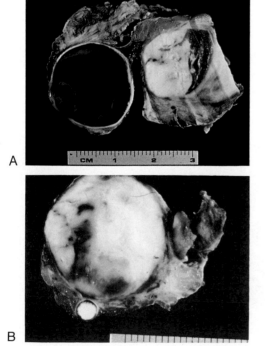

Figure 174–8. *A*, Recurrent orbital schwannoma that was misinterpreted as a benign lesion, leading to an exenteration. Note that the mass is extremely well circumscribed but it has an area of internal hemorrhagic cyst formation. *B*, The variegated cut surface of the lesion exhibits areas of yellow xanthomatous transformation, brown-black areas of hemorrhage, and at the periphery an attenuated perineurial capsule. The optic nerve is present below. (*A* and *B*, Courtesy of Elise Torczynski, M.D.)

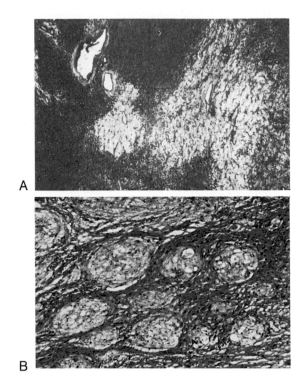

A

B

Figure 174–9. Orbital schwannoma. *A,* Schwannomas often display alternating areas of more compactly arranged cells, shown on the left (Antoni A pattern), along with looser myxoid foci, shown toward the right (Antoni B pattern). *B,* Small islands of Antoni B tissue are separated by slender strands of Antoni A tissue. Some of the Antoni B cells have undergone secondary lipidization with xanthoma cell transformation.

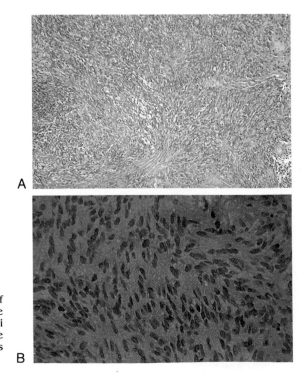

A

B

Figure 174–10. Orbital schwannoma. *A,* Schwannomas have a population of short fascicles of cells with an eosinophilic cystoplasmic background. In the center of the field are small clusters of lipidized xanthoma cells. *B,* The nuclei have a delicate chromatin pattern. There is a background neuropil appearance of interweaving cytoplasmic cellular processes. The Masson trichrome was negative, indicating the paucity of interstitial collagen.

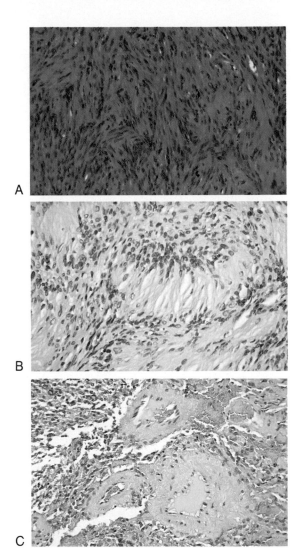

Figure 174–11. Orbital schwannoma. *A*, There is a tendency for lateral regimentation of the nuclei, so-called nuclear palisading. Note the delicate eosinophilic fibrillary background as the cytoplasmic processes interdigitate. *B*, This highly regimented arrangement of delicate eosinophilic cytoplasmic processes bordered on each side by clusters of nuclei is a pattern referred to as *Verocay body formation.* (Courtesy of A. R. Rosenberg, M.D., and Ben Pilch, M.D.) *C*, Several small blood vessels have a distinctive eosinophilic cuff of redundant basement membrane, highly suggestive of schwannoma and not manifested by most other orbital tumors.

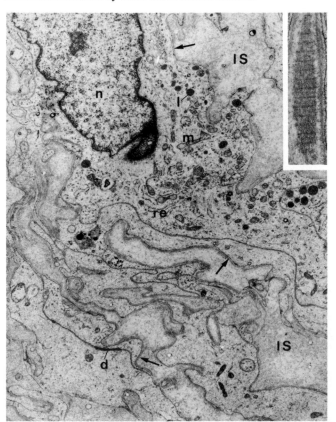

Figure 174–12. Transmission electron micrograph of an orbital schwannoma. The cells are electron-lucent and extend myriad processes, which are ensheathed with uninterrupted basement membranes *(arrows)*. Sometimes the basement membrane material may assume a banded character as indicated in the *inset,* a configuration referred to as *Luse bodies.* Occasional interweaving cell processes are connected by a desmosome (d). The intercellular space (IS) contains flocculent material. The cytoplasm is endowed with electron-dense lysosomes (l), scattered mitochondria (m), and short profiles of rough-surfaced endoplasmic reticulum (re). (n, nucleus with a small nucleolus.) (Courtesy of Takeo Iwamoto, M.D.)

conglutination of the actin filaments during fixation. Because of basement membrane production in a leiomyoma, both PAS-positive and reticulin-staining fibers can be detected, such as in a schwannoma.

MANAGEMENT

Schwannomas are typically isolated and well-circumscribed adult orbital tumors that are amenable to local excision. The presence of a capsule aids in complete extirpation. However, difficulties may arise due to the fish-flesh character of the tumor, owing to a variable but generally minimal content of scaffolding collagen. These tumors can burst and break up into many pieces if the capsule should be rent or rendered highly attenuated in the course of surgical dissection through cleavage planes. If most of the tumor is removed, it may be wisest to wait for a recurrence than to attempt a complete removal of the tumor, particularly if there is a risk of producing damage to orbital nerves, the optic nerve, or the extraocular muscles. Fortunately, it may take many years for a schwannoma to recur, and the risk of malignant degeneration is negligible.

Surgical approaches depend primarily on tumor location, and the choice of superior, anterior, lateral, medial, or inferior orbitomy is usually straightforward. Because of the encapsulation, tumors that extend posteriorly beyond the orbit may occasionally be managed by an orbital approach alone[15]; this is generally not feasible for diffuse or plexiform neurofibromas or for malignant peripheral nerve sheath tumors. Since schwannomas are of Schwann cell origin, they typically occur on the periphery of the involved nerve, and axons are not included within the lesion. Therefore, it is often possible to strip the tumor away from the nerve.[8] The more elongated tumors may spread within the perineural spaces preferentially and can even protrude through the superior orbital fissure.

Schwannomas are held to be relatively immune to malignant transformation, even upon recurrence. We have seen cases, however, of recurrent schwannoma in which there is hypercellularity and minimal to moderate mitotic activity. Such cases, in the absence of frank nuclear pleomorphism, probably represent locally aggressive tumors rather than metastasizing tumors; nevertheless, a much more vigorous effort at total extirpation should be undertaken. There is one report in the literature of an orbital schwannoma that appears to have undergone a malignant transformation in a patient with neurofibromatosis.[16]

Neurofibroma

Histologically, neurofibromas are quite distinct from schwannomas. Schwannomas are pure proliferations of Schwann cells, whereas neurofibromas consist of a mixture of Schwann cells, peripheral nerve axons, endoneural fibroblasts, and perineural cells. They represent from 0.5 to 2.4 percent of orbital tumors (see Table 174–1). There are three typical types of orbital neurofibromas. The *localized* neurofibroma, usually not associated with neurofibromatosis type 1, behaves clinically and radiographically like a schwannoma, in that it is a solitary soft tissue mass that is relatively well circumscribed, although lacking encapsulation. The *plexiform* neurofibroma, which is the most common subtype, diffusely invades orbital tissues, with each unit surrounded by its own perineurium; it is usually associated with neurofibromatosis type 1. The *diffuse* neurofibroma invades orbital tissues, is not ensheathed in repeating perineuria like the plexiform neurofibroma, and is variably associated with neurofibromatosis type 1.

Localized Neurofibroma

CLINICAL FEATURES

From the clinical point of view, the features of localized neurofibroma and schwannomas are virtually indistinguishable (Fig. 174–13A and B); they are somewhat more likely than schwannomas to be associated with neurofibromatosis (in about 10 percent of cases).[17] Like the schwannoma, the localized neurofibroma presents as a localized soft tissue orbital mass, often causing painless or mildly painful proptosis in young to middle-aged adults. Pain may result from involvement of a sensory nerve by the tumor. Corneal exposure from proptosis may be symptomatic unless there is concurrent corneal anesthesia. Alternatively, severe pain may suggest either an amputation neuroma or adenoid cystic carcinoma of the lacrimal gland.

Other symptoms and signs may be seen in patients with localized neurofibroma. If located posteriorly, optic neuropathy, with accompanying decreased acuity, color vision, field changes, an afferent pupillary defect, and optic atrophy may be present. In general, however, visual changes are less common. Diplopia, especially when referrable to one or more extraocular muscles innervated by an involved orbital nerve, may be diagnostic but most likely is secondary to mechanical disturbance, as with a wide variety of non-neural orbital tumors.

Localized neurofibroma is not encapsulated, but its CT and MRI appearance is similar to that of a schwannoma (see Fig. 174–13C and D). It is most commonly seen in the superior orbit, but may also present in the inferior orbit, arising from the infraorbital nerve.[18] Neurofibromas may be seen in the lacrimal fossa region (see Fig. 174–13E),[5] whereas a schwannoma has not been described in this locale. The localized form of neurofibroma is capable of presenting as multiple small individual tumors in the orbit. This should prompt the diagnosis of neurofibromas with associated neurofibromatosis type 1, although multiple separate neurofibromas have been reported in patients with no evidence of neurofibromatosis-1.[17, 19] Rarely, cavernous hemangioma may also have several rounded, isolated but concurrent tumors at the time of presentation.[20]

PATHOLOGY

At the time of surgery, localized neurofibromas are white to tan, depending on the amount of interstitial

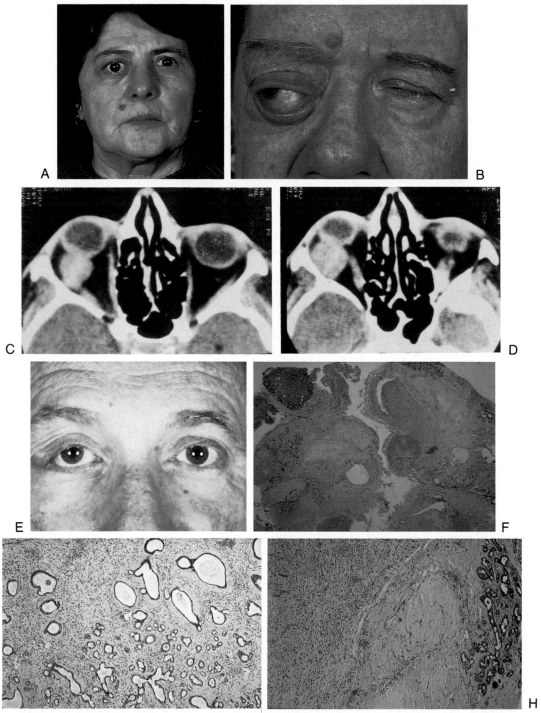

Figure 174–13. Localized orbital neurofibroma. *A,* Note how quiet the eyeball looks and the overall normal configuration of the eyelids with 6 mm of well-tolerated proptosis. *B,* A 40-yr history of a neglected right orbital neurofibroma has led to stretching of the eyelids with minimal congestion of the surface of the globe and an absence of corneal exposure. The eyelids were able voluntarily to completely close on the globe. *C* and *D,* Two axial CT scans in somewhat different planes of a localized and isolated neurofibroma exhibiting slight irregularities of the outline of the lesion, which is not as elegantly well encapsulated as the typical schwannoma (a lesion delineated by the perineurium of the nerve of origin, whereas the neurofibroma acquires a fibrous compression pseudocapsule). *E,* An unusual neurofibroma of the lacrimal gland producing a lateral ptosis of the right upper eyelid. *F,* The excised specimen obtained from the patient shown in *E* is a myxoid lesion that has infiltrated the parenchyma of the lacrimal gland, relatively undisturbed portions of which are shown toward the upper left, but islands of ductular tissue are also scattered throughout. *G,* Ectatic ductules of the lacrimal gland are separated by myxoid neurofibromatous tissue. Such an appearance might be easily confused with that of a benign mixed tumor (pleomorphic adenoma). The ductular units lack the characteristic splaying off of an outer myoepithelial layer, as seen in benign mixed tumors. *H,* Very watery myxoid tissue is shown immediately to the left of surviving ducts of preexistent lacrimal gland on the right. A somewhat more cellular but still loose proliferation of spindle cells is present on the far left.

collagen. On the cut surface, they are variably firm to mucinous but do not offer the yellow discoloration and cystification that are characteristic of many schwannomas.

Microscopically, neurofibromas consist of wavy cells, dispersed typically in small bundles (Fig. 174–14A), but occasionally widely dispersed in a highly myxoid matrix (see Fig. 174–13F to H). The cell nuclei resemble those of fibroblasts, except that they are more undulating (see Fig. 174–14B and C). There is a moderate background of capillaries, which helps to distinguish the myxoid variant (see Fig. 174–14D to F) from a pure myxoma, the latter being for the most part bereft of small blood vessels. A highly distinctive organization of neurofibromas is in small packets of wavy cells, which on occasion can be demonstrated to possess axon cylinders with the Bodian stain. These bundles or fascicles may be rhythmically distributed throughout the lesion and separated from each other by a looser myxoid stroma. The latter is rich in hyaluronic acid, as brought out with the alcian blue stain. Occasional organoid laminations of Schwann cells and endoneural fibroblasts can be observed, mimicking cutaneous sensory corpuscles (Fig. 174–14G). The tumors are relatively cohesive on the gross level owing to the variably prominent deposition of collagen, and they have a compression pseudocapsule.

Electron microscopy reveals a mixture of cell types, including Schwann cells and putative perineural cells with basement membranes, and often a more prominent constituency of endoneural fibroblasts (Fig. 174–15), which are devoid of basement membrane production. Immunohistochemical stains are unpredictably helpful; the S100 stain is usefully positive in fewer than 50 percent of cases, because of the variable population of participatory Schwann cells (see Fig. 174–14H). The Leu-19 antibody to the CD56 antigen stains neurofibromas, schwannomas, and malignant schwannomas, but also stains rhabdomyosarcomas.[21] Antibodies to epithelial membrane antigen (EMA), which is present in perineural cells, may distinguish the better differentiated of these tumors, which differ in their perineural sheathing.[22]

MANAGEMENT

Localized neurofibromas, although not encapsulated, are often otherwise circumscribed and may be excised using approaches similar to those employed for other solitary orbital tumors. Most of these tumors reside in the superior orbit and are well reached by a superior orbitotomy, either transeptally through a lid crease incision if the tumor is anterior or extraperiosteally through a brow or lid crease incision if the tumor is more posterior. A transcranial approach is generally not necessary.[23]

There are two important differences between schwannomas and localized neurofibromas that affect their management. As mentioned previously, the localized form of neurofibroma may present as several small orbital tumors. Although this is relatively unusual, when found, these lesions should be carefully and independently removed. In some circumstances very small tumors may be left behind until a later date, when they are larger and more easily removed. Second, the neurofibroma is capable of undergoing malignant transformation into a malignant peripheral nerve sheath tumor (neurofibrosarcoma or malignant schwannoma); although neurofibromas elsewhere in the body may have a 10 percent probability of malignant transformation, this has not been verified for orbital neurofibromas. The diagnosis and management of this tumor are briefly discussed later, and at greater length in Chapter 178.

Plexiform and Diffuse Neurofibromas

CLINICAL FEATURES

Many clinicians and pathologists do not accurately distinguish between plexiform (Fig. 174–16) and diffuse (Fig. 174–17) neurofibromas, both of which are expressions of neurofibromatosis type 1, the latter more variably than the former. Both the plexiform and diffuse neurofibromas make their appearance within the first decade of life (often from age 2 to 5[17]) in contradistinction to the isolated and circumscribed peripheral nerve sheath tumors that are not associated with neurofibromatosis type 1 and that present in early to middle adulthood.

In comparison with the localized neurofibroma of adults, there is no circumscription to either of these tumors. Clinically, there may be massive overgrowth of the lids, along with similar infiltration of the orbit and facial tissues (elephantiasis neuromatosa) (Fig. 174–18). On palpating the eyelids in a plexiform neurofibroma, one may feel a vermiform collection of individual units (bag of worms), and if there is lacrimal gland involvement, one may see an S-shaped lid with a more prominent lateral ptosis or drooping of the outer lid. In the diffuse neurofibroma, the lids are thickened but one does not detect any underlying individualized units. In patients with either the typical S-shaped eyelid contour or a diffusely invasive mass, or with the suspicion of a plexiform or diffuse neurofibroma, a careful survey should be pursued for café-au-lait spots (Fig. 174–19A), skin neurofibromas (fibroma molluscum) (Fig. 174–19B and C), Lisch iris nodules, axillary freckles, and other ocular stigmata of neurofibromatosis type 1 such as ectropion uveae, pigmented fundus lesions, uveal melanocytic and ganglioneuromatous diffuse thickening, and glaucoma. Thickened corneal nerves, once thought to be part of neurofibromatosis type 1, are now believed to be more commonly associated with multiple endocrine neoplasia syndrome type IIa[24] and IIb.[25] Pulsatile proptosis may be indicative of dysplasia of one or more of the orbital bones, most commonly the greater wing of the sphenoid. The arterial pulsation of the cerebrospinal fluid is thus transmitted to the globe via the bone defect, and this is accentuated with the Valsalva maneuver. In the absence of signs of vascular engorgement, this sign may be pathognomonic of neurofibromatosis type 1 and help to make the diagnosis of a questionable orbital lesion. The radiographic findings of plexiform

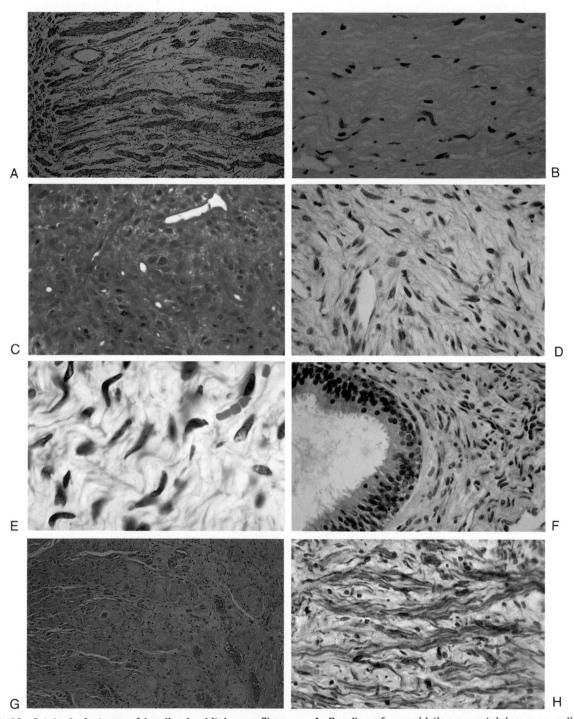

Figure 174–14. Cytologic features of localized orbital neurofibromas. *A,* Bundles of neuroid tissue containing axon cylinders are separated by a myxoid matrix. *B,* Wavy cells with curved nuclei and undulating processes are widely distributed within an eosinophilic matrix that was rich in collagen, as demonstrated by the Masson trichrome. *C,* Compactly arranged cells are widely separated by a collagen-rich interstitial matrix. Note that the cells are ovoid and tend to have nuclei with pointed ends. The capillaries are not thickened with redundant basement membrane, as in a schwannoma. *D,* Wavy cells in a less compact arrangement in comparison with *C. E,* Comma-shaped and undulating nuclei are highly typical of neurofibroma. *F,* Undulating neurofibromatous tissue embraces a draining duct of the lacrimal gland, from the case illustrated in Figure 174–13*E* and *F. G,* Laminated sensory-type corpuscles are not unusual in focal areas of neurofibroma. *H,* Wavy bundles of cells are stained positive for S100 protein, but the cells in between these bundles are negative-staining. Neurofibromas are heterogeneous in their immunohistochemical reactions because of a multiplicity of participating cell types, only the Schwann cells being S100-positive.

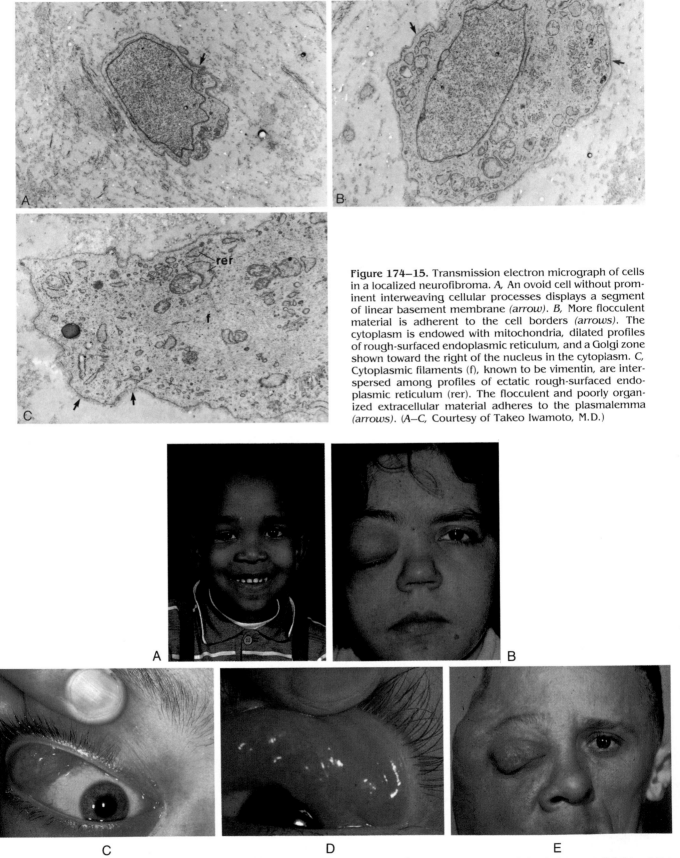

Figure 174–15. Transmission electron micrograph of cells in a localized neurofibroma. A, An ovoid cell without prominent interweaving cellular processes displays a segment of linear basement membrane (arrow). B, More flocculent material is adherent to the cell borders (arrows). The cytoplasm is endowed with mitochondria, dilated profiles of rough-surfaced endoplasmic reticulum, and a Golgi zone shown toward the right of the nucleus in the cytoplasm. C, Cytoplasmic filaments (f), known to be vimentin, are interspersed among profiles of ectatic rough-surfaced endoplasmic reticulum (rer). The flocculent and poorly organized extracellular material adheres to the plasmalemma (arrows). (A–C, Courtesy of Takeo Iwamoto, M.D.)

Figure 174–16. Plexiform orbital and eyelid neurofibromas in neurofibromatosis type 1 (NF1). A, Minimal degree of right orbital involvement with a plexiform neurofibroma has caused infiltration of the lacrimal gland and the lateral aspect of the right upper lid. B, More extensive eyelid and orbital infiltration. C, Eversion of the upper eyelid reveals massive enlargement of the palpebral lobe of the lacrimal gland from infiltration by plexiform neurofibroma. (Courtesy of Frederick Blodi, M.D.) D, Eversion reveals multiple small translucent submucosal neurofibromatous units of the superior tarsal and forniceal conjunctiva. E, This adult had massive facial deformity resulting from an extensive plexiform neurofibroma involving the eyelid and orbit. (B and E, Courtesy of Martha Farber, M.D., and Morton Smith, M.D.)

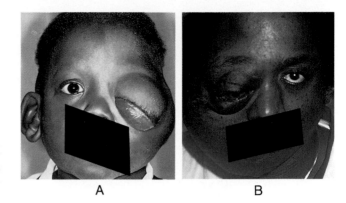

Figure 174–17. Massive orbital, eyelid, and facial deformity from infiltration with diffuse neurofibroma in NF1. *A,* A child had a very full upper eyelid and massive infiltration of the orbit. *B,* An adult had more extensive overgrowth of the ocular adnexal and facial tissues. (Courtesy of Dr. Sterkers.)

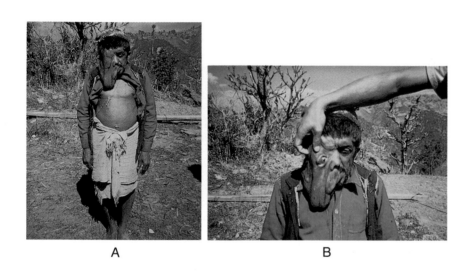

Figure 174–18. Elephantiasis neuromatosa of the face in NF1. *A,* A pendulous mass obscures the eyeball and also involves the right hemifacial structures. *B,* By elevating the redundant skin of the upper eyelid, a nonfunctioning globe is revealed. (*A* and *B,* Courtesy of William N. Hawks, M.D.)

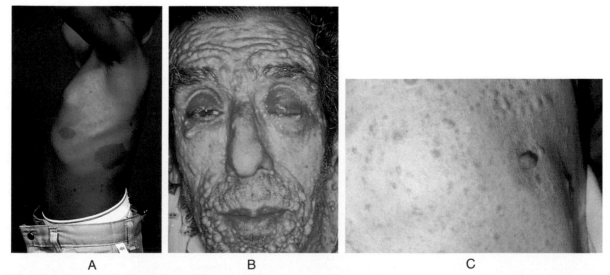

Figure 174–19. Cutaneous manifestations of NF1. *A,* Different-sized café-au-lait flat patches appear in the lateral abdominal skin. *B,* Myriad cutaneous neurofibromas (fibroma molluscum) involve the facial tissues, including the eyelids. There is no involvement of the deeper orbital tissues. The more severe the superficial subcutaneous involvement with these tumors, the less likely there will be deep orbital lesions. (Courtesy of Martha Farber, M.D., and Morton Smith, M.D.) *C,* Fibroma molluscum of the chest wall skin.

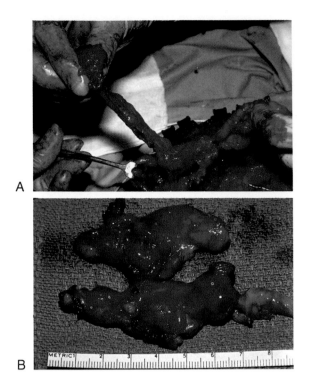

Figure 174–20. Plexiform neurofibroma in NF1. *A,* Spaghetti-like structures are being excised from the orbit. *B,* Interconnecting units of neurofibromatous tissue are removed by decompressive orbital surgery. (*A* and *B,* Courtesy of Arthur Grove, M.D.)

and diffuse neurofibromas are discussed in a later section.

PATHOLOGY

In the plexiform neurofibroma, which is pathognomonic for neurofibromatosis type 1, the tissues are expanded by recognizable neural units (Fig. 174–20), each of which possesses an outer multilaminar perineural sheath and variably cellular to myxoid endoneural compartments that feature Schwann cells, endoneural fibroblasts, and axons that can be brought out with the Bodian stain (Fig. 174–21). Luxol fast blue may reveal axonal myelination by Schwann cells. The perineural

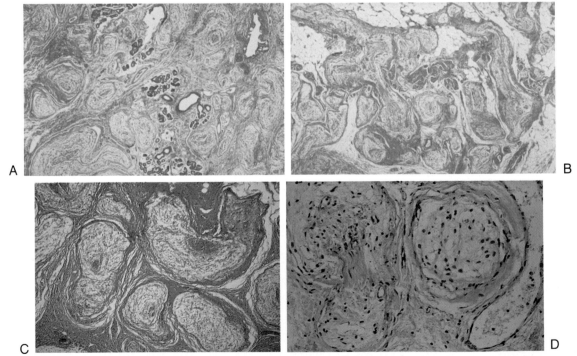

Figure 174–21. Plexiform orbital neurofibroma. *A,* Individual units of the neurofibromatous tissue that infiltrate the lacrimal grand. *B,* Similar units within the orbital fat. (*A* and *B,* Courtesy of Martha Farber, M.D. and William Frayer, M.D.) *C,* The loose neurofibromatous units are each individually ensheathed by a multilaminar and fibrotic perineurium. (Courtesy of Martha Farber, M.D., and Morton Smith, M.D.) *D,* The endoneurial compartments of the neurofibromatous units are variably cellular and myxoid.

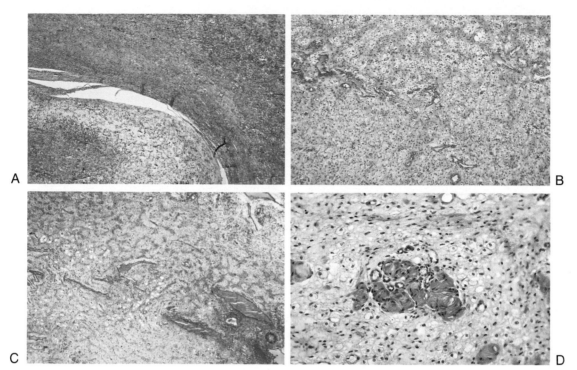

Figure 174–22. Diffuse neurofibroma in NF1. *A,* Compact neurofibromatous tissue is shown toward the upper right; it has separated through a cleavage plane with a malformed nerve shown toward the bottom left. *B,* Vascularized and compactly arranged tissues are present toward the bottom, and paler-staining cells are separated by a capillary network above. *C,* Most of this portion of the tumor is pale-staining owing to xanthomatous change of the tumor cells. The tumor tissue is subdivided by a luxuriant capillary network. *D,* A focus of tactile corpuscle formation. Note that the surrounding cells are vacuolated xanthoma cells, probably a transformation of the tumor cells themselves rather than infiltrating histiocytic cells.

cells will be epithelial membrane antigen positive, whereas the variably conspicuous Schwann cells will be S100 positive. The perineural cell may be identified ultrastructurally in these tumors[13]; basement membrane formation, pinocytic vesicles, subplasmalemmal plaque-like densities, and actin filaments are featured.

In contradistinction, the diffuse neurofibroma is not subdivided or demarcated by perineural units and may occasionally be seen in isolation from neurofibromatosis type 1. One observes a monotonous spindle cell proliferation that replaces all of the involved tissues (Fig. 174–22 *A* and *B*); there is a variable amount of collagen, and myxoid stromal changes are usually inconspicuous. The tumor cells are wavy, but not as frequently bundled into individual units as in an isolated neurofibroma. Xanthomatous changes can be detected in older lesions (Fig. 174–22*C*). Many of the cells will not be stained for the S100 protein, suggesting that they are endoneural fibroblasts. Laminated corpuscular structures may also be seen (Fig. 174–22*D*).

The major differential diagnosis of the plexiform neurofibroma is a post-amputation neuroma (see later), in which individual compact units of Schwann cells are separated by a fibrous stroma, but in which a distinct multilaminar perineurium cannot be observed.

MANAGEMENT

The management of both plexiform and diffuse neurofibroma is often highly unsatisfactory. Diffuse and plexiform neurofibromas are much more difficult to excise than are localized neurofibromas or schwannomas, since they intercalate between important ocular tissues such as the muscles, nerves, and lacrimal gland. Complete excision is the exception, not the rule; one should anticipate robust bleeding during surgery because these lesions are richly vascularized, and it might be advisable to type and cross-match blood preoperatively in case a blood transfusion is required. After debulking operations there will almost always be regrowth of tumor. In many cases, expectant management is advisable. Sometimes there is a relative quiescence after the growth spurt of adolescence. Although those neurofibromas elsewhere in the body in association with neurofibromatosis type 1 have about a 10 percent probability of malignant transformation, this has not quantified for orbital neurofibromas and is relatively uncommon.

In cases with massive disfigurement and a blind eye, enucleation, partial exenteration, or complete exenteration may become necessary, especially if intracranial invasion is likely. Collaboration among the orbital surgeon, neurosurgeon, and plastic surgeon may be necessary to deal with some of the more extensive lesions in which imaginative approaches are often used.[26] The carbon dioxide laser has been resorted to for performing subtotal ablation of plexiform neurofibromas.[27, 28] It allows ablation of soft tissue with relatively precise margins and to a controllable depth with good hemostasis. It does not differentiate, however, between a tumor and normal tissue. Initial experience is encouraging, but it has not been widely applied, and its benefit over standard techniques remains to be clarified.

It should be remembered that patients with plexiform and diffuse neurofibromas are also likely to suffer other vision-threatening tumors of the optic nerve that can accompany neurofibromatosis type 1, most typically either a pilocytic astrocytoma, or less commonly a primary nerve sheath meningioma.

Malignant Peripheral Nerve Sheath Tumors

Also called malignant schwannoma or neurofibrosarcoma, this tumor is described in greater detail in Chapter 178 but will be succinctly discussed here. Malignant peripheral nerve sheath tumors (MPNST) are rare tumors of the orbit that arise from the peripheral nerve sheath but do not always betray a Schwann cell origin ultrastructurally. Like isolated neurofibromas and schwannomas, these tumors appear to preferentially arise from branches of the trigeminal nerve (Fig. 174–23A). They are encountered in both the presence and the absence of neurofibromatosis type 1.

In one study of eight malignant peripheral nerve sheath tumors encountered in the orbit,[29] two arose in the setting of von Recklinghausen's neurofibromatosis. MPNST are seen in older individuals, although when encountered in a setting of orbital plexiform or diffuse neurofibroma of von Recklinghausen's disease, they can be discovered in the second and third decades. There is a remarkable case of an orbital MPNST arising in a 5-year-old child in an association with a myxoid neurofibroma, but with no evidence of neurofibromatosis type 1 (see Fig. 174–23B and C); the patient has survived with a functioning globe 9 yr after local excision.[30]

Microscopically, the tumors can consist of spindle cells (Fig. 174–24), epithelioid cells, or a mixture of both (biphasic pattern). MPNST can even have a heteroplastic component of cartilaginous cells. The tumors have been reported to occur in patients with a preexisting benign-appearing lesion, suggesting a sarcomatous transformation.[7, 31] Striated muscle components have been described in some MPNST ("Triton tumors"); although this entity has not yet been described as a primary orbital lesion, there is a reported case of a sinus tumor that invaded the orbit (Fig. 174–25).[32]

A typical presentation of these tumors is as a circumscribed deep lid nodule, often in the superomedial anterior orbital quadrant (see Fig. 174–23A), consistent with an origin from the supraorbital nerve. However, other orbital nerves may be involved.[31] They may feel cystic on palpation. Hypophthalmos may be evident due to their mass effect. Pain can be produced spontaneously, as well as hypesthesia of the skin in the distribution of the involved nerve.[17] These tumors display inexorable growth, with a predilection for intraneural growth posteriorly through the superior orbital fissure into the middle cranial fossa up to the trigeminal ganglion; there are even autopsy cases showing further spread of the tumor along the trigeminal nerve roots to the pons.[29] The only chance for cure in these patients, once the diagnosis is intimated by pain and hypesthesia, is accurate pathologic diagnosis and early radical surgery. Failure to diagnose the tumor leads to delays in definitive therapy and recurrence, by which time the tumor may already have reached the brain and may be inescapably fatal. Alternatively, metastasis to regional lymph nodes, the lungs, or the bony skeleton may occur. The prognosis in malignant schwannoma is poor. Of 13 patients reported in the literature, only four patients

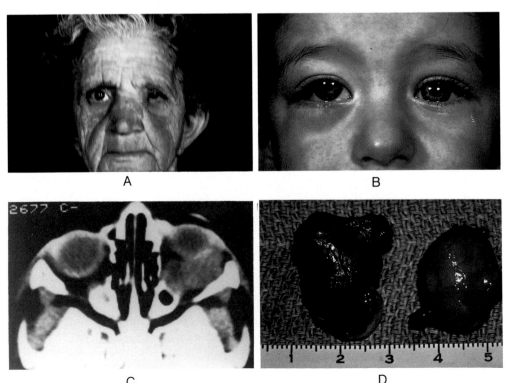

Figure 174–23. Malignant peripheral nerve sheath tumors (malignant schwannoma). A, An elderly patient had a left superonasal orbital mass that had produced hypesthesia in the distribution of the supraorbital nerve. B, A 5-year-old boy presented with a rapidly developing right orbital mass, presumed clinically to be a rhabdomyosarcoma. C, The axial CT scan of the patient shown in B revealed a bilobed lesion, the lobe in the more nasal and posterior orbit having a looser texture, whereas the more lateral and larger unit in this projection appeared to be solid. D, At the time of surgery the bilobed tumor consisted of a myxoid neurofibroma, shown on the left, and a more solid malignant schwannoma, shown on the right. Nine years after local excision the patient had a functioning globe, no orbital recurrence, and no distant metastases. (B–D, Courtesy of Albert Hornblass, M.D.)

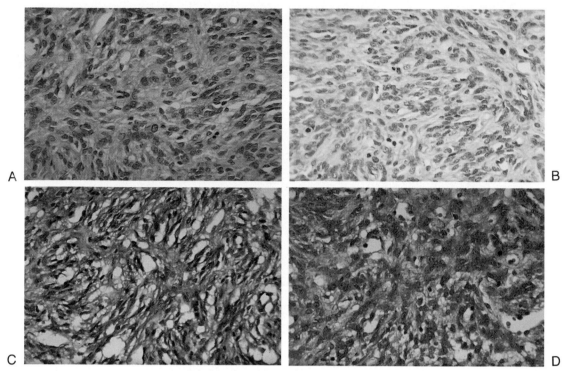

Figure 174–24. Malignant peripheral nerve sheath tumor (MPNST) of the orbit. *A* and *B,* These mitotically active spindle cells have only a faintly fascicular arrangement. There is a delicate fibrillary background consisting of interweaving cellular processes. In *B,* there is a suggestion of nuclear palisading. The tumor cells were S100-negative and vimentin-positive. Many tumors deemed to be MPNSTs are S100-negative, either because they did not originate from Schwann cells or because the MPNST lost this property in the process of malignant transformation. *C,* A more myxoid area in which small clusters of cells are separated by watery extracellular matrix material. *D,* Because of the nuclear palisading, consideration was given to the lesion being a leiomyosarcoma, but the Masson trichrome shown here failed to demonstrate cytoplasmic filamentation, nor was desmin or smooth muscle specification identifiable. The red-staining structures are the nuclei; note also the absence of blue-staining extracellular collagen.

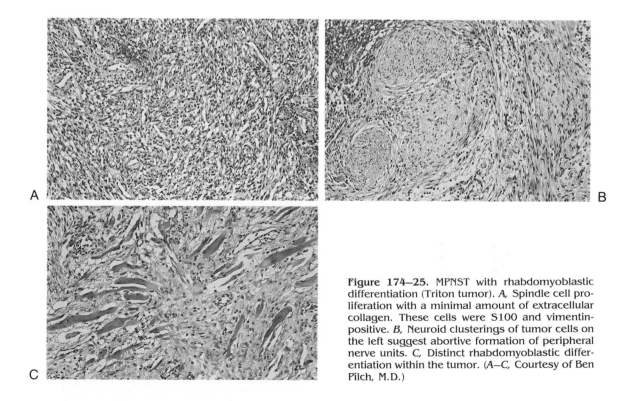

Figure 174–25. MPNST with rhabdomyoblastic differentiation (Triton tumor). *A,* Spindle cell proliferation with a minimal amount of extracellular collagen. These cells were S100 and vimentin-positive. *B,* Neuroid clusterings of tumor cells on the left suggest abortive formation of peripheral nerve units. *C,* Distinct rhabdomyoblastic differentiation within the tumor. (*A–C,* Courtesy of Ben Pilch, M.D.)

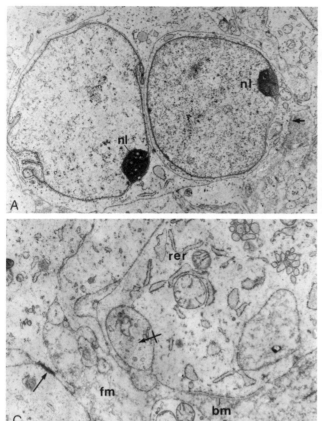

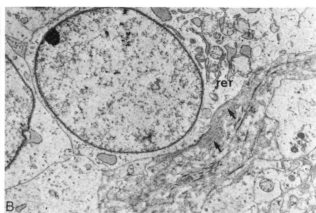

Figure 174–26. Transmission electron micrographs of an MPNST. *A,* The tumor cells are electron-lucent and only focally demonstrate basement membrane material *(arrow).* The nucleoli (nl) are large and peripherally placed at the nuclear membrane. *B,* The electron-lucent cells possess rough-surfaced endoplasmic reticulum (rer). There is a focal deposition of redundant-based membrane material *(arrows).* *C,* Cellular processes enfold one another *(crossed arrow).* The *uncrossed arrow* indicates an intercellular desmosome. Partial basement membrane (bm) is apparent, and most of the extracellular matrix is composed of flocculent material (fm). The electron-lucent cytoplasm contains short profiles of rough-surfaced endoplasmic reticulum (rer). (*A–C,* Courtesy of Takeo Iwamoto, M.D.)

survived for more than 5 yr.[31] Radiotherapy and chemotherapy have been used for palliation.

The pathologic and ultrastructural patterns of malignant peripheral nerve sheath tumor are somewhat heterogeneous (Fig. 174–26). Some of these tumors arise from Schwann cells and are therefore S100 positive, but others may arise from perineural cells or endoneural fibroblasts, or from Schwann cells that no longer express Schwann cell characteristics. For this reason, it is probably best to refer to these tumors with the more noncommittal term of malignant peripheral nerve sheath tumor rather than malignant schwannoma. It should not be forgotten that amelanotic melanomas (both primary orbital and metastatic) are typically S100 positive and can closely simulate an MPNST; antimelanoma monoclonal antibodies or the ultrastructural demonstration of melanosomes would be useful in making this diagnosis.

OTHER NEURAL AND NEUROID TUMORS

Amputation Neuroma

Amputation neuromas (Fig. 174–27) are localized proliferations of Schwann cells, axons, and fibroblasts occurring after an amputation of a peripheral nerve. The injury may be from transection or crush. In the orbit they are usually reported after surgical trauma,[33] particularly enucleation or other periocular surgery, but they may also occur after blunt trauma.[34] Pain and "phantom limb" sensations can accompany these tumors; there are two remarkable cases of conjunctival inclusion cysts having an amputation neuroma in their walls.[35] As mentioned earlier, Schwann cell units are separated by a fibrous stroma, but there is no clear-cut multilaminar perineurium. Amputation neuromas are treated with excision.

Recent research is helpful in understanding the putative pathophysiology of amputation neuroma, as well as other Schwann cell proliferations. There is evidence that chemical signals from axons increase Schwann cell mitosis. For example, fractions from growth cones, which are present at the leading edge of extending neurites, cause proliferation of cultured Schwann cells.[36] A variety of growth factors act in vitro on Schwann cells, including platelet-derived growth factor, basic fibroblast growth factor, and glial growth factor.[37, 38] Myelin basic protein, as well as other myelin components, may cause Schwann cell proliferation.[39] Cytokines, such as interleukin-1, have been implicated in control of Schwann cell proliferation.[40] Alternatively, Schwann cell proliferation in schwannomas may be a result of a loss of an autocrine inhibitory activity, such as is expressed in short-term Schwann cell cultures.[41, 42] One such candidate factor is a fraction of fibronectin.[43] Finally, there is some evidence that neurofibromas contain mitogens[44] and inhibitors[45] of Schwann cells.

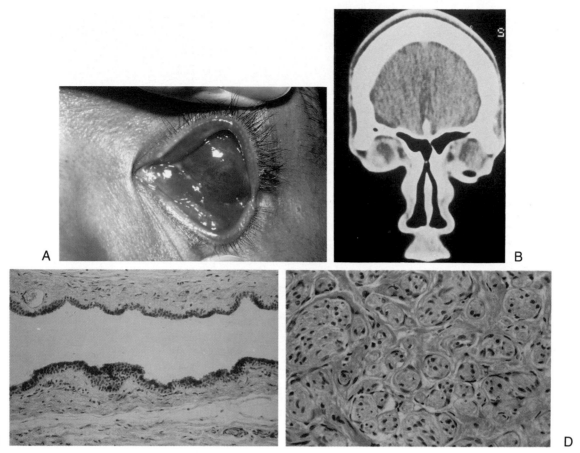

Figure 174–27. Postamputation orbital neuroma. *A,* Twenty-five years after removal of a phthisical eye, a transilluminable cystic lesion is present in the orbit. *B,* Coronal CT scan reveals a cystic lesion in the orbit with an adjacent round density at its inferonasal border. *C,* The excised cyst is lined by nonkeratinizing squamous epithelium containing mucus-producing goblet cells. *D,* In the inferonasal solid nodule, there is a proliferation of neuromatous tissue. An indistinct perineurium surrounds each unit and fuses with a fibrotic stroma. (*A–D,* From Messmer EP, Camara J, Boniuk M, Font R: Amputation neuroma of the orbit. A report of two cases and review of the literature. Published courtesy of Ophthalmology 91:1420–1423, 1984.)

Optic Nerve Tumors

Optic nerve gliomas (Fig. 174–28), which are more properly referred to as juvenile pilocytic astrocytomas, are fusiform, ordinarily benign enlargements of the optic nerve, contained within an intact but sometimes attenuated dural sheath.[46–48] These tumors usually become symptomatic in the first decade, before most benign peripheral nerve sheath tumors manifest themselves. Pilocytic astrocytomas consist of spindle cells and may frequently exhibit mucinous changes that could invite the mistaken diagnosis of a schwannoma or neurofibroma. In a pilocytic astrocytoma there is a distinct sparseness of extracellular collagen; both the reticulin and the periodic acid–Schiff (PAS) stains fail to reveal intercellular linear deposits of fibrillar material. This material, which on the ultrastructural level corresponds to basement membranes in schwannomas and other tumors, is not elaborated by astrocytoma cells, except when they abut stroma. Pilocytic astrocytomas contain cytoplasmic glial intermediate filaments, which can be stained positively with immunohistochemical methods

Figure 174–28. Primary optic nerve glioma (juvenile pilocytic astrocytoma). *A,* Coronal CT scan discloses a well-defined mass lesion behind the globe that is indissociable from the optic nerve shadow. *B,* The tumor is restrained by a thinned dural sheath, shown on the right. The subdural proliferation of tumor tissue is beset with numerous carrot-shaped eosinophilic structures (Verhoeff bodies or Rosenthal fibers), which are not seen in peripheral nerve sheath neurofibromas or schwannomas.

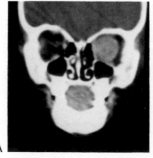

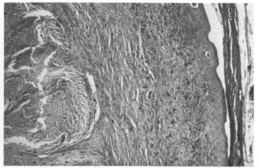

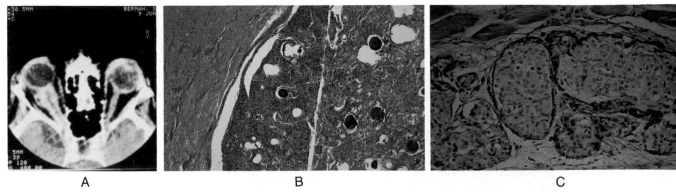

Figure 174–29. Primary optic nerve sheath meningioma. *A,* Axial CT scan reveals a central radiolucent shadow running down the middle of an irregularly thickened optic nerve (railroad tracking). The irregularity of the margins of the swollen optic nerve suggests infiltration of the dura and invasion of the surrounding orbital soft tissues. *B,* Numerous dark-staining psammoma bodies are present in a transitional cell meningioma of the optic nerve meninges. The optic nerve is compressed on the left. *C,* Meningothelial nests and whorls of cells are infiltrating the orbital extraocular muscles, fibers of which are shown above. Some of the tumor cells have intranuclear vacuoles of herniated cytoplasm. The nesting pattern might invite the mistaken diagnosis of squamous cell carcinoma.

for glial fibrillary acidic protein (GFAP). In contradistinction, schwannomas and neurofibromas are GFAP-negative but are positive for the intermediate filament vimentin. Rosenthal fibers are astrocytic cytoplasmic inclusions seen in gliomas, Alexander's disease, and other disorders; they contain α-B-crystallin, which is probably ubiquitinated.[49, 50] Their appearance may be helpful in diagnosing optic nerve gliomas.

Meningiomas (Fig. 174–29) have a predilection for women in their forties. They arise primarily from the meningothelial cells of the arachnoid of the optic nerve and often invade the dura.[46-48] They may exceedingly rarely develop in ectopias of meningothelial cells entrapped within the perineurium or epineurium of orbital nerves (and therefore would be primary within the soft tissues of the orbit and totally separate from the optic nerve). They may also secondarily invade the orbit from the cranial side, most typically from the sphenoid bone, from the paramedian and basofrontal regions of the skull, and most rarely, from ectopias in the paranasal sinuses or the glabellar region of the nose. Meningiomas arising from the sinuses must be distinguished from squamous cell carcinoma. Virtually all primary optic nerve meningiomas consist of polyhedral meningothelial cells, with a tendency to form whorls, and sometimes there may be interspersed spindle cells, which in combination with the meningothelial cells are assigned to the category of transitional meningioma. They are characterized by the pathognomonic psammoma bodies, the origin of which probably is adjacent to or at small vessels, based on the presence of type IV collagen,[51, 52] and which typically acquire calcium deposits. Purely fibroblastic meningiomas arise hardly ever in the optic nerve but may be observed in secondary invasion from the cranial side. Meningioma cells frequently have intranuclear vacuoles; contain the cytoplasmic intermediate filament vimentin, often in copious amounts; and may display surface membrane positivity for EMA. Although both meningiomas and squamous cell carcinomas have desmosomes and are EMA-positive, the former is cytokeratin-negative, in contradistinction to the latter.

Esthesioneuroblastoma

Esthesioneuroblastoma is an uncommon neuroectodermal tumor of olfactory epithelium, typically of the superior nasal cavity; it rarely involves the orbit.[53] The orbit is invaded as the tumor destroys bone locally and transgresses the sinus walls to intrude on the orbital soft tissues. Radiographically, the lesion appears as a homogeneous soft tissue mass with bone erosion, molding, or rarely hyperostosis (Fig. 174–30).[54] Pathologically, the diagnosis of esthesioneuroblastoma may be difficult. The tumor consists of small round neuroblastic cells (not unlike those in a retinoblastoma) that exhibit mitotic activity. The cells grow in cords, islands, and lobules, divided by a variably pronounced fibrovascular stroma. Within the trabecular units, the tumor cells are often dyscohesive but may demonstrate an eosinophilic background of interweaving cytoplasmic processes in the better differentiated forms, which can also form rosettes and neuroepithelial structures (Fig. 174–31). The nuclei have a distinctive finely stippled appearance, as not infrequently encountered in neural crest and neuroectodermal tumors.

Immunohistochemical studies are quite valuable in making the diagnosis of esthesioneuroblastoma in questionable cases, when the differential diagnosis includes other primitive round-cell tumors, including occasionally lymphoma. Staining for neuron-specific enolase, neurofilaments, S100, or HNK-1 (with the Leu-7 antibody) and not for epithelial, lymphoid, or muscle markers may be diagnostic.[55, 56] Neurosecretory dense core granules are seen on electron microscopy. Esthesioneuroblastoma is aggressive, recurring locally, as well as metastasizing to distant sites. Treatment is a combination of excision, radiotherapy, and sometimes chemotherapy.

Neuroblastoma

Neuroblastoma, while commonly metastatic to the orbit of children, is extremely unusual as a primary

Figure 174–30. Esthesioneuroblastoma. A, Axial CT scan demonstrates involvement of the ethmoid sinuses, with bowing of the medial lamina papyracea on one side and definite invasion of the orbital soft tissues on the other. B, Coronal projection of case shown in A, indicating also destruction of the roof of the nose in the region of the lamina cribrosa. C, Axial CT scan of another case with prominent destruction of the nasal and medial orbital bones and with soft tissue replacement of the anterior and medial orbit. D, Higher in the orbit another axial CT scan shows invasion of the anterior cranial fossa along with massive medial orbital bone destruction. (A–D, Courtesy of Michael Joseph, M.D.)

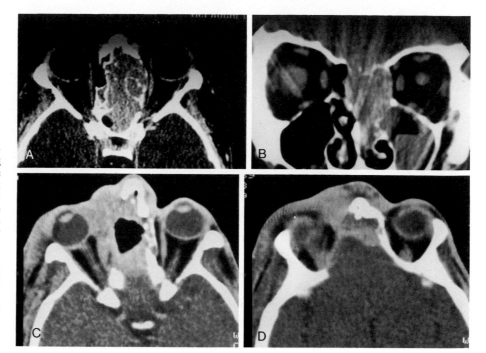

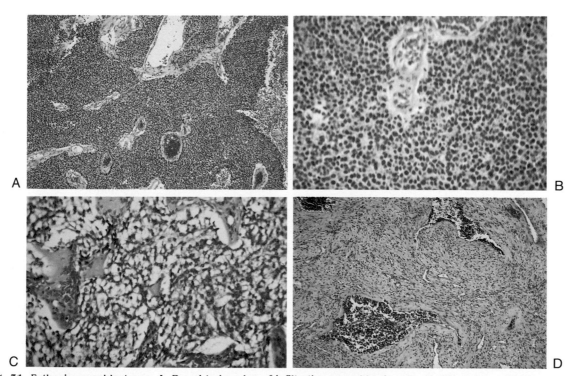

Figure 174–31. Esthesioneuroblastoma. A, Broad trabeculae of infiltrating neuroblastic cells. B, The tumor cells are generally round and mitotically active. C, In some tumors, there may be a more delicate background neuropil of interweaving eosinophilic processes. D, Smaller clusters of neuroblastic cells are separated by a more abundant fibrotic stroma. (A–D, Courtesy of Ben Pilch, M.D.)

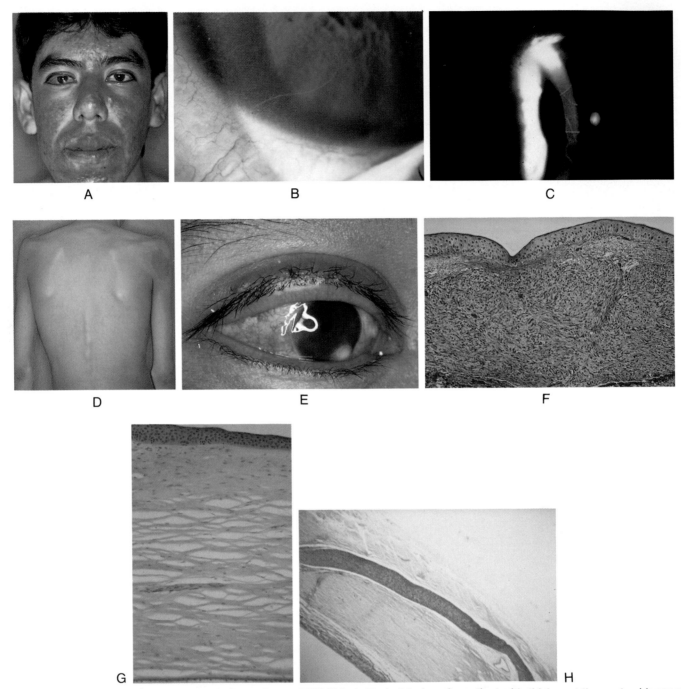

Figure 174–32. Multiple endocrine neoplasia syndrome (MEN IIb). *A,* Typical facies of a patient with thickened lips and evidence of ocular irritation, particularly on the right. *B,* Several thickened corneal nerves are entering toward the bottom left. *C,* Slit-lamp view of criss-crossing thickened nerves in the paraxial cornea. *D,* The patient has a marfanoid habitus, with a café-au-lait spot in the right periaxillary deltoid region. *E,* Conjunctival irritation, along with a white peripheral conjunctival-corneal neurofibroma. Note the thickening of the eyelid margin and the rostral displacement of the eyelashes into several rows. *F,* A biopsy of the white corneal lesion displays wavy bundles of neurofibromatous tissue beneath the nonkeratinizing conjunctival squamous epithelium. (*A, B, D–F,* Courtesy of Narsing Rao, M.D.) *G,* A thickened corneal nerve is shown in the lower third of the corneal button. Electron microscopy revealed that the nerves are not myelinated. (*C* and *G,* Courtesy of Gordon Klintworth, M.D.) *H,* A massively thickened long posterior ciliary nerve in a scleral canal. (Courtesy of Alan Friedman, M.D.)

tumor in this location. In one report of a well-differentiated primary orbital neuroblastoma that was recurrent and resistant to radiation, orbital exenteration was eventually necessary because of the potential for extension intracranially.[57] This tumor, with cells containing neurosecretory granules on a fine neurophil, forming perivascular and Wright rosettes, and not destructive of bone, should be distinguished from neuroendocrine carcinomas, which typically present in the orbit after invasion from the paranasal sinuses.[58, 59] In the latter tumor, the neurosecretory granules are typically larger than neuroblastoma, and the tumor cells grouped in lobules on a background of fibrous stroma, rather than a neuropil.[57, 59]

Multiple Endocrine Neoplasia Type IIb

Multiple endocrine neoplasia (MEN) type IIb (Fig. 174–32) is an autosomal dominantly inherited syndrome consisting of thickened corneal nerves (presenting in the first decade), medullary cancer of the thyroid (presenting in the second decade), pheochromocytoma (presenting in the third decade), a marfanoid habitus, and mucosal neuromas. In addition to thickened corneal nerves, other intraocular nerves and probably orbital nerves are also enlarged, but not in sufficient proportion to cause proptosis. There is a distinctive thickening of the lid margin with rostral displacement of the eyelashes, multiple epibulbar neuromas, and thickened lips. Axillary café-au-lait spots and lingual, bowel, and periungual neuromas are frequently seen. These neuromas consist of proliferating perineural and Schwann cell elements,[60] and may include subconjunctival neuromas.[61] This syndrome has been confused with neurofibromatosis type 1 because of the overlap of several clinical features. The bowel and uveal tract may also be diffusely thickened from a diffuse ganglioneuromatosis, another feature not uncommonly seen in neurofibromatosis type 1. Many patients with MEN IIb die at early ages, usually because of the development of amyloid-producing medullary carcinoma of the thyroid. These tumors, which may be bilateral and secrete calcitonin, develop in the second decade or after and are often diagnosed too late, with local and distant metastases eventuating. It is rare for an ophthalmologist to be able to alert a patient and an internist to the possibility of a fatal disease from such a singular finding as thickening of the corneal nerves.

Other Neuroid Tumors

Paraganglioma, or chemodectoma, is a well-vascularized tumor arising from nonchromaffin (chemosensory) paraganglion cells, which in the orbit are presumed to be those of the ciliary ganglion, or ectopically associated with peripheral nerves. Treatment is excisional. The malignant counterpart has traditionally been considered to be the alveolar soft part sarcoma, which is highly aggressive, may metastasize, and is treated with radical excision; support for a neural origin of this tumor,

however, is tenuous. Granular cell schwannoma, or myoblastoma, is a rare tumor consisting of cords of round or polygonal cells containing PAS-positive granules, possibly arising from Schwann cells that have become facultative phagocytes,[62] although some believe that they are of mesodermal origin.[63] Treatment is excisional. These tumors are more thoroughly discussed in Chapter 178.

COMPARATIVE OVERVIEW OF RADIOGRAPHIC AND ULTRASONOGRAPHIC DIAGNOSIS

Radiographic modalities may be useful in studying the anatomic extent and tissue nature of peripheral nerve tumors. Unfortunately, they are not always diagnostic, either in distinguishing these tumors from other solid tumors of the orbit or in determining whether they are benign or malignant.[64] In many cases, a combination of modalities may also be insufficient.[65]

The CT appearance of schwannomas and localized neurofibromas is relatively nonspecific, typically revealing a single intraconal or extraconal rounded mass that does not extend to the orbital apex,[8] unlike what is seen in optic nerve neoplasms.[66] Because these lesions arise from peripheral nerves, an ovoid or fusiform shape, with the long axis in the direction of the involved nerve, may be seen.[62] Calcification may be present within the tumor. Erosion and expansion, but not invasion, of the bone orbit may be demonstrated.[8, 66, 67] The tumor may enhance early with contrast, although perhaps not as much as in hemangiopericytoma; the cavernous hemangioma does not enhance early because it is a stagnant vascular lesion rather isolated from the orbital vessels. In certain cases, contrast enhancement may be absent in peripheral nerve tumors.[68]

MRI was heralded by its ability to distinguish types of tumors on the basis of differences in signals from protons in different microenvironments. It is now clear that a wide variety of orbital tumors appear very similar on MRI. Similar to fibrous histiocytoma, hemangiopericytoma, and cavernous hemangioma, both neurofibroma and schwannoma display low signal on T_1-weighted images and high signal on T_2-weighted images[10, 67, 69]; however, if blood-breakdown products or a substantial amount of lipid accumulation is present in the lesion, there may be foci of high signal on T_1-weighted images.

High-resolution MRI may help to distinguish between schwannoma and neurofibroma on the basis of the peripheral location of the originating nerve with respect to the tumor in the former and the more common absence of a capsule in the latter.[69] The use of the paramagnetic contrast agent gadolinium diethylenetriaminepentaacetic acid with T_1-weighted images may best delineate the anatomy of these tumors.[70] Whereas localized neurofibromas and schwannomas on imaging studies offer a round or ovoid shape in most cases, each may also have internal soft tissue variegations on both CT scanning and MRI. In the case of neurofibromas, these textural density gradients are the result of the

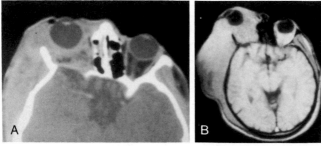

Figure 174–33. Diffuse orbital and periorbital neurofibroma in a patient with NF1. *A,* The soft tissue mass shows a homogeneous density in this axial CT scan. *B,* In a T₁-weighted MRI study, the lesion is also displayed as a homogeneous mass extending into the temple and cheek regions. Rather than having low signal intensity, as occurs in most orbital tumors in T₁-weighted images, this lesion has a surprising degree of signal intensity comparable to the fat shown in the contralateral retroorbital space. The reason for the high signal intensities in this case was the widespread and heavy deposition of xanthomatous cells throughout the lesion. The study depicted in both *A* and *B* corresponds to the patient shown in Figure 174–13A. *(A* and *B,* Courtesy of Dr. Sterkers.)

formation, intense xanthomatization of some of the tumor cells, and even hemosiderin-laden macrophages resulting from blood-breakdown products from the leaky tumor microvasculature. Distinguishing malignant schwannoma from more benign orbital schwannomas or neurofibromas is difficult. In three cases for which CT was performed, a circumscribed homogeneous mass was thought to be nonspecific for distinguishing the former from the latter.[31] Sophisticated MR image analysis techniques may help to separate benign peripheral nerve tumors from those that are malignant.[71] Finally, in the differential diagnosis of circumscribed cystic lesions in the retrobulbar or peripheral orbital compartments without an osseous defect (thus ruling out most dermoid cysts), the possibilities are primarily limited to schwannoma, respiratory choristoma, focal hemorrhagic lymphangioma, necrosis in a primary orbital melanoma, and necrosis in a metastasis.

While localized neurofibromas will have smooth borders with some surface irregularities or may appear identical to schwannomas on CT scanning, the plexiform and diffuse neurofibromas are typically diffusely invasive, with irregular contours. CT and MRI scanning may be helpful in differentiating plexiform from diffuse neurofibromas in the setting of neurofibromatosis type 1. Although both of these conditions may be associated with defects in the sphenoid bone, the diffuse neurofibroma has a homogeneous soft tissue texture in which

variably intense deposition of mucopolysaccharides, such as hyaluronic acid. If large pockets are present within the lesion, the overall density of the corresponding region on MRI would be isointense with muscle. In the case of schwannoma, there may also be major cyst

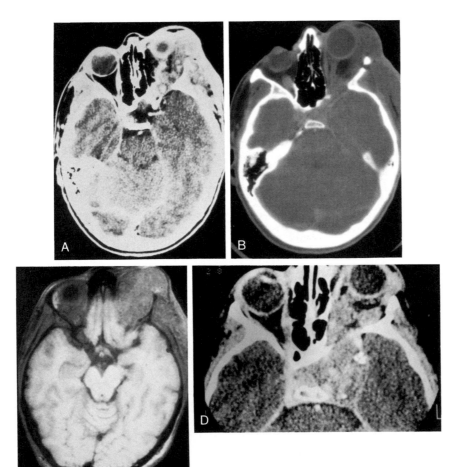

Figure 174–34. Plexiform neurofibroma in NF1. *A,* Axial CT scan discloses heterogeneous subunits of the lesional tissue. *B,* A bone window demonstrates the characteristic defect in the sphenoid bone, which can lead to pulsatile exophthalmos. *C,* MRI study in the axial plane also discloses subunits within the lesion, but less clearly than in the CT scan in *A.* Bone abnormalities are less well shown in MRI studies compared with CT scanning. *(A–C,* Courtesy of Arthur Grove, M.D.) *D,* A plexiform neurofibroma with orbital involvement and a sphenoid bone defect. Note especially the involvement of the texturally variegated tissue in the cavernous sinus region. This is due to extension of the plexiform neurofibromatous tissue from the orbit into the cavernous sinus through the superior orbital fissure. (Courtesy of Nancy Newman, M.D.)

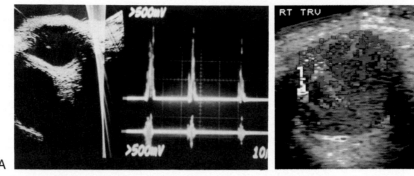

Figure 174–35. Ultrasonographic studies of orbital tumors. *A,* B-scan of an orbital schwannoma is shown in the left half of the study. Notice the circumscription of the lesion and the excellent transmission of sound to the posterior orbit. A portion of the orbital wall reflection is shown toward the bottom left. The A-scan ultrasonogram on the right demonstrates few internal acoustic interfaces. (Courtesy of D. Jackson Coleman, M.D.) *B,* A Doppler ultrasonogram of an orbital hemangiopericytoma reveals a high degree of blood flow throughout the lesion. Both neurofibroma and schwannoma would be expected to have less flow. The color coding does not reflect arterial or venous flow, but rather flow in various directions. (Courtesy of Gerald Harris, M.D.)

the infiltrating tumor replaces the fat and other orbital structures (Fig. 174–33). The plexiform neurofibroma, on the other hand, will be disclosed to have heterogeneous soft tissue characteristics (Fig. 174–34) bespeaking the variably sized nerve thickenings and tumoral subunits. Particularly in the case of the plexiform neurofibroma, there may be an extension of lesional tissue through the superior orbital fissure into the cavernous sinus region, which should not be interpreted as reflecting a malignant transformation. If the patient acquires the rapid onset of new symptoms, which by radiographic means can be correlated with the appearance of a more solid mass lesion in the otherwise more heterogeneous nature of the soft tissue swelling, then one should suspect such an event.

Echographic characteristics (Fig. 174–35*A*) of schwannoma and localized neurofibroma may be helpful in preoperatively distinguishing these tumors from other slow-growing rounded tumors of the orbit. For example, ultrasonography reveals many acoustic interfaces in cavernous hemangioma, whereas there will be an attenuation of the reflected echos in the benign peripheral nerve sheath tumors, with low internal reflectivity, good transmission, and rounded contour characteristically present.[67] However, multiply cystic peripheral nerve sheath tumors may demonstrate tissue interfaces with signal attenuation.[8] The cystic areas may be surrounded by smaller cysts with variably reflectivity.[68] Doppler ultrasonography (see Fig. 174–35*B*) may also be useful in diagnosis by disclosing minimal to moderate blood flow, unlike the higher velocity blood flow typical of well-circumscribed hemangiopericytomas and well-vascularized fibrous histiocytomas.

Angiography of peripheral nerve tumors of the head and neck has been systematically described; moderate vascularity with tortuous tumor vessels, puddling of contrast medium, and multiple feeding vessels were thought to be characteristic.[72]

REFERENCES

1. Shields JA, Guibor P: Neurilemoma of the eyelid resembling a recurrent chalazion. Arch Ophthalmol 102:1650, 1984.

2. Smith PA, Damato BE, Ko MK, et al: Anterior uveal neurilemmoma—A rare neoplasm simulating malignant melanoma. Br J Ophthalmol 71:34, 1987.
3. Graham CM, McCartney AC, Buckley RJ: Intrascleral neurilemmoma. Br J Ophthalmol 73:378, 1989.
4. Woog JJ, Albert DM, Solt LC, et al: Neurofibromatosis of the eyelid and orbit. Int Ophthalmol Clin 22:157, 1982.
5. McDonald P, Jakobiec FA, Hornblass A, et al: Benign peripheral nerve sheath tumors (neurofibromas) of the lacrimal gland. Ophthalmology 90:1403, 1983.
6. Knowles DM, Jakobiec FA, McNally L, et al: Lymphoid hyperplasia and malignant lymphoma occurring in the ocular adnexa (orbit, conjunctiva, and eyelids): A prospective multiparametric analysis of 108 cases during 1977 to 1987. Hum Pathol 21:959, 1990.
7. Jakobiec FA, Jones IS: Neurogenic tumors. *In* Duane TS (ed): Clinical Ophthalmology, Chapter 41, Vol 2. Philadelphia, JB Lippincott, 1976.
8. Rootman J, Goldberg C, Robertson W: Primary orbital schwannomas. Br J Ophthalmol 66:194, 1982.
9. Bickler-Bluth ME, Custer PL, Smith ME: Neurilemoma as a presenting feature of neurofibromatosis. Arch Ophthalmol 106:665, 1988.
10. Capps DH, Brodsky MC, Rice CD, et al: Orbital intramuscular schwannoma. Am J Ophthalmol 110:535, 1990.
11. Freedman SF, Elner VM, Donev I, et al: Intraocular neurilemmoma arising from the posterior ciliary nerve in neurofibromatosis: Pathologic findings. Ophthalmology 95:1559, 1988.
12. Faucett DC, Dutton JJ, Bullard DE: Gasserian ganglion schwannoma with orbital extension. Ophthal Plast Reconstr Surg 5:235, 1989.
13. Erlandson RA, Woodruff JM: Peripheral nerve sheath tumors: An electron microscopic study of 43 cases. Cancer 49:273, 1982.
14. White W, Shiu MH, Rosenblum MK, et al: Cellular schwannoma: A clinicopathologic study of 57 patients and 58 tumors. Cancer 66:1266, 1990.
15. Shields JA, Kapustiak J, Arbizo V, et al: Orbital neurilemoma with extension through the superior orbital fissure. Arch Ophthalmol 104:871, 1986.
16. Schatz H: Benign orbital neurilemoma: Sarcomatous transformation in von Recklinghausen's disease. Arch Ophthalmol 86:268, 1971.
17. Krohel GB, Rosenberg PN, Wright JE, et al: Localized orbital neurofibromas. Am J Ophthalmol 100:458, 1985.
18. Della Rocca RC, Roen J, Labay GR, et al: Isolated neurofibroma of the orbit. Ophthalmic Surg 16:634, 1985.
19. Shields JA, Shields CL, Lieb WE, et al: Multiple orbital neurofibromas unassociated with von Recklinghausen's disease. Arch Ophthalmol 108:80, 1990.
20. Harris GJ, Jakobiec FA: Cavernous hemangioma of the orbit: A clinicopathological analysis of sixty-six cases. *In* Jakobiec FA (ed): Ocular and Adnexal Tumors. Birmingham, AL, Aesculapius Publishing Company, 1978.

21. Mechtersheimer G, Staudter M, Moller P: Expression of the natural killer cell-associated antigens CD56 and CD57 in human neural and striated muscle cells and in their tumors. Cancer Res 51:1300, 1991.

22. Ariza A, Bilbao JM, Rosai J: Immunohistochemical detection of epithelial membrane antigen in normal perineurial cells and perineurioma. Am J Surg Pathol 12:678, 1988.

23. Heesen J, Grote W, Schettler D, et al: Choice of surgical approach in orbital space occupations—An interdisciplinary problem. Neurosurg Rev 11:239, 1988.

24. Kinoshita S, Tanaka F, Ohashi Y, et al: Incidence of prominent corneal nerves in multiple endocrine neoplasia type 2A. Am J Ophthalmol 111:307, 1991.

25. Vasen HF, van der Feltz M, Raue F, et al: The natural course of multiple endocrine neoplasia type IIb: A study of 18 cases. Arch Intern Med 152:1250, 1992.

26. van der Meulen J: Orbital neurofibromatosis. Clin Plast Surg 14:123, 1987.

27. Kennerdell JS, Maroon JC: Use of the carbon dioxide laser in the management of orbital plexiform neurofibromas. Ophthalmic Surg 21:138, 1990.

28. Mamalis N, Apple DJ, Williams RD, et al: Surgical removal of an "inoperable" neurofibroma. Ophthalmic Surg 19:37, 1988.

29. Jakobiec FA, Font RL, Zimmerman LE: Malignant peripheral nerve sheath tumors of the orbit: A clinicopathologic study of eight cases. Trans Am Ophthalmol Soc 83:332, 1985.

30. Eviatar JE, Hornblass AH, Hirschorn BH, et al: Malignant peripheral nerve sheath tumor of the orbit: A report of a nine year survival following local excision. Ophthalmology (In press.)

31. Lyons CJ, McNab AA, Garner A, et al: Orbital malignant peripheral nerve sheath tumours. Br J Ophthalmol 73:731, 1989.

32. Bhatt S, Graeme CF, Joseph MP, et al: Malignant Triton tumor of the head and neck. Otolaryngol Head Neck Surg 105:738, 1991.

33. Blodi FC: Amputation neuroma in the orbit. Am J Ophthalmol 32:929, 1949.

34. Okubo K, Asai T, Sera Y, et al: A case of amputation neuroma presenting proptosis. Ophthalmologica 194:5, 1987.

35. Messmer EP, Camara J, Boniuk M, et al: Amputation neuroma of the orbit: Report of two cases and review of the literature. Ophthalmology 91:1420, 1984.

36. Dent EW, Ida JA, Yoshino JE: Isolated growth cones stimulate proliferation of cultured Schwann cells. Glia 5:105, 1992.

37. Hardy M, Reddy UR, Pleasure D: Platelet-derived growth factor and regulation of Schwann cell proliferation in vivo. J Neurosci Res 31:254, 1992.

38. Stewart HJ, Eccleston PA, Jessen KR, et al: Interaction between cAMP elevation, identified growth factors, and serum components in regulating Schwann cell growth. J Neurosci Res 30:346, 1991.

39. Komiyama A, Suzuki K: Normal rate of Schwann cell proliferation in the MBP-deficient shiverer mouse during wallerian degeneration. Brain Res 563:345, 1991.

40. Lisak RP, Bealmear B: Antibodies to interleukin-1 inhibit cytokine-induced proliferation of neonatal rat Schwann cells in vitro. J Neuroimmunol 31:123, 1991.

41. Eccleston PA, Mirsky R, Jessen KR: Spontaneous immortalization of Schwann cells in culture: Short-term cultured Schwann cells secrete growth inhibitory activity. Development 112:33, 1991.

42. Muir D, Varon S, Manthorpe M: Schwann cell proliferation in vitro is under negative autocrine control. J Cell Biol 111(2663):71, 1990.

43. Muir D, Manthorpe M: Stromelysin generates a fibronectin fragment that inhibits Schwann cell proliferation. J Cell Biol 116:177, 1992.

44. Ratner N, Lieberman MA, Riccardi VM, et al: Mitogen accumulation in von Recklinghausen neurofibromatosis. Ann Neurol 27:298, 1990.

45. Asai K, Hotta T, Nakanishi K, et al: von Recklinghausen neurofibroma produces neuronal and glial growth-modulating factors. Brain Res 556:344, 1991.

46. Jakobiec FA, Depot MJ, Kennerdell JS, et al: Combined clinical and computed tomographic diagnosis of orbital glioma and meningioma. Ophthalmology 91:137, 1984.

47. Eggers H, Jakobiec FA, Jones IS: Tumors of the optic nerve. Doc Ophthalmol 41:43, 1976.

48. Levin LA, Jakobiec FA: Optic nerve tumors of childhood: A decision-analytical approach to their diagnosis. Int Ophthalmol Clin 32:223, 1992.

49. Goldman JE, Corbin E: Rosenthal fibers contain ubiquitinated alpha B-crystallin. Am J Pathol 139:933, 1991.

50. Iwaki T, Wisniewski T, Iwaki A, et al: Accumulation of alpha B-crystallin in central nervous system glia and neurons in pathologic conditions. Am J Pathol 140:345, 1992.

51. Bellon G, Caulet T, Cam Y, et al: Immunohistochemical localisation of macromolecules of the basement membrane and extracellular matrix of human gliomas and meningiomas. Acta Neuropathol (Berl) 66:245, 1985.

52. Ogawa K, Oguchi M, Nakashima Y, et al: Distribution of collagen type IV in brain tumors: An immunohistochemical study. J Neurooncol 7:357, 1989.

53. Lindquist TD, Orcutt JC, Gown AM: Monoclonal antibodies to intermediate filament proteins: Diagnostic specificity in orbital pathology. Surv Ophthalmol 32:421, 1988.

54. Regenbogen VS, Zinreich SJ, Kim KS, et al: Hyperostotic esthesioneuroblastoma: CT and MR findings. J Comput Assist Tomogr 12:52, 1988.

55. Axe S, Kuhajda FP: Esthesioneuroblastoma: Intermediate filaments, neuroendocrine, and tissue-specific antigens. Am J Clin Pathol 88:139, 1987.

56. Perentes E, Rubinstein LJ: Immunohistochemical recognition of human neuroepithelial tumors by anti-Leu 7 (HNK-1) monoclonal antibody. Acta Neuropathol (Berl) 69:227, 1986.

57. Jakobiec FA, Klepach GL, Crissman JD, et al: Primary differentiated neuroblastoma of the orbit. Ophthalmology 94:255, 1987.

58. Silva EG, Butler JJ, Mackay B, et al: Neuroblastomas and neuroendocrine carcinomas of the nasal cavity: A proposed new classification. Cancer 50:2388, 1982.

59. Kameya T, Shimosato Y, Adachi I, et al: Neuroendocrine carcinoma of the paranasal sinus: A morphological and endocrinological study. Cancer 45:330, 1980.

60. Van Zyl JA, Muller GS, Rossouw DJ, et al: Multiple endocrine neoplasia type IIb: a clinicopathological report. J Surg Oncol 45:282, 1990.

61. Nasir MA, Yee RW, Piest KL, et al: Multiple endocrine neoplasia type III. Cornea 10:454, 1991.

62. Shields JA: Diagnosis and Management of Orbital Tumors. Philadelphia, WB Saunders, 1989.

63. Muller W, Dahmen HG: Granular cell tumor of the optic nerve. Graefes Arch Clin Exp Ophthalmol 207:181, 1978.

64. Levin LA, Rubin PAD: Advances in orbital imaging. Int Ophthalmol Clin 32:1–25, 1992.

65. Allman MI, Frayer WC, Hedges TRJ: Orbital neurilemoma. Ann Ophthalmol 9:1409, 1977.

66. Dervin JE, Beaconsfield M, Wright JE, et al: CT findings in orbital tumours of nerve sheath origin. Clin Radiol 40:475, 1989.

67. Bergin DJ, Parmley V: Orbital neurilemoma. Arch Ophthalmol 106:414, 1988.

68. Byrne BM, van Heuven WA, Lawton AW: Echographic characteristics of benign orbital schwannomas (neurilemomas). Am J Ophthalmol 106:194, 1988.

69. Cerofolini E, Landi A, DeSantis G, et al: MR of benign peripheral nerve sheath tumors. J Comput Assist Tomogr 15:593, 1991.

70. Tien RD, Hesselink JR, Chu PK, et al: Improved detection and delineation of head and neck lesions with fat suppression spin-echo MR imaging. Am J Neuroradiol 12:19, 1991.

71. Mann FA, Murphy WA, Totty WG, et al: Magnetic resonance imaging of peripheral nerve sheath tumors: Assessment by numerical visual fuzzy cluster analysis. Invest Radiol 25:1238, 1990.

72. Abramowitz J, Dion JE, Jensen ME, et al: Angiographic diagnosis and management of head and neck schwannomas. AJNR Am J Neuroradiol 12:977, 1991.

73. Henderson JW: Orbital Tumors. New York, Thieme-Stratton, 1980.

74. Rootman J: Diseases of the Orbit. Philadelphia, JB Lippincott, 1988.

75. Kennedy RE: An evaluation of 820 orbital cases. Trans Am Ophthalmol Soc 82:134, 1984.

Chapter 175

■

Orbital and Ocular Adnexal Lymphoid Tumors

PETER A. D. RUBIN and FREDERICK A. JAKOBIEC

Over the past decade a great deal of progress has been made in understanding the clinicopathologic features of benign and malignant ocular adnexal and orbital lymphoid tumors. The advent of immunologic and molecular genetic techniques has helped to unravel some of the biology and most of the immunocytic composition of these tumors. It is now possible to provide a reliable description of the major findings in the archetypical patient with an orbital lymphoid tumor: an older individual; characteristic molded and angulated soft tissue contours without bone destruction on computed tomography (CT) scan; general preservation of ocular function with painless proptosis and sometimes diplopia; benign or favorable cytologic composition in most lesions featuring small or intermediate lymphocytes (Fig. 175–1); overwhelming B-lymphocytic lineage for the "malignant" monoclonal proliferations or T-cell preponderance in the pseudolymphomas; more often than not limitation of the lesion to the ocular adnexa without systemic lymphoma (which fortunately occurs in only 30 to 35 percent of patients); and readily treatable disease when localized to the orbit with low doses of fractionated radiotherapy (1500 to 2000 rads).

Regardless of whether the patient has a diagnosis of a benign or malignant proliferation after a biopsy and an immunopathologic evaluation, all patients should have a noninvasive systemic work-up, because a significant minority (approximately 25 percent) of apparently benign lesions may still be associated with systemic lymphoma. To date there has been no single histologic, immunologic, or molecular genetic parameter, or even a group of parameters, that has enabled prediction with almost total accuracy of which lesions are localized or part of a systemic disease. The fact that orbital well-differentiated monoclonal lesions have about the same association of systemic disease as the "benign" polyclonal lesions suggests that there may be an in situ evolutionary relationship between these two processes.

For the systemic oncologist, the development of a lymphoid tumor in extranodal sites during the course of a nodal lymphoma represents a worsening of the condition and a deterioration of the prognosis. The systemic oncologist, however, is also aware that lesions beginning in "extranodal" sites may have a different biology from lymphomas that originate primarily in lymph nodes. Many oncologists and indeed ophthalmologists are not aware that the extranodal sites constituted by the conjunctiva, orbit, lacrimal gland, and eyelids endow lymphoproliferations with different behaviors and prognoses that cannot be inferred from knowledge derived only from the study of systemic nodal lymphomas. For example, in the ocular adnexa the worst prognosis for associated systemic lymphoma is attached to tumors that are located exclusively in the preseptal lid skin without orbital involvement, whereas more favorable prognoses are associated with conjunctival, orbital, and lacrimal gland tumors.

Patients who present with bilateral orbital or lacrimal gland masses do not have a significantly increased incidence of systemic lymphoma in comparison with those who present with strictly unilateral disease, and bilaterality itself in the absence of systemic disease definitely does not warrant systemic chemotherapy. It is also now understood that a careful histopathologic evaluation of lesions is just as accurate (but by no means flawless) in predicting the possibility of systemic disease as immunologic data. For routine diagnostic purposes we have concluded that immunophenotypic analysis of the con-

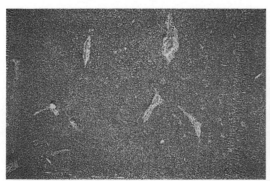
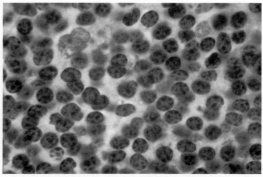

Figure 175–1. *A,* Low-power histopathology of a diffuse proliferation of lymphocytes. In contrast to pseudotumors, there is scant interstitial stroma. *B,* A high-power view reveals a tightly packed array of well-differentiated lymphocytes.

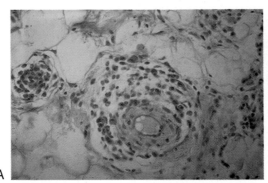 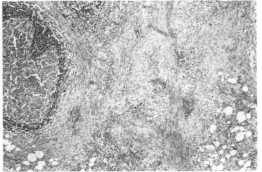

Figure 175–2. Pseudotumor histopathology. *A,* The infiltrate is relatively hypocellular. In the perivascular region there is a characteristic polymorphous infiltrate, including eosinophils, plasma cells, and lymphocytes. *B,* A more advanced pseudotumor demonstrates fibrous replacement of orbital fat. There is a light interspersal of inflammatory cells in the fibrous tissue and a germinal center on the left.

stituent cell populations does not contribute very much to patient management. Another important discovery has been that not all polyclonal lesions are necessarily restricted to the ocular adnexa, whereas most monoclonal lesions remain localized. The equation of *benign = polyclonal and malignant = monoclonal* should therefore not be automatically or rigidly applied to ocular adnexal lesions, because we cannot determine the metastasizability of these lesions from their immunophenotypic composition.

In several large orbital series, lymphoid tumors of benign and malignant character represent approximately 10 percent of biopsy-proven orbital disorders.[1–5] Conversely, among patients with systemic lymphoma, initial orbital presentation manifested by proptosis is rare. In an extensive review of autopsy cases in 1269 patients with systemic lymphoma, only three patients (0.24 percent) initially presented with orbital involvement whereas 13 patients (1.3 percent) developed orbital lymphoma during the course of the disease.[6] Despite their frequency, the topic of orbital lymphoid tumors seems to perplex many ophthalmologists as well as medical oncologists. The source of this confusion can be attributed to many factors, including a lack of understanding of the nature of ocular and orbital immune cell populations; confusion among orbital lymphoid tumors, pseudolymphomas, and the separate and distinct entity of orbital pseudotumor; unfamiliarity with the immunologic and histologic interpretation of orbital lymphoid tumors; and the lack of experience in application of this information to guide a systemic work-up of patients and to predict the course of their diseases.

Unlike orbital lymphoid tumors, which are clinically insidious in their onset and typically present over months, orbital pseudotumors have a more explosive onset that is characterized by pain and discomfort. Pathologically, biopsies of orbital pseudotumors demonstrate a polymorphous infiltrate that is relatively hypocellular with interstitial edema and perivascular lymphocytic, eosinophilic, and polymorphonuclear leukocytic infiltration.[7] Subacute and chronic presentations of pseudotumor are characterized by more extensive fibrosis and further decreased cellularity (Fig. 175–2). Although pseudotu-

mors can extensively involve the orbit and globe itself,[8] these lesions are cytologically benign and should not be categorized with the hypercellular orbital lymphomas. In fact, when this disorder is associated with systemic disease, it is usually associated with an underlying autoimmune disorder, typically Wegener's granulomatosis, polyarteritis nodosa, rheumatoid arthritis, systemic lupus erythematosus (SLE), dermatomyositis, or Crohn's disease, whereas the systemically associated orbital lymphoid lesion is nearly always disseminated lymphoma.

OCULAR ADNEXAL LYMPHOCYTIC POPULATIONS

The orbit is devoid of formed lymph nodes; thus, by definition, lymphoid lesions arising within the orbit are considered extranodal. Anatomic and immunologic studies revealed[9–11] that the only native orbital population of lymphocytes lie within the substantia propria of the conjunctiva and in the interstitium of the lacrimal gland (Fig. 175–3). The presence of this indigenous population of lymphocytes, which are capable of undergoing hyperplasia, may help to account for the relative infrequency with which proliferations within the conjunctiva and lacrimal gland are associated with systemic diseases, apart from Sjögren's syndrome.

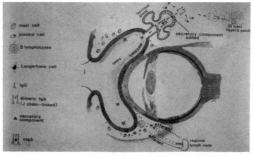

Figure 175–3. A schematic representation of the distribution of immunocytes within the orbit and adnexal structures.

CLINICAL PRESENTATION

The typical age of presentation is 50 to 70 yr, with a median age within the 60s and a female predominance that was observed in two large studies.[12, 13] These lesions are rare in children, and patients with inflammatory pseudotumor present at an earlier age (30 to 40 yr) and exhibit a slight male predominance. Lymphoid tumors of the orbit typically present very insidiously and are devoid of symptoms of pain, inflammatory features (injection, chemosis), or functional deficit. Clinical signs may include proptosis, ptosis, diplopia, mild motility disorder, visual decline,[14] or even rarely bilateral blindness.[15] The anatomic localization of these lesions to the lid, conjunctiva, lacrimal gland, or other orbital compartments is critical because of the different prognostic features associated with each locus. Given the native population of lymphocytes within the conjunctiva, proliferations within the substantia propria are less likely to be associated with systemic disease. Localization of lesions is usually possible after skilled clinical evaluation and adjunctive diagnostic imaging.

EXAMINATION FEATURES

When present within the conjunctiva, lymphoid lesions appear as salmon-colored patches attributable to the dense cellularity, fine microvasculature, and scant interstitial matrix (Fig. 175–4).

These lesions, when confined to the conjunctival substantia propria, are readily movable over the epibulbar surface and do not result in proptosis or extraocular motility deficits, which are signs more suggestive of orbital involvement. It is important to determine if the conjunctival lesion represents an epibulbar extension from an orbital process (Fig. 175–5).[16] If the lesion appears fixed to the globe in the absence of other orbital signs, it may represent an extraocular extension of an intraocular uveal lymphocytic proliferation.[17]

Lesions confined to the preseptal portion of the eyelid represent the rarest presentation of orbital and adnexal lymphoid proliferations. In these cases it is typically possible to easily palpate the posterior extent of the

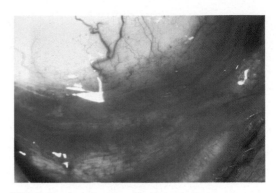

Figure 175–4. Conjunctival lymphoid "salmon-patch" lesion. This lymphoid tissue is located within the substantia propria of the conjunctiva and is freely mobile over the underlying tunics.

mass. The anterior, preseptal location of the mass can be confirmed by a CT scan (Fig. 175–6).

The orbital lesions most frequently involve the superior and anterior orbits and are probably attributable to the native population of lymphocytes within the lacrimal gland. These lesions clinically result in proptosis and downward displacement of the globe. When located within the anterior orbit, these lesions can mold to the septum and orbital rim and can be palpated as a rubbery to firm mass. If the lesion arises within the lacrimal gland and expands its normal surrounding structure, or if there is a prominent follicular organization to the lesion, a pebbly or micronodular surface can be appreciated (Fig. 175–7). Bilateral or recurrent orbital lesions were once thought to imply local malignancy, yet bilaterality does not increase the incidence of past, concurrent, or future nonocular disease.[18] Extraocular muscles can serve as a focus for lymphoid tumors (Fig. 175–8);[19] the levator/superior rectus complex is most commonly involved. The muscle may surprisingly retain considerable contractility because of the paucity of collagen deposition. This common finding enables these infiltrates to be distinguished from the more common causes of extraocular muscle enlargement, such as thyroid orbitopathy and idiopathic myositis (pseudotumor). Late presentations of orbital lymphoid lesions, particularly when associated with advanced systemic disease, can extensively involve all of the orbital and adnexal structures (Fig. 175–9).

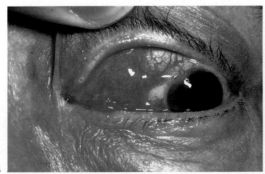
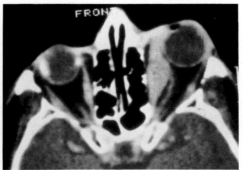

A

B

Figure 175–5. A, Anterior epibulbar extension of a deeper orbital lymphoma. The lesion's adherence to the surface of the globe, lack of salmon appearance to the conjunctiva, and the associated proptosis are all suggestive of its deeper and more posterior origin. B, The CT scan reveals a large molding soft tissue mass tracking along the medial orbit and extending onto the epibulbar surface of the left eye.

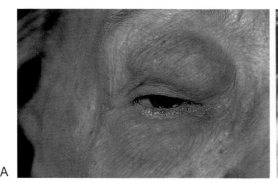
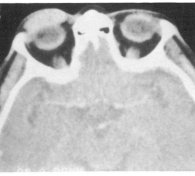

Figure 175–6. *A,* Lymphoid lesion of the preseptal portion of the eyelid. On palpation, the lesion had a doughy consistency. *B,* The accompanying CT scan further delineates the lesion to the preseptal anterior adnexal structures.

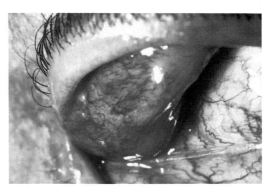

Figure 175–7. Lymphoid infiltrate of the lacrimal gland with resulting diffuse, uniform oblong enlargement of the lacrimal gland. The enlarged portion of the palpebral lobe is readily visualized in the superior fornix.

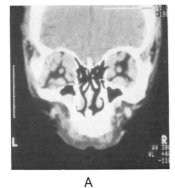
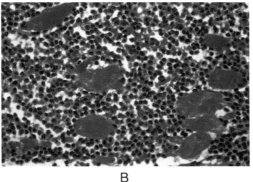

A
B

Figure 175–8. Lymphomatous infiltration of the extraocular muscles. *A,* A coronal CT scan shows bilateral diffuse enlargement of all the extraocular muscles, most typically suggestive of thyroid orbitopathy or a pseudotumor. *B,* The histopathology reveals a lymphoid tumor within the striated extraocular muscle, splaying apart the muscle fibers. (Courtesy of M. Boniuk, M.D.)

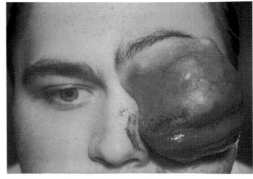

Figure 175–9. Systemically advanced anaplastic lymphoma with extensive orbital involvement. The patient succumbed to the systemic disease shortly after this picture was taken.

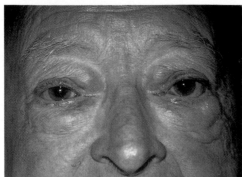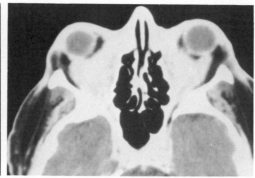

Figure 175–10. Bilateral orbital lymphoma. *A,* The clinical appearance of this patient is consistent with involutionary dermatochalasis, yet palpation of the lids demonstrated firm rubbery masses, not consistent with herniated orbital fat. *B,* The CT scan of this orbital lymphoma demonstrates bilateral symmetric soft tissue masses with exquisite molding to the globe.

RADIOLOGIC APPEARANCE

Orbital plain films provide a low yield of detection of lymphoid lesions, owing to their inherent poor soft tissue resolution. Ultrasound provides improved efficiency of detection of ocular, anterior orbital, and intraconal lesions; however, a CT scan greatly improves diagnostic sensitivity of these soft tissue orbital lesions. A CT scan of orbital lymphoid tumors reveals characteristic findings and permits the accurate determination of anatomic extent of these lesions. The radiologic appearance of these lymphoid tumors is best understood by remaining cognizant of the stroma-free and relatively monomorphous composition of the lesion, without encapsulation. Thus, these lesions tend to mold themselves to preexisting orbital structures, without eroding bone or enlarging the orbit.[20] When the lesions contact orbital structures that offer at least moderate resistance, including bone, globe, muscle, or optic nerve, then smooth sharply demarcated contours with abutment—not invasion of these barriers—result (Fig. 175–10). When orbital lymphoid tumors propagate within the orbital fat, which offers minimal resistance to their growth, fine irregular serrations occur, corresponding to the fine septations of the microfascial structure within orbital fat.[21] These

findings are most convincingly seen when viewing both the axial and coronal images. Given the superior and anterior predilection of these orbital lesions, it is natural that potential confusion with primary epithelial tumors of the lacrimal gland is experienced (Figs. 175–11 and 175–12). Primary lacrimal gland epithelial tumors possess a firmer stroma and are likely to cause adjacent erosive or possibly destructive bone changes; appear more globular or rounded with a posterior arclike (rather than perpendicular) take-off from bone; and are less likely to involve the anterior palpebral lobe of the lacrimal gland, which is typically involved along with the orbital lobe in lymphoid tumors.[22] Magnetic resonance imaging (MRI) possesses good soft tissue definition like a CT scan (Fig. 175–13) but lacks the specificity to differentiate benign from malignant neoplasms and does not give good definition to the bony perimeters of the orbit. Therefore, at this time, orbital MRI does not offer any additional advantage over a CT scan in the evaluation of these lesions.

PATHOLOGIC FEATURES

Clinically it is impossible to distinguish between benign and malignant orbital lymphoid infiltrates. Since there are no preformed lymph nodes in the orbit, gross

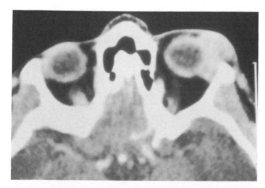

Figure 175–11. An axial CT scan of a lymphoma primarily within the lacrimal gland. The origin of the lesion within the lacrimal fossa with a perpendicular take-off posteriorly without bone erosion, involvement of both the palpebral and orbital lobes of the lacrimal gland, and the fine serrations at the interface with the surrounding orbital fat are all characteristic of lymphocytic infiltrates of the lacrimal gland.

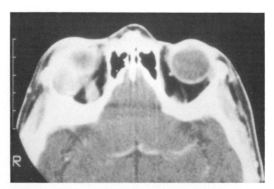

Figure 175–12. An axial CT scan of a pleomorphic adenoma of the lacrimal gland. In contrast to the lymphoid infiltrate of the lacrimal gland, this lesion is situated primarily posteriorly within the orbital lobe of the lacrimal gland, and bone erosion with fossa formation is present.

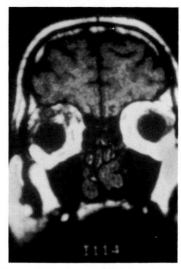

Figure 175–13. An MRI of an orbital lymphoma more clearly illustrates its diffuse infiltration within the orbital fat.

features including effacement of nodal structures or invasion of the lymph node's capsule, which are useful in studying nodal lymphoid lesions, are not applicable within the orbit. Even after careful histopathologic review of the cytomorphology of these lesions, a significant amount of ambiguity remains. Histologically, lymphoid infiltrates consisting of a monomorphous, cytologically atypical population of cells are readily identified as malignant lymphoma (Fig. 175–14), whereas infiltrates featuring large benign-appearing lymphoid follicles with reactive germinal centers and a heterogeneous cell population including lymphocytes, histiocytes, and plasma cells are clearly cytologically benign and are classified as reactive lymphoid hyperplasia or pseudolymphoma (Fig. 175–15).

On low power, inspection of these lymphoid proliferations provides a general sense of the overall architecture. Well-defined germinal centers with a clear mantle zone, in which the germinal center cells are larger than those in the mantle zone, are pseudolymphomas (Fig. 175–16). In contrast, in faint nodular patterns that characterize certain lymphomas, the cells in the pseu-

dogerminal center are of the same composition as those in the mantle zone. Despite the lack of ambiguity at the ends of the histopathologic spectrum, a large percentage of these lesions are histologically indeterminant or borderline. They often feature dense and diffuse homogeneous infiltrates of small lymphocytes with absent to minimal cytologic atypia (Fig. 175–17).

In some cases, intracellular eosinophilic inclusions consisting of immunoglobulins may cause characteristic morphologic changes of the lymphocyte. These include the Dutcher body (see Fig. 175–20), which is an eosinophilic pseudointranuclear inclusion that consists of immunoglobulin and is commonly associated with systemic plasma cell dyscrasias. A rare morphologic variant, reported only once in the orbit,[23] is the signet ring cell in which intracytoplasmic vacuolated or eosinophilic material displaces the nucleus to the side of the cell.[24] Immunocytochemical techniques are often necessary to distinguish this lymphocyte variant from morphologically similar-appearing adenocarcinoma or liposarcoma. In another rare morphologic variant, the tumor cells may elaborate surface villi, mimicking hairy cell leukemia.[25]

In the past, idiopathic orbital inflammations or pseudotumors have been mistakenly classified within the pool of lymphoproliferations. These inflammatory lesions are hypocellular in comparison with lymphoid tumors; stated conversely, lymphoid tumors are hypercellular and display a distinct sparsity of collagen. There are, however, extremely rare sclerosing lymphomas of the orbit, in which large atypical cells are separated into clusters or small lobules by tracts of collagen. Multiple schemata for classifying lymphoid lesions have been proposed. The most widely used system for catagorizing systemic lymphomas is the modified Rappaport classification (Table 175–1). A classification system for non-Hodgkin's orbital lymphoid lesions is listed in Table 175–2.

Immunologic Criteria

The introduction of immunohistochemical methods to study the subpopulations of these orbital lymphoid infil-

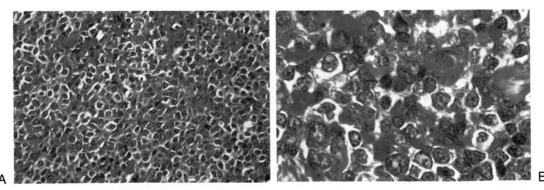

Figure 175–14. Malignant lymphoma histopathology: A, low power, and B, high power. The high-power view (B) clearly demonstrates the high-grade nature of this lesion with its large irregularly round anaplastic cells.

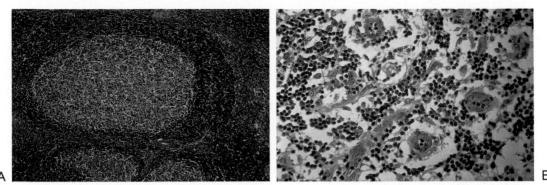

Figure 175–15. Histopathology: reactive hyperplasia or pseudolymphoma. A, Well-defined germinal center with a clear mantle zone. Such lesions are typically polyclonal with a T-cell predominance. B, Capillary endothelial proliferation, typical of a pseudolymphoma.

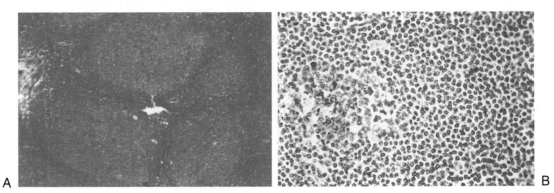

Figure 175–16. Low-power lymphomatous patterns. A, Follicular or nodular lymphoma. This differs from the germinal centers of pseudolymphoma by virtue of its indistinctness between the core of the follicle and the mantle zone. B, Pseudofollicle or residual germinal center on the left in an otherwise diffuse proliferation of lymphocytes.

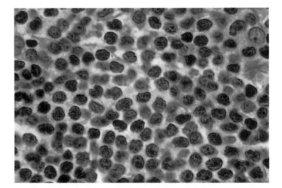

Figure 175–17. Intermediate cell lymphoma histopathology. In contrast to the large cell lymphoma, these nuclei are smaller, yet they possess an irregularity in the contour of the nuclear cell membrane. Pseudofollicles, Dutcher bodies, and polykaryocytes are all histologic features indicating monoclonality in intermediate lymphomas.

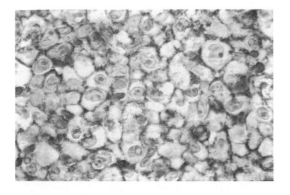

Figure 175–18. Large cell lymphoma. Immunoperoxidase staining for common leukocytic antigen (CLA) establishes the diagnosis of lymphoma and rules out other possible anaplastic carcinomas. (Courtesy of Ralph Eagle, M.D.)

Table 175–1. NON-HODGKIN'S LYMPHOMA: INTERNATIONAL FORMULATION (MODIFIED RAPPAPORT CLASSIFICATION)

Low Grade
Small lymphocytic (well-differentiated lymphocytic)
  With or without chronic lymphatic leukemia
  With or without plasmacytoid features
Follicular, small cleaved cell (nodular, poorly differentiated lymphocytic)*
Follicular, mixed small cleaved and large cell (nodular, mixed lymphocytic-histiocytic)*

Intermediate Grade
Follicular, large cell (nodular, histiocytic)*
Diffuse, small cleaved cell (diffuse, poorly differentiated lymphocytic)*
Diffuse, mixed small and large cell (diffuse mixed lymphocytic-histiocytic)*
Diffuse, large cell (diffuse, histiocytic)*

High Grade
Immunoblastic-plasmacytoid, clear cell, polymorphous types (histiocytic)
Lymphoblastic-convoluted and nonconvoluted cell types (lymphoblastic)
Small noncleaved cell, Burkitt's type

Miscellaneous
Mycosis fungoides
Hairy cell leukemia
Malignant histiocytosis
Unclassified

From Rosenberg S: National Cancer Institute–sponsored study of classifications of non-Hodgkin's lymphomas: Summary and description of a working formulation for clinical usage. Cancer 49:2112–2135, 1982.
*Exclusively or predominantly of follicle center cell origin.

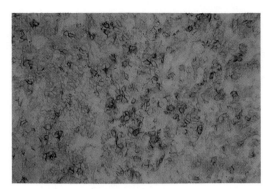

Figure 175–19. Immunoperoxidase stain for kappa light chain establishes the diagnosis of a B-cell monoclonal proliferation.

trates has permitted determination of diverse subpopulations of lymphocytes that appear identical by light microscopy (Fig. 175–18).[26] It is generally accepted that monoclonal immunoglobulin expression is diagnostic for malignancy. Almost all of the malignant orbital lymphoid proliferations have been shown to consist primarily of B-cell lymphocytes,[12, 13] and clonality is best assessed by determination of a predominant monotypic surface light chain immunoglobulin (Fig. 175–19 and Table 175–3). The preferred classification of lymphocyte surface antigens is by the "CD" (Tables 175–4 and 175–5) antigen system rather than by commercial monoclonal antibodies. Large studies have independently found that approximately two thirds of all ocular adnexal infiltrates had monotypic B-cell expression.[12, 13] Interestingly, among lesions histopathologically classified as reactive lymphoid hyperplasia, or pseudolymphoma, there is a preponderance of T-cell lymphocytic expression (see Table 175–3).

About half of these malignant (monotypic) lesions in one series[12] possessed indeterminant or borderline histopathology, so that the immunophenotypic analysis of these lesions provided additional diagnostic sensitivity. Of the indeterminant cases that proved to be malignant (monotypic) by immunophenotypic criteria, the only histologic feature studied that correlated highly with monotypia among this group was the presence of Dutcher bodies (Fig. 175–20). This feature was found in one third of the lesions that were shown to be lymphomas, whereas it was never detected in polytypic or polyclonal proliferations. Multinucleated cells (polykaryocytes) (Fig. 175–21) and abortive or residual germinal centers have also been frequently detected in small cell monoclonal proliferations.

Genetic Analysis

Recombinant molecular genetics provides newer, more sensitive techniques for detecting monoclonality

Table 175–2. CLASSIFICATION SYSTEM FOR NON-HODGKIN'S ORBITAL LYMPHOID NEOPLASMS

Histopathologic Category	Definition
Reactive lymphoid hyperplasia (pseudolymphoma)	Hypercellular lesion with sheets of mature lymphocytes and scattered plasma cells and histiocytes devoid of a significant reactive stroma; may display a diffuse, patternless character or follicular organization in which the follicular center cells exhibit varying morphologic features and prominent mitotic activity and are accompanied by tingible body macrophages
Atypical lymphoid hyperplasia (borderline lesions)	A diffuse or follicular lymphoid proliferation in which the cells manifest borderline maturity or in which a subpopulation of atypical cells with large hyperchromatic nuclei is scattered among more mature lymphocytes and plasma cells
Plasmacytoma (including myeloma)	A diffuse infiltrate of variably differentiated plasma cells consisting of plasmacytoid lymphocytes, immunoblasts, and mature plasma cells
Malignant lymphoma (Rappaport)	Lymphocytic, well differentiated, diffuse Lymphocytic, intermediately differentiated, diffuse Lymphocytic, poorly differentiated, diffuse or nodular Histiocytic, diffuse, or nodular Mixed lymphocytic and histiocytic, diffuse or nodular Undifferentiated, diffuse Burkitt's type

Modified from Knowles DM, Jakobiec FA: Orbital lymphoid neoplasms: A clinicopathologic study of 60 cases. Cancer 46:576–589, 1980.

Table 175–3. ORBITAL LYMPHOMATOUS TUMORS: IMMUNOPHENOTYPE PROFILE

Type of Cell	%
Monoclonal B cell	65–70
Polyclonal (mostly T cell)	30
Indeterminate	2
T cell, Hodgkin's, plasma cell, Burkitt's	<1

Table 175–4. MONOCLONAL ANTIBODIES AND CELL MARKERS FOR LYMPHOCYTES, NATURAL KILLER CELLS, AND MONOCYTES-HISTIOCYTES

Type of Cell	Monoclonal or Marker
T lymphocytes	OKT 1
	OKT 3
	OKT 11 (E rosette receptor)
	LEU 1
T-suppressor/cytotoxic cells	OKT 5
	OKT 8
	LEU 2a
T-helper/inducer cells	OKT 4
	LEU 3a
Natural killer cells	OKM 1
	OKT 10
	LEU 7
B lymphocytes	LEU 14
	B1
	OKB 2
	OKB 7
	BA-1
	Cell surface immunoglobulin
Plasma cells	OKT 10
	Cytoplasmic immunoglobulin
Monocytes-histiocytes	OKM 1
	OKM 5
	OKT 6 (Langerhans' cells)
	M 221

From Jakobiec FA, Lefkowitch J, Knowles DM: B- and T-lymphocytes in ocular disease. Ophthalmology 91:635–654, 1984.

OKT, OKB, and OKM series: Ortho Diagnostic System, Inc, Raritan, NJ. Leu and M series: Becton-Dickinson, Sunnyvale, CA.

of lymphoid lesions, because molecular genetic transformations occur prior to the phenotypic surface expression that are detectable by immunohistochemical methods, and the sensitivity for detecting small monoclonal subpopulations is enhanced. These genetic recombinations (e.g., in the immunoglobulin loci) can be analyzed by Southern blotting[27] after endonuclease treatment of the DNA or by polymerase chain reaction (PCR) techniques.[28] Since these rearrangements occur in accordance with a developmental hierarchy in B-cell differentiation,[29] in which heavy chain genes are modified prior to kappa and lambda light chain genes, early genetic detection preceding surface immunoglobulin expression is possible.

The ability to detect subtle immunoglobulin gene rearrangements has permitted the identification of previously undetectable small clonal B-cell proliferations.[30, 31] Interestingly, this method of analysis demonstrated that even orbital lymphoid tumors, classified as benign histopathologically and polyclonal immunophenotypically, typically have gene arrangements in subpopulations of cells suggestive of an emerging B-cell clonality.[30] Clearly, molecular genetics provides a new level of diagnostic sensitivity; however, its promise as a prognostic tool has not been as clearly established. These findings do suggest that polyclonal proliferations may evolve locally in the orbit into monoclonal lesions.

Histopathologic Correlation With Systemic Disease

The central issue facing the physician in the management of these patients is what criteria—histology, immunophenotype, location, or bilaterality—are most use-

ful in predicting concurrent or future likelihood of developing systemic lymphoma. Although higher grade orbital lymphomatous malignancies are increasingly associated with systemic disease, a proportion of patients even with the most benign pathology can have systemic disease (Table 175–6). Cell type has at least some predictive importance, because the highest percentage of systemic disease (46 percent) occurred in the highest grades of lymphoma (large cell and follicular center cleaved cell lesions) in a large study of 108 patients by Knowles and associates.[13] Even patients with lymphoid hyperplasia (pseudolymphoma) have approximately a 25

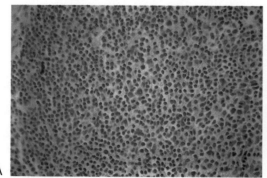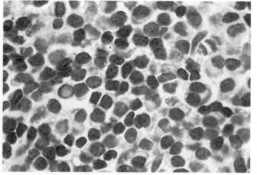

Figure 175–20. Lymphoplasmacytoid proliferation of lymphocytes. *A,* Low power. The small nuclei are widely spaced secondary to the relatively rich eosinophilic cytoplasm. *B,* Dutcher body, which is an intranuclear inclusion of immunoglobulin (left of center). Many of the cells have ample cytoplasm with perinuclear halos due to the abundant immunoglobulin-producing Golgi bodies in these cells.

Table 175–5. WORLD HEALTH ORGANIZATION-RECOMMENDED NOMENCLATURE FOR HUMAN LEUKOCYTE DIFFERENTIATION ANTIGENS

Antigen	Antigen Molecular Weight	Monoclonal Antibodies	Positive Cells
CD1	P45/12	Leu 6, T6, OKT6	Thymocytes, Langerhans' cells
CD2	P50	Leu 5B, T11, OKT11	E-rosette receptor, T and NK cells
CD3	P19-29	Leu 4, T3, OKT3	T cells
CD4	P55	Leu 3, T4, OKT4	Helper-inducer T cells, monocytes
CD5	P67	Leu 1, T, T101	T cells, B-cell subset, CLL cells
CD6	P120	T12	T cells
CD7	P41	Leu 9, 3A1	T, T-ALL, and NK cells
CD8	P32-33	Leu 2, T8, OKT8	Suppressor-cytotoxic T cells, NK subset
CD9	P24	BA-2	Lymphoid leukemia-associated antigen
CD10	P100	CALLA, J5	PMN, pre–B leukemia cells
CD11	P170/95	CR3/Leu 15, OKM1 MO1	Monocytes, PMN, NK cells, T subset (C_3bi receptor)
CD15	LNFP-III	Leu M1	Monocytes, PMN, activated T cells
CD16	P50-70	Leu 11	NK cells, PMN (IgG Fc receptor cells)
CD19	P95	Leu 12, B4	B, CLL, and pre–B-ALL cells
CD20	P35	Leu 16, B1	B cells
CD21	P140	CR2, B2	B cells, C_3d receptor cells
CD22	P135	Leu 14	B, CLL, and hairy cell leukemia cells
CD23	P45	Blast-2	
CD24	P45, P55, P65	BA-1	B, CLL, and pre–B-ALL cells
CD25	P55	IL-2 receptor	Mitogen-activated T cells, HTLV-I– and HTLV-II–infected T cells

Adapted from Jackson AL, Warner NL: Preparation and analysis by flow cytometry of peripheral blood leukocytes. *In* Rose NR, Friedman H, Fahey JL (eds): Manual of Clinical Laboratory Immunology, 3rd ed. Washington, DC, American Society of Microbiology, 1986, p 227.

Leu, CALLA, CR, IL2: Becton Dickinson Immunocytometry Systems, Mountain View, CA. T series: Coulter Electronics, Inc, Hialeah, FL. OKT & OKM series: Ortho Diagnostic, Inc, Raritan, NJ. BA: Hybritech, San Diego, CA. CLL: Chronic lymphocytic leukemia. T-ALL: T-cell acute lymphocytic leukemia. LNFP-III: Lacto-N-fucopentaose III. IL-2: interleukin 2. HTLV-I and HTLV-II: human T-cell leukemia virus types I and II. NK: natural killer. B-ALL: B-cell acute lymphocytic leukemia.

percent chance of developing systemic disease when followed for 5 yr. Although there is a loose correlation relating histopathologic/immunophenotypic findings with systemic disease, the association is not great enough to permit the clinician to systemically evaluate some patients while deferring complete medical work-up in others. Therefore, all patients with ocular adnexal lymphoid lesions should have a systemic evaluation.

Site as a Predictor of Histopathology and of Systemic Disease

Using combined histopathologic and immunophenotypic criteria, most lymphoid neoplasms possess malignant features (monoclonality) independent of their location. Lesions of the eyelid carry the highest incidence of histopathologic malignancy.[13] The most common site of ocular adnexal presentation for lymphoid neoplasms is the orbital soft tissues, muscle, and fat, followed by the lacrimal gland and conjunctiva, and least often within the eyelids in the absence of orbital disease. The overall incidence of systemic disease associated with ocular adnexal lymphoid proliferations is approximately 30 to 35 percent (Table 175–7). Orbital soft tissue lesions (including the lacrimal gland) and conjunctival lesions are associated with systemic disease in one fifth to one third of cases, respectively. Alternatively, lesions localized only to the preseptal portion of the eyelids (not an anterior extension of a deeper orbital process) are associated with systemic lymphoma in about two thirds of cases (see Table 175–7). It is important to keep in mind that this final grouping of cases limited to the eyelids is the most rare clinical presentation, comprising approximately 5 to 10 percent of cases. This finding of

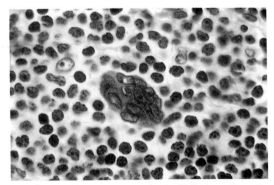

Figure 175–21. Polykaryocyte *(center)* within a proliferation of an intermediate cell lymphoma.

Table 175–6. ORBITAL LYMPHOMATOUS TUMORS: CORRELATION WITH SYSTEMIC DISEASE

Histopathology	Incidence of Systemic Disease (%)
High grade, large, cleaved	46
Reactive lymphoid hyperplasia	27
Immunophenotype	
B-cell monoclonal	35
Polyclonal	29

From Jakobiec FA, Knowles DM: An overview of ocular adnexal lymphoid tumors. Trans Am Ophthalmol Soc 87:420, 1989.

Table 175–7. ORBITAL LYMPHOMATOUS TUMORS: CORRELATION WITH SYSTEMIC DISEASE

Location	Incidence of Systemic Disease
Orbit	35% (24/69)
Conjunctiva	20% (6/30)
Eyelid	67% (6/9)
Bilateral	35% (6/17)

From Jakobiec FA, Knowles DM: An overview of ocular adnexal lymphoid tumors. Trans Am Ophthalmol Soc 87:420, 1989.

a differential incidence of systemic disease, associated most notably with cases limited to the preseptal portion of the eyelid, underscores the clinical importance of establishing the locus of the lymphoid proliferation through the clinical examination and adjunctive imaging during the initial assessment of patients with orbital and adnexal lymphoid proliferations.

Interestingly, among bilateral orbital lymphoid lesions the incidence of association with systemic disease is about 35 percent, approximating the overall association with systemic disease seen among all new patients presenting with orbital and adnexal lymphoid tumors.[18] Although perhaps counterintuitive, the presence of bilateral disease does not imply the presence of clinically significant systemic disease and does not mandate systemic chemotherapy.

SYSTEMIC EVALUATION

Whether or not malignant lymphomas actually originate in the orbit and disseminate to other sites in the body, or whether they represent metastatic deposits where they are more readily detected, thus signaling systemic disease, is still a source of controversy.[32–35] In large series, approximately 13 to 19 percent of patients have documented past history of nonocular lymphoma at the time of presentation.[12, 13] These lesions are commonly found within the orbit, lacrimal gland, or eyelids, whereas the conjunctival presentation is rarely associated with antecedent systemic disease. Over the course of follow-up it could be anticipated that approximately 20 to 25 percent of patients not known previously to have systemic lymphoma will develop evidence of disseminated disease within 5 yr.[13] Patients who demonstrate no evidence of prior or coexistent systemic involvement of lymphoma at presentation (clinically stage I) and continue to be free of evidence of systemic disease at 6 mo and 1 yr follow-up have a very high likelihood (87 percent) of remaining free of systemic disease.[13] Therefore, careful early clinical staging has become the best prognosticator for the later development of systemic lymphoma. Due to the utility of clinical staging, systemic evaluations of patients with orbital lymphoid lesions are best conducted by clinical oncologists with an interest in lymphomas. These physicians can initiate a search upon orbital presentation for occult systemic disease. The hematologic work-up should include a complete blood count (CBC), serum protein immunoelectropho-

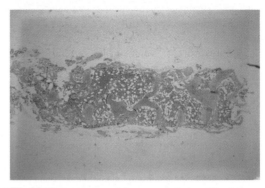

Figure 175–22. Bone marrow biopsy specimen. The bone marrow preserves the trabeculae of bone, with some cellular aggregates. Unless those lymphoid aggregates are reflected in a hematologic disturbance, they should not be treated.

resis (SPIEP) (especially in patients with lymphoplasmacytoid lesions), antinuclear antibodies (ANAs), rheumatoid factor (RF) (indicated in patients suspected of Sjögren's syndrome who may also have lymphoid lesions of the lacrimal gland), erythrocyte sedimentation rate (ESR), and bone marrow biopsy (Fig. 175–22). In addition to an orbital CT scan, the radiologic evaluation should include a chest roentgenogram or chest CT scan and an abdominal CT scan, thus screening for other systemic lymphoid proliferations. A bone scan, especially if bone pain is present upon presentation, and a liver-spleen scan may also be useful.

SURGICAL MANAGEMENT

Upon establishing suspicion of an ocular adnexal lymphoid lesion, biopsy of the lesion is essential. The diffuse infiltrating nature of orbital lesions makes their total excision challenging and risky. Additionally, their excellent response to local low-dose irradiation obviates the need for attempted excision of the orbital lesions. Conjunctival, epibulbar, and some lacrimal gland lesions can be easily accessed for direct incisional biopsy (Fig. 175–23). Most orbital lesions are in the anterior/superior orbit, and their surgical exposure through the lid (Fig. 175–24) or through a subperiosteal brow incision pro-

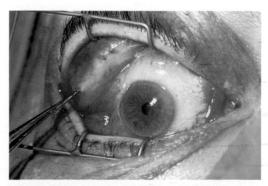

Figure 175–23. Biopsy of the lacrimal gland. This can usually be obtained transconjunctivally in lesions that are clinically and radiographically suggestive of a lymphoid process.

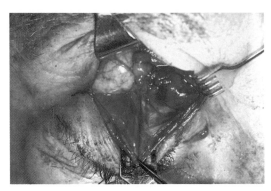

Figure 175–24. Lid crease approach to anterior orbitotomy. The normal orbital fat *(left)* is seen juxtapositioned to an orbital lymphoid infiltrate *(right)*.

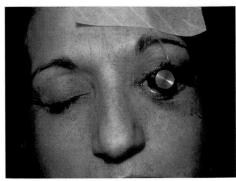

Figure 175–26. During orbital irradiation, the globe and lens are protected with a metallic shield mounted on a suction contact lens.

vides adequate exposure for biopsy. In rare cases when the lesion is more posterior in the orbit, a lateral orbitotomy with bone removal may be necessary to obtain access and a representative biopsy. Alternatively, fine-needle biopsy coupled with specific cell surface marker studies of the cytologic sample can provide sufficient diagnostic material and avoid the need for incisional surgery.

If the lesion is situated primarily within the lacrimal gland, careful preoperative assessment focusing upon the previously addressed radiologic and clinical findings seen with lymphoid tumors is essential to establish a presumptive diagnosis. In these cases, it is possible to obtain an incisional biopsy of the lacrimal gland. However, if following the preoperative evaluation there is a significant concern that the lesion may represent an epithelial tumor of the lacrimal gland, a lateral orbitotomy with complete removal of the entire intact lacrimal gland should be performed in an effort to avoid the risk associated with a percutaneous incisional biopsy into a benign, mixed tumor.

Conjunctival lesions are typically diffuse, and an adequate biopsy should provide enough diagnostic tissue. However, in selected cases, a localized conjunctival lesion may be easily excised without significantly sacrificing the conjunctival surface. In these cases a complete excision coupled with close postoperative follow-up may prevent the need for orbital irradiation.

In cases of bilateral lymphoid tumors, only one side needs to be biopsied, because identical histology and immunophenotype are typically found bilaterally in these cases.[18]

The gross specimens typically appear salmon-colored and are fish-flesh consistency (Fig. 175–25). Surgical specimens for histopathologic review should be placed in formalin. Additional specimens, if possible, should be prepared as frozen sections[36, 37] or cell suspensions to permit immunophenotypic or genetic analysis. Although more data are made available with adjunctive immunologic evaluation, a careful histologic evaluation of lymphoid specimens is economically preferable, because the histopathologic findings seem to be just as good in terms of predicting systemic disease.

TREATMENT

If upon completing a systemic survey no evidence of extraorbital disease is discovered, then local orbital radiotherapy with appropriate shielding of the globe is advised (Fig. 175–26). For cytologically benign lesions, 1500 to 2000 rads in divided doses is sufficient treatment, whereas 2000 to 3000 rads is recommended (Table 175–

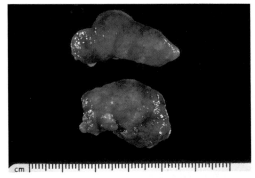

Figure 175–25. Gross fresh appearance of a lacrimal gland tumor, demonstrating the fish-flesh character of the lymphoid proliferation.

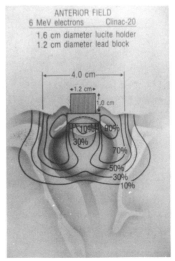

Figure 175–27. Dosimetry for anterior orbital irradiation.

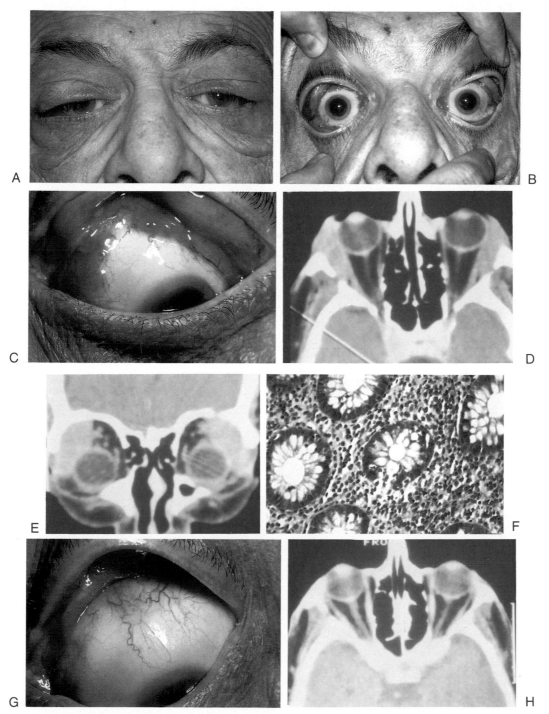

Figure 175–28. Case presentation. *A,* A 63-year-old man presented with a 6-mo history of gradual ptosis bilaterally. *B,* Retraction of the upper eyelids revealed diffusely enlarged, tan-colored lacrimal glands. *C,* The superior epibulbar surface possessed a salmon-colored fleshy mobile mass, classic for a lymphoid proliferation. *D,* The axial CT scan and *E,* the coronal CT scan demonstrated exquisitely symmetric enlargement of the lacrimal glands. A biopsy of the lesion confirmed the diagnosis of a lymphoid tumor. *F,* The systemic work-up uncovered a lymphoid infiltration in the proximal gastrointestinal (GI) tract. A GI biopsy demonstrates the interstitial proliferation of lymphocytes. The disruption of the secretory acini *(center),* termed a lymphoepithelial lesion, is more commonly associated with monoclonal proliferations. Since the patient was found to have systemic disease and non–vision-threatening orbital disease, he was treated only with systemic chemotherapy. *G,* Clinically, there was complete regression of the conjunctival and lacrimal masses following the chemotherapy. *H,* The follow-up CT scan also highlights the impressive regression of the deeper orbital components.

Table 175–8. TREATMENT OF ORBITAL LYMPHOMATOUS TUMORS

Type of Disease	Treatment
Systemic Disease	
Mild orbital involvement	Systemic chemotherapy
Vision-threatening orbital disease	Chemotherapy and orbital irradiation
Isolated Orbital Disease	*Orbital Irradiation*
Benign histopathology	1500–2000 rads
Malignant histopathology	2000–3000 rads

8) for histopathologically or immunophenotypically malignant lesions (Fig. 175–27).[38, 39] Close clinical follow-up at least every 6 mo for 2 yr upon completion of radiation treatment in coordination with an ongoing medical oncologic screen is advised. Complications of radiation treatment, when given in these low doses in a fractionated fashion including dry eye and lenticular changes, are typically minimal.[40]

If systemic disease is discovered at the time of presentation, then appropriate systemic chemotherapy should be administered (Fig. 175–28). The effects of systemic treatment on the orbital or lid lesion should be assessed before instituting orbital irradiation. If massive orbital involvement threatening vision in association with systemic lymphoma is found on presentation, then systemic chemotherapy and localized orbital irradiation may be instituted concurrently. It is important to be aware that chemotherapy potentiates the cytotoxic effect of irradiation. Therefore, this small subset patient population needs to be particularly carefully followed for ocular radiation sequelae (i.e., retinopathy, cataract), which may not appear for several years following treatment. In no case should systemic chemotherapy be given for an isolated orbital lesion. If a patient is discovered to have systemic lymphoma, the outlook is still quite favorable because many of the lymphomas are comparatively indolent and may consist of fewer malignant cell types.

Systemic steroids are useful in treating inflammatory pseudotumors; but when used in the presence of orbital lymphoid lesions, they invariably result in a temporary reduction of the mass, followed by a clinical rebound upon cessation of the steroids. Lymphoid lesions should, therefore, not be treated with a diagnostic trial of systemic steroids, and other lesions treated as "pseudotumors" that do not respond well to steroid therapy should be biopsied.

REFERENCES

1. Jones IS, Jakobiec FA: Diseases of the Orbit. Hagerstown, MD, Harper & Row, 1979, pp 135–44, 187–262, 309–416.
2. Henderson JW: Orbital Tumors, 2nd ed. New York, BC Decker, 1980, pp 67–114, 344–376.
3. Shields JA, Bakewell B, Augsburger JJ, Flanagan JC: Classification and incidence of space occupying lesions of the orbit: A survey of 645 biopsies. Arch Ophthalmol 102:1606–1611, 1984.
4. Jakobiec FA, Font RL: Orbit. In Spencer WH, Font RL, Green WR, et al (eds): Ophthalmic Pathology: An Atlas and Textbook, 3rd ed, vol. 3. Philadelphia, WB Saunders, 1986, pp 2459–8660.
5. Rootman J: Diseases of the Orbit: A Multidisciplinary Approach. Philadelphia, JB Lippincott, 1988, pp 143–197, 205–240, 293–305, 481–492.
6. Rosenburg SA, Diamond HD, Jaslowitz B, Craver LF: Lymphosarcoma: A review of 1269 cases. Medicine 40:31–84, 1961.
7. Jakobiec FA, Font RL: Orbit: Lymphoid tumors. In Spencer WH, Font RL, Green WR, et al (eds): Ophthalmic Pathology: An Atlas and Textbook, 3rd ed. Philadelphia, WB Saunders, 1986, vol. 3, pp 2663–2711, 2777–2795.
8. Ryan SJ, Zimmerman LE, King FM: Reactive lymphoid hyperplasia: An unusual form of intraocular pseudotumor. Trans Am Ophthalmol Otolaryngol 76:652–671, 1972.
9. Jakobiec FA, Iwamoto T: The ocular adnexa. In Jakobiec FA (ed): Ocular Anatomy, Embryology, and Teratology. Philadelphia, Harper & Row, 1982, pp 677–732.
10. Wieczorak R, Jakobiec FA, Sacks EH, Knowles DM: The immunoarchitecture of the normal lacrimal gland: Relevancy for understanding pathologic conditions. Ophthalmology 95:100–109, 1988.
11. Sacks EH, Wieczorek R, Jakobiec FA, Knowles DM: Lymphocytic subpopulations in the normal human conjunctiva: A monoclonal antibody study. Ophthalmology 93:1276–1283, 1986.
12. Mederios LJ, Harris NL: Lymphoid infiltrates of the orbit and conjunctiva: A morphologic and immunophenotypic study of 99 cases. Am J Surg Pathol 13:459–471, 1989.
13. Knowles DM, Jakobiec FA, McNally L, Burke JS: Lymphoid hyperplasia and malignant lymphoma occurring in the ocular adnexa (orbit, conjunctiva, and eyelids): A prospective multiparametric analysis of 108 cases during 1977 to 1987. Hum Pathol 21:959–973, 1990.
14. Henderson JW: Orbital Tumors, 2nd ed. New York, BC Dekker, 1980.
15. Harris GJ: Bilateral blindness due to orbital lymphoma. Ann Ophthalmol 13:427–430, 1981.
16. Malis N, Mackman G, Holds J, et al: Simultaneous and bilateral conjunctival and orbital lymphoma presenting as a conjunctival lesion. Ophthalmol Surg 19:662–663, 1988.
17. Jakobiec FA, Sacks E, Kronish JW, Weiss T, Smith M. Multifocal static creamy choroidal infiltrates: An early sign of lymphoid neoplasia. Ophthalmology 94:397–406, 1987.
18. McNally L, Jakobiec FA, Knowles DM: Clinical, morphologic, immunophenotypic, and molecular genetic analysis of bilateral ocular adnexal lymphoid neoplasms in 17 patients. Am J Ophthalmol 103:555–568, 1987.
19. Hornblass A, Jakobiec FA, Riefler DM, et al: Orbital lymphoid tumors located predominantly within extraocular muscles. Ophthalmology 94:688–697, 1987.
20. Yeo JH, Jakobiec FA, Abbott GF, Trokel SL: Combined clinical and computed tomographic diagnosis of orbital lymphoid tumors. Am J Ophthalmol 94:235–245, 1982.
21. Koorneef L: New insights into human orbital connective tissue. Arch Ophthalmol 95:1269–1273, 1977.
22. Jakobiec FA, Yeo JH, Trokel SL, et al: Combined clinical and computed tomographic diagnosis of lacrimal fossa lesions. Am J Ophthalmol 94:785–807, 1982.
23. Dolman PJ, Rootman J, Quenville NF: Signet-ring cell lymphoma in the orbit: A case report and review. Can J Ophthalmol 21:242–245, 1986.
24. Kim H, Dorfman RF, Rappaport H: Signet cell lymphoma: A rare morphologic and functional expression of nodular (follicular) lymphoma. Am J Surg Pathol 2:119–132, 1978.
25. Font RL, Shields J: Large cell lymphoma of the orbit with microvillous projections ("porcupine lymphoma"). Arch Ophthalmol 103:1715–1719, 1985.
26. Knowles DM, Jakobiec FA: Ocular adnexal lymphoid neoplasms: clinical, histopathologic, electron microscopic, and immunologic characteristics. Hum Pathol 13:148–162, 1982.
27. Southern EM: Detection of specific sequences among DNA fragments separated by gel electrophoresis. J Mol Biol 98:503–517, 1975.
28. Lardelli P, Swaby RF, Medeiros LJ, et al: Determination of lineage and clonality in diffuse lymphomas using polymerase chain reaction technique. Hum Pathol 22:685–689, 1991.
29. Tonegawa S: Somatic generation of antibody diversity. Nature 302:575–581, 1983.

30. Jakobiec FA, Neri A, Knowles DM: Genotypic monoclonality in immunophenotypically polyclonal orbital lymphoid tumors: A new model of tumor progression in the lymphoid system. Ophthalmology 94:980–994, 1987.
31. Mederios LJ, Andrade RE, Harris NL, Cossman J: Lymphoid infiltrates of the orbit and conjunctiva: comparison of immunologic and gene rearrangement data. Lab Invest 660:614, 1989.
32. Ellis JH, Banks PM, Campbell RJ, et al: Lymphoid tumors of the ocular adnexa: Clinical correlation with the working formulation classification and immunoperoxidase staining of paraffin sections. Ophthalmology 92:1311–1324, 1985.
33. Lazzarino M, Mora E, Rosso R, et al: Clinicopathologic and immunologic characteristics of non-Hodgkin's lymphomas presenting in the orbit: A report of eight cases. Cancer 55:1907–1912, 1985.
34. Jakobiec FA, Knowles DM: An overview of ocular adnexal lymphoid tumors. Trans Am Ophthalmol Soc 87:420–444, 1989.
35. Knowles DM, Jakobiec FA: Orbital lymphoid neoplasms: A clinicopathologic study of 60 patients. Cancer 46:576–589, 1980.
36. Harris NL, Harmon DC, Pilch B, et al: Immunohistologic diagnosis of orbital lymphoid infiltrates. Am J Surg Pathol 18:83–91, 1984.
37. Turner RR, Egbert P, Warnke RA: Lymphocytic infiltrates of the conjunctiva and orbit: Immunohistochemical staining of 16 cases. Am J Clin Pathol 81:447–452, 1984.
38. Bessell EM, Henk JM, Wright JE, et al: Orbital and conjunctival lymphoma treatment and prognosis. Radiother Oncol 13:2237–2244, 1988.
39. Reddy EK, Bhata P, Evans RG: Primary orbital lymphomas. Int J Radiat Oncol Biol Phys 15:1239–1241, 1988.
40. Bessell EM, Henk JM, Whitelocke RAF, et al: Ocular morbidity after radiotherapy of orbital and conjunctival lymphoma. Eye 1:90–96, 1987.

Chapter 176

■

Other Lymphocytic Disease Processes

PETER A. D. RUBIN and FREDERICK A. JAKOBIEC

PLASMA CELL PROLIFERATIONS

Multiple myeloma and its related disorders (plasma cell dyscrasias) are all characterized by an abnormal proliferation of a single clone of highly specialized B lymphocytes engaged in the production of a specific immunoglobulin. This monoclonal immunoglobulin, which is often referred to as the M protein or myeloma protein, involves one class of heavy chains (γ, α, μ, δ, or ϵ) that characterize one of the five major immunoglobulins (IgG, IgA, IgM, IgD, or IgE) or one of the light chains (κ or λ).

Clinically, multiple myeloma typically arises between 40 and 70 yr, peaking in the seventh decade. Bone pain, fatigue, and a normocytic-normochromic anemia are the most common presenting symptoms and signs. Serum hyperviscosity can result from elevated serum immunoglobulins and may be manifested clinically with decreased visual acuity from a central retinal vein occlusion (Fig. 176–1). Some evidence of renal insufficiency attributable to Bence Jones protein obstructing the distal and collecting tubules is present in approximately half of the patients.[1]

Not all plasma cell proliferations are multiple myelomas. Isolated plasma cell proliferations either within bone or in an extramedullary location are also seen. In cases of solitary plasmacytomas of bone, the diagnosis depends on histologic confirmation, no evidence of other lesions in the skeleton, the absence of or only small amounts of M protein in the serum or urine, and the lack of significant constitutional findings. More than half of these patients demonstrate lesions within the verte-

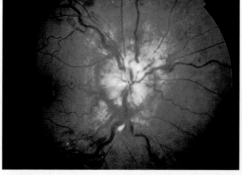
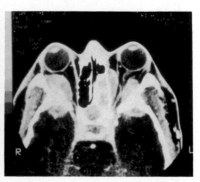

Figure 176–1. *A,* Fundus photograph of a patient with multiple myeloma. The retinal venous tortuosity and optic nerve swelling are reflective of the hyperviscosity encountered in this disorder. Additionally, the large orbital masses *(B)* cause orbital apical compression and contribute to the fundus findings. *B,* The CT scan shows extensive bilateral orbital involvement. Following systemic chemotherapy, there was marked resolution of the orbital masses. (Courtesy of Mark Balles, M.D.)

A   B

bral column. Treatment consists of local irradiation to the lesion of approximately 4500 rads. These patients must be followed very closely, because more than half of them will develop overt multiple myeloma and a smaller proportion of patients will demonstrate new bone lesions.

Extramedullary plasmacytomas arise outside of the bone marrow and represent about 3 percent of plasma cell proliferations.[2, 3] These lesions most commonly occur within the upper respiratory tract, including the nasal cavity and the sinuses. As with isolated plasmacytomas of bone, diagnostically these lesions cannot be distinguished from multiple myeloma except in the presence of a negative systemic work-up, including a skeletal survey and bone marrow biopsy. Irradiation is the recommended treatment for isolated lesions, and follow-up is mandated to assess for recurrences or systemic involvement.

Although rare, ranging from 0.1 to 0.5 percent of all orbital tumors,[5] each of these plasma cell proliferations has been observed in the orbit. Orbital involvement can occur as part of systemic multiple myeloma (Fig. 176–2),[4–11] with local bone destruction; from an isolated plasmacytoma involving one of the orbital walls[4, 10, 14]; or as an extramedullary plasmacytoma arising from either the orbital soft tissue[12, 13, 15–17] or from secondary extension to the orbit of a sinus or pharyngeal extramedullary soft tissue plasmacytoma.

The plasma cell proliferations arising in the bone marrow frequently involve the orbital roof or lateral wall and result in the clinical presentation of progressive proptosis, pain, downward or medial displacement of the globe, and occasionally diplopia. Soft tissue presentation, including lacrimal gland involvement[18–20] or infiltration of the extraocular muscles,[21] results in similar findings. An isolated case of bilateral orbital extramedullary plasmacytoma has also been reported.[22]

Lytic lesions arising within the orbital bone should raise the possibility in an older individual of a plasma cell proliferation based on radiographic findings. A metastatic carcinoma would be a reasonable differential diagnostic possibility. In rare plasmacytic lesions primarily involving the orbital soft tissue, the CT appearance featuring a regular contoured and uniformly dense mass molding to the surface of the globe is nonspecific

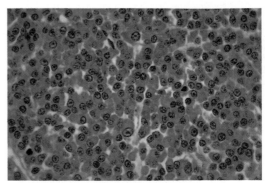

Figure 176–3. Plasmacytoid features in a reasonably well-differentiated myelomatous deposit.

and shared with other lymphoproliferations; thus, the specific preoperative diagnosis is rarely suspected.

Upon establishing the diagnosis with biopsy (Fig. 176–3), isolated orbital lesions respond impressively to local irradiation in the range of 2000 to 4000 rads.[5, 10, 14] Close vigilance for evidence of systemic involvement, local recurrence, or additional plasmacytomas is advised. Systemic involvement is best treated with systemic chemotherapy and possibly adjunctive radiotherapy.

HODGKIN'S LYMPHOMA

Although as much 25 percent of all nodal lymphomas are of the Hodgkin's histologic subtype, orbital Hodgkin's lymphoma is very rare. This is due to a large extent to the fact that the orbit is devoid of formed lymph nodes, and when present in the orbit, lymphomas are almost always of the non-Hodgkin histologic subtype.

Hodgkin's lymphoma is characterized by the diagnostic Reed-Sternberg cell found on biopsy (Fig. 176–4), which features a large bilobed or multilobate nucleus with prominent nucleoli, and a nuclear clear zone, surrounding the acidophilic nucleoli, which impart an "owl-eyed" appearance to this cell. Although necessary for establishing the diagnosis of Hodgkin's lymphoma, these Reed-Sternberg cells typically comprise less than 1 percent of the total cell population. Most of the cells

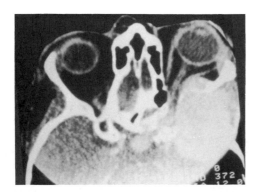

Figure 176–2. Axial CT scan in a case of multiple myeloma. There is destruction of the lateral orbital wall with prominent soft tissue involvement in the orbit and middle cranial fossa.

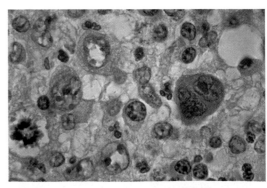

Figure 176–4. Hodgkin's lymphoma and its histopathology. A diagnostic Reed-Sternberg cell is present in the center of the field. An atypical star-burst mitotic figure is shown on the left.

are normal reactive cells that consist of a mixture of lymphocytes, plasma cells, fibroblasts, and eosinophils. The sparse presence of the Reed-Sternberg cell in Hodgkin's infiltrates requires a close review of multiple cuts of the histologic specimen in suspicious cases. Interestingly, Reed-Sternberg cells are not pathognomonic for Hodgkin's disease, because they are also found in other conditions—including infectious mononucleosis, toxoplasmosis, and cytomegalovirus infections—thus fueling the speculation that Hodgkin's disease might have an infectious origin.

Clinically, Hodgkin's disease is notable among the lymphomas for its orderly progression to anatomically adjacent lymphatic foci; therefore, meticulous clinical staging, often including a chest and abdominal computed tomography (CT) scan, bone marrow biopsy, lymphangiography, and an exploratory laparotomy/splenectomy, is recommended in order to establish a prognosis and to direct appropriate therapy.[23]

The rarity of orbital involvement with Hodgkin's disease limits its documentation to several isolated case reports.[24–31] In these unusual cases the orbital presentation typically occurs in the terminal process of the disease or following apparently successful treatment of disease initially presenting in a nonorbital location.[24, 31] Involvement of the superficial adnexal structures may result in a more aggressive clinical appearance with focal tissue necrosis (Fig. 176–5). Involvement of the orbital bones can cause hyperostosis or no detectable changes with adjacent soft tissue masses; osteolysis as with myeloma is rarer. Intracranial involvement of Hodgkin's lymphoma is similarly rare,[35] and in some cases may have adjacent intraorbital involvement (Fig. 176–6).[24, 25] Alternatively, orbital disease without apparent intracranial extension has been observed.[26–28] In disseminated cases, bilateral orbital involvement may occur.[29, 30]

Intraocular involvement in patients with known Hodgkin's disease, manifested by posterior uveitis, periphlebitis, and papillitis, has been reported,[32–34] but in these cases there was no involvement of the ocular adnexa or orbit.

Fortunately, Hodgkin's disease has become a model for curable neoplasms. The mainstay of treatment has included radiotherapy alone or with adjunctive chemotherapy. The orbital disease is typically sensitive to local irradiation. However, when Hodgkin's disease appears

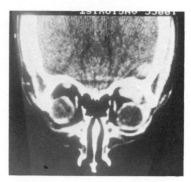

Figure 176–6. A coronal CT scan of Hodgkin's lymphoma with intracranial involvement extending through the orbital roof. (From Case Records of the Massachusetts General Hospital (Case 7–1989.) (Reprinted by permission of the New England Journal of Medicine 320:447–457, 1989.)

in the orbit, it is typically late in the course of the disease and reflects widespread extranodal involvement, which portends a worse clinical prognosis. This underscores the need for clinical follow-up of patients with Hodgkin's disease to include an assessment of the orbit and ocular adnexa for evidence of occult recurrent disease.

T-CELL LYMPHOMAS

Orbital T-cell lymphomas are extremely rare. Well-characterized T-cell lymphomas of the orbit and ocular adnexa are usually limited to case reports. Interestingly, in cases of inflammatory pseudotumor and of pseudolymphoma, the lesions consist mainly of polyclonal T cells (approximately 50 to 70 percent of constituent cells).

More commonly, although still rarely, lesions can be associated with T-cell cutaneous lymphomas, which are also known as *Mycosis fungoides*. Clinically, these lesions may present as eczematoid or psoriasiform plaques, universal erythroderma (Fig. 176–7), nodules, or ulcers (Fig. 176–8). These lesions are suspected clinically, especially when they grossly resemble fungal lesions, and the diagnosis is confirmed at biopsy, which reveals characteristic cerebriform T lymphocytes (Fig. 176–9). At the time of diagnosis, peripheral lymphade-

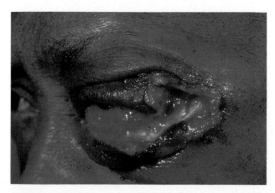

Figure 176–5. Eyelid involvement and tissue necrosis in Hodgkin's lymphoma.

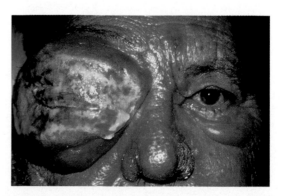

Figure 176–7. *Mycosis fungoides* with universal erythroderma. (Courtesy of Alan Proia, M.D.)

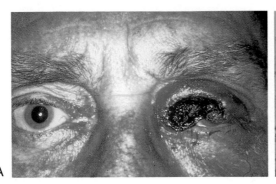

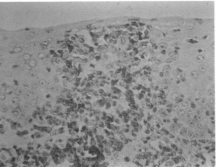

Figure 176–8. *A,* T-cell lymphoma limited to the eyelid with ulceration. *B,* The histopathology demonstrates the Pautrier-like microabscess from the epidermotropism of the T lymphocytes. (Courtesy of Seymour Brownstein, M.D.)

nopathy is common and visceral involvement is unusual. When detected in the orbit, the lesions of cutaneous T-cell lymphomas are commonly associated with a previously recognized systemic disease.[36] More rarely, these lesions may be limited to the orbit[37] or may have an initial systemic presentation as an orbital mass.[38]

Adult T-cell leukemia-lymphoma (ATLL) resembles cutaneous T-cell lymphoma; however, it has a much more aggressive course. ATLL is characterized by generalized lymphadenopathy typically sparing the mediastinum, osteolytic bone lesions, hypercalcemia, and a leukemic phase with bone marrow involvement.[39] Treatment usually involves local irradiation in conjunction with systemic chemotherapy. This T-cell lymphoma has been found to be caused by the retrovirus human T-cell leukemia virus (HTLV-I).[40] Additionally, HTLV-I is also associated with tropical spastic paraparesis.[41] The HTLV-I virus is endemic in the southeastern United States, Japan, Africa, and the Caribbean[42]—the sites of increased prevalence of ATLL. In some regions of Japan, the incidence of seropositivity for HTLV-I is greater than 25 percent, yet only a small proportion of seropositive patients (1 to 2 percent) seem to ultimately develop a malignancy.[43]

Orbital ATLL has been convincingly reported in only one patient.[44] With the increasing frequency of neoplasms observed arising from lymphotropic viruses (i.e., HTLV-III), more frequent observations are anticipated in the future. We have treated one patient with orbital involvement with HTLV-I manifested by proptosis and multiple cranial nerve palsies, in the terminal course of disease in association with intracranial involvement (Fig. 176–10). The therapies for HTLV-I lymphomas are still experimental. Systemic and, if indicated, intrathecal chemotherapy constitute the typical treatment modalities. Limited response has been reported with the use of a monoclonal antibody to the receptor of interleukin 2.[45] Despite these treatments, no long-term remissions have been reported.

AIDS AND ORBITAL LYMPHOMA

Lymphomas appear among the myriad of neoplastic disorders encountered in patients with AIDS. In general the lymphomas in the setting of AIDS are typically high grade, of B-cell origin, and extranodal. In one large study of non-Hodgkin's lymphomas in homosexual men with either AIDS, generalized lymphadenopathy, or no prodromal signs, 60 of 62 patients had an extranodal lymphoma, with the central nervous system, bone marrow, gastrointestinal tract, and mucocutaneous sites involved in order of decreasing frequency.[46] Other lymphoproliferative neoplasms (although much less common) found in patients with or at high risk for AIDS include Hodgkin's lymphoma and lymphocytic leukemia.

Orbital involvement among these AIDS-related lymphomas is unusual and limited to isolated reports and inclusion in large series.[46–49] Given the rapid evolution of some of these orbital neoplasms, an opportunistic infectious process is usually the other leading diagnostic

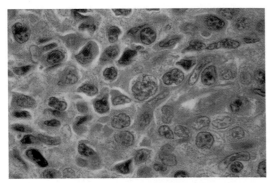

Figure 176–9. Histopathology of T-cell lymphoma demonstrating the characteristic cerebriform hyperconvoluted cleaved nuclei.

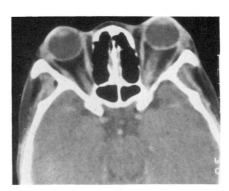

Figure 176–10. A CT scan of HTLV-I lymphoma with infiltration of the left optic nerve.

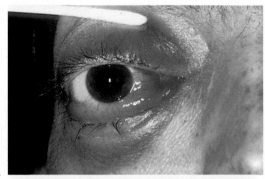

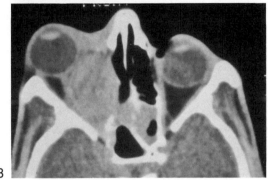

Figure 176–11. Orbital B-cell lymphoma in a patient with known AIDS. *A,* This patient presented with painless proptosis and anterior orbital congestion. *B,* The CT scan demonstrated an infiltrating orbital soft tissue mass that was consistent with a neoplastic or opportunistic infectious mass. An orbital biopsy and cell surface marker studies established the diagnosis of an orbital lymphoma.

concern in the patient with AIDS presenting with an orbital mass. CT imaging helps to delineate the extent of orbital involvement as well as evaluate the adjacent sinuses (Fig. 176–11). The diagnosis can be established most definitively by an open biopsy, although a preliminary attempt with a fine-needle aspirational biopsy and cytologic analysis may be an appropriate initial alternative.

In cases with isolated orbital involvement, local irradiation may be effective, especially in the presence of vision-threatening massive proptosis. Not surprisingly, these patients may concomitantly possess opportunistic ocular infections that portend a worse prognosis for vision. Overall, the prognosis is predictably poor despite irradiation or chemotherapy.

BURKITT'S LYMPHOMA

Burkitt's lymphoma is a rare B-cell monoclonal malignant lymphoma with characteristic clinical, histologic, epidemiologic, and genetic findings. The first definitive description of this disorder was made by Burkitt in 1958, when he described an unusual clustering of jaw tumors associated with abdominal visceral tumors in Ugandan children.[50] Jaw tumors occur on presentation in approximately 50 percent of endemic (African) cases, with a slight predominance of lesions within the maxilla. Understandably, the maxillary tumors may frequently present with a secondary orbital mass. Orbital involvement

is manifested by painless proptosis, superior globe displacement, and chemosis. Rare cases involving primarily the superior orbit, particularly the lacrimal gland, have also been described.[51]

Due to the short doubling time of the tumor (less than 3 days), the clinical picture progresses very rapidly, and the tumor often reaches massive hideous proportions at the time of presentation. Meningeal infiltration with malignant pleocytosis occurs at presentation in 20 to 30 percent of patients and is associated with the clinical findings of cranial nerve palsies or epidural mass with spinal compression.

The greatest incidence of Burkitt's lymphoma is in the African region spanning 15 degrees north to 15 degrees south of the equator. In this "endemic" belt, the incidence is approximately 5 to 15/100,000. In nonendemic areas (e.g., North America, Europe) the incidence is 20 to 100 times less. Interestingly, nonendemic cases possess different clinical and genetic features. In endemic cases, the median age of presentation is 7 to 8 yr and in nonendemic cases 11 to 12 yr. We have seen cases in adults that presented with either intraocular or ocular adnexal masses in the absence of bone destruction (Fig. 176–12). Facial tumors account for two thirds of new presentations in endemic cases, whereas in nonendemic regions abdominal mass presentation predominates and only one third involve the jaw. In 96 percent of endemic cases, Epstein-Barr virus (EBV) DNA is present within the genome of some tumor cells, whereas only 10 to 20 percent of nonendemic cases possess viral incorporation into the host DNA.[52]

Despite these discordant features, both the endemic

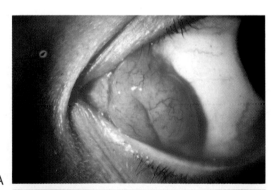

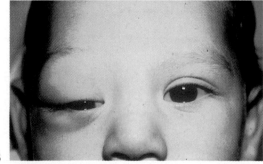

Figure 176–12. Nonendemic Burkitt's lymphoma. Unusual clinical presentations may include: *A,* Salmon-colored caruncular mass. (Courtesy of Barbara Streeten, M.D.) *B,* Rapidly growing orbital mass in the absence of bone destruction. (Courtesy of Charles Lee, M.D.)

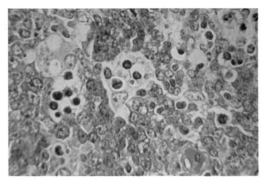

Figure 176–13. Burkitt's lymphoma histopathologically displays large histiocytes ("starry sky pattern") with clear cytoplasmic debris ("tingible bodies") scattered among an aggregate of large neoplastic lymphocytes.

and nonendemic tumors usually express cell surface immunoglobulin that is characterized by a cytogenetic translocation between the c-*myc* oncogene located on band q 24 of chromosome 8 (8 q 24) and at one of the immunoglobulin loci. This occurs most frequently at the immunoglobulin heavy chain gene located on chromosome 14 (14 q 32), or else at one of the genes for light chain kappa (2 p12) or lambda (22q11).[53] In the process of these translocations involving the c-*myc* oncogene, there is deregulation of c-*myc* that is an essential component in tumorigenesis.[54]

Histopathologically, the appearance of Burkitt's lymphoma is characterized by a uniform background of large round or oval lymphocytes with regularly shaped or cleaved nuclei and multiple prominent nucleoli. Interspersed within the collection of neoplastic lymphocytes are large, pale-staining, benign phagocytic histiocytes or macrophages. These cells produce the characteristic "starry sky" appearance (Fig. 176–13). Outside

of Africa this disease and particularly its orbital manifestations are especially uncommon, and it is rarely suspected clinically when the characteristic jaw lesion is absent. There have been increasing reports of this tumor arising in patients with AIDS.[49, 55]

In nonendemic areas another disorder, granulocytic sarcoma, is more likely to be encountered clinically in children. Granulocytic sarcoma, previously referred to as chloroma, is a soft tissue or visceral focus of infiltrating leukemic cells in the absence of peripheral blood and occasionally bone marrow involvement. Similar to Burkitt's lymphoma, the median age of presentation is 7 yr with a slight male predominance.[56] In these patients, the soft tissue deposits in the ocular adnexa are characteristically the initial manifestation of an impending systemic leukemia (Fig. 176–14A). On histopathologic examination, the Leder stain for cytoplasmic esterase or immunohistochemical muramidase stain for lysozyme permits an accurate diagnosis (Fig. 176–14B and C). Electron microscopy revealing myelogenous lysosomal granules or specific monoclonal antibodies can also be useful in establishing the diagnosis. In this age range, rhabdomyosarcoma, the most common pediatric primary malignant tumor of the orbit, presents with a similar clinical fulminance to Burkitt's lymphoma and granulocytic sarcoma, and it must also be considered.

The established treatment of choice for Burkitt's lymphoma is chemotherapy due to the typically disseminated nature of the disease upon presentation and the exquisite sensitivity of the rapidly dividing tumor cells to pharmacologic agents. A combined chemotherapy regimen including cyclophosphamide, vincristine, methotrexate, and corticosteroids is successful in achieving remission in more than 50 percent of cases.[57] Occasionally, before the initiation of chemotherapy, the primary tumor is debulked or resected. Prophylactic irradiation to the brain is occasionally administered in patients with

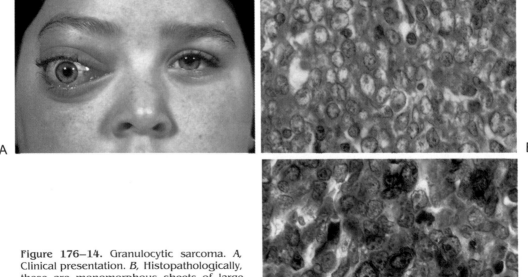

Figure 176–14. Granulocytic sarcoma. *A,* Clinical presentation. *B,* Histopathologically, these are monomorphous sheets of large cells with fine nucleoli. H&E ×450. *C,* Muramidase stain for lysosomal granules. The Leder stain for esterase requiring formalin-fixed tissue can also help with the diagnosis.

bone marrow involvement. The tumor volume and the extent of systemic involvement are the best prognostic features. Naturally, early recognition and rapid initiation of chemotherapy provide the best chances for enhancing survival.

LYMPHOMATOID GRANULOMATOSIS

Lymphomatoid granulomatosis, another very rare lymphoreticular disease, typically exhibits pulmonary involvement. This is a distinct disorder that lies within the clinical spectrum between Wegener's granulomatosis and malignant lymphoma. In addition to bilateral pulmonary infiltrates that may be seen in 80 percent of cases, 40 percent of patients have cutaneous manifestations.[58] The skin findings commonly appear as erythematous noduloulcerative lesions. When involving the eye and its adnexa, ocular findings of uveitis, scleritis, and vasculitis predominate.[58–60] Even less commonly, cutaneous lesions may appear in the periorbital region.[58, 61] The skin lesions are reminiscent of the cutaneous ulcerations found in T-cell lymphomas. Interestingly, immunohistochemical analysis has been suggestive of a T-cell disorder.[62]

On pathologic examination, a polymorphic lymphoreticular infiltrate with plasmacytoid cells and a necrotizing vasculitis is characteristically encountered. This disorder is distinguished from Wegener's granulomatosis histopathologically by the absence of multinucleated giant cells.

The primary differential considerations are infectious processes, other vasculitides, and central facial lymphomas (i.e., lethal midline granuloma). Central nervous system findings, particularly cranial nerve palsies, are found in about 20 percent of patients with lymphomatoid granulomatosis. Systemic lymphoma with nodal involvement occurs in approximately 10 to 50 percent of patients.[58, 59] Despite treatment about two thirds of patients with lymphomatoid granulomatosis succumb to their disease, most commonly as a result of pulmonary complications.

ANGIOLYMPHOID HYPERPLASIA WITH EOSINOPHILIA (KIMURA'S DISEASE)

Angiolymphoid hyperplasia with eosinophilia (ALHE) is a rare benign disorder involving primarily the face and scalp and is characterized by isolated or multiple papular to nodular lesions within the skin and subcutaneous tissues. This condition, which was initially described by Kimura and associates in 1948[63] in a Japanese population, was commonly associated with lymphadenopathy and peripheral blood eosinophilia. Interestingly, in nonoriental patients there is a lower incidence of these systemic findings.[64] A varied nomenclature has been applied to this condition, including atypical pyogenic granuloma,[65] histiocytoid hemangioma,[66] subcutaneous angiolymphoid hyperplasia,[67] and Kimura's disease.

Ocular adnexal and orbital involvement is rare and is limited to isolated case reports and to one small series.[68] Characteristic presentation is in the fourth to seventh decades, with slight male predominance and a subacute to chronic history of proptosis, ptosis, or eyelid mass. These lesions are typically isolated. Simultaneous systemic findings of lymphadenopathy and peripheral blood eosinophilia have not been reported, although in one case associated with obstructive airway disease, there was a delayed, transient eosinophilia.[69]

Grossly, the lesions are commonly well-circumscribed firm reddish brown masses due to their high vascularity. Histopathologic examination of this tissue features an abnormal proliferation of small blood vessels lined by plump vacuolated endothelial cells and surrounded by a chronic inflammatory infiltrate that is rich in eosinophils and variably intense lymphocytes with scattered lymphoid follicles (Fig. 176–15). Evidence of vasculitis can sometimes be identified. Given the rarity of this lesion, the histopathologic diagnosis can be challenging and the condition must often be distinguished from angiosarcoma, Kaposi's sarcoma, epithelioid hemangioendothelioma, eosinophilic granuloma, insect bite, pyogenic granuloma, lymphomatous proliferation, and inflammatory pseudotumor.

The etiology of this condition remains unclear, although most agree that it represents a reactive inflammatory process rather than a true neoplasm. The pres-

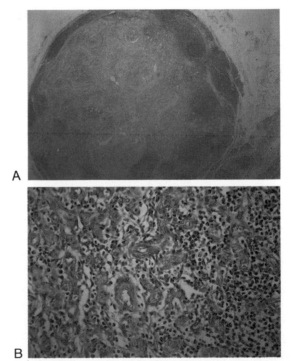

Figure 176–15. Angiolymphoid hyperplasia with eosinophilia (Kimura's disease). *A,* A circumscribed but nonencapsulated orbital mass features a zonal pattern, with hyperplastic lymphoid elements concentrated at the periphery, while in the center there is a proliferation of blood vessels. *B,* Prominent capillary proliferation with an accompanying intense eosinophilic leukocytic infiltration. (*A* and *B,* Courtesy of Ahmed A. Hidayat, M.D.)

ence of eosinophilia and in some cases elevated IgE or increased antibodies to *Candida albicans* fueled speculation that the lesion represents an allergic type I hypersensitivity reaction or an infectious process.[70]

In one anophthalmic orbital presentation, a polymethylmethacrylate Iowa enucleation implant may have provided an inciting stimulus.[71]

The treatment modality of choice is complete surgical excision. Intralesional or systemic corticosteroids alone, or adjunctively to subtotal surgical excision, have also proven effective.

REFERENCES

1. Bergsagel DE: Lymphocytic disorders: Malignant proliferative response and/or abnormal immunoglobulin synthesis—plasma cell dyscrasias. *In* Williams WJ, Beutler E, Ersler AJ, et al (eds): Hematology, 4th ed. New York, McGraw-Hill, 1990.
2. Knowling MA, Harwood AR, Bergsagel DE: Comparison of extramedullary plasmacytomas with solitary and multiple plasma cell tumors of bone. J Clin Oncol 1:255–262, 1983.
3. Woodruff RK, Whittle JM, Malpas JS: Solitary plasmacytoma: Extramedullary soft tissue plasmacytoma. Cancer 43:2340–2343, 1979.
4. deSmet MD, Rootman J: Orbital manifestations of plasmacytic lymphoproliferations. Ophthalmology 94:995–1003, 1987.
5. Rodman HI, Font RL: Orbital involvement in multiple myeloma. Arch Ophthalmol 87:30–35, 1972.
6. Knapp AJ, Gartner S, Henkind P: Multiple myeloma and its ocular manifestations. Surv Ophthalmol 31:343–351, 1987.
7. Benjamin I, Taylor H, Spindler J: Orbital and conjunctival involvement in multiple myeloma: Report of a case. Am J Clin Pathol 63:811–817, 1975.
8. Jain BS: Solitary myeloma of the orbit. Am J Ophthalmol 58:855–858, 1964.
9. Rose D, Taylor C: Multiple myelomatosis affecting the orbit. Br J Ophthalmol 41:438–439, 1957.
10. Handrousa A: Multiple myelomatosis with proptosis. Br J Ophthalmol 39:41–43, 1955.
11. Knowles DM, Halper JA, Trokel S, Jakobiec FA: Immunofluorescent and immunoperoxidase characteristics of IgD-lambda myeloma involving the orbit. Am J Ophthalmol 85:485–494, 1978.
12. Nikoskelainen E, Dellaporta A, Rice T, et al: Orbital involvement by plasmacytoma: A report of two cases. Acta Ophthalmol 54:755–761, 1976.
13. Bjornberg K: Extramedullary plasmacytoma in the orbit. Acta Ophthalmol 40:330–335, 1962.
14. Levin SR, Spaulding AG, Wirman JA: Multiple myeloma: Orbital involvement in a youth. Arch Ophthalmol 95:642–644, 1977.
15. McEvoy J: Plasma cell myeloma of orbit. Am J Ophthalmol 32:1745–1746, 1949.
16. Jonasson F: Orbital plasma cell tumors. Ophthalmologica 177:152–157, 1978.
17. Khalil MK, Huang S, Viloria J, et al: Extramedullary plasmacytoma of the orbit: Case report with results of immunocytochemical studies. Can J Ophthalmol 16:39–42, 1981.
18. Gould L, Ostrove R: Extramedullary myeloma of the lacrimal gland. Am J Ophthalmol 60:1125–1126, 1965.
19. Rubenzik R, Tenzel R: Multiple myeloma involving the lacrimal gland. Ann Ophthalmol 7:1077–1078, 1975.
20. Shields JA, Cooper H, Donoso LA, et al: Immunohistochemical and ultrasound study of unusual IgM lambda lymphoplasmacytic tumor of the lacrimal gland. Am J Ophthalmol 101:451–457, 1986.
21. Raflo GT, Farel TA, Sioussat RS: Complete ophthalmoplegia secondary to amyloidosis associated with multiple myeloma. Am J Ophthalmol 92:221–224, 1981.
22. Gonnering RS: Bilateral primary extramedullary orbital plasmacytomas. Ophthalmology 94:267–270, 1987.
23. Rosenburg S, Kaplan H: Evidence for an orderly progression in the spread of Hodgkin's disease. Cancer Res 26:1225–1231, 1966.
24. Case Records of the Massachusetts General Hospital (case 7—1989). N Engl J Med 320:447–457, 1989.
25. Sapozinak MD, Kaplan HS: Intracranial Hodgkin's disease: A report of 12 cases and review of the literature. Cancer 52:1301–1307, 1983.
26. Sen DK, Mohan H, Catterjee PK: Hodgkin's disease in the orbit. Int Surg 55:183–186, 1971.
27. Papaleo G, Gallo AB, Zito G, et al: Su di un caso di molattia di Hodgkin con localizzazione endoorbitaria. Haematologica 62:95–97, 1977.
28. Patel S, Rootman J: Nodular sclerosing Hodgkin's disease of the orbit. Ophthalmology 90:1433–1436, 1983.
29. Ordonez-Gallego A, Montero-Garcia JM, Mate-Benito I, et al: Formas clinicas insolitas de la enfermedad de Hodgkin. Rev Clin Esp 122:313–322, 1976.
30. Fratkin JD, Shammas HF, Miller SD: Disseminated Hodgkin's disease with orbital involvement. Arch Ophthalmol 96:102–104, 1978.
31. Kremer I, Loven D, Mor C, Lurie H: A solitary conjunctival relapse of Hodgkin's disease treated by radiotherapy. Ophthal Surg 20:494–496, 1989.
32. Bishop JE, Salmonsen PC: Presumed intraocular Hodgkin's disease. Ann Ophthalmol 17:589–592, 1985.
33. Mosteller MW, Margo CE, Hesse RJ: Hodgkin's disease and granulomatous uveitis. Ann Ophthalmol 17:787–790, 1985.
34. Barr CC, Joondeph HC: Retinal periphlebitis as the initial clinical finding in a patient with Hodgkin's disease. Retina 3:253–257, 1983.
35. Cuttner J, Meyer R, Huang YP: Intracerebral involvement in Hodgkin's disease: A report of 6 cases and review of the literature. Cancer 43:1497–1506, 1979.
36. Stenson S, Ramsay DL: Ocular findings in *Mycosis fungoides*. Arch Ophthalmol 99:272–277, 1981.
37. Laroche L, Laroche L, Pavlakis E, Saraux H: Immunologic characterization of an ocular adnexal lymphoid T tumor by monoclonal antibodies. Ophthalmologica 187:43–49, 1983.
38. Meekins B, Proia AD, Klintworth GK: Cutaneous T-cell lymphoma presenting as a rapidly enlarging ocular adnexal tumor. Ophthalmology 92:1288–1293, 1985.
39. Uchiyama T, Yodoi J, Sagawa F, et al: Adult T-cell leukemia: Clinical and hematologic features of 16 cases. Blood 50:481–492, 1977.
40. Gallo RC, Kalyanaraman VS, Sarngaadharan MG, et al: Association of human type C retrovirus with a subset of adult T-cell cancers. Cancer Res 43:3892–3899, 1983.
41. Kim JH, Durack DT: Manifestations of human T-lymphotropic virus type I infection. Am J Med 84:919–928, 1988.
42. Blattner WA, Blayney DW, Robert-Guroff M, et al: Epidemiology of human T-cell leukemia/lymphoma virus. J Infect Dis 147:406–416, 1983.
43. Hinoma Y: Seroepidemiology of adult origin of virus carriers in Japan. AIDS Res 2:517–522, 1986.
44. Lauer SA, Fischer J, Jones J, et al: Orbital T-cell lymphoma in human T-cell leukemia virus I infection. Ophthalmology 95:110–115, 1988.
45. Waldman TA, Goldma CK, Bongiovanni KF, et al: Therapy of patients with human T-cell lymphotropic virus I induced adult T-cell leukemia with anti-tac, a monoclonal antibody to the receptor for interleukin-2. Blood 72:1805–1816, 1988.
46. Ziegler JL, Beckstead JA, Volberding PA, et al: Non-Hodgkin's lymphoma in 90 homosexual men: Relation to generalized lymphadenopathy and the acquired immunodeficiency syndrome. N Engl J Med 311:565–570, 1984.
47. Khojasteh A, Reynolds RD, Khojasteh CA: Malignant lymphoreticular lesions in patients with immune disorders resembling acquired immunodeficiency syndrome (AIDS): Review of 80 cases. South Med J 79:1070–1075, 1986.
48. Antle CM, White VA, Horsman DE, Rootman J: Large cell orbital lymphoma in a patient with acquired immunodeficiency syndrome: Case report and review. Ophthalmology 97:1494–1498, 1990.
49. Ziegler JL, Drew WL, Miner RC, et al: Outbreak of Burkitt's-like lymphoma in homosexual men. Lancet 2:631–633, 1982.
50. Burkitt D: A sarcoma involving the jaws in African children. Br J Surg 46:218–223, 1958.
51. Burkitt DP: General features and facial tumors. *In* Burkitt DP, Wright DH (eds): Burkitt's Lymphoma. Edinburgh, E&S Livingstone, 1970.

52. Magrath I: The pathogenesis of Burkitt's lymphoma. Adv Cancer Res 55:133–270, 1990.
53. Dalla-Favera R, Bregni M, Erickson J, et al: Human *c-myc* oncogene is located on the region of chromosome 8 that is translocated in Burkitt lymphoma cells. Proc Natl Acad Sci USA 79:7824, 1982.
54. Lombardi L, Newcomb E, Dalla-Favera R: Pathogenesis of Burkitt lymphoma: Expression of an activated *c-myc* oncogene causes the tumorigenic conversion of EBV-infected human B lymphoblasts. Cell 49:161, 1987.
55. Young SA, Crocker DW: Burkitt's lymphoma in a child with AIDS. Pediatr Pathol 11:115–122, 1991.
56. Zimmerman LE, Font RL: Ophthalmic manifestations of granulocytic sarcoma (myeloid sarcoma or chloroma). Am J Ophthalmol 80:975–990, 1975.
57. Ziegler JL: Treatment results of 54 American patients with Burkitt's lymphoma are similar to the African experience. N Engl J Med 297:75–80, 1977.
58. Katzenstein AA, Carrington CB, Liebow AA: Lymphomatoid granulomatosis: A clinicopathologic study of 152 cases. Cancer 43:360–373, 1979.
59. Fauci AS, Haynes BF, Costa J, et al: Lymphomatoid granulomatosis: Prospective clinical and therapeutic experience over 10 years. N Engl J Med 306:68–74, 1982.
60. Tse DT, Mandelbaum S, Chuck DA, et al: Lymphomatoid granulomatosis with ocular involvement. Retina 5:94–97, 1985.
61. Font RL, Rosenbaum PS, Smith JL: Lymphomatoid granulomatosis of the eyelid and brow with progression to lymphoma. J Am Acad Dermatol 23:334–337, 1990.
62. Nichols PW, Koss M, Levine AM, et al: Lymphomatoid granulomatosis: A T-cell disorder? Am J Med 72:467–471, 1982.
63. Kimura T, Yoshimura S, Ishikawa E: On the unusual granulation combined with hyperplastic changes of the lymphatic tissues. Trans Soc Pathol Jap 37:179–180, 1948.
64. Henry PG, Burnett JW: Angiolymphoid hyperplasia with eosinophilia. Arch Dermatol 114:1168–1172, 1978.
65. Jones EW, Bleehan SS: Inflammatory angiomatous nodules with abnormal blood vessels occuring about the ears and scalp (pseudo or atypical pyogenic granuloma). Br J Dermatol 81:804–816, 1969.
66. Rosai J, Gold J, Landy R: The histiocytoid hemangiomas: A unifying concept embracing several previously described entities of the skin, soft tissue, large vessels, bone, and heart. Hum Pathol 10:707, 1979.
67. Reed RJ, Tarazakis N: Subcutaneous angioblastic lymphoid hyperplasia with hyperplasia (Kimura's disease). Cancer 29:489–497, 1972.
68. Hidayat AA, Cameron JD, Font RL, et al: Angiolymphoid hyperplasia with eosinophilia (Kimura's disease) of the orbit and ocular adnexae. Am J Ophthalmol 96:176–189, 1983.
69. Sheren SB, Custer PL, Smith M: Angiolymphoid hyperplasia with eosinophilia of the orbit with obstructive airway disease. Am J Ophthalmol 108:167–169, 1989.
70. Takenaka T, Okuda M, Usami A, et al: Histochemical and immunological studies on eosinophilic granuloma of soft tissue, so-called Kimura's disease. Clin Allergy 6:27–39, 1976.
71. Smith DL, Kincaid MC, Nicolitz E: Angiolymphoid hyperplasia with eosinophilia (Kimura's disease) of the orbit. Arch Ophthalmol 106:793–795, 1988.

Chapter 177

■

Metastatic and Secondary Orbital Tumors

NICHOLAS J. VOLPE and DANIEL M. ALBERT

ORBITAL METASTATIC TUMORS

Patients with cancer die because of the ability of their tumors to invade and metastasize. Metastatic and secondary cancers of the eye and its adnexa are rare compared with other secondary sites but are now being recognized with much greater frequency as patients with malignancies treated with modern therapies survive longer. In fact, metastatic and secondary tumors are the most common malignancies to involve the eye and orbit.[1-3] Recognition of this entity, therefore, has become more important for both internists and ophthalmologists. They must be able to recognize the protean clinical presentations of these many different metastasizing tumors and the possible sites of origin and to utilize the appropriate management strategies.

The orbit is the second most common site for metastatic disease to the eye and its adnexa, with the uveal tract involved more frequently. Unfortunately, after identification of a metastatic tumor to the uvea or orbit the prognosis for survival is uniformly bad, and few patients survive for more than 1 yr.[1] Prompt recognition

of this condition may help in the detection of a previously unrecognized systemic malignancy or allow for early treatment. In many cases, treatment can be only palliative; however, in other cases, using modern combined modality therapies, patient survival can be prolonged.

Incidence and Prevalence

The first reported case of metastatic disease of the orbit was by Horner in 1864.[4] Since then the disease has been recognized with increasing frequency. In a comprehensive review,[5] Goldberg, Rootman, and Cline identified 245 reported cases of metastatic tumors to the orbit in the literature. Of those 245 cases almost half were reported in the last decade. They point out that, although the disease is possibly becoming more common as cancer patients survive longer and their tumors are altered immunologically by therapy, this dramatic increase in reported cases also reflects the overall proliferation of the medical literature. The consideration of the incidence and prevalence of this condition must be approached in two different ways: first, is the question of how many people with carcinomas will develop orbital metastases and second, what percentage of orbital disease is caused by metastatic lesions?

The percentage of patients with known systemic malignancies who have clinically documented metastases to the eye and its adnexa is not as high as the incidence of identification of tumor foci in autopsy studies of patients who have succumbed to their malignancies. Godtfredsen,[6] in 1944, found ophthalmoscopic evidence of metastatic tumors to the eye in 6 of 8712 (0.07 percent) patients referred for radiation therapy. With increasing sophistication and better examination techniques, Albert and associates,[7] in 1967, found an incidence of 4.7 percent of eye or orbital involvement in 213 patients with known malignancies.

In their autopsy study of 230 patients with proven carcinomas, Bloch and Gartner[3] found 12 percent (28 patients) with pathologic evidence of metastases to the eye and orbit. Five patients had orbital metastases representing 2 percent of patients autopsied; however, the entire orbital contents were not examined. This bias is built into all histopathologic studies that examine this problem; that is, most autopsy studies[1, 2, 8, 9] examine the globe completely and only parts of the orbital contents. Therefore, these studies have estimated that intraocular metastases are three to eight times more likely to occur than are orbital metastases. It may be that because the choroid is the most vascular tissue of the eye and its adnexa, it is most likely to be the site of blood-borne metastases. However, Freedman and Folk[10] reviewed 112 patients presenting with ocular and orbital metastases that were evaluated clinically with modern methods and found that 56 had choroidal involvement, 49 had orbital involvement, and 5 had both sites involved. The remaining two patients had lesions involving the optic nerve and retina. This question cannot be addressed adequately until an autopsy study of the entire orbital contents of patients with systemic malignancies is performed. Suffice it to say that orbital lesions are likely to occur almost as frequently as intraocular metastases. It has been estimated that 25,000 patients/yr who die of systemic malignancies also have ocular involvement. With increased clinical awareness and sophistication as well as more sensitive diagnostic modalities, increasing numbers of patients with metastatic orbital lesions will be identified.

The incidence of metastatic tumors as the cause of orbital disease ranges in various series from 1 to 3 percent. Rootman[11] found 29 (2.1 percent) cases of metastatic tumors in 1409 consecutive patients with orbital disease of any kind, evaluated by various modalities. Shields and associates[12] found metastatic tumors in 16 (2.5 percent) of 645 orbital biopsies performed. Moss,[13] reporting the series of Reese and Jones in 1962, found 3 (1.3 percent) metastatic tumors among 230 patients with expanding lesions of the orbit who were diagnosed clinically, pathologically, and radiologically. In Reese's entire series of 877 cases of orbital neoplasms, 29 (3.3 percent) were metastatic lesions.[14] In a biopsy series of 300 patients with expanding orbital lesions, Silva,[15] reported 7 cases (2.3 percent) of metastatic tumors.

If one considers only orbital neoplasms, metastatic disease represents a more significant percentage. Henderson[16] found that 56 (10.1 percent) of 552 patients with neoplasms had metastatic tumors. Furthermore, Goldberg and associates[5] found that 38 (12 percent) of 314 patients with orbital neoplasms had metastatic tumors.

In summary, metastatic orbital tumors are being recognized with increased frequency. If one extrapolates from autopsy studies of ocular metastases, it is likely that subclinical disease frequently goes unrecognized. Generally, orbital disease is uncommon and is only caused by metastatic tumors in a relatively small percentage of cases. However, it is essential that all ophthalmologists be familiar with this entity and the spectrum of disease for which it is responsible. Familiarity aids in prompt diagnosis and treatment, affording patients improved quality of life and possibly an increased rate of survival.

Pathogenesis of Metastatic Orbital Tumors

TRAVEL TO THE ORBIT

The orbit, posterior to the septum, does not contain any lymphatic channels. Therefore, it is presumed that all metastatic tumors reach the eye and its adnexa via the blood stream. It follows that all tumor emboli that are to reach the eye must have passed through the pulmonary circulation and seeded the lungs with tumor emboli. However, in one study, 15 percent of cases with ocular metastases had no demonstrable pulmonary metastases at the time of autopsy.[17] It is likely that some of the pulmonary foci are microscopic and are not detected but also that some of the emboli reach the arterial circulation by passing through the Batson vertebral system of vessels, thus bypassing the pulmonary circulation. Tumor cells subsequently travel in the carotid system to reach the orbit via the ophthalmic artery. Several early review studies suggested that there was a left-sided predilection for metastatic tumors.[9, 18, 19] It was postulated that because the left carotid artery arises directly from the aorta and the right carotid artery arises off the inominate artery, metastatic emboli have a more direct path to the left side. Other studies have failed to demonstrate a left-sided predilection.[1-3, 7, 20] In fact, in their recent and most comprehensive review of the world's literature on orbital metastases, Goldberg and associates[5] found a slight right-sided predilection for orbital metastases and bilateral disease in approximately 10 percent of patients.

The majority of the blood supply to the orbit is through the ophthalmic artery. It arises acutely off the internal carotid and this, along with the relatively small percentage of the body's blood flow that travels through the ophthalmic artery, is the reason why ocular and adnexa metastases occur relatively infrequently. In addition, a small amount of blood flow reaches the orbit via branches (facial, maxillary, and temporal) of the external carotid artery. After seeding through the vascular system, tumor emboli arrest in the microvasculature of the different ocular tissues. Areas of increased vasculature (particularly the choroid in the posterior pole of the globe) receive the most emboli and are frequently involved with metastatic disease. However, there are also important local or "soil" factors, possibly immunologic, that determine whether the embolic tumor cell is able to divide and proliferate.[21, 22]

LOCALIZATION IN THE ORBIT

After travel through the carotid system, the tissue-specific localization of tumor emboli within the orbit has been considered in several series.[16, 18, 23, 24] Hart[18] found that the medial orbit was the most frequently involved, whereas Font and Ferry,[24] found no predilection. In reviewing the literature, Goldberg and associates found that approximately 40 percent of tumors involved the lateral orbit, and only 12 percent involved the inferior orbit. In this series, 30 percent occurred in the superior orbit and 20 percent occurred in the medial orbit.[5]

At the time of diagnosis, there is often unencapsulated tumor growth with diffuse involvement of the various orbital tissues (Fig. 177–1). However, certain localizing generalizations can be made. Initial tumor emboli can lodge in muscle, fat, or bone or involve the orbit diffusely. In clinical studies in which tumor localization can be accomplished by high-resolution computed tomography (CT) scanning, the bone and fat are each

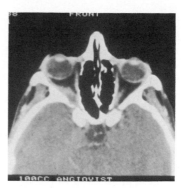

Figure 177–2. Metastatic lung carcinoma to the right orbit presenting as a "bumpy" and enlarged lateral rectus muscle. (Courtesy of N. Snebold, M.D.)

involved twice as often as metastatic lesions to the muscle.[5] Breast carcinoma most frequently involves the fat initially, and prostate carcinoma has a strong predilection for bone. In their literature review of 31 cases of metastatic tumors to the extraocular muscles, Capone and Slamovits[25] found that 16 cases arose from the breast and that six cases arose from melanoma. After initial seeding, most tumors go on to infiltrative unencapsulated growth. Occasionally, thyroid and renal metastases grow as discrete nodules.

Metastatic lesions that discretely involve the muscles (Fig. 177–2) can be the most challenging lesions to diagnose.[22, 26, 27] In these situations, the numerous inflammatory and infiltrative conditions that cause enlargement or "bumpy" muscles[28] must be considered, and metastatic disease frequently masquerades as other more common inflammatory conditions.[29] Among these diseases are Graves' disease, idiopathic inflammatory pseudotumor, acromegaly, amyloidosis, trichinosis, carotid-cavernous fistula, rhabdomyosarcoma, orbital lymphoid tumors, and systemic vasculitic diseases. In a CT scan review study, Rothfus and Curtin found 10 cases of metastases in 137 patients with CT scan evidence of extraocular muscle enlargement.[30] Clinical suspicion must remain high, and all "atypical" inflammatory orbital disease must be biopsied promptly—even if there has been some clinical response with use of systemic steroids.

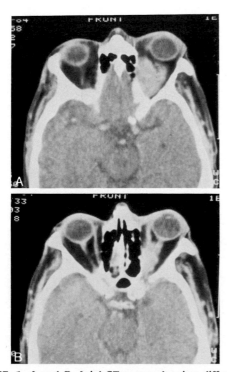

Figure 177–1. A and B, Axial CT scans showing diffuse involvement of orbital tissues by metastatic adenocarcinoma.

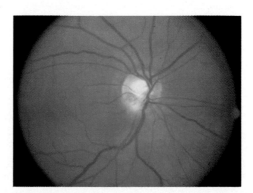

Figure 177–3. Metastatic adrenal cell carcinoma to the inferior pole of the optic nerve. (Courtesy of S. Lessell, M.D.)

Metastases can travel directly to the optic nerve head (Fig. 177–3). Ferry and Font found that 3 of 227 cases (1.3 percent) of metastases to the eye and orbit involved only the optic nerve or its sheath.[1] Metastases can occur anywhere along the course of the nerve. In addition, optic nerve involvement can develop secondary to choroidal metastases. In 1970, Ginsberg and associates[31] reviewed 115 cases of metastatic carcinoma to the optic nerve and found that 39 percent developed secondary to intraocular metastases, 33 percent from direct hematogenous spread to the optic nerve itself, and 20 percent from meningeal carcinomatosis with optic nerve involvement. In an autopsy review study of 169 secondary optic nerve tumors, Christmas and associates[32] found that metastatic tumors were the cause in 20 (12 percent) of the cases. As with other secondary sites, the most common source of the primary tumor is breast carcinoma followed by lung carcinoma.[31–33] Ginsberg and associates[31] found other primary sites in their review, including the stomach, pancreas, mediastinum, melanoma, uterus, and ovary.

The optic nerve can also be involved with diffuse meningeal carcinomatosis (Fig. 177–4), and here, in addition to carcinomas, lymphoma and myloma may also be the primary source. The prevalence of meningeal carcinomatosis is approximately 5 percent, but this varies with the type of primary tumor.[34, 35] Meningeal involvement has been reported as high as 28 percent in small cell carcinoma of the lung.[36] In a review of cases at the Mayo Clinic, Little and associates found that the optic nerve was involved in 14 percent (4/29) of cases of meningeal carcinomatosis.[37] Redman and associates examined patients with meningeal carcinomatosis secondary to head and neck tumors and found that the optic nerve was the most commonly involved nerve.[38] Visual loss can occur in up to one third of patients with meningeal carcinomatosis.[39] Visual loss appears late in the disease and frequently occurs abruptly.[40]

Metastatic tumors have can travel directly to the eyelid.[41, 42] Hood, Font, and Zimmerman noted a peculiar "histiocytoid" histopathologic appearance in most patients with metastatic breast carcinoma to the eyelid, which often makes pathologic diagnosis difficult.[42]

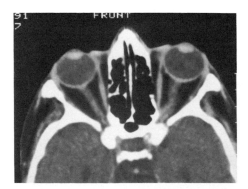

Figure 177–4. CT scan appearance of diffuse thickening of the left optic nerve secondary to meningeal involvement by metastatic oat cell carcinoma.

Table 177–1. COMMON PRIMARY SOURCES OF METASTATIC ORBITAL TUMORS

Primary Tumor Site	%
Breast	42
Lung	11
Prostate	8
Melanoma	5
Unknown primary	11

From Goldberg RA, Rootman J, Cline RA: Tumors metastatic to the orbit: A changing picture. Surv Ophthalmol 35:1, 1990.

PRIMARY SOURCE OF METASTATIC ORBITAL TUMORS

Virtually all tumors have been reported to metastasize to the orbit. The most accurate estimate of the relative frequencies can be made from the existing clinical review studies (Table 177–1). Goldberg and associates,[5] in combining the data in nine large clinical series, found that the breast is the most common source of metastatic tumor to the orbit, representing 42 percent of cases.[7, 10, 16, 19, 24, 43–46] Metastatic lung and unknown primary source each comprised 11 percent. Prostate (8.3 percent) and melanoma (5.2 percent) were the next most frequent sources. Interestingly, gastrointestinal malignancy, one of the most common adult cancers responsible for morbidity and mortality, was the primary source in only 4.4 percent of the combined cases. There is a built-in bias to these large clinical studies because the more aggressive and lethal tumors (e.g., lung carcinoma) are likely to be underrepresented given their more fulminant course leading to early death prior to evaluation for orbital signs and symptoms.

A significant portion (13 percent) of the cases were caused by a variety of other tumors that occur much less frequently individually. Included in these series, as well as in various case reports, are primary sources including liposarcoma,[47] thyroid,[48–50] testicle, adrenal, carcinoid,[51–54] bladder,[55] pheochromocytoma,[56] pancreas,[57] fibrous histiocytoma,[58] liver,[59, 60] uterus,[61] parotid,[62] ovary, bile duct, fibrosarcoma male breast,[63] and choroidal melanoma.[64]

TIMING OF METASTATIC DISEASE

The timing of metastatic disease in relation to diagnosis of systemic malignancy and average patient survival is interesting and generally reflects the overall behavior of the primary tumor; that is, more indolent tumors tend to be diagnosed before orbital metastases and are associated with longer patient survival. Unfortunately, metastatic disease to the eye and its adnexa is associated with a uniformly bad prognosis. At the time of onset of orbital symptoms most patients have a known primary malignancy, and approximately one half have widespread metastatic disease. Various studies reflect different incidences of orbital metastases heralding systemic malignancies, depending on the type of study. In the Mayo Clinic series,[16] Henderson found that 30 percent of patients had orbital signs and symptoms as the initial manifestation of their malignancy. Font and Ferry found in a clinical pathologic series an incidence of about 60 percent (17/28) without known malignancies.[24] This high ratio most likely reflects a built-in bias to a pathologic review series that seemingly is more likely to include patients who died of unknown causes. In their cumulative review of the literature, Goldberg and associates[5] found an overall incidence of 42 percent of patients who had orbital disease before the detection of a systemic malignancy. The trend over time seemed to be a decrease in the frequency in which metastatic cancer presented as an orbital lesion. Overall, patient and physician sophistication and effective screening methods have most likely been responsible for the earlier diagnosis of primary malignancies in the last 2 decades. The spectrum is wide, and in almost one third of cases, systemic malignancy will often be diagnosed by orbital biopsy. On the other hand, situations arise in which an orbital mass is diagnosed in patients with only a very distant history of malignancy, and these may represent metastatic disease. Often after a 5-yr disease-free interval, patients believe that they are cured of their cancer and will not volunteer this prior history of malignancy.

Temporal patterns are more distinctive when each of the primary sources is considered separately. In general, patients with orbital metastases survive longer than do patients with the same primary source metastatic to the uveal tract.[1, 10, 24] More indolent primary sources associated with long patient survival metastasize late and are therefore rarely seen in the orbit as a presenting sign. Most notable in this group is breast carcinoma, which is the most common source of metastatic orbital disease. The majority (75 percent) of cases of breast carcinoma have a known primary source diagnosed approximately 3 yr earlier. In fact, Henderson had only one patient in whom orbital disease preceded detection of the primary breast tumor.[16] One case of orbital metastases occurred 20 yrs after the diagnosis of the primary tumor.[1] The relatively less aggressive growth pattern of breast carcinoma, as well as the available hormonal therapies, also allow for the longest patient survival among the different primary sources. Similar behavior with years prior to metastases to the orbit and prolonged survival measured in years after ophthalmic diagnosis are seen with thyroid carcinoma.[16, 29, 50, 65]

Another primary source frequently diagnosed prior to orbital metastases is malignant melanoma of the skin. Unfortunately, in this case although the primary site is often (90 percent) well known for about 2 yr, the metastases represent a fulminant dissemination of disease and are associated with poor survival. In their review, Orcutt and Char[66] found that a mean interval of survival in patients with melanoma metastatic to the orbit was 4 mo and that no patients survived for longer than 6 mo.

Prostate carcinoma is known for its relatively indolent growth. On average, patients with orbital lesions are diagnosed 6 mo after the primary tumor. Boldt and Nerad[67] had three of eight patients in whom the primary

tumor was unknown at the time of diagnosis. The median survival in their group of eight patients was 26 mo, although Goldberg and associates found that the median was 6 to 8 mo.[5]

More aggressive clinical behavior is observed in patients with gastrointestinal, kidney, and lung primary sites. In these patients, early orbital metastases (before detection of the primary site) and short survival constitute the rule. Patients with metastatic lung carcinoma are generally considered to have the worst prognosis.[5, 10, 45]

The average time of patient survival after diagnosis of orbital metastases is approximately 9 mo.[5] Ferry and Font compared patients with ocular metastases versus those with orbital metastases and found that survival was 5.4 mo versus 15.4 mo for anterior segment versus orbital metastases.[1] However, not all patients do poorly. There are many reports of patients, particularly those concerning patients with breast, prostate, and carcinoid tumors, who have survived for many years with their metastatic orbital tumors.[52, 68] As described earlier, one would expect that hematogenous orbital metastases are associated with disseminated disease and that, in most cases, pulmonary metastases should occur commonly with orbital metastases since the emboli most frequently reach the orbit only after passing through the pulmonary circulation. Henderson found that in 51 of 55 patients, other signs of metastatic disease were present at the time of orbital diagnosis.[16] In Goldberg's series,[5] only 47 percent of patients were diagnosed with simultaneous systemic and orbital metastases. This discrepancy may reflect how thoroughly clinicians searched for other metastatic foci, given the fact that some are likely to be subclinical and microscopic.

The significance of isolated versus disseminated disease becomes apparent in certain situations. First, the clinician must direct treatment to all affected areas to improve the patient's quality of life. Second, in certain situations, particularly carcinoid and renal cell carcinoma, which occasionally may have solitary metastases, removal of an isolated metastatic lesion can be part of a surgical cure of the carcinoma.

Clinical Characteristics

SIGNS AND SYMPTOMS

Orbital metastases can be accompanied by any of the common signs and symptoms of orbital disease. The clinical syndromes are usually diverse, but there are certain recurrent themes. The presentation also depends on the histologic type and growth pattern of the primary tumor and on the type of orbital tissue involved. Most important is the relative abruptness and disproportionate amount of symptoms that these lesions cause compared with other space-occupying orbital lesions.[5, 16, 69, 70] Patients most frequently complain of diplopia,[5, 45, 46] ptosis,[71] proptosis,[45] eyelid swelling,[16] and pain[5] (Table 177–2). Henderson points out that because they frequently lodge in or are adjacent to the extraocular

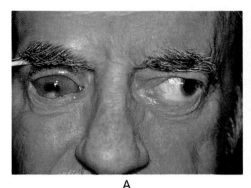 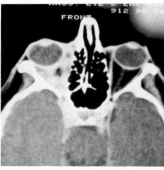 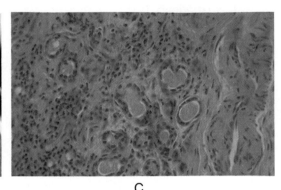

A   B   C

Figure 177–5. Sixty-year-old man (A) presented with the acute onset of proptosis, frozen globe, and exposure keratitis resulting in corneal ulceration. The CT scan (B) shows diffuse involvement of orbital tissue. The biopsy (C) shows metastatic squamous cell carcinoma. The primary source of tumor was unknown. (Courtesy of J. Shore, M.D.)

muscles, diplopia and acquired eye deviation are more common and are frequently an earlier manifestation of metastatic disease compared with primary orbital tumors.[16] Other commonly reported symptoms include a palpable mass and decreased vision. Frequently noted signs are exophthalmos, noncomitant eye deviation, conjunctival infection, palpable mass, subnormal visual acuity, disc edema, retinal folds, and enophthalmos (Figs. 177–5 and 177–6). Classically, metastatic breast carcinoma causes enophthalmos (Fig. 177–7) secondary to contraction induced by the scirrhous histologic nature of the tumor (Fig. 177–8).[72] This phenomenon has also been seen in cases of metastatic lung and gastric carcinoma.

Goldberg and associates divide the clinical syndromes produced by metastatic lesions into five broad categories, all of which overlap.[5] The first is a mass presentation in which displacement of the globe calls the orbital tumor to attention (Fig. 177–9). The second is the infiltrative pattern (see Fig. 177–7) in which diplopia, enophthalmos, and a firm orbit are characteristic. The functional presentation represents patients in whom decreased acuity or ophthalmoplegia secondary to a cranial neuropathy are the dominant signs and symptoms (Figs. 177–10 and 177–11). The inflammatory syndrome is dominated by signs and symptoms of chemosis, injection, lid swelling, and pain that is aggravated by eye movements (see Fig. 177–5). Occasionally, the tumor presents silently with no signs or symptoms and is discovered on incidental clinical or radiologic examination. It is rare that any single patient fits completely into one of these categories, but there is usually a dominant pattern. In a series of 38 patients, Goldberg and Rootman found that 24 patients could easily be categorized by one of the patterns.[46] They went on to separate the reviewed case reports into these categories and found that 66 percent fitted into the mass presentation and that 24 percent fitted into the infiltrative pattern.[5] Metastatic breast carcinoma was seen to present approximately half of the time in each of the aforementioned categories, whereas prostate (76 percent of cases) and melanoma (82 percent of cases) almost always fit into the mass presentation group. They concluded that except for breast and gastrointestinal tumors the mass presentation was the most common, although they point out that pain, inflammation, and a secondary motility disturbance often accompany the mass presentation.

Henderson emphasizes that the location of the tumor determines the type of clinical syndrome.[16] Anterior lesions are more likely to have swelling, ptosis, and a palpable mass and later go on to cause progressive motility disturbances. Posterior lesions may be characterized by proptosis, visual loss, papilledema, and pressure on the globe. This group of patients also go on to severe restriction of motility.

DIAGNOSIS

Metastatic tumors have been misdiagnosed as virtually any of the common orbital diseases (Table 177–3).

Table 177–2. COMMON SYMPTOMS OF METASTATIC ORBITAL DISEASE*

Diplopia	Proptosis
Ptosis	Eyelid swelling
Blurred vision	Pain

*All occur abruptly with a disproportionate amount of symptoms compared with primary orbital lesions.

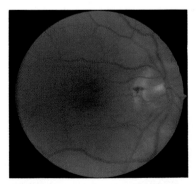

Figure 177–6. Chorioretinal folds secondary to metastatic renal cell carcinoma to the orbit.

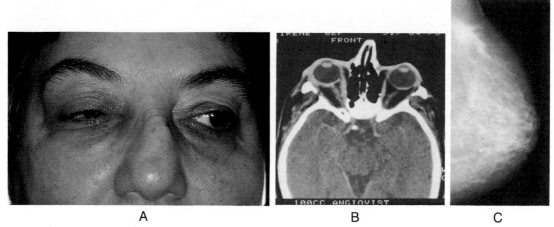

Figure 177–7. Fifty-year-old woman *(A)* presented with an inflamed orbit, enophthalmos, and restricted motility. The CT scan *(B)* shows irregular enlargement of the right medial rectus and diffuse infiltration of the anterior orbital tissues. Mammography *(C)* disclosed a calcified breast mass. *(A–C, Courtesy of J. Shore, M.D.)*

Goldberg and associates identified 24 cases of misdiagnosed orbital metastatic lesions and found that the inflammatory presentation was the most commonly misdiagnosed.[5] In these cases, pseudotumor[24, 49, 73, 74] and orbital cellulitis[46, 75] were the most common misdiagnoses. Breast carcinoma is notorious for an "inflammatory" presentation (see Fig. 177–7) and misdiagnosis.[76]

The next most likely misdiagnosis was in the group of patients with a dysfunctional presentation secondary to ophthalmoplegia. In this group, myasthenia gravis was the incorrect diagnosis in three patients.[26, 77, 78] Finally, the mass lesion presentation of metastatic tumors was misdiagnosed on three occasions as lacrimal gland tumor.[79, 80] Meningiomas are thought to occur more frequently in patients with breast carcinoma. Situations arise in which metsatatic breast carcinoma must be distinguished from sphenoid wing meningioma (Fig. 177–12). Finally, metastases can imitate the radiographic appearance of benign, primary orbital tumors such as cavernous hemangionas (Fig. 177–13).

If, after complete history and eye examination the clinician suspects metastatic disease, he or she should proceed with a complete physical examination, including an examination of the breasts in a woman, the prostate in a man, and a test of the stool for occult blood in both sexes. Ancillary laboratory tests may also prove to be helpful. A complete blood count may demonstrate a microcytic anemia secondary to a bleeding gastrointestinal tumor. Carcinoembryonic antigen (CEA) may be elevated in certain patients, particularly those with gastrointestinal malignancies. This was found by Bullock[77] to be specific for metastatic disease in patients with orbital masses. This test is not nearly as sensitive as it is specific, and therefore a negative CEA would not rule out a metastatic lesion. In elderly men, a prostate acid phosphatase level elevation would point to a metastatic prostate lesion.

A unique syndrome is seen in men with seminoma who can present with an acute orbital inflammatory syndrome[81, 82] that responds to steroids and in whom no orbital mass is found. These patients often have elevated human chorionic gonadotropin (HCG) levels. The clinician should not dismiss a mass lesion without a proper work-up since seminoma has been reported to metastasize to the orbit.[83, 84]

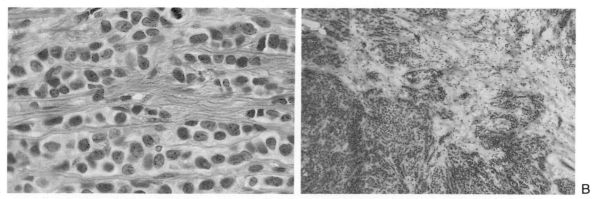

Figure 177–8. Histopathology of the patient (also in Fig. 177–7) shows typical "indian file" organization of metastatic breast carcinoma cells *(A)* and scirrhous changes *(B)* responsible for enophthalmos. *(A and B, Courtesy of J. Shore, M.D.)*

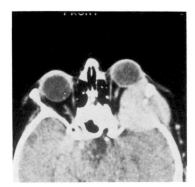

Figure 177–9. CT scan appearance of metastatic oat cell carcinoma to the left orbit, presenting with the acute onset of proptosis. Note the extensive bone destruction and indentation of the globe. (Courtesy of A. Weber, M.D.)

Table 177–3. DIFFERENTIAL DIAGNOSIS OF METASTATIC ORBITAL TUMORS

Orbital cellulitis	Primary lacrimal gland tumor
Pseudotumor	Lymphoma
Thyroid orbitopathy	Sphenoid wing meningioma
Dural sinus fistula	Primary vascular or neural
Myasthenia gravis	orbital tumors

The "gold standard" for noninvasive orbital diagnosis is CT scanning, and coronal and axial contrast-enhanced studies should be obtained on all patients with orbital disease in whom metastatic disease is suspected. The diversity of CT scan appearance reflects the differences in clinical presentation. Generally, the lesions appear poorly defined and relatively dense compared with the surrounding fat, with similar intensity as the extraocular muscles (Fig. 177–14) and vascular structures.[85, 86] Healy reviewed 22 cases of orbital metastases evaluated by CT scan.[71] In two thirds of these patients, there was some evidence of adjacent bone destruction. Sixty percent of lesions were extraconal; 20 percent were intraconal; and 20 percent were both. Contrast enhancement was seen in all cases examined before and after contrast. Interestingly, two thirds of patients had evidence of intracranial disease, either by direct extension or discrete metastases. Lesions involving the intraconal space can be diffuse or discrete. The globe is usually indented, and the lesions are rarely calcified.[5] Involvement of the extraocular muscles classically shows a focal enlargement of one area of muscle with an irregular border against adjacent fat.[25, 28, 86] Cases of diffuse enlargement of single (see Fig. 177–2) or multiple muscles (including the tendon in one case) have also been described.[25] Contiguous bone involvement can be seen. Goldberg and associates looked at the spectrum of CT scan features reported in the literature and found that a mass lesion followed by bone involvement was the most common CT scan feature.[5] Prostatic carcinoma is notorious for bone involvement (Fig. 177–15) and is typically associated with osteoblastic lesions.[66] Thyroid and renal cell cancer are most frequently associated with osteolytic lesions (Fig. 177–16). However, these are only generalizations, and any of the three can be associated with either type of bone lesion.

More information can be obtained from other diagnostic modalities. B-scan ultrasonography can be used to better characterize extraocular muscle enlargement. With the increasing availability of magnetic resonance imaging (MRI), clinicians are becoming more familiar with the more detailed anatomic information that can be obtained, particularly from the sagittal sections. MRI may prove useful as an adjunctive diagnostic modality.[86, 87] For example, MRI scan T_1-weighted images show sharp contrast between enlarged muscles and the high signal intensity of the surrounding fat. When lesions are separate from the muscles in the extraconal space, they are easily seen in contradistinction to the high signal intensity of the surrounding fat on T_1-weighted images. Images weighted toward T_2 are less sensitive, because the fat is less distinctive. As is true of bone disease in general, MRI is not adequate for evaluating bony metastases.[88, 89]

The definitive diagnosis of metastatic tumors can be made only with a tissue biopsy. In cases of disseminated disease, metastatic disease to the orbit can occasionally be presumed and treatment given. Ideally, some tissue should be obtained prior to treatment. It is this situation, the diagnosis of malignant, nonresectable orbital tu-

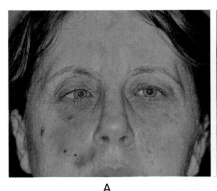
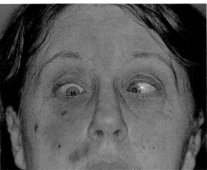
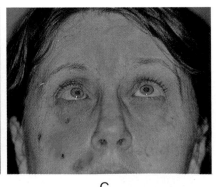

A   B   C

Figure 177–10. This 63-year-old woman with a history of breast carcinoma presented with diplopia and esotropia (A). The examination showed impaired abduction consistent with a right sixth-nerve palsy (B) and impaired elevation (C) consistent with a partial right third-nerve palsy. (Courtesy of N. Snebold, M.D.)

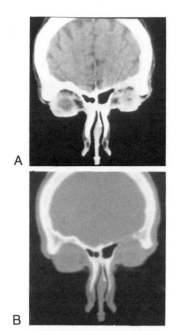

Figure 177–11. CT scan appearance of the patient in Figure 177–10 revealed diffuse infiltration of the superior and lateral orbit (B) and destruction of the bony roof (A). Tumor extended into the cavernous sinus. The biopsy was consistent with metastatic breast carcinoma. (Courtesy of N. Snebold, M.D.)

scirrhous breast carcinoma and gastrointestinal malignancies in which needle biopsies are often nondiagnostic.[5, 92, 93] Complications are minimized when performed by experienced surgeons.[94] Finally, orbital biopsy and subsequent histochemical analysis have been shown to be adequate in predicting estrogen receptor positivity in metastatic breast carcinoma.[95]

TREATMENT

The main goal of treatment of metastatic orbital tumors is palliative, and it is directed toward the patient's comfort and preservation of vision whenever possible. Several different treatment options exist (Table 177–4). If the patient is comfortable and has normal visual function, there is a role for conservative management with observation alone on systemic hormonal or chemotherapy. As systemic therapies improve, patients are surviving longer with systemic metastases. In these patients whose quality of life begins to be affected and in whom good vision and pain free eyes are essential, treatment must be instituted. In situations in which the cause of the orbital mass is unclear or if pathologic diagnosis of the orbital tumor is needed to identify primary source, biopsy and, if possible, excision of the mass is indicated. In most situations the clinician will be treating a patient either after incisional or needle biopsy or presumably based on systemic metastases. Rarely, situations arise in which complete excision can be attempted to effect a cure. This may be the case with metastatic carcinoid tumor (Fig. 177–17) or renal cell carcinoma, in which the orbital metastasis is the sole manifestation of secondary disease. Only rarely is disease so poorly controlled by medical modalities that surgical debulking is required.

The mainstay of treatment is radiotherapy. The recommended treatment is 3000 to 5000 cGy for 2 wk, in divided doses delivered through the lateral orbital wall, and care is taken to avoid the anterior segment of the

mors, that is one of the most important applications of the orbital fine needle biopsy. Accuracy rates up to 80 percent have been described in these situations, but even proponents of the technique acknowledge the frequent limitation to cytologic not histologic diagnosis.[90–92] Thus, although the cells can be identified as malignant (e.g., undifferentiated carcinoma), the primary source of the tissue is less easily determined. The technique is therefore less useful in cases of unknown primary disease when orbital biopsy can be used to diagnose the primary source. The needle biopsy is most unpredictable in situations of sclerosing tumors, such as

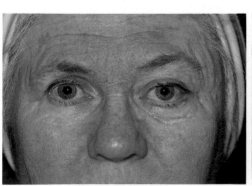
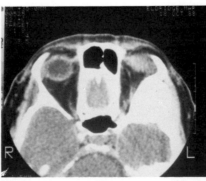
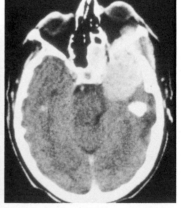

A   B   C

Figure 177–12. A 58-year-old woman with a history of breast carcinoma presented with the gradual onset of proptosis (A). The CT scan (B) was consistent with left sphenoid wing meningioma. Note the hyperostosis of the lateral orbit wall. The CT scan of a different patient (C) shows the typical appearance of metastatic breast carcinoma to the sphenoid wing with bony destruction. (Courtesy of J. Shore, M.D.)

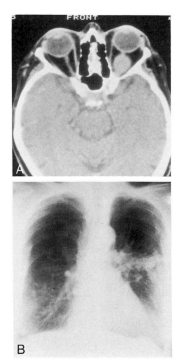

Figure 177–13. An elderly man presented with proptosis of the left eye. The CT scan *(A)* was possibly consistent with cavernous hemangioma. The orbital biopsy and chest x-ray *(B)* were diagnostic of metastatic lung carcinoma to the orbit.

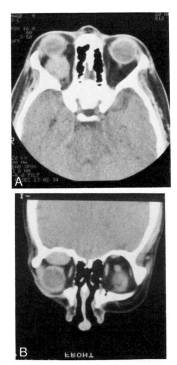

Figure 177–14. Axial *(A)* and coronal *(B)* CT scans of metastatic uterine carcinoma to the right orbit. The lesion has the same intensity as the surrounding muscles and optic nerve. (Courtesy of N. Snebold, M.D.)

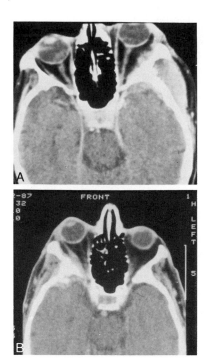

Figure 177–15. *(A)* Metastatic prostate carcinoma to the left orbit, showing an osteoblastic lesion *(B)*. Another case of metastatic prostate carcinoma to the orbit. In this case, the bone lesion is lytic.

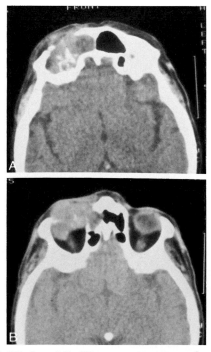

Figure 177–16. *A* and *B,* CT scan appearance of massive bone destruction of the superior and medial orbit secondary to metastatic renal cell carcinoma. (Courtesy of A. Weber, M.D.)

eye. The eye should be shielded whenever possible. Patients usually experience significant improvement in mass effect, pain, and congestion (Fig. 177–18). The success rates are reported to be 70 to 90 percent for

relief of symptoms and improvement of ocular function.[96, 97] Goldberg and associates[5] found a success rate of 73 percent in their combined series, including their own patients and those reported to date in the literature. Significant radiation side effects can occur in all of the ocular tissues.[98] Fortunately, most patients do not have radiation sequelae, as they normally occur in

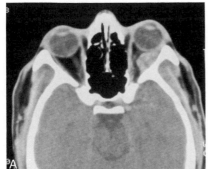

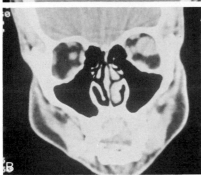

Figure 177–17. *A* and *B*, CT scan appearance of a solitary metastatic lesion to the orbit in a patient with carcinoid tumor of the lung. Occasionally, the metastases is isolated and discrete and resection for cure can be attempted.

a time frame beyond the average survival of these patients. In Huh's series of 70 patients, no serious side effects were observed.[97]

There are no specific chemotherapies or hormonal therapies that are designed for treatment of metastatic orbital disease. However, the orbit is equally likely to respond to systemic therapies as is the primary tumor or other areas of dissemination. Thus, patients with metastatic orbital disease from estrogen receptor positive breast carcinoma responsive to antiestrogens, prostate carcinoma responsive to orchiectomy or diethylstilbesterol, and small cell carcinoma of the lung responsive to chemotherapy should all be treated aggressively with these modalities. These patients frequently enjoy improvement and temporary control of their disease.

Table 177–4. TREATMENT OF METASTATIC ORBITAL TUMORS

Observation
Systemic hormonal or chemotherapy
Radiation
Surgical excision
Exenteration

Pediatric Metastatic Orbital Tumors

This disease is very different from the type that occurs in adults (Table 177–5). In children, metastatic disease to the eye and its adnexa almost exclusively involve the orbit. Metastatic disease to the uvea is extremely uncommon. Also, metastases commonly do not arise from carcinomas, such as in adults, but from sarcomas. Neuroblastoma and Ewing's sarcoma are the most common sources of metastatic disease to the orbit. Neuroblastoma is second only to rhabdomyosarcoma as the most frequent malignant tumor of the orbit that occurs in children. Medulloblastoma and Wilms' tumor metastasize to the orbit less frequently.[20, 70, 99, 100] Musarella found that 20 percent of children with neuroblastoma had ocular involvement and that three quarters of these patients had proptosis or ecchymoses.[100] The typical presentation for children with neuroblastoma is that of rapidly expanding exophthalmos with eyelid ecchymoses (Fig. 177–19). The disease is frequently bilateral, and the temporal orbit is typically involved with a lytic bone lesion (Fig. 177–20).[99] The most common site of primary tumor is the adrenal gland for cases with orbital involvement. It is unclear whether the metastases arise in the orbital soft tissue or in the bone with contiguous spread.[20] Most cases (90 percent) occur before 5 yr of age, and the prognosis is best in children younger than 1 yr of age. Neuroblastoma can also be associated with the paraneoplastic syndrome of opsoclonus and myoclonus.

Metastatic Ewing's sarcoma is a disease of the second decade and can present as a sudden onset of proptosis due to a hemorrhagic metastasis from the long bones. The disease has also been seen to arise primarily in the soft tissues or bone of the orbit.[101] Albert and associates

Figure 177–18. Pre- *(A)* and post- *(B)* radiation photographs of metastatic breast carcinoma to the left zygoma and orbit. Mass effect and proptosis were dramatically reduced.

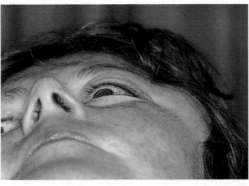

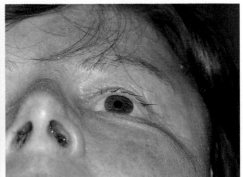

A

B

<table>
<tr><td colspan="1">

**Table 177–5. PEDIATRIC METASTATIC
ORBITAL TUMORS**

Embryonal or undifferentiated sarcomas
Rarely carcinoma
Orbit involved more commonly than uvea
Neuroblastoma and Ewing's most common
Wilms' tumor rare
Proptosis and ecchymoses
Commonly bilateral
Poor prognosis
Management with combined therapy
</td></tr>
</table>

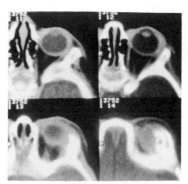

Figure 177–20. CT scan appearance of the patient in Figure 177–19 shows a lytic bone lesion of the temporal orbit. (Courtesy of J. Woog, M.D.)

found that the disease was unilateral in all 12 of their patients.[20] The pathology is usually undifferentiated and, like neuroblastoma, the prognosis is poor despite combined treatment with radiation and chemotherapy.

The orbit is more commonly involved by leukemia in children than it is in adults. Rootman found that in his series of orbital tumors, leukemia was the cause of acute proptosis in children in 11 percent of the malignant cases.[11] Granulocytic sarcoma or the extramedullary form of acute myloblastic leukemia can present initially as an orbital mass.[102] The average age of presentation is 7 yr of age, and the disease can be bilateral. With appropriate systemic chemotherapy the prognosis is good, and the disease can be arrested before the development of disseminated disease. In addition to arising primarily in the orbit of infants, teratomas can secondarily involve the orbit by direct extension from surrounding structures.[103] In children, lymphomas infrequently involve the orbit.

SECONDARY ORBITAL TUMORS

Secondary orbital tumors involve the orbit by direct extension and can arise in any of the adjacent structures including the sinuses and nasopharynx, the meninges and brain, the eye, the conjunctiva and lids, and the lacrimal sac (Table 177–6). Most of these primary lesions are addressed elsewhere in the text, and what follows is a discussion of these lesions as orbital diseases. Rootman found that secondary neoplasias represented one third of all cases of orbital neoplasias.[11] Henderson's series,[104]

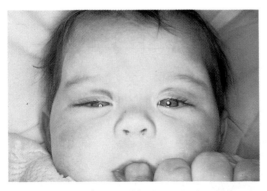

Figure 177–19. Metastatic neuroblastoma to the orbit, presenting with bilateral eyelid ecchymoses. (Courtesy of J. Woog, M.D.)

which did not include orbital bone lesions, found that these cases represented 15 percent of orbital neoplasias. Shields and associates found that secondary tumors represented 11 percent of biopsied orbital lesions and that more than one third of these represented contiguous spread from intraocular disease.[12] Therefore, secondary tumors are a common cause of orbital disease. It is important that the ophthalmologist be familiar with these lesions because they frequently present with orbital signs, and their management often involves a multidisciplinary approach involving the several services of a surgeon specializing in the head and neck, an oncologist, and a radiation therapist.

Paranasal Sinus Tumors

Most orbital secondary neoplasms arise from the paranasal sinus cavities. More than 50 percent of patients with sinus and nasal tumors can have signs and symptoms related to the eye or orbit.[105] The sinuses are cavities formed within the maxilla, frontal, sphenoid, and ethmoid bones and are lined with mucous membrane. The maxillary and sphenoid sinuses are present at birth, and all of the sinuses develop throughout

**Table 177–6. TYPES OF SECONDARY
ORBITAL TUMORS**

Paranasal Sinus Tumors	Conjunctival Tumors
Benign	Squamous cell carcinoma
Mucocele	Melanoma
Osteoma	
Inverted papilloma	Eyelid Tumors
Malignant	Basal cell carcinoma
Squamous cell carcinoma	Squamous cell carcinoma
Adenocarcinoma	Sebaceous cell carcinoma
Adenoid cystic carcinoma	
Melanoma	Intraocular Tumors
Esthesioneuroblastoma	Uveal melanoma
	Retinoblastoma
Nasopharyngeal Tumors	
Squamous cell carcinoma	Intracranial Tumors
Lymphoepithelioma	Meningioma
	Glioblastoma
Lacrimal Sac Tumors	Chordoma
Epithelial tumors	
Melanoma	

childhood until they reach their final size in adolescence. Each sinus communicates with the nasal pharynx by a bony osteum, and each is directly adjacent to the orbit. The primary mode of extension of sinus tumors to the orbit is via direct extension. This can be accomplished by bone erosion, extension along normal neurovascular bundles, and extension through preexisting bone canals. In the case of the maxillary sinus, which is the most common origin of these secondary orbital tumors, only thin bone separates the inferior orbital fissure from the mucosa of the sinus.

Benign Tumors

The sinus tumors invading the orbit can be benign or malignant. Benign lesions include inverting papilloma, osteomas, juvenile angiofibroma, and unusual neuroectodermal tumors. In one series,[105] although considered to be benign, inverting papilloma was the second most common lesion to invade the orbit after squamous cell carcinoma. These papillomas typically arise in the lateral nasal wall or in the mucosa of the ethmoid sinus.[105, 106] Although nonmetastasizing, these lesions can extend locally to involve the orbit. They typically grow through the middle meatus into the maxillary sinus. The most common orbital presenting signs and symptoms are nasal congestion, pain, epiphora, lid swelling, and headache.[104] They more typically are detected before this when the patient has only epistaxis or nasal obstruction. These lesions are notorious for recurrences and are associated with squamous cell carcinoma of the sinus in 5 to 10 percent of cases. Therefore, aggressive and complete excision must be accomplished to prevent a recurrence.

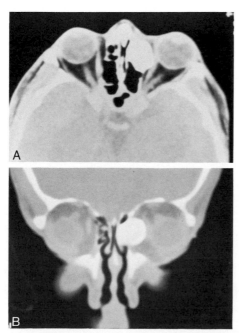

Figure 177–21. *A* and *B,* CT scan appearance of osteoma with an extension into the left orbit. Bone windows *(A)* show compact bone. (Courtesy of M. Joseph, M.D.)

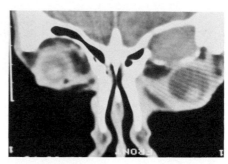

Figure 177–22. A large frontal sinus mucocele is shown extending into the left orbit. (Courtesy of M. Joseph, M.D.)

Osteoma was the second most common benign lesion to involve the orbit and was studied by Johnson.[105] Osteomas are benign tumors that arise in the paranasal sinuses. The most common location is the frontal sinus. These can involve the orbit by direct slow growth into the orbital cavity (Fig. 177–21) or indirectly by blocking a sinus drainage ostia and subsequently causing a mucocele with orbital involvement. Osteomas frequently enlarge most during rapid skeletal growth, and therefore they are an important consideration in children and adolescents. Some consider that these occur secondarily in patients who have had orbital trauma or sinus infections. Others believe that they represent a developmental lesion occurring at the site of fusion of membranous and cartilaginous bone. Common presenting signs include sinus congestion and proptosis. The lesion represents compact bone (without fibrovascular stroma) and is managed by simple excision.

Mucoceles of the paranasal sinuses are benign lesions that are capable of invading the orbit and causing orbital disease. Henderson identified mucoceles in 65 of 764 patients with orbital tumors.[104] This represented 19 percent of the secondary orbital tumors. Mucoceles are thought to arise when the sinus ostia are obstructed and the mucous-secreting respiratory epithelium is trapped giving rise to fluid-filled cysts (Fig. 177–22). Mucoceles are not thought to be associated with malignancy; however, Weaver and Bartley reported seven patients in whom a malignancy was found incidentally in association with the mucocele at the time of surgery.[107] Other authors have reported cases in which the malignancy was thought to occlude the sinus ostia, and subsequently this resulted in mucocele formation.[108, 109]

SQUAMOUS CELL CARCINOMA

Squamous cell carcinoma is the most common sinus malignancy to involve the orbit.[11, 104, 105, 110, 111] These tumors arise, in most cases, from the maxillary sinus and occasionally from the nasal cavity, ethmoids, or frontal sinus. Up to two thirds of patients with antral squamous cell carcinoma present at advanced stages with orbital involvement.[105, 106, 112, 113] The disease is twice as common in men and occurs most commonly from 40 to 60 yr of age. Patients often have a history of chronic sinusitis and cigarette smoking. Unfortunately, because most patients have symptoms that are not dissimilar

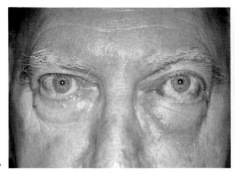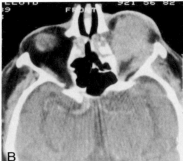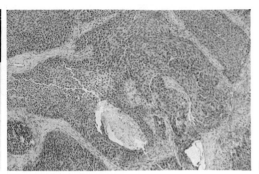

Figure 177–23. Upward displacement of the left globe *(A)* secondary to antral carcinoma. The CT scan *(B)* shows an extension of the tumor into the inferior orbit. The biopsy *(C)* revealed nonkeratinizing squamous cell carcinoma. (Courtesy of P. Rubin, M.D.)

from those of chronic sinusitis, many patients present having had disease for longer than 6 mo. Because the tumors often do not invade the orbit in the retrobulbar space, these patients present with nonaxial displacement of the globe; that is, the eye is pushed upward (Fig. 177–23) in antral carcinoma and down and outward in ethmoid carcinoma. Other common presenting symptoms include (Table 177–7) chronic pain (particularly in the distribution of one of the cranial nerves), epiphora, proptosis, facial swelling (particularly of the lower lid), nasal obstruction, and epistaxis. Visual loss and diplopia also occur. Involvement of the structures of the lower orbit can cause massive congestion and chemosis mimicking an inflammatory process. Other signs include proptosis, strabismus, hypesthesia, and a mass on nasal examination (Table 177–8). When comparing metastatic to secondary orbital tumors, Rootman found that in metastatic carcinomas the disease was not painful and that proptosis was axial in most cases (75 percent). This was in contradistinction to secondary malignancy in which pain and paresthesias were present in 74 percent of cases, and nonaxial displacement occurred in 53 percent.[114] Carcinomas arising from the floor of the maxillary sinus are less likely than those from the roof of the sinus to involve the orbit. Tumors involving the floor can spread to the pterygoid region and present with pain in the teeth. Further extension of these tumors to the base of the skull can cause multiple cranial nerve palsies. Malignant disease of the sphenoid sinus is rare. However, because the optic canal forms part of the wall of the sphenoid sinus, tumors arising in the sinus can occasionally invade the optic nerve. Harbison and associates reviewed 42 cases of sphenoid sinus carcinoma and found that five patients (12 percent) had optic nerve and chiasmal invasion.[115]

Tumors involving the ethmoid sinuses are less common and represent approximately 5 to 6 percent of all sinus carcinomas. These patients more commonly present with nasal congestion and epistaxis than do patients with antral carcinoma. Intracranial spread occurs earlier than in antral carcinoma. Despite its lower incidence, Mohan and associates found these tumors invading the orbit as frequently as antral carcinoma.[110] This may be explained by its easy access to the orbit from the ethmoids, given the relative thinness of the lamina papyracea (Fig. 177–24). Frontal sinus malignancies are rare but can involve the frontal lobe and the structures around the sella turcica at a very early stage.

The sinus tumor mass can usually be identified with conventional radiographs of the sinuses that reveal a clouding of the normal lucent areas and destruction of the bony sinus walls. However, the referring diagnosis based on the initial radiographs is often chronic sinusitis, and this can lead to a delay in diagnosis of 3 to 5 mo.[104] Conley emphasized that because these tumors demonstrate perineural spread through preexisting foramina, extension can occur to the orbit without evidence of bone erosion.[116] CT scans help to better define what is frequently a large mass involving the orbit, and there is often extensive bone destruction (Fig. 177–25). The study should include coronal and axial views and should extend to the base of the skull, which can frequently be involved by these tumors.

The overall prognosis for these patients is poor, and the treating team of physicians often finds therapy geared primarily at palliation. The 5-yr survival rate is 25 to 35 percent for squamous cell carcinoma with orbital disease. Overall, 5-yr survival has been reported to be

Table 177–7. SYMPTOMS OF SINUS TUMORS WITH ORBITAL INVOLVEMENT

Chronic sinusitis
Nasal obstruction and epistaxis
Pain
Nonaxial displacement of the globe
Lower lid swelling
Diplopia
Blurred vision
Epiphora

Table 177–8. SIGNS OF SINUS TUMORS WITH ORBITAL INVOLVEMENT

Proptosis and displacement of the globe
Congestion and chemosis
Strabismus
Decreased acuity
Hypesthesia
Nasal mass

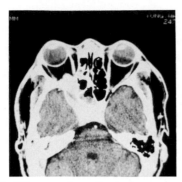

Figure 177–24. CT scan of a patient who presented with acute loss of vision secondary to optic neuropathy, showing squamous cell carcinoma of the right ethmoid extending into the orbital apex. (Courtesy of M. Joseph, M.D.)

as high as 74.4 percent (all sinus tumors) when a combination of radiation and radical surgery is used.[117] This difference in survival is consistent with the fact that orbital involvement represents an advanced state of disease. In many cases, the tumors, because of inability to excise them at initial surgery, continue to cause morbidity and mortality through local invasion, and only at a very late stage do they metastasize. Distant spread is to lymph nodes and the lung most commonly. The recommended treatment dose of radiation is 5000 to 6000 cGy for 3 to 5 wk. Disease that is limited to the nodes (without distant metastases) may be curable in certain cases by combined surgery and radiation therapy.

Management begins with the biopsy material taken, usually by a transnasal biopsy. In some cases in which the tumor involves the orbit, tissue sampling can be accomplished by fine-needle orbital biopsy.[91, 92, 118] Histopathologically, most tumors consist of squamous cells, which result from carcinomatous transition in areas of metaplasia of the normal ciliated columnar epithelium that lines the sinuses. Most tumors are poorly differentiated and therefore do not produce keratin.

Radical surgery is the procedure of choice, but often the physician and the patient are unwilling to accept the disfiguring consequences that may be required to extirpate the tumor completely. Among the most important factors affecting the treatment plan is the fate of the eye. Exenteration is frequently part of the plan when attempting to completely excise tumors involving the orbit, especially if bone erosion has been demonstrated.[119–122] The necessity of removing the eye has been addressed by many authors[119–121, 123] and has been most affected by better preoperative radiologic evaluation with CT scanning and the combination of less radical surgery with radiation therapy. Perry and associates, in a series that was somewhat nonrepresentative because of the large numbers of esthesioneuroblastomas included, found that with the use of preoperative radiation therapy and careful examination of the periorbita at the time of surgery with frozen section control, only 5 of 41 patients required exenteration.[121] Local disease recurrence was not a problem in patients managed in this way. Interestingly, they had 14 patients in whom the CT scan demonstrated gross orbital involvement but

were found at surgery to have intact periorbita, therefore the eye was saved. Of these patients, 11 patients were free of local recurrence and the other three patients had advanced disease involving the base of the skull, which could not have been cured by exenteration. They concluded by recommending that if, after radiation, the periosteum is not extensively involved, the eye can be saved during paranasal sinus cancer surgery without increased incidence of a local recurrence. Johnson and associates noted that in addition to providing tumor control, cisplatin significantly ameliorated pain in terminal patients with extensive sinus and orbital disease.[105]

Other Malignant Tumors of the Paranasal Sinuses

In addition to squamous cell carcinoma, adenocarcinoma, adenoid cystic carcinoma, esthesioneuroblastoma and melanoma can occur in the paranasal sinus and invade the orbit. In Johnson's series, four of the five patients with adenocarcinoma had involvement of the orbit on initial evaluation.[105] Adenocarcinoma is thought to arise from the minor salivary glands in the respiratory epithelium or perhaps from pluripotential precursor stem cells of the basal epithelium. These tumors are thought to occur more commonly in wood workers.[114, 124] Although thought to occur more typically in the ethmoids, Johnson found tumors originated commonly in both the maxillary and ethmoid sinuses.[105] Significant bone destruction is usually present on x-ray studies. Since these tumors are less radiosensitive, radical surgery, possibly combined with chemotherapy, is the procedure of choice.

Adenoid cystic carcinoma (Fig. 177–26; see also Fig. 177–25) arises from the minor salivary glands of the respiratory epithelium and is locally aggressive much like its counterpart in the lacrimal gland. This tumor is a secondary invader of the orbit as frequently as it is primary in the lacrimal gland.[104] It can reach the orbit secondarily from the sinus, nasopharynx, salivary gland, or the oral cavity. Patients are typically younger than those who develop squamous cell carcinoma. Although the oldest patient was 72 yr old, Henderson found that

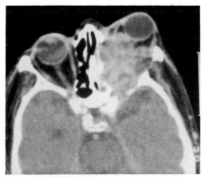

Figure 177–25. CT scan appearance of a patient with adenoid cystic carcinoma invading the orbit with massive bone destruction. (Courtesy of M. Joseph, M.D.)

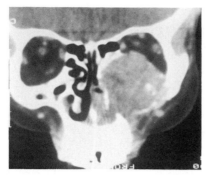

Figure 177–26. CT scan appearance of a patient with adenoid cystic carcinoma of the ethmoid sinus with massive orbital involvement. (Courtesy of M. Joseph, M.D.)

six of ten patients with secondary adenoid cystic carcinoma of the orbit were less than 37 yr of age.[104] The tumor has a tendency to advanced spread perineurally, which is often not apparent on initial resection attempts, and this in turn leads to frequent local recurrences. Henderson noted that even with infiltrative orbital involvement, these patients better tolerated the infiltration with less inflammatory signs and symptoms compared with patients who had other secondary orbital tumors.[104] Patients, usually after numerous surgeries, and a protracted course (7 to 21 yr in four of Henderson's patients[104]) succumb to localized disease, and up to 40 percent[114] develop hematogenous metastases. The treatment involves a combination of radical surgery, high-dose radiation, and chemotherapy.

Esthesioneuroblastoma is a rare neoplasm that arises from neuroepithelium of the olfactory tract and can spread secondarily to the sinus and then to the orbit. These tumors are histopathologically similar to neuroblastoma. Presenting symptoms are typical of other sinus lesions and include nasal obstruction, epistaxis, and anosmia. The tumor occurs in children and young adults, is slow growing, and usually has a protracted course. In fact, one of the patients in Johnson's series had a recurrence and orbital involvement 27 yr after initial surgery and irradiation.[105] Distant metastases occur in the lung and cervical lymph nodes. Treatment involves surgery, chemotherapy, and irradiation. The 5-yr survival rate is 50 percent, but the 5-yr disease-free rate is only 18 percent.

Pigmented melanocytes exist in the epithelium of the nose, mouth, and sinuses, and therefore malignant melanomas can arise in these tissues. Orientals may have a propensity to develop this tumor because of mucosal melanosis.[125] Identification of the primary site can be difficult in these cases and often leads to an inadequate initial surgery (Fig. 177–27). These tumors are almost impossible to cure, and patients succumb from local and metastatic disease.

Other tumors that can rarely invade the orbit include odontogenic tumors, including ameblastoma[126, 127] and ameloblastic fibrosarcoma. Ameblastoma is a benign tumor that arises most commonly from the mandible and is treated by resection. Rhabdomyosarcoma may also arise primarily in the sinuses (particularly ethmoid)

and secondarily involves the orbit. As with primary orbital rhabdomyosarcoma, early diagnosis is crucial to the patient's survival, and the mainstay of therapy is not wide resection but involves a combination of chemotherapy and radiation therapy. Other malignant sinus tumors that have been reported to invade the orbit include fibrosarcoma, chondrosarcoma (Fig. 177–28), sinus glioblastoma multiforme, and mucoepidermoid carcinoma.[104, 105]

Orbital Extension of Tumors of the Nasopharynx

Squamous cell carcinoma of the nasopharynx is the primary site in approximately 15 percent of patients with secondary orbital tumors. Henderson believed that these cases were more disappointing than their sinus counterparts with even further delay in diagnosis.[104] Five-yr survival is estimated at 0 to 10 percent.[128] These patients are more likely to have inadequate biopsies and inadequate initial surgeries. Distant metastases and direct invasion into the brain are common, and orbital invasion is only a late manifestation. Lesions in the nose can occur on the turbinate and gain access to the orbit via the nasolacrimal system. Similar carcinomas can arise in the pharynx and hypopharynx and occur with increased frequency in Chinese patients. These tumors invade in all directions and metastasize to regional lymph nodes earlier than do their sinus counterparts. Nonsquamous cell tumors can arise in these areas, as they do in the sinuses from the epithelium of the minor salivary glands. A rare variant of squamous cell carcinoma in the naso-

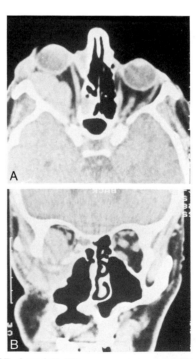

Figure 177–27. A and B, CT scan appearance of the invasion of the right orbit by melanoma. The primary site of the tumor could not be determined. (Courtesy of M. Joseph, M.D.)

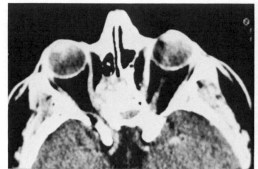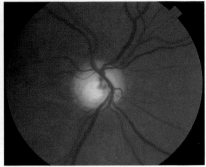

Figure 177–28. Chondrosarcoma of the right ethmoid sinus. The CT scan *(A)* shows an extension into the orbit with resultant compressive optic neuropathy and optic atrophy *(B)*.

pharynx is lymphoepithelioma. This tumor consists of poorly differentiated, nonkeratizing epithelial cells that proliferate in a background of a benign lymphoid stroma. The tumor has two histologic variants—the Regaud and Schmincke types. Metastatic lesions to the lymph nodes occur in up to 70 percent of cases, and bone destruction is common at the base of the skull with associated cranial nerve palsies.[129] The tumor is highly radiosensitive, and 5-yr survival may be as high as 35 percent.[129] Finally, invasive carcinomas of the nasopharynx are important considerations in patients with cavernous sinus syndrome and painful ophthalmoplegia.

Orbital Extension From Lacrimal Sac Tumors

The lacrimal sac can be involved by a wide variety of tumors,[130, 131] including epithelial tumors, lymphoma, schwannoma, hemangiopericytoma, fibrous histiocytoma, and melanoma.[132] In addition, up to 25 percent of lacrimal sac tumors are inflammatory masses of both granulomatous and nonspecific inflammatory lesions.[114] Ryan and Font,[133] in their study of 27 patients, divided the epithelial tumors into papillomas, papillomas with foci of carcinoma, and frank carcinoma. The average age of patients with these carcinomas was 55 yr of age, and all had a chronic course with indolent bouts of inflammation and epiphora. The treatment is resection, and the tumor is not known to metastasize. However, when a tumor with aggressive histopathologic features occurs, resection should include the surrounding bone; furthermore, when the orbital septum is violated, exenteration should be performed. Postoperative radiotherapy is advocated for aggressive lesions. Inverted papilloma should be treated with wide excision and careful surveillance for recurrence. The nonepithelial tumors, schwannoma, hemangiopericytoma, fibrous histiocytoma, and melanoma should be treated in a similar manner with wide local excision and exenteration, if necessary. Cases of lymphoma are best managed with radiation therapy and systemic chemotherapy.

Orbital Extension From Conjunctival Tumors

Conjunctival epithelium can be involved by both squamous cell carcinoma and malignant melanoma. The majority of these cases are squamous cell carcinomas that arise in the perilimbal conjunctiva in areas of preexisting dysplasia, solar keratosis, or carcinoma in situ.[134] The disease is seen mostly in elderly men, and because of its association with solar exposure and chronic irritation, it is seen in younger patients from the tropics. These tumors are discussed in detail elsewhere in the text and are typically indolent, slow growing, and occasionally exophytic tumors that only invade superficially. Histopathologically they are well-differentiated squamous cell carcinomas. Aggressive spindle cell and mucoepidermoid varieties have been described. Ocular invasion, nodal metastases, and orbital invasion each occur in approximately 10 percent of patients.[114] Iliff and associates[135] reviewed 27 cases and found that four had orbital invasion. They emphasized that because the tumors are low-grade recurrences, if diagnosed early, they can be managed successfully with local resection guided by map biopsies and local cryotherapy. In fact, even after repeated recurrences and progressive invasion into the orbit, there is a low rate of nodal metastases. Orbital invasion is managed by exenteration and less satisfactorily with radiation therapy in patients who are not amenable to exenteration. Rootman reported two cases of orbital invasion—one that presented with a picture similar to orbital cellulitis and another that presented with a fistula on the lower eyelid.[114]

Malignant melanoma of the conjunctiva is a much more lethal disease. In Rootman's series,[114] orbital invasion by conjunctival melanoma represented 0.5 percent of all orbital cases and 7.4 percent of secondary orbital tumors. The lesions can arise de novo in preexistent nevi, but they occur most commonly in areas of primary acquired melanosis.[136, 137] As with uveal melanoma, the cells may be spindle, intermediate, or epithelioid. In lesions that occur in primary acquired melanosis, atypical histologic changes that may be premalignant can be identified.[138] The management of the conjunctival lesions is simple excision and involves close surveillance until recurrences occur, at which time exenteration may be required. Some success has been reported with the adjuvant use of cryotherapy and radiation therapy.

Orbital Extension of Eyelid Tumors

Most tumors arising in the periocular skin are basal cell carcinomas. Basal cell carcinoma has been found to

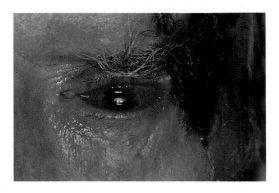

Figure 177–29. Basal cell carcinoma of the left temporal fossa with invasion of the superior orbit, causing cicatrization and fixation to the bone of the left upper lid. This resulted in exposure and a sterile corneal melt. The patient had the lesion for at least 9 yr and had three prior resections.

represent approximately 80 percent of eyelid neoplasms, whereas squamous cell carcinoma represents approximately 7 percent of cases.[139] Although basal cell carcinoma is more common, the number of cases with orbital extension is about equal for the two types of tumor. This is true because of the more indolent course of basal cell carcinoma compared with the less frequent, more aggressive squamous cell carcinoma. Basal cell carcinoma may present with orbital involvement because of neglect and delayed presentation or recurrences after incomplete excisions (Fig. 177–29). The lesions are locally invasive (particularly the morpheaform variety) and almost never metastasize. The lesions most often involve the sun-exposed lower eyelid (50 percent) and the medial canthal region (25 percent). The medial canthal lesions are the most likely to invade the orbit, not because of different tumor behavior but because of the close proximity of the tumor to the bone and lacrimal system and the tendency of surgeons to be less aggressive in these areas.[114]

Henderson found that basal cell carcinoma invading the orbit represented 2.3 percent of his findings in 764 patients with orbital tumors.[104] All except three of the 18 cases originated in the eyelids. The average patient was 50 to 80 yr of age and reported the lid lesion anywhere from 2 to 32 yr prior to presentation with orbital disease. Although orbital invasion may not be apparent, Henderson emphasizes that fixation of the underlying lesion to the orbital bone (see Fig. 177–29) is an important clue that suggests orbital invasion.[104] There is not a strong inflammatory component, and the invasion typically extends circumferentially around the anterior orbital structures, with deep orbital penetration being rare (Fig. 177–30). Pain is uncommon and occurs only when the nerves of the periorbita become involved. With early involvement of the extraocular muscles, patients develop diplopia in extremes of gaze.

The options for treatment of basal cell carcinoma include irradiation, surgical excision, or both. There are no clear guidelines, and the treatment plan must be tailored to suit each patient. One of the most important decisions to make at an early stage is whether the eye can be saved and whether the patient is willing to lose the eye and undergo an operation that may be disfiguring. If the patient is amenable to the surgery and is medically able to undergo major surgery, radical en-bloc surgery including exenteration, removal of all periorbita and periosteum as well as all suspicious bones is required and offers the best chance for survival (Fig. 177–31). Margins can be established with frozen sections, either during surgery or before resection under local anesthesia using the Mohs technique.

Others have emphasized the efficacy of radiation therapy, with 5-yr tumor control rates of up to 95

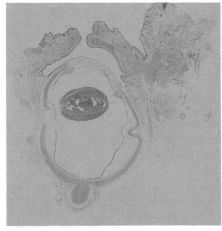
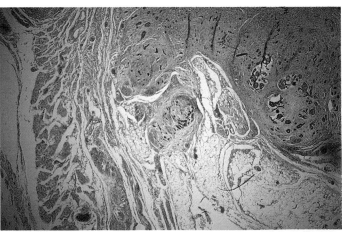

A   B

Figure 177–30. Low-power view (A) of an exenteration specimen from the patient in Figure 177–29. The upper right part of the field shows the invasion of the anterior orbit. A higher-power view (B) shows foci of morpheaform basal cell carcinoma extending into the orbital fat.

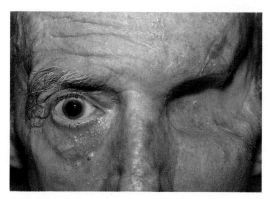

Figure 177–31. The same patient is free of disease after exenteration and skin graft.

percent.[140] However, less than optimal results may occur when the surgeon and the patient elect to use radiation therapy in order to preserve the function of the eye. In these situations, when eye shielding cannot always be reliably accomplished, patients may frequently end up with a nonfunctional, painful eye because of radiation-induced side effects including keratitis, cataract, retinopathy, optic neuropathy, or loss of adnexal structures. Certainly, high-dose radiation therapy may be an excellent alternative for elderly debilitated patients who cannot or will not undergo radical surgery. Additionally, some success has been reported with the use of systemic chemotherapy in these patients.[141]

Squamous cell carcinoma, although much less common than basal cell carcinoma, is more aggressive and invasive and is capable of metastases to regional lymph nodes. In their review of the literature, Riefler and Hornblass found that squamous cell carcinoma represented 9 percent of reported cases of eyelid malignancy, and Aurora and Blodi found squamous cell carcinoma in 7 percent of cases.[139, 142] The tumor occurs in sun-exposed areas of fair-skinned people, and there is a well-established genetic predisposition in patients with xeroderma pigmentosum. There is a slight lower lid predilection, but the upper lid (not the medial canthal area as in basal cell carcinoma) is the second most common site. In general, squamous cell carcinoma arising in the eyelid skin has a more indolent course than that beginning in the paranasal sinuses or in the nasopharynx. The presentation is more acute compared with basal cell carcinoma, and most patients can date the onset of signs and symptoms to within 1 yr of presentation. Orbital invasion occurs late, either after multiple excisions and recurrences or after neglect. Early perineural invasion makes ophthalmoplegia and pain more common than basal cell carcinoma. Because of its metastatic capability, the tumors must be treated radically by surgical excision with control of margins or with radiation therapy in patients who are unwilling or unable to undergo exenteration or radical surgery.

Sebaceous cell carcinoma can arise in any of the oil-producing adnexal structures including the meibomian glands, the glands of Zeis, and the sebaceous appendages of the hair follicles in the skin of the eyelid. Fortunately, the tumor is rare. Henderson found only three patients with orbital extension in a series of 745 orbital tumors.[104] The incidence of orbital invasion of sebaceous cell carcinoma was 6 percent[143] and 17 percent[144] in two large series. The tumor is more common in females, and most frequently involves the upper eyelid. Orientals may be more likely to develop this disease, and it typically occurs late in life.[144] Usually patients with orbital involvement present with a painless lump on the eyelid that has recurred after excision of a "chalazion." Doxonas and Green found the most common presentations included a localized tumor and blepharoconjunctivitis.[145] The disease receives much attention from ophthalmologists because of the importance of recognizing it at an early stage. If recognized within 6 mo of onset, mortality is 13 percent versus 43 percent in cases recognized after 6 mo.[114] Misdiagnosis in the past frequently occurred at the histopathologic level as well as at the clinical level. With increased suspicion and early diagnosis, patient survival has greatly increased since 1970.[145]

Unlike basal cell carcinoma, the lesions do not usually ulcerate. Orbital invasion, which occurs in 6 to 35 percent[143–145] of cases, may be associated (in 70 percent of cases[114]) with metastases to regional lymph nodes. In addition to metastases and orbital invasion, sebaceous cell carcinoma can spread in pagetoid fashion along the skin and conjunctiva. This is particularly common in patients with "blepharoconjunctivitis" presentation. Because of this ability to spread in numerous ways, radical and complete excision with frozen section control of margins is recommended for the management of these tumors. Since metastatic disease to the regional lymph nodes is the most common form of extension, a careful search for these nodes should be made so that radical lymph node dissection can be included in the surgical plan, if necessary. Death from generalized metastases (particularly the liver and the lung) can occur, and the survival rate is only about 30 percent in patients with orbital involvement. Radiotherapy is usually only palliative and is used for unresectable recurrences, although satisfactory tumor control has been reported with doses of about 4500 rads in patients who refuse or are unable to undergo radical surgery.[146]

Other eyelid and adnexal tumors have been reported to involve the orbit. The apocrine glands of Moll can be a source of adenocarcinoma of the eyelid with orbital invasion.[147] Eccrine and mucinous sweat glands can also be the source of invading eyelid adenocarcinoma.[148] Oncocytoma or oncocytic carcinoma have been reported to invade the orbit from both the caruncle[149] and the ethmoid sinus.[150] In all cases, clinicians and pathologists must be careful to rule out the more common possibility of a metastatic adenocarcinoma to the eyelid.

Eyelid skin melanoma was a source of orbital invasive tumor in one patient in Rootman's series.[114] Although most arise de novo, it is important for clinicians to recognize the various precursor lesions that can give rise to melanoma, including lentigo maligna (Hutchinson's melanotic freckle), the dysplastic nevus syndrome (autosomal dominant), and the giant nevocytic nevi. The important treatment emphasis of melanoma should be on prevention (ultraviolet light exposure) and on early

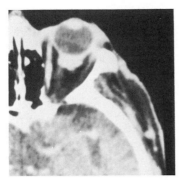

Figure 177–32. CT scan appearance of nodular extrascleral extension of uveal melanoma.

identification with complete excision given its propensity to widespread metastases.

Extrascleral and Orbital Extension From Intraocular Tumors

MELANOMA

The management of uveal melanoma and, more particularly, the extent that tumor spread can result from surgical manipulation remain controversial topics in ophthalmology. Extrascleral extension occurs in 10 to 15 percent of patients with uveal melanoma,[151, 152] and patients with uveal melanoma that extends into the orbit have a dismal prognosis regardless of the therapy chosen, with two thirds of patients dying of metastatic disease.[153] A number of risk factors have been identified that worsen the prognosis, including large tumor size, rupture of Bruch's membrane, pathologic type (mixed and epithelioid worse than spindle cell), and extension beyond the sclera. The management of orbital extension is also controversial and for the most part depends on personal and institutional philosophy and on how early the extrascleral extension and orbital involvement are detected.[104, 154, 155]

Shammas and Blodi in 1977 reported that seven of eight patients undergoing exenteration early on for the management of extrascleral extension achieved 5-yr survival.[153] However, Kersten and associates[154] in a retrospective study reevaluated the same patients and others and concluded that, in the long term, early exenteration did not improve survival in 16 patients with extrascleral extension compared with those undergoing enucleation alone. However, they did believe that it may have an impact on survival in patients with obvious tumor transection at the time of enucleation. Shields and associates have proposed a scheme that they use to manage patients with extrascleral extension.[155] Although there are numerous subtleties, they advocate resection of the surrounding tenon's tissue at the time of enucleation with radiotherapy for flat lesions. In cases in which nodular extension is diagnosed preoperatively, they prefer preoperative radiation before enucleation and tenonectomy. In cases of larger nodular extrascleral exten-

sion (Fig. 177–32), preoperative radiotherapy should be followed by exenteration and systemic chemotherapy or immunotherapy. Unfortunately, patients with orbital recurrence after enucleation almost all have coexisting metastatic disease, and the prognosis is uniformly poor.

RETINOBLASTOMA

Retinoblastoma is the most common intraocular tumor of childhood. Extension beyond the confines of the globe can occur via blood-borne metastases to distant sites, extension through the choroid and sclera into the orbit, and extension via the optic nerve to the central nervous system. Orbital extension occurs in 8 percent of patients with retinoblastoma. Although intraocular retinoblastoma can now be treated successfully with a 90 percent 5-yr survival, the prognosis for patients with orbital extension remains grim, and virtually 90 percent succumb to their disease.[156, 157] Although Bruch's membrane remains relatively resistant to penetration, once the tumor reaches the choroid, growth becomes more rapid and the tumor becomes more virulent. The tumor reaches the orbit through the loose connective tissue surrounding the vessels and nerves and enters the sclera. The connective tissue surrounding the eye must be carefully evaluated microscopically to identify tumor cells that are likely to result in orbital recurrence. Upon reaching the orbit, the tumor cells grow quickly as undifferentiated neuroblastic cells without Flexner Wintersteiner rosettes.[128]

The average age of onset of orbital involvement is 22 mo. Only 9 percent of these patients survive, and death typically occurs within 1 yr. In neglected primary cases, retinoblastoma can have an orbital presentation with progressive proptosis, lid swelling, and ecchymoses. The patient with a secondarily involved orbit typically presents with a lump or bump in an anophthalmic socket (Fig. 177–33). In patients in whom an orbital implant is placed, the recurrence may be more difficult to detect. The masses are nontender and prominently vascularized. Their growth is slow and measured in months compared with rhabdomyosarcoma, which grows in days. The tumor can gain access to the central nervous system either through direct extension through the optic nerve or, more rarely, via the posterior ciliary emissaries into

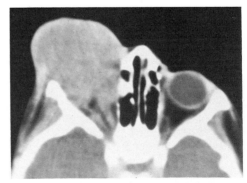

Figure 177–33. CT scan appearance of massive retinoblastoma recurrence in the anophthalmic socket.

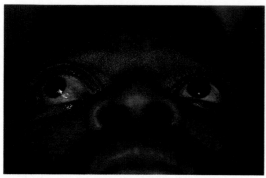
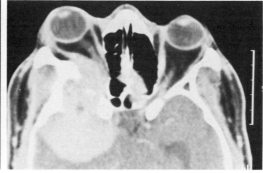

Figure 177–34. Proptosis and congestion of the right globe (A) secondary to a large sphenoid wing meningioma with an extension into the orbit (B).

the subarachnoid space. The amount of direct optic nerve extension has clearly been correlated with patient survival. Patients who have extension to the cut nerve margin have the worst prognosis. After enucleation and careful microscopic evaluation of the globe, the team must decide what are the relative risks of orbital, central nervous system, and distant spread. Although some patients have cytology performed on the cerebrospinal fluid, extension to the cut optic nerve margin or evidence of retinoblastoma cells near the pia mandates an evaluation of the cerebrospinal fluid. Treatment after enucleation often combines systemic chemotherapy and radiation therapy to the orbit if there is extrabulbar extension, orbital recurrence, massive posterior choroidal extension with periemissarial invasion, or iatrogenic rupture of the globe at the time of surgery. Treatment of central nervous system disease is based on cerebrospinal fluid evaluation and on the presence of tumor at the cut margin of the optic nerve. Orbital involvement in the past has been associated with a high death rate. However, because of increasing success in the management of retinoblastoma with disease outside of the globe using chemotherapy, orbital disease must be treated aggressively. Radiation therapy and occasionally surgical debulking are used to limit the chances of central nervous system and distant spread and to improve the chances for survival. The management should be done by a multidisciplinary team consisting of an ophthalmologist, an oncologist, and a radiotherapist.

Orbital Extension of Intracranial Tumors

Orbital involvement by intracranial tumors is rare and for the most part is seen mainly with meningiomas, particularly those that involve the sphenoid bone (Fig. 177–34). They can present after numerous resections and recurrences or primarily because of extension along the lateral orbital wall and posterior orbit causing proptosis and lid swelling. Additionally, if growing more medially or in the lesser wing of the sphenoid, the tumors can involve the structures in the posterior orbit, causing ophthalmoplegia and visual loss with only minimal proptosis.

Other tumors occurring in the region of the sella and the base of the skull can also invade the orbit. It is virtually unheard of for pituitary tumors to invade the orbit and cause proptosis. Craniopharyngiomas located in the suprasellar region do not usually invade the orbit. High-grade astrocytomas of the frontal lobe can invade the roof of the orbit (Fig. 177–35).[158] Clivus tumors including chordoma have also been reported to extend into the orbit.[159–161] Typically, proptosis occurs late and is a manifestation of advanced stage of disease (Fig. 177–36). Orbital involvement can also occur with extension of tumors, especially lymphoma and meningeal carcinomatosis, through the subarachnoid space into the optic nerve sheath.[114]

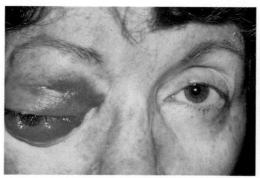
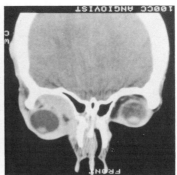

Figure 177–35. Clinical (A) and CT scan (B) appearance of chemosis and orbital congestion secondary to glioblastoma invading the orbit. (Courtesy of P. Rubin, M.D.)

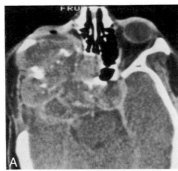
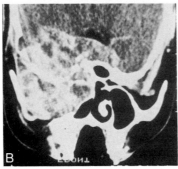

Figure 177–36. Axial *(A)* and coronal *(B)* CT scans of large recurrent chorodoma with bone destruction and extension into the orbit. The eye was enucleated at a previous resection.

REFERENCES

1. Ferry AP, Font RL: Carcinoma metastatic to the eye and orbit. I: A clinicopathologic study of 227 cases. Arch Ophthalmol 92:276, 1974.
2. Castro PA, Albert DM, Wang WJ, Ni C: Tumors metastatic to the eye and adnexa. Int Ophthalmol Clin 22:189, 1982.
3. Bloch RS, Gartner S: The incidence of ocular metastatic carcinoma. Arch Ophthalmol 85:673, 1971.
4. Horner F: Carcinoma der Dura Mater Exophthalmus. Klin Monatsbl Augenheilkd 2:186, 1864.
5. Goldberg RA, Rootman J, Cline RA: Tumors metastatic to the orbit: A changing picture. Surv Ophthalmol 35:1, 1990.
6. Godtfredsen E: On the frequency of secondary carcinoma of the choroid. Acta Ophthalmol 22:394, 1944.
7. Albert DM, Rubenstein RA, Scheie HG: Tumor metastases to the eye. I: Incidence in 213 patients with generalized malignancy. Am J Ophthalmol 63:723, 1967.
8. Nelson CC, Hertzberg BS, Klintworth GK: A histopathologic study of 716 eyes in patients with cancer at the time of death. Am J Ophthalmol 95:788, 1983.
9. Jensen OA: Metastatic tumors of the eye and orbit: A histopathologic analysis of a Danish series. Acta Pathol Microbiol Scand 212 (Suppl):201, 1970.
10. Freedman MI, Folk JC: Metastatic tumors to the eye and orbit: Patient survival and clinical characteristics. Arch Ophthalmol 105:1215, 1987.
11. Rootman J: Frequency and differential diagnosis of orbital disease. *In* Rootman J (ed): Diseases of the Orbit. Philadelphia, JB Lippincott, 1988.
12. Shields JA, Bakewell B, Augsberger JJ, Flanagan JC: Classification and incidence of space-occupying lesions of the orbit: A survey of 645 biopsies. Arch Ophthalmol 102:1606, 1984.
13. Moss HM: Expanding lesions of the orbit: A clinical study of 230 consecutive cases. Am J Ophthalmol 54:761, 1962.
14. Reese AB: Expanding lesions of the orbit. Trans Ophthalmol Soc UK 91:85, 1971.
15. Silva D: Orbital tumors. Am J Ophthalmol 65:318, 1968.
16. Henderson JW, Farrow GM: Metastatic carcinoma. *In* Henderson JW: Orbital Tumors, 2nd ed. New York, BC Decker, 1980.
17. Ferry AP: Metastatic carcinoma of the eye and ocular adnexa. Int Ophthalmol Clin 7:615, 1967.
18. Hart WM: Metastatic carcinoma to the eye and orbit. Int Ophthalmol Clin 2:465, 1962.
19. Stephens RF, Shields JA: Diagnosis and management of cancer metastatic to the uvea: A study of 70 cases. Ophthalmology 86:1336, 1979.
20. Albert DM, Rubenstein RA, Scheie HG: Tumor metastases to the eye. II: Clinical study in infants and children. Am J Ophthalmol 63:727, 1967.
21. Albert DM, Zimmerman AW, Zeidman I: Tumor metastases to the eye. III: Fate of circulating tumor cells to the eye. Am J Ophthalmol 63:733, 1967.
22. Fidler IJ, Balch CM: The biology of cancer metastasis and the implications for therapy. Curr Probl Surg 24:129, 1987.
23. Ferry AP: The biological behavior and pathologic features of carcinoma metastatic to the eye and orbit. Trans Am Ophthalmol Soc 71:373, 1973.
24. Font RL, Ferry AP: Carcinoma metastatic to the eye and orbit. III: A clinicopathologic study of 28 cases metastatic to the orbit. Cancer 38:1326, 1976.
25. Capone A, Slamovits TL: Discrete metastasis of solid tumors to extraocular muscles. Arch Ophthalmol 108:237, 1990.
26. Ashton N, Morgan G: Discrete carcinomatous metastases in the extraocular muscles. Br J Ophthalmol 58:112, 1974.
27. Trokel SL, Hilal SK: Recognition and differential diagnosis of enlarged extraocular muscles in computed tomography. Am J Ophthalmol 87:503, 1979.
28. Slamovits TL, Burde RM: Bumpy muscles. Surv Ophthalmol 33:189, 1988.
29. Divine RD, Anderson RL: Metastatic small cell carcinoma masquerading as orbital myositis. Ophthalmic Surg 14:483, 1982.
30. Rothfus WE, Curtin HD: Extraocular muscle enlargement: A CT review. Radiology 151:677, 1984.
31. Ginsberg J, Freemond AS, Calhoun JB: Optic nerve involvement in metastatic tumors. Ann Ophthalmol 2:604, 1970.
32. Christmas NJ, Mead M, Richardson EP, et al: Secondary optic nerve tumors. Surv Ophthalmol (in press).
33. Arnold AC, Hepler RS, Foos RY: Isolated metastases to the optic nerve. Surv Ophthalmol 26:75, 1981.
34. Amer MH, Al-Sarraf M, Baker IH, et al: Malignant melanoma and central nervous system metastases. Cancer 42:660, 1978.
35. Yap HY, Yap BS, Tashima CK, et al: Meningeal carcinomatosis in breast cancer. Cancer 42:283, 1978.
36. Aroney RS, Dalley DN, Chan WK: Meningeal carcinomatosis in small cell carcinoma of the lung. Am J Med 71:26, 1981.
37. Little JR, Dale AJD, Okazaki H: Meningeal carcinomatosis: Clinical manifestations. Arch Neurol 30:138, 1984.
38. Redman BG, Tapazoglou E, Al-Sarraf M: Meningeal carcinomatosis in head and neck cancer. Cancer 58:2656, 1986.
39. Altrocchi PA, Reinhardt PH, Eckman PB: Blindness and meningeal carcinomatosis. Arch Ophthalmol 88:508, 1972.
40. Susac JO, Smith JL, Powell JO: Carcinomatous optic neuropathy. Am J Ophthalmol 76:672, 1973.
41. Riley FC: Metastatic tumors of the eyelids. Am J Ophthalmol 69:259, 1970.
42. Hood CI, Font RL, Zimmerman LE: Metastatic mammary carcinoma in the eyelid with histiocytoid appearance. Cancer 31:793, 1973.
43. Bullock JD, Yanes B: Metastatic tumors of the orbit. Ann Ophthalmol 12:1392, 1980.
44. Kennedy RE: An evaluation of 820 orbital cases. Trans Am Ophthalmol Soc 82:134, 1984.
45. Shields CL, Shields JA, Peggs M: Tumors metastatic to the orbit. Ophthalmic Plast Reconstr Surg 4:73, 1988.
46. Goldberg RA, Rootman J: Clinical characteristics of metastatic orbital tumors. Ophthalmology 97:620, 1990.
47. Abdalla MI, Ghaly AF, Hosni F: Liposarcoma with orbital metastases: Case report. Br J Ophthalmol 50:426, 1966.
48. Betharia SM: Metastatic orbital carcinoma of the thyroid. Ind J Ophthalmol 33:191, 1985.
49. Hornblass A, Kass LG, Reich R: Thyroid carcinoma metastatic to the orbit. Ophthalmology 94:1004, 1987.
50. Knapp A: Metastatic thyroid tumor in the orbit. Arch Ophthalmol 52:68, 1923.

51. Harris AL, Montgomery A: Orbital carcinoid tumor. Am J Ophthalmol 90:875, 1980.
52. Riddle PJ, Font RL, Zimmerman LE: Carcinoid tumors of the eye and orbit: A clinicopathologic study of 15 cases, with histochemical and electron microscopic observations. Hum Pathol 13:459, 1982.
53. Rush JA, Walker RR, Campbell RJ: Orbital carcinoid tumor metastatic from the colon. Am J Ophthalmol 89:636, 1980.
54. Shetlar DJ, Font RL, Ordonez N, et al: A clinicopathologic study of three carcinoid tumors metastatic to the orbit. Ophthalmology 97:257, 1990.
55. Smiley SS: An orbital metastasis from the urinary bladder. Arch Ophthalmol 74:809, 1965.
56. Scharf Y, Ben Arieh Y, et al: Orbital metastases from extra-adrenal pheochromcytoma. Am J Ophthalmol 69:638, 1970.
57. Snidermann HR: Orbital metastases from tumor of the pancreas: Report of two cases with necropsy findings. Am J Ophthalmol 25:1215, 1942.
58. Stewart WB, Newman NM, Cavender JC, et al: Fibrous histiocytoma metastatic to the orbit. Arch Ophthalmol 96:871, 1978.
59. Lubin JR, Grove AS Jr, Zakov ZN, et al: Hepatoma metastatic to the orbit. Am J Ophthalmol 89:268, 1980.
60. Zubler MA, Rivera R, Lane M: Hepatoma presenting as a retro-orbital metastasis. Cancer 48:1883, 1981.
61. Drake ET, Dobben GD: Leiomyosarcoma of the uterus with unusual metastases. JAMA 170:1294, 1959.
62. Saxena RB, Mathur RN, Sonani SZ: Orbital metastasis of mixed parotid tumor. Ind J Ophthalmol 23:23, 1975.
63. Schlaen ND, Naves AE: Orbital and choroidal metastases from carcinoma of the male breast. Arch Ophthalmol 104:1344, 1986.
64. Shields JA, Shields CL, Shakin EP, Kobetz LE: Metastasis of choroidal melanoma to the contralateral choroid, orbit and eyelid. Br J Ophthalmol 72:456, 1988.
65. Oberman HA, Fayos JV, Lampe I: Pathology-radiation therapy conference: Unusual orbital tumor. U Mich Med 35:36, 1969.
66. Orcutt JC, Char DH: Melanoma metastatic to the orbit. Ophthalmology 95:1033, 1988.
67. Boldt HC, Nerad JA: Orbital metastasis from prostate carcinoma. Arch Ophthalmol 106:1403, 1988.
68. Rosenbluth J, Laval J, Weil JV: Metastasis of bronchial adenoma to the eye. Arch Ophthalmol 63:47, 1960.
69. Spaide RF, Granger E, Hammer BD, et al: Rapidly expanding exophthalmos: An unusual presentation of small cell lung cancer. Br J Ophthalmol 73:461, 1989.
70. Jakobiec FA, Font RL: Orbit. In Spencer WH (ed): Ophthalmic Pathology: An Atlas and Textbook, 3rd ed., vol. 3. Philadelphia, WB Saunders, 1985.
71. Healy JF: Computed tomographic evaluation of metastases to the orbit. Ann Ophthalmol 15:1026, 1983.
72. Cline RA, Rootman J: Enophthalmos: A clinical review. Ophthalmology 91:229, 1984.
73. Sher JH, Weinstock SJ: Orbital metastasis of prostatic carcinoma. Can J Ophthalmol 18:248, 1983.
74. Yeo JH, Jakobiec FA, Iwamoto T, et al: Metastatic carcinoma masquerading as scleritis. Ophthalmology 90:184, 1983.
75. Whyte AM: Bronchogenic carcinoma metastasizing to the orbit: A case report. J Maxillofac Surg 6:277, 1978.
76. Mottow-Lippa L, Jakobiec FA, Iwamoto T: Pseudoinflammatory metastatic breast carcinoma of the orbit and lids. Ophthalmology 88:575, 1981.
77. Bullock JD, Yanes B: Ophthalmic manifestations of metastatic breast cancer. Ophthalmology 87:961, 1980.
78. Seretan EL: Metastatic adenocarcinoma from the stomach to the orbit. Arch Ophthalmol 99:1469, 1981.
79. Denby P, Harvey L, English MG: Solitary metastasis from an occult renal cell carcinoma presenting as a primary lacrimal gland tumor. Orbit 5:21, 1986.
80. Divina RD, Anderson RL, Ossoinig KC: Metastatic carcinoid unresponsive to radiation therapy presenting as a lacrimal fossa mass. Ophthalmology 89:516, 1982.
81. Mann AS: Bilateral exophthalmos and seminoma. J Clin Endocrinol Metab 27:1500, 1867.
82. Taylor JB, Solomon BH, Levine RE, et al: Exophthalmos in seminoma: Regression with steroids and orchiectomy. JAMA 240:860, 1978.
83. Rush JA, Older JJ, Richman AV: Testicular seminoma metastatic to the orbit. Am J Ophthalmol 91:258, 1981.
84. Ballinger WH Jr, Wesley RE: Seminoma metastatic to the orbit. Ophthalmic Surg 15:120, 1984.
85. Hesselink JR, Davis KR, Weber AL, et al: Radiologic evaluation of orbital metastasis with emphasis on computed tomography. Radiology 137:363, 1980.
86. Peyster RG, Shapiro MD, Haik BG: Orbital metastasis: Role of magnetic resonance imaging and computed tomography. Radiol Clin North Am 25:647, 1987.
87. Shields CL, Shields JA, Eagle RC, et al: Orbital metastases from a carcinoid tumor: Computed tomography, magnetic resonance imaging and electron microscopic findings. Arch Ophthalmol 105:968, 1987.
88. Han JS, Benson JE, Bonstelle CT, et al: Magnetic resonance imaging of the orbit: A preliminary experience. Radiology 150:755, 1984.
89. Li KC, Poon PY, Hinton P, et al: MR imaging of orbital tumors with CT and ultrasound correlations. J Comput Assist Tomogr 8:1039, 1984.
90. Dresner SD, Kennerdell JS, Dekker A: Fine needle aspiration biopsy of metastatic orbital tumors. Surv Ophthalmol 27:397, 1983.
91. Kennerdell JS, Dekker A, Johnson BL, et al: Fine needle aspiration biopsy: A report of its use in orbital tumors. Arch Ophthalmol 97:1315, 1979.
92. Kennerdell JS, Slamovits TL, Dekker A, et al: Orbital fine needle aspiration biopsy. Am J Ophthalmol 99:547, 1985.
93. Krohel GB, Tobin DR, Chavis RM: Inaccuracy of fine needle aspiration biopsy. Ophthalmology 92:666, 1985.
94. Liu D: Complications of fine needle aspiration biopsy of the orbit. Ophthalmology 92:1768, 1985.
95. Reifler DM, Davidson P: Histochemical analysis of breast carcinoma metastatic to the orbit. Ophthalmology 93:254, 1986.
96. Glasburn JR, Klionsky M, Brady LW: Radiation therapy for metastatic diseases involving the orbit. Am J Clin Oncol 7:145, 1984.
97. Huh SH, Nisce LZ, Simpson LD, et al: Valve of radiation therapy in the treatment of orbital metastasis. Am J Roentgenol Radium Ther Nucl Med 120:589, 1974.
98. Moss WT: The orbit. In Moss WT, Cox JD (eds): Radiation Oncology: Rationale, Technique, Results. St. Louis, CV Mosby, 1989.
99. Fatkin JD, Purcell JJ, Krachmer JH, et al: Wilms' tumor metastatic to the orbit. JAMA 238:1841, 1977.
100. Musarella MA, Chen HSL, DeBoer G, Gallie BL: Ocular involvement in neuroblastoma: Prognostic implications. Ophthalmology 91:936, 1984.
101. Rootman J, Chan KW: Tumors. In Rootman J: Diseases of the Orbit. Philadelphia, JB Lippincott, 1988.
102. Davis JL, Parke DW, Font RL: Granulocytic sarcoma of the orbit: A clinicopathologic study. Ophthalmology 92:1758, 1985.
103. Weiss AH, Greenwald MJ, Margo CE, Myers W: Primary and secondary orbital teratomas. J Pediatr Ophthalmol Strab 26:44, 1989.
104. Henderson JW: Secondary epithelial neoplasms. In Henderson JW: Orbital Tumors, 2nd ed. New York, BC Decker, 1980.
105. Johnson LN, Krohel GB, Yeon EB, Parnes SM: Sinus tumors invading the orbit. Ophthalmology 91:209, 1984.
106. Vrabec DP: The inverted schneiderian papilloma: A clinical and pathologic study. Laryngoscope 85:186, 1975.
107. Weaver DT, Bartley GB: Malignant neoplasia of the paranasal sinuses associated with mucocele. Ophthalmology 98:342, 1991.
108. Robinson JM: Frontal sinus cancer manifested as a frontal mucocele. Arch Otolaryngol 101:718, 1975.
109. Guerry RK, Smith JL: Paranasal sinus carcinoma causing orbital mucocele. Am J Ophthalmol 80:943, 1975.
110. Mohan H, Sen D, Gupta D: Orbital affection in nasal and paranasal neoplasms. Acta Ophthalmol 47:289, 1969.
111. Weber AL, Stanton AC: Malignant tumors of the paranasal sinuses: Radiologic, clinical and histopathologic evaluation of 200 cases. Otolaryngol Head Neck Surg 6:761, 1984.
112. Gullane PJ, Conley J: Carcinoma of the maxillary sinus: A correlation of the clinical course with orbital involvement, pterygoid erosion, or pterygopalatine invasion and cervical metastases. J Otolaryngol 12:141, 1983.

113. Conley JJ: The risk to the orbit in head and neck cancer. Laryngoscope 95:515, 1985.

114. Rootman J: Secondary tumors of the orbit. *In* Rootman J: Diseases of the Orbit. Philadelphia, JB Lippincott, 1988.

115. Harbison JW, Lessell S, Selhorst JB: Neuro-ophthalmology of sphenoid sinus carcinoma. Brain 107:855, 1984.

116. Conley JJ: Sinus tumors invading the orbit. Trans Am Acad Ophthalmol Otolaryngol 70:615, 1976.

117. Flores AD, Anderson DW, Doyle PJ, et al: Paranasal sinus malignancy: A retrospective analysis of treatment methods. J Otolaryngol 13:141, 1984.

118. Osguthorpe JD, Saunders RA, Adkins WY: Evaluation of and access to posterior orbital tumors. Laryngoscope 93:766, 1983.

119. Sisson GA: Symposium. III: Treatment of malignancies of paranasal sinuses: Discussion and summary. Laryngoscope 80:945, 1970.

120. Harrison DFN: Problems in surgical management of neoplasms arising in the paranasal sinus. J Laryngol Otol 90:649, 1976.

121. Perry C, Levine PA, Williamson BR, Cantrell RW: Preservation of the eye in paranasal sinus cancer surgery. Arch Otolaryngol Head Neck Surg 114:632, 1988.

122. Som ML: Surgical management of carcinoma of the maxilla. Arch Otolaryngol Head Neck Surg 99:20, 1974.

123. Larson DL, Christ JE, Jesse RH: Preservation of the orbital contents in cancer of the maxillary sinus. Arch Otolaryngol Head Neck Surg 108:370, 1982.

124. Jakobiec FA, Rootman J, Jones IS: Secondary and metastatic tumors of the orbit. *In* Jones IS, Jakobiec FA (eds): Diseases of the Orbit. New York, Harper & Row, 1979.

125. Takagi M, Ishikawa G, Mori W: Primary malignant melanoma of the oral cavity in Japan with special reference to mucosal melanosis. Cancer 34:358, 1974.

126. Komisar A: Plexiform ameloblastoma of the maxilla with extension to the skull base. Head Neck Surg 7:172, 1984.

127. Weiss JS, Bressler SB, Jacobs EF, et al: Maxillary ameloblastoma with orbital invasion. Ophthalmology 92:710, 1985.

128. Jakobiec FA, Rootman J, Jones IS: Secondary and metastatic tumors of the orbit. *In* Duane TD (ed): Clinical Ophthalmology, vol. 2. New York, Harper & Row, 1978.

129. Batsakis J: Tumors of the Head and Neck. Baltimore, Williams & Wilkins, 1974.

130. Ashton N, Choyce DP, Fison LG: Carcinoma of the lacrimal sac. Br J Ophthalmol 35:366, 1951.

131. Flanagan JC, Stokes DDP: Lacrimal sac tumors. Ophthalmology 85:1282, 1978.

132. Lloyd WC III, Leone CR Jr: Malignant melanoma of the lacrimal sac. Arch Ophthalmol 102:104, 1984.

133. Ryan S, Font R: Primary epithelial neoplasms of the lacrimal sac. Am J Opthalmol 76:73, 1973.

134. Zimmerman L: Squamous cell carcinoma and related lesions of the bulbar conjunctiva. *In* Boniuk M (ed): Ocular and Adnexal Tumors. St. Louis, CV Mosby, 1964.

135. Iliff W, Marback R, Green WR: Invasive squamous cell carcinoma of the conjunctiva. Arch Ophthalmol 93:119, 1975.

136. Folberg R, McClean WI, Zimmerman LE: Malignant melanoma of the conjunctiva. Hum Pathol 16:129, 1985.

137. Lederman M, Wybar K, Busby E: Malignant epibulbarmelanoma: Natural history and treatment by radiation therapy. Br J Ophthalmol 68:605, 1984.

138. Jakobiec FA, Folberg R, Iwamoto T: Clinicopathologic characteristics of premalignant and malignant melanocytic lesions of the conjunctiva. Ophthalmology 96:147, 1989.

139. Aurora A, Blodi F: Lesions of the eyelid: A clinicopathologic study. Surv Ophthalmol 15:94, 1970.

140. Fitzpatrick PJ, Thompson GA, Easterbrook WM, et al: Basal and squamous cell carcinoma of the eyelids and their treatment by radiotherapy. Int J Radiat Oncol Biol Phys 10:449, 1984.

141. Luxemberg M, Guthrie T Jr: Chemotherapy of eyelid and periorbital tumors. Trans Am Ophthalmol Soc 83:162, 1985.

142. Reifler DM, Hornblass A: Squamous cell carcinoma of the eyelid. Surv Ophthalmol 30:349, 1986.

143. Ginsberg J: Present status of meibomian gland carcinoma. Arch Ophthalmol 73:271, 1965.

144. Boniuk M, Zimmerman LE: Sebaceous carcinoma of the eyelid, eyebrow, caruncle and orbit. Trans Am Acad Ophthalmol Otolaryngol 72:619, 1978.

145. Doxanas MT, Green WR: Sebaceous gland carcinoma: Review of 40 cases. Arch Ophthalmol 102:245, 1984.

146. Hendley RL, Rieser JC, Cavanagh HD, et al: Primary radiation therapy for meibomian gland carcinoma. Am J Ophthalmol 87:206, 1979.

147. Ni C, Kuo PK, Dryja TP, et al: Sweat gland tumors of the eyelids: A clinicopathologic analysis of 55 cases. *In* Ni C, Albert DM (eds): Tumors of the Eyelid and Orbit: A Chinese-American Collaborative Study. Boston, Little, Brown, 1982.

148. Khalil M, Brownstein S, Codere F, Nicolle D: Eccrine sweat gland carcinoma of the eyelid with orbital involvement. Arch Ophthalmol 98:2210, 1980.

149. Gonnering RS, Sonneland PR: Oncocytic carcinoma of the plica semilunaris with orbital extension. Ophthalmic Surg 18:604, 1987.

150. Chui RTK, Liao SY, Bosworth H: Recurrent oncocytoma of the ethmoid sinus with orbital invasion. Otolaryngol Head Neck Surg 93:267; 1985.

151. Shammas HF, Blodi FC: Orbital extension of choroidal and ciliary body melanomas. Arch Ophthalmol 95:2002, 1977.

152. Starr HJ, Zimmerman LE: Extrascleral extension and orbital recurrence of malignant melanomas of the choroid and ciliary body. Ophthalmol Clin 2:369, 1962.

153. Affeldt JC, Minckler DS, Azen SP, Yeh L: Prognosis in uveal melanoma with extrascleral extension. Arch Ophthalmol 98:1975, 1980.

154. Kersten RC, Tse DT, Anderson RL, Blodi FC: The role of orbital exenteration in choroidal melanoma with extrascleral extension. Ophthalmology 92:436, 1985.

155. Shields JA, Augsburger JJ, Corwin S, et al: The management of uveal melanomas with extrascleral extension. Orbit 5:31, 1986.

156. Ellsworth RM: Orbital retinoblastoma. Trans Am Ophthalmol Soc 72:79, 1974.

157. Rootman J, Ellsworth RM, Hofbauer J, et al: Orbital extension of retinoblastoma: A clinicopathologic study. Can J Ophthalmol 13:72, 1978.

158. Blodi F: Unusual orbital tumors and their treatments. *In* Symposium on Surgery of the Orbit and Adnexa. St Louis, CV Mosby, 1974.

159. Ferry AP, Haddad HM, Goldman JL: Orbital invasion by an intracranial chordoma. Am J Ophthalmol 92:7, 1981.

160. Daicker BC: Chordom der Orbita. Ophthalmologica (Basel) 176:236, 1978.

161. Flament J, Forest M: Envahissement osteolytique massif de l'orbite par un chordome: Discussion d'une observation privilegiée et revue de la littérature. J Fr Ophthalmol 2:647, 1979.

Chapter 178

∎

Rare Intraosseous and Primary Orbital Tumors

PETER A. NETLAND, RAMON L. FONT, and
FREDERICK A. JAKOBIEC

Certain rare primary orbital tumors are not easily categorized among other orbital tumors. Some of these tumors, including endodermal sinus tumor or primary orbital melanoma, are unique in their histogenesis. In other tumors, including alveolar soft part sarcoma and the pigmented retinal choristoma (formerly called retinal anlage tumor), the origin is disputed, and the tumors cannot be grouped with other orbital tumors with known histogenesis. The diagnosis of these rare orbital tumors is frequently elusive clinically and is typically made by histopathologic examination. Table 178–1 lists the tumors in the order they are covered in this chapter.

ENDODERMAL SINUS TUMOR

The endodermal sinus tumor is a malignant germ cell neoplasm that usually appears in the gonads but on rare occasions can occur in extragonadal locations, including the orbit. Because of similarities to certain structures in the rat placenta, the tumor was labeled as endodermal sinus tumor.[1] Other terms for this tumor include infantile embryonal carcinoma[2] and yolk sac tumor.[3] Endodermal sinus tumor is a germ cell tumor, as is the case with germinoma (seminoma), embryonal carcinoma, chorio-

Table 178–1. RARE INTRAOSSEOUS AND PRIMARY ORBITAL TUMORS

Endodermal sinus tumor
Alveolar soft part sarcoma
Granular cell tumor
Pigmented retinal choristoma
Nonchromaffin paraganglioma
Primary carcinoid tumor
Primary melanoma
Ectomesenchymal tumors
Neuroepithelioma
Primary orbital neuroblastoma
Malignant rhabdoid tumor
Mesenchymal chondrosarcoma
Angiosarcoma
Intravascular papillary endothelial hyperplasia
Malignant peripheral nerve sheath tumor
Paget's disease
Hereditary diaphyseal dysplasia
Infantile cortical hyperostosis
Brown tumor
Intraosseous myxoma
Primary intraosseous hemangioma
Lethal midline granuloma

carcinoma, and teratoma. In humans and other mammals, the germ cells originate in the yolk sac endoderm and migrate through the mesentery to the genital ridge to become the undifferentiated gonad.[4] Midline extragonadal sites, including intracranial and orbital locations, may receive aberrantly migrating cells. In the chick embryo, it has been demonstrated that germ cells may also gain access to the circulation.[5] Although these germ cells usually disappear as development progresses, some may persist and give rise to extragonadal germ cell tumors.

The clinical and pathologic features of five cases of endodermal sinus tumor of the orbit have been reported from the Armed Forces Institute of Pathology (AFIP),[6] including a case previously published in a case report.[7] Clinically, the mean age at time of presentation was 13 mo, with a range of 3 mo to 4 yr. In contrast, patients with nonorbital extragonadal yolk sac tumors tend to be older, with an average age of 14 yr at presentation in a series of 19 patients with such tumors.[6] All patients with orbital yolk sac tumors in the AFIP series presented with proptosis of the affected eye, and one patient presented with ipsilateral visual loss and papilledema. Two patients in this series showed extraorbital extension, one of whom acquired intracranial extension with metastatic disease and died 10 mo after the onset of proptosis. Because of the age of the patients and the rapid onset of proptosis, the tumor is likely to be mistaken for rhabdomyosarcoma, which is much more common in this clinical setting.

Endodermal sinus tumors are always malignant in contrast with teratomas of the orbit that have a similar germ cell origin but show benign clinical behavior. Ovarian endodermal sinus tumor has a poor prognosis and requires aggressive treatment.[5, 8] Triple-drug chemotherapy combined with surgery offers superior results to surgery alone or a combination of surgery and radiation therapy. Testicular yolk sac tumors have an age-dependent prognosis, with a better prognosis in children younger than 2 yr.[3] Most extragonadal endodermal sinus tumors are fatal; however, aggressive treatment of orbital tumors can result in long-term survival.[6] This may be related to the anatomic location of the orbital tumors that results in noticeable proptosis when the tumor mass is relatively small, permitting recognition and treatment of orbital tumors at a comparatively early stage. Similarly, orbital rhabdomyosarcomas have a better prognosis than rhabdomyosarcomas in other sites, probably because the tumor is manifested clinically at an earlier time than in most other sites.[9]

Microscopic examination of these tumors shows characteristic histologic features. The tumor may be circumscribed but is not encapsulated. There is a pseudopapillary pattern with many intertwining slitlike spaces lined with a flat to cuboidal epithelium and a scant intervening stroma. The epithelial cells demonstrate marked anaplasia and frequent mitoses. Occasional cystic spaces with invaginating folds of epithelium are found that resemble glomeruli (Schiller-Duval bodies), which are perithelial accumulations of the embryonal epithelium around central vascular cores (Fig. 178–1). Areas of necrosis and hemorrhage are often observed. Some cases may show focal areas of myxomatous stroma. Both tumor cells and the stroma may contain numerous hyalin globules that stain with PAS and are resistant to diastase predigestion.

The immunoperoxidase reaction for α-fetoprotein is positive, with staining localized to the cytoplasm of tumor cells (see Fig. 178–1C). The hyaline globules do not contain α-fetoprotein, but there may be occasional staining at the margins of these globules. Metastatic lesions or tumors treated with chemotherapy may lose their α-fetoprotein positivity.[6] Staining for α-fetoprotein can be helpful in distinguishing this tumor from orbital rhabdomyosarcoma, which is relatively common in the affected age group. Although serum levels of α-fetoprotein have not been measured in children with orbital yolk sac tumors, endodermal sinus tumors in other locations are associated with elevated serum α-fetoprotein levels.[4, 10, 11] These serum levels have been used to monitor therapeutic response[12, 13] and presumably would be useful in primary orbital yolk sac tumors. It is possible, however, that orbital lesions with their smaller volumes may not produce enough secreted antigen to be detectable in the blood.

ALVEOLAR SOFT PART SARCOMA

Alveolar soft part sarcoma is a rare soft tissue tumor of uncertain histologic origin that usually appears in the extremities but can appear in the orbit. Christopherson and colleagues first used the term alveolar soft part sarcoma based on the unique histologic appearance and pattern of clinical behavior.[14] In addition to vascularized compact cellular aggregates, the tumor cells may be arranged in an alveolar form with a central space lacking organized material, hence the descriptive term soft part. Because of its rarity, this tumor is usually misdiagnosed clinically.[15–17]

There has been debate regarding the histologic origin of alveolar soft part sarcoma. The three principal hypotheses of origin are neural crest (particularly Schwann cell and paraganglia), vascular, and myogenic. Smetana and Scott reported 14 cases of alveolar soft part sarcoma in the extremities, which they characterized as malignant tumors of nonchromaffin paraganglioma (chemodectoma) based on light microscopic appearance.[18] Welch and associates noted that both paragangliomas and alveolar soft part sarcoma had been identified in the orbit and suggested a similar histologic origin.[19] However, nonchromaffin paragangliomas have not been identified in the extremities, and catecholamines considered typical of paraganglial tissue have not been detected in any alveolar soft part sarcoma. The Schwann cell hypothesis is based on an ultrastructural study of a case of alveolar soft part sarcoma in which myelinated structures were observed.[20] The application of immunohistochemical techniques has failed to provide evidence supporting a neural crest origin. No immunoreactivity has been documented when tumors are examined with antibody directed to S100, cytokeratin, glial filament acidic pro-

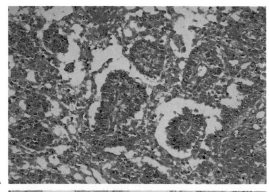

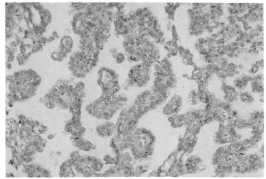

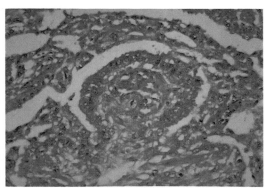

Figure 178–1. Endodermal sinus tumor. *A,* Light microscopy shows anastomosing cords of cuboidal cells with a scanty stroma. Also note several Schiller-Duval bodies, which are organoid invaginations of epithelial cells around central vascular cores resembling glomeruli (H&E, ×157). *B,* Higher magnification of Schiller-Duval body. These organoid structures resemble glomeruli, with a layer of embryonal epithelium surrounding a vascular core. (*A* and *B,* Courtesy of C. E. Margo, M.D., University of Florida.) *C,* Tumor cells demonstrate intracytoplasmic brown staining in immunoperoxidase reaction for α-fetoprotein (×100). Published courtesy of *Ophthalmology* 90:1426–1432, 1983.

tein, chromogranin, and neural filaments.[20] Immunohistochemical examination of nonorbital alveolar soft part sarcoma has shown that the granules in the cytoplasm as well as the larger crystals stain positively for renin, which is normally found in the renal juxtaglomerular cells.[21] An interesting possibility is that these tumor cells are derived from mural cells of vascular spaces, which produce ectopic renin. On the basis of these results, the term malignant angioreninoma has been proposed as an alternative to alveolar soft part sarcoma. However, the material is apparently not released into the serum because hypertension is not associated with the tumor. Also these findings have not been confirmed by other investigators.[22, 23]

Although not proven at this time, several lines of evidence support the myogenic hypothesis of histogenesis. First, the tumor arises clinically in skeletal muscle and shares certain clinical features with rhabdomyosarcoma.[14, 20] Second, the characteristic cytoplasmic crystalloids found in alveolar soft part sarcoma are similar morphologically to rods observed in cells of benign rhabdomyoma and nemaline myopathy[24] as well as to actin filaments.[25] Third, there is immunohistochemical evidence supporting the myogenic hypothesis. Examination of alveolar soft part sarcoma has shown a high proportion of positive reactivity with antibodies directed to B-enolase, actin, desmin, and vimentin, whereas staining for myoglobin has been negative.[20, 26-28] Also the characteristic crystalloids contain Z-protein antigen. These findings suggest a nonstriated myogenic origin of alveolar soft part sarcoma. As suggested by Christopherson and colleagues,[14] alveolar soft part sarcoma might represent a variant of rhabdomyosarcoma, possibly arising from muscle spindle[14, 20] or could be considered a malignant counterpart of granular cell tumor (myoblastoma).

The frequency of alveolar soft part sarcoma has been estimated between 0.04 and 1.0 percent of all soft tissue sarcomas.[29] In a review of 143 cases from the AFIP, there were 39 cases (27.3 percent) in the head and neck region, with the orbit and tongue the most frequently affected.[29] The tumor predominately affects the extremities in adults (especially the buttocks and thighs), whereas in children it occurs more frequently in the head and neck region. Although alveolar soft part sarcoma is malignant, the growth and spread of the tumor can be indolent. In a study of 53 cases of alveolar soft part sarcoma of the extremities, Lieberman and associates identified prolonged disease-free intervals in females younger than 20 yr but found the disease to be uniformly fatal within 20 yr.[30] The 2-, 5-, and 10-yr survivals were 83 percent, 59 percent, and 47 percent, respectively. In another series, Evans found a median survival of 79 mo in patients with nonorbital alveolar soft part sarcoma.[31] In uncontrolled clinical studies to date, the tumor appears relatively insensitive to radiotherapy or chemotherapy.

In the largest orbital series, Font and associates[32] noted that orbital lesions present most commonly with proptosis of approximately 4 mo duration, lid swelling, and dilation of conjunctival vessels. Up to one third of patients with alveolar soft part sarcoma of the extremi-

ties may present with metastatic disease, which typically develops in the lungs, bones, and brain. Cerebral metastases may be the first sign of disease and are more common in alveolar soft part sarcoma than other types of soft tissue sarcomas.[29] In contrast, there have been no reports of metastatic disease at presentation in orbital alveolar soft part sarcoma. In both orbital and nonorbital alveolar soft part sarcoma, women are affected more commonly than men with a ratio of more than 3:1. Because of the tendency for young females to be affected and the occurrence of cases during pregnancy, a hormonal influence has been suggested but is unproved.[33] In nonorbital sites, alveolar soft part sarcoma presents over a wide age range and is found most often in adolescents and young adults between 15 and 35 yr of age.[29] Similarly, in the orbital series reported by Font and colleagues,[32] the average age was 23 yr, the age range was 11 mo to 69 yr, and 13 of 17 patients were affected within the first three decades of life. Although the right side of the body has been more commonly affected in reports of nonorbital alveolar soft part sarcoma, there does not appear to be a preference for one orbit over the other. Longer disease-free intervals have been documented for patients with orbital compared with nonorbital alveolar soft part sarcoma,[20, 32] which may be related to earlier diagnosis, smaller size, and treatment of orbital lesions. In the series described by Font and associates,[32] only 2 of the 15 patients with complete clinical follow-up had died from metastatic disease after a protracted course of 14 and 21 yr, respectively, after initial surgery.

Grossly, the tumor is usually well-circumscribed and may even have a partial capsule. These tumors may bleed profusely when undergoing biopsy because of the presence of numerous endothelial-lined vascular channels. On sectioning, the tumor may be rubbery and pink, tan, or reddish-brown. There are frequently large areas of necrosis or hemorrhage.

The microscopic appearance of this tumor is characteristic (Fig. 178–2). There may be a pseudocapsule, and dense fibrous trabeculas divide the tumor into irregular-sized compartments. The tumor cells line up along delicate fibrovascular trabeculae and may delaminate into the cavities within these tumor cell nests. The central degeneration and loss of cohesion in these tumor cell islands gives a pseudoalveolar or organoid pattern. The large polyhedral tumor cells have an acidophilic cytoplasm with distinct cell boundaries. The darkly staining vesicular nucleus contains a prominent nucleolus and is usually located paracentrally or eccentrically within the cytoplasm. Mitotic figures and nuclear pleomorphism are rare. In contrast, vascular invasion is common, which explains the tendency toward early metastasis. There may be numerous dilated veins at the margin of the tumor, which probably arise because of multiple arteriovenous shunts.

The diagnostic features can be demonstrated with the PAS stain. This stain reveals the characteristic PAS-positive crystalline structures that resist diastase predigestion and have rectangular, rhomboidal, and needle-like appearances (see Fig. 178–2C). The crystals may also be demonstrated with methylene blue stain. These

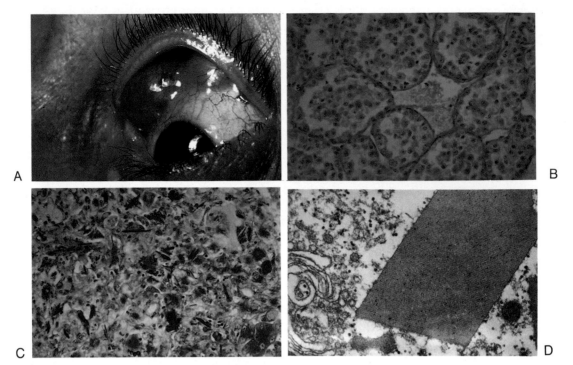

Figure 178-2. Alveolar soft part sarcoma of the orbit. *A,* Clinical photograph of the left eye of a 54-year-old woman with proptosis and tearing for several months. A bilobed and yellowish-red subconjunctival mass was present supranasally. The patient had an excisional biopsy performed followed by exenteration and was alive and well 5 yr and 2 mo after surgery. *B,* The tumor cells show a distinctive pseudoalveolar or organoid pattern, with nests of polyhedral tumor cells separated by thin fibrovascular septa. The tumor cells in the center of the pseudoalveolar cavities or "soft part" may be loosely cohesive or degenerating. These cells may have granular acidophilic cytoplasm and eccentric paracentral nuclei, many of which contain a prominent single nucleolus. *C,* Many of the tumor cells contain the characteristic crystalline material positive for periodic acid–Schiff stain in the cytoplasm. These crystals are resistant to diastase predigestion (periodic acid–Schiff stain). *D,* Electron micrograph shows a crystalline inclusion with a regular periodicity of 8 to 10 nm. Well-developed Golgi lamellae are present on the left, and many small round electron-dense glycogen granules are present, especially in the upper left.

crystals are present in at least 80 percent of these tumors and have not been demonstrated in any other neoplasm.[29] Also careful examination of the cytoplasm reveals a fine granularity, more noticeable on PAS than H&E staining, that is resistant to diastase predigestion. This material is present even in tumors without formed crystals and may be a precursor of the crystals.[29] In addition, PAS-positive glycogen particles that are sensitive to diastase predigestion are frequently present. The histologic features of alveolar soft part sarcoma may vary, which may cause confusion with other tumors. The tumor may resemble metastatic renal cell carcinoma, and angiosarcoma-like patterns caused by degeneration of tumor cells in pseudoalveolar cavities or pericytoma-like patterns with irregular branching channels have been described.[32] However, the presence of the characteristic PAS-positive crystalline material confirms the diagnosis of alveolar soft part sarcoma.

Electron microscopic examination of the crystals shows a regular lattice pattern of 80 to 100 angstrom internal periodicity (see Fig. 178–2*D*).[34] These appear to arise from moderately electron-dense smaller membrane-limited granules that fuse to create the larger crystalline inclusions. There are also abundant parallel stacks of rough-surfaced endoplasmic reticulum, lipid droplets, glycogen granules, numerous mitochondria, and a well-developed Golgi system. In addition, desmosomes and hemidesmosomes have been observed.[35]

The differential diagnosis includes metastatic renal cell carcinoma, paraganglioma, and granular cell tumor. These tumors primarily affect patients older than 40 yr and are rare in patients younger than 25 yr, unlike alveolar soft part sarcoma.[29] Renal cell carcinoma may have an organoid nestlike pattern, and tumor cells may contain lipid and glycogen, but PAS-positive and diastase-resistant crystalline material is absent. Glycogen is absent in both granular cell tumor and paraganglioma. Granular cell tumor has a characteristic cellular morphology and does not show the pseudoalveolar or organoid pattern. Paraganglioma shows prominent nonspecific lipid and phospholipid, whereas there is less prominent lipid and no elevated phospholipid in alveolar soft part sarcoma.[35] Rarely, the tumor is confused with alveolar rhabdomyosarcoma and angiosarcoma.

Because of the rarity of this tumor, the best mode of therapy is not known. However, most authors recommend wide surgical excision as the primary therapy. In some patients, surgical treatment has been followed with radiotherapy or chemotherapy, usually with a minimal or poor response.[20] In one study of nonorbital alveolar soft part sarcoma, the radiosensitivity was low, with a marked response in only 3 of 16 patients.[30] In the event of recurrence or metastasis, most authors recommend adjunctive chemotherapy with or without radiotherapy. Exenteration is reserved only for extremely bulky lesions that cannot be excised or for local recurrences.

GRANULAR CELL TUMOR

Granular cell tumor occurs most frequently in the tongue and subcutaneous tissues but rarely occurs in other parts of the body including the orbit and adnexa.[36] The reported ophthalmic sites include the orbit, periorbital skin and eyelids, extraocular muscles, lacrimal sac, ciliary body, conjunctiva, and caruncle.[37] After the initial description of this tumor by Abrikossoff in 1926,[38] the tumor has been known by many names, most of which have made reference to a putative cell of origin. Because the histogenesis is not well-understood at this time, the noncommittal descriptive term granular cell tumor is preferred.

Proposed cell types of origin have included skeletal muscle cell, smooth muscle cell, fibroblast, histiocyte, undifferentiated mesenchymal cell, neural cell, and Schwann cell.[37] An origin from striated muscle was first proposed by Abrikossoff and was supported by tissue culture studies performed by Murray.[39] The tumor was previously called granular cell myoblastoma because of a presumed origin from striated muscle. However, this theory has been largely discounted because the tumor develops in areas lacking muscle, and there has been no supporting evidence from ultrastructural or immunohistochemical studies. A histiocytic origin has been proposed[40, 41] but is considered unlikely because the tumor cells lack specific histiocytic markers such as lysozyme and α_1-antitrypsin.[42] In one case, immunochemical stains revealed the presence of carcinoembryonic antigen, which was interpreted as a sign of a primitive cell of origin, probably related to mesenchymal cells.[43]

Initially suggested in 1935,[44] the possibility of neural origin has gained popularity with various cellular candidates including perineural fibroblasts,[45] Schwann cells,[46] and primitive mesenchymal cells with the potential to differentiate into Schwann or granular cells.[37, 42] Schwann cell origin, in particular, has been supported by ultrastructural studies that have demonstrated a close relationship of axons and tumor cells, the presence of intracytoplasmic myelin figures, so-called angulate bodies, and the presence of basement membrane.[37] Immunohistochemical studies provide additional evidence for a neural origin of granular cell tumor. Granular cell tumor cells stain positively for S100 protein,[47–49] a protein initially identified in neural tissue and subsequently identified in other tissues. More recently, both granular cell tumor cells and Schwann cells were found to contain only the β-subunit of S100 protein.[50] Variable results have been reported with stains for neuron-specific enolase, which is present in nerve cells and absent in Schwann cells.[51, 52] It should be remembered that Schwann cells can become facultative histiocytes in the course of wallerian degeneration and may phagocytose myelin debris and display lysosomal hyperplasia. It has been suggested that granular cell tumors represent a neoplastic form of this cellular behavior.[53]

The largest series of patients with granular cell tumor of the orbit and ocular adnexa was reported by Jaeger and coworkers, who reviewed 25 previously reported cases and added 6 additional cases of their own.[37] The age of the patients ranged from 3 to 74 yr, with an average age of 39.8 yr, which is similar to the age range in reported studies of granular cell tumors occurring in other locations. The sex distribution was almost equal, with 16 males and 14 females (the sex of one patient in the series was not reported). The duration of signs or symptoms before diagnosis varied from 2 wk to 5 yr. These orbital tumors most commonly present with exophthalmos or diplopia but can also present with decreased visual acuity resulting from optic nerve involvement.[37, 52] In nonorbital granular cell tumors, between 10 and 15 percent are multicentric and 1 to 3 percent are malignant.[52] Although granular cell tumors are generally considered to be benign, invasion of local tissues has been demonstrated in orbital granular cell tumors.[52–54] Because the clinical behavior is usually benign, the treatment is wide local excision. If not completely excised, the lesions can recur. Because wide local excision of infiltrative orbital tumors is technically difficult, frozen-section control is recommended.

Grossly, the tumor is white to gray-tan and is generally well-encapsulated. Microscopically, the tumor cells are round to oval-shaped with a small basophilic nucleus that may contain a prominent eosinophilic nucleus (Fig. 178–3). The nuclei are usually centrally located, and there is no mitotic activity. There is an abundant gran-

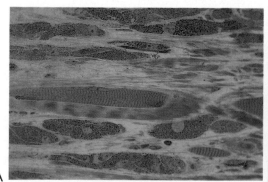
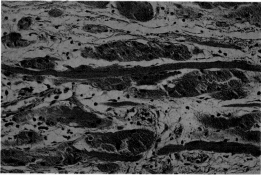

Figure 178–3. Granular cell tumor of the orbit. A, Clusters of tumor cells infiltrate among normal skeletal muscle fibers. Tumor cells are large polygonal cells with myriad cytoplasmic granules, small eccentric or paracentral nuclei, and prominent nucleoli (toluidine blue, ×265). B, Tumor cells are found in clusters between strands of muscle and collagenous tissue. The cytoplasmic granules stain postitively with periodic acid–Schiff, Sudan black B, Indian red, Masson's trichrome, and immunohistochemical stains for S100 protein (Masson's trichrome).

ular eosinophilic cytoplasm that stains with PAS that is not altered by diastase predigestion. The granules also stain positively with Sudan black B, Indian red, and Masson's trichrome and may stain with oil red O. The cytoplasm of the tumor cells also reacts positively for S100 protein. The tumor cells are arranged in clusters or ribbons between strands of collagenous tissue, normal skin adnexa, or skeletal muscle cells. There may also be exuberant pseudocarcinomatous hyperplasia of the overlying surface epithelium when the tumor is located close to the epidermis or to a mucous membrane.[55]

Electron microscopic examination shows individual cells or groups of cells surrounded by a basal lamina.[42, 52] The cytoplasm is distended by numerous pleomorphic, round, lysosomal-type cytoplasmic inclusions that are often membrane-bound, lined by single and occasionally double-limiting membrane (Fig. 178–4). These inclusions are heterogeneous and may contain electron-dense and electron-lucent cores and granular and lamellar material. More immature, spindled mesenchymal cells are frequently interspersed among the primary tumor cells. These cells may contain dense ovoid filamentous membrane-bound aggregates termed angulate or Bangle bodies.[56]

PIGMENTED RETINAL CHORISTOMA (RETINAL ANLAGE TUMOR, MELANOTIC NEUROECTODERMAL TUMOR OF INFANCY)

The pigmented retinal choristoma, also known as the retinal anlage tumor or the melanotic neuroectodermal tumor of infancy, is a rare tumor that usually involves the head and neck region. In a review of 158 cases, 92.8 percent occurred in the head and neck region, with the maxilla being the most frequently involved site.[57] Other sites that have been reported are the mandible, mediastinum, scapula, skull, brain, femur, epididymis, oropharynx, and shoulder. Orbital invasion is rare and is usually a result of secondary extension from a tumor arising in the maxilla or zygoma.[58–61] Since the initial description of the tumor by Krompecher in 1918,[62] the tumor has been known by a variety of outdated terms, including congenital melanocarcinoma, retinoblastic teratoma, melanotic progonoma, pigmented or melanotic ameloblastoma, melanotic adamantinoma, pigmented epulis, and melanotic neuroectodermal tumor of infancy.[63] Halpert and Patzer were the first to use the term retinal anlage tumor, stating that the folded, pigmented, cuboidal epithelium resembled the ciliary process of the eye, and the sheets of small hyperchromatic cells were comparable to the nuclear layers of the retina.[64] The variety of terms for this tumor has resulted largely from uncertainty regarding its histogenesis. Zimmerman proposed the term pigmented retinal choristoma, which is a descriptive term indicating that the tumor is melanotic and has the appearance of a retinal-derived tumor without assuming derivation from retinal anlage.[63]

Various tissues or cells of origin have been proposed, including congenital melanocytes, odontogenic, retinal anlage, neuroectodermal development, teratoma, and neural crest origin.[65] Of these possibilities, the most widely accepted has been neural crest origin.[61] Elevated levels of vanillymandelic acid have been reported.[66, 67] Ultrastructural studies have also supported the possibility of neural crest origin.[57, 67] Cytoplasmic processes have been identified that contain neurosecretory granules and microtubules.[68] Also histochemical studies have demonstrated some similarities to neural crest-derived tumors.[58]

The relatively large, elongated melanosomes in the pigmented cells of this tumor were emphasized by Zimmerman.[63] He noted that these melanosomes are not encountered in cutaneous or uveal nevi or melanomas of neural crest derivation. Instead, they are similar to the pigment granules of the retinal pigment epithelium, a tissue of neuroectodermal origin. This morphologic feature suggests an origin from displaced neuroepithelium rather than neural crest. Others favored the concept of a one-sided differentiation of a teratoma from germ cell origin.[69] Further work is necessary to distinguish among these possibilities.

The tumor usually occurs in infants younger than 1 yr, although it can occur in older children and adults.[61] There is no sexual predilection.[57] Catecholamine release has been reported.[67] Computed tomography and particularly magnetic resonance imaging (MRI) results may indicate preoperatively a melanin-containing tumor, with a high signal intensity in MRI T_1-weighted images.[70] The tumor usually is benign; however, 4 percent have been classified as malignant.[57, 68] The local recurrence rate has been reported to range from 10 to 15 percent,[57] and the tumor can be multifocal.[71] Simple rather than radical surgical excision is usually sufficient therapy, and chemotherapy and radiotherapy are usually not recommended.[72] Repeated local excision may be required for recurrence.

On gross examination, the tumor is usually firm, lobulated, and well-circumscribed and may have a darkly pigmented appearance. Microscopically, two populations of tumor cells can be identified (Fig. 178–5). There are cells with abundant cytoplasm containing varying numbers of pigment granules and larger, more vesicular nuclei. As noted by Zimmerman,[63] the pigment granules in these cells are relatively large and conspicuously elongated comparable to those found in retinal pigment epithelial cells. These cells line alveolar spaces and small clefts and may infold as papillae into the central lumens. There are also small basophilic cells ("neuroblastic cells") with scant cytoplasm and round or oval hyperchromatic nuclei that occur in nests or cords, sometimes suspended in the luminal areas. Mitotic figures are rare. A variably dense fibrotic stroma separates these complex adenomatous units. Electron microscopic examination shows membrane-bound electron-dense melanosomes in the pigmented cells that are heterogeneous and often elliptical with a lamellar internal structure (Fig. 178–6). The neuroblastic cells may have long, thin cytoplasmic processes with microtubules and dense-core granules.

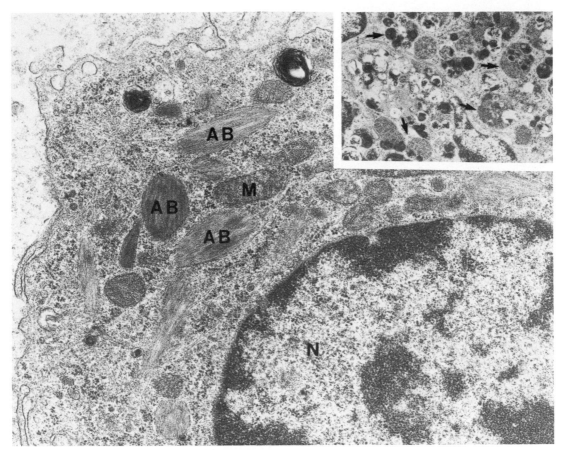

Figure 178–4. Granular cell tumor. Electron microscopy shows mesenchymal cells, which may contain fusiform filamentous structures termed angulated or Bangle bodies (AB). (M, mitochondria; N, nucleus.) Inset shows complex lysosomal-type inclusions *(arrows)* within the cytoplasm.

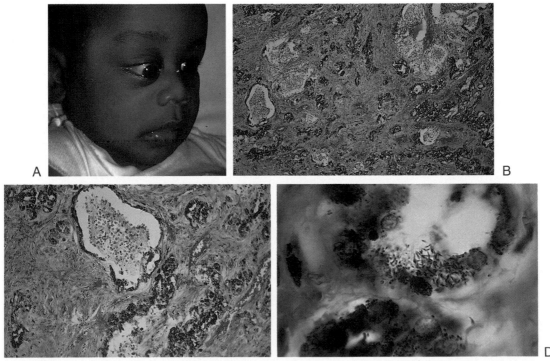

Figure 178–5. Pigmented retinal choristoma. *A,* A 4-month-old boy with right exophthalmos caused by orbital pigmented retinal choristoma (retinal anlage tumor). (Reproduced with permission from Lamping KA, Albert DA, Lack E, et al: Melanotic neuroectodermal tumor of infancy [retinal anlage tumor]. Ophthalmology 92:144, 1985.) *B,* Vascularized fibrous stroma contains numerous nests and cords of cells and irregular slitlike alveolar spaces (H&E). *C,* The alveolar spaces contain two cell types: large pigmented cuboidal cells that line the alveolar spaces and basophilic cells with scanty cytoplasm filling the cavities of large spaces (H&E). *D,* Higher magnification of the pigmented cells shows large vesicular nuclei and abundant cytoplasm containing varying amounts of elongated pigment granules (H&E). *(B–D,* Courtesy of L. E. Zimmerman, M.D.)

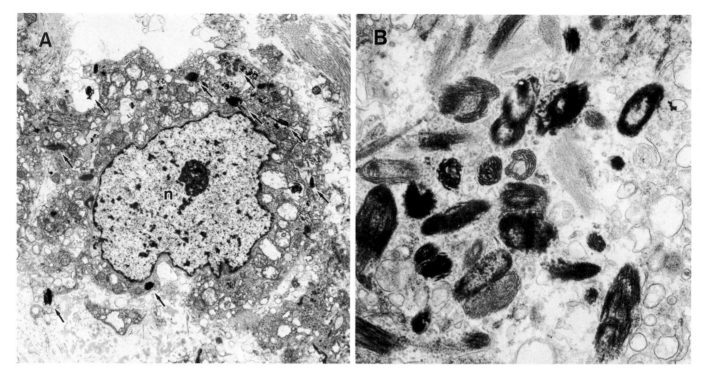

Figure 178–6. Pigmented retinal choristoma (retinal anlage tumor). *A,* Electron micrograph of a pigmented tumor cell containing a central nucleus (n) and large, electron-dense melanin granules (*arrows*) that are present in the cytoplasm (×10,500). *B,* Higher magnification of the cytoplasmic granules. When cut longitudinally the granules may appear elliptical, whereas when cut transversely the granules appear round or ovoid. Although not seen in this micrograph, some of the granules may possess a limiting membrane. The granules show varying degrees of electron density and have a heterogeneous internal structure consisting of longitudinally directed lamellae and irregularly shaped globules (×37,000). (Courtesy of G. Richard Dickersin, M.D., Department of Pathology, Massachusetts General Hospital.)

NONCHROMAFFIN PARAGANGLIOMA

Nonchromaffin paraganglioma most frequently occurs as glomus jugulare (middle ear and mastoid) and carotid body tumors; however, this tumor may arise from paraganglion cells anywhere in the body, with rare occurrences in the paranasal sinuses, nasal cavity, larynx, nasopharynx, and orbit.[73] Nonchromaffin paraganglioma is also called chemodectoma, sympathoblastoma, and chromaffinoma. This tumor is a neural crest tumor that appears to arise from chemoreceptor cells, although there has been no definite demonstration of chemoreceptor function. Orbital paragangliomas presumably arise from local paraganglia but can also result from an invading intracranial tumor.[74] The presence of paraganglionic tissue in the human orbit is not well-established. Paraganglionic cells have been described near the ciliary ganglion of the chimpanzee,[75, 76] and a structure termed infraorbital paraganglion has been identified on the orbital floor in serial orbital sections from a newborn infant.[75, 77] However, subsequent attempts to identify paraganglial tissue in human adults have been unsuccessful.[78]

In 1952, Fisher and Hazard published the first case of orbital nonchromaffin paraganglioma.[78] However, 16 of the initial 29 reported cases have been reclassified as alveolar soft part sarcoma.[32] Archer and associates reviewed the remaining 13 reported cases and included a case of their own.[79] In their series, the age range on presentation was 3 to 68 yr, with an average age of 36 yr. Six patients were female and eight were male. Duration of symptoms ranged from 2 mo to 17 yr, with the majority being only a few months. This differs from nonchromaffin paragangliomas in other head and neck locations, in which the onset and progression of symptoms may occur over years rather than months. Most patients present with unilateral proptosis but may also exhibit diplopia, decreased visual acuity, and papilledema. In nonorbital paragangliomas, multiple-site involvement occurs in 10 to 20 percent and metastasis in 5 to 10 percent.[73] The behavior of orbital nonchromaffin paraganglioma may be less predictable than paragangliomas occurring in other locations, and the prognosis is uncertain. In the series by Archer and colleagues, most patients (8/14) were treated surgically by exenteration, yet 37 percent (3/8) of patients undergoing exenteration had a recurrence of orbital disease within 6 wk to 15 mo.[79] The therapy is surgical excision with frozen-section control. Nonchromaffin paraganglioma is also a radiosensitive tumor; recurrence after irradiation is uncommon.[73]

Grossly, the tumor is usually well-circumscribed without a true capsule and is vascular, often having prominent feeding vessels. Histopathologically, the tumor is composed of clusters of cells sometimes referred to as "zellballen," which are separated from each other by a rich vascular or sinusoidal pattern (Fig. 178–7). The

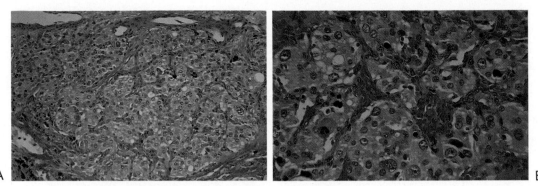

Figure 178–7. Nonchromaffin paraganglioma. *A,* Light microscopy shows tumor cells in an alveolar pattern (H&E, ×40). *B,* Tumor cells grow in clusters called zellballen. These cells have abundant eosinophilic cytoplasm, and their nuclei show moderate nuclear pleomorphism with a distinctive stippling of the nuclear chromatin. (H&E, ×100). (Courtesy of A. Morales, M.D.)

pattern may resemble alveolar soft part sarcoma, with an alveolar or organoid arrangement of epithelioid cells within a reticulin framework containing thin-walled blood vessels, and dense fibrous bands may occur (Fig. 178–8). The tumor cells are polygonal and contain round or oval monotonous, stippled nuclei. There is no mitotic activity. An important negative finding is the absence of cytoplasmic PAS-positive inclusions, such as those encountered in alveolar soft part sarcoma. There may be argentaffin or argyrophilic granules in the cytoplasm, which can be demonstrated with the argentaffin or long Fontana reactions.

Immunohistochemical stains display positive staining for neuron-specific enolase, neurofilament protein, chromogranin, and synaptophysin, whereas staining is negative for glial fibrillary acidic protein (GFAP), S100 protein, and vimentin.[80] Electron microscopic examination can be helpful in the histopathologic differentiation of nonchromaffin paraganglioma from other alveolar orbital tumors. Ultrastructurally, there are interdigitating cell membranes and neurosecretory granules characterized as spheric, membrane-bound cytoplasmic inclusions ranging from 80 to 250 nm (Fig. 178–9). There may be two cell populations: those containing evenly

distributed chromatin with relatively lucent cytoplasm, and another with irregularly condensed nuclei, occasional nuclear indentations, and dense cytoplasm endowed with numerous mitochondria and filaments. Melanosomes have been identified in the cells of one tumor, termed melanotic paraganglioma.[80]

PRIMARY CARCINOID TUMOR

Carcinoid tumors are slow-growing, potentially malignant neoplasms that usually arise in the gastrointestinal tract but may occur in the bronchial tree, thymus, or other sites. These tumors are derived from neuroendocrine cells termed enterochromaffin or Kulchitsky's cells. Because the tumor may release serotonin and other vasoactive substances, a minority of patients may acquire the carcinoid syndrome. Ophthalmic manifestations of the carcinoid syndrome include lacrimation, conjunctival injection, and retinal and choroidal vasospasm with perivascular pigment clumping.[81] One case of bilateral orbital involvement in a patient with extensive metastatic carcinoid tumor showed the unusual feature of reproducible hypertension with orbital pal-

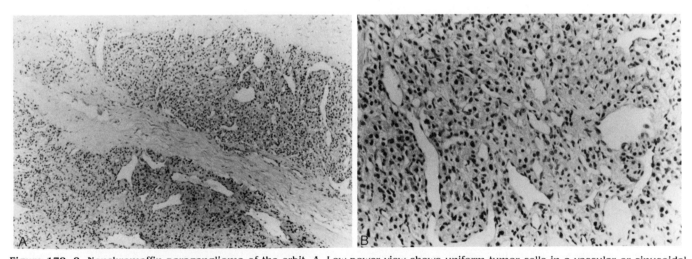

Figure 178–8. Nonchromaffin paraganglioma of the orbit. *A,* Low-power view shows uniform tumor cells in a vascular or sinusoidal pattern with a fibrous band (H&E, ×80). *B,* Higher power view shows groups of tumor cells with minimal nuclear pleomorphism separated by vascular spaces (H&E, ×320). From Archer KF, Hurwitz JJ, Balogh JM, et al: Orbital nonchromaffin paraganglioma. Published courtesy of *Ophthalmology* 96:1659–1666, 1989.

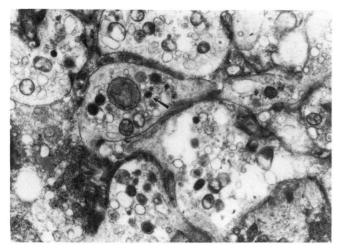

Figure 178–9. Electron micrograph of nonchromaffin paraganglioma demonstrates interdigitating cell membranes and cytoplasmic membrane–bound electron-dense neurosecretory granules (*arrow*) (original magnification ×30,000). From Archer KF, Hurwitz JJ, Balogh JM, et al: Orbital nonchromaffin paraganglioma. Published courtesy of *Ophthalmology* 96:1659–1666, 1989.

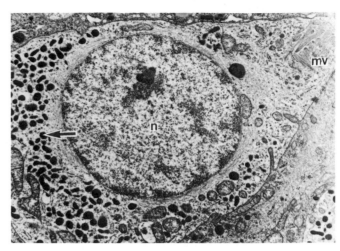

Figure 178–11. Orbital carcinoid tumor. Transmission electron microscopy demonstrating tumor cell with large nucleus (n), apical microvilli (mv), and pleomorphic neurosecretory granules (*arrow*) concentrated in the basal cytoplasm (×14,000). (Reproduced with permission from Shields CL, Shields JA, Eagle RC Jr, et al: Orbital metastasis from a carcinoid tumor. Arch Ophthalmol 105:970, 1987. Copyright 1987, American Medical Association.)

pation, thought to be due to systemic release of vasoactive substances.[82] The diagnosis of carcinoid syndrome may be established by demonstrating elevated levels of 5-hydroxyindoleacetic acid (5-HIAA) in the urine.

Microscopically, carcinoid tumor cells may be arranged in solid lobules, cordlike or trabecular patterns, rosette or tubular formations, or a combination of these patterns. The large polygonal tumor cells contain hyperchromatic, delicately stippled, eccentric nuclei with eosinophilic granular cytoplasm. The tumor cells contain neurosecretory granules in their basal cytoplasm that can be demonstrated with Grimelius (argyrophilic) stain (Fig. 178–10). Fontana-Masson (argentaffin) stain may be positive, particularly in ileal carcinoids that are metastatic to the orbit. Ultrastructural studies show both

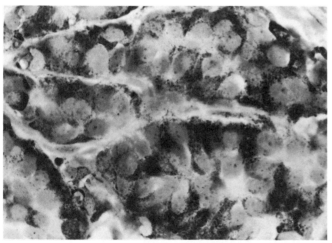

Figure 178–10. Orbital carcinoid tumor cells show intensely positive cytoplasmic reaction when stained for argyrophilic neurosecretory granules (Grimelius, ×400). (Reproduced with permission from Shields CL, Shields JA, Eagle RC Jr, et al: Orbital metastasis from a carcinoid tumor. Arch Ophthalmol 105:970, 1987. Copyright 1987, American Medical Association.)

light and dark cells possessing apical microvilli. Microtubules and microfilaments are loosely packed in the light cells in contrast with the densely packed microtubules and microfilaments in dark cells. Cytoplasmic neurosecretory granules are prominent in the basal cytoplasm (Fig. 178–11).

In rare cases, carcinoid tumor may metastasize to the orbit or uvea (Fig. 178–12).[83] Interestingly, uveal metastases originate preferentially from bronchial carcinoids, whereas the vast majority of orbital metastases arise from ileal carcinoids.[83, 84] It is possible to distinguish bronchial and ileal carcinoid tumors because the histologic patterns, histochemical staining properties, and ultrastructural findings vary according to the embryonic site of origin.[85, 86] Although the standard treatment of orbital metastatic disease is radiation and chemotherapy, orbital metastasis from carcinoid tumors is an exception to this therapeutic rule.[86] Radiotherapy can be beneficial[87]; however, total surgical excision may be recommended because the tumor can demonstrate indolent growth and radioresistance, and patient survival may be prolonged after removal of the tumor.[88, 89]

Zimmerman and coworkers described a patient believed to have a primary orbital carcinoid tumor (Fig. 178–13).[90] Their patient was observed for 15 yr without evidence of a nonorbital primary site. The patient presented with marked proptosis and visual loss resulting from compressive optic neuropathy. There were no symptoms of carcinoid syndrome, and after treatment with orbital exenteration, the urinary 5-HIAA levels were normal. Another tumor initially described as primary orbital neuroblastoma was diagnosed as an orbital carcinoid tumor using immunohistochemical techniques.[91] Because the patient was asymptomatic during the 8 yr after removal of the tumor and the systemic evaluation was negative, this case may represent a primary orbital carcinoid tumor. However, it should be remembered that primary lesions of metastatic carcinoid

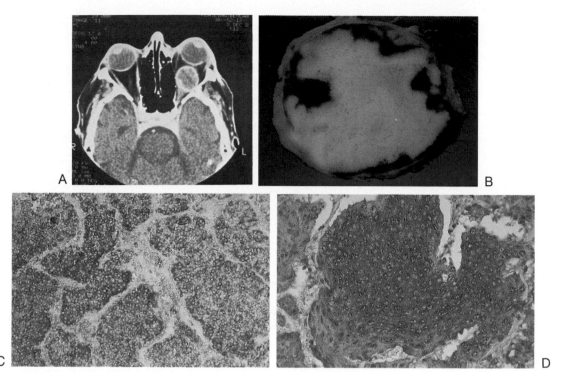

Figure 178–12. Orbital carcinoid tumor. A 71-year-old woman with metastatic carcinoid tumor of unknown primary site acquired proptosis and cranial nerve III palsy on the left side. *A,* Computed tomographic scan shows a well-circumscribed intraconal mass in the left orbit. *B,* Gross specimen shows pale yellow central area of ischemic necrosis surrounded by rim of viable reddish-brown tissue. *C,* Tumor cells show immunoreactivity for chromogranin A (×64). *D,* Tumor cells demonstrate immunoreactivity for synaptophysin (×100). (Reproduced with permission from Shetlar DJ, Font RL, Ordonez N, et al: A clinicopathologic study of three carcinoid tumors metastatic to the orbit. Published courtesy of *Ophthalmology* 97:260, 1990.)

tumors may be clinically undetectable until autopsy.[86, 92] Careful follow-up and meticulous autopsy studies are necessary to establish with certainty whether these cases represent primary or secondary orbital lesions.

PRIMARY MELANOMA

Primary orbital melanoma is much less common than secondary tumors, which can develop from ocular or cutaneous melanoma.[93] Primary orbital melanoma accounts for less than 1 percent of primary orbital neoplasms.[94, 95] These primary tumors arise from orbital melanocytes of neural crest origin, which may be located along ciliary nerves, scleral emissary vessels, or optic nerve leptomeninges.[93, 94] These cells may represent deep hamartomatous persistences that are deposited during neural crest migration.[96] Primary melanoma may also originate from anomalous deposits of melanocytes associated with periorbital pigmentary disorders.[96–98] Nearly one half of primary orbital melanomas have been associated with pigmentary disorders, such as oculodermal melanocytosis (nevus of Ota), ocular melanocytosis, and blue nevi.[98] Patients should be examined carefully for deep cutaneous periocular pigmentation, including above the hairline, that may indicate an excess of neural

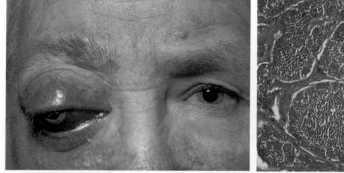
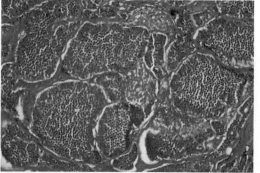

Figure 178–13. Primary orbital carcinoid tumor. *A,* A 71-year-old woman presented with slowly progressive proptosis of 11 yr of duration. *B,* Low-power magnification shows lobules of basaloid tumor cells. The large tumor cells have eccentric nuclei displaying stippling of nuclear chromatin (H&E, ×60). (Courtesy of Lorenz E. Zimmerman, M.D., Armed Forces Institute of Pathology, Washington, DC.)

crest cells in the distribution of the trigeminal nerve. Because primary orbital melanoma has a tendency to spread along nerves through the superior and inferior orbital fissures, melanocytosis of the contiguous bone and meninges may be observed. The prognosis for these lesions is poor.

In a review of 30 documented cases of primary orbital melanoma, 23 (77 percent) developed in adults, whereas 7 (23 percent) were found in children or adolescents.[98] Patients presented most commonly with painless proptosis, with the duration of symptoms varying from 1 mo to several years. There was no sexual predilection, and the tumor was usually found in whites, with two cases reported in blacks. This is of interest because periocular pigment disorders such as nevus of Ota are found predominantly in Asian and black patients.[97]

On computed tomography, the tumor often has a circumscribed appearance, whereas occasional cystic areas may be seen that correspond to areas of necrosis (Fig. 178–14). In contrast, operative findings of 30 documented primary orbital melanomas showed that only 4 were encapsulated and treatable by primary resection.[98] The degree of encapsulation does not correlate with the histologic types. One clinical feature that may aid the clinician in suspecting primary orbital melanoma is associated ocular, cutaneous, or orbital pigmentary lesions, which are present in approximately 40 percent of primary orbital melanomas.[98]

Grossly, most of the lesions are partially pigmented and may even appear to be hematomas if completely pigmented. Histopathologically, the tumor shows pleomorphism, enlargement of nuclei, necrosis, and the presence of mitotic figures. The cell type may be spindled, mixed, or epithelioid. The tumors may be associated with nevus of Ota, blue nevus, or cellular blue nevus. If there is an associated nevus of Ota or blue nevus, there are dendritic melanocytes interspersed in the stromal or fibrous tissue. When a cellular blue nevus is present, there is a discrete nodule of closely packed, nonpigmented, schwannian-type spindle cells without intervening stroma.

On electron microscopic examination, the melanoma cells are virtually indistinguishable from those of a choroidal melanoma, particularly with reference to the granular type of melanosome that is found in choroidal melanoma (Fig. 178–15).[96] There may be desmosome-like cell junctions and cytoplasmic nuclear indentations or pockets. Cutaneous origin or metastasis should be considered if the melanosomal morphology resembles that of the dendritic melanocyte, which has distinctive elongated or football-shaped melanosomes with internal melanofilamentary cross-linkages producing periodicity.[99] Although not described in the orbit, melanotic Schwann cell tumors can be distinguished by their Schwann cell features, including basement membrane production, elongated and tangled cell processes, and mesaxon and pseudomesaxon formation.[100]

When the tumor is well-circumscribed, primary resection may be sufficient, and disease-free follow-up periods of up to 32 yr have been reported.[98] Most of these tumors have been treated with exenteration. Because there is a tendency for tumor cells to grow along the nerves through the superior and inferior orbital fissures, attention should be directed at discovering any pigmented tissue in this area. With intracranial extension, a craniotomy may be required for complete resection of

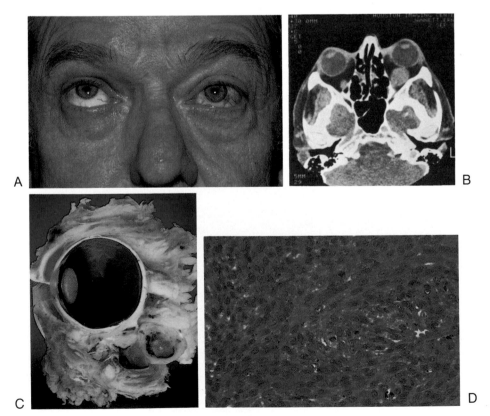

Figure 178–14. Primary orbital melanoma. *A,* A 50-year-old man with a restrictive myopathy of the left inferior rectus muscle. *B,* Computed tomographic scan shows the tumor mass involving the left inferior rectus muscle. (Courtesy of R. Wilkins, M.D.) *C,* Exenterated orbital contents show the tumor associated with the inferior rectus muscle, which has several variably pigmented solid areas. *D,* This melanoma was composed predominantly of spindle cells (H&E, ×100).

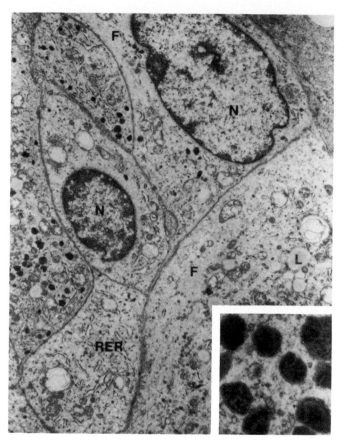

Figure 178–15. Primary orbital melanoma. Electron micrograph of epithelioid tumor cells showing scattered cytoplasmic filaments (F), rough-surfaced endoplasmic reticulum (RER), nuclei (N), and scattered lipid droplets (L). The inset demonstrates the granular nature of the melanosomes in contrast to the filamentary and striated appearance of cutaneous melanosomes.

tumor. Surgical resection may also be necessary in large or painful tumors. Adjuvant therapy (radiation therapy and chemotherapy) should be considered in diffuse lesions or in lesions that are incompletely excised, recurrent, or metastatic.

ECTOMESENCHYMAL TUMORS

Because there are no true mesodermal paraxial somites in the head and neck region, the neural crest contributes most of the connective tissues in the orbital and facial areas. These connective tissues are referred to as ectomesenchyme or mesectoderm. Fibroblasts and smooth muscle cells in the orbit and face may demonstrate unusual neurogenic differentiations because of their neural crest origin.[101, 102] Thus, a smooth muscle tumor of the antrum that secondarily invaded the orbit had the appearance by light microscopy of a neurogenic or peripheral nerve sheath tumor; however, this tumor was identified as mesectodermal leiomyosarcoma by ultrastructural features including cytoplasmic actin filaments.[103]

It is also possible for neurogenic tumors to modulate toward mesenchyme, reflecting the "ectomesenchymal" differentiation capacity ascribed to neural crest tissue.

For example, in the so-called Triton tumor, striated muscle has been identified in some malignant peripheral nerve sheath tumors.[104, 105] Also there are complex masses of heterologous tissues termed ectomesenchymomas, which contain neurogenic tissue, pigmented tissue, and mesenchymal elements including rhabdomyoblastic differentiation.[106]

NEUROEPITHELIOMA

In 1965, Howard described a malignant neuroepithelioma in the orbit of a child that proved resistant to surgery and radiotherapy.[107] Tumor cells lined elongated trabeculae or neurotubular units and also formed nests filling the central cavities. These cells had a neuroblastic appearance and were mitotically active. Other primary orbital neuroepithelial or primitive neuroectodermal tumors have been described.[108, 109] These tumors are malignant and may demonstrate various neuronal or neuroglial features. Pathologically, Homer-Wright rosettes, true rosettes, and perivascular pseudorosettes may be present. Also the tumor may show a prominent mesenchymal or neuroglial component, which can be demonstrated by special stains such as immunohistochemical stain for GFAP. Neuroepitheliomas of nonorbital soft tissues have been described[29] as well as the so-called extraosseous Ewing's sarcoma, which is actually a tumor of primitive neuroectodermal origin.[110] It is uncertain whether these tumors arise from neural crest or from true ectoderm that detaches from the anterior neural tube. Most cases of Ewing's sarcoma of the orbit represent metastases, but a case of primary Ewing's sarcoma arising in the orbital roof has been described.[111]

These tumors may be distinguished from neuroblastoma by light and electron microscopy. By light microscopy, the cells lack the imbrication of delicate cytoplasmic processes (neuropil) of neuronal and schwannian differentiation. Ultrastructurally, the cells lack the abundant elongated neuritic processes and prominent neurosecretory granules of neuroblastoma.[110] Several observations provide additional evidence that peripheral neuroepitheliomas are distinct from neuroblastoma. Some peripheral neuroepitheliomas have a specific chromosomal translocation (11;22) not found in neuroblastoma, and there is no evidence that these tumors have the n-*myc* gene amplification characteristic of some neuroblastomas.[112, 113]

PRIMARY ORBITAL NEUROBLASTOMA

Primary differentiated neuroblastoma of the orbit has been reported.[114, 115] In one case report, primary orbital neuroblastoma was described in a 37-year-old woman. This patient was treated with surgical excision and radiotherapy, resulting in long-term survival without recurrence during the 12-yr follow-up period.[114] In another reported case, the tumor had histologic and ultrastructural features of esthesioneuroblastoma, which usually arises from the olfactory epithelium in the nasal cavity, nasopharynx, or paranasal sinuses.[115] It should be remembered, in attempting to identify the site of origin of these tumors, that esthesioneuroblastoma, arising from the olfactory sensory epithelium, may invade the orbit. Although this tumor usually presents with nasal obstruction, loss of smell, or epistaxis, the tumor may present to the ophthalmologist with ophthalmic manifestations such as periorbital pain, tearing, eyelid edema, proptosis, globe injection, and ptosis.[116]

Microscopic examination of primary orbital neuroblastoma shows spindle and ovoid cells that extend delicate eosinophilic processes (Fig. 178–16). These processes imbricate to form a dense fibrillary neuropil background. Tumor cells may display certain patterns, including perivascular rosettes with cytoplasmic processes oriented perpendicular to vessel walls as well as aggregated neurites with an annulus of nuclei called Homer-Wright rosettes. Palisading of nuclei may be identified, and there is little or no mitotic activity. Immunohistochemical staining for neuron-specific enolase is positive, which can aid in establishing the diagnosis of a neuroblastic lesion. Also ultrastructural studies show small, catecholamine-type, dense-core neurosecretory granules in the perikaryon region of the tumor cells and in the cytoplasmic processes (neurites). Although occasionally elliptical in shape, most of these granules are round and measure approximately 140 nm in diameter. The neuropil background, ultrastructurally, is composed of the interweaving of myriad cytoplasmic processes containing neurosecretory granules and neurotubules (Fig. 178–17).

MALIGNANT RHABDOID TUMOR

Malignant rhabdoid tumor is rare and usually presents as a highly malignant renal tumor in infants. This tumor has been identified in several extrarenal locations, including the orbit.[117–119] Because these tumors have been identified in several different sites, a number of histogenetic theories have been proposed, including origin from pluripotential mesenchymal cells, neural crest cells, primitive neuroectodermal cells, histiocytic cells, epithelial cells, and lymphohematopoietic progenitor cells.[118] It appears that the malignant rhabdoid tumor may be a phenotypic expression of many different cellular lines, and currently there is no unifying theory of histogenesis.

Rootman and colleagues reported the first orbital case in a 6-week-old male infant with a rapidly progressive retrobulbar lesion.[117] The patient was treated with subtotal resection followed by radiotherapy and chemotherapy and was alive 2 yr after surgery without local recurrence or metastasis. Malignant rhabdoid tumor of the orbit has also been reported in adults.[118, 119] In one case report, malignant rhabdoid tumor arising from the lacrimal gland was described in a 50-year-old man.[118] This patient survived without evidence of tumor recurrence or metastasis during the 15-mo follow-up period after orbital exenteration coupled with adjunctive chemotherapy and radiotherapy. Another case report described a 47-year-old man with orbital malignant rhabdoid tumor who was alive 18 mo after surgery and orbital irradiation.[119] An intraocular metastatic malignant rhabdoid tumor in an infant showed orbital extension and was treated with exenteration.[120] The comparatively favorable survival in these cases may be due to earlier detection of orbital lesions or confinement of the tumor by the bony walls of the orbit.

Histologically, the tumor exhibits sheets of loosely cohesive epithelioid cells with abundant eosinophilic cytoplasm (Fig. 178–18). Other, less common, architectural patterns may be found, including sclerosing, cartilaginous, osteosarcomatous, alveolar, lymphomatoid, histiocytoid, spindled, hemangiopericytomatous, organoid or paragangliomatous, and pseudopapillary or pseudoglandular patterns. In areas containing globoid (rhabdoid) tumor cells, mitotic figures are readily identified, and many of the tumor cells contain eosinophilic cytoplasmic inclusions. The eosinophilic inclusions may displace notched or vesicular nuclei with prominent "owl-eye" nucleoli. Ultrastructural and immunohistochemical studies have shown that these cytoplasmic inclusions contain the intermediate filament vimentin.[118] Unlike rhabdomyosarcoma, immunohistochemical and ultrastructural studies fail to reveal any evidence of myoblastic differentiation in malignant rhabdoid tumor.

MESENCHYMAL CHONDROSARCOMA

Mesenchymal chondrosarcoma is a rare malignancy that was first described in 1959 by Lichtenstein and Bernstein.[121] The term mesenchymal chondrosarcoma is derived from the distinctive histologic appearance of the tumor, with a background of primitive undifferentiated mesenchymal cells containing scattered islands of well-differentiated cartilage. Because the tumor may demonstrate a hemangiopericytoma-like growth pattern, this tumor has also been described as hemangiopericytoma with cartilaginous differentiation.[122, 123] The incidence of mesenchymal chondrosarcoma is higher in the skeleton than in the soft tissues,[124] with extraskeletal tumors showing a predilection for the extremities, meninges, and the head and neck, particularly the orbit.[122, 125–130] One case has also been reported as originating in the eyelid, with local recurrence after primary excision.[131]

Because the tumor contains two distinct cell populations, the histogenesis of this tumor is uncertain. One possibility is differentiation of mesenchymal sarcoma, with transformation of anaplastic cells into chondrocytes. The other possibility is dedifferentiation of chondrosarcoma, with transformation of chondrocytes into anaplastic cells. In support of the former possibility, the tumor arises in areas such as the orbit where cartilage is absent. Other mesenchymal tumors of the orbit are discussed in Chapter 187.

Although a wide range of ages have been reported, the peak incidence of mesenchymal chondrosarcoma is in the second and third decades of life.[125] Overall, there is no sexual predilection; however, the reported tumors arising in the orbit show a preponderance of women. Patients with orbital tumors usually present with unilateral progressive proptosis. Pain, diplopia, and headache are variable features. Plain films and computed tomog-

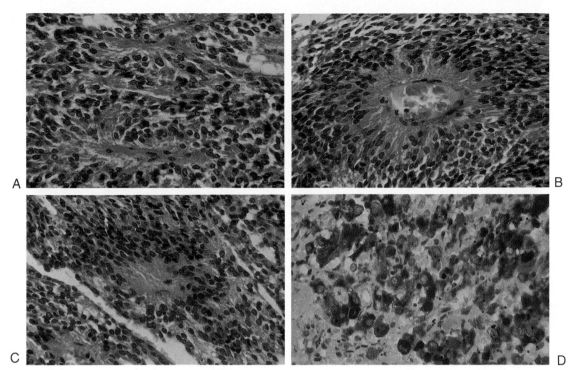

Figure 178–16. Primary orbital neuroblastoma. *A,* Tumor cells have orthochromatic nuclei and extend delicate eosinophilic processes to form a neuropil background (H&E, original magnification ×320). *B,* Perivascular rosette with interwoven cytoplasmic processes directed perpendicularly to the wall of a capillary (H&E, original magnification ×320). *C,* A Wright rosette composed of centrally directed cellular processes (neurites) with a surrounding annulus of nuclei (H&E, original magnification ×320). *D,* Immunohistochemical staining for neuron-specific enolase is positive as indicated by cytoplasmic brown reaction product (immunoperoxidase reaction, original magnification ×320). Published courtesy of *Ophthalmology* 94:255–266, 1987.

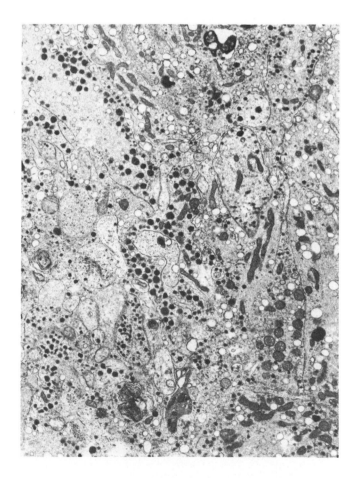

Figure 178–17. Primary orbital neuroblastoma. Electron micrograph showing dense interweaving cellular processes (neurites) containing cytoplasmic neurosecretory granules, which correspond to the fibrillary neuropil background observed by light microscopy (original magnification ×10,000). Published courtesy of *Ophthalmology* 94:255–266, 1987.

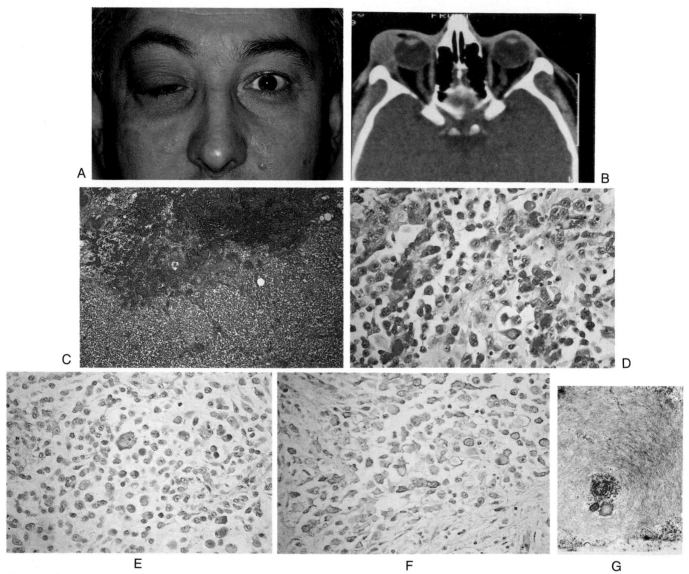

Figure 178–18. Malignant rhabdoid tumor. *A,* A 50-year-old man presented with a 1-mo history of erythema and swelling of the right eyelids and proptosis. *B,* Computed axial tomogram shows a rounded mass lateral to the globe projecting anterior to the orbital rim. *C,* Microscopically, most of the tumor contained sheets of dyscohesive tumor cells. In the upper area of this photomicrograph, tumor cells infiltrate preexisting elements of the lacrimal gland (H&E, ×60). *D,* Higher power magnification shows dyscohesive epithelioid or globoid (rhabdoid) cells with occasional prominent cytoplasmic eosinophilic inclusions (H&E, ×240). *E,* Immunohistochemical staining of the tumor cells shows positive staining for cytoplasmic vimentin filaments (immunoperoxidase reaction, ×220). *F,* Cell membranes of tumor cells stain positively for epithelial membrane antigen (immunoperoxidase reaction, ×220). *G,* Transmission electron microscopy demonstrates whorls of cytoplasmic intermediate filaments (×41,000). (Reproduced with permission from Niffenegger JH, Jakobiec FA, Shore JW, et al: Adult extrarenal rhabdoid tumor of the lacrimal gland. Published courtesy of *Ophthalmology* 99:568, 570, 573, 1992.)

raphy may show an irregular mass containing punctate calcifications and gray cloud-like opacities as a result of the cartilaginous component of the tumor.

On gross examination, the tumor is pale and firm and contains coalescing blue-gray nodules of cartilage, with occasional hard yellowish-tan areas of osteoid and bone. On microscopic examination, the tumor has a bimorphic appearance, containing two distinct cellular elements (Fig. 178–19). There are both islands of well-differentiated cartilage and a background of undifferentiated mesenchymal cells. The mesenchymal cells are small, have scanty cytoplasm, and contain round to spindle-shaped hyperchromatic nuclei with variable mitotic activity. Reticulin stain reveals reticulin fibers among the anaplastic mesenchymal cells suggestive of hemangiopericytoma. The cartilage stains strongly for hyaluronidase-resistant mucopolysaccharide with the colloidal iron stain. There may be areas of necrosis or hemorrhage. Also areas of calcification and even ossification may be found in the tumor.

When examined under low-power magnification, the mesenchymal cells may aggregate around vascular channels in a hemangioma-like pattern. Focal areas of cartilaginous and osseous metaplasia may occur in hemangiopericytoma; however, the diffuse distribution of islands of well-differentiated cells with the typical features of chondrocytes identifies the tumor as mesenchymal chondrosarcoma. Synovial sarcoma may be distinguished from mesenchymal chondrosarcoma by the presence of the characteristic biphasic epithelial and spindle-cell pattern in the synovial sarcoma. Also synovial sarcoma rarely demonstrates cartilaginous metaplasia. Mesenchymal chondrosarcoma usually can be readily distinguished from the usual chondrosarcoma. Chondrosarcoma contains larger and more pleomorphic cartilaginous elements than the mesenchymal chondrosarcoma. More important, chondrosarcoma does not contain the areas of anaplastic mesenchymal cells typical of mesenchymal chondrosarcoma and usually arises in the orbital and sinus bones.

Ultrastructural studies are not crucial for the diagnosis of mesenchymal chondrosarcoma, but they confirm the bimorphic pattern.[131] The well-differentiated cells have typical features of chondrocytes, including an ovoid nucleus, cytoplasmic lipid vacuoles, glycogen, rough endoplasmic reticulum, and abundant matrix. In contrast, anaplastic cells have round to ovoid nuclei, no cytoplasmic droplets, scanty rough endoplasmic reticulum, and sparse matrix. Immunohistochemical studies show that the chondromatous tumor cells stain positively for S100 protein.

Mesenchymal chondrosarcoma is a highly malignant tumor with a poor prognosis. Local recurrences are common, and metastases occur, predominantly in the lung. Of the 10 cases of extraskeletal chondrosarcoma reported by Guccion and colleagues, only 1 patient survived more than 5 yr.[125] This patient had an orbital tumor treated by orbital exenteration. A few patients have been reported with long-term survival of more than 20 yr.[127, 128] The therapy is with radical excision. Patients are frequently treated with chemotherapy or radiotherapy, but the value of these adjunctive treatments is not known.

ANGIOSARCOMA

Angiosarcoma and other soft tissue sarcomas are malignant tumors that are derived from cells of mesenchymal origin. Angiosarcoma accounts for less than 1

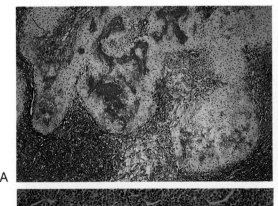
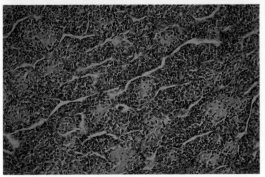
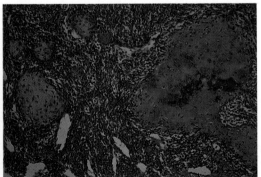

Figure 178–19. Orbital mesenchymal chondrosarcoma. A, The tumor contains sheets of undifferentiated mesenchymal cells, well-differentiated cartilage, and osteoid (H&E, ×70). B, Islands of well-differentiated cartilage in a background of undifferentiated mesenchymal cells and numerous dilated vascular spaces. The island of cartilage on the right contains central calcification (H&E, ×115). C, In this section, the tumor shows gradual transitions from undifferentiated mesenchymal cells to cartilage. The tumor cells are arranged along slitlike vascular spaces (H&E, ×165).

percent of soft tissue sarcomas and has a predilection for the skin and superficial soft tissues.[132] Localization of angiosarcoma in the orbit is very rare, accounting for less than 3 percent of angiosarcomas. The term angiosarcoma reflects the derivation of this tumor from vascular endothelial cells. Other terms in the literature that are synonymous with angiosarcoma include malignant hemangioendothelioma, angioendothelioma, malignant angioma, angiofibrosarcoma, angioblastic sarcoma, hemangioblastoma, hemangioendothelioblastoma, hemangioendotheliosarcoma, intravascular endothelioma, and malignant endothelioma.[133] Descriptions of other vascular tumors of the orbit may be found in Chapter 173.

The clinical features of orbital angiosarcoma were described in a review of 15 cases by Hufnagel and colleagues.[134] There was a preponderance of pediatric cases in this group, accounting for two thirds of the lesions. The median age at the time of diagnosis was 11 yr, with ages ranging from 2 wk to 66 yr. There was no sexual predilection among the adult or pediatric patients. Although the patients had similar clinical presentations, the median duration of signs and symptoms was shorter for the pediatric patients (3 mo) compared with the adult group (1.5 yr). Patients most frequently presented with proptosis, eyelid swelling, and ptosis resulting from a propensity for anterosuperior orbital involvement. One patient presented with a subconjunctival mass.[134] Patients with posterior orbital involvement usually present with proptosis. One unusual patient with a posterior orbital tumor mimicking Tolosa-Hunt syndrome presented with facial pain and diplopia.[135] Because the tumor is poorly circumscribed, may be multifocal, and has a tendency to metastasize, it is difficult to establish the extent of orbital involvement of periorbital lesions. Thus, whether or not an eyelid tumor has extended into the orbit may be difficult to ascertain. Computed tomography shows an infiltrative or circumscribed mass that enhances with contrast.

Angiosarcoma is a highly malignant tumor associated the a poor prognosis. In a series of head and neck angiosarcomas from the Mayo Clinic, the 2- and 5-yr survivals were 53 and 41 percent, respectively.[136] In the series reviewed by Hufnagel and colleagues, angiosarcoma of the orbit was associated with a poor prognosis.[134] Two of five adult patients were alive and tumor-free with fewer than 2 yr follow-up, whereas in the pediatric group 1 patient of 10 was alive and disease-free with fewer than 3 yr follow-up. Involvement of the posterior orbit is associated with a bleak prognosis, with all reported patients ultimately acquiring recurrent or metastatic tumor. Because the tumor is poorly circumscribed and local control appears to be important for favorable clinical outcome, treatment usually involves radical excision, most commonly exenteration. Radiation therapy and chemotherapy are often combined with surgical therapy, but there is no established benefit with these adjunctive treatments.

Microscopically, there are several distinct patterns, including angiomatous, spindle-cell, and undifferentiated patterns.[137] The angiomatous pattern is the most characteristic, with irregular lumina and clefts forming a network of sinusoids (Fig. 178–20). These lumina often contain erythrocytes and may be lined with anaplastic endothelial cells. Because these tumor cells form aggregates, they may form intraluminal buds or papillary projections. The tumor cells may show a range of differentiation; the differentiated tumors exhibit proliferating endothelial cells outlined with reticulin fibers. Spindle cells may be found with indistinct cell outlines and small nucleoli. Areas containing spindle cells do not form obvious vascular channels; however, the clefts between tumor cells may contain erythrocytes, representing abortive attempts to form vascular structures. The spindle cells may also form compact bundles. Undifferentiated areas are composed of pleomorphic polygonal cells, which resemble epithelial or melanocytic cells.

Ultrastructural features vary depending on the degree of differentiation of the endothelial tumor cells. They may show luminal pinocytotic vesicles, polarized basal lamina, intercellular tight junctions, and intercellular canaliculi. Occasionally, Weibel-Palade bodies may be seen. Immunohistochemical stains for endothelial cell markers may confirm the diagnosis of angiosarcoma. One of the most reliable markers for endothelial cells is Factor VIII/von Willebrand antigen (antihemophilic factor antigen),[138] which is usually positive in angiosarcoma. Lectins are animal or plant proteins that demonstrate specific binding to certain glycoproteins. Ulex europaeus agglutinin I (UEAI) lectin is a useful marker for endothelial cells[139] and has shown positive staining of angiosarcoma cells.[140] Angiotensin converting enzyme shows a high degree of specificity for endothelial cells[138, 141] and, although not yet shown clinically, might be a useful label for angiosarcoma. Similarly, if the diagnosis of angiosarcoma was uncertain, labeling of fresh tissue with fluorescent acetylated low-density lipoprotein could provide evidence for an endothelial cell origin of the tumor.[141]

The epithelioid variant, which represents a small fraction of angiosarcomas, has distinct histologic and biologic features.[142, 143] This variant has been termed epithelioid hemangioendothelioma or histiocytic hemangioma. The tumor is found in adults and is characterized by an epithelioid or histiocytoid endothelial cell component. The neoplastic endothelial cells display prominent cytoplasmic vacuolization. This variant is malignant but appears to have lower metastatic potential and exhibits a "borderline" behavior compared with the typical angiosarcoma.

The differential diagnosis of angiosarcoma includes other vascular tumors, particularly intravascular papillary endothelial hyperplasia, hemangiopericytoma, and Kaposi's sarcoma. Hemangiopericytoma, which is derived from pericytes that surround blood vessels, has a predilection for the orbit.[144] Microscopically, these tumors usually exhibit distinctive ramifying "staghorn" vascular structures, but occasionally they may be confused with angiosarcoma. Immunohistochemical stains are most helpful, because hemangiopericytoma tumor cells do not stain with Factor VIII or UEAI. Although reticulin stain has been recommended, it is rarely pos-

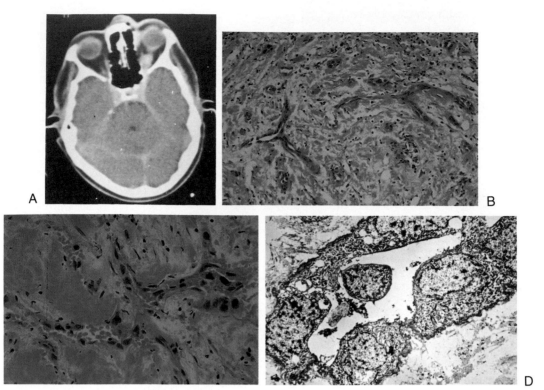

Figure 178–20. Orbital angiosarcoma. *A,* Computed tomographic scan demonstrates a poorly defined mass near the orbital apex. *B,* Tumor cells form cords and tubular structures that display a tendency to form lumens (H&E, × 64). *C,* Some tubular structures contain erythrocytes, indicating their vascular origin (H&E, × 100). Malignant endothelial cells may also appear in dyscohesive clusters and contain hyperchromatic, pleomorphic nuclei with eosinophilic cytoplasm. *D,* Transmission electron microscopy of tubule lined by neoplastic endothelial cells shows endothelial cells containing numerous vacuoles and surrounded by basal lamina (uranyl acetate and lead citrate, × 22,800).

sible to distinguish the hemangiopericytoma with tumor cells outside the reticulin network from angiosarcoma with tumor cells within the reticulin network. Kaposi's sarcoma also may be confused with angiosarcoma. However, the presence of sinusoidal channels lined by pleomorphic endothelial cells is unusual in Kaposi's sarcoma. Also eosinophilic intracytoplasmic globules may be found in Kaposi's sarcoma tumor cells, whereas staining of the spindle-tumor cells is negative for Factor VIII antigen and UEAI.[145] Primary orbital Kaposi's sarcoma has not been convincingly documented, even in patients with AIDS, although a primary conjunctival tumor might extend into the orbit. It should be remembered that angiosarcoma may reach the orbit by extension from adjacent structures such as the maxillary sinus[146] or by metastasis from another primary site.[147]

INTRAVASCULAR PAPILLARY ENDOTHELIAL HYPERPLASIA

Intravascular papillary endothelial hyperplasia is a rare benign vascular tumor that may superficially resemble angiosarcoma. Since the first description by Masson of "hemangioendotheliome vegetant intravasculaire" in 1923,[148] the tumor has been described under a variety of outdated names, including Masson's vegetant intravascular hemangioendothelioma, intravascular angio-

matosis, Masson's pseudoangiosarcoma, intravascular endothelial proliferation, and endovascularite proliferante thrombopoietique.[149] This tumor usually arises in the subcutaneous tissues of the extremities and fingers, trunk, or head and neck region and has been reported in the eyelids[149–153] and orbit.[153–155] Involvement of the orbit by local extension of a tumor arising in the maxillary sinus, resulting in proptosis and facial pain, has been reported.[156] Although this tumor usually develops within the vascular channels of the deep dermis or subcutis, it may arise in varices, hemangiomas, or hematomas and other deep soft tissue vascular abnormalities. In the orbit, the tumor usually develops within the lumens of thrombosed orbital varices and may rarely arise within arteries.

Orbital intravascular papillary endothelial hyperplasia usually causes progressive proptosis and has a well-circumscribed appearance on computed tomography. Grossly, the tumor may appear encapsulated and may be dusky blue or purple (Fig. 178–21). Microscopically, there may be remnants of the preexistent vein or artery at the periphery of the tumor. Early in the course of evolution of the lesion, there is an exuberant proliferation of endothelial cells over cores of fibrin that stain intensely with the trichrome stain. Later the fibrinous material is converted to collagenized cores. The fronds of endothelial cells usually form a single layer but may form several concentric layers around the cores of fibrin

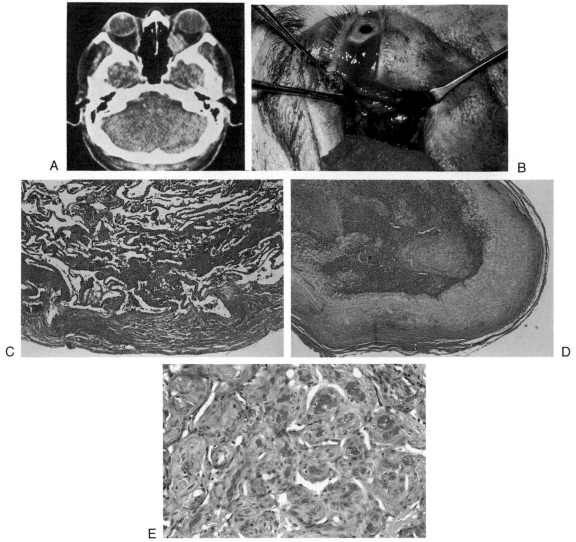

Figure 178–21. Intravascular papillary endothelial hyperplasia. A 55-year-old man acquired proptosis, conjunctival infection and chemosis, restricted motility, and pain in the right eye. *A,* Computed tomography shows a well-circumscribed retrobulbar mass. *B,* Orbital exploration shows a large blue-black apparently encapsulated mass. *C,* The lumen of the vein is filed with papillary fronds composed of endothelial cells around collagenous cores (H&E, ×60). *D,* In unusual cases, the tumor may be surrounded by the thickened wall of an artery. The lumen is occluded by organizing the thrombus with areas of papillary hyperplasia (H&E, ×25). *E,* Higher magnification shows endothelial cells surrounding the central cores of fibrin and collagenous tissue (H&E, ×250).

or collagen. Electron microscopy demonstrates spindle-shaped cells with features of endothelial cells forming a polarized basement membrane and containing numerous micropinocytotic vesicles on the plasmalemma.[153] Some cells show ultrastructural features of pericytes, including bundles of actin-like cytoplasmic filaments and fusiform densities, some of which insert onto the plasmalemma.

The differential diagnosis of this lesion includes angiosarcoma, hemangiopericytoma, Kaposi's sarcoma, intravenous pyogenic granuloma, intravascular fasciitis, intravenous atypical vascular proliferation, malignant endovascular papillary cutaneous angioendothelioma of childhood, and angiolymphoid hyperplasia with eosinophilia (Kimura's disease).[149, 153] Clearkin and Enzinger described features of intravascular papillary endothelial hyperplasia that distinguish this lesion from angiosarcoma.[157] In contrast with angiosarcoma, intravascular papillary endothelial hyperplasia usually demonstrates

an intravascular location, central thrombotic zone, minimal cellular pleomorphism, and rare mitotic figures, and it is uncommon to observe solid areas, piling up of the endothelium, and necrosis. Although it has been suggested that this lesion represents a primary endothelial proliferation with secondary thrombosis, most cases are probably the result of a reactive process secondary to a thrombosis that forms in a preexisting vascular lesion.[149, 153, 157] Clinically, intravascular papillary endothelial hyperplasia usually is benign; however, intracranial extension of an orbital tumor has been reported.[155]

MALIGNANT PERIPHERAL NERVE SHEATH TUMOR

The term malignant peripheral nerve sheath tumor indicates that these tumors arise from nerve sheath elements but does not specifically identify the cell of origin. Similarly, these tumors have also been named neurogenic sarcoma, malignant neurilemoma, neurilemmosarcoma, and malignant neuroma. Other synonymous terms imply a more specific cell of origin, including malignant schwannoma, fibromyxosarcoma of nerve, neurofibrosarcoma, fibrosarcoma of nerve, and malignant peripheral glioma. Although not all tumors arise from Schwann cells, many authors prefer the term malignant schwannoma for this group of tumors.

Depending on the cell of origin, peripheral nerve sheath tumors are of either neural crest or mesodermal derivation. Neural crest tumors arise from Schwann cells or perineural cells. Although perineural cells do not produce myelin, they histologically resemble Schwann cells.[158] Nerve sheath tumors of mesodermal origin arise from the epineural fibroblast. Unlike Schwann cells, these fibrocytes do not produce myelin and lack a basement membrane.

In general, malignant nerve sheath tumors are uncommon, representing approximately 10 percent of all soft tissue sarcomas.[159] Nearly half of these tumors are associated with von Recklinghausen's disease or with an antecedent neurofibroma but usually not with a benign schwannoma. Patients with neurofibromatosis reportedly have a 3 to 13 percent chance of acquiring a malignant nerve sheath tumor; however, these figures may be exaggerated. Although patients with von Recklinghausen's disease may present at an earlier age, most of the patients with peripheral nerve sheath tumor range in age from 20 to 50 yr at presentation. There is no consistent sex predilection, except for a male predominance in tumors associated with von Recklinghausen's disease. These tumors typically arise in the major nerve trunks, such as the sciatic nerve, the brachial plexus, and the sacral plexus. Thus, the tumors characteristically develop in the proximal portions of the upper and lower extremities and the trunk.

Primary orbital malignant nerve sheath tumor is very rare. Isolated case reports have appeared describing orbital tumors in patients with and without neurofibromatosis.[160–164] The largest series was reported by Jakobiec, Font, and Zimmerman, who described eight cases from the AFIP.[165] Other studies reported extension into the orbit from adjacent soft tissues or sinuses.[166–168] Also discovery of an orbital tumor should initiate a search for an alternative primary site, because orbital malignant nerve sheath tumor may be metastatic.[169]

Orbital primary malignant nerve sheath tumor has a distinct tendency to develop in the anterior supranasal orbit from the supraorbital branch of the trigeminal ophthalmic nerve. Clinically, the appearance of a mass under the uneroded skin of the supranasal quadrant suggests the possibility of a malignant nerve sheath tumor. There may be pain, hypesthesia, or anesthesia in the distribution of the involved nerve.

In the series of orbital malignant nerve sheath tumors reported by Jakobiec and coworkers,[165] the patients ranged in age from 19 to 75 yr, with half the patients younger than 50 yr. There was no strong sex predilection, with 5 men and 3 women in the series. Two of the eight patients had von Recklinghausen's neurofibromatosis. Patients with malignant nerve sheath tumor had a poor prognosis, with an especially rapid and unfavorable clinical course after incomplete excision. The tumor exhibited locally aggressive behavior and a strong neurotropism frequently extending along the trigeminal nerve toward the middle cranial fossa, with involvement to the pons demonstrated at autopsy in two cases. The tumor may also extend anteriorly along the supraorbital nerve and may be observed clinically as a palpable or visible mass across the forehead.

Patients with malignant nerve sheath tumor have a high mortality rate as a result of both intracranial extension and distant metastasis. The primary treatment of these tumors is complete excision, usually exenteration for orbital tumors. Because of the proclivity for extension along nerves, examination of margins with frozen sections may indicate the need for craniotomy. Although the tumor may be resistant to adjuvant therapy, chemotherapy or radiotherapy is often combined with surgical excision of the tumor. Despite the poor prognosis, one 15-month-old boy was free of tumor 9 yr after local excision of a malignant nerve sheath tumor.[170] This patient is unusual because of his age, and he is one of the few known long-term survivors.

Microscopically, the most common pattern is the spindle cell-fascicular type.[159] The plump spindle cells generally have abundant cytoplasm and oval nuclei, with fine nuclear chromatin stippling and small nucleoli (Fig. 178–22). These cells also exhibit a high mitotic rate and nuclear pleomorphism, suggesting the malignant behavior of the tumor. Besides the spindle cell-fascicular pattern, orbital tumors may demonstrate malignant plexiform, alveolar-organoid, pseudoglandular, neurotubular (Fig. 178–23), and epithelioid variants.[165] These tumors also may be biphasic, including both spindle and epithelioid cells. Palisading may be present, and necrosis may be noted. Myxoid areas can be found, particularly in association with neurofibromatosis. Heterotopic elements may be present, including bone, cartilage, muscle, and glandular tissue.

Ultrastructural studies may distinguish features of perineural cells and Schwann cells in these tumors.[165] More commonly, perineural cell characteristics may be seen, including an overall bipolar spindle shape, interrupted segments of basement membrane, pinocytotic vesicles at the plasmalemma, cytoplasmic filaments, and short segments of rough-surfaced endoplasmic reticulum with few mitochondria. Typical Schwann cell characteristics are often absent; however, some cells may demonstrate intertwining, slender cellular processes and basement membranes. Although typical of Schwann cells, banded basement membrane material (Luse bodies) is usually not observed in malignant nerve sheath tumor.

Immunohistochemical staining for S100 protein, which is found in the cytoplasm of Schwann cells, is sometimes positive in malignant nerve sheath tumor. Although not helpful when tumor cells do not stain, positive staining with antibody to S100 protein may help to distinguish these tumors from other epithelioid and spindle-cell tumors. CD56 and CD57 antigens show sequence homologies to the neural cell adhesion molecule (N-CAM)

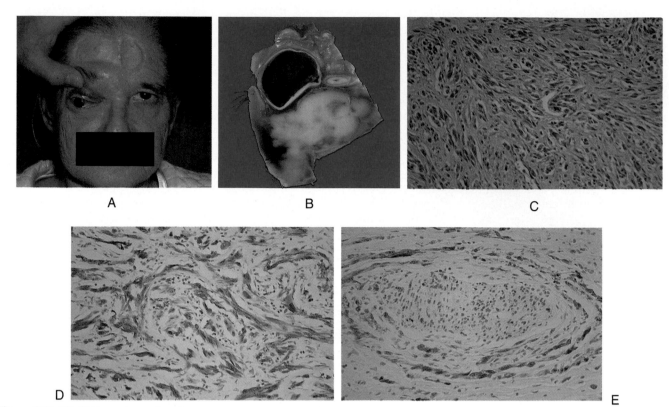

Figure 178–22. Malignant peripheral nerve sheath tumor. *A,* A 79-year-old woman had three recurrences of mass located in the right periorbital region supranasally. She subsequently underwent orbital exenteration with resection of the frontal bone but acquired intracranial invasion of the tumor and died approximately 1 yr later. *B,* Exenterated orbital contents show a tumor involving the superior orbit. *C,* The tumor is composed of interlacing fascicles of spindle-shaped cells intermixed with scattered plumper epithelioid cells (H&E, ×51). *D,* Immunohistochemical staining for S100 protein demonstrates positive staining of the tumor cells (immunoperoxidase reaction, ×51). *E,* Tumor cells extending along nerve (perineural invasion) show positive staining for S100 protein (immunoperoxidase reaction, ×64).

and can be demonstrated immunohistochemically in benign and malignant schwannomas.[171] Epithelial membrane antigen (EMA) is an immunohistochemical marker that can identify normal and neoplastic perineural cells.[172] In conjunction with S100 protein (a Schwann cell marker), EMA may be useful in distinguishing tumors of perineural cell origin. Although immunohistochemical staining for CD56, CD57, and EMA are not as widely available as S100 protein, markers such as these are promising clinical and research tools.

Other peripheral nerve tumors of the orbit are described in Chapter 174.

PAGET'S DISEASE AND MISCELLANEOUS INTRAOSSEOUS LESIONS

Paget's disease of bone (osteitis deformans) may affect the orbit. Radiologic changes of the orbit and skull reflect the lytic, mixed, or sclerotic phases of the disease. The diagnosis is made by the characteristic x-ray findings, and an elevated serum alkaline phosphatase may be found. Ophthalmic manifestations can include angioid streaks, choroidal sclerosis, and extraocular muscle palsies. In rare cases, unilateral or bilateral exophthal-

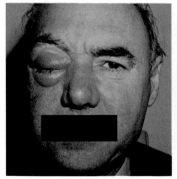

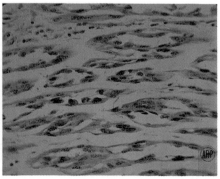

Figure 178–23. Malignant peripheral nerve sheath tumor. *A,* A 50-year-old man presented with swollen eyelids 1 yr after removal of a supranasal subcutaneous lesion misinterpreted as a sweat gland carcinoma. The patient had diminished sensation in the distribution of the ophthalmic division of the trigeminal nerve because of involvement with tumor. *B,* An area of tumor showing a neurotubular pattern composed of plump spindle cells lining elongated pseudolumens. There were no axon cylinders in this area (H&E, ×220).

mos may be due to Paget's disease. One interesting patient presented with a 5-yr history of progressive proptosis and limitation of ocular motility.[173] Calcitonin injections produced no improvement; however, the proptosis and ocular motility disturbances markedly improved after treatment with 3-aminohydroxypropylidene-1,1-bisphosphonate.

Hereditary diaphyseal dysplasia (Engelmann's disease) is a rare systemic dystrophy of bone associated with osteosclerosis.[174] Ophthalmic manifestations include proptosis, optic disc edema, and optic atrophy. Infantile cortical hyperostosis (Caffey's disease) usually affects the mandible but can involve the orbit, causing proptosis.[175] Radiographic studies show thickening of the soft tissues around the affected bone, and histopathologic findings show a periostitis. This thickening develops in affected infants and then subsides over several months without causing permanent ocular damage.

The brown tumor is a focal lesion of bone associated with hyperparathyroidism, which may develop in the orbit.[176–179] This tumor is found more commonly in primary hyperparathyroidism and less frequently in secondary hyperparathyroidism. In the brown tumor, increased osteoclastic activity leads to bone resorption, trabecular fibrosis, microfractures, and hemorrhage (Fig. 178–24). This tumor may be located in bone or soft tissue. Grossly, the tumors have a brown appearance because of hemosiderin pigment deposits. Diagnosis of a brown tumor should initiate a search for the cause of the hyperparathyroidism, and a bone survey may show evidence of demineralization. In the case of primary hyperparathyroidism associated with brown tumor, treatment is excision of the tumor followed by exploration and removal of the parathyroid.

Intraosseous myxoma may affect the orbital walls (Fig. 178–25).[180, 181] Myxomas are benign neoplasms of mesenchymal origin that, histologically, contain stellate cells and delicate reticulin fibers in a loose mucoid stroma devoid of blood vessels. Although the tumor is benign, inadequate removal may result in local recurrence; therefore, treatment is with wide local resection. An interesting entity is Carney's complex, comprised of eyelid myxoma, potentially fatal cardiac myxoma, gonadal tumors, and other metabolic abnormalities.

Primary intraosseous hemangioma is an uncommon benign lesion that usually involves the vertebrae.[182, 183] The most common extravertebral site is the skull, usually the frontal or parietal bones. Involvement of the orbital bones is rare. In the orbit, the tumor usually presents with slowly progressive proptosis. Women are more commonly affected than men, and the tumor usually occurs in the fourth or fifth decades of life. Radiographically, there is a lytic lesion often exhibiting a honeycombed appearance or sunburst pattern with fine reticulated lines radiating from the center of the mass.[183] Most hemangiomas are the cavernous type, whereas the capillary type is quite rare (Fig. 178–26). Treatment consists of surgical excision.

When considering lesions of the bony walls of the

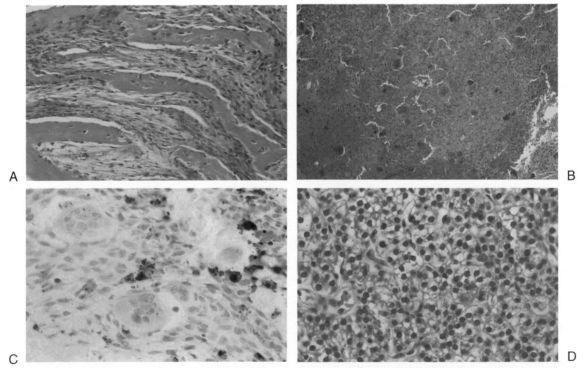

A

B

C

D

Figure 178–24. Brown tumor of the orbit. This tumor may show prominent osteoblastic and osteoclastic activity with fibrovascular proliferation and hemorrhage. *A*, Reactive bone at the edge of the lesion (H&E). *B*, Adjacent to an area of hemorrhage, there are histiocytes, fibroblasts, and randomly dispersed multinucleated giant cells. *C*, Mono- and multinucleated histiocytes and intracellular and extracellular blood-breakdown products that stain positively for iron (Prussian blue stain). *D*, In this patient, there was an associated parathyroid adenoma composed principally of sheets of chief cells (H&E). (Courtesy of A. Friedman, M.D.)

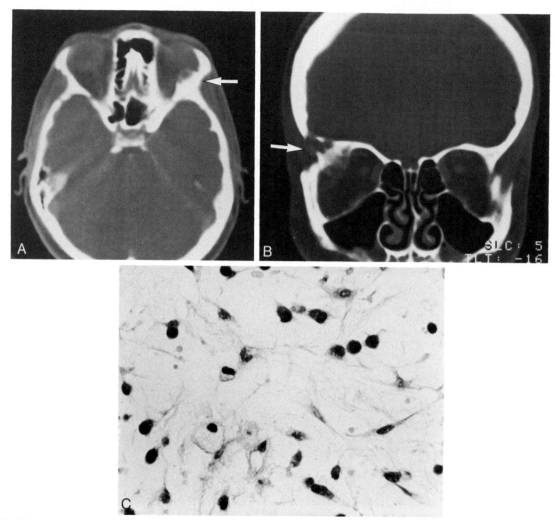

Figure 178–25. Myxoma of bone involving the orbit. Axial *(A)* and coronal *(B)* computed tomographic scans show a mass arising from bone extending into the orbit and posteriorly involving the pterion and greater wing of sphenoid. There is focal destruction of the left lateral orbital wall *(arrows).* C, Photomicrograph showing stellate, spindled, and sometimes vacuolated cells in a loose network of reticulin fibers and mucoid material, with a paucity of blood vessels. (Reproduced with permission from Candy EJ, Miller NR, Carson BS: Myxoma of bone involving the orbit. Arch Ophthalmol 109:919, 1991. Copyright 1991, American Medical Association.)

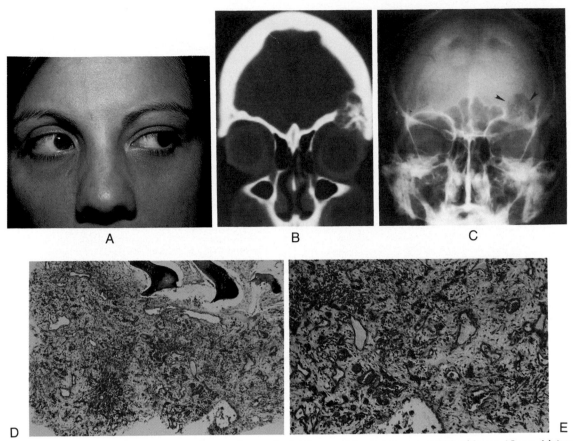

Figure 178–26. Primary intraosseous capillary hemangioma. *A,* A 31-year-old woman presented with an 18-mo history of slowly progressive blepharoptosis and proptosis of the left eye. The clinical photograph shows mild blepharoptosis of the left eyelid with subtle fullness between the superior eyelid sulcus and the eyebrow. Results of the motility examination were normal. *B,* Plain x-ray film of the skull shows a well-circumscribed lytic lesion with fine radiating reticulated pattern (*arrowheads*). *C,* Computed tomographic scan displays a lytic lesion with coarse, internal, bone reticulations. *D,* There is a loose stroma with prominent capillary proliferation and extravasation of erythrocytes resembling granulation tissue. In the upper right, several blue-stained bony trabeculae are present (Masson's trichrome, ×20). *E,* The tumor shows a proliferation of capillaries that display variable caliber of their lumens. These vascular lumens are lined by low cuboidal endothelial-like cells (Masson's trichrome, ×40).

orbit, the differential diagnosis includes osteoma (and Gardner's syndrome), osteosarcoma, chondrosarcoma, ossifying fibroma, and fibrous dysplasia. Postmortem examination of one patient who had been observed for 17 yr with the erroneous clinical diagnosis of fibrous dysplasia demonstrated a rare intraosseous lipoma involving the orbital portion of the frontal bone.[184] The chondroma is a rare tumor that can arise from the cartilaginous trochlea.[185] A cartilagenous hemartoma has also been described, which originated in a portion of the orbit away from the trochlea.[186] Multiple enchondromatosis (Ollier's disease), an idiopathic disease usually involving the long bones, has been described in the ethmoid sinus and can secondarily invade the orbit.[187] Other rare lesions of orbital bones including giant cell reparative granuloma, aneurysmal bone cyst, and orbital cholesterol granuloma, which are discussed in Chapter 179.

LETHAL MIDLINE GRANULOMA

Patients affected with lethal midline granuloma have a relentless destructive process of unknown cause that involves the nose, paranasal sinuses, palate, and facial soft tissues.[188, 189] This destructive granulomatous inflammatory process involves soft tissue, cartilage, and bone, with erosion through contiguous structures such as the orbit (Fig. 178–27).[190] Untreated, the patients frequently die as a result of erosion into major vessels of the head and neck with resulting exsanguination. Patients may be treated with radiotherapy, with prolonged disease-free intervals.

Previous reports of lethal midline granuloma have been classified into at least four categories: idiopathic midline destructive disease, Wegener's granulomatosis, polymorphic reticulosis, and lymphoma.[188] Idiopathic midline destructive disease is a diagnosis of exclusion. On histologic examination, idiopathic midline destructive disease shows acute and chronic inflammation with variable degrees of focal necrosis. There is no cellular atypia, and signs of granulomatous vasculitis or fibrinoid necrosis of the vessel walls are absent, although giant cells may be seen occasionally. Clinically, it is important to distinguish Wegener's granulomatosis from lethal midline granuloma, because the therapy for the former involves cytotoxic and immunosuppressive medication, whereas the latter is usually treated with radiation.

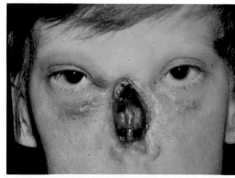

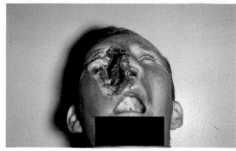

Figure 178–27. Lethal midline granuloma. *A,* A 25-year-old man with advanced lesions of lethal midline granuloma with total loss of the external nose. The nasopharynx was exposed, and there was brawny erythema of the surrounding central face, including the eyelids, cheeks, and upper lip. This patient had evidence of nasal disfigurement and skin changes beginning at age 13. (Courtesy of D. Cogan, M.D.) *B,* Midline destructive process involving the nose, palate, sinuses, and the adjacent orbit. The patient acquired a free communication between the mouth and the nasal cavity.

Osteolytic lesions that are caused by lymphoreticular malignancies feature either large anaplastic lymphocytes or highly pleomorphic cells (polymorphic reticulosis) with a background inflammatory population of mixed (polymorphic) cell types.

REFERENCES

1. Telium G: Endodermal sinus tumors of the ovary and testis: Comparative morphogenesis of the so called mesonephroma ovarii (Schiller) and extraembryonic (yolk sac-allantoic) structures of the rat's placenta. Cancer 12:1092, 1959.
2. Mostofi FK: Infantile testicular tumors. Bull N Y Acad Med 18:684, 1952.
3. Pierce BG, Bullock WK, Huntington RW Jr: Yolk sac tumors of the testis. Cancer 25:644, 1970.
4. Huntington RW Jr, Bullock WK: Yolk-sac tumors of extragonadal origin. Cancer 25:1368, 1970.
5. Fox H, Langley FA: Tumors of the Ovary. Chicago: Yearbook Medical Publishers, 1976.
6. Margo CE, Folberg R, Zimmerman LE, et al: Endodermal sinus tumor (yolk sac tumor) of the orbit. Ophthalmology 90:1426, 1983.
7. Katz NNK, Ruymann FB, Margo CE, et al: Endodermal sinus tumor (yolk-sac carcinoma) of the orbit. J Pediatr Ophthalmol Strabismus 19:270, 1982.
8. Kurman RJ, Norris HJ: Endodermal sinus tumor of the ovary: A clinical and pathologic analysis of 71 cases. Cancer 38:2404, 1976.
9. Porterfield JF, Zimmerman LE: Rhabdomyosarcoma of the orbit: A clinicopathologic study of 55 cases. Virchows Arch [A] 335:329, 1962.
10. Palmer PE, Safai H, Wolfe AJ: Alpha-1 antitrypsin and alpha-fetoprotein: Protein markers in endodermal sinus (yolk sac) tumors. Am J Clin Pathol 65:575, 1976.
11. Talerman A, Haije WG: Alpha-fetoprotein and germ cell tumors: A possible role of yolk sac tumor in production of alpha-fetoprotein. Cancer 34:1722, 1974.
12. Tsuchida Y, Kaneko M, Yokomuri K, et al: Alpha-fetoprotein, prealbumin, albumin, alpha-1-antitrypsin and transferrin as diagnostic and therapeutic markers for endodermal sinus tumors. J Pediatr Surg 13:25, 1978.
13. Tsuchida Y, Saito S, Ishida M, et al: Yolk sac tumor (endodermal sinus tumor) and alpha-fetoprotein: A report of three cases. Cancer 32:917, 1973.
14. Christopherson W, Foote F, Stewart F: Alveolar soft part sarcomas: Structurally characteristic tumors of uncertain histogenesis. Cancer 5:100, 1952.
15. Abrahams IW, Fenton RH, Vidone R: Alveolar soft-part sarcoma of the orbit. Arch Ophthalmol 79:185, 1968.
16. Grant GD, Shields JA, Flanagan JC, et al: The ultrasonographic and radiologic features of a histologically proven case of alveolar soft-part sarcoma of the orbit. Am J Ophthalmol 87:773, 1979.
17. Bunt AH, Bensinger RE: Alveolar soft part sarcoma of the orbit. Ophthalmology 88:1339, 1981.
18. Smetana H, Scott W: Malignant tumors of non-chromaffin paraganglia. Milit Surg 109:330, 1951.
19. Welsh R, Bray D, Shipkey F, et al: Histogenesis of alveolar soft part sarcoma. Cancer 29:191, 1972.
20. Simmons WB, Haggerty HS, Ngan B, et al: Alveolar soft part sarcoma of the head and neck. A disease of children and young adults. Int J Pediatr Otorhinolaryngol 17:139, 1989.
21. Deschryves-Kecskemeti K, Kraus FT, Engleman W, et al: Alveolar soft part sarcoma—A malignant angioreninoma. Am J Surg Pathol 6:5, 1982.
22. Auerbach H, Brooks J: Alveolar soft part sarcoma: More evidence against a myogenic origin. Lab Invest 52:4A, 1985.
23. Mukai M, Iri H, Nakajima T, et al: Alveolar soft part sarcoma. A review on its histogenesis and further studies based on electron microscopy, immunohistochemistry, and biochemistry. Am J Surg Pathol 7:679, 1983.
24. Fisher E, Reidbord H: Electron microscopic evidence suggesting the myogenous derivation of the so-called alveolar soft part sarcoma. Cancer 27:151, 1971.
25. Mukai M, Torikata C, Iri H, et al: Alveolar soft part sarcoma: An elaboration of a three-dimensional configuration of the crystalloids by digital image processing. Am J Pathol 116:398, 1984.
26. Mukai M, Torikata C, Iri H, et al: Histogenesis of alveolar soft part sarcoma: An immunohistochemical and biochemical study. Am J Surg Pathol 10:212, 1986.
27. Auerbach H, Brooks J: Alveolar soft part sarcoma: A clinicopathologic and immunohistochemical study. Cancer 609:66, 1987.
28. Ogawa K, Nakashima Y, Yamabe H: Alveolar soft part sarcoma, granular cell tumor, and paraganglioma: An immunohistochemical comparative study. Acta Pathol Jpn 36:895, 1986.
29. Enzinger FM, Weiss SW: Malignant tumors of uncertain histogenesis. *In* Enzinger FM, Weiss SW (eds.): Soft Tissue Tumors, 2nd ed. St Louis, CV Mosby, 1988, pp 929–965.
30. Lieberman P, Foote F, Stewart F, et al: Alveolar soft-part sarcoma. JAMA 198:1047, 1966.
31. Evans HL: Alveolar soft-part sarcoma. A study of 13 typical examples and one with a histologically atypical component. Cancer 55:912, 1985.
32. Font RL, Jurco S, Zimmerman LE: Alveolar soft-part sarcoma of the orbit: A clinicopathologic analysis of seventeen cases and a review of the literature. Hum Pathol 13:569, 1982.
33. Spector R, Travis L, Smith J: Alveolar soft part sarcoma of the head and neck. Laryngoscope 89:1301, 1979.
34. Shipkey FH, Lieberman PH, Foote FW, et al: Ultrastructure of alveolar soft part sarcoma. Cancer 17:821, 1964.
35. Welsh RA, Beam DM, Shipkey FH, et al: Histogenesis of soft part sarcoma. Cancer 29:191, 1972.
36. Garancis JC, Komorowski RA, Kuzma JF: Granular cell myoblastoma. Cancer 25:542, 1970.
37. Jaeger MJ, Green WR, Miller NR, et al: Granular cell tumor of the orbit and ocular adnexae. Surv Ophthalmol 31:417, 1987.
38. Abrikossoff A: Uber myome ausgehend non der goergestreiften willkurlichen muskulatur. Virch Arch [A] 260:215, 1926.

39. Murray MR: Cultural characteristics of three granular cell myoblastoma. Cancer 4:857, 1951.
40. Azzopardi JG: Histogenesis of granular cell myoblastoma. J Pathol Bacteriol 71:85, 1956.
41. Leroux R, Delarve J: Sur trois cas de tumeurs a cellules granuleuses de la cavite buccale. Bull Assoc Fr Etude Cancer 28:427, 1939.
42. Miettinen M, Lehtonen E, Lehtola H, et al: Histogenesis of granular cell tumor—An immunohistochemical and ultrastructural study. J Pathol 142:221, 1984.
43. Moriarty P, Garner A, Wright JE: Case report of granular cell myoblastoma arising within the medial rectus muscle. Br J Ophthalmol 67:17, 1983.
44. Feyrter F: Uber eine eigenartige geschwulstform des nervengewebes im menschlichen verdauungsschlauch. Virch Arch [A] 295:480, 1935.
45. Constanzi G, Bosincu L, Denti S, et al: Evidence for collagen fibrils inside the cells of granular cell myoblastomas. Pathol Res Pract 170:61, 1980.
46. Fisher ER, Wechsler H: Granular cell myoblastoma—A misnomer. Electron microscopic and histochemical evidence concerning its Schwann cell derivation and nature (granular cell schwannoma). Cancer 15:936, 1962.
47. Stefansson K, Wollmann RL: S-100 protein in granular cell tumors (granular cell myoblastomas). Cancer 49:1834, 1982.
48. Nakasoto Y, Ishizeki J, Takahashi K, et al: Immuno-histochemical localization of S-100 protein in granular cell myoblastoma. Am J Surg Pathol 49:1624, 1982.
49. Armin A, Conelly E, Rawden G: An immunoperoxidase investigation of S-100 protein in granular cell myoblastomas: Evidence for Schwann cell derivation. Am J Clin Pathol 79:37, 1983.
50. Takahashi K, Isobe T, Ohtsuki Y, et al: Immunohistochemical study on the distribution of alpha and beta subunits of S100 protein in human neoplasm and normal tissues. Virchows Arch [B] 45:385, 1984.
51. Rode J, Dhillon AP, Papadaki L: Immunohistochemical staining of granular cell tumour for neurone-specific enolase: Evidence in support of a neural origin. Diagn Histopathol 5:205, 1982.
52. Dolman PJ, Rootman J, Dolman CL: Infiltrating orbital granular cell tumour: A case report and literature review. Br J Ophthalmol 71:47, 1987.
53. Spencer WH: Ophthalmic Pathology: An Atlas and Textbook, vol. 3. Philadelphia, WB Saunders, 1986.
54. Dunnington JH: Granular cell myoblastoma of the orbit. Arch Ophthalmol 40:14, 1948.
55. Ferry AP: Granular cell tumor (myoblastoma) of the palpebral conjunctiva causing pseudoepitheliomatous hyperplasia of the conjunctival epithelium. Am J Ophthalmol 91:234, 1981.
56. Bangle R Jr: A morphological and histochemical study of the granular cell myoblastoma. Cancer 5:950, 1952.
57. Cutler LS, Chaudhry AP, Topazian R: Melanotic neuroectodermal tumor of infancy: An ultrastructural study, literature review, and reevaluation. Cancer 48:257, 1981.
58. Koudstaal J, Oldhoff J, Panders AK, et al: Melanotic neuroectodermal tumor of infancy. Cancer 22:151, 1968.
59. Hall WC, O'Day DM, Glick AD: Melanotic neuroectodermal tumor of infancy: An ophthalmic appearance. Arch Ophthalmol 97:922, 1979.
60. Templeton AC: Orbital tumours in african children. Br J Ophthalmol 55:254, 1971.
61. Lamping KA, Albert DM, Lack E, et al: Melanotic neuroectodermal tumor of infancy (retinal anlage tumor). Ophthalmology 92:143, 1985.
62. Krompecher E. Zur histogenese und morphogie der adamantinome und sonstiger kiefergeschwulste. Beitr Pathol Anat 64:165, 1918.
63. Zimmerman LE: Discussion of melanotic neuroectodermal tumor of infancy (retinal anlage tumor). Ophthalmology 92:148, 1985.
64. Halpert B, Patzer R: Maxillary tumor of retinal anlage. Surgery 22:837, 1947.
65. Allen MS, Harrison W, Jahrsdoerfer RA: Retinal anlage tumors. Am J Clin Pathol 51:309, 1969.
66. Borello ED, Gorlin RJ: Melanotic neuroectodermal tumor of infancy—A neoplasm of neural crest origin: Report of a case associated with high urinary excretion of vanillylmandelic acid. Cancer 19:196, 1966.
67. Dehner LP, Sibley RK, Sank JJ Jr, et al: Malignant melanotic neuroectodermal tumor of infancy: A clinical, pathologic, ultrastructural, and tissue culture study. Cancer 43:1389, 1979.
68. Navas Palacios JJ: Malignant melanotic neuroectodermal tumor; light and electron microscopic study. Cancer 46:529, 1980.
69. Tobo M, Sumiyoshi A, Yamakawa Y: Sellar teratoma with melanotic progonoma. Acta Neuropathol (Berl) 55:71, 1981.
70. Atkinson GO Jr, Davis PC, Patrick LE, et al: Melanotic neuroectodermal tumor of infancy: MR findings and review of the literature. Pediatr Radiol 20:20, 1989.
71. Jones P, Williams A: A case of multicentric melanotic adamantinoma. Br J Surg 48:282, 1960/61.
72. Thoma GW: Ameloblastic tumors. Cancer Bull (Houston) 24:98, 1972.
73. Devita VT, Hellman S, Rosenberg SA, et al: Cancer: Principles and Practice of Oncology, 3rd ed. Philadelphia, JB Lippincott, 1989.
74. Prabhakar S, Sawhney IMS, Chopra JS, et al: Hemibase syndrome: An unusual presentation of intracranial paraganglioma. Surg Neurol 22:39, 1984.
75. Ahmed A, Dodge OG, Kirk RS: Chemodectoma of the orbit. J Clin Pathol 22:584, 1969.
76. Botar J, Pribek L: Corpuscle paraganglionnaire dans l'orbit. Ann Anat Pathol 12:227, 1935.
77. Mawas J: Sur un organe épithélial non décrit, le paraganglioma intraorbitaire. C R Hebol Séances Acad Sci (Paris) 202:977, 1936.
78. Fisher ER, Hazard JB: Nonchromaffin paraganglioma of the orbit. Cancer 5:521, 1952.
79. Archer KF, Hurwitz JJ, Balogh JM, et al: Orbital nonchromaffin paraganglioma: A case report and review of the literature. Ophthalmology 96:1659, 1989.
80. Paulus W, Jellinger K, Brenner H: Melanotic paraganglioma of the orbit: A case report. Acta Neuropathol 79:340, 1989.
81. Wong VG, Melmon KL: Ophthalmic manifestations of the carcinoid flush. N Engl J Med 277:406, 1967.
82. Kroheal GB, Perry S, Hepler RS: Acute hypertension with orbital carcinoid tumor. Arch Ophthalmol 100:106, 1982.
83. Shetlar DJ, Font RL, Ordonez N, et al: A clinicopathologic study of three carcinoid tumors metastatic to the orbit: Immunohistochemical, ultrastructural, and DNA flow cytometric studies. Ophthalmology 97:257, 1990.
84. Archer DB, Bardiner TA: An ultrastructural study of carcinoid tumor of the iris. Am J Ophthalmol 94:357, 1982.
85. Williams ED, Sandler M: Classification of carcinoid tumours. Lancet 1:238, 1963.
86. Shields CL, Shields JA, Eagle RC Jr, et al: Orbital metastasis from a carcinoid tumor. Computed tomography, magnetic resonance imaging, and electron microscopic findings. Arch Ophthalmol 105:968, 1987.
87. Rush JA, Waller RR, Campbell RJ: Orbital carcinoid tumor metastatic from the colon. Am J Ophthalmol 89:636, 1980.
88. Divine RD, Anderson RL, Ossoinig KC: Metastatic carcinoid unresponsive to radiation therapy presenting as a lacrimal fossa mass. Ophthalmology 89:516, 1982.
89. Martin RG: Management of carcinoid tumors. Cancer 26:547, 1970.
90. Zimmerman LE, Stangl R, Riddle PJ: Primary carcinoid tumor of the orbit. A clinicopathologic study with histochemical and electron microscopic observations. Arch Ophthalmol 101:1395, 1983.
91. Font RL, Battifora H, Jakobiec FA, et al: Orbital carcinoid tumor. Arch Ophthalmol 109:315, 1991.
92. Riddle PJ, Font RL, Zimmerman LE: Carcinoid tumors of the eye and orbit: A clinicopathologic study of 15 cases with histochemical and electron microscopic observations. Hum Pathol 13:459, 1982.
93. Shields JA: Primary melanocytic tumors. In Diagnosis and Management of Orbital Tumors. Philadelphia, WB Saunders, 1989, pp 275–287.
94. Reese AB: Orbital neoplasms and lesions simulating them. In Tumors of the Eye, 3rd ed. New York, Harper & Row, 1976, pp 434–466.

95. Shields JS, Bakewell B, Augsburger JJ, Flanagan JC: Classification and incidence of space-occupying lesions of the orbit. Arch Ophthalmol 102:1606, 1984.

96. Jakobiec FA, Ellsworth R, Tannenbaum M: Primary orbital melanoma. Am J Ophthalmol 78:24, 1974.

97. Dutton JJ, Anderson RL, Schelper RL, et al: Orbital malignant melanoma and oculodermal melanocytosis: Report of two cases and review of the literature. Ophthalmology 91:497, 1984.

98. Rice CD, Brown HH: Primary orbital melanoma associated with orbital melanocytosis. Arch Ophthalmol 108: 1130, 1990.

99. Jakobiec FA: The ultrastructure of conjunctival melanocytic tumors. Trans Am Ophthalmol Soc 82:599, 1984.

100. Font RL, Truong L: Melanotic schwannoma of soft tissues. Electron-microscopic observations and review of literature. Am J Surg Pathol 8:129, 1984.

101. Jakobiec FA, Font RL, Tso MOM, et al: Mesectodermal leiomyoma of the ciliary body: A tumor of presumed neural crest origin. Cancer 39:2102, 1977.

102. Jakobiec FA, Iwamoto T: Mesectodermal leiomyoma of the ciliary body associated with a nevus. Arch Ophthalmol 96:692, 1978.

103. Jakobiec FA, Mitchell JP, Chauhan PM, et al: Mesectodermal leiomyosarcoma of the antrum and orbit. Am J Ophthalmol 85:51, 1978.

104. Woodruff JM, Chernik NL, Smith MC, et al: Peripheral nerve tumors with rhabdomyosarcomatous differentiation (malignant "Triton" tumors). Cancer 32:426, 1973.

105. Ducatman BS, Scheithauer BW: Malignant peripheral nerve sheath tumors with divergent differentiation. Cancer 54:1049, 1984.

106. Karcioglu ZA, Someren A, Mathes SJ: Ectomesenchymoma: A malignant tumor of migratory neural crest (ectomesenchyme) remnants showing ganglionic, schwannian, melanocytic, and rhabdomyoblastic differentiation. Cancer 39:2486, 1977.

107. Howard GM: Neuroepithelioma of the orbit. Am J Ophthalmol 59:934, 1965.

108. Shuangshoti S, Menakanit W, Changwaivit W, et al: Primary intraorbital extraocular primitive neuroectodermal (neuroepithelial) tumour. Br J Ophthalmol 70:543, 1986.

109. Wilson BW, Roloff J, Wilson HL: Primary peripheral neuroepithelioma of the orbit with intracranial extension. Cancer 62:2595, 1988.

110. Mierau GW: Extraskeletal Ewing's sarcoma (peripheral neuroepithelioma). Ultrastruct Pathol 9:91, 1985.

111. Alvarez-Berdecia A, Schut L, Bruce DA: Localized primary Ewing's sarcoma of the orbital roof, case report. J Neurosurg 50:811, 1979.

112. Griffin CA, McKean C, Israel MA, et al: Comparison of constitutional and tumor associated 11;22 translocations. Non-identical break points on chromosomes 11 and 22. Proc Natl Acad Sci USA 83:6122, 1986.

113. Schwab M, Alitalo K, Klempnauer KH, et al: Amplified DNA with limited homology to my cellular oncogene is shared by human neuroblastoma cell lines and a neuroblastoma tumor. Nature 305:245, 1983.

114. Jakobiec FA, Klepach GL, Crissman JD, et al: Primary differentiated neuroblastoma of the orbit. Ophthalmology 94:255, 1987.

115. Shehata WM: Primary esthesioneuroblastoma of the orbit. IMJ 172:427, 1987.

116. Rakes SM, Yeatts RP, Campbell RJ: Ophthalmic manifestations of esthesioneuroblastoma. Ophthalmology 92:1749, 1985.

117. Rootman J, Damji KF, Dimmick JE: Malignant rhabdoid tumor of the orbit. Ophthalmology 96:1650, 1989.

118. Niffenegger JH, Jakobiec FA, Shore JW, et al: Adult extrarenal rhabdoid tumor of the lacrimal gland. Ophthalmology 99:567, 1992.

119. Johnson LN, Sexton M, Goldberg SH: Poorly differentiated primary orbital sarcoma (presumed malignant rhabdoid tumor). Arch Ophthalmol 109:1275, 1991.

120. Akhtar M, Ali MA, Sackey K, et al: Malignant rhabdoid tumor of the kidney presenting as intraocular metastasis. Pediatr Hematol Oncol 8:33, 1991.

121. Lichtenstein L, Bernstein D: Unusual benign and malignant chondroid tumors of bone: A survey of some mesenchymal cartilage tumors and malignant chondroblastic tumors, including a few multicentric ones, as well as many atypical benign chondroblastomas and chondromyxoid fibromas. Cancer 12:1142, 1959.

122. Reeh MJ: Hemangiopericytoma with cartilaginous differentiation involving orbit. Arch Ophthalmol 75:82, 1966.

123. Fisher ER, Davis JS, Lemmen LJ: Meningeal hemangiopericytoma. Arch Neurol Psychiatr 79:40, 1958.

124. Bertoni F, Picci P, Bacchini P, et al: Mesenchymal chondrosarcoma of bone and soft tissues. Cancer 52:533, 1983.

125. Guccion JG, Font RL, Enzinger FM, et al: Extraskeletal mesenchymal chondrosarcoma. Arch Pathol 95:336, 1973.

126. Cardenas-Ramirez L, Albores-Saavedra J, de Buen S: Mesenchymal chondrosarcoma of the orbit. Arch Ophthalmol 86:410, 1971.

127. Nakashima Y, Unni KK, Shives TC, et al: Mesenchymal chondrosarcoma of bone and soft tissue: A review of 111 cases. Cancer 57:2444, 1986.

128. Salvador AH, Beabout JW, Dahlin DC: Mesenchymal chondrosarcoma—Observations on 30 new cases. Cancer 28:605, 1971.

129. Sevel D: Mesenchymal chondrosarcoma of the orbit. Br J Ophthalmol 58:882, 1974.

130. Shimo-Oku M, Okamoto N, Ogita Y, et al: A case of mesenchymal chondrosarcoma of the orbit. Acta Ophthalmol (Copenh) 58:831, 1980.

131. Rohrbach JM, Steuhl KP, Pressler H, et al: Primary extraskeletal mesenchymal chondrosarcoma of the lid. Graefes Arch Clin Exp Ophthalmol 229:172, 1991.

132. Enzinger FM, Weiss SW: Malignant vascular tumors. In Enzinger FM, Weiss SW (eds): Soft Tissue Tumors, 2nd ed. St Louis, CV Mosby, 1988, pp 545–580.

133. Shuangshoti S, Chayapum P, Suwanwela N, et al: Unilateral proptosis as a clinical presentation in primary angiosarcoma of skull. Br J Ophthalmol 72:713, 1988.

134. Hufnagel T, Ma L, Kuo T-T: Orbital angiosarcoma with subconjunctival presentation: Report of a case and literature review. Ophthalmology 94:72, 1987.

135. Messmer EP, Font RL, McCrary JA III, et al: Epithelioid angiosarcoma of the orbit presenting as Tolosa-Hunt syndrome: A clinicopathologic case report with review of the literature. Ophthalmology 90:1414, 1983.

136. Freedman AM, Reiman IIM, Woods JE: Soft-tissue sarcomas of the head and neck. Am J Surg 158:367, 1989.

137. Rosai J, Sumner HW, Kostianovsky M, et al: Angiosarcoma of the skin: A clinicopathologic and fine structural study. Hum Pathol 7:83, 1976.

138. Zetter BR: Culture of capillary endothelial cells. In Jaffe EA (ed): Biology of Endothelial Cells. Boston, Martinus Nijhoff, 1984, pp 14–26.

139. Holthofer H, Virtanen I, Kariniemi A-L, et al: Ulex europaeus I lectin as a marker for vascular endothelium in human tissues. Lab Invest 47:60, 1982.

140. Ordonez NG, Batsakis JG: Comparison of Ulex europaeus I lectin and factor VIII-related antigen in vascular lesions. Arch Pathol Lab Med 108:129, 1984.

141. Netland PA, Zetter BR, Via DP, et al: In situ labelling of vascular endothelium with fluorescent acetylated low density lipoprotein. Histochem J 17:1309, 1985.

142. Weiss SW, Enzinger FM: Epithelioid hemangioendothelioma: A vascular tumor often mistaken for a carcinoma. Cancer 50:970, 1982.

143. Rosai J, Gold J, Landry R: The histiocytoid hemangiomas: A unifying concept embracing several previously described entities of skin, soft tissue, large vessels, bone and heart. Hum Pathol 10:707, 1979.

144. Croxatto JO, Font RL: Hemangiopericytoma of the orbit: A clinicopathologic study of 30 cases. Hum Pathol 13:210, 1982.

145. Miettinen M, Holthofer H, Lehto VP, et al: Ulex europaeus I lectin as a marker for tumors derived from endothelial cells. Am J Clin Pathol 79:32, 1983.

146. Bankaci M, Myers EN, Barnes L, et al: Angiosarcoma of the maxillary sinus: Literature review and case report. Otolaryngol Head Neck Surg 1:274, 1979.

147. Jakobiec FA, Jones IS: Vascular tumors, malformations and degenerations. In Tasman W, Jaeger EA (eds): Duane's Clinical

Ophthalmology, vol. 2. Philadelphia, JB Lippincott, 1991, pp 1–40.

148. Masson MP: Hemangioendotheliome vegetant intravasculaire. Bull Soc Anat (Paris) 93:517, 1923.
149. Sorenson RL, Spencer WH, Stewart WB, et al: Intravascular papillary endothelial hyperplasia of the eyelid. Arch Ophthalmol 101:1728, 1983.
150. Dhermy P, Offret H, Saraux H: Localisation palpebrale de l'hemangioendotheliome vegetant intra-vasculaire. J Fr Ophthalmol 1:361, 1978.
151. Amerigo J, Berry CL: Intravascular papillary endothelial hyperplasia in the skin and subcutaneous tissue. Virch Arch [A] 387:81, 1980.
152. Wolter JR, Lewis RG: Endovascular hemangioendothelioma of the eyelid. Am J Ophthalmol 78:727, 1974.
153. Font RL, Wheeler TM, Boniuk M: Intravascular papillary endothelial hyperplasia of the orbit and ocular adnexa: A report of five cases. Arch Ophthalmol 101:1731, 1983.
154. Hofeldt AJ, Zaret CR, Jakobiec FA, et al: Orbitofacial angiomatosis. Arch Ophthalmol 97:484, 1979.
155. Weber FL, Babel J: Intravascular papillary endothelial hyperplasia of the orbit. Br J Ophthalmol 65:18, 1981.
156. Stern Y, Braslavsky D, Segal K, et al: Intravascular papillary endothelial hyperplasia in the maxillary sinus: A benign lesion that may be mistaken for angiosarcoma. Otolaryngol Head Neck Surg 117:1182, 1991.
157. Clearkin KP, Enzinger FM: Intravascular papillary endothelial hyperplasia. Arch Pathol Lab Med 100:441, 1976.
158. Harkin JD, Reid RJ: Tumors of the peripheral nervous system. Washington, DC, Armed Forces Institute of Pathology, 1968.
159. Enzinger FM, Weiss SW: Soft Tissue Tumors. St Louis, CV Mosby, 1983.
160. Schatz H: Benign orbital neurilemmoma: Sarcomatous transformation in von Recklinghausen's disease. Arch Ophthalmol 86:268, 1971.
161. Grinberg MA, Levy NS: Malignant neurilemoma of the supraorbital nerve. Am J Ophthalmol 78:489, 1974.
162. Henderson JW: Orbital Tumors, 2nd ed. New York, BC Decker, 1980.
163. Nieuwenhuis I, Witschel H: Das benigne und das maligne Schwannom der orbita—Klinisches bild und histopathologische diagnose. Fortschr Ophthalmol 85:782, 1988.
164. Lyons CJ, McNab AA, Garner A, et al: Orbital malignant peripheral nerve sheath tumours. Br J Ophthalmol 73:731, 1989.
165. Jakobiec FA, Font RL, Zimmerman LE: Malignant peripheral nerve sheath tumors of the orbit: A clinicopathologic study of eight cases. Trans Am Ophthalmol Soc 83:332, 1985.
166. Gullane PJ, Gilbert RW, van Nostrand AWP, et al: Malignant schwannoma in the head and neck. J Otolaryngol 14:171, 1985.
167. Rootman J, Robertson WD: Neurogenic tumors. In Rootman J (ed): Diseases of the Orbit. Philadelphia, JB Lippincott, 1988, pp 281–334.
168. Bleach NR, Keen CE, Dixon JA: Superficial malignant schwannoma on the face: A case for early radical surgery. J Laryngol Otol 103:316, 1989.
169. Jaais F, Sivanesan S: Metastatic malignant schwannoma of orbit: A case report. Med J Malaysia 41:356, 1986.

170. Eviatar JA, Hornblass A, Herschorn B, et al: Malignant peripheral nerve sheath tumor of the orbit in a 15-month-old child—Nine year survival after local excision. Ophthalmology 99:1595, 1992.
171. Mechtersheimer G, Staudter M, Moller P: Expression of the natural killer cell-associated antigens CD56 and CD57 in human neural and striated muscle cells and their tumors. Cancer Res 51:1300, 1991.
172. Ariza A, Bilbao JM, Rosai J: Immunohistochemical detection of epithelial membrane antigen in normal perineurial cells and perineurioma. Am J Surg Pathol 12:678, 1988.
173. Buckler HM, Cantrill JA, Klimiuk PS, et al: Paget's disease of the orbit: Before and after APD. Br Med J 295:1655, 1987.
174. Morse PH, Walsh FB, McCormick JR: Ocular findings in hereditary diaphyseal dysplasia (Englemann's disease). Am J Ophthalmol 68:100, 1969.
175. Minton LR, Elliott JH: Ocular manifestations of infantile cortical hyperostosis. Am J Ophthalmol 64:902, 1967.
176. Weiss RR, Schoeneman MJ, Primack W, et al: Maxillary brown tumor of secondary hyperparathyroidism in a hemodialysis patient. JAMA 243:1929, 1980.
177. Naiman J, Green WR, D'Heurle D, et al: Brown tumor of the orbit associated with primary hyperparathyroidism. Am J Ophthalmol 90:565, 1980.
178. Parrish CM, O'Day DM: Brown tumor of the orbit: Case report and review of the literature. Arch Ophthalmol 104:1199, 1986.
179. Levine MR, Chu A, Abdul-Karim FW: Brown tumor and secondary hyperparathyroidism. Arch Ophthalmol 109:847, 1991.
180. Maiuri F, Corriero G, Galicchio B, et al: Myxoma of the skull and orbit. Neurochirurgia [Stuttg] 31:136, 1988.
181. Candy EJ, Miller NR, Carson BS: Myxoma of bone involving the orbit. Arch Ophthalmol 109:919, 1991.
182. Relf SJ, Bartley GB, Unni KK: Primary orbital intraosseous hemangioma. Ophthalmology 98:541, 1991.
183. Hook SR, Font RL, McCrary JA, et al: Intraosseous capillary hemangioma of the frontal bone. Am J Ophthalmol 103:824, 1987.
184. Small ML, Green R, Johnson LC: Lipoma of the frontal bone. Arch Ophthalmol 97:129, 1979.
185. Jepson CN, Wetzig PC: Pure chondroma of the trochlea: A case report. Surv Ophthalmol 11:656, 1966.
186. Bowen JH, Christensen FH, Klintworth GK, et al: A clinicopathologic study of a cartilaginous hemartoma of the orbit: A rare case of proptosis. Ophthalmology 88:138, 1981.
187. DeLaey JJ, DeSchryver A, Kluyskens P, et al: Orbital involvement in Ollier's disease (multiple echondromatosis). Int Ophthalmol 5:149, 1982.
188. Pickens JP, Modica L: Current concepts of the lethal midline granuloma syndrome. Otolaryngol Head Neck Surg 100:623, 1989.
189. Kornblut AD, Fanci AS: Idiopathic midline granuloma. Otolaryngol Clin North Am 15:685, 1982.
190. Chu FC, Rodrigues MM, Cogan DG, et al: The pathology of idiopathic midline destructive disease (IMDD) in the eyelid. Ophthalmology 90:1385, 1983.

Chapter 179

■

Orbital Histiocytic Disorders

PETER A. NETLAND, RAMON L. FONT, and
FREDERICK A. JAKOBIEC

The orbit may be affected by various granulomatous inflammatory processes. The term *granulomatous inflammation* refers to chronic inflammatory processes that are characterized histologically by the conspicuous predominance of cells of the macrophage or histiocyte series, especially by their modified forms called *epithelioid cells* and *giant cells*. These disease processes may be localized (unifocal) or systemic (multifocal). In this chapter, the chalazion and granulomatous diseases due to infections, such as tuberculosis and aspergillosis, are not reviewed. This chapter focuses on histiocytic disorders and systemic diseases of undetermined etiology, some of which have quasineoplastic properties. These histiocytic disorders include Langerhans' cell histiocytosis, cholesterol granuloma, giant cell reparative granuloma of bone, sinus histiocytosis, juvenile xanthogranuloma, Erdheim-Chester disease, pseudorheumatoid nodules, necrobiotic xanthogranuloma, sarcoidosis, tuberous xanthoma, and unusual foreign body reactions to injected material such as silicone. The intraosseous conditions commence within the diploë of the involved bone but eventually erode through the cancellous cortices, ultimately to be restrained on the cranial side by the dura and on the orbital side by the periorbital lining membrane.

LANGERHANS' CELL HISTIOCYTOSIS (HISTIOCYTOSIS X)

The term *histiocytosis X* was proposed by Lichtenstein in 1953 to include three related disorders (eosinophilic granuloma, Hand-Schüller-Christian disease, and Letterer-Siwe disease), which he believed were different clinical expressions of a single nosologic entity.[1] Although *eosinophilic granuloma* was first coined by Lichtenstein and Jaffe to describe a single histiocytic lesion in bone,[2] the term is now used to describe histiocytic mass lesions that are unifocal or multifocal and generally originate in bone sites. The original description of Hand-Schüller-Christian disease was of the triad of exophthalmos, bony defects of the skull, and diabetes insipidus. This combination is rare, but the eponym has been used to describe the chronic disseminated form of histiocytosis X involving both bone and soft tissues.[3] Letterer-Siwe disease was initially described as a disease of infancy with widespread soft tissue and visceral involvement with or without bone lesions and an acute or subacute and sometimes fatal course. It is the closest to a true neoplastic disorder.

The three disorders included in histiocytosis X cannot be reliably distinguished by the histopathologic appearance of affected tissues, and there is considerable clinical overlap among these three conditions. Although the term *eosinophilic granuloma* is frequently used for unifocal or multifocal masses, the eponymic terms for disseminated disease *(Hand-Schüller-Christian* and *Letterer-Siwe diseases)* are not widely used at present. The three syndromes are probably not distinct entities but rather represent a spectrum of disease from least to greatest aggressiveness.[3] Because the histiocyte within the characteristic lesions has been shown to be the Langerhans' cell, there is increasing use of the more contemporary term: *Langerhans' cell histiocytosis*.[4, 5]

Eosinophilic granuloma occurs in older children and young adults and has an excellent prognosis. Because of the possibility of systemic involvement or progression to more disseminated forms of histiocytosis X, a thorough systemic evaluation and close follow-up are required.[6] The chronic form of histiocytosis X (Hand-Schüller-Christian syndrome or multifocal eosinophilic granuloma) usually occurs in children but not in infants and has been described in adult patients. This form is characterized by involvement of bone (including the skull) and soft tissue sites, including the viscera, lymph nodes, and skin. This disease usually has a chronic, protracted course and a favorable prognosis, but short bursts of disease progression may occur. The most acute and virulent form of histiocytosis X (Letterer-Siwe syndrome) usually occurs in infants or children less than 3 yr of age. Patients often have marked constitutional symptoms and involvement of the skin and mucous membranes. Most patients rapidly deteriorate, with progressive involvement of bone marrow or vital organs, and death may occur within 1 or 2 yr after the onset of the disease.

In patients with histiocytosis X, orbital involvement is common, particularly in patients with eosinophilic granuloma. The overall incidence of orbital involvement in patients with histiocytosis X in larger series ranges from 1 to 20 percent.[7-9] In one series of 76 children with histiocytosis X, 18 (24 percent) had orbital involvement.[10] In this series, the most common ophthalmic problem was bilateral or unilateral proptosis, followed by ptosis, papilledema, optic atrophy, and seventh-nerve palsy. Proptosis may be severe, and globe luxation has been reported.[11] Neuroophthalmic complications are rare,[10] but a case of cavernous sinus syndrome has been reported.[12] Intraocular involvement is also rare but may occur in infants with the more aggressive, subacute form of the disease.[10] It should be remembered that histiocytosis X is an uncommon disease, thus the overall

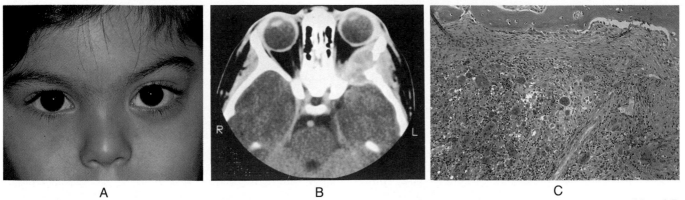

Figure 179–1. Histiocytosis X. *A*, A 4-year-old boy presented with a 3-wk history of swelling and ptosis of the left upper eyelid and 3-day history of proptosis of the left eye. *B*, Computed tomography shows a lytic lesion with irregular borders involving the superotemporal orbit. *C*, Microscopic examination shows multinucleated giant cells with a background of histiocytes, eosinophils, and lymphocytes (H&E, ×40). (*A–C*, Courtesy of J. A. Shields, M.D., Wills Eye Hospital.)

contribution to orbital disease in the general population is low, accounting for less than 1 percent of orbital tumefactions in most series.[6, 7, 10]

In patients with localized orbital involvement, the eosinophilic granuloma has a distinct predilection for the superotemporal orbital bone at the rim of the orbit (Figs. 179–1 and 179–2).[13–15] Radiographically, an irregular, serrated lytic lesion may be detected. As the lesion grows out of the diploë and through the periorbita, an inflammatory response may ensue, suggesting a dacryoadenitis clinically. Orbital involvement is almost invariably associated with a lytic lesion of the orbital wall. Disease confined to orbital soft tissues without bone involvement is rare, and in these cases, it is important to rule out other lesions that may contain eosinophils, such as granulocytic sarcoma and pediatric orbital pseudotumor.[15, 16]

Histopathologic examination demonstrates the unifying features of the different forms of Langerhans' cell histiocytosis. From a single biopsy, it is not possible to distinguish unifocal and multifocal or acute and chronic disease. Light microscopy shows sheets of large histiocytes with a variable number of eosinophils, plasma cells, and lymphocytes. The histiocytes contain large ovoid, indented, or folded nuclei with distinct chromatin and nuclear membranes. Immunofluorescence studies have demonstrated the extracellular deposition of the eosinophil core granule protein (major basic protein), which may have some role in the pathogenesis of the disease.[17] Because hemorrhage is frequent within the tumors, hemosiderin-laden macrophages may be observed. In older lesions, the cells may be vacuolated and accumulate cholesterol (foam cells). Multinucleated giant cells, fibrosis, and areas of necrosis may also be present within the lesion.

Ultrastructural studies have revealed a characteristic cytoplasmic inclusion that is identical to the Birbeck granule of Langerhans' cells, referred to as the *racket body, Birbeck granule, Langerhans' granule,* or *X body* (see Fig. 179–2).[15, 18, 19] The multinucleated giant cells contain abundant mitochondria and profiles of smooth-surfaced endoplasmic reticulum but do not contain Langerhans' granules. Examination of a number of histiocytes may be necessary to reveal Langerhans' granules, because as few as 2 percent of histiocytes may contain these granules.[20] These cells also stain positively with monoclonal antibody OKT-6 and with antibody for S100 protein.[21] Various ultrastructural and immunohisto-

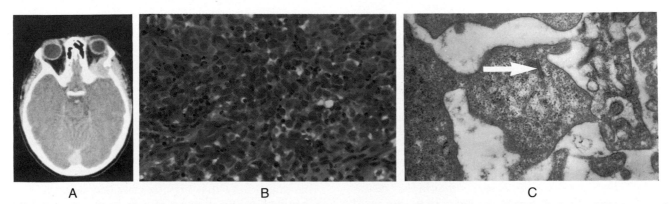

Figure 179–2. Histiocytosis X. A 13-year-old male with eosinophilic granuloma in the superior-lateral orbit. *A*, Computed tomography shows a lytic lesion with irregular borders involving the superotemporal orbit. *B*, Microscopic examination demonstrates sheets of histiocytes admixed with eosinophils and occasional lymphocytes. H&E, ×100. *C*, Electron microscopic examination of the histiocytes may show the cytoplasmic racket-shaped or cylindrical Birbeck granule (racket body, Langerhans' granule, or X body). ×27,000.

chemical studies have demonstrated that the abnormal proliferation of histiocytes in histiocytosis X is derived from Langerhans' cells.[3, 6, 20, 22]

Unfavorable prognostic signs include bone marrow involvement (as suggested by anemia and thrombocytopenia), pulmonary dysfunction or respiratory insufficiency, and absence of osteolytic lesions.[3] In general, the prognosis improves with increasing age: Younger patients are more likely to have multifocal involvement. Treatment of localized lesions, which have a favorable prognosis, is usually conservative, with limited surgery or curettage. Spontaneous remissions have been reported, probably by progressive fibrous replacement.[23] Prompt healing has been reported after intralesional corticosteroid injections in extraorbital[24] and orbital[25, 26] sites. Low-dose radiation therapy, from 300 to 1000 rad in divided doses, is effective for lesions in inaccessible areas or in sites associated with high morbidity.[15, 27] For disseminated disease, prednisone may be helpful, with the addition of chemotherapeutic agents if the response to steroids is inadequate.[3, 6, 10, 28]

GIANT CELL REPARATIVE GRANULOMA OF BONE, GIANT CELL TUMOR OF BONE, AND ANEURYSMAL BONE CYST

Giant cell reparative granuloma of bone, giant cell tumor of bone, and aneurysmal bone cyst are intraosseous lesions that contain histiocytes and may occur around the orbit, in certain cases clinically resembling orbital eosinophilic granuloma. Giant cell reparative granuloma of bone is thought to be related to trauma or intraosseous hemorrhage and originates usually in flat bones of the skull and mandible.[29–31] This lesion predominantly affects patients between the ages of 10 and 25 yr. They may report a history of trauma, but the lesions can occur without antecedent trauma. Thus, the term *reparative* may not apply, and the lesion can be referred to as *giant cell granuloma of bone*.[31] The lesions may resolve spontaneously, but definitive treatment consists of surgery or, in resistant cases, radiotherapy. The condition is benign, and healing with new bone formation follows surgical curettage. Sudden hemorrhage within the lesion may lead to rapid clinical progression. Histopathologically, these granulomas display a zonal pattern, with areas of hemorrhage, fibrosis, and osteoblastic multinucleated giant cells. Deposits of hemosiderin may be noted, as well as areas of new osteoid production and bone resorption. Multinucleated giant cells may be present and are usually found at the periphery of hemorrhagic areas. An important feature that distinguishes this lesion from eosinophilic granuloma is the absence of eosinophils.

Giant cell reparative granuloma should be distinguished from giant cell tumor of bone. In a true giant cell tumor, the giant cells are uniformly dispersed and dominate the entire field. Hemorrhage is a less promi-

nent feature. The giant cells are generally larger and more rounded, with a greater number of nuclei. The stroma is composed of predominantly plump round cells. The tumor usually does not produce new bone formation. Clinically, the two lesions can also be distinguished. Patients with giant cell tumor of bone are generally older (third and fourth decades), and it is unusual to encounter the tumor in a patient less than 20 yr old. Also, giant cell tumors have a high local recurrence rate and may metastasize.

Aneurysmal bone cyst is distinguished from giant cell reparative granuloma by the presence of large blood-filled channels in the aneurysmal bone cyst. First described by Jaffe and Lichtenstein in 1942,[32] aneurysmal bone cyst can be observed anywhere in the skeleton. This condition usually affects the metaphyses of the long bones and vertebrae but rarely may affect the bony orbit. It is a nonneoplastic lesion, which nonetheless expands and destroys bone. The overwhelming majority of patients have been adolescents and young adults, and there may be a slight predominance of females over males.[33] Most patients present with proptosis, which may be precipitous owing to intralesional hemorrhage and rapid expansion of the lesion.

The cause of these lesions is unknown. One possibility includes primary lesions of bone such as venous thrombosis or an arteriovenous communication leading to increased venous pressure within the affected area of bone. Faulty bone formation and organization of hemorrhage are other possibilities. Fibrous dysplasia has been associated with aneurysmal bone cyst,[34] possibly because of mechanical closure of venous outflow in affected areas. In addition to fibrous dysplasia, aneurysmal bone cyst–like areas may be observed in giant cell reparative granuloma, nonossifying fibroma, chondroblastoma, osteosarcoma, and fibromyxoma.[35]

The radiologic appearance of aneurysmal bone cyst may suggest the diagnosis. The affected area of bone may have a blown-out appearance, but several radiologic phases have been identified, including osteolysis, rapid growth, stabilization, and healing, with progressive ossification.[36] Computed tomography reveals a destructive lesion with patchy or rimlike enhancement surrounding a central cavity. Magnetic resonance imaging may suggest the presence of blood-breakdown products in these cavities by displaying intense signals in T_1-weighted images.[37] Angiography usually shows a mass effect, but a tumor-like blush has been observed.[37]

Microscopic examination of aneurysmal bone cyst shows a cystic appearance with non–endothelium-lined spaces that are empty or filled with blood.[38] Also seen are a fibrous stroma and a capsule containing spindle cells, hemosiderin, and often osteoid formation. Histiocytes and multinucleated giant cells are present in areas of bone resorption and repair. Treatment is usually with curettage alone; radiotherapy has been advocated for recurrent lesions.

Another entity that may be classified with this group of histiocytic intraosseous lesions is the brown tumor. This tumor, which may occur in bone or soft tissue, is discussed in Chapter 178.

HEMATIC PSEUDOCYST, CHOLESTEROL GRANULOMA, AND CHOLESTEATOMA

The terminology used in connection with accumulations of blood and blood-breakdown products has been confusing; identical terms have sometimes been used for apparently different pathologic and clinical entities. An *ecchymosis* represents the extravasation of fresh blood throughout tissues and tissue planes, which are expanded, but the blood does not loculate into a single space, real or potential. On the other hand, a *hematoma* is a focal collection of blood, which may be delimited by fascial and periorbital membranes from its inception. In the orbit, most hematomas occur subperiosteally after trauma but rarely may develop within the soft tissues of the orbit itself.

Others have used the term *blood cyst* for collections of blood in preexisting lesions, such as in a dermoid cyst or within the expanded spaces of a lymphangioma (these lesions are sometimes called *chocolate cysts*). Blood cysts are usually intraconal in location. Also, blood cysts associated with lymphangioma typically occur in patients younger than 10 yr, and the very rare blood cysts that may be associated with cavernous hemangioma are usually found in patients in their second to fourth decades. We believe that retention of the term *blood cyst* when associated with preexisting structures that have or have had a distinct epithelial or nonepithelial lining that can still be at least partially recognized is useful, and the term has the virtue of distinguishing such collections from idiopathic or posttraumatic collections of blood in spaces that are not endowed with either an epithelial or endothelial lining. The term *hematocoele* has been used for various blood-containing entities but is so indefinite in its meaning that we recommend discontinuation of its use.

The term *hematic cyst* has been used by some workers for intraosseous cholesterol granuloma formation (probably resulting from the accumulation of blood-breakdown products within the bone), as well as for a unifocal subperiosteal or soft tissue loculated chronic collection of blood and its breakdown products.[39, 40] Other terms in use have included *orbital blood cyst* without epithelial lining or *chronic hematic cysts*. For the intraosseous idiopathic or posttraumatic granuloma formation, we prefer the term *cholesterol granuloma*; for chronic subperiosteal or intraorbital soft tissue accumulations of blood-breakdown products (which often have less prominent cholesterol granulomas), we recommend the term *hematic pseudocyst*, because these lesions are not endowed with a lining of some type, which is necessary for the categorization of all true cysts. A hematic pseudocyst has a fibrous condensation or pseudocapsule without a preexistent or acquired endothelial or epithelial lining.

Hematic pseudocysts are typically located peripherally in the orbit, usually in the superotemporal orbit adjacent to or involving the frontal bone. These pseudocysts often occur in a subperiosteal location and may resemble subdural hematomas in their behavior. A rare case of an intraconal hematic pseudocyst has been reported in a 35-year-old man who suffered orbital trauma (Fig. 179–3).[41] Clinically, patients usually present with painless proptosis, frequently with diplopia, usually over a period of months to years. They may occasionally present with acute proptosis and may develop visual loss due to optic nerve compression.[42] The age of diagnosis varies widely, ranging from 5 to 54 yr,[39] and affected patients are predominantly male. Treatment of hematic pseudocyst is with surgical curettage.

Radiographic findings may be very helpful in the diagnosis of hematic pseudocyst. Computed tomography shows a well-defined nonenhancing mass usually superiorly and subperiosteally. These masses are usually extraconal and may show erosion of the surrounding bone. B-scan ultrasonography shows low internal reflectivity of the cystic cavity.[43] Arteriography, which is rarely necessary clinically, shows a mass with no blush. Although the computed tomographic findings are nonspecific, the magnetic resonance imaging findings can be characteristic but may vary temporally after acute hemorrhage. Chronic hematic pseudocysts show increased signal equal to orbital fat on T_1-weighted images and hyperintense signals to fat on T_2-weighted images.[44, 45]

The cause of hematic pseudocysts is uncertain, and the initial event is often subclinical. Trauma is the likely cause in most patients, although the trauma may not be readily associated with the symptoms of the hematic pseudocyst in the patient's view. Other possible causes of hematic pseudocyst include origination from eosinophilic granuloma, venous engorgement (such as during heavy exercise or Valsalva's maneuver), and systemic illnesses such as bleeding diatheses, scurvy, rickets, leukemia, or systemic vascular disease.[39, 40] The frontal bone is the largest concave bony surface in the orbit, and the periosteum is not as firmly attached in this area as it is elsewhere in the orbit, which may explain the preferential subperiosteal location of the hematic pseudocyst in the superior orbit.[46]

Microscopically, the hematic pseudocyst has a fibrous pseudocapsule that is not lined by epithelium or endothelium. Cholesterol clefts, chronic inflammatory cells, giant cells, lipid-laden histiocytes, and hemosiderin-containing macrophages may be present. Hematoidin bodies or crystals may be identified—red-brown birefringent crystals seen among cholesterol clefts. Hematoidin is a hemoglobin-derived pigment closely related to bilirubin, which stains with the Gmelin reaction for bile pigments (and does not stain with Prussian blue).[47] Hemosiderin in the pseudocyst may react with Prussian blue, which stains for free iron.

The cholesterol granuloma superficially resembles the hematic pseudocyst clinically and morphologically (Figs. 179–4 and 179–5).[48] Other terms for cholesterol granuloma include *lipid-containing granuloma* and *nonepithelium-containing cholesteatoma*. The term *cholesterol granuloma* is more aptly applied to often intraosseous and predominantly solid lesions, whereas the term *hematic pseudocyst* suggests at least a partially fluid-containing lesion. Both hematic pseudocyst and cholesterol

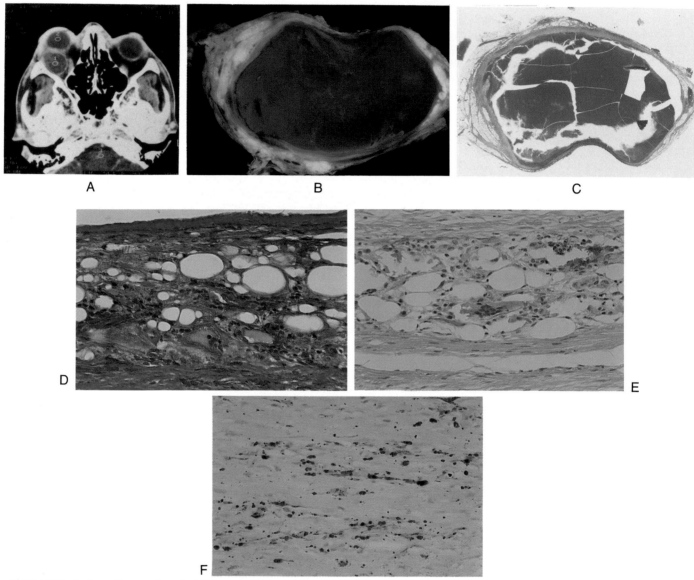

Figure 179–3. Hematic pseudocyst. A 35-year-old man with an orbital mass 2 wk after blunt trauma to the right eye. *A,* Axial computed tomography shows a well-circumscribed, cystic orbital mass (1) displacing the globe anteriorly (2). *B,* Longitudinal cut section of the orbital pseudocyst demonstrating a fibrous pseudocapsule containing blood. *C,* Low-power photomicrograph shows the blood-filled cystic mass surrounded by a fibrous pseudocapsule with adherent orbital fat. Masson's trichrome, original magnification ×1.2. *D,* Lumen (*above*) with blue-stained fibrous condensation or pseudocapsule and variable-sized clear spaces due to lipid removed during tissue processing. Masson's trichrome, ×80. *E,* Fibrous pseudocyst wall contains histiocytes and occasional multinucleated giant cells. H&E, ×62. *F,* Particulate material stains positively for iron in the pseudocyst wall. Prussian blue, ×80. This unusual hematic pseudocyst was in the orbital soft tissues rather than in the more common subperiosteal location. (*A–F,* Courtesy of J. W. Sassani, M.D., and S. Goldberg, M.D., Pennsylvania State University College of Medicine.)

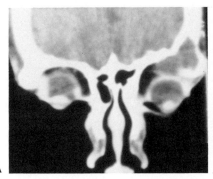 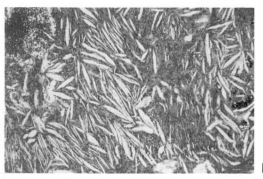

Figure 179–4. Orbital cholesterol granuloma. A 39-year-old man presented with a 1-yr history of slowly progressive left proptosis and vertical diplopia on upgaze. A, Computed tomography demonstrating erosion of bone in the superotemporal orbit with relatively smooth borders. The lesion extends into the orbit superiorly and posteriorly. B, Histologic examination shows many cholesterol clefts. H&E. (A and B, Courtesy of Peter A.D. Rubin, M.D., Massachusetts Eye and Ear Infirmary.)

granuloma are xanthomatous reactive lesions that are probably closely related or the same entity in different stages of development and organization.

Although cholesteatomas in the temporal bone are well known to otolaryngologists, cholesteatoma may occur around the orbit, especially in the frontoethmoid area.[48, 49] These lesions have also been referred to as *epidermoid cysts*.[50] The characteristic microscopic feature of this cyst is a capsule lined with hyperkeratotic squamous epithelium, which proliferates exuberantly and may extend outside of the cyst lumen. The primary orbital cholesteatoma usually originates in the frontal, sphenoid, and ethmoid diploë and may extend into neighboring structures. The primary orbital cholesteatoma probably is derived from ectodermal remnants that stay within the cranial bones during embryonic development. More rarely, secondary cholesteatoma may develop after trauma or surgery. These lesions create a well-corticated lytic defect in the bone. Magnetic resonance images of cholesteatoma and cholesterol granuloma are similar, with both lesions showing a high signal intensity in T_1-weighted images.[51] Cholesteatomas may have a typical bone defect with smooth demarcated edges associated with a sclerotic margin, which can be demonstrated by computed tomography with a bone

window setting.[50] Histopathologically, these cysts are lined by keratinizing squamous epithelium and may contain cholesterol crystals and histiocytes, but eosinophils are absent. Cholesteatomas may be distinguished from dermoid cysts by the absence of mesodermal structures such as hair follicles and sebaceous glands. Unlike cholesterol granuloma, simple cavity drainage is not adequate therapy. Complete surgical excision of the cyst lining is mandatory; otherwise, the epithelial lining continues to desquamate and expand, leading to erosion of surrounding structures. Other lesions that may resemble cholesteatoma are mucocele and chronic osteomyelitis of the frontal bone.

SINUS HISTIOCYTOSIS WITH MASSIVE LYMPHADENOPATHY

This disease is most frequent in children and young adults and is more common in blacks.[52–54] Approximately 10 percent of patients may develop ocular adnexal involvement.[55] Orbital soft tissue swelling may cause unilateral or bilateral proptosis, which can be severe in some cases. In contrast to classic proptosis, ophthalmic involvement may present with epibulbar or lid lesions,

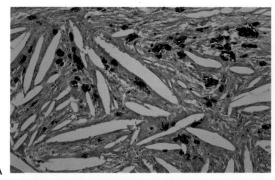 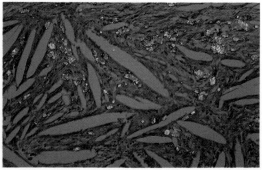

Figure 179–5. Cholesterol granuloma. A 35-year-old man presented with a 3-wk history of proptosis and downward displacement of the right eye. The patient underwent lateral orbitotomy with removal of a friable mass in the superior orbit. A, Microscopic examination showed numerous cholesterol clefts surrounded by histiocytes and occasional multinucleated foreign body–type giant cells. Numerous reddish-brown hematoidin crystals are interspersed among the cholesterol clefts. H&E, ×270. B, Under polarized light, the hematoidin crystals are highly birefringent. H&E, ×270.

with sometimes mild systemic manifestations.[55] The outstanding clinical feature is massive cervical lymphadenopathy. The retroperitoneal lymph nodes may also be involved; however, unlike other histiocytic disorders, the viscera and skin are generally unaffected. In unusual cases, the disease may present in older patients with minimal or absent lymphadenopathy.[55] The disease usually has a protracted course but is self-limited. Although the overall prognosis is favorable, the clinical course is relatively unaffected by therapy, with no proven benefit of radiotherapy or chemotherapy, which may actually worsen the condition. In a small percentage of patients, the disease can be fatal.[55] Patients may die of locally infiltrative lesions involving a vital organ, advanced multifocal disease, immunologic abnormalities, or infections. Immunologic abnormalities that can accompany the disease include autoimmune joint disease, Coombs-positive anemia, systemic amyloidosis, Wiskott-Aldrich syndrome, immunologic pancytopenia, asthma, glomerulonephritis, nephrotic syndrome, and anti–factor VIII antibodies.[55]

On gross examination, the affected orbital soft tissue may have a white cut surface, caused by abundant fibrous tissue. Low-power microscopic examination shows pale-staining areas containing histiocytes subdivided by trabeculas of connective tissue (Fig. 179–6). The histiocytes form sheets of cells and may contain engulfed erythrocytes (erythrophagocytosis), plasma cells, or lymphocytes (emperipolesis, lymphophagocytosis). Mature lymphocytes are also scattered throughout the lesion, sometimes demonstrating follicular organization.

In lymph nodes, the histiocytes are distinctively localized along the sinus channels, in both subcapsular and central medullary regions. Because there are no lymph nodes in the orbit, the affected areas contain randomly dispersed lymphocytes and histiocytes, without an organized topography. Ultrastructural studies have failed to demonstrate the cytoplasmic inclusions typical of Langerhans' cells, suggesting that this lesion has a histiocytic heritage that is distinct from eosinophilic granuloma[56, 57]; the cells, however, are S100-positive but OKT6-negative.

JUVENILE XANTHOGRANULOMA

Although juvenile xanthogranuloma most commonly affects the skin, the eyes are the most common location for extracutaneous lesions.[58] The disease is familiar to ophthalmologists because it usually is manifested in the eye as a xanthogranulomatous infiltration of the iris, which can cause hyphema and glaucoma. Primary orbital involvement with juvenile xanthogranuloma is rare. Zimmerman reported five patients with orbital involvement, four of whom had no skin involvement.[59] The lesion was present at birth in three of the cases and at 2 to 3 mo of age in the other cases. Bone erosion was noted in one of the cases, the details of which were published subsequently.[60–62] Gaynes and Cohen described an 8-month-old girl with massive proptosis and no skin lesions.[63] A patient with congenital macronodular juvenile xanthogranuloma affecting the eyelids and

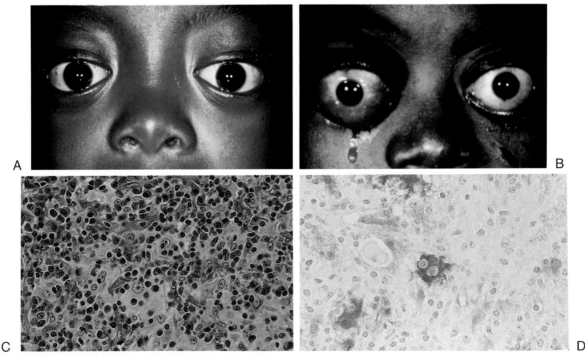

Figure 179–6. Sinus histiocytosis with massive lymphadenopathy. *A,* A 4-year-old boy with bilateral symmetric proptosis. (Courtesy of David S. Friendly, M.D.) *B,* Bilateral proptosis, with a visible subconjunctival mass in the right eye. Microscopically, the orbital lesions are composed of lobules of histiocytes admixed with mononuclear inflammatory cells separated by dense bands of connective tissue. (Courtesy of Pierre Dhermy, M.D.) *C,* High-power view shows polymorphic infiltrate of histiocytes, lymphocytes, and plasma cells. The cytoplasm of the histiocytes may contain lymphocytes, erythrocytes, or plasma cells, as demonstrated in this photomicrograph. H&E, ×128. *D,* The histiocytes stain positively for S100 antigen (immunoperoxidase stain).

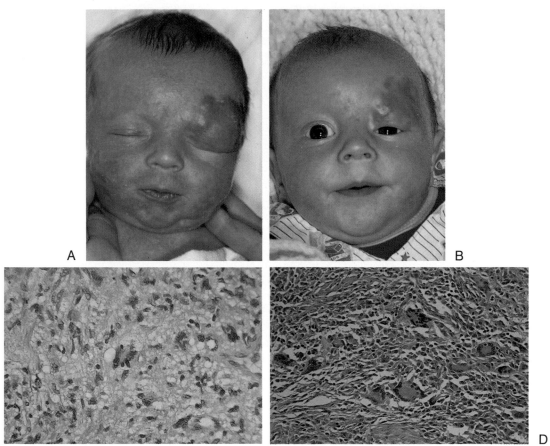

Figure 179–7. Juvenile xanthogranuloma. A full-term male infant presented with a congenital left upper eyelid lesion. Biopsy of the yellowish-red nodular mass showed juvenile xanthogranuloma. *A*, Complete ptosis of the left upper eyelid before therapy. *B*, Two weeks after intralesional corticosteroid injection, the lesion has significantly regressed and the eyelid is elevated above the pupil. The lesion continued to improve and nearly completely disappeared 1 yr after treatment. *C*, Microscopic examination shows vacuolated histiocytes with a Touton giant cell in the center of the field. H&E, ×100. (*A–C*, From Schwartz TL, Carter KD, Judisch GF, et al: Congenital macronodular juvenile xanthogranuloma of the eyelid. Ophthalmology 98:1230, 1991.) *D*, Photomicrograph of another orbital lesion shows sheets of benign-appearing histiocytes with occasional Touton giant cells. (Courtesy of C. L. Shields, Wills Eye Hospital.)

anterior orbit has been reported (Fig. 179–7).[64] Shields and coworkers reported a patient with solitary orbital involvement with juvenile xanthogranuloma that was present at birth (Fig. 179–8).[65] This patient had a superonasal orbital and preseptal mass but no skin lesions. Because there are no unique or totally reliable clinical features, although cutaneous lesions are usually orange or yellow, the diagnosis is made after biopsy. Once the diagnosis is confirmed by biopsy, the lesion may be observed, because spontaneous resolution can be expected to occur. Systemic corticosteroids may be used when the mass is large or causes damage to ocular structures.[63] Low-dose radiotherapy may be attempted in refractory cases.

Microscopic examination reveals sheets of histiocytes and the diagnostic cell of juvenile xanthogranuloma, the Touton giant cell. In this cell, a central annulus of nuclei encloses a central eosinophilic cytoplasm, and the outer cytoplasm is pale and vacuolated. The background stroma is composed of lymphocytes, plasma cells, and occasional eosinophils admixed with the mononucleated polygonal and spindled histiocytes. Electron microscopic examination fails to reveal Langerhans' granules, as found in the eosinophilic granuloma group of conditions, and the cells are S100-negative.

ERDHEIM-CHESTER DISEASE

Erdheim-Chester disease is a rare and potentially fatal lipogranulomatous disorder that was reported by Chester in 1930.[66] Most patients with Erdheim-Chester disease do not have orbital involvement; however, Alper and colleagues reported the first two orbital cases in 1983.[67] More recently, Shields and associates have reported two cases.[68] Patients with orbital involvement present with progressive bilateral exophthalmos, which may lead to ophthalmoplegia and visual loss due to compressive optic neuropathy (Fig. 179–9). Xanthelasma-type lid lesions are noted; they are more indurated than the ordinary velvety xanthelasma (Fig. 179–10). The presence of these indurated xanthelasma-type lesions and bilateral proptosis should bring to mind the possibility of Erdheim-Chester disease.

Biopsy of the orbital lesion shows fibrosing xanthogranulomas that exhibit xanthomatous histiocytes, fibro-

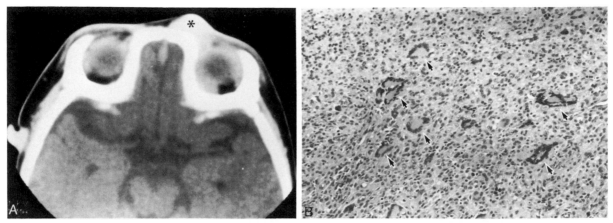

Figure 179–8. Orbital juvenile xanthogranuloma. *A,* Computed tomography shows an extraconal soft tissue density that extends from the left preseptal region *(asterisk)* posteriorly along the medial orbital wall back to the orbital apex. *B,* Photomicrograph demonstrates dense background of benign histiocytes containing occasional Touton giant cells. Several Touton giant cells are designated by arrows. H&E, ×50. (From Shields CL, Shields JA, Buchanon HW: Solitary orbital involvement with juvenile xanthogranuloma. Arch Ophthalmol 108:1588, 1990. Copyright 1990, American Medical Association.)

sis with collagenation, and Touton giant cells. Unlike the histiocytosis X group, the histiocytes do not stain for S100 protein, and no Langerhans' granules are seen.[67] Mononuclear inflammatory cells, such as lymphocytes, may be admixed in the sheets of xanthoma cells. These xanthoma cells have small central nuclei and abundant vacuolated pale cytoplasm, which is due to loss of lipid during routine paraffin embedding. The xanthoma cells are histiocytes with imbibed lipid, which in Erdheim-Chester disease is predominantly choles-

terol. In Erdheim-Chester disease, abnormalities of the lipid profile of peripheral blood are generally not found. Although the cause of this disorder is unknown, the abnormality in histiocytes may be in cellular metabolism or processing of ingested lipid.

Touton giant cells are also found in necrobiotic xanthogranuloma, in juvenile xanthogranuloma, and rarely in liposarcoma. In considering this differential diagnosis, no necrobiotic foci are found in Erdheim-Chester disease as they are in necrobiotic xanthogranuloma. Pa-

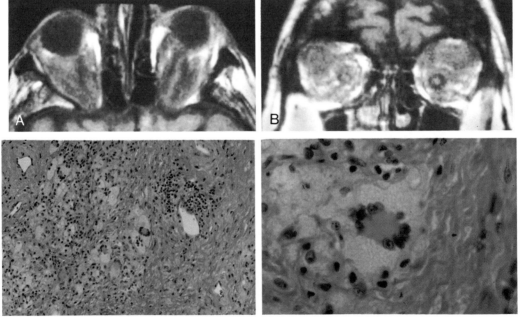

Figure 179–9. Erdheim-Chester disease. A 68-year-old white man developed shortness of breath and also noted progressive bilateral proptosis, visual loss, and ophthalmoplegia over 1 mo. He was found to have diabetes insipidus, pericardial and pleural effusions, hydronephrosis, and ascites, with bilateral orbital masses and disc edema. Radiographically, patchy lytic and sclerotic lesions were noted in the long bones. The patient's vision improved rapidly after orbital decompression, and he improved transiently after treatment with systemic steroids but died 6 mo later. Axial *(A)* and coronal *(B)* computed tomography demonstrating bilateral soft tissue infiltrating masses. *C,* Low-power microscopy shows xanthomatous histiocytes *(left)* and fibrosis (more prominent to the *right*) admixed with Touton giant cells and mononuclear inflammatory cells. H&E. *D,* Higher power shows xanthomatous histiocytes, lymphocytes, and a Touton giant cell. H&E. *(A–D,* Courtesy of Irma M. Lessell, M.D., Lahey Clinic.)

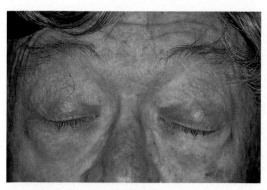

Figure 179–10. Firm yellow lesions of the eyelid in a patient with Erdheim-Chester disease. Although they superficially resemble xanthelasma, these lid lesions are more indurated than ordinary xanthelasma. (Courtesy of J.A. Shields, M.D., Ocular Oncology Service, Wills Eye Hospital.)

tients with juvenile xanthogranuloma are typically young, whereas Erdheim-Chester disease has been reported in older patients. Also, some morphologic differences in the histiocytes are reported among these disorders.[67] Although they contain lipids, the histiocytes in juvenile xanthogranuloma may be smaller and are not xanthomatous. The most important difference is that it is rare for patients with juvenile xanthogranuloma to have serious systemic involvement. In contrast, systemic involvement is characteristic of Erdheim-Chester disease.

In Erdheim-Chester disease, pathognomonic radiographic changes in the skeleton consist of symmetric bilateral patchy lytic and sclerotic lesions and thickening of metaphyses. Nuclear medicine studies show symmetric bilateral radionuclide uptake in areas of bony abnormality. These areas of bone involvement may be painful or they may be asymptomatic. Other possible systemic manifestations of Erdheim-Chester disease include pleural and pericardial effusion, pulmonary fibrosis, cardiac decompensation, atherosclerosis, cerebrovascular accident, retroperitoneal xanthogranuloma or fibrosis, and bilateral hydronephrosis. Systemic corticosteroid therapy may cause transient improvement of orbital and extraorbital disease, but such therapy is often ineffective.

ADULT ORBITAL XANTHOGRANULOMA

Identification of orbital xanthogranuloma should initiate a search for involvement of bone and other organ systems, in order to establish the diagnosis of Erdheim-Chester disease. In the absence of systemic findings, an orbital xanthogranuloma in an adult would be comparable to the isolated orbital juvenile or infantile xanthogranuloma. Such an isolated orbital lesion has been described in a 38-year-old woman with painless progressive bilateral proptosis of 16-yr duration (Fig. 179–11).[69] Biopsy demonstrated xanthogranuloma, and systemic evaluation showed no involvement of bones or other organ systems. In this patient, the bilateral orbital lesions were resistant to corticosteroid therapy, but total

remission was achieved with a combination of systemic corticosteroid therapy and orbital radiation therapy, without evidence of recurrence during a 3-yr follow-up period. Three additional cases of orbital xanthogranuloma in adults have been described.[70] These patients presented with yellow cutaneous periorbital plaques and anterior-superior orbital involvement. They were treated with systemic chemotherapy, causing a marked improvement clinically.

We have identified two patients at the Massachusetts Eye and Ear Infirmary with isolated orbital xanthogranuloma. One was a 54-year-old man who presented with a 6-yr history of proptosis and who then developed diplopia and subcutaneous waxy yellow nodules on the eyelids bilaterally. Systemic evaluation was unrevealing, and biopsy showed large polyhedral xanthoma cells, Touton giant cells, and lymphoid follicles. Another patient was a 43-year-old man with a 6-mo history of progressive eyelid swelling. Biopsy showed the typical findings of xanthogranuloma with Touton giant cells, and a thorough systemic evaluation was unrevealing. These patients developed asthma coincident with the onset of orbital disease (Mills M, Dallow R, and Jakobiec F: Personal communication, 1992). This phenomenon may be similar to sinus histiocytosis with massive lymphadenopathy, in which immunologic abnormalities such as asthma can accompany the disease.[55]

This adult-onset primary orbital xanthogranuloma should be distinguished from Erdheim-Chester disease, which is characterized by systemic involvement. Necrobiotic xanthogranuloma may be distinguished by dysproteinemia and histologic findings. Careful analysis of additional adult patients with isolated orbital involvement will help to establish adult orbital xanthogranuloma as a separate nosologic entity.

PSEUDORHEUMATOID NODULES

Pseudorheumatoid subcutaneous nodules resemble rheumatoid nodules in their microscopic appearance but occur in children who are otherwise healthy and have no evidence of systemic rheumatic disease. Rarely, these lesions can occur in adults and are usually found on the extremities and scalp. They have been reported less commonly in the periocular skin near the orbital rim.[71, 72] Although trauma is probably not an important factor, some history of trauma is reported in less than 25 percent of reported cases.[71] One study described 21 cases in children and young adults who had lesions usually in the lateral upper eyelid and outer canthal region.[73] The lesions were multiple in five cases, and some lesions clinically appeared to be "cystic" because they were soft and fluctuant. Local recurrences developed in 20 percent of cases, but by definition, none of the patients developed rheumatoid fever, rheumatoid arthritis, or any evidence of systemic disease. The lesions were treated with simple excision.

Histologically, the lesions are necrobiotic granulomas that contain stellate areas of necrobiosis surrounded by palisading reactive fibroblasts and histiocytes (Fig. 179–12). The necrobiotic areas contain homogenized colla-

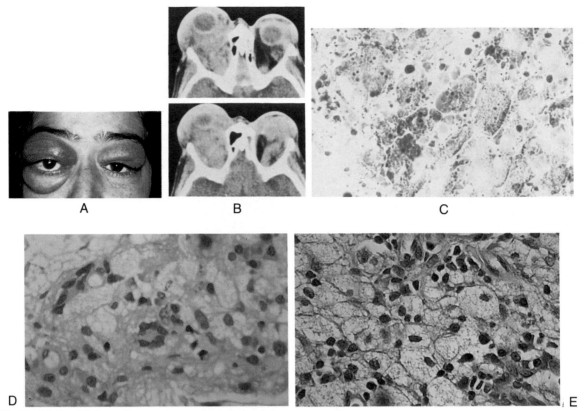

Figure 179–11. Adult orbital xanthogranuloma. *A,* Patient with severe bilateral proptosis and swollen eyelids; the right side is more severely affected than the left. Systemic evaluation showed no involvement of bones or other organs. *B,* Axial computed tomography showing dense bilateral soft tissue mass lesions; the right orbit is more severely affected than the left. *C,* Frozen section of xanthoma cells containing intracytoplasmic lipid, which is stained red. Oil red O, ×350. *D,* A Touton giant cell is present centrally, with a background of mononucleated xanthoma cells. *E,* Xanthoma cells with foamy vacuolated, pale cytoplasm and small nuclei. (*A–E,* Courtesy of A. Hidayat, Armed Forces Institute of Pathology.)

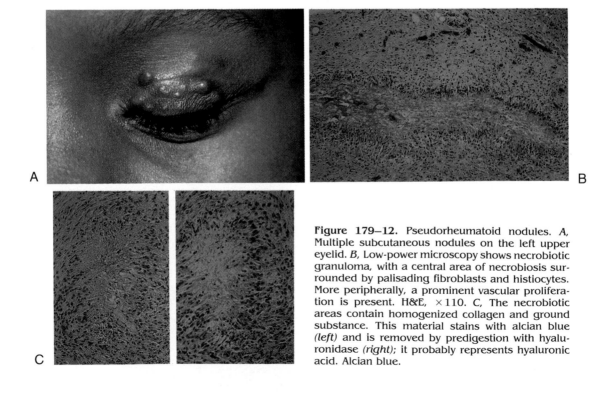

Figure 179–12. Pseudorheumatoid nodules. *A,* Multiple subcutaneous nodules on the left upper eyelid. *B,* Low-power microscopy shows necrobiotic granuloma, with a central area of necrobiosis surrounded by palisading fibroblasts and histiocytes. More peripherally, a prominent vascular proliferation is present. H&E, ×110. *C,* The necrobiotic areas contain homogenized collagen and ground substance. This material stains with alcian blue *(left)* and is removed by predigestion with hyaluronidase *(right)*; it probably represents hyaluronic acid. Alcian blue.

gen and increased amounts of ground substance, which is sensitive to hyaluronidase and probably represents hyaluronic acid. Phosphotungstic acid–hematoxylin staining shows no evidence of fibrinoid necrosis or fibrinous material in the necrobiotic areas. A variable mononuclear lymphocytic and plasmacytic infiltrate is present. Occasional eosinophils and multinucleated giant cells can be seen but are not typical. There may be changes suggestive of focal arteritis, with endothelial proliferation in some areas. This entity can be distinguished clinically and histopathologically from other similar lesions, including systemic lupus erythematosus, rheumatoid nodules, granuloma annulare, and necrobiosis lipoidica diabeticorum.[72]

NECROBIOTIC XANTHOGRANULOMA

Necrobiotic xanthogranuloma with paraproteinemia is an unusual histiocytic disorder that was first described by Kossard and Winkelmann in 1980.[74] Subsequent reports have emphasized the ophthalmic features of this disease.[75–79] It is characterized by dysproteinemia and multiple yellow xanthomatous skin lesions, which show a predilection for the periorbital area, face, trunk, and proximal part of the limbs.[80] In a study of 22 patients, 13 (59 percent) were women and 9 (41 percent) were men.[80] The mean age of the patients at diagnosis was 53 yr, with a range of 26 to 71 yr.

The condition is accompanied by hematologic abnormalities, particularly dysproteinemia. In the cases in which immunoelectrophoresis was performed, the dysproteinemia was frequently due to a monoclonal IgG paraprotein.[74] Other inconstant findings include a low serum complement level, cryoglobulinemia, anemia, leukopenia, and hyperlipidemia. The erythrocyte sedimentation rate is typically elevated. Myeloma and other lymphoproliferative disorders may be present.

Periocular involvement is found in nearly all cases and is usually manifested by the development of multiple painless nonpruritic nodules or plaques involving the eyelid skin. These lesions may appear as either waxy xanthomatous plaques, deeper violaceous plaques, or flesh-colored nodules, which can undergo ulceration and scarring. The subcutaneous lid lesions may extend into the anterior orbit, and there may be an orbital mass associated with proptosis.[80] Other less common ophthalmic findings include conjunctival involvement, keratitis, scleritis or episcleritis, glaucoma, and anterior uveitis.[76, 80] One patient has been reported to have associated Cogan's syndrome (interstitial keratitis with vestibuloauditory dysfunction).[79] The eyelid lesions may be so severe that they cause eyelid dysfunction such as lagophthalmos,[75] which can lead to corneal ulceration and loss of the eye.[74, 80]

Histopathologically, the lesions are characterized by areas of eosinophilic collagen degeneration or necrobiosis and granuloma formation (Fig. 179–13). Broad bands of hyaline necrobiosis, which separate granulomatous masses, are found. Cellular masses consist of

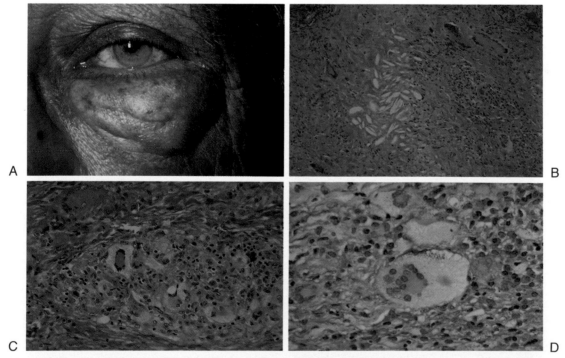

Figure 179–13. Necrobiotic xanthogranuloma. *A,* Yellowish mass in the left lower lid. *B,* An area of eosinophilic collagen degeneration (necrobiosis) is surrounded by histiocytes, giant cells, and lymphocytes. *C,* Areas of xanthomatous histiocytes, lymphocytes, and multinucleated giant cells (Touton and foreign-body types) are separated by bands of hyaline necrobiosis. *D,* Higher power micrograph of a Touton giant cell with a background of xanthoma cells.

sheets of histiocytes as well as giant cells and lesser numbers of lymphocytes. A prominent finding is numerous giant cells, both Touton and foreign-body types. Foci of xanthomatization confer a foamy appearance to the cytoplasm of the histiocytes and giant cells. Involvement of the skin from the middermis through the panniculus is common, with an apparent "Touton cell panniculitis."[80] Lymphoid nodules, foci of plasma cells, and cholesterol clefts may also be noted. The histiocytes and giant cells fail to show significant anti–S100 protein immunohistochemical staining.

Several diseases may cause xanthomatous deposits in the periorbital area. Included in the clinical differential diagnosis are xanthelasma (xanthoma planum), xanthoma tuberosum, generalized plane normolipemic xanthoma, xanthoma disseminatum, the various xanthomas of hyperlipidemia, Erdheim-Chester disease, juvenile xanthogranuloma, and necrobiosis lipoidica.[80] Necrobiosis lipoidica, which tends to affect the pretibial areas in diabetic patients, can in unusual instances produce xanthomatous lesions in the periorbital region.[81, 82] In addition to necrobiosis lipoidica, other conditions that may share similar histopathologic findings include granuloma annulare, subcutaneous rheumatoid nodules, and pseudorheumatoid nodules. These disorders can be distinguished on the basis of their associated clinical findings.[75, 80] Pseudorheumatoid nodules, for example, generally affect children, whereas necrobiotic xanthogranuloma generally affects patients in their fifth and sixth decades.

The clinical course of necrobiotic xanthogranuloma is characterized by progressive local tissue destruction, with rare spontaneous remissions. The response to local therapy, with surgical excision and intralesional or topical steroids, is usually poor.[80] Surgical excision has been associated with recurrence and increased disease activity.[76] Local radiotherapy has been beneficial in cutaneous disease[80] and has been reported to cause stable remission in one patient with orbital disease.[78] The systemic disease may cause death in up to half of affected individuals.[74, 76, 79, 80] Systemic corticosteroids have shown variable success rates. The most favorable response has been with low doses of systemically administered chemotherapeutic agents.

GIANT CELL POLYMYOSITIS

Orbital involvement may occur in giant cell polymyositis, which is a severe and potentially fatal disorder. In one case report, extraocular muscle inflammation was described as the initial and most prominent manifestation of the disease.[83] A 37-year-old Costa Rican woman developed severe bilateral painful proptosis and ophthalmoplegia. She subsequently had facial, pharyngeal, laryngeal, and cardiac muscle involvement. After a partial and temporary response to a combination of steroids and chemotherapy, the patient developed a cardiac arrhythmia and died 18 mo after the onset of symptoms. Klein and colleagues reported a similar case of severe granulomatous myositis.[84] Their patient was a 65-year-old woman who also died of a cardiac arrhythmia.

Although histologic findings showed extraocular muscle inflammation without giant cells, examination of the myocardium showed severe giant cell myocarditis, suggesting that this case represents a variant of giant cell polymyositis.

As illustrated by these cases, giant cell polymyositis is often refractory to therapy with corticosteroids or other medications. Myocardial involvement is characterized by a short clinical course, with frequent occurrence of sudden death due to arrhythmia or fulminating congestive heart failure. Histologic features include diffuse destruction of muscle fibers with infiltration by histiocytes, lymphocytes, and multinucleated giant cells (Fig. 179–14). Both polymyositis and dermatomyositis can cause ophthalmoplegia[85]; however, biopsy specimens demonstrate absence of granulomatous inflammation with giant cells in the latter. In contrast to the more common form of idiopathic orbital myositis, orbital granulomatous myositis is in the spectrum of giant cell polymyositis and is associated with a guarded prognosis.

SARCOIDOSIS

Sarcoidosis is a multisystem granulomatous disease of unknown origin, often affecting young adults. The most common manifestations are bilateral hilar adenopathy, pulmonary infiltrates, skin lesions, and ocular or ocular adnexal involvement. The black population of the United States has the highest rate of sarcoidosis in the world, followed by the white populations of Norway, Sweden, and Ireland.[86] The risk of sarcoidosis is ten times higher in black adults than in whites in the United States. Women are at two to three times greater risk for the development of sarcoidosis than men. The disease usually presents in adults between 20 and 40 yr of age but can rarely occur in children[87, 88]; it is usually sporadic but can be familial.

The term sarcoidosis refers to a disseminated multisystem disease, whereas the term sarcoid may be used to describe an isolated focal lesion.[89] Because sarcoidosis is by definition a multisystem disease, Jakobiec and Jones consider the rare cases of isolated orbital involvement to be examples of granulomatous pseudotumor rather than true sarcoidosis.[90] Alternatively, Jakobiec has referred to these patients as having a sarcoidal reaction pattern limited to the orbit.[91] Such patients are often women in late middle age. True orbital sarcoidosis may be defined as a spontaneously arising mass of the orbit that histologically demonstrates the characteristic granulomatous reaction and occurs in the context of systemic sarcoidosis involving at least one other remote body site. Most patients who present with orbital sarcoid are subsequently found to have systemic sarcoidosis when they undergo complete physical, laboratory, and radiologic examinations, although isolated orbital "sarcoid" granulomas can rarely occur.[92] The rare patient with orbital sarcoidal granulomas but no other systemic findings should be questioned about previous orbital trauma, and polarized microscopy should be performed to rule out granulomatous response to a retained foreign body.

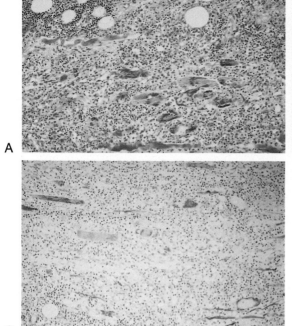

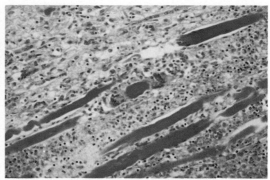

Figure 179–14. Giant cell polymyositis. *A,* Microscopic examination of a biopsy specimen shows replacement of most of the muscle tissue with a chronic inflammatory infiltrate consisting of histiocytes, eosinophils, lymphocytes, and multinucleated giant cells. H&E. *B,* Higher power shows remnants of degenerated skeletal muscle with giant cells on both sides of one fragment. There is a dense background infiltrate of histiocytic cells and lymphocytes. *C,* Immunohistochemical staining for muscle-specific actin shows that the small fragments are remnants of degenerated muscle cells. (*A–C,* Courtesy of L. E. Zimmerman, M.D.)

In the orbit, the most frequent site of involvement is the lacrimal gland, typically bilaterally (Fig. 179–15).[93–96] Only 7 to 15 percent of patients with systemic sarcoidosis have clinically detectable enlargement of the lacrimal gland,[97] although special imaging studies reveal a higher proportion of involvement. The typical computed tomographic appearance is that of a molded, V-shaped lesion of the superotemporal orbit extending beyond the orbital rim.[94] The V or wedge configuration is due to superimposition of the enlarged palpebral and orbital lobes. Gallium scanning is a highly sensitive but nonspecific method for demonstrating lacrimal gland involvement; it can be diagnostically helpful, particularly in patients with recent onset of disease.[98] In one series, the gallium images showed increased activity in 80 percent of lacrimal glands, whether or not they were clinically detectably enlarged.[99]

Orbital sarcoid granulomas may present with proptosis, lid swelling, pain, reduced visual acuity, or less commonly diplopia and ptosis.[88] In addition to lacrimal gland disease, granulomas may quite atypically be found in the fibroadipose tissue and extraocular muscles of the orbit. It should be remembered that the most common sign of ophthalmic involvement with sarcoidosis is uveitis. However, rare soft tissue orbital lesions may have extraocular muscle or optic nerve involvement and involvement of adjacent paranasal sinuses.[100–105] Radiographs show evidence of bone destruction.[103] Clinically, orbital involvement is usually unilateral and is more likely to occur in adults, although it has been reported in children.[88]

If sarcoidosis is suspected and the patient has visible nodules in the conjunctiva, a conjunctival biopsy can be diagnostic.[101, 106] If a lacrimal gland biopsy is necessary, it is preferable to sample the deeper orbital lobe through the lid, concealing the scar in a lid fold. The superficial lobe contains the ducts that drain from the deeper orbital lobe; therefore, a minimal amount of tissue should be sampled or, preferably, biopsy of the palpebral lobe should be avoided. Chest radiographs should be taken to identify the presence of typical hilar adenopathy or pulmonary infiltrates. Radiographs of the hands may

Figure 179–15. Sarcoidosis. *A,* Axial computed tomography shows bilateral enlargement of the lacrimal glands, more prominently on the right. The lesions show the characteristic molded V shape extending beyond the orbital rim. *B,* Biopsy demonstrates noncaseating granuloma with epithelioid histiocytes and mononuclear inflammatory cells. A dense mononuclear inflammatory infiltrate is seen at the periphery, admixed with lacrimal gland. H&E, ×40.

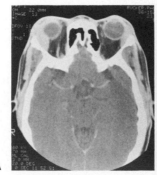

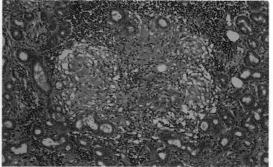

show small lytic lesions. Laboratory evaluation should include angiotensin converting enzyme, lysozyme, and calcium levels. Intracutaneous injection of sarcoidal antigen in the Kveim test can confirm the diagnosis. Gallium scanning can be helpful in demonstrating uptake over the orbits, parotid glands, and lungs. The association of sarcoid uveitis with parotid involvement and facial nerve palsy is referred to as *Heerfordt's syndrome* (uveoparotid fever).

Histologically, the lesions are noncaseating granulomas. The absence of caseation necrosis is evidence against the diagnosis of tuberculosis. The granulomas consist of collections of epithelioid histiocytes with scattered mononuclear inflammatory cells. The term *naked granulomas* is used when mononuclear inflammatory cells are sparse or nearly absent. Multinucleated giant cells and cytoplasmic inclusions (asteroid bodies and conchoid bodies) may be observed. These giant cells have nuclei present at the periphery of the cytoplasm. No specific ultrastructural features have been described, except that the histiocytes lack Langerhans' granules or other inclusions. Studies of T-cell subsets have demonstrated a zonal distribution within the granulomas, with helper T cells locating preferentially in the central areas and suppressor T cells locating at the periphery, possibly helping to contain the outward extension of the granulomas.[21]

Spontaneous resolution of orbital lesions is rare. Systemic corticosteroid therapy is the mainstay of treatment, with initial prednisone doses usually in the range of 60 to 100 mg/day. Improvement may occur within days but occurs usually by 3 to 6 wk. Recurrences following cessation of steroid therapy are common. In chronic cases, progressive fibrosis may occur, and treatment may require surgical excision.

TUBEROUS XANTHOMA

Tuberous xanthomas may occur in association with familial hypercholesterolemia, broad-beta disease, cerebrotendinous xanthomatosis, and β-sitosterolemia but may occur in apparently normolipemic patients.[107] These usually large subcutaneous lesions have a predilection for the fingers, elbows, knees, and buttocks; however, they may occur in the periorbital area (Fig. 179–16).[108] Histologically, sheets of lipid-laden histiocytes are found, as well as cholesterol clefts and multinucleated giant cells. In chronic lesions, proliferation of fibroblasts may occur. The marked fibrosis observed in long-standing tuberous xanthomas may be related to the fibrogenic properties of extracellular cholesterol, which may extravasate from abnormally permeable blood vessels in these lesions. These lesions differ from xanthelasma in that they are more deeply located and contain foamy histiocytes and multinucleated giant cells as well as extracellular cholesterol deposits, fibrosis, and inflammatory cells.

It may be difficult to distinguish tuberous xanthoma from fibrous histiocytoma. Cutaneous fibrous histiocytoma can occur anywhere but frequently afflicts the lower extremities. The eyelids are an unusual location for the cutaneous type of fibrous histiocytoma.[109] The deep type of fibrous histiocytoma has a predilection for

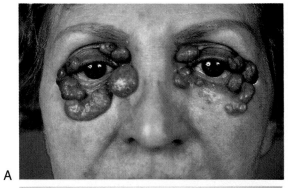

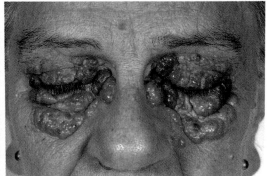

Figure 179–16. Tuberous xanthoma. *A*, Multiple firm, nontender yellowish nodules of 6-yr duration involving upper and lower eyelids bilaterally. (Courtesy of M.O.M. Tso, M.D.) *B*, Long-standing bilateral firm yellowish masses of the upper and lower eyelids. (Courtesy of F. Buffam, M.D., and J. Rootman, M.D.) *C*, Microscopic examination shows multinucleated giant cells and histiocytes with a fibrous background.

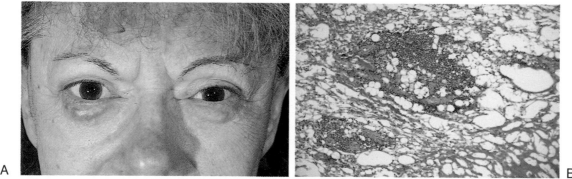

Figure 179–17. Lipogranuloma. *A,* Chronic bilateral lower eyelid masses following cosmetic silicone injections. *B,* Histologically, spaces of various sizes are surrounded by collagen and mononuclear inflammatory cells, with few remaining histiocytes. The clear spaces contained silicone removed during tissue processing. (*A* and *B,* Courtesy of E. H. Sacks, M.D.)

the orbit.[110–113] Cutaneous fibrous histiocytoma is a poorly demarcated lesion consisting of interlacing fascicles of fibroblastic cells that exhibit a vague storiform pattern admixed with histiocytic cells and multinucleated giant cells. Epidermal hyperplasia and basal cell layer hyperpigmentation may be found. Deep fibrous histiocytomas are similar, but they may demonstrate a more marked storiform pattern and may contain focal collections of lipid-laden histiocytes. The stroma may also exhibit myxoid changes and areas of hyalinization, and transitional stages between the histiocytic and fibroblastic cells may be observed. Patients with hyperlipidemia may have a more prominent histiocytic component and cholesterol clefts, potentially causing confusion with

tuberous xanthoma.[114] Similarly, chronic tuberous xanthomas may show increased fibrosis and may be difficult to distinguish morphologically from fibrous histiocytoma.

ORBITAL LIPOGRANULOMA

Orbital lipogranuloma represents the response of mononucleated or multinucleated histiocytes to extracellular lipid. The lipogranuloma may be caused by exogenous material, such as silicone or paraffin. Alternatively, damage to orbital lipocytes by trauma or inflammation or even fat necrosis due to vasculitis may

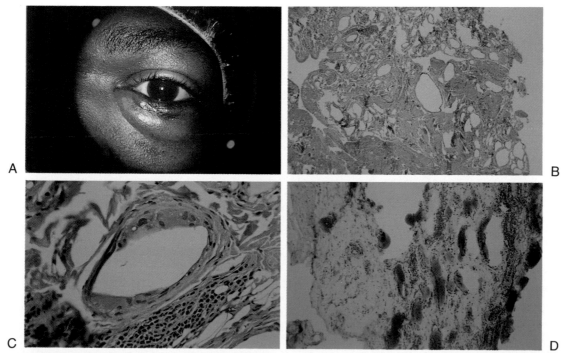

Figure 179–18. Oleogranuloma. A 22-year-old black man injected himself with petroleum jelly in the lower eyelids to attempt cosmetic improvement. *A,* Lower eyelid mass several weeks after injection of petroleum jelly. *B,* Histologically, muscle and subcutaneous tissue are infiltrated with chronic nongranulomatous inflammatory cells and numerous clear spaces of various sizes. H&E. *C,* Clear spaces are lined with epithelioid cells containing foamy cytoplasm; some of the cells are multinucleated. H&E. (*A–C,* Courtesy of S. S. Searl, M.D., Rochester, NY.) *D,* Frozen section stained with oil red O demonstrates lipid material in the spaces. Oil red O. (From Boynton JR, Searl SS, Heimer JL, et al: Eyelid oleogranulomas caused by petroleum jelly injection. Arch Ophthalmol 106:551, 1988. Copyright 1988, American Medical Association.)

lead to lipogranuloma formation. Rupture of a dermoid cyst may also release oily material into the orbit, inciting lipogranuloma formation. A lipogranuloma should be distinguished from a xanthogranuloma. In a lipogranuloma, histiocytes surround prominent extracellular collections of lipid, which may leave empty spaces of various sizes during tissue processing (Fig. 179–17). In contrast, a xanthogranuloma contains histiocytes with myriad intracytoplasmic vacuoles. When the cytoplasm is honeycombed and rarefied by these vacuoles, the xanthoma cells are called *foam cells*.

Several unusual cases of lipogranuloma caused by exogenous material have been reported. Paraffin has been injected around the eye, with an undesirable cosmetic result.[115] In one patient, injection of silicone oil caused lipogranulomas and eyelid deformities.[116] In another patient, silicone oil was injected into a postenucleation socket, causing an exuberant response that ultimately led to debulking surgery (Chavis R, Zimmerman LE: Personal communication, 1987). We have seen a 57-year-old woman who had silicone injection into both lower eyelids for cosmetic reasons, resulting in progressive lipogranuloma formation over a 15-yr period. Boynton and coworkers described a 22-year-old black man who injected himself in the lower lids with petroleum jelly (Vaseline) in an attempt to improve his appearance.[117] He developed prominent oleogranulomas, which were removed 4 mo after the initial injection (Fig. 179–18). Lipogranulomas due to exogenous materials in the orbit resemble those found in other body areas that have been augmented or altered by oily materials, usually for attempted cosmetic improvement.

REFERENCES

1. Lichtenstein L: Histiocytosis X: Integration of eosinophilic granuloma of bone, "Letterer-Siwe disease" and "Schüller-Christian disease" as related manifestations of single nosologic entity. Arch Pathol 56:84, 1953.
2. Lichtenstein L, Jaffe HL: Eosinophilic granuloma of bone with report of a case. Am J Pathol 16:595, 1940.
3. Nolph MB, Luikin GA: Histiocytosis X. Otolaryngol Clin North Am 15:635, 1982.
4. Favara BE, Jaffe R: Pathology of Langerhans' cell histiocytosis. Hematol Oncol Clin North Am 1:75, 1987.
5. McClelland J, Pritchard J, Chu AC: Current controversies. Hematol Oncol Clin North Am 1:147, 1987.
6. Char DH, Ablin A, Beckstead J: Histiocytic disorders of the orbit. Ann Ophthalmol 16:867, 1984.
7. Shields JA: Histiocytic tumors and pseudotumors. *In* Shields JA (ed): Diagnosis and Management of Orbital Tumors. Philadelphia, WB Saunders, 1989.
8. Oberman HA: Idiopathic histiocytosis: A correlative review of eosinophilic granuloma, Hand-Schüller-Christian disease and Letterer-Siwe disease. J Pediatr Ophthalmol 5:86, 1968.
9. Bray PT: Histiocytosis X. *In* Deeley TJ (ed): Modern Radiotherapy and Oncology: Malignant Disease in Childhood. London, Butterworth, 1974.
10. Moore AT, Pritchard J, Taylor DSI: Histiocytosis X: An ophthalmological review. Br J Ophthalmol 69:7, 1985.
11. Wood CM, Pearson ADJ, Craft AD, et al: Globe luxation in histiocytosis X. Br J Ophthalmol 72:631, 1988.
12. Gross FJ, Waxman JS, Rosenblatt MA, et al: Eosinophilic granuloma of the cavernous sinus and orbital apex in an HIV-positive patient. Ophthalmology 96:462, 1989.
13. Baghdassarian SA, Shammas HF: Eosinophilic granuloma of the orbit. Ann Ophthalmol 9:1247, 1977.
14. Feldman RB, Moore DM, Hood CI, et al: Solitary eosinophilic granuloma of the lateral orbital mass. Am J Ophthalmol 100:318, 1985.
15. Jakobiec FL, Trokel SL, Aron-Rosa D, et al: Localized eosinophilic granuloma (Langerhans' cell histiocytosis) of the orbital frontal bone. Arch Ophthalmol 98:1814, 1980.
16. Jakobiec FA, Mottow L: Pediatric orbital pseudotumor. *In* Jakobiec FA (ed): Ocular and Adnexal Tumors. Birmingham, AL, Aesculapius, 1978.
17. Trocme SD, Baker RH, Bartley GB, et al: Extracellular deposition of eosinophil major basic protein in orbital histiocytosis X. Ophthalmology 98:353, 1991.
18. Hashimoto K: Langerhans' cell granule: An endocytotic organelle. Arch Dermatol 104:148, 1971.
19. Anemiya T, Yoshida H: Electron microscopic study of the orbital lesion of Hand-Schüller-Christian disease. J Pediatr Ophthalmol 14:242, 1977.
20. Mierau GW, Favara BE, Branman JM: Electron microscopy in histiocytosis X. Ultrastruct Pathol 3:137, 1982.
21. Jakobiec FA, Lefkowitch J, Knowles DM II: B- and T-lymphocytes in ocular disease. Ophthalmology 91:635, 1984.
22. Beckstead JH, Woods GS, Turner RR: Histiocytosis-X cells and Langerhans' cells: Enzyme histochemical and immunological similarities. Hum Pathol 15:826, 1984.
23. Glover AT, Grove AS Jr: Eosinophilic granuloma of the orbit with spontaneous healing. Ophthalmology 94:1008, 1987.
24. Cohen M, Zornoza J, Cangir A, et al: Direct injection of methylprednisolone sodium succinate in the treatment of solitary eosinophilic granuloma of the bone: A report of 9 cases. Radiology 136:289, 1980.
25. Wirtschaffer JD, Nesbit M, Anderson P, et al: Intralesional methylprednisolone for Langerhans' cell histiocytosis of the orbit and cranium. J Pediatr Ophthalmol Strabismus 24:194, 1987.
26. Kindy-Degnan NA, LaFlamme P, Duprat G, et al: Intralesional steroid in the treatment of an orbital eosinophilic granuloma. Arch Ophthalmol 109:617, 1991.
27. Harnett AN, Doughty D, Hirst A, et al: Radiotherapy in benign orbital disease. II: Ophthalmic Graves' disease and orbital histiocytosis X. Br J Ophthalmol 72:289, 1988.
28. Favara BE, McCarthy RL, Milerau GW: Histiocytosis X. Hum Pathol 14:663, 1983.
29. Hirschl S, Katz A: Giant cell reparative granuloma outside the jaw bone. Hum Pathol 5:171, 1974.
30. Scully RE, Mark EJ, McNeely BU. Case Records of the Massachusetts General Hospital: Case 10–1984. N Engl J Med 310:642, 1984.
31. Hoopes PC, Anderson RL, Blodi FC: Giant cell (reparative) granuloma of the orbit. Ophthalmology 88:1361, 1981.
32. Jaffe HL, Lichtenstein L: Solitary unicameral bone cyst with emphasis on the roentgen picture, the pathologic appearance and the pathogenesis. Arch Surg 44:1004, 1942.
33. Ronner HJ, Jones IS: Aneurysmal bone cyst of the orbit: A review. Ann Ophthalmol 15:626, 1983.
34. Buraczewski J, Dabska M: Pathogenesis of aneurysmal bone cyst: Relationship between the aneurysmal bone cyst and fibrous dysplasia of bone. Cancer 28:597, 1971.
35. Biesecker JL, Marcove RC, Huvos AG, et al: Aneurysmal bone cysts. Cancer 26:615, 1970.
36. Dabska M, Buraczewski J: Aneurysmal bone cyst. Cancer 23:371, 1969.
37. Hunter JV, Yokoyama C, Moseley IF, et al: Aneurysmal bone cyst of the sphenoid with orbital involvement. Br J Ophthalmol 74:505, 1990.
38. Johnson TE, Bergin DJ, McCord CD: Aneurysmal bone cyst of the orbit. Ophthalmology 95:86, 1988.
39. Milne HL III, Leone CR, Kincaid MC, et al: Chronic hematic cyst of the orbit. Ophthalmology 94:271, 1987.
40. Bergin DJ, McCord CD, Dutton JJ, et al: Chronic hematic cyst of the orbit. Ophthalmic Plast Reconstr Surg 4:31, 1988.
41. Goldberg SH, Sassani JW, Parnes RE: Traumatic intraconal hematic cyst of the orbit. Arch Ophthalmol 110:378, 1992.
42. Amrith S, Baratham G, Khoo CY, et al: Spontaneous hematic cysts of the orbit presenting with acute proptosis: A report of three cases. Ophthalmic Plast Reconstr Surg 6:273, 1990.
43. Cameron JD, Letson RD, Summers CG: Clinical significance of

hematic cyst of the orbit. Ophthalmic Plast Reconstr Surg 4:95, 1988.

44. Kersten RC, Derten JL, Bloom HR, et al: Chronic hematic cyst of the orbit: Role of magnetic resonance imaging in diagnosis. Ophthalmology 95:1549, 1988.

45. Loeffler M, Hornblass A: Hematic cyst of the orbit. Arch Ophthalmol 108:886, 1990.

46. Wolter JR: Subperiosteal hematomas of the orbit in young males: A serious complication of trauma or surgery in the eye region. Trans Am Ophthalmol Soc 77:104, 1979.

47. Shapiro A, Tso MOM, Putterman AM, et al: A clinicopathologic study of hematic cysts of the orbit. Am J Ophthalmol 102:237, 1986.

48. Parke DW II, Font RL, Boniuk M, et al: "Cholesteatoma" of the orbit. Arch Ophthalmol 100:612, 1982.

49. Campanella RS, Caldarelli DD, Friedberg SA: Cholesteatoma of the frontal and ethmoid areas. Ann Otol Rhinol Laryngol 88:518, 1979.

50. Eijpe AA, Koornneef L, Verbeeten B Jr: Intradiploic epidermoid cysts of the bony orbit. Ophthalmology 98:1737, 1991.

51. Fukuta K, Jackson IT: Epidermoid cyst and cholesterol granuloma of the orbit. Br J Plast Surg 43:521, 1990.

52. Codling BW, Soni KC, Barry DR, et al: Histiocytosis presenting as swelling of orbit and eyelid. Br J Ophthalmol 56:517, 1972.

53. Friendly DS, Font RL, Rao NA: Orbital involvement in "sinus" histiocytosis: A report of four cases. Arch Ophthalmol 95:2006, 1977.

54. Foucar E, Rosai J, Dorfman RF: The ophthalmologic manifestations of sinus histiocytosis with massive lymphadenopathy. Am J Ophthalmol 87:354, 1979.

55. Zimmerman LE, Hidayat AA, Grantham RL, et al: Atypical cases of sinus histiocytosis (Rosai-Dorfman disease) with ophthalmological manifestations. Trans Am Ophthalmol Soc 86:113, 1988.

56. Sanchez R, Sibley RK, Rosai J: The electron microscopic features of sinus histiocytosis with massive lymphadenopathy: A study of eleven cases. Ultrastruct Pathol 2:101, 1981.

57. Ngendagayo P, Roels H, Quatacker J, et al: Sinus histiocytosis with massive lymphadenopathy in Rwanda: Report of 8 cases with immunohistochemical and ultrastructural studies. Histopathology 7:49, 1983.

58. Lever WF, Schaumburg-Lever G: Histopathology of the Skin, 6th ed. Philadelphia, JB Lippincott, 1983.

59. Zimmerman LE: Ocular lesions of juvenile xanthogranuloma. Trans Am Acad Ophthalmol Otolaryngol 69:412, 1965.

60. Sanders TE, Miller JE: Infantile xanthogranuloma of the orbit. Trans Am Acad Ophthalmol Otolaryngol 69:458, 1965.

61. Sanders TE: Infantile xanthogranuloma of the orbit: A report of three cases. Am J Ophthalmol 61:1299, 1966.

62. Staple TW, McAlister WH, Sanders TE, et al: Juvenile xanthogranuloma of the orbit: Report of a case with bone destruction. Am J Roentgenol 91:629, 1964.

63. Gaynes PM, Cohen GS: Juvenile xanthogranuloma of the orbit. Am J Ophthalmol 63:755, 1967.

64. Schwartz TL, Carter KD, Judisch GF, et al: Congenital macronodular juvenile xanthogranuloma of the eyelid. Ophthalmology 98:1230, 1991.

65. Shields CL, Shields JA, Buchanon HW: Solitary orbital involvement with juvenile xanthogranuloma. Arch Ophthalmol 108:1587, 1990.

66. Chester W: Uber lipoidgranulomatose. Virchows Arch Pathol Anat 279:561, 1930.

67. Alper MG, Zimmerman LE, LaPiana FG: Orbital manifestations of Erdheim-Chester disease. Trans Am Ophthalmol Soc 81:64, 1983.

68. Shields JA, Karcioglu ZA, Shields CL, et al: Orbital and eyelid involvement with Erdheim-Chester disease. Arch Ophthalmol 109:850, 1991.

69. Nasr AM, Johnson T, Hidayat A: Adult onset primary bilateral orbital xanthogranuloma: Clinical, diagnostic, and histopathologic correlations. Orbit 10:13, 1991.

70. Rose GE, Patel BC, Garner A, et al: Orbital xanthogranuloma in adults. Br J Ophthalmol 75:681, 1991.

71. Floyd BB, Brown B, Isaacs H, Minckler DS: Pseudorheumatoid nodule involving the orbit. Arch Ophthalmol 100:1478, 1982.

72. Ross MJ, Cohen KL, Peiffer RL, et al: Episcleral and orbital pseudorheumatoid nodules. Arch Ophthalmol 101:418, 1983.

73. Rao NA, Font RL: Pseudorheumatoid nodules of the ocular adnexa. Am J Ophthalmol 79:471, 1975.

74. Kossard S, Winkelmann RK: Necrobiotic xanthogranuloma with paraproteinemia. J Am Acad Dermatol 3:257, 1980.

75. Codere F, Lee RD, Anderson RL: Necrobiotic xanthogranuloma of the eyelid. Arch Ophthalmol 101:60, 1983.

76. Robertson DM, Winkelmann RK: Ophthalmic features of necrobiotic xanthogranuloma with paraproteinemia. Am J Ophthalmol 97:173, 1984.

77. Bullock JD, Bartley GB, Campbell RJ, et al: Necrobiotic xanthogranuloma with paraproteinemia: Case report and a pathogenetic theory. Ophthalmology 93:1233, 1986.

78. Char DH, LeBoit PE, Ljung BE, et al: Radiation therapy for ocular necrobiotic xanthogranuloma. Arch Ophthalmol 105:174, 1987.

79. Cornblath WT, Dotan SA, Trobe JD, et al: Varied clinical spectrum of necrobiotic xanthogranuloma. Ophthalmology 99:103, 1992.

80. Finan MC, Winkelmann RK: Necrobiotic xanthogranuloma with paraproteinemia: A review of 22 cases. Medicine 65:376, 1986.

81. Bowling GB, Wilson JE: Atypical (annular) necrobiosis lipoidica of the face and scalp. Dermatologica 135:11, 1967.

82. Mackey JP: Necrobiosis lipoidica diabeticorum involving scalp and face. Br J Dermatol 93:729, 1975.

83. Kattah JC, Zimmerman LE, Kolsky MP, et al: Bilateral orbital involvement in fatal giant cell polymyositis. Ophthalmology 97:520, 1990.

84. Klein BR, Hedges TR III, Dayal Y, et al: Orbital myositis and giant cell myocarditis. Neurology 39:988, 1989.

85. Susac JO, Garcia-Mullin R, Glaser JS: Ophthalmoplegia in dermatomyositis. Neurology 23:305, 1973.

86. Bresnitz EA, Strom BL: Epidemiology of sarcoidosis. Epidemiol Rev 5:124, 1983.

87. Hoover DL, Khan JA, Giangiacomo J: Pediatric ocular sarcoidosis. Surv Ophthalmol 30:215, 1986.

88. Khan JA, Hoover DL, Giangiacomo J, et al: Orbital and childhood sarcoidosis. J Pediatr Ophthalmol Strabismus 23:190, 1986.

89. Henderson J: Orbital vasculitis, Wegener's granulomatosis, and orbital sarcoidosis. In Henderson J (ed): Orbital Tumors, 2nd ed. New York, Thieme-Stratton, 1980.

90. Jakobiec FA, Jones I: Orbital inflammations. In Jakobiec FA, Jones I (eds): Diseases of the Orbit. New York, Harper & Row, 1979.

91. Spencer WH: Ophthalmic Pathology: An Atlas and Textbook, vol. 3. Philadelphia, WB Saunders, 1986.

92. Collison JMT, Miller NR, Green WR: Involvement of orbital tissues by sarcoid. Am J Ophthalmol 102:302, 1986.

93. Melmon KL, Goldberg JS: Sarcoidosis with bilateral exophthalmos as the initial symptom. Am J Med 33:158, 1960.

94. Jakobiec FA, Yeo JH, Trokel SL, et al: Combined clinical and computed tomographic diagnosis of lacrimal fossa lesions. Am J Ophthalmol 74:785, 1982.

95. Nowinski T, Flanagan J, Ruchman M: Lacrimal gland enlargement in familial sarcoidosis. Ophthalmology 90:909, 1983.

96. Sacher M, Lanzieri CF, Sobel LI, et al: Computed tomography of bilateral lacrimal gland sarcoidosis. J Comput Assist Tomogr 8:213, 1984.

97. James DG, Anderson R, Langley D, et al: Ocular sarcoidosis. Br J Ophthalmol 48:461, 1964.

98. Karma A, Poukkula AA, Ruokonen AO: Assessment of activity of ocular sarcoidosis by gallium scanning. Br J Ophthalmol 71:361, 1987.

99. Weinreb RN, Yavitz EQ, O'Conner GR, et al: Lacrimal gland uptake of gallium citrate (Ga-67). Am J Ophthalmol 92:16, 1981.

100. Paport I, Beltrami CA, Salvoline U, et al: Sarcoidosis simulating a glioma of the optic nerve. Surg Neurol 8:353, 1977.

101. Nichols CW, Eagle RC Jr, Yanoff M, et al: Conjunctival biopsy as an aid in the evaluation of the patient with suspected sarcoidosis. Ophthalmology 87:287, 1980.

102. Stannard K, Spalton DJ. Sarcoidosis with infiltration of the external ocular muscles. Br J Ophthalmol 69:562, 1985.

103. Wolk RB: Sarcoidosis of the orbit with bone destruction. Am J Neuroradiol 5:204, 1984.

104. Rider JA, Dodson JW: Sarcoidosis: Report of a case manifested by retrobulbar mass, proptosis, destruction of orbit, and infiltration of paranasal sinuses. Am J Ophthalmol 33:117, 1950.

105. Bronson LJ, Fisher YL: Sarcoidosis of the paranasal sinuses with orbital extension. Arch Ophthalmol 94:243, 1976.

106. Karcioglu ZA, Brear R: Conjunctival biopsy in sarcoidosis. Am J Ophthalmol 99:68, 1985.

107. Fleischmajer R, Tint GS, Bennett HD: Normolipemic tendon and tuberous xanthomas. J Am Acad Dermatol 5:290, 1981.

108. Shukla Y, Ratnawat PS: Tuberous xanthoma of upper eye lids (a case report). Indian J Ophthalmol 30:161, 1982.

109. John T, Yanoff M, Scheie HG: Eyelid fibrous histiocytoma. Ophthalmology 88:1193, 1981.

110. Jakobiec FA, Klapper D, Maher E, et al: Infantile subconjunctival and anterior orbital fibrous histiocytoma. Ophthalmology 95:516, 1988.

111. Jakobiec FA, Howard G, Jones I, et al: Fibrous histiocytoma of the orbit. Am J Ophthalmol 77:333, 1974.

112. Font RL, Hidayat AA: Fibrous histiocytoma of the orbit: A clinicopathologic study of 150 cases. Hum Pathol 13:199, 1982.

113. Biedner B, Rothkoff L: Orbital fibrous histiocytoma in an infant. Am J Ophthalmol 85:548, 1978.

114. Hunt SJ, Santa Cruz DJ, Miller CW: Cholesterotic fibrous histiocytoma: Its association with hyperlipoproteinemia. Arch Dermatol 126:506, 1990.

115. Heidingsfeld ML: Histopathology of paraffin prosthesis. J Cutan Dis 24:513, 1906.

116. Rees TD, Ballantyne DL Jr, Seidman I: Eyelid deformities caused by the injection of silicone fluid. Br J Plastic Surg 24:125, 1971.

117. Boynton JR, Searl SS, Heimer JL, et al: Eyelid oleogranulomas caused by petroleum jelly injection. Arch Ophthalmol 106:550, 1988.

Index

Index

Note: Page numbers in *italics* refer to illustrations; page numbers followed by t refer to tables.

Body dysmorphic disorder, symptoms of, 3748–3749, 3749t
Bone, aneurysmal cyst of, 1904
    vs. giant cell reparative granuloma, 2082
  blastomycosis of, 3059–3060
  coccidioidomycosis of, 3055–3056
  cryptococcosis of, 3047
  disorders of, in ocular inflammation, 471–472
    orbital, radiology of, *3540*, 3540–3542, *3541*
    visual system in, 3559
  giant cell reparative granuloma of, 2082
    vs. giant cell tumor of bone, 2082
  healing of, 2110
  in sarcoidosis, 3137
  radiation effects on, 3295–3296
Bone graft, in orbital fracture, 3442, 3445, *3445*, 3454
Bone marrow, plasma cell proliferations of, 2020
  transplantation of, graft-versus-host disease after, 214–215
Bonnet sign, 799
Bonnet's syndrome, hallucinations in, 3734
Book of Selection of Eye Diseases, 608
Borrelia burgdorferi, 403, 2159, 3085–3089. See also *Lyme disease.*
  ocular, 169, 452, *452*
  transplacental transmission of, 3086
Borrelia recurrentis, 3088
Boston's sign, 2945t
Botfly, sheep, 1709
Botryomycosis, orbital, 1944
Botulinum toxin, action of, *2755*, 2755–2758, *2756*, 2756t, 2757t
  in dysthyroid eyelid retraction, 1837
  in infantile esotropia, 2759, *2759*
  in thyroid ophthalmopathy, 1916
  strabismus treatment with, 2755–2760
    complications of, 2758
    diplopia in, 2758
    indications for, 2758–2759, *2759*
    pupillary dilatation in, 2758
    results of, 2755–2757, *2756*, 2757t
      long-term, 2755, *2755*
    side effects of, 2758
    systemic effects of, 2758
    technique of, 2760
    vs. surgery, 2759–2760
Botulism, 3009
  ocular motor nerves in, 2462
Bourneville's syndrome, 2270t, 3307–3310. See also *Tuberous sclerosis.*
Bowel cancer, sebaceous adenoma and, 1766. See also *Muir-Torre syndrome.*
Bowen's disease, 1735, *1735*, 2293
Bowman's layer, anterior mosaic crocodile shagreen of, 33
  calcium deposits on, 68
  dystrophy of, 30, *32–33*
  in central crystalline dystrophy, 41, *46*
  in chronic herpetic keratitis, 129
  in hereditary anterior dystrophy, 30
  in keratoconus, 59
Boxing, ocular injury in, 3496t, 3497t
Brachium conjunctivum, in vertical eye movements, 2396, *2397*
Bradycardia, intraoperative, 2856–2857
  perioperative, 2852
Brain, degenerative disease of, magnetic resonance imaging of, 3581, *3582*

Brain *(Continued)*
  edema of, posterior cerebral artery occlusion after, 2636
    visual system in, 3560
  lesions of, ischemic, 2658
    radiology of, 3554–3588, *3587*
    sites of, 3556
  lingual/fusiform gyri of, *2643*
  penetrating injury to, imaging of, 3375
  tumors of, 2669–2682
    classification of, 2670, 2670t
    clinical manifestations of, 2670–2671, 2671t
    computed tomography of, 2671–2672, *2672*
    diagnosis of, surgical, 2672
    incidence of, 2670
    laboratory studies in, 2671–2672, *2672*
    magnetic resonance imaging of, 2672, *2672*
    metastatic, 3559–3560, *3560*
    primary, 2673–2675, *2674*
    symptoms of, 2670
    transfemoral angiography of, 2672
    treatment of, acute, 2672–2673
      corticosteroids in, 2672–2673
  visual areas of, corticocortical connections of, 2641, *2643*
  visual information streams of, *2644*
Brain stem, anesthesia of, local anesthetic spread and, 2862
  arteriovenous malformation of, magnetic resonance imaging of, 3575, *3577*
  astrocytoma of, 2675
  at inferior colliculi, *2448*
  glioma of, magnetic resonance imaging of, 3581–3582, *3583*
  in saccade generation, *2398*, 2398–2399
  infarction of, symptoms of, 2663t
  lesions of, abducens paresis in, 3473
    ipsilateral gaze palsy and, 2395–2396
    ischemic, 2662–2666
    pupillary light reflex in, 2476
  pontomedullary junction of, in horizontal eye movements, 2396
Brain stones, in neurofibromatosis, 3303–3304
  in tuberous sclerosis, 3308–3309
Branch retinal artery occlusion, 718–720, 720t, *728*, 728, *729*, *730*
  antiphospholipid antibodies in, *2524*, 2525
  atheromatous, 2666
  calcific emboli and, 729, *729*
  cholesterol emboli and, 729
  clinical manifestations of, 2514
  neovascular glaucoma and, 1498
  ocular infarction and, 2656
  ocular infarction from, 2656
  optic neuropathy from, 2364–2365, *2365*
  platelet-fibrin emboli and, 729
  Purtscher's retinopathy and, 729, *730*
  recurrent, auditory symptoms in, 2516
  retinal emboli and, 729, *729*, *730*
  talc emboli and, 729, *730*
  treatment of, 729, 2514
Branch retinal vein occlusion, 735, 740–743, *741–743*
  aneurysms in, 742
  collateral vessels in, 742, *743*
  complications of, 741–742
  diseases associated with, 741
  evaluation of, 741

Branch retinal vein occlusion *(Continued)*
  fluorescein angiography in, 741, *742*
  fundus findings in, 741, *741*
  hemorrhage in, 742
  in Eales disease, 793
  in polycythemia, 998
  in systemic lupus erythematosus, 2898
  ischemia in, 742
  laser photocoagulation in, 743
  macroaneurysm formation and, 799
  macular edema in, 742
  neovascular glaucoma and, 1494
  neovascularization in, 742, *742*
  pathophysiology of, 740–741
  retinal detachment in, 742
  treatment of, 743
  vessel sheathing in, 742, *743*
  visual acuity in, 741
  vs. Leber's idiopathic stellate neuroretinitis, 812
Breast cancer, ataxia-telangiectasia and, 3320
  in Cowden's syndrome, 1789
  metastases from, *2679*, 3517
    computed tomography of, 3534, *3535*
    glaucoma and, 1558
    pathology of, *2339*, 2340t
    to choroid, 723, 1460, 3214, 3216, *3216*
    to ciliary body, 1459–1460
    to eyelid, 1792, *1793*, 1819
      vs. primary signet ring carcinoma, 1785
    to iris, 1459, 3204, 3262, *3262*
    to orbit, 3521
    to uvea, 3260, 3261, 3262, *3262*, *3264*, *3266*
    ultrasonography of, 3549, *3549*
  tamoxifen in, retinal toxicity of, 1047, *1048*
Bridle suture, in glaucoma filtration surgery, *1625*, 1625–1626, *1626*
Bright-light test, in angle-closure glaucoma, 1337
Brightness Acuity Tester, glare assessment with, 675–676
Briquet's syndrome, 3190
Brisseau, Michel Pierre, 607
Broad-beta disease, 301
Brodmann's areas, functional zones in, 2640, *2641*
  in saccade control, 2400–2401
Brolene, in *Acanthamoeba* keratitis, 187
  ocular toxicity of, 91
Bromocriptine, in pituitary adenoma, 2620
  in pituitary tumors, 2677
  in thyroid ophthalmopathy, 1909
Bronchoalveolar lavage, in sarcoidosis, 3140
Bronchopulmonary aspergillosis, 3038–3039
  diagnosis of, 3040
  treatment of, 3040
Bronchospasm, surgical risk and, 2853
Bronchus, carcinoid tumor of, 2060
Bronson electromagnet, 1174, *1174*
Brooke's tumor, 1791, *1792*
Broomball, ocular injury in, 3496t
Brown tumor, orbital, 2073, *2073*
Brown's syndrome, of superior oblique tendon sheath, 2743, *2743*
  trochlear nerve palsy in, 2455
Brubaker, Richard, 610
Brucella, 452–453, 3008–3009
Brucella abortus, 3008, 3009
Brucella canis, 3008
Brucella melitensis, 3008, 3009

Choroidal neovascularization *(Continued)*
    occult appearance on, *836*, 836–837, *837*
    retinal pigment epithelium tears on, 838,
        839
    in age-related macular degeneration, 721–
        722, *722*
    in presumed ocular histoplasmosis syn-
        drome, 490, *491*, 493–494, 493t, *494*
    in subretinal fibrosis and uveitis syndrome,
        974
    juxtafoveal, treatment of, 841–843, *843*,
        844t, 847
    occult, in age-related macular degenera-
        tion, 723
    pathogenesis of, 834–835
    pathology of, 2170–2171
    recurrence of, 849–850
    serpiginous choroiditis and, 519, 522
    signs of, 835, *835*
    subfoveal, treatment of, 843–845, *845*, 847
    symptoms of, 835
    treatment of, 844–848
        laser photocoagulation in, 844–847, *846*,
            846t
            evaluation of, 847–848, *848*
            precautions in, 846–847
            preparation for, 845
            protocol for, 845–846, *846*, 846t
            wavelength selection in, 846
        low-vision aids in, 850
    visual acuity and, 849–850
    vitreous hemorrhage from, 839
    vs. serpiginous choroiditis, 522
Choroidal nevus (nevi), 3244–3248
    amelanotic, 3246
    cell types in, 3246–3247
    classification of, 3247
    clinical aspects of, 3245–3246, *3246*
    diagnosis of, 3248
    drusen in, 3246, *3246*, 3247
    dysplastic nevus syndrome and, 3245
    epidemiology of, 3245
    etiology of, 3245
    fluorescein angiography in, 3246, *3246*
    hemorrhage in, 3246, *3247*
    histogenesis of, 3245
    histopathology of, 3246–3247
    malignant transformation of, 3247–3248
    management of, 3248
    natural history of, 3247–3248
    pigmentation of, 3246
    prognosis for, 3247–3248
    size of, 3245–3246
    tissue changes in, 3246, 3247
    topography of, 3245–3246
    treatment of, 3248
    vs. choroidal melanoma, 3212, *3213*
Choroidal osteoma, vs. choroidal melanoma,
    3214, *3215*
Choroidal veins, indocyanine green
    angiography of, 720, *720*, *721*
Choroideremia, *1225*, 1225–1226
    carriers of, 1225
    fundus photograph in, *1215*
    pathology of, 2174–2175, *2175*
Choroiditis, *Aspergillus fumigatus* infection
    and, 2164
    birdshot. See *Retinochoroiditis, birdshot.*
    cryptococcal, 2163
        in acquired immunodeficiency syndrome,
            941
    definition of, 407

Choroiditis *(Continued)*
    disseminated, ocular histoplasmosis syn-
        drome and, 866
    Epstein-Barr virus and, 433
    fungal, in intravenous drug abusers, 473,
        473
    geographic, 517
    granulomatous, in presumed ocular histo-
        plasmosis, 2163, *2163*
    guttate, 1254
    honeycomb, Doyne's, 1254, *1254*
    Hutchinson-Tay, 1254
    in sympathetic ophthalmia, 498, *500*
    in uveal effusion, 550, *551*
    juxtapapillary, in ocular histoplasmosis
        syndrome, 864, *865*, 866
    lymphocytic, in presumed ocular histoplas-
        mosis syndrome, 491
    multifocal. See also *Subretinal fibrosis and
        uveitis syndrome.*
        disciform macular degeneration and, 974
        panuveitis and, 973
        vs. birdshot retinochoroiditis, 479
        vs. ocular histoplasmosis syndrome, 868
        vs. presumed ocular histoplasmosis syn-
            drome, 493
    peripheral, in Fuchs' heterochromic irido-
        cyclitis, 512
    pneumocystic, 460, *460*, 3067
        in acquired immunodeficiency syndrome,
            939, *939*, 3112, *3112*
        treatment of, 3068
    septic, abdominal abscess and, 470, *470*
    serpiginous, 517–523
        active lesions in, 517, *517*, *518*
            fluorescein angiography of, *518*, 518–
                519
        clinical findings in, 519–520
        differential diagnosis of, 521–522
        electroretinography of, 517
        etiology of, 520–521
        fluorescein angiography of, *518*, 518–519
        fovea in, 517–518
        histopathology of, 520
        indocyanine green angiography in, 723–
            724, *724*
        macular, 517–518, *517–519*
        monitoring of, 523
        neurologic disease and, 520
        pathology of, 2167
        peripapillary, 517, *517–519*
        prognosis for, 522
        recurrent, 517, *518*, *519*
        resolution of, 517, *519*, *520*
            fluorescein angiography of, 519
        scotoma in, 517
        treatment of, laser photocoagulation in,
            523
            medical, 522–523
        vision blurring in, 517
        vs. acute posterior multifocal placoid
            pigment epitheliopathy, 521–522
    syphilitic, 970, *971*
    tuberculous, 453, *453*
        in acquired immunodeficiency syndrome,
            941
    vitiliginous, 475. See also *Retinochoroidi-
        tis, birdshot.*
    vs. retinoblastoma, 2266
Choroidopathy, birdshot, 404. See also
    Retinochoroiditis, birdshot.
    geographic, 517

Choroidopathy *(Continued)*
    in scleroderma, 2923, *2923*
    in systemic lupus erythematosus, 2898–
        2899
    Pneumocystis carinii and, 2158–2159
Choroidoretinopathy, birdshot. See
    Retinochoroiditis, birdshot.
Chromaffinoma, 2058–2059, *2059*, *2060*
Chromatic sensitivity, in normal-tension
    glaucoma, 1352
Chromatolysis, injury and, 2120t
Chromatopsia, 1247
Chromogranin, immunohistochemical
    staining with, 2376t
Chromophore, 584–585
    absorption spectrum of, 578
    fluorescent, 584
    ultraviolet absorption by, in intraocular
        lens, 644
    visible light absorption by, 583
Chromosome, abnormalities of, lens
    abnormalities and, 2787t
    polymerase chain reaction in, 2122–2123
Chromosome 2, in aniridia, 3351
    in retinitis pigmentosa, 1219
Chromosome 3, in retinitis pigmentosa, 1219
    in von Hippel–Lindau disease, 3310
Chromosome 5, in Gardner's syndrome, 3352
Chromosome 6, in retinitis pigmentosa, 1221
Chromosome 11, in aniridia, 3351
    in diabetes mellitus, 2927
    map of, *3351*
Chromosome 17, in neurofibromatosis, 3302
Chromosome 22, in neurofibromatosis, 3302
Chronic obstructive pulmonary disease,
    surgical risk and, 2853
Chrysiasis, gold compounds and, 2142
    in rheumatoid arthritis, 2893
    lens in, 2210
Chrysops infection, 3072–3073
Chymase, mast cell, 80–81
α-Chymotrypsin, glaucoma and, 1293
    in intracapsular cataract extraction, 617,
        617
Cicatricial pemphigoid, 3164–3165, 3164t.
    See also *Pemphigoid, cicatricial.*
Cicatrization, in antiviral therapy, 90
    in trachoma, 180
Cigarette smoking, choroidal
    neovascularization and, 834
    in pars planitis syndrome, 467
Cilia. See *Eyelashes.*
Ciliary artery (arteries), *1875*
    anterior, 389
    in uveal metastases, 3261
    posterior, long, 389
        short, *389*, 389–390, *390*
        thrombosis of, 390–391
        trauma to, 392
Ciliary block glaucoma, 1522. See also
    Glaucoma, malignant.
Ciliary body, chemotherapy toxicity to, 2995t
    cyst of, angle closure in, 1396
        in dysproteinemia, 2999
    hyposecretion of, in angle-closure glau-
        coma, 1373
    in glaucoma filtration surgery, 1647–1648,
        1648
    in secondary open-angle glaucoma, 2281–
        2282, *2282*
    medulloepithelioma of, 545
        glaucoma and, 1457

Deoxyribonucleic acid (DNA), analysis of, polymerase chain reaction in, 2122
  in chronic progressive external ophthalmoplegia, 2493
  in hereditary retinal disease, *1190*, 1190–1191, 1191t
  in hereditary retinoblastoma, 3271–3278
  in Kearns-Sayre syndrome, 2493
  in Leber's optic neuropathy, 2597
  in progressive ophthalmoplegia, 2491–2492
  in retinitis pigmentosa, 1218–1222, *1220*, 1220t, *1221*, 1232
  ultraviolet B radiation of, 581
Depigmentation, of cilia, 1858, *1858*
Depo-Medrol. See *Methylprednisolone acetate (Depo-Medrol)*.
Deposition, legal, definition of, 3785
  in malpractice, 3798–3799
Depression, 3735–3736, 3735t
  antidepressants for, 3736
  diagnosis of, 3735–3736, 3735t
  drug-induced, 3736, 3736t
  in birdshot retinochoroiditis, 477
  in blindness, 3735–3736, 3735t, 3736t
  in cataract removal, 607, *607*
  in iritis, 473
  in vision loss, 3185, 3669, 3693, 3735–3736, 3735t, 3736t
  medical conditions and, 3736, 3736t
  neurovegetative symptoms of, 3735, 3735t
Dermatitis, 3154–3159
  atopic, 3155–3157, 3155t
    allergy in, 111–112, *112*
    blepharitis with, 109–112, *110–112*
    cataract in, 2216
    characteristics of, 2119t
    clinical features of, 3155–3156, 3155t
    etiology of, 3156–3157
    keratoconjunctivitis with, 93
    lid taping in, 111, *111*
    ocular manifestations of, 3156, *3156*
    pathogenesis of, 3156–3157
    prednisolone acetate for, 111
    Staphylococcus aureus and, *110*, 111
    treatment of, 3157
    viral infection in, 111, *111*, 3156
  chronic, madarosis and, 1853, *1853*
  contact, 3157–3159, *3158*, 3158t
    characteristics of, 2119t
    clinical features of, 3158
    drugs and, 213, *213*
    etiology of, 3158
    ocular manifestations of, 3158, *3158*
    of eyelids, 112, 2301
    pathogenesis of, 3158
    treatment of, 3158–3159
  eczematous, drug-related, characteristics of, 2119t
  infantile, iridocyclitis with, 472
  of eyelids, 133, *133*, 1704
  in herpes zoster ophthalmicus, 138, *138*
  rosacea. See *Rosacea*.
  seborrheic, *3154*, 3154–3155, 3154t
    clinical features of, *3154*, 3154–3155, 3154t
    etiology of, 3154–3155
    in ataxia-telangiectasia, 3321
    ocular, 3154, *3154*
    pathogenesis of, 3154–3155
    treatment of, 3155
  Staphylococcus pyogenes infection in, 2832
Dermatitis herpetiformis, ocular, 200

Dermatobia hominis, 1709, *1710*
Dermatome, thoracic, herpes zoster virus and, 137
Dermatomyositis, eyelid in, 1863, *1864*, 2300
  periorbital, 113, *113*
  retinal manifestations of, 989–990
Dermatosis, inflammatory, 2118–2119, 2119t
  acute, 2118, 2119t
  chronic, 2118
  radiation, 1735–1736
Dermatosis papulosa nigra, of eyelid, 1716, *1717*
Dermis, connective tissue of, 2117
Dermoid tumor, 1896–1898, *1897*
  clinical presentation of, 1896
  computed tomography of, 1897, *1897*
  conjunctival, 277, *277*
    pathology of, 2127, *2127*
  dumbbell, 1896, *1897*
  histology of, 1897
  magnetic resonance imaging of, 1897
  pediatric, 2792–2793, *2794*
  radiographic analysis of, 1897
  treatment of, 1897–1898
  vs. epidermoid tumor, 1896
  vs. teratoma, 1896
Dermolipoma, conjunctival, 277–278, *278*
  pathology of, 2127
Descemet's membrane, in Chandler's syndrome, *58*, *59*
  in chronic herpetic keratitis, 129
  in congenital hereditary endothelial dystrophy, *50*, *51*, *51*
  in cornea guttata, 51, *52*
  in Fuchs' dystrophy, *53*, 54
  in glaucoma, 1297
  in keratoconus, 15, *18*, 59, *60*
  in macular dystrophy, 40, *44*
  in Peters' anomaly, 19, *20*, *21*
  in posterior polymorphous dystrophy, 54, *54*, *57*
  in sclerocornea, 19, *22*, *23*
  Kayser-Fleischer rings in, 312, *313*
  rupture of, 3490, *3490*
Desmin, immunohistochemical staining with, 2376t
Detachment. See specific types, e.g., *Retinal detachment*.
Deuteranomaly, 1242t. See also *Color vision, abnormal*.
Deuteranopia, 1238, 1242t. See also *Color vision, abnormal*.
Devic's disease, bilateral optic neuritis in, 2554–2555
  visual system in, 3557
Dexamethasone. See also *Corticosteroids*.
  in postoperative endophthalmitis, 1163, 1163t
  topical, intraocular pressure and, 1462
Dexamethasone provocative test, in open-angle glaucoma, 1339
Dextrose, in perioperative diabetes management, 663
DHPG. See *Ganciclovir* entry.
Diabetes mellitus, 2925–2934
  acquired parafoveolar telangiectasia and, 808
  branch retinal vein occlusion and, 741
  cardiovascular disease with, 2931
  cataract in, 570–571, 2212
  cataract surgery in, 776–777
  central retinal vein occlusion and, 737

Diabetes mellitus *(Continued)*
  classification of, 2925–2926, 2925t
  complications of, acute, 2930
    chronic, 2931–2932
  diagnosis of, 2926
  epidemiology of, 2926–2927
  eye care in, 779
  eye disease with, 2932, 2932t. See also specific types, e.g., *Diabetic retinopathy*.
  genetics of, 2927
  gestational, 2925, 2932–2933, 2933t
  glaucoma and, 1292, 1556
  glucose control in, 777
  glucose in, preoperative, 667
  human leukocyte antigens in, 2927, 2928
  hyperglycemia in, 2928
  insulin-dependent (type I), 1495, 2925
    pathogenesis of, 2928
    perioperative management of, 662–663, 663t
  iris neovascularization and, 1495–1496
  iris pigment epithelium in, vacuolization of, 383, *383*
  iritis with, 472
  ischemic optic neuropathy and, 2572, 2575, 2657
  juvenile, optic atrophy in, 2595, 2598
    papillopathy in, 2575, *2576*
  ketoacidosis with, 2930
  lens abnormalities in, 2787t
  myopia and, 3616
  neurologic disease with, 2932
  neuroretinitis secondary to, vs. Leber's idiopathic stellate neuroretinitis, 812
  non–insulin-dependent (type II), 2925, 2928
  nonketotic hyperosmolar syndrome with, 2930
  oculomotor nerve palsy in, 2454
  open-angle glaucoma with, 1556
  optic atrophy in, 2595, 2598
  optic neuritis in, 2575
  papillopathy in, 2575, *2576*
  pathogenesis of, 2927–2928
    glucose metabolism in, 2927–2928
    insulin in, 2927–2928
  pediatric, cataract in, 2763
    diagnosis of, 2926
  penetrating artery disease in, 2666
  perioperative management of, 662–663, 663t, 2853
    dextrose in, 663
    diet in, 663
    insulin in, 663, 663t
    preoperative evaluation and, 662
  pregnancy and, 777–778, 2932–2933, 2933t
  renal disease in, 2931–2932
  retinal blood flow in, 758
  retinopathy of. See *Diabetic retinopathy*.
  treatment of, 2928–2930
    complications of, 2929–2930
    diet in, 2928–2929
    glucose normalization in, 2928
    insulin in, 2929
    oral hypoglycemic agents in, 2929
    pancreas transplantation in, 2933–2934
  uveal, 2167–2168
  vasculopathy in, 2931
  visual findings in, 3557
Diabetic ketoacidosis, 2930
Diabetic nephropathy, diabetic retinopathy and, 778–779

Glaucoma *(Continued)*
    pupillary dilation in, 1370
  retinitis pigmentosa and, 1555
  sequelae of, 1393–1394, *1394*
  subacute, 1385, 1389, 1390
    treatment of, 1385
  synechial, 1366, 1372
    chamber-deepening procedure in, 1378
    indentation gonioscopy in, 1377–1378
    trabecular meshwork changes in, 1373–1374
  treatment of, 1380–1385
    chamber deepening in, 1382, 1621–1622
    conjunctiva changes in, 1296–1297
    corneal indentation in, 1383
    filtration surgery in, 1383. See also *Filtration surgery.*
    goniosynechialysis in, 1382–1383, *1383*
    intraoperative gonioscopy in, 1621–1622
    laser gonioplasty in, *1605*, 1605–1607
      complications of, 1607, 1607t
      indications for, 1605, 1605t
      postoperative management for, 1606
      technique of, 1606, *1606*, 1606t
    laser iridectomy in, 1597–1604
      complications of, 1604, 1604t
      indications for, 1598, 1598t
      performance of, *1601*, 1601–1604, *1602*, 1602t, *1603*
      postlaser treatment in, 1604, 1604t
      technique of, *1599*, 1599–1600, *1600*, 1600t
    laser iridotomy in, 1336
    lens extraction in, 1383
    paracentesis in, 1383
    peripheral iridectomy for, prone provocative test after, 1338
    peripheral iridectomy in, 1618–1621. See also *Iridectomy, peripheral.*
    peripheral iridoplasty in, 1382
    peripheral iridotomy in, 1382
    peripheral laser synechialysis in, 1382
    pharmacologic, 1380–1382
      aqueous formation in, 1381
      miotics in, 1380–1381
      mydriatic-cycloplegic therapy in, 1382
      ocular pressure reduction in, 1381–1382
      pain reduction in, 1382
      parasympathomimetic agents in, 1380–1381
    pilocarpine in, 1380–1381
    pupilloplasty in, 1382
    sector iridectomy in, 1621, *1621*
  unilateral, 1384
  vs. ghost cell glaucoma, 1384
  vs. inflammatory glaucoma, 1384
  vs. neovascular glaucoma, 1384
  vs. phacolytic glaucoma, 1384
  vs. phacomorphic glaucoma, 1447
  vs. primary open-angle glaucoma, 1366

Glaucoma *(Continued)*
    vs. secondary angle-closure glaucoma, 1365
    pseudotumor and, 1925
    scleral buckling surgery and, 1105
  secondary, acquired immunodeficiency syndrome and, 1559
    age-related macular degeneration and, 1558–1559
    carotid cavernous fistula and, 1470–1472, *1471, 1472*
    choroidal hemangioma and, 1558
    choroidal melanoma and, 1458–1459
    choroidal metastases and, 1460
    ciliary body medulloepithelioma and, 1457
    ciliochoroidal effusion and, 1562, *1562*
    congenital syphilis and, 1433
    intravitreal gas tamponade and, 1563–1565
    iris tumors and, 1455–1456
    metastases and, 1558
    nanophthalmos and, 1530, 1531–1532
    panretinal photocoagulation and, 1563
    pathology of, 2286
    primary ciliary body tumors and, 1456–1458
    retinal detachment repair and, *1562*, 1562–1563
    retinoblastoma and, 1458, 3280, *3280*
    retinopathy of prematurity and, 1554
    uveitic, 1458, 1560, 1564t
      choroidal melanoma and, 1458–1459
      retinoblastoma and, 1458
      symptoms of, 1294
    vs. neovascular glaucoma, 1489, *1489*
    vs. primary angle-closure glaucoma, 1365
    tonography in, *1333*, 1333–1335, *1334*
  angle-recession, 1439–1440, *1440*. See also *Glaucoma, traumatic.*
  Axenfeld's anomaly with, 15
  burned-out, 1357
  cataract and, 1304, 1552, 1641–1645
  choroidal malignant melanoma and, 1458–1459
  ciliary block, 1522. See also *Glaucoma, malignant.*
  ciliary body malignant melanoma and, *1457*, 1457–1458
  ciliary body medulloepithelioma and, 1457
  ciliary body melanocytoma and, 1457
  color vision in, 1302
  combined-mechanism, 1389–1399
    anterior chamber depth in, 1391
    classification of, 1391
    clinical course of, 1390–1393, *1390–1394*
    clinical manifestations of, 1389, *1390*
    differential diagnosis of, 1393–1396, *1394–1397*
    epidemiology of, 1396–1397
    gonioscopy in, 1391–1393, *1392, 1393*
    management of, *1398*, 1398–1399, *1399*
    pathophysiology of, 1397–1398, *1398*
    peripheral anterior synechiae in, 1395, *1395*
    slit-lamp examination in, 1391, *1391*
    vs. open-angle glaucoma, 1395
  congenital, goniotomy for, lens notch from, 2185, *2188*
    in neurofibromatosis, 3304
    pathology of, 2286, *2286*

Glaucoma *(Continued)*
  retinitis pigmentosa and, 1555
    vs. juvenile-onset open-angle glaucoma, 1347
    vs. megalocornea, 14
  congestive. See *Glaucoma, neovascular.*
  contrast sensitivity in, 1302
  corticosteroid-induced, 1294, 1462–1465
    administration routes and, 1463–1464, 1463t
    cataract surgery and, 1512
    clinical course of, 1464
    clinical findings in, 1464
    differential diagnosis of, 1464–1465
    endogenous route in, 1463–1464, 1463t
    epidemiology of, 1462–1463
    genetic basis of, 1462
    in juvenile rheumatoid arthritis, 2790
    management of, 1465
    pathogenesis of, 1464
    periocular route in, 1463, 1463t
    systemic route in, 1463, 1463t
    topical route in, 1463, 1463t
  diabetic. See *Glaucoma, neovascular.*
  Doppler velocimetry in, 1312
  enzyme, 1293
  episcleral venous pressure and, Sturge-Weber syndrome and, 3316
  epithelial edema with, intraocular pressure reduction in, 254
  etiology of, 1295–1296, 1296t
    inflammation in, 1293
    optic atrophy in, 1293
    penetrating keratoplasty in, 1293
    scleral buckling in, 1293
    trauma in, 1293
  exfoliative. See *Exfoliation syndrome.*
  fibrous proliferation and, 1483
  filtration surgery in, 1623–1639. See also *Filtration surgery.*
  ghost cell, 1514, 1561
    etiology of, 1293
    pathology of, 2282, *2283*
    traumatic, 1441, *1441*
    vitrectomy and, 775
    vs. angle-closure glaucoma, 1384
    vs. neovascular glaucoma, 1489
  Goldmann perimetry in, 1301–1302
  hemolytic, 2282, *2282*
  hemorrhagic. See *Glaucoma, neovascular.*
  herpes zoster virus and, 142
  histiocytosis and, 1461
  in aniridia, 369, 2146
  in Axenfeld-Rieger syndrome, 378
  in Behçet's disease, 1022
  in Chandler's syndrome, 54, *58*
  in corneal graft failure, 334–335
  in Fuchs' heterochromic iridocyclitis, 411, 507, 515
  in intermediate uveitis, 426
  in keratoprosthesis, 341
  in Lowe's syndrome, 2189
  in nanophthalmos, 549
  in penetrating keratoplasty, 326, 335
  in retinopathy of prematurity, 2810
  in sarcoidosis, 446
  inflammatory, 1426–1434, 1426t
    episcleritis and, 1433–1434
    Fuchs' heterochromic iridocyclitis and, *1428*, 1428–1429
    glaucomatocyclitis crisis and, 1429–1430
    herpes simplex virus and, 1430–1431, *1431*

Guanosine diphosphatase–activating protein, in neurofibromatosis, 3302
Guanosine monophosphate, cyclic (cGMP), in cone dysfunction, 1244
  in mast cell activation, 79
  in neurofibromatosis, 3302
Guillain-Barré syndrome, ocular motor nerves in, 2462, 2463
  ophthalmoplegia with, 2438–2439
  upper eyelid retraction in, 1833
Guilt, in vision loss, 3669
Gumma, in syphilis, 3079, 3081
Gunn's sign, in branch retinal vein occlusion, 740
Gunn's syndrome, 1831
  in congenital fibrosis syndrome, 2495
  synkinesis in, 2432
Guttate choroiditis, 1254
Guyton-Minkowski potential acuity meter, 677
Gyrate atrophy, choroidal, 1226, *1226*
  fundus photograph in, *1215*
  myopia and, 3147
  ornithine-δ-aminotransferase deficiency and, 2983
  pathology of, 2175
  pediatric, 2788
  retinal, 1226, *1226*
    fundus photograph in, *1215*
Gyrus, fusiform, 2641, *2643*
  lingual, 2641, *2643*
  temporal, middle, organization of, 2641

Haab's striae, in glaucoma, 1297, 2286, *2286*
Haag-Streit AC pachymeter, 1374
Haemophilus, 162
  in mucopurulent conjunctivitis, 163
  orbital infection with, 1943
Haemophilus aegyptius, 162
Haemophilus aphrophilus, 3006
Haemophilus influenzae, 1943, 1944
  in endogenous endophthalmitis, 417, 3122
  in postoperative endophthalmitis, 1162
  in preseptal cellulitis, 2831
Haemophilus parainfluenzae, 3006
Hailey-Hailey disease, syringoma in, 1779
Hair. See also *Eyebrow(s); Eyelashes.*
  growth of, 1851–1852, *1852*. See also *Hypertrichosis.*
  lanugo-type, 1851
  loss of, 1852–1855, *1853, 1854*
    chemicals and, 1853
    drugs and, 1853
    endocrine disorders and, 1853
    infection and, 1853
    local factors in, 1853–1854, *1854*
    neoplastic, 1854, *1854*
    neurosis and, 1854
    systemic diseases and, 1853, *1853*
    trauma and, 1854, *1854*
    treatment of, 1854–1855
      surgical, 1854–1855
  misdirection of, *1855*, 1855–1858, 1855t, *1856–1858*
  pigmentary disorders of, 1858, *1858*
  textural disorders of, 1858
Hair follicles, histology of, 2117, *2118*
  pilomatrixoma of, *1788*, 1788–1789
  trichilemmoma of, 1789, *1790*
  trichoepithelioma of, 1791, *1792*
  trichofilliculoma of, 1789, 1791, *1791*

Hair follicles *(Continued)*
  tumors of, *1788*, 1788–1792, *1790–1792*, 2296–2297
Haliwa Indians, benign hereditary intraepithelial dyskeratosis in, *281*, 281–282
Hallermann-Streiff syndrome, 2196
Hallopeau, localized acrodermatitis continua of, 3153
Hallucinations, ictal, 2649
  occipital lobe disease and, 2636
  release, 2649
  visual, 2649
    in Bonnet's syndrome, 3734
    in vision loss, 3734–3735, 3735t
    organic vs. functional, 3735t
Halo, chorioscleral, in normal-tension glaucoma, 1354
Halo nevus, of eyelid, *1800*, 1800–1801
Halothane, intraocular pressure and, 2859
  visually evoked potentials and, 2865
Hamartoma, 2270t, 3300
  astrocytic, in neurofibromatosis, 3305, *3305*
    in tuberous sclerosis, 3309, *3309*
    vs. retinoblastoma, 2266, 3281, *3281*
  blood vessel, 2270t
  cartilaginous, orbital, 2304
  choroidal, in neurofibromatosis, 3304–3305, *3305*
  in phakomatoses, 2271t
  iridic. See *Lisch's nodules.*
  neural, 2268t
  of retina and retinal pigment epithelium, 3254–3256, *3255, 3256*
  orbital, 2333–2334
  vascular, 2268t
    conjunctival, 2127
Hamartomatous polyposis syndromes, 2977t, 2978–2979
Hand-foot-and-mouth disease, 3026, *3026*
Hand-Schüller-Christian disease, 2080, 3333. See also *Langerhans' cell histiocytosis.*
Hansen's disease. See *Leprosy.*
Hara, T., 612
Harada-Ito procedure, 2751
Harada's disease, 481
  exudative retinal detachment and, 1088
  fluorescein angiography in, *705*
  vs. central serous chorioretinopathy, 822
  vs. Vogt-Koyanagi syndrome, 481t
Hassall-Henle warts, 51, 2139
Head, movement of, examination of, 2415–2416
    vestibuloocular reflex and, 2401
  pain in, vs. cluster headache, 2694
  posture of, examination of, 2415–2416
    nystagmus and, 2743–2744
  trauma to, carotid cavernous sinus fistula and, 1470
    oculomotor nerve injury and, 3470–3472, *3471*
Headache, 2693–2695
  cluster, 2693–2694
    differential diagnosis of, 2694
    treatment of, 2694–2695
  in acute posterior multifocal placoid pigment epitheliopathy, 909
  in brain tumors, 2670
  in idiopathic intracranial hypertension, 2700, *2700*, 2704, 2705–2706
  in temporal arteritis, 2902

Headache *(Continued)*
  ischemic cerebrovascular accident and, 2695
  neuroophthalmology and, 2389
  sexual activity and, 2695
  stabbing, 2695
  tension-type, 2693
  vascular disorders and, 2695
Healon (sodium hyaluronate), as vitreous substitute, 1143–1144
Health Care Quality Improvement Act, disciplinary proceedings and, 3788
Health maintenance organizations, 3791
Hearing, examination of, 2415–2416
  loss of, in congenital rubella syndrome, 963
    in Eales disease, 795
Heart disease, antihypertensive therapy in, 2872
  atherosclerotic. See *Atherosclerosis.*
  in amyloidosis, 2959
  in Kearns-Sayre syndrome, 2493
  in Lyme disease, 3085
  in sarcoidosis, 3137
  in syphilis, 3079
  surgical risk and, 2853
Heart failure, episcleral venous pressure with, 1475
  hypertension and, 2873
  in amyloidosis, 2959
  surgical risk and, 2852
  timolol effects on, 1575
Heart murmurs, surgical risk and, 2853
Heart rate, levobunolol effect on, 1576
  timolol effect on, 1575
Heat stroke, upward gaze deviation in, 2502, *2502*
Heavy metal, intoxication with, visual system in, 3560
  lens deposition of, cataract and, 2210–2211, *2211*
Heerfordt's syndrome, 1954, 2094, 3135
Heidelberg laser tomographic scanner, 1318, *1319*
Heinz bodies, in ghost cell glaucoma, 1514
Helmet, protective, 3501, *3501*
Helmholtz, Herrmann, 1265–1266, *1266*
Hemangioblastoma, cerebellar, in von Hippel–Lindau disease, 3311
  orbital, 2067–2069, *2069*, 2268t
Hemangioendothelioblastoma, 2067–2069, *2069*
Hemangioendothelioma, 2067–2069, *2069*
  malignant, 1972–1973
Hemangioendotheliosarcoma, 1972–1973, 2067–2069, *2069*
Hemangioma, 1967–1973
  capillary, axial myopia and, 3145
    of eyelid, 2297
    orbital, 1967–1969, *1968*
      computed tomography of, 1968, *1968*, 3525
      differential diagnosis of, 1968
      magnetic resonance imaging of, 3525, *3526*
      management of, 1969
      pathology of, 2333, *2333*, 2349t
  cavernous, chiasmal, 2620
    location of, 3522
    of eyelid, 2297
    orbital, 1970–1973, *1971, 1972*, 1973t
      histology of, 1971, *1971*

Hyphema *(Continued)*
  complications of, 3388–3389
    corneal bloodstaining after, 3389
    glaucoma and, 1437–1438, *1438*, 3389
    laboratory evaluation of, 3386
    pathophysiology of, 3386
    prognosis for, 3390
    rebleeding after, 3388–3389
    sickle cell disease and, 3389–3390
    treatment of, 3386–3387
      antifibrinolytic agents in, 3387, *3387*
      cycloplegics in, 3386–3387
      inpatient, 3386
      medical, 3386–3387
      miotics in, 3386–3387
      salicylates in, 3386
      steroids in, 3387
      supportive, 3386
      surgical, 3387–3388, *3388*
        indications for, 3387–3388
        techniques of, 3388, *3388*
    treatment of, 1438, *1438*, 3386–3387
      anterior chamber washout in, 1438,
        1438, 3388, *3388*
      limbal clot delivery in, 3388
  visual acuity with, 3390
Hypocalcemia, cataracts in, 2214
Hypochondriasis, 265
  symptoms of, 3747, 3749t
Hypochromia, iridic, in Fuchs' heterochromic
  iridocyclitis, 504–505, *505*
Hypoderma bovis, 1709
Hypoemotionality, visual, 2648–2649
Hypofluorescence. See at *Fluorescein
  angiography.*
Hypogammaglobulinemia, in ataxia-
  telangiectasia, 3322
Hypoglycemia, 2929
  in serpiginous choroiditis, 520
  lens abnormalities in, 2787t
  perioperative management of, 662
Hypoglycemic agents, 2929, 2929t
Hypokalemia, carbonic anhydrase inhibitor
    therapy and, 1583
  controversy over, 667–668
  diuretics and, 667
  electrocardiographic changes in, 667–668
  preoperative, 668
Hypolipoproteinemia, ocular manifestations
  of, 301–303, *302*, 302t, *303*
Hypoparathyroidism, cataracts in, 2214
Hypophyseal-pharyngeal duct,
    craniopharyngioma of, 2621
Hypophysis, chiasm and, 2616
Hypophysitis, lymphoid, 2624
Hypopituitarism, adenoma and, 2619
Hypoplasia, dermal, coloboma in, 2794
  familial, in pediatric glaucoma, 2774
  iridic, 2146, *2147*, *2148*
  optic nerve, congenital, 2795, 2797, *2797*
    neonatal, 2835, *2835*
    septum pellucidum absence in, 2797,
      2797
Hypoproinsulinemia, familial, 2928
Hypopyon, black, in metastatic malignant
    melanoma, 1459
  in Behçet's disease, 1020, *1021*, 3129, *3129*
  in systemic non-Hodgkin's lymphoma, 536,
    537
Hypotension, glaucoma and, 1292
  ocular, in pathologic myopia, 881
  perioperative, 2856

Hypotensive episode, vs. normal-tension
    glaucoma, 1358
Hypothalamus, in optic tract disease, 2630
Hypothermia, in central retinal artery
    occlusion, 732
  intraocular, 1143
Hypothyroidism, thyroid-stimulating
    hormone assay in, 2947–2948, *2948*
  visual field defects in, 2624
Hypotony, after Molteno implant, 1663–1664
  after vitreoretinal surgery, 1135–1136
  choroidal folds and, 895
  in penetrating keratoplasty, 326–327
  in uveal effusion, 553–554
Hypotropia, in Graves' disease, 2742, *2742*
  in oculomotor nerve palsy, 2738, *2738*
Hypoxia, cellular, 2102t
  central retinal artery injury with, 731–732
  contact lens–induced, 3624–3625
    clinical manifestations of, *3625*, 3625–
      3627
  in neovascularization, 1492
  intraoperative, 2856
Hysterectomy, idiopathic macular hole and,
    883
Hysteria, horizontal gaze deviation in, 2502
Hysterical visual loss, 3189–3191

I cell, in mucolipidosis type II, 304
I-cell disease, corneal abnormalities in, 2786
  ocular manifestations of, 2780
  skeletal/facial changes in, 2783
Ichthyosis, congenital, cataract in, 2216
Ichthyosis vulgaris, 3156
Idiopathic blind spot enlargement syndrome,
    vs. multiple evanescent white dot
    syndrome, 917–918
Idiopathic flat detachment of the macula. See
    Central serous chorioretinopathy.
Idiopathic inflammatory pseudotumor. See
    Pseudotumor.
Idiopathic macular serous detachment. See
    Central serous chorioretinopathy.
Idiopathic orbital inflammation. See
    Pseudotumor.
Idiopathic thrombocytopenic purpura,
    retinopathy in, 999
Idoxuridine, 3028
  in ocular viral disease, 118–119, 119t, 136
  ocular toxicity of, 90–92
Ignipuncture, in retinal detachment, 1092–
    1093, *1276*, 1276–1277, *1277*
Ileum, carcinoid tumor of, 2060
Illness, denial of, 3747
  psychologic-physiologic features of, con-
    ceptual model for, 3750–3751
Illumination, instrumentation for, 1122t
Image, real, optics of, 3603–3604, *3604*
  virtual, optics of, 3603–3604, *3604*
Imaging. See also *Computed tomography;
    Magnetic resonance imaging;
    Ultrasonography.*
  radiographic anatomy and, 3505–3511
Imidazole, for fungal infections, 176t, 177
Immune system, 2110–2111
  disorders of, 2102t
    autoantibodies in, 2895–2896, 2896t
    pathology of, 2110–2112, 2112t, 2113t
  in ataxia-telangiectasia, 3322
  in atopic dermatitis, 111, 3156–3157

Immune system *(Continued)*
  in atopic keratoconjunctivitis, 95
  in Behçet's disease, 992, 1019, 3130
  in birdshot retinochoroiditis, 475
  in blepharitis, 104
  in candidiasis, 3031
  in CAR syndrome, 3353, *3353*
  in coccidioidomycosis, 3055
  in corneal transplant rejection, 213
  in dermatomyositis, 989–990
  in Eales disease, 795
  in erythema multiforme, 3169
  in experimental acute retinal necrosis,
    954–955
  in Fuchs' heterochromic iridocyclitis, 510,
    512
  in human immunodeficiency virus infec-
    tion, 3104–3105
  in juvenile rheumatoid arthritis, 987
  in keratoacanthoma, 1717
  in ocular histoplasmosis syndrome, 491,
    863–864
  in ocular toxoplasmosis, 930–931, *931*
  in pemphigus, 3167–3168
  in polymyositis, 989–990
  in progressive systemic sclerosis, 989
  in recurrent ocular herpes simplex, 124–
    125
  in relapsing polychondritis, 993
  in rheumatoid arthritis, 986
  in scleroderma, 2920–2921
  in subretinal fibrosis and uveitis syndrome,
    975–976
  in sympathetic ophthalmia, 500
  in systemic lupus erythematosus, 988
  in temporal arteritis, 2902
  in thyroid ophthalmopathy, 2941
  in tissue injury, 2112, 2113t
  in uveitis, 1445–1446, 2150–2151, 2164
  in Vogt-Koyanagi-Harada syndrome, 484
  in Wegener's granulomatosis, 990, 2909–
    2910
Immunization, parainfectious optic neuritis
    in, 2611
Immunoglobulin, immunohistochemical
    staining with, 2376t
Immunoglobulin A, in nephropathy, 420
Immunoglobulin E, in atopic
    keratoconjunctivitis, 95
  in giant papillary conjunctivitis, 88
  in ocular allergy, 82
  in vernal conjunctivitis, 84
  receptors for, mast cell, 79
Immunoglobulin E pentapeptide, in allergic
    conjunctivitis, 83
Immunoglobulin E suppressive factor, in
    atopic keratoconjunctivitis, 96–97
Immunoglobulin G, in Fuchs' heterochromic
    iridocyclitis, 512
  in giant papillary conjunctivitis, 88–89
  in vernal conjunctivitis, 84
Immunoglobulin light chains, staining for,
    2381–2382
Immunoglobulin M, in giant papillary
    conjunctivitis, 89
Immunohistochemistry, 2372–2385
  antigen–antibody interaction in, 2372–2373
  autolysis in, 2372
  controls in, 2374–2375
  detection systems in, 2373
    avidin-biotin peroxidase in, 2374, *2374*
    direct method, 2373, *2373*

Keratoconjunctivitis sicca *(Continued)*
  in rosacea, 106
  in scleroderma, 2922, *2922*
  in Sjögren's syndrome, 993, 1938
  in systemic lupus erythematosus, 2897
  late, 266, *266*
  mechanisms of, *260*, 260–263, *261–263*
  ocular surface disease in, pathology of,
    259–260
  rose bengal staining in, 267–268, *268*
  tear lactoferrin immunoassay in, 10
  tear lysozyme test in, 9–10
Keratoconus, 15, *18*, 59, *60*
  contact lenses for, fitting of, *3641*, 3641–
    3642
    diagnostic lenses in, 3642
    visual acuity after, 3642
    indications for, 3641
  corneal opacity in, 2185, *2188*
  epikeratoplasty for, 356
  keratoglobus and, 61
  pathology of, 2141
  thermokeratoplasty for, 356, *357*
Keratocytes, collagen secretion of, 985–986
  in corneal chemical injury, *235*
  in fleck dystrophy, 45, *48*
  in Grayson-Wilbrandt dystrophy, 49, *49*
Keratoepithelioplasty, in corneal ulcer, 230,
  232
Keratoglobus, 61, *62*, 2141
Keratolysis, in rheumatoid arthritis, 2891
Keratomalacia, vitamin A deficiency and,
  2982
Keratometry, 7, *7*, 344
  intraocular lens power on, 605, 3657
  validation of, 606t
Keratomileusis, hyperopic, 351, *352*
  in myopia, 351–352
Keratomycosis, antifungals for, 176–178, 178t
  aspergillar, 1707
  corneal biopsy in, 174–176, *175*, *176*
  paracentesis in, 176
  penetrating keratoplasty in, 178–179
  suspicion for, 174
Keratoneuritis, radial, in *Acanthamoeba*
  keratitis, 185, *186*
Keratopathy, actinic, 68, *69*
  band, 68, *70*, 70–71
    calcific, 2141, *2141*
    disease causes of, 70
    idiopathic, 33
    in gout, *311*, 311–312
    in juvenile rheumatoid arthritis–associ-
      ated uveitis, 2794
    in sarcoidosis, 445–446
    noncalcific, 2142
    pathology of, 2142
    urate, in gout, *311*, 311–312
    vitamin D excess and, 2984
  bullous, aphakic, 2134, *2134*, *2135*
    in corneal edema, 245, *247*
    keratoscopy of, *7*
    pseudophakic, in anterior chamber intra-
      ocular lens, 642, *642*
    soft contact lenses and, 255
  crystalline, infectious, 167, *167*
  droplet, climatic, 68, *69*, 2142
  epithelial, charged particle irradiation and,
    3239
  in toxic epidermal necrolysis, 212, *212*
  Labrador, 68, *69*, 2142
  lagophthalmic, 2142

Keratopathy *(Continued)*
  lipid, after corneal hydrops, 66
    pathology of, 2142
  neuroparalytic, 2142
  proliferative vitreoretinopathy treatment
    and, 1118
  punctate, fluorescein staining of, 10, *10*
    in atopic keratoconjunctivitis, 94
    in toxic reactions, 90
Keratophakia, 352, *352*
  in aphakia, 641
Keratoplasty, 3
  in cataract surgery, 252, 252t
  in corneal edema, 255
  in Fuchs' dystrophy, 54
  in granular dystrophy, 36
  lamellar, 319–325, 345t
    automated, 321, *321*
    complications of, 325
    freehand, 321–322, *322*
    graft-host neovascularization in, 325
    history of, 319–320
    in chemical injury, 229–230, *231*, 242
    in noninfected corneal ulcer, 232–233
    in ocular herpes simplex, 134
    indications for, *320*, 320–321, 345t
    inlay, donor preparation in, 322–323,
      322–324
      for stromal pathology, 320
      for tectonic purposes, 320
      recipient preparation in, *321*, 321–322,
        322
      technique of, 321–323, *321–324*
    onlay, *320*, 320–321
      technique of, 323–325, *324*
    perforation in, 323, *324*, 325
    pseudo anterior chamber in, 325
    suturing in, 322–323, *323*
    tectonic, 320
  penetrating, 325–336
    astigmatism in, 335
    cataract extraction with, 331–332
    coloboma repair with, 330, *331*
    complications of, 333–334, 1541
      operative, 333
      postoperative, immediate, 333–334
      late, 334
    concomitant procedure with, 330–332,
      331, *332*
    corticosteroids after, 332
    cytoid macular edema after, 902
    donor material in, epithelium of, 327
      preservation of, 328
      selection of, 327–328
    glaucoma and, 332–333, 335, 1293,
      1541–1550, 1541t
      assessment in, 1541–1542
      graft size in, 1543t, 1544
      intraocular pressure in, 1542–1545
      mechanisms of, 1542–1545, 1546t
      peripheral anterior synechiae in,
        1544–1545
      phakic status in, 1543–1544
      postoperative factors in, 1543t, 1544–
        1545
      preoperative, 1543t, 1544
      preoperative factors in, 1543–1544,
        1543t
      risk factors for, 1542
      steroids in, 1544t, 1545
      treatment of, 1545–1549
      α-agonists in, 1546

Keratoplasty *(Continued)*
      beta-blockers in, 1546
      carbonic anhydrase inhibitors in,
        1546
      ciliodestructive procedures in, 1549
      cryotherapy in, 1549, 1549t
      cyclodialysis in, 1548
      epinephrine in, 1546
      filtration surgery in, 1547–1548,
        1547t
      high-intensity ultrasound in, 1549
      laser, 1546–1547, 1549
      medical, 1546
      Molteno's implant in, 1548, *1548*
      parasympathomimetics in, 1546
      prosthetic devices in, 1548
      Schocket's tube in, 1548–1549
      steroids in, 1546
      surgical, 1547–1549, 1547t
      synechialysis in, 1548
    graft failure in, 334–335
    graft rejection in, *335*, 335–336, *336*
    history of, 325–326
    in *Acanthamoeba* keratitis, 187–188
    in corneal ulcer, 232–233
    in herpes zoster ophthalmicus, 146
    in keratomycosis, 178–179
    in ocular herpes simplex, *134*, 134–135
    in trauma, 3399
    indications for, 326, 345t, 1541
    infection in, 334
    intraocular pressure after, 1542
    iridectomy with, 330, *331*, *332*
    lens extraction with, 330–332
    postoperative care in, 332, 332–333
    preoperative considerations in, 327–328
    procedure for, 328–332, *331*, *332*
      anterior chamber assessment in, 330
      graft size in, 328–329
      suturing in, 329–330
        complications of, 334
      technique of, 345t
      trephinization in, 329
    prognosis of, 326–327
    rhegmatogenous retinal detachment and,
      1086
    rigid gas-permeable contact lenses after,
      3644
    superficial punctate keratitis after, *333*
    vitreoretinal procedures with, 332
    vitreous removal with, 332
    wound leakage in, 333
  viral infection and, 117
Keratoprosthesis, 3, 338–341
  buried membrane, 338, *339*
  complications of, *340*, 340–341
  contact lens, 338, *339*
  cornea and, 339, *340*
  fluid-barrier procedure and, 338, *339*
  glaucoma and, 341
  in noninfected corneal ulcer, 233
  indications for, 340
  intrastromal membrane, 338, *339*
  materials for, 338
  necrosis and, *340*, 341
  nonpenetrating membrane, 338, *339*
  penetrating, 338–340, *339*, *340*
  posterior membrane, 338, *339*
  results of, 340–341, *341*
  retroprosthesis membrane formation and,
    341
  through-and-through, 338–339, *339*

Occipital lobe *(Continued)*
  blindness from, 2636, 2638
    causes of, 2636, 2637t
    cerebrovascular accident and, 2636,
      2637t
  clinical manifestations of, 2671t
  in color anomia, 2645–2646
  in pure alexia, 2646
  neuroophthalmologic findings in, *2634*,
    2634–2636, *2635*, 2637t, 2638
  tumors and, 2371t
  visual defects in, *2634*, 2634–2635, *2635*
  visual field defects in, 2636
  visual field loss in, 2635–2636
  posterior cerebral arterial supply to, *2661*
  visual area 1 of, 2640–2641, *2641*, *2642*
Occipitofugal syndromes, ventral, 2645–2649
Occipitoparietal areas, in Balint's syndrome,
  2650
Occipitotemporal cortex, infarction of, in
  prosopagnosia, 2647
Occlusion therapy, in chemical injury, 240
  in early infantile esotropia, 2731
  in pediatric strabismic amblyopia, 2730,
    2730
  in vernal conjunctivitis, 86
Occupational therapy, in low vision
  rehabilitation, 3671–3672, 3683–3686,
    3683t. See also *Low vision, rehabilitation
    of.*
Ochronosis, 296–297
  corneal findings in, 297, *297*
Octafluorocyclobutane (C₄F₈), 1149
Octofluorocyclopropane (C₃F₈), intravitreal
  tamponade with, glaucoma after, 1563–
    1565
Octopus perimetry, in glaucoma, 1304, *1304*
Ocular bobbing, in coma, 2505, *2505*
Ocular flutter, burst neuron inhibition defect
  and, 2399
  opsoclonus and, 2430
Ocular histoplasmosis syndrome, 488–495,
  860–876, 2163, 3049, 3051, 3052
  amphotericin B in, 869
  antihistamines in, 869
  clinical features of, 489–490, *490*, *491*,
    864–867, 864t, *865–867*
  desensitization in, 869
  diagnostic testing in, 492, 492t
  differential diagnosis of, 492–493, 493t,
    868–869, 869t
  disseminated choroiditis, 866, *867*
  epidemiology of, 488–489, 489t, 860–861,
    861
  exogenous histoplasmic endophthalmitis in,
    867
  experimental animal model of, 863
  extrafoveal subretinal neovascular mem-
    brane and, laser photocoagulation in,
    869–870, *870*, 872, *873*
  fellow eye in, 861, 875
  fluorescein angiography in, 455, *455*, 867–
    868, 867t, *868*
  histocompatibility antigens in, 864
  histopathology of, 861–863, *862*, *863*
  Histoplasma capsulatum in, 455, *455*, 489,
    489t
  history of, 488
  immunology of, 863–864
  indocyanine green angiography in, 724

Ocular histoplasmosis syndrome *(Continued)*
  juxtafoveal subretinal neovascular mem-
    brane and, laser photocoagulation in,
    871, 871–872, *873*
  juxtapapillary chorioretinal atrophy in,
    864, *865*, *866*
  laser photocoagulation in, 869–873, *870*,
    871, *873*
    guidelines for, 872
  lymphocyte hyperreactivity in, 864
  macular lesions in, 864–866, *866*
  optic disc edema in, 866
  organism in, 861–862
  pathology of, 2163, *2163*
  pathophysiology of, 490–492
  pigment epithelial detachments in, 866
  prognosis for, 492
  pseudo, 404–405
  punched-out chorioretinal lesions in, 864,
    865
  steroids in, 869
  subretinal neovascular membrane in, re-
    currence of, 873–874
    definition of, 873
    etiology of, 874, *874*
    incidence of, 873
    presentation of, 874, *875*
    treatment of, 874
      complications of, 874, 874t, *875*
  systemic features of, 489t
  systemic infection in, 861–862
  treatment of, 493–494, 493t, *494*, 869, 3053
    complications of, 874, 874t, *875*
    fluorescein angiography after, 875–876
    follow-up for, 875
    visual recovery after, 876
  vitreous hemorrhage in, 867
  vs. acute posterior multifocal placoid pig-
    ment epitheliopathy, 868
  vs. Behçet's disease, 868–869
  vs. birdshot choroidopathy, 868
  vs. central serous chorioretinopathy, 822
  vs. diffuse unilateral subacute neuroreti-
    nopathy, 868
  vs. multifocal choroiditis, 868
  vs. panuveitis, 868
  vs. vitritis, 866
  vs. Vogt-Koyanagi syndrome, 868–869
Ocular infarction, 2655–2657
  anterior ischemic optic neuropathy and,
    2656–2657
  branch retinal artery occlusion and, 2656
  central retinal artery occlusion and, 2655–
    2656
  definition of, 2654
Ocular ischemia, 2653–2657. See also specific
  types, e.g, *Transient monocular visual
  loss.*
Ocular ischemic syndrome. See also *Ischemic
  ocular syndrome.*
Ocular larva migrans, 3072
Ocular motility. See also *Eye movements.*
  disorders of, 1883, 3474, 3474t
  in chiasmal disorders, 2618
  in nonorganic visual disorders, 2708
  in thyroid ophthalmopathy, 2946, *2946*
  in trauma treatment, 3367
  neuroophthalmologic examination of,
    2389, 2391
  orbital fracture and, 3469–3470
  trauma and, 3468–3471
Ocular motor nerves. See *Cranial nerve(s).*

Ocular pulse amplitude, in carotid cavernous
  fistula, 1471
Ocular rigidity, coefficient of, in tonometry,
  1330
  in tonography, 1333
Ocular surface, 3, 257
  diseases of, tear secretion and, 261–262
  epithelium of, electrolytes and, 270
  in chemical injury, 235–236, 237
  in dry eye disorders, 259–260
  physiology of, 257
Ocular syndrome, ischemic. See *Ischemic
  ocular syndrome.*
Ocular tilt reaction, 2420
  contraversive, tonic, 2420, *2421*
  in coma, 2506
  ipsilesional, tonic, 2421
  vs. unilateral superior oblique palsy, 2420
Ocular tracking, smooth pursuit defects and,
  2404
Oculinum. See *Botulinum toxin.*
Oculocerebral syndrome, 2779, *2779*
Oculocerebrorenal syndrome, lens pathology
  in, 2188–2189, *2189*
  ocular manifestations of, 2779, *2779*
  rickets in, 2783
  visual system in, 3561
Oculodermal melanocytosis, 1802, *1802*
  congenital, 2147, 2149
    hyperchromic heterochromia iridum in,
      372, 372–373, *373*
  in neurofibromatosis, 3305
Oculography, of eye movement disorders,
  2413–2414, *2414*
Oculomotor nerve, *1876*, *1879*
  aberrant regeneration of, 2452–2453, *2453*,
    2477
  abnormalities of, 2449–2454, *2451*, 2451t,
    2453, 2453t
  anatomy of, 2444, *2445–2449*
  fascicle of, 2444, *2446*
  inferior, *1875*, *1880*
  lesions of, 2413
  neuromyotonia of, 2453
  palsy of, aberrant nerve regeneration in,
    2738
    acquired, 2450–2452, *2451*, 2451t
    adduction, 2417
    Benedikt's syndrome from, 2451, *2451*
    botulinum toxin in, 2758
    causes of, 2451–2452
    congenital, 2450
      cyclic paresis in, 2452
    evaluation of, 2449, *2450*, 2453–2454,
      2453t
    fascicular, 2450–2451, *2451*
    in cavernous sinus, 2452
    in subarachnoid space, 2451, 2451–2452
    intracranial aneurysm and, *2451*, 2451–
      2452
    paralytic strabismus in, 2737, 2737–2738
    pupillary sparing, 2452
    treatment of, 2453–2454
    Weber's syndrome from, 2451, *2451*
  paresis of, in coma, 2503
  superior, *1875*, *1880*, 2444, *2447*
  synkinesis of, 2452–2453
  traumatic lesions of, *3471*, 3471–3472
  vascular supply of, 2444, *2446*
  within cavernous sinus, 2444, *2447*
Oculomotor nucleus, in horizontal eye
  movements, 2394–2395, *2395*

Pediatric patient *(Continued)*
    visual acuity testing in, *2719–2722,*
        2719–2723
        after age 6, 2722
        age 3 to 6, 2721, *2722*
        alternative techniques in, *2722,* 2722–
          2723
        birth to age 3, *2719–2721, 2720, 2721*
        error in, 2719, *2719*
        fixation responses in, CSM method
          for, *2720,* 2720–2721
        motor responses in, 2720
        optotypes for, 2721, *2722*
        preferential looking in, 2722, *2722*
        visual evoked potentials in, 2723
    visual development and, 2718t
    visual field testing in, 2724
    visual function testing in, 2719–2728
    eye of, schematic representation of, 3286,
      3286
    glaucoma in, 2769–2777. See also *Glau-*
      coma, pediatric.
    gross motor development in, 2718t
    herpes simplex virus infection in, 964–965,
      965
    Hurler's syndrome in. See *Hurler's syn-*
      drome.
    hyperopia in, correction of, 3616–3617
    hypophyseal stalk glioma in, 3567
    inherited metabolic disease in, ocular man-
      ifestations of, 2777–2791. See also
      Metabolic disease, inherited.
    intermittent exotropia in, 2732–2733, *2733*
    low vision in, 3665
      rehabilitation of, 3682–3683
    migraine in, 2692–2693
    motor responses in, 2720
    myopia in, correction of, 3615
    ocular trauma in, *3490,* 3490–3493, 3490t,
      3491, 3492
    ophthalmologist for, 2715
    optic nerve glioma in, 2578, 2579t, *2580–*
      2583, 2581, 2583–2584, 2622. See also
      Glioma, optic nerve, pediatric.
    orbital cellulitis in, *2832,* 2832–2833
    orbital disorders in, frequency of, 1888–
      1889, 1888t, 1889t
      radiology of, 3521
    orbital mucormycosis in, 2834, *2834*
    pineoblastoma in, 3568
    pineocytoma in, 3568
    preseptal cellulitis in, 2831–2832, *2832*
    retinal function assessment in, 2837
    retinal viral infection in, 962–967
    retinitis pigmentosa in, 1230
    retinoblastoma in. See *Retinoblastoma.*
    retinopathy of prematurity in. See *Retinop-*
      athy of prematurity.
    sarcoidosis in, ocular findings in, 448
    shaken baby syndrome in, 1030–1031, *1031*
    small blue cell tumor in, 2329–2330
    strabismus in, 2730–2760. See also *Esotro-*
      pia; Exotropia.
    subacute sclerosing panencephalitis in,
      965–966
    subperiosteal abscess in, 2832–2833
    superior oblique weakness in, correction
      of, 2750
    treatment of, adjustment issues in, 3700–
      3706
      communicating diagnosis in, 3703

Pediatric patient *(Continued)*
    emergency surgery/hospitalization in,
      3703
    enucleation in, team-family approach to,
      3703–3706, *3704, 3705*
    office set-up in, 3702, 3702t
    preadmission preparation in, 3702–3703
    presurgical preparation in, 3702–3703
    varicella-zoster virus in, *966,* 966–967
    visually impaired, development of, 3707–
      3708
      early intervention services for, 3712,
        3712t
      educational assessment of, 3711–3712
      educational needs of, 3710, 3711t
      educational services for, 3712–3713
      growth/development issues of, 3707–
        3713
      public laws for, 3710–3711
      rehabilitation of, 3692–3693
      resources for, 3771
      services for, 3775, 3775t
Pediculus humanus, 3088
Peer Review Organizations, in ambulatory
    cataract surgery, 657
Pelizaeus-Merzbacher disease, ocular
    movement abnormalities in, 2788t
    pediatric, 2779
Pellagra, 114, 1798
Pelli-Robson chart, contrast sensitivity
    testing with, 674, *676,* 2545
Pelvic inflammatory disease, 3093. See also
    Chlamydia trachomatis.
Pemphigoid, 3162–3165
    bullous, 2119, 3162–3164, 3162t
      clinical features of, 3162, *3162*
      etiology of, 3162–3163, *3163*
      pathogenesis of, 3162–3163, *3163*
      treatment of, 3163
    cicatricial, 3164–3165, 3164t
      autoantibodies in, 196
      biopsy in, 198, *199*
      Brusting-Perry dermatitis of, 196
      clinical features of, *197,* 197–198, 3164,
        3164
      conjunctival findings in, 2129–2130
      diagnosis of, 198, *199*
      differential diagnosis of, 199t
      distichiasis in, 1855
      drug-induced, 90, 196, 3165
      epidemiology of, 196
      etiology of, 3165
      genetic predisposition to, 196
      glaucoma medication and, 90–91
      mast cells in, 88
      ocular manifestations of, 196–200, 3164,
        3164
      pathogenesis of, 196–197, 3165
      skin involvement in, 3164
      staging of, *197,* 197–198
      treatment of, 3165
        adjunctive, 199
        systemic, 198–199, 199t
      upper eyelid entropion in, 1838
    end-stage, keratoprosthesis for, *341*
Pemphigus, 2119, 3165–3168, 3165t
    clinical features of, 3165–3167, *3166*
    drug-induced, 3167
    etiology of, 3167–3168
    paraneoplastic, 3167
    pathogenesis of, 3167–3168
    treatment of, 3168

Pemphigus erythematosus, *3166,* 3166–3167
Pemphigus foliaceus, clinical features of,
    3166, 3166–3167
    myasthenia gravis and, 3167
    thymoma and, 3167
Pemphigus vegetans, 3165–3166
Pemphigus vulgaris, 199–200, 2119
    clinical features of, 3165–3166, *3166*
Pencil magnet, 1174, *1174*
Penetrating artery disease, 2666–2667
    causes of, 2666–2667
    diagnosis of, 2666–2667
    evaluation of, 2666–2667
    symptoms of, 2666
Penicillamine, in rheumatoid arthritis, 2893
    pemphigus with, 3167
Penicillin, in corneal infections, 170t
    in leptospirosis, 3090
    in neonatal conjunctivitis, 165, 2829
    in ocular syphilis, 972–973
    in purulent gonococcal conjunctivitis, 164
    ocular toxicity of, 91
Pentamidine, in *Pneumocystis carinii*
    infection, 939, 3068
Pentyde, in atopic keratoconjunctivitis, 96–
    97
Peptic ulcer disease, ocular inflammation in,
    467–468
Peptococcus, 168
Peptostreptococcus, 162, 168
Perfluorocarbon gases, 1149
Perfluorocarbon liquids, in retinal breaks,
    1130
    low-viscosity, as vitreous substitutes, 1144–
      1147, *1145–1147,* 1145t
      characteristics of, 1144–1145, *1145,*
        1145t
      in foreign body treatment, 1147
      in proliferative diabetic retinopathy,
        1146
      in proliferative vitreoretinopathy, 1145–
        1146, *1146*
      in traumatic retinal detachment, 1147
      indications for, 1145–1147, 1145t, *1146,*
        1147
      physical properties of, 1145, 1145t
      removal of, 1146
      specific gravity of, 1144
      techniques for, 1145–1147, *1146, 1147*
Perfluorodecalin ($C_{10}F_{18}$), 1145, *1145*
Perfluoroethane (C_2F_6), 1149
    in giant retinal tear repair, 1150
    in pneumatic retinopexy, 1100, 1101t
    in retinal detachment repair, 1150
Perfluoromethane (CF_4), 1149
Perfluoro-*n*-butane (C_4F_{10}), 1149
Perfluoro-*n*-octane (C_8F_{18}), 1145
Perfluorooctane, *1145*
Perfluorooctylbromide, 1145
Perfluorophenanthrene ($C_{14}F_{24}$), 1145, *1145,*
    1154
Perfluoropropane (C_3F_8), 1149, 1279
    in pneumatic retinopexy, 1100, 1101t
Perfluorotributylamine ($C_{12}F_{27}N$), 1145
Perfluorooethylcyclohexane (C_8F_{16}), 1145
Perfusion pressure, definition of, 1368
Periarteritis nodosa, 1936–1937, *2115*
Pericallosal artery, *2661*
Pericarditis, *Candida,* 3032–3033
Pericytes, angiogenesis inhibition by, 1493
    capillary, in diabetic retinopathy, 2259

Perimetry, Goldmann, in glaucoma, 1301–1302
  in idiopathic intracranial hypertension, 2700–2701, *2701*
  Octopus, in glaucoma, 1304, *1304*, 1307
  Tubingen, in glaucoma, 1302, 1307
Periorbita, *1877*
Peripapillary veins, inflammatory sheathing of, in Leber's idiopathic stellate neuroretinitis, 811
Peripheral anterior synechiae, traumatic, 1440–1441
Peripheral cystoid degeneration, retinal, 1067–1068
Peripheral nerve, orbital, vs. optic nerve, 1978
Peripheral nerve sheath tumor, orbital, 1978–2003, 2070–2072, *2072*. See also specific types, e.g., *Orbital schwannoma*.
  differential diagnosis of, 1979
  malignant, *1994*, 1994–1996, *1995*, *1996*
  pathology of, 2324–2325, *2325–2326*, 2348t
  presentation of, 1979
  prevalence of, 1980t
Peripheral neuropathy, 2932
  in amyloidosis, 2959
Peripheral ulcerative keratitis, in rheumatoid arthritis, 2891, *2891*
Peripherin, gene for, 1221
Periphlebitis, retinal, 792. See also *Eales disease*.
  acute, diffuse. See *Frosted branch angiitis*.
Periscleritis, 1924. See also *Pseudotumor*.
Peritonitis, *Candida*, 3033, 3036
Perkins tonometer, 1332, *1332*
  in pediatric eye exam, 2725, *2725–2726*
Perls' stain, of lens epithelium, 2210, *2211*
Peroxidase-antiperoxidase, in diagnostic immunohistochemistry, 2374
Perphenazine, in postherpetic neuralgia, 146
Persistent hyperplastic primary vitreous, *2185*, *2797*, 2797–2798, *2798*
  cataract in, *2197*, 2198
  computed tomography of, 3514
  fibrovascular plaque in, 2242, *2242*
  glaucoma with, 1555
  magnetic resonance imaging of, 3514
  pathology of, *2197*, 2197–2198, *2242*, 2242–2243
  pediatric, *2797*, 2797, *2798*
    cataract in, *2762*, 2762
  surgery for, 2797–2798
  vs. retinoblastoma, 2266
Personality, borderline, 3733
  compulsive, 3731–3732, 3732t
  dependent, 3731, 3732t
  dramatizing, 3732, 3732t
  illness response and, 3731–3733, 3732t
  in central serous chorioretinopathy, 818, 821
  masochistic, 3732, 3732t
  medical care and, 3733
  narcissistic, 3732, 3732t
  paranoid, 3732, 3732t
  schizoid, 3732–3733, 3732t
  styles of, illness response and, 3731–3733, 3732t
  type A, in central serous chorioretinopathy, 818, 821

Personality *(Continued)*
  types of, 3731–3733, 3732t
  vision loss and, 3180–3181
Peters' anomaly, cataract in, 2185, *2188*
  in Axenfeld-Rieger syndrome, 378, *378*
  in pediatric glaucoma, 2774
  pathology of, 2135
  type I, *18*, 19
  type II, 19, *20–21*
  vs. juvenile-onset open-angle glaucoma, 1347
Petroleum jelly (Vaseline), cosmetic injection of, *2095*, 2096
Petrosal nerve, *1877*
Petrous ridge, abducens nerve palsy at, 2458–2459
Peutz-Jeghers syndrome, 2977t, 2978
  lentigo simplex of, 1798, *1798*
Phacoanaphylaxis, 1445–1446
Phacoemulsification, anterior chamber, 635, *635*
  anterior chamber incision in, 633, *634*
  aqueous-viscoelastic exchange in, 633, *634*
  calipers in, 633, *633*
  capsulorhexis in, 633, *634*
  in cataract surgery, 621
  Kelman technique of, 610–611
  limbal incisions in, 633, *634*
  nucleus emulsification in, 633, *635*, 635
  nucleus prolapse in, 633, *635*
  nucleus sculpting in, 633, *634*
  posterior chamber, 633, *634*, *635*, 635
  posterior chamber lens implantation and, in nanophthalmos, 1539
  systems for, 624–625, *625*
  wound closure in, 639, *639*
Phacofiltration technique, in nanophthalmos, 1539
Phacofragmentation, irrigation with, 611
Phagocytes, mononuclear, in acute inflammation, 2105–2106
Phagocytosis, in acute inflammation, 2105, *2106*
  in corticosteroid-induced glaucoma, 1464
  pigment, in sympathetic ophthalmia, 498, *500*
Phagolysosomes, degradation by, 2105
Phagosomes, engulfment by, 2105
  injury to, 2103t
Phakitis, infectious, lens abscess in, 2217, *2217*
Phakomatosis, 3298–3323. See also specific disorders, e.g., *Neurofibromatosis*.
  classification of, 3300–3301, 3300t
  history of, 3298–3301
  pathology of, 2268t–2271t
  retinoschisis in, 1083
Pharyngoconjunctival fever, adenovirus and, *149*, 149–150, *150*
  vs. adult inclusion conjunctivitis, 183
Phenothiazide, cataracts from, 2216
Phenothiazine(s), corneal epithelium and, 305–306
  in postherpetic neuralgia, 146
  intoxication with, upward gaze deviation in, 2502
  ophthalmologic effects of, 3738–3739, 3738t
  retinal toxicity of, 1044–1046, *1045*
Phenylalanine, lens, ultraviolet B radiation absorption by, 576, *577*
Phenylbutazone, leukemia and, 2988

Phenylephrine, cyclopentolate with, in cataract extraction, 626, 627t
  in angle-closure glaucoma testing, 1337
  in malignant glaucoma, 1524
  in nanophthalmos, 1533
  pupillary effects of, 2472
  toxicity of, in retinopathy of prematurity, 2806
Phenylephrine-pilocarpine test, in angle-closure glaucoma, 1337
Phenylephrine test, in acquired aponeurogenic ptosis, 1827
Pheochromocytoma, 2871
  hypertension in, 2870
  in neurofibromatosis, 3304
  in von Hippel-Lindau disease, 3311
Philadelphia chromosome, in chronic myelogenous leukemia, 2990
Phlebolith, in orbital varix, 1472
Phlyctenule, allergic response and, 2129
  limbal, varicella, 135, *135*
Phlyctenulosis, 212–213, *212–213*
Phosphate, conjunctival deposition of, 2129
Phosphenes, movement, in optic neuritis, 2540–2541
  sound-induced, in optic neuritis, 2541
Phosphodiesterase, cAMP degradation by, 79
  nucleotide, in cone dysfunction, 1244
Phosphodiesterase inhibitors, in allergic disorders, 79
Photic retinopathy, 1032–1036, 2257
  ophthalmic instruments in, 1034–1035, *1035*
Photoablation, 1615
Photoactive dyes, in retinoblastoma, 3283
Photochemical reaction, 578
Photocoagulation, carbon dioxide, in neovascular glaucoma, 1505
  in retinoblastoma, 3282–3283
  in retinopathy of prematurity, 2807
  injury in, 3416
  laser, burns from, 1036
    complications of, 753t
    in acquired retinoschisis, 1076, 1077–1078, *1078*
    in acute retinal necrosis, 959, *959*
    in age-related macular degeneration, 841–849, *846*, 846t
    in angioid streaks, 857
    in Behçet's disease, 1025
    in branch retinal vein occlusion, 743
    in central retinal vein occlusion, 740
    in Coats' disease, *805*, 806, *806*
    in congenital retinoschisis, 1081
    in cytomegalovirus retinitis, 3110
    in diabetic retinopathy, 748, 749t, 752t, 753t, 755–757
    in Eales disease, 794, *794*
    in epiretinal macular membranes, 922
    in macular holes, 888
    in ocular histoplasmosis syndrome, 869–873, *870*, *871*, *873*
    in ocular toxoplasmosis, 933
    in presumed ocular histoplasmosis syndrome, *491*, 493
    in proliferative diabetic retinopathy, 766–773, 769t, *771*, *772*, 772t
    in proliferative sickle cell retinopathy, *1015*, *1016*, 1016–1017
    in retinal angioma, 3312–3313
    in retinal arterial macroaneurysms, 799–800, *800*

Retinoschisis *(Continued)*
  macular abnormality in, 1078–1079, *1079*
  pathology of, 2244
  pigment clumps in, 1080, *1080*
  retinal detachment and, *1081*, 1081–1082, *1082*
  treatment of, *1081*, 1081–1082, *1082*, 1082t
  vs. acquired retinoschisis, 1082t
  degenerative, retinal holes and, 1061, *1061*
  foveal, familial, 1256
  in child abuse, 1083
  in vitreoretinal degeneration, 2243
  optic pit and, 1083
  retinopathy of prematurity and, 1083
  senile. See *Retinoschisis, acquired.*
  X-linked, 1078–1082, *1079–1082*, 1082t
    juvenile, full-field electroretinography in, 1196, *1197*
      neovascular glaucoma in, 1499
      rhegmatogenous retinal detachment and, 1087
    vs. retinal detachment, 1101
Retinoscopy, 343–344
  axis refinement in, 3613–3614
  pediatric, 2728, *2728*
  power refinement in, 3613–3614
  streak, 344
    in objective refraction, 3613–3614
Retrobulbar hemorrhage, trauma and, 3377–3378, *3378*
Retrobulbar neuritis, vs. multiple evanescent white dot syndrome, 917
Retrobulbar tumor, episcleral venous pressure with, 1475
Retrochiasm, disorders of, 2629–2639
  traumatic lesions of, 3467
Retrocorneal membrane, 1483. See also *Fibrous proliferation.*
Retroviruses, 3104
  replication of, 3021–3022
Reuling, G., 608–609
Reversal reaction, in leprosy, 3017–3018
Rhabdoid tumor, orbital, malignant, 2065, *2066*, 2335, *2335*, 2337, 2349t
Rhabdomyosarcoma, iridic, 3259
  orbital, 2042
    computed tomography of, 3529, 3531, *3531*
    evaluation of, 3531t
    magnetic resonance imaging of, 3531
    pathology of, 2329–2330, *2331*, 2348t
    vs. capillary hemangioma, 1968
Rheumatic disease, pediatric. See also *Rheumatoid arthritis, juvenile.*
  differential diagnosis of, 2784, 2785t
Rheumatism, palindromic, 472
Rheumatoid arthritis, 2887–2893
  amyloidosis in, 2963
  anterior uveitis in, 410–411
  articular manifestations of, 2888–2889, 2888t
  blindness in, 2893
  chloroquine toxicity in, 2893
  clinical features of, 2888–2893
  corneal degeneration with, 63, *63*
  corneal furrows in, 205–206
  corneal manifestations of, *2890*, 2890–2891
  corneal ulceration in, 206
  criteria for, 2887t
  episcleral manifestations of, 2891
  episcleritis in, 204, *204*

Rheumatoid arthritis *(Continued)*
  extraarticular manifestations of, 2889, 2889t
  joint involvement in, 2888t
  juvenile, 2783–2794
    clinical presentation of, 2785–2788, 2787t
    complications of, 2787t
    definition of, 2785
    differential diagnosis of, 2783–2785, 2784t, 2785t
    emotional conflict in, 473
    incidence of, 2785
    inflammatory glaucoma and, 1433
    ocular inflammation in, 471
    pauciarticular, 2785t, 2786
    polyarticular, 2785t, 2786
    prognosis for, 2788–2789, 2789t
    retinal manifestations of, 987–988
    subclassification of, 2784–2785, 2785t
    systemic, 2785t, 2786
    treatment of, 2789–2794
      band keratopathy chelation in, 2794
      cataract extraction in, 2792–2793
      corticosteroids in, 2789–2790
      cytotoxic agents in, 2790–2792
      glaucoma surgery in, 2793–2794
      medical, 2789–2792
      mydriatic cycloplegics in, 2790
      nonsteroidal anti-inflammatory agents in, 2790
      surgical, 2792–2794
    uveitis in, 2166
    vs. childhood sarcoid arthritis, 3135t
  keratoconjunctivitis sicca in, 203, *203*
  laboratory findings in, 2890
  major histocompatibility antigens in, 2888
  ocular chrysiasis in, 2893
  ocular findings in, 203
  ophthalmic manifestations of, *2890*, 2890–2893, *2891*, *2892*
  pathogenesis of, 2888
  prednisone for, posterior subcapsular cataracts from, 2216
  retinal manifestations of, 986–987, *987*
  scleral manifestations of, 2891–2893, *2892*
  scleritis in, 204, *204*, 471
  sclerosis in, 206
  ulcerative keratitis in, 205, *205*
  venous stasis retinopathy in, 2893
Rheumatoid factor, 2890
Rhinophyma, in rosacea, 106, *107*, 3159
Rhinoscleroma, orbital, 2310
Rhinosporidiosis, conjunctival, 2128
Rhizomucor, 3041. See also *Zygomycosis.*
Rhizopus, 3041. See also *Zygomycosis.*
  orbital, 1948–1949
Rhodopsin density, assessment of, 1194, *1194*
  normal values for, 1194
Rhodopsin gene, in retinitis pigmentosa, 1219–1222, *1220*, 1220t, *1221*
  mutations in, 1219, 1220t
  nonsense mutation of, in retinitis pigmentosa, 1221–1222
  nucleotide sequences of, *1220*
  structure of, 1221, *1221*
  vitamin A pocket of, 1221, *1221*
Ribavirin, 3030
Riboflavin, deficiency of, 114
Rickets, 2984
Rieger's anomaly, vs. juvenile-onset open-angle glaucoma, 1347

Rieger's syndrome, nonocular abnormalities in, 377–378
  pathology of, 2135
  pediatric glaucoma in, 2774
  vs. juvenile-onset open-angle glaucoma, 1347
Riesman's sign, 2945t
Rifampin, in leprosy, 3019t
  in tuberculosis, 417, 3015–3016, 3015t
Riley–Day syndrome, corneal findings in, *315*, 315–316
  pediatric, 2785
  retinal ganglion cell loss in, *2522*
Rimantadine, 3030
River blindness, 463
Rocky Mountain spotted fever, anterior uveitis in, 419
Rod(s), distribution of, 1183–1184, *1184*
  spectral sensitivity testing of, 1185, *1185*
Rodenstock confocal scanning laser ophthalmoscope, 1318
Rodenstock Optic Nerve Head Analyzer, for optic nerve head imaging, 1315–1316, *1316*
Rodenstock's panfunduscopic lens, in slit-lamp biomicroscopy, *695*, *696*
Rodent ulcer. See *Basal cell carcinoma.*
Romaña's sign, 3074
Romberg's disease, vs. scleroderma, 2922
Rosacea, 106–108, *3159*, 3159–3160, 3159t
  blood vessels in, clinical features of, 3159, *3159*, 3159t
  etiology of, 3159–3160
  facial, 106, *106*, *107*
  ocular manifestations of, 3159, *3159*
  pathogenesis of, 107–108, 3159–3160
  treatment of, 3160
    dry eye in, 108
    lid hygiene in, 108, *108*
    metronidazole in, 109, *110*
    tetracycline in, 108–109, 109t
Rosai-Dorfman disease, 3333
Rose bengal staining, in dry eye disorders, 267
  in keratoconjunctivitis sicca, 267–268, *268*
  in meibomitis/meibomian gland dysfunction, 268, *268*
  in nocturnal lagophthalmos, 268, *268*
  in vernal conjunctivitis, 85
  of epithelial defects, 11, *11*
  scoring system for, 267
Rosenbach's sign, 2945t
Rosenthal's fibers, in astrocytic processes, 2121
Roth's spot, in bacterial endocarditis, 3007
  in leukemia, *2991*, 2991–2992
  in metastatic bacterial endophthalmitis, 2157
Rubbing, of eyes, 2119t
  in keratoconus, 59
Rubella (German measles), 155, 3021t, 3024t, 3025, *3026*
  cataracts and, 2193–2194, *2194*, 2762–2763
  cataracts of, 2189
  in subacute sclerosing panencephalitis, 459, *459*, *460*
  myopia and, 3147–3148
  ocular, 155
  retinal, 963, *963*
    in pediatric patient, 962–963, *963*
  retinopathy in, 459, *459*

Syphilis *(Continued)*
　clinical manifestations of, 3080–3081,
　　3080t, *3081*
　corneal manifestations of, 970–971
　diagnosis of, 971–972, *972*
　epidemiology of, 969
　etiology of, 969
　human immunodeficiency virus infection
　　and, 972
　interstitial keratitis in, 970–971, *971*,
　　971t
　neuroophthalmic manifestations of, 970
　pathology of, *2157*, 2158
　scleral manifestations of, 970–971
　transmission of, 969
　treatment of, 972–973
　uveal manifestations of, 969–970, *970*,
　　971
　vasculitis of, 984
　vs. frosted branch angiitis, 983t, 984
　vs. Leber's idiopathic stellate neuroretin-
　　itis, 812, *813*
　of eyelids, 1704
　optic neuritis in, 2554
　optic neuropathy in, 2608–2609
　oral lesions in, 451, *451*
　primary, 3078–3079
　prognosis for, 3082
　secondary, 3079
　tertiary, 3079
　transmission of, 969
　treatment of, 3082t, 3083
Syringocystadenoma papilliferum, light
　microscopy of, *1774*, 1775
　of eyelid, *1774*, 1774–1775
　pathology of, 2296
Syringoma, of eyelid, 1779, *1780*, 1781, *1781*,
　2295
Syringomatous carcinoma, of eyelid, 1785,
　1787, 1787–1788
Systemic lupus erythematosus, 2894–2900
　autoantibodies in, 2895–2896, 2896t
　chorioidopathy in, 2898–2899, 2899t
　classification of, 2895t, 2899–2900
　clinical features of, 2895, 2896t
　corticosteroids in, 3736
　cutaneous lesions of, 2897, *2897*
　diagnosis of, 1938
　drug-induced, 2895
　episcleritis in, 206
　keratitis in, 206
　keratoconjunctivitis sicca in, 2897
　laboratory findings in, 2895–2896
　neuroophthalmologic manifestations of,
　　2899, 2899t
　ocular manifestations of, 1937
　of eyelid, 1863, *1864*
　of eyelids, 114, *114*
　orbital manifestations of, 2899
　orbital vasculitis in, 1938
　pathogenesis of, 2897
　retinal manifestations of, 988, *989*
　retinopathy in, 2897–2898, *2898*, 2899t
　scleritis in, 206
　treatment of, 2896
　vs. frosted branch angiitis, 983t, 984
Systemic sclerosis, progressive. See
　Scleroderma.

T cell:B cell ratio, in intermediate uveitis,
　436

Tabes dorsalis, 3079–3080
Taches de bougie, in sarcoidosis, 446, *447*
Tachycardia, supraventricular, intra-
　operative, 2852
　ventricular, intraoperative, 2856
Taenia multiceps, 3074
Taenia solium, 1711, 3073
　larva of, 462
Taeniasis, 3073
Takayasu's syndrome, 2114
　retina-ocular ischemia in, 1498
Talc embolus, branch retinal artery occlusion
　and, 729, *730*
Tamoxifen, ocular toxicity of, 2996t
　retinal toxicity of, 1047, *1048*
Tamponade, in retinal break treatment,
　1129–1130
　instrumentation for, 1122t
Tangier disease, corneal findings in, 302–303,
　302t, *303*
　pediatric, corneal abnormalities in, 2786
　ocular manifestations of, 2783
Tapetochoroid dystrophy, progressive, 2174–
　2175, *2175*
Taping, eyelid, in atopic dermatitis, 111, *111*
Tarsal glands, *1689*
　excretory ducts of. See *Meibomian
　　gland(s).*
Tarsal kink syndrome, 1845
　horizontal, 1698–1699
Tarsal plate, *1876*
　superior, *1877*
Tarsal strip procedure, in lower eyelid
　entropion, *1847*, 1847–1848, *1848*, *1849*
Tarsorrhaphy, in chemical injury, 240
　in dry eye disorders, 274
　in noninfected corneal ulcer, 229
　lateral, in herpes zoster ophthalmicus, 146,
　　146
　in ocular herpes simplex, 133–134
Tarsus, lower lid, 1691
　upper lid, 1691
　with meibomian gland, 2288, *2288*
Tax Equity and Fiscal Responsibility Act,
　cataract surgery and, 657
Tay-Sachs disease, cherry-red spots in, 2522
　GM$_1$-ganglioside in, 307
　pediatric, ocular manifestations of, *2778*,
　　2778–2779
T-cell leukemia-lymphoma, orbital, 2022,
　2022
T-cell lymphoma, orbital, *2021*, 2021–2022,
　2022
Tear compartment, optics of, contact lens
　and, 3622–3623
Tear duct, obstruction of, neonatal, 2769
Tear film, anatomy of, 257–259
　aqueous layer of, 258
　blinking and, 259
　break up of, in keratoconjunctivitis sicca,
　　260
　definition of, 257
　electrolyte composition of, 258
　epithelial interactions with, 7–10, *8*, *9*
　evaluation of, 7–10, *8*, *9*
　breakup time in, 8, *8*
　dye dilution test in, 8, *9*
　lactoferrin test in, 10
　lysozyme test in, 9–10
　marginal tear film strip measurement in,
　　9
　osmolarity in, 9, *9*, *10*

Tear film *(Continued)*
　Schirmer test in, 7–8, *8*
　thickness in, 258
　volume in, 7–8, *8*
　evaporation in, 262
　fluorescein staining of, *99*
　lacrimal gland secretion and, 258
　lipid layer of, 259
　marginal, measurement of, 9
　mucous layer of, 257–258
　ocular surface and, 257
　osmolarity of, 258
　　evaporation and, 261, *261*
　　in keratoconjunctivitis sicca, 259–260
　　increased, mechanisms for, *260*, 260–
　　　261, *261*
　　measurement of, 268–269, *269*
　　punctum occlusion and, 272, *272*
　physiology of, 257–259
　proteins in, 258
　stability of, 259
　　in keratoconjunctivitis sicca, 260
　volume of, punctum occlusion and, 272
Tear substitutes, in chemical injury, 240
Tears, 258
　flow of, 258
　flow rate of, 261, *261*
　histamine in, 80
　human immunodeficiency virus in, 1332
　lactoferrin in, in dry eye disorders, 269–
　　270
　production of, 258
　　decreased, 260–261, *261*
　　dye dilution testing of, 8, *9*
　tumor shedding into, in sebaceous carci-
　　noma, 1759
　volume of, 258
Tegmentum, central, *2446*
　medullary, lateral, ischemia of, 2664
Teichopsia, in migraine, 2690
Telangiectasia, 2270t. See also *Ataxia-
　telangiectasia.*
　conjunctival, 2127
　　in Fabry's disease, 306, *306*
　parafoveolar, acquired, 807
　　congenital, 806–807, *807*
　　idiopathic, 807
　perifoveolar, idiopathic, 808
　retinal, exudative retinal detachment and,
　　1089
Telecanthus, 1700, *1700*
　in epicanthus inversus, 2841
　vs. hypertelorism, 1700
Telescope, astronomical, in low vision optical
　devices, 3676–3677, *3677*
　Galilean, angular magnification of, 3608,
　　3610
　　in contact lens aphakia correction, 3622,
　　　3622
　　in low vision optical devices, 3676, *3677*
Television, closed circuit, in low vision
　rehabilitation, 3681, *3681*
Temperature, multiple sclerosis and, 2684,
　2685
Temporal arteritis, 2901–2907. See also
　Arteritis, temporal.
Temporal artery, anatomy of, *2661*
　biopsy of, in temporal arteritis, 2904–2905,
　　2905
Temporal lobe, cavernous hemangioma of,
　magnetic resonance imaging of, 3575,
　3578